General Anaesthesia

Fourth edition

General Anaesthesia

Fourth edition
Volume 1

Editors

T. Cecil Gray, MD, FRCP, FRCS, FFARCS
Formerly Dean of the Faculty of Medicine
and Professor of Anaesthesia,
University of Liverpool

J. E. Utting, MA, MB, BChir, FFARCS
Professor of Anaesthesia,
University of Liverpool

John F. Nunn, MD, PhD, FFARCS
Head, Division of Anaesthesia,
Clinical Research Centre, and
Hon. Consultant Anaesthetist,
Northwick Park Hospital,
Harrow, Middlesex
Dean, Faculty of Anaesthetists of the
Royal College of Surgeons of England

Butterworths
London Boston
Sydney Wellington Durban Toronto

United Kingdom London	**Butterworth & Co (Publishers) Ltd** 88 Kingsway, WC2 6AB
Australia Sydney	**Butterworths Pty Ltd** 586 Pacific Highway, Chatsworth, NSW 2067 Also at Melbourne, Brisbane, Adelaide and Perth
Canada Toronto	**Butterworth & Co (Canada) Ltd** 2265 Midland Avenue, Scarborough, Ontario, M1P 4S1
New Zealand Wellington	**Butterworths of New Zealand Ltd** T & W Young Building, 77—85 Customhouse Quay, 1, CPO Box 472
South Africa Durban	**Butterworth & Co (South Africa) (Pty) Ltd** 152—154 Gale Street
USA Boston	**Butterworth (Publishers) Inc** 10 Tower Office Park, Woburn, Massachusetts 01801

First published 1959
Second edition 1965
Third edition 1971
Reprinted 1974

© Butterworth & Co (Publishers) Ltd, 1980

ISBN 0 407 00144 1   individual volume
     0 407 00146 8   set of two volumes

British Library Cataloguing in Publication Data

General anaesthesia — 4th ed.
   1. Anesthesia
   I. Gray, Thomas Cecil   II. Nunn, John Francis
   III. Utting, J E
   617'.96   RD81   79-42889

   ISBN 0-407-00146-8 Set
   ISBN 0-407-00144-1 (Vol. 1)
   ISBN 0-407-00145-X (Vol. 2)

Typeset by Butterworths Litho Preparation Department
Origination by Adroit Photolitho Ltd, Birmingham
Printed and bound by Wm Clowes & Sons Ltd, London and Beccles

Preface to the fourth edition

It is eight years since the publication of the third edition of this work. The fact that it is still in demand may be taken as a tribute to the foresight and contemporary approach of the authors. However, anaesthesia has not stood still and it would be generally agreed that a new edition is required.

It is interesting that over these years the 'comprehensive' text has more than held its own against the specialized monograph. Indeed, the pendulum of taste and student opinion seems to have swung rather more toward it. The qualified specialist no less than the student often prefers one book for reference rather than a library.

This edition comprises mostly new material and involves many new authors. By reinserting chapters on 'Anaesthesia for . . .' there is rather more emphasis on practical aspects than in previous editions but, the Editors hope, with no detriment to the theoretical basis of practice. Experience in the medicolegal field persuades one that it is fault in practice and slackness in technique which result in disaster more often than does lack of theoretical knowledge.

As its title implies, this work is concerned primarily with 'General Anaesthesia', but we have come to believe that there must be some reference to local and regional anaesthesia. We have aimed to indicate the theoretical background of these techniques, their indications and their dangers, rather than to provide a detailed exposition of nerve block techniques, which are so well described elsewhere.

Intensive therapy has now become an essential field of activity for anaesthetists and Professor John Utting is warmly welcomed as having a special responsibility for this section of the work. Indeed, he has played a large part in determining principles and in the planning of the whole.

Once again the Editors have allowed different styles of presentation. It seems desirable that within acceptable limits authors should be given freedom to express their views in the way they think best. Some of the authors also prefer not to use detailed references but to indicate the bibliographic sources which they have used. The Editors have respected this viewpoint.

We are greatly indebted to all our authors, all of whom are fully occupied with their professional work and must find it difficult to give time to contribute in this way to the literature. May they find reward for their effort in the help that these volumes will give to anaesthetists all over the world, both those established and those training in their specialty.

Finally, we are grateful to the Publishers and especially to the staff who have been closely connected with this work and have throughout been helpful and co-operative.

This will be the final edition for the senior Editor who with complete confidence hands on this work, which he inherited from the late Dr Frankis Evans, to those who have played the greater part in bringing to fruition this present edition.

July 1979
TCG. JFN

Preface to the first edition

The editors approached the task of revising *Modern Practice in Anaesthesia* and of bringing it up to date with trepidation. The field of anaesthesia is expanding so widely and developments are taking place so rapidly that a 'textbook' appeared impracticable. Up to now the student has had to rely on a series of special monographs, many excellent examples of which have been published over the last few years. Yet those of us who deal with postgraduate students are aware that the need is still felt for a book suitable for both study and reference and as comprehensive as it is practicable to make it. This accounts for the considerable popularity of a famous synopsis. We present these two volumes on *General Anaesthesia,* therefore, hoping to fill this need.

Accepted authorities on the various aspects of medicine touching on anaesthetic practice have written on their special subjects. Such diverse authorship must lead inevitably to varying literary styles and modes of presentation, and in many places emphasis is achieved by the overlapping of text between two chapters; this emphasis is intended to drive home the important points and teaching. A variety of views are expressed on some subjects or techniques. Here we have permitted freedom of expression where the teaching propounded would be acceptable to a reasonable body of opinion — even though we ourselves were not always in agreement. When necessary the authors have been asked to incorporate at least some reference to other acceptable points of view.

An early decision was taken to omit detailed consideration of local anaesthetics. This field is amply covered elsewhere.

One further point which has concerned us is the place of anatomy and physiology in a textbook of anaesthesia. In these basic sciences the knowledge demanded of the modern anaesthetist is so extensive that it would appear as if only the original textbooks would cover the ground. However, we feel that there is a place for chapters dealing in detail with many specialized parts of these subjects, knowledge of which is of immediate importance to anaesthetists in their everyday work. The chapters on physiology and anatomy were written with this guiding principle in mind.

The chapter on neurophysiology is by design somewhat more comprehensive, as this information is not readily available to anaesthetists, especially those who are not within reach of a medical library.

We would like to acknowledge our gratitude to our Publishers for their assistance. We are deeply indebted and most grateful to all those who, despite the pressure of their own work and publications, have added to the value of these pages by the teaching and wisdom contained in their contributions.

September 1959
Frankis T. Evans
T. Cecil Gray

Contributors

Clive P. Aber, BSc, MD, FRCP
Consultant Physician/Cardiologist, Department of Cardiology,
Hull Royal Infirmary, and Kingston General Hospital, Hull

Aileen K. Adams, MB, ChB, FFARCS
Consultant Anaesthetist, Addenbrooke's Hospital, Cambridge;
Associate Lecturer, University of Cambridge

R. S. Ahearn, MB, BS, FFARCS, FFARACS
Consultant Anaesthetist, Royal Liverpool Hospital

A. C. Allison, MA, DPhil, BM, BCh, FRCPath
Director, International Laboratory for Research on Animal Diseases,
Nairobi, Kenya

A. Angel, BSc, PhD
Reader in Physiology, University of Sheffield

Herbert G. R. Balmer, MA, MD, FFARCS, FFARCS(I)
Consultant Anaesthetist, Plymouth General Hospitals

Peter Baylis
Solicitor of the Supreme Court

Norman A. Bergman, MD, FFARCS
Professor and Chairman, Department of Anesthesiology,
University of Oregon Medical School, Portland, Oregon

D. R. Bevan, MA, MB, BChir, MRCP, FFARCS
Associate Professor, Department of Anaesthesia, McGill University,
Royal Victoria Hospital, Montreal, Quebec
Formerly Senior Lecturer/Consultant Anaesthetist, St Mary's Hospital,
London

Gerald W. Black, MD, PhD, FRCP(I), FFARCS
Consultant Anaesthetist, The Royal Belfast Hospital for Sick Children,
and Royal Victoria Hospital, Belfast

Malcolm Brown, BSc(Eng), PhD, MInstP, MIEE, CEng
Principal Physicist, Liverpool Area Health Authority (Teaching);
Hon. Lecturer in Medical Electronics, University of Liverpool

R. Bryce-Smith, MA, DM, FFARCS
Consultant Anaesthetist, Nuffield Department of Anaesthetics, Oxford;
Lecturer in Anaesthetics, University of Oxford

Geoffrey W. Burton, BSc, MB, ChB, FFARCS, DA
Consultant Anaesthetist, Bristol Health District (Teaching);
Clinical Lecturer in Anaesthetics, University of Bristol

Gordon H. Bush, MA, DM, FFARCS, DA
Consultant Anaesthetist, Alder Hey Children's Hospital, Liverpool

T. N. Calvey, BSc, MD, PhD
Senior Lecturer in Pharmacology, University of Liverpool;
Hon. Consultant, Whiston Hospital, Prescot, Merseyside

Donald Campbell, MB, ChB, FFARCS
Professor of Anaesthesia, University of Glasgow;
Hon. Consultant Anaesthetist, Royal Infirmary, Glasgow

Ian W. Carson, MD, FFARCS
Consultant Anaesthetist, Cardiac Surgical Unit, Royal Victoria Hospital,
Belfast

R. S. J. Clarke, BSc, MD, PhD, FFARCS
Reader in Anaesthetics, Queen's University of Belfast

D. F. Cochrane, MB, ChB, MRCS, LRCP, FFARCS, DA
Consultant Anaesthetist to Avon Area Health Authority (Teaching),
Frenchay Hospital, Bristol

R. S. Cormack, BA, BSc, BM, BCh, FFARCS
Consultant Anaesthetist, Northwick Park Hospital, Harrow, Middlesex;
Hon. contract with Clinical Research Centre, Harrow, Middlesex

J. Selwyn Crawford, MB, ChB, DA(London), MD(Illinois), FFARCS, FRCOG
Consultant Anaesthetist, Birmingham Maternity Hospital;
Hon. Lecturer in Obstetric Anaesthesia and Analgesia,
University of Birmingham

A. Cuschieri, MD, ChM, FRCS, FRCS(Ed)
Professor and Head of the Department of Surgery,
Ninewells Hospital and Medical School, Dundee

Harold T. Davenport, MB, ChB, FRCP(C), FFARCS
Consultant Anaesthetist, Northwick Park Hospital,
and Clinical Research Centre, Harrow, Middlesex

A. R. de C. Deacock, FFARCS, FRCP(C), FACA
Consultant Anaesthetist, The Royal Free Hospital,
and The Royal National Orthopaedic Hospital, London

A. W. Diamond, FFARCS
Consultant Anaesthetist, Frenchay Hospital, Bristol

P. M. E. Drury, MA, MB, BChir, FFARCS
Consultant Anaesthetist, Royal Liverpool Hospital, and
Part-time Lecturer, Department of Anaesthesia, University of Liverpool

John W. Dundee, MD, PhD, MRCP, FFARCS
Professor of Anaesthetics, Queen's University of Belfast

Edmond I. Eger, II, MD
Professor and Vice Chairman for Research, Department of Anesthesia,
University of California, San Francisco

G. E. Hale Enderby, FFARCS
Senior Consultant Anaesthetist, Queen Victoria Hospital, East Grinstead,
Sussex

Anne McKenzie Florence, MB, ChB, FFARCS
Consultant Anaesthetist, Broadgreen Hospital, Liverpool;
Clinical Lecturer, Department of Anaesthesia, University of Liverpool

I. C. Geddes, MD, FFARCS, DA
Senior Lecturer, Anaesthetic Unit, The London Hospital

A. A. Gilbertson, MB, ChB, FFARCS
Director, General Intensive Therapy Unit, Royal Liverpool Hospital;
Lecturer in Anaesthesia, University of Liverpool

H. J. Goldsmith, MD, FRCP
Consultant Physician, Royal Liverpool Hospital and
Liverpool Regional Nephrological Centre

T. Cecil Gray, MD, FRCP, FRCS, FFARCS
Formerly Dean of the Faculty of Medicine and Professor of Anaesthesia,
University of Liverpool

V. A. Grimshaw, MA, MB, BChir, FFARCS
Consultant Anaesthetist, The General Infirmary at Leeds

M. J. Halsey, MA, DPhil
Member of Scientific Staff, Division of Anaesthesia,
Clinical Research Centre, Harrow, Middlesex

C. D. Hanning, BSc, MB, BS, FFARCS
Research Fellow, Shock Study Group, Department of Surgery,
University of Glasgow;
Senior Registrar in Anaesthesia, Department of Anaesthetics,
Western Infirmary, Glasgow

M. D. Hargreaves, MB, ChB, FFARCS
Consultant Anaesthetist, The General Infirmary at Leeds

A. M. Hewlett, MB, ChB(Otago), FFARCS
Consultant Anaesthetist, Northwick Park Hospital, Harrow, Middlesex

B. C. Hovell, MB, ChB, FFARCS
Consultant Anaesthetist, Department of Anaesthesia, Hull Royal Infirmary

Gough Hughes, MD, MRCS, LRCP, FFARCS, DA
Consultant Anaesthetist, Liverpool Area (Teaching) and
Liverpool Regional Hospital Board; Lecturer in Anaesthesia,
University of Liverpool

G. H. Hulands, MB, ChB, FFARCS
Consultant Anaesthetist, Northwick Park Hospital, Harrow, Middlesex

A. R. Hunter, MD, FRCS, FFARCS
Professor of Anaesthetics, University of Manchester

Jennifer M. Hunter, MB, ChB, FFARCS
Senior Lecturer in Anaesthesia, University of Liverpool

Bryan Jennett, MD, FRCS
Professor of Neurosurgery, University of Glasgow and
Institute of Neurological Sciences, Southern General Hospital, Glasgow

Clive Jolly, MB, BS(Lond), FFARCS, DA
Consultant Anaesthetist, Ipswich Hospitals, Suffolk

Leon Kaufman, MD, FFARCS
Consultant Anaesthetist, University College Hospital and
St. Mark's Hospital, London; Senior Lecturer in Anaesthesia,
University College Hospital Medical School, London

Joan J. Kendig, PhD
Associate Professor of Biology in Anesthesia, Stanford
University School of Medicine, California

P. G. Lawler, MA, BM, BCh, MRCP, FFARCS
Scientific Officer, Division of Anaesthesia, Clinical Research Centre and
Hon. Senior Registrar, Division of Anaesthetics, Northwick Park Hospital,
Harrow, Middlesex

I. McA. Ledingham, MD, FRCS(Ed)
Reader, Department of Surgery, University of Glasgow;
Hon. Consultant Clinical Physiologist, Intensive Therapy Unit and
Surgical Director, Accident and Emergency Department, Western Infirmary,
Glasgow

H. A. Lee, MB, BS, BSc, FRCP, MRCS
Professor of Metabolic Medicine, University of Southampton;
Deputy Director, Wessex Regional Renal Unit;
Co-Director, Wessex Transplant Unit; Physician to St. Mary's Hospital,
Portsmouth

Julian M. Leigh, MD, FFARCS
Director, Intensive Care Unit, Royal Surrey County Hospital, Guildford

R. J. Linden, MB, ChB, PhD, DSc, FRCP
British Heart Foundation Professor of Cardiovascular Studies,
University of Leeds

S. Lipton, MB, ChB, FFARCS
Director, Centre for Pain Relief, Mersey Regional Department of Medical
and Surgical Neurology, Walton Hospital, Liverpool;
Visiting Fellow, Bio-Engineering Unit, Salford University;
Clinical Lecturer, Department of Anaesthesia, University of Liverpool

W. McCaughey, MB, FFARCS, FFARCS(I)
Consultant Anaesthetist, Craigavon Area Hospital, Co. Armagh;
Lecturer, Department of Anaesthetics, Queen's University of Belfast

D. G. McDowall, MD(Ed), FFARCS
Professor of Anaesthesia, University of Leeds;
Hon. Consultant Anaesthetist, The General Infirmary at Leeds,
and St James's University Hospital, Leeds

Ronald A. Millar, MD, PhD(Ed), MSc(McGill), FFARCS, FACA, FRCP(C)
Professor and Chairman, Department of Anesthesia,
Health Sciences and Memorial University, St John's, Newfoundland

James S. Milledge, MD, FRCP(E)
Consultant in Respiratory Medicine, Northwick Park Hospital,
and Member of Scientific Staff, Medical Research Council,
Clinical Research Centre, Harrow, Middlesex

John F. Nunn, MD, PhD, FFARCS
Head, Division of Anaesthesia, Clinical Research Centre,
and Hon. Consultant Anaesthetist, Northwick Park Hospital, Harrow,
Middlesex

Cedric Prys-Roberts, MA, DM, PhD, FFARCS
Professor of Anaesthetics, University of Bristol;
Hon. Consultant Anaesthetist, Bristol Royal Infirmary

E. B. Raftery, MD, BSc, FRCP
Consultant Cardiologist, Northwick Park Hospital,
and Clinical Research Centre, Harrow, Middlesex

G. Jackson Rees, MB, ChB, FFARCS, FFARACS, DA
Consultant Anaesthetist, Royal Liverpool Children's Hospital and
Alder Hey Children's Hospital, Liverpool;
Director of Paediatric Anaesthetic Studies, University of Liverpool

J. C. Richardson, MB, ChB(Hons), DA, FFARCS
Clinical Lecturer and Consultant Anaesthetist,
Liverpool Regional Cardiothoracic Surgical Centre, Broadgreen Hospital,
Liverpool

D. V. Roberts, BSc, MD
Senior Lecturer in Physiology, University of Liverpool

Frank L. Robertshaw, MB, ChB(St Andrews), FFARCS, DObstRCOG, DA
Chairman and Senior Consultant, Department of Anaesthesia,
Park Hospital, Trafford Area Health Authority, Manchester

James D. Robertson, MD, FRCP(Ed), FRCS(Ed), FFARCS, DA
Professor of Anaesthetics, University of Edinburgh

P. J. Sanderson, PhD, DipBact, MB, BS, MRCPath
Consultant Microbiologist, Northwick Park Hospital, Harrow, Middlesex

Graham Smith, BSc, MD, FFARCS
Senior Lecturer in Anaesthesia, University of Glasgow;
Hon. Consultant Anaesthetist, Western Infirmary, Glasgow

Steven Lewis Snowdon, MB, ChB, FFARCS
Senior Lecturer, Department of Anaesthesia, University of Liverpool;
Consultant Anaesthetist, Royal Liverpool Hospital

Alastair A. Spence, MD, FFARCS
Reader in Anaesthesia, University of Glasgow;
Head of University Department of Anaesthesia, Western Infirmary, Glasgow

Norman C. Staub, MD
Professor of Physiology, Cardiovascular Research Institute, and
Department of Physiology, University of California, San Francisco,
California

J. C. Stoddart, MD, BS, FFARCS
Consultant in Charge, Intensive Therapy Unit, Royal Victoria Hospital,
Newcastle upon Tyne;
Regional Consultant in Intensive Therapy (Northern Region)

Leo Strunin, MD, FFARCS
Professor of Anaesthetics, King's College Hospital and Medical School,
London

Jean Sturrock, BA, MPhil
Member of Hon. Scientific Staff, Division of Anaesthesia,
Clinical Research Centre, Harrow, Middlesex

Edward Sumner, MA, BM, BCh(Oxon), FFARCS
Consultant Anaesthetist, The Hospital for Sick Children, London

John Andrew Thornton, MRCS, LRCP, MD, FFARCS, DA
Professor and Head of Department of Anaesthetics, University of Sheffield

M. E. Tunstall, MB, BS, FFARCS, DObstRCOG
Consultant Anaesthetist, Aberdeen Royal Infirmary

J. E. Utting, MA, MB, BChir, FFARCS
Professor of Anaesthesia, University of Liverpool

H. B. Valman, MA, MD, FRCP, DCH, DRCOG
Consultant Paediatrician, Northwick Park Hospital, and
Clinical Research Centre, Harrow, Middlesex

B. A. Walker, MD, FRCP
Consultant Physician, Royal Liverpool Hospital

Richard William Ernest Watts, MD, DSc, PhD, FRCP, FRIC
Head, Division of Inherited Metabolic Diseases, Clinical Research Centre,
Harrow, Middlesex;
Hon. Consultant Physician, Northwick Park Hospital, Harrow, Middlesex

D. C. White, MB, BS, FFRACS
Consultant Anaesthetist, Northwick Park Hospital, Harrow, Middlesex

Norton E. Williams, MB, ChB, FFARCS
Consultant Anaesthetist, Whiston Hospital, Prescot, Merseyside;
Lecturer (part-time) in Clinical Pharmacology, University of Liverpool

H. Wilson, MD, PhD
Senior Lecturer in Pharmacology, University of Liverpool

T. N. P. Wilton, MA, MRCS, LRCP, FFARCS, DA
Emeritus Consultant Anaesthetist to Avon Area Health Authority
(Teaching)

Contents of this volume

Contents of volume 2

Fundamentals of anaesthetic action

1 Functions and structure of cell components in relation to action of anaesthetics
A.C. Allison

The physicochemical studies reviewed in Chapter 3 show that anaesthetics can interact with lipid bilayers and with proteins. The interactions occur mainly with hydrophobic sites of a variety of biological macromolecules. It is not surprising that anaesthetics can influence the permeability of cellular membranes and the activities of some enzymes and other proteins. It has long been known that anaesthetics have a wide range of effects on cells, from unicellular organisms to the human cerebral cortex. In his classic monograph *Anesthésiques et l'asphyxie* Claude Bernard (1875) described the reversible inhibition by anaesthetics of phagocytosis, spore germination and growth of yeast. Other general effects of anaesthetics have been summarized by Winterstein (1919) and Heilbrunn (1952). Inhibition of cerebral cortical respiration by barbiturates was described by Quastel and Wheatley (1932) and arrest of mitosis in plant cells by anaesthetics was reported by Östergren (1944).

These and other observations have given rise to many theories of the mode of action of anaesthetics. The purpose of this chapter is to present a brief review of what is known of the structure and function of different cell constituents, and then to consider in outline the evidence that these functions are affected by anaesthetics. One important question is what effects occur with concentrations of anaesthetics approximately equivalent to those attained in the blood and tissues during the course of clinical anaesthesia. Many of the effects described are seen only with higher concentrations of anaesthetics, and are unlikely to have clinical relevance.

THE CELL MEMBRANE

The cell membrane, also known as the plasma membrane or plasmalemma, has as its outstanding property selective permeability. Cytoplasmic protein is kept within the membrane, and with it an osmotic balance is maintained. The membrane couples the release of energy by adenosine triphosphatases with the selective transport of ions and other small molecules across the membrane against a concentration gradient. Specialized functions carried out by certain membranes include the efficient propagation of electrical impulses by nerve cell membranes and the provision of electrical insulation by the myelin sheath.

The basic structure of a membrane is that of a bilayer of phospholipids with their polar groups facing outwards and their hydrophobic lipid chains facing inwards (Finean *et al.*, 1966). Membrane proteins float in the phospholipid bilayer. At physiological temperature some of the lipid bilayer is in a liquid state, allowing lateral diffusion of phospholipid and protein molecules, or complexes of molecules, within the plane of the membrane (Singer and Nicolson, 1972). On the basis of solubility and other physical factors, membrane proteins have been divided into intrinsic proteins, which are found within the membrane bilayer, and extrinsic proteins, which are water soluble and located on the aqueous faces of the membrane.

The phospholipids, including phosphatidylcholine, phosphatidylserine, phosphatidylethanolamine and sphingomyelin, comprise more than 70% of membrane lipid. These molecules have specific melting points, determined by the degree of unsaturation and length of the hydrocarbon chain as well as the structure of the head group. Unsaturated phospholipids have a lower melting point than saturated, and at body temperature can exist in a semiliquid state. Thus the ratio of unsaturated to saturated phospholipids is one important factor determining how much of the bilayer exists in the fluid state. In this fluid environment, lateral diffusion of the phospholipid molecules and other membrane components can occur. The kinetics of phospholipid exchange at temperatures that 'melt' the hydrocarbon chains show that exchange reactions between laterally adjacent phospholipid molecules occur in less than 10^{-6} seconds. On the other hand, the measured half-time for 'flip-flop' of membrane phospholipids from one lamella of the bilayer to the other is several orders of magnitude lower than the rate of lateral phospholipid diffusion (Kornberg and McConnell, 1971).

The concept of membrane fluidity has been supported by three lines of evidence: the redistribution or capping of membrane markers; aggregation and disaggregation of intramembranous particles visualized by freeze-fracture electron microscopy; and membrane fusion. When divalent or multivalent ligands bind to membrane glycoprotein or other receptors, the latter undergo a topographical redistribution from a random dispersion to localization in patches and, finally, a cap at one pole of the cell. The complex surface is then endocytosed or shed from the surface of the cell (Taylor *et al.*, 1971).

Fusion of membranes is required for a variety of cell functions, including the fusion of secretory granules containing neurotransmitters at neuromuscular junctions and synapses (Poste and Allison, 1973). Four stages in membrane fusion can be recognized: contact between cell membranes; induction of fusion, involving the displacement of calcium and ATP from the membrane; the actual fusion event, with interdigitation of adjacent lipid bilayers; and finally stabilization, in which the membranes return to their normal state.

Membrane receptors

Receptors can be broadly defined as a class of molecules (which can exist independently or in the form of a complex) with stereochemical configurations, net electrostatic charges or other physicochemical properties that favour specific interactions with complementary molecules, which can result in a biological response. Receptors in the membrane represent normal functional complexes which may participate in active transport of metabolites and recognition phenomena. Specific receptors on the plasma membranes of mammalian cells are known for neurotransmitters, peptide hormones, bacterial toxins, viruses, lectins and components of the immune system (e.g. the Fc component of immunoglobin and the complement cleavage product C3b). Membrane receptors can be protein, glycoprotein, lipid or glycolipid in composition, and they are in dynamic equilibrium with other membrane components. Molecular interactions between receptors and specific membrane phospholipids may be essential for proper receptor conformation.

The receptor for acetylcholine has not yet been isolated from mammalian cells, but from the electric organ of the fishes *Electrophorus* or *Torpedo*. The receptor is characterized by its binding of the protein α-bungarotoxin; although its lipid solubility and tendency to aggregate make the receptor protein difficult to work with, a lot of information has been obtained about its properties (Eldefrawi and Eldefrawi, 1977). The whole receptor complex has a molecular weight of the order of 270 000 to to 330 000. The smallest molecular weight subunit (about 40 000) carries binding sites for agonists and antagonists.

The acetylcholine receptor protein has a very high affinity for Ca^{2+}, and evidence has accumulated that Ca^{2+} may play a role in the reaction of the receptor with the corresponding agonist. Displacement of Ca^{2+} from the receptor by acetylcholine or agonists may be directly responsible for receptor-mediated changes in permeability of neural membranes to inorganic ions.

THE SYNAPSE

A specialized area of the plasma membranes of two adjacent nerve cells is the synapse. This description is of the structure of the synapse; effects of anaesthetics on synaptic functions are discussed in Chapter 5. Electron microscopic observations show a distinct gap of 0.2—0.3 nm between the pre- and postsynaptic membranes. In the presynaptic cytoplasms are many small globules called synaptic vesicles, each about 50 nm in diameter (*Figure 1.1*). They occur in groups near the presynaptic membrane. Mitochondria are also numerous in the presynaptic cytoplasm, providing a local supply of ATP. Each of the synaptic vesicles is thought to contain a package or quantum of neurotransmitter. Both synapses and motor end-plates contain similar vesicles; the end-plate has been studied in detail. There are frequent miniature end-plate potentials, and the amount of acetylcholine in a quantum can be calculated by injecting known amounts

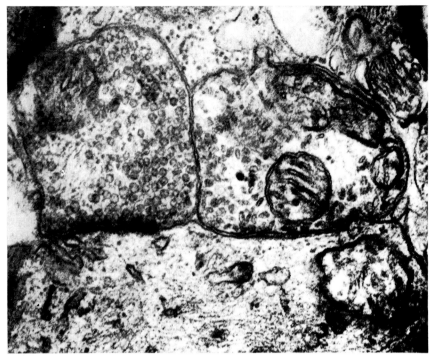

Figure 1.1
Electron micrograph (aldehyde fixation × 36 000) of two spinal
cord synapses on a dendrite. One contains round synaptic vesicles
and the other flat synaptic vesicles and a mitochondrion; the former
is thought to be excitatory and the other inhibitory. Note the dark
staining of the apposed membranes. (By courtesy of E. G. Gray)

into the synapse and measuring the response with microelectrodes. The
synaptic vesicle is about the correct size to contain this quantity. Fractions
from homogenized brains rich in synaptic vesicles (synaptosomes) are
rich in neurotransmitters. In adrenergic nerve endings synaptic vesicles
contain a dense particle thought to be a reaction product between noradrenaline and the fixative. In animals treated with reserpine, which
depletes stores of noradrenaline, vesicles containing granules disappear.

When the impulse reaches the presynaptic membrane, calcium ions
enter (Katz, 1965; Llinas, Blinks and Nicholson, 1972); this is necessary
for transmitter release. Since calcium ions promote fusion of membranes
(Poste and Allison, 1973), fusion of the synaptic vesicle membrane with
the plasma membrane may be one of the initial events for which calcium
is required.

The origin of synaptic vesicles and the way they arrive at the presynaptic
membrane are still uncertain. The vesicles may form, at least in part, by
infolding of the plasma membrane near the site of release (membrane
recycling). Alternatively, or additionally, the synaptic vesicles may pass
down the axon from the cell body. In suitably prepared sections of brain,
synaptic vesicles are often seen in association with microtubules; presumably these are labile since they are not seen by conventional techniques

(Smith, Järlfors and Beránek, 1970; Gray, 1977). Microtubules are involved in movement of other cellular organelles, such as chromosomes, and they may be involved in the translocation of synaptic vesicles to the plasma membrane. The short time interval between depolarization and transmitter release shows that this must take place with vesicles already alongside the plasma membrane, ready to fuse with it. Chemical synapses have a synaptic delay of about one-thousandth of a second (1 ms). Since the cleft is only about 20 nm wide (50 nm at the motor end-plate), diffusion of transmitter across it requires only a few millionths of a second (μs). The delay must be due mainly to the time required for mobilization and release of neurotransmitter.

It has long been known that synapses on dendritic spines of cerebral cortical neurons are excitatory while those on the soma of the neurons are inhibitory. The synapses on the dendritic spines (type 1) have a more pronounced postsynaptic thickening and a wider synaptic cleft than synapses on the somas (type 2 (Gray, 1969); *Figure 1.1*). In other sites also type 1 synapses are excitatory and those of type 2 are inhibitory. Uchizono (1965) noted that after initial fixation with aldehyde followed by osmium tetroxide, the synaptic vesicles of excitatory synapses appear round, while those at inhibitory synapses are flattened or elongated (*Figure 1.1*).

A further type of synapse is electrically transmitting. This may be a specialization of the 'functional coupling' between various cell types other than nerve cells, in which an action potential in either of two cells will generate an action potential in the other. This occurs in regions of close apposition of the cell membranes, which have lower resistivity than the surrounding membranes (Bennet, 1966). At the motor giant synapses of the crayfish, however, the junctional region is so specialized that it will transmit electrically from one cell to the other but not *vice versa* (Furshpan and Potter, 1959). In the central nervous system of fish, where combined functional and morphological studies have been made, some synapses are formed by fusion of the apposed pre- and postsynaptic membranes. Although presynaptic vesicles and thickenings may be present, the vesicles are less numerous and clustered around the thickenings than those seen in chemically transmitting synapses (Bennet, Nakajima and Pappas, 1967). Nothing is known about effects of anaesthetics on electrically transmitting synapses.

INTERACTION OF ANAESTHETICS WITH MEMBRANES

Local anaesthetics

Local anaesthetics block nerve impulse conduction by preventing influx of sodium ions (Taylor, 1959). They do this by affecting the membrane permeability increase, hence the sodium channels, and not by altering the ionic gradients or the resting membrane potential of the nerve. Many local anaesthetic molecules have a tertiary amine group and lipophilic hydro-carbon group. At about physiological pH the molecules are partly protonated and partly uncharged; the latter can penetrate through the hydrocarbon region of cell membranes. Two questions which have long concerned neurophysiologists are whether the protonated or uncharged form of the local anaesthetic is active and whether the main activity is on the inner or the outer side of the cell membrane. Measurements of the rate of onset and efficiency of anaesthetic action as a function of external pH suggest that local anaesthetics are most effective on the inside of the membrane in a cationic form (Narahashi, Frazier and Yamada, 1970; Strobel and Bianchi, 1970). This difference is not absolute: the uncharged form of local anaesthetics is also able to block nerve impulses (Ritchie and Ritchie, 1968), and, unlike water-soluble blocking agents, local anaesthetics are effective when applied to either side of the nerve cell membrane (Narahashi, Andersen and Moore, 1967).

Three general mechanisms of the action of local anaesthetics have been put forward. Seeman (1972) suggested that penetration of anaesthetics into the hydrocarbon region of the membrane expands the membrane volume, thereby blocking the sodium channel. McLaughlin (1975) proposed that local anaesthetics act in their positively charged form at the membrane surface, increasing the surface potential and affecting the voltage-measuring system of the sodium channels. According to Strichartz (1975), local anaesthetics combine with specific receptors in the nerve membrane. Anaesthetic molecules form a complex with sodium channels in the membranes. The channels must be open for sodium ion flow before this complex can be formed; and when it is formed, ions cannot flow through this channel.

The initial interaction may be with the acidic phospholipid phosphatidyl-serine, which is known to be concentrated in the inner lamella of the bilayer of the plasma membrane in those cells which have been studied (Bretscher, 1972). Specificity of interaction of local anaesthetics with phospholipids was shown by Hauser, Penkett and Chapman (1969). High-resolution nuclear magnetic resonance spectroscopy showed that procaine and tetracaine interact preferentially with the acidic phospholipid phosphatidylserine, the main interaction being electrostatic with the hydrophilic head of the phospholipid. Sax and Pletcher (1969) have suggested that formation of a hydrogen bond between local anaesthetics and acceptor groups in membranes may be a feature in the interaction of local anaesthetics. One of the properties of these local anaesthetics is that they displace calcium ions bound to phospholipid (Blaustein and Goldman, 1966). Either of these mechanisms might perturb the functioning of the sodium channel.

Actions of local anaesthetics are considered further in Chapter 17.

Alcohol and inhalational anaesthetics

The observations quoted above raised the possibility that alcohol and inhalational anaesthetics might block axonal conduction by increasing ion permeability through the nerve cell membrane. However, it is unlikely that this is the explanation of their mode of action. Halsey, Smith and Wood (1970) found that the concentrations of ether and chloroform required to change the rate of Na^+ or K^+ transport in red blood cells significantly, to alter the rate of passive leakage of cations or to produce haemolysis, are about ten times higher than the mean arterial blood concentrations occurring in clinical anaesthesia. The authors conclude that their results throw doubt on theories relating effects of anaesthetics to perturbation of cation transport through biological membranes in general, and suggest that the effects of anaesthetics are more specific than has frequently been assumed. Further evidence for specificity comes from the fact that synaptic transmission is more sensitive to inhalational anaesthetics than is axonal conduction (see below).

Higher concentrations of general anaesthetics do block axonal conduction, but this is due to decreased rather than increased cation permeability. Recent studies have confirmed earlier reports that alcohol and ether depress sodium conductance and that their effects can be overcome by increasing extracellular sodium (Inoue and Frank, 1967). Studies of membrane currents with the sucrose gap technique and voltage clamp (Moore, Ulbricht and Takata, 1964) have shown that ethanol reduces maximum sodium and potassium conductances; Armstrong and Binstock (1964), using coaxial electrodes, found conductance of sodium more depressed than that of potassium.

All these results suggest that local anaesthetics may well act by decreasing cation permeability across nerve cell membranes, and that general anaesthetics in concentrations above the clinical range have a similar effect. General anaesthetics in the clinical range probably have only minor effects, if any, on cation mobility through membranes and, therefore, on axonal transmission.

CYTOPLASMIC STRUCTURE AND MOTILITY

The distinctive organelles of the cytoplasm lie in protoplasmic ground substance called hyaloplasm, the composition of which varies in different parts of the cell. Alongside the nucleus is a highly gelated region containing the centriole and centrosphere and surrounded by the Golgi system. Peripheral to this is a relatively solated region — known as endoplasm — containing mitochondria, lysosomes, endoplasmic reticulum and vacuoles (*Figures 1.2* and *1.3*). Active cytoplasmic streaming, carrying organelles, occurs in this region. In some cells the most peripheral cytoplasm, known as ectoplasm, is gelated and free of organelles. Areas of gelation in the ectoplasm may break down, especially where pseudopodia are being extended, and endoplasm bearing organelles floods in. It is now recognized that fibrous structures (microtubules and microfilaments) contribute to the rigidity and viscosity of cytoplasm as well as to the movement (see Porter, 1966; Ishikawa, Bischoff and Holtzer, 1969). Reversible transitions, such as the formation and breakdown of microtubules, contribute to changes in cytoplasmic viscosity and motility.

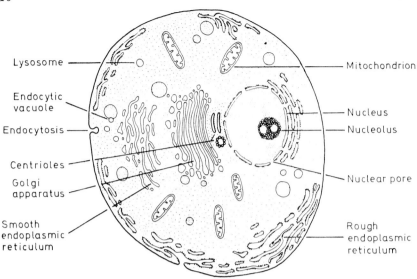

Figure 1.2
Diagrammatic representation of a cell, showing the major constituents

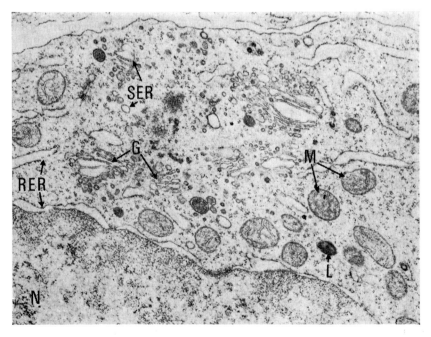

Figure 1.3
Electron micrograph (× 16 000) of a lymphoid cell, showing the major constituents. N, nucleus; RER, rough-surface endoplasmic reticulum; SER, smooth-surface endoplasmic reticulum; G, Golgi system on either side of the centriole, which is cut tangentially; M, mitochondria; L, lysosome. (By courtesy of S. de Petris)

Claude Bernard (1875) believed that anaesthesia is due to a reversible 'semicoagulation' of protoplasm. However, Heilbrunn (1920) found that the cytoplasm of sea-urchin eggs becomes less viscous after exposure to anaesthetics (including ether, chloroform, paraldehyde, chloral hydrate and urethane) in the relatively low concentrations required to prevent cell division; higher concentrations of anaesthetics brought about irreversible coagulation of cytoplasm. The decreased viscosity was shown by the ease with which cytoplasmic granules could be sedimented by centrifugation, and it could also be produced by cold (-3 to $6°C$). Heilbrunn (1952) quotes several observations that viscosity of the cytoplasm of slime moulds, algae, *Elodea* cells, bean cells, and *Sempervivum* cells is decreased by low and increased by high concentrations of anaesthetics. Brinley (1928) reported that brownian movement increased when amoebae were exposed to ether, chloroform or alcohol, indicating a decrease in viscosity.

In contrast, Seifriz (1941) showed that chloroform and cyclopropane reversibly stop cytoplasmic streaming in the slime mould *Physarum polycephalum* and found this to be due to a rapid and reversible thixotropic setting, or gelatinization, of the cytoplasm. The altered cytoplasm could not be deformed by pressures sufficient to bring about deformation of normal cytoplasm. Seifriz suggested that the thixotropic setting of protoplasm is due to a rapid and readily reversible locking of linear protein molecules.

Goldacre (1952) and Bruce and Christiansen (1965) reported that amoebae (*Amoeba* spp.) and giant amoebae (*Chaos chaos*) exposed to anaesthetics (20% saturation with ether or 10% saturation with halothane) stop moving and no longer respond to stimuli. Their cytoplasm divides into a broad, peripheral clear zone and a central zone containing cytoplasmic granules. These changes were attributed to tight cross-linking of the colloidal constituents of the plasmagel. There is evidence for disturbance of microfilament-mediated locomotion by halothane in the slime mould *Dictyostelium discoideum* (Wiklund and Allison, 1972).

Motility

Inhalational anaesthetics cause a reversible decrease of motility in a wide range of cell species. The observations of Claude Bernard (1875) on *Paramoecium* can readily be confirmed on laboratory strains of the ciliate *Tetrahymena pyriformis* which can be brought to a standstill by 5% halothane, with good recovery on withdrawing the agent. The slime mould *Physarum polycephalum* stops its rhythmic streaming under the influence of a range of anaesthetics (Seifriz, 1941), and it is also possible to arrest the cyclosis of *Elodea canadensis* (Nunn, unpublished). There is a striking cessation of movement of mammalian lymphocytes in culture on exposure to 2% halothane and this effect is fully reversible (Nunn, Sharp and Kimball, 1970). In contrast, the motility of macrophages in culture is not influenced by the same concentration of halothane. There is indirect evidence that movement of polymorphs is reduced by anaesthetics (Bruce, 1966) but direct observations do not appear to have been reported.

MICROTUBULAR SYSTEMS

Electron micrographs of suitably fixed material show small tubular structures in the cytoplasm of most cells. The tubules are about 200—240 Å in diameter and of indefinite length. In cross-section there are 13 subunits 40 Å in diameter, and these are regularly arranged as superimposed rings to make up the microtubule. The protein subunits have a molecular weight of 60 000 with 1 mole of guanine nucleotide per mole of protein (Stephens, 1968); they have no demonstrable lipid. Microtubules are best known in cilia and flagella, in which they are characteristically arranged in the form

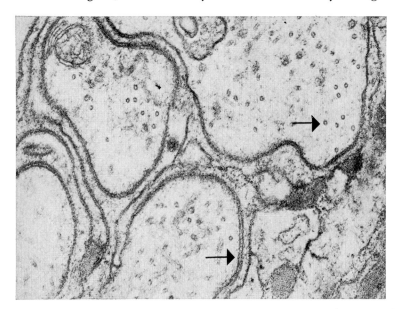

Figure 1.4
Electron micrograph of three nerve axis cylinders (× 60 000),
showing microtubules in transverse section (upper arrow) and in
longitudinal section. The lower arrow shows the trilaminar unit
membrane structure of the cell membrane when cut transversely.
(In collaboration with S. de Petris)

of two central tubules surrounded by nine pairs of tubules. This arrangement is common to the flagella and cilia of motile bacteria, and plant and animal cells. As Behnke and Forer (1967) have pointed out, the microtubules of flagella and cilia are relatively stable to treatments that break down the structure of labile cytoplasmic microtubules. These are numerous in the mitotic spindle (Porter, 1966), the circumferential band in blood platelets (Behnke, 1965) and in neurons (*Figure 1.4*), especially in the axon hillock (Palay *et al.,* 1968). Microtubules are thought to provide rigidity in cytoplasm and are often concentrated in regions where movement is taking place, as in feeding protozoa, the mitotic spindle and contracting melanophore (Porter, 1966), motile lymphocytes (Hirsch and Fedorko, 1968) and streaming slime moulds (Crawley, 1966). Microtubules resemble actin in composition, and it has been suggested that they may form a contractile actomyosin-like system (see Porter, 1966). Another set of fibrous proteins in cells, known as microfilaments, has the capacity to interact with heavy meromyosin (Ishikawa, Bischoff and Holtzer, 1969).

Labile microtubules, including those of the mitotic spindle, disappear when exposed to colchicine, cold or high pressure (Marsland, 1968; Tilney, 1968); the effects of cold and pressure are readily reversible. Allison and Nunn (1968) suggested that general anaesthetics might bring about reversible breakdown of microtubules, and clear evidence has been obtained that this is the case in two classic situations. The protozoon *Actinosphaerium nucleofilum* has ray-like projections or axopods which are supported by a helical arrangement of microtubules. On exposure to inhalational anaesthetics in clinical concentrations, the axopods collapse and are retracted, and the microtubules are no longer recognizable in electron micrographs; this is readily reversible on withdrawal of the anaesthetic (Allison *et al.*, 1970). Within a few minutes of exposure to halothane (2% in air), the mitotic spindles in fertilized eggs of the sea-urchin (*Echinus esculentis*) disappear, as shown by the observations with the polarizing microscope, and reappear soon after withdrawal of the anaesthetic (*Figure 1.5*).

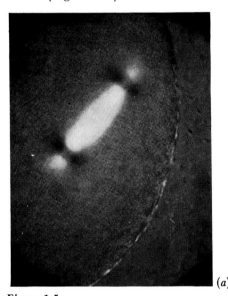 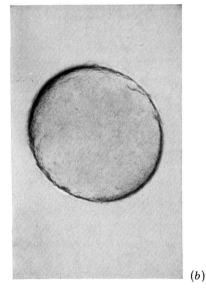

(a) (b)

Figure 1.5
Fertilized eggs of the sea-urchin (*Echinus*) seen with the polarizing microscope, showing in (a) a normal egg a birefringent spindle and in (b) an egg exposed to 2% halothane no mitotic spindle but weak residual birefringence of the peripheral fertilization membrane. (Unpublished observations in collaboration with A. Forer and J. F. Nunn)

It seems likely that the anaesthetics interact with non-polar sites in microtubular protein, and that this interferes with the hydrophobic bonding which holds the subunits together in the assembled microtubule. Dispersal of microtubules could explain many of the observed effects of anaesthetics in clinical concentrations on cellular structure and behaviour, including decreased cytoplasmic viscosity and movement and the colchicine-like arrest of mitosis described by Östergren (1944). However, this does not appear to be a major factor in the inhibition of mammalian cell multiplication by inhalational anaesthetics (see Chapter 10). It is also uncertain whether effects on microtubules play any role in the induction of clinical anaesthesia. The labile microtubules associated with synaptic vesicles are difficult to study, although those in the axons themselves are easily observed (see *Figure 1.4*) and are still demonstrable in the optic nerves of animals anaesthetized with halothane (Saubermann and Gallagher, 1973). The role of microtubules in axonal transport is discussed in the next section, but it seems unlikely that inhibition of this process could account for the extreme rapidity with which anaesthesia follows exposure of the brain to the anaesthetic agent. It might, however, explain some delayed effects of prolonged anaesthesia. Some evidence has been presented that microtubules may participate in the release of insulin from pancreatic islet cells (Lacy *et al.*, 1968) and of histamine from mast cells (Gillespie, Levine and Malawista, 1968). It is conceivable that effects on microtubules or some other anaesthetic-sensitive contractile system could inhibit the release of transmitter at critical synapses. Moreover, microtubules could play a part in maintaining the configuration of neuronal processes, so that if they are dispersed the close apposition of nerve cell membranes which is required for synaptic transmission may be altered. The finding that animals treated with colchicine are unusually sensitive to anaesthetics (Ferguson and Theodore, 1952) would be consistent with a role of micro-tubular changes in anaesthesia, but more direct evidence of their involvement is still required.

Axonal transport

There is now substantial evidence that proteins are synthesized in nerve cell bodies and transported down axons (Barondes, 1967). This has been shown by autoradiography and other techniques. If nerves are ligated, they swell on the proximal side of the ligature, and these swellings also contain relatively large quantities of noradrenaline (Dahlström, 1967). Hence this transmitter appears to be transported down the axon also, although it is not yet clear what proportion of transmitters are synthesized locally and what proportion come from the cell body. Axonal transport of proteins and noradrenaline is reduced in animals treated with colchicine, which selectively binds to microtubular protein (see Sjöstrand, Frizell and Hasselgren, 1970); this suggests that microtubules may play a part in axonal transport.

Other drugs which bind microtubular protein are the *Vinca* alkaloids, vincristine and vinblastine, which are used in cancer chemotherapy (Bensch and Malawista, 1969). One of the complications of vincristine therapy is peripheral neuropathy, which is readily reproduced in experimental animals (Uy *et al.*, 1967). Repeated administration of colchicine induces a rather similar neuropathy in experimental animals, with extreme muscular weakness (Ferguson and Theodore, 1952). It is tempting to conclude that these slowly developing abnormalities result from failure of transport from the nerve cell bodies to the periphery of proteins or other materials required for functional integrity; but this interpretation is still speculative.

MITOCHONDRIA AND OXIDATIVE METABOLISM

Mitochondria are visible in living cells by phase-contrast microscopy as short or long filaments carried about by cytoplasmic movement. In electron micrographs they are seen to be bounded by an outer membrane and to have characteristic foldings or cristae of an inner membrane. As discussed by Geddes in Chapter 2, these organelles contain the major oxidative enzymes of the cell, including the tricarboxylic acid cycle, the system for fatty acid oxidation and the respiratory chain. The important oxidative phosphorylation reaction gives a high yield of ATP, most of which passes out of the mitochondria for provision of energy elsewhere in the cell.

Recently evidence has accumulated that mitochondria have some measure of genetic and biochemical autonomy. Mitochondria contain DNA in a circular double-helical form, transcribe their own specific messenger RNA and synthesize some proteins of the inner mitochondrial membrane (see Nass, 1969; Ashwell and Work, 1970). The mitochondrial system for synthesizing protein resembles that in bacteria rather than that in mammalian cells: the ribosomes in mitochondria are small and protein synthesis is inhibited by drugs such as chloramphenicol. These facts have lent some support to the long-held view that mitochondria have evolved from symbiotic bacteria and have retained some features of eukaryotic metabolism. Since bacteria are remarkably resistant to gaseous anaesthetics (Wardley-Smith and Nunn, 1970), it might perhaps be expected that most anaesthetics in clinical concentrations would have only slight effects on mitochondrial function.

Barbiturates certainly inhibit mitochondrial metabolism. Quastel and Wheatley (1932) found decreased oxygen consumption in cerebral cortex preparations treated with barbiturates, and amylobarbitone is widely used to inhibit the mitochondrial respiratory chain at a point between bound NAD and flavoprotein (Lehninger, 1965). Inhibition of the respiratory pathway in isolated mitochondria by halothane has also been reported (Cohen and Marshall, 1968). However, it is likely that this effect was seen at partial pressures higher than those used clinically. The mitochondria were equilibrated with dilute halothane vapour at $0°C$, after which the preparations were sealed and oxygen consumption studied at $25°C$. The increase in temperature would cause a marked reduction in solubility of halothane in the media with a consequent increase in partial pressure, since the concentration of halothane was not allowed to change. The effective partial pressure of halothane in these experiments was therefore considerably higher than the cited value which refers to equilibration at $0°C$.

Several groups of investigators have found the oxygen consumption of anaesthetized humans to be only about 10% below basal and close to the level observed after sedation (Robertson and Reid, 1952). Cerebral oxygen consumption is reduced proportionately after inhalational anaesthesia by 10–20% (McDowall, 1965), but during barbiturate anaesthesia it is much more strongly inhibited, to about half of control values (Pierce *et al.*, 1962).

If anaesthetics markedly affect the generation or utilization of high-energy compounds in the brain, it would be expected that these would be depleted or would accumulate during anaesthesia. Several studies, carefully undertaken to avoid *post mortem* changes and other artefacts, have failed to reveal changes in the levels of ATP, creatine phosphate, NADH or NAD^+ in brains of animals anaesthesized with ether, halothane, nitrous oxide or cyclopropane (McIlwain, 1959; Michenfelder, Van Dyke and Theye, 1970; Nilsson and Siesjö, 1970; Biebuyck, Dedrick and Scherer, 1975); in animals made hypoxic, falls in cerebral ATP levels were readily demonstrable. Barbiturates had no effects on ATP levels (Gatfield *et al.*, 1966; Michenfelder, Van Dyke and Theye, 1970; Nilsson and Siesjö, 1970), although changes in oxygen consumption and in levels of lactate and pyruvate, as well as in the $NADH/NAD^+$ ratio, were reported.

The conclusion drawn from these studies is that anaesthesia does not interfere to a measurable extent with energy-yielding or energy-utilizing reactions. With the exception of barbiturate anaesthesia, the slight depression in oxygen consumption observed follows changes in over-all metabolic activity without any changes in the levels of high-energy compounds in the brain. These results provide no support for the asphyxial theory of narcosis, according to which anaesthetics produce loss of consciousness in the same way as does hypoxia. The possibility is not excluded that changes in energy production or utilization in particular neuronal compartments, or in a minority of critical cells, could take place without this being apparent in over-all metabolite levels in the brain. However, there is no evidence for this at present.

THE GOLGI APPARATUS

The Golgi apparatus, which is well developed in neurons, consists of stacks of flattened cisternae bounded by membranes and pinched off at the edges to form vesicles. Two functions are now attributed to the Golgi apparatus. The first is the accumulation and packaging for transportation of proteins synthesized in the rough endoplasmic reticulum. Caro and Palade (1964) have shown that radioactive amino acids are first incorporated into the endoplasmic reticulum, and then pass through the Golgi apparatus before being localized in secretory granules. The same sequence of events has been observed in the formation of lysosomes in developing white blood cells (Fedorko and Hirsch, 1966). The second function of the Golgi apparatus is the synthesis of polysaccharides and attachment of these to proteins, as originally shown by Neutra and Leblond (1966) and Northcote and Pickett-Heaps (1966). Effects of anaesthetics on these processes have not been investigated.

THE ENDOPLASMIC RETICULUM (otherwise known as microsomes)

The endoplasmic reticulum (ER) is a membranous cytoplasmic system of canals or vesicles, some of which are smooth surfaced while the remainder are rough surfaced or granular because numerous ribosomes are embedded within their limiting membranes.

ROUGH-SURFACED ENDOPLASMIC RETICULUM

Rough-surfaced ER is the site of synthesis of proteins which are hydrophobic and released directly into membranes without passing through an aqueous phase, and of proteins which are enclosed in membranes for export (secreting granules) or storage within the cell (for example, lysosomes). Effects of anaesthetics on this system do not appear to have been studied.

SMOOTH-SURFACED ENDOPLASMIC RETICULUM

Smooth-surfaced ER contains drug-metabolizing enzymes and in liver cells undergoes dramatic proliferation after exposure to barbiturates (see Chapters 2 and 7). Metabolism of certain compounds in endoplasmic reticulum gives rise to more toxic forms; for example, carbon tetrachloride is converted to a highly reactive chloroform radical (see Slater, 1968).

LYSOSOMES

Lysosomes are organelles containing hydrolytic enzymes present in all cells except mature non-nucleated erythrocytes. Primary lysosomes bud off the Golgi apparatus to form the storage granules which are especially numerous in some cells such as peripheral blood granulocytes. When bacteria, foreign proteins or other materials are taken into cells by infolding of the plasma membrane (endocytosis), primary lysosomes fuse with the endocytic vacuole and discharge their enzymes into it. These digest the contents of the vacuole more or less completely, and what is left is termed a residual body. Many drugs, including anti-inflammatory and antimalarial compounds, when taken up by living cells are concentrated in lysosomes (Allison and Young, 1969). Treatment of living cells with some agents, such as vitamin A or anticellular antibody, brings about discharge of lysosomal enzymes into the exterior without damaging the cell. These important factor in the pathogenesis of arthritis (Dingle and Fell, 1969). Lysosomes play an important role in cytotoxicity, although this may in many cases be secondary to damage occurring in other organelles (Slater, 1968). Anaesthetics in toxic concentrations may well have effects on lysosomes, although these have not been adequately studied.

Bruce (1967) has reported that phagocytosis of bacteria is inhibited by halothane, confirming old observations with ether (Graham, 1911) and chloroform (Hamburger, 1916). Prolonged exposure to anaesthetics might therefore impair defence against bacteria, and there is some evidence that this occurs (Bruce, 1967). Many species of bacteria are remarkably resistant to anaesthetics, and several non-pathogens were found to divide at almost the control rate during exposure to 3% halothane (Wardley-Smith and Nunn, 1970).

CALCIUM IONS

In view of the postulated role of Ca^{2+} in neurotransmitter release, effects of anaesthetics on the influx of Ca^{2+} through membranes or release from membrane components are of special interest. Calcium pumps in mitochondria (and sarcoplasmic reticulum of muscle cells) ensure that intracellular Ca^{2+} concentrations are of the order of 10^{-7} mol/l (Baker, 1972), a concentration so low that it is never attained outside living cells unless a chelating agent such as EDTA or EGTA is used. The low figure is thought to be determined by the need to keep actomyosin ATPase activity turned off (Weber and Murray, 1973). Specific channels allowing Ca^{2+} to enter the cytoplasm are probably widespread in living organisms; for example, in the membranes of the sarcoplasmic reticulum and other intracellular calcium stores. In some cells there are, in addition, Ca^{2+}-mediated action currents in some smooth muscles, crustacean muscles and heart muscles (Durham, 1974). The speed and direction of the beating of the cilia of *Paramoecium* are controlled by Ca^{2+} entry into the cell (Eckert, 1972), and a mutant with a defect in the Ca^{2+}-permeation mechanism has been found (Satow and Kung, 1974).

Baker (1974) has pointed out that in the well characterized squid axon, Ca^{2+} can enter through Na^+ channels as well as through independent Ca^{2+} channels. This second route is qualitatively similar to synaptic transmitter release in its sensitivity to other metal ions and to various drugs, and in its slow rate of rise. Ca^{2+} entry is sensitive to small changes in membrane potential insufficient to produce an action potential.

It has long been known that Ca^{2+} (or Ba^{2+} or Sr^{2+}) is required for neurotransmitter release (Katz, 1966). Studies with the luminescent protein aequorin* have shown, in stimulated presynaptic nerves, a rise in cytoplasmic Ca^{2+} concentration accompanying neurotransmitter release (Llinas, Blinks and Nicholson, 1972). This is just one of many examples

---

*Aequorin is luminescent in the presence of Ca^{2+} and may be used as an intracellular Ca^{2+} detector. *Ed.*

enzymes break down intercellular matrix, and this is believed to be an of the role of increased cytoplasmic Ca^{2+} concentration triggering the release of packaged secretions (see Allison and Davies, 1974). In rat mast cells, Foreman, Mongar and Gomperts (1973) have shown that exposure to cell-bound (reaginic) antibody and antigens raises the influx of Ca^{2+} and brings about selective release of histamine without loss of cell viability. Moreover, using an ionophore (A23187) which increases the permeability of the plasma membrane to Ca^{2+}, these investigators have shown that raising the cytoplasmic concentration of Ca^{2+} (or Sr^{2+}) triggers an energy-dependent reaction, discharging histamine from the cells. Analogous evidence in other systems is summarized by Gomperts (1976).

Durham (1974) has reviewed evidence that rhythmic activity in a variety of biological systems, from streaming in slime moulds to discharge in nerve and muscle, is due to cyclical variations in Ca^{2+} permeability through membranes. This concept can be extended to rhythmic activity in the central nervous system which maintains consciousness. If that is the case, small changes in Ca^{2+} permeability through membranes could be responsible for anaesthesia. Some of the effects of anaesthesia on cardiac and skeletal muscle could have a similar basis, as well as occasional complications of anaesthesia, such as hyperthermia following exposure to halothane (Harrison *et al.*, 1969; Kalow *et al.*, 1970; see also Chapter 45). If the sarcoplasmic reticulum of Landrace pigs and a few sensitive humans were especially sensitive to Ca^{2+} release by halothane, tonic muscular contraction could result. Pollard and Millar (1973) found that halothane increases twitch height of electrically stimulated skeletal muscle; this could reflect increased Ca^{2+} release from the sarcoplasmic reticulum.

Such varying sensitivities of Ca^{2+} permeability in different membranes might explain the selectivity of action of anaesthetics. Some membranes in certain neurons of the central nervous system would be highly sensitive, while others might be moderately sensitive, and so forth. Differential sensitivity of synapses in the central nervous system has in fact been demonstrated (see Chapter 6). Effects on other systems such as cardiac and skeletal muscle, and on submammalian cells, likewise would be observed at varying concentrations of anaesthetics.

There is evidence that Ca^{2+} is required for the binding to specific receptor molecules of acetylcholine (Eldefrawi and Eldefrawi, 1977), and the same may be true of other neurotransmitters.

In general, events which could be relevant to biological effects of anaesthetics, including those on contractile systems, membrane fusion and neurotransmitter binding, depend on permeability of Ca^{2+} through membranes and displacement of calcium from membrane constituents. This could be a prime target of anaesthetic action. The involvement of Ca^{2+} in local anaesthetic action has long been postulated (Ritchie and Greengard, 1966); for example, procaine and other local anaesthetics displace Ca^{2+} from phospholipids (Blaustein and Goldman, 1966). Effects on calcium ion availability at specific sites could be a common link in the observed effects of anaesthetics on a wide range of cell functions in various forms of life.

References

Allison, A. C. and Davies, P. (1974). Interactions of membranes, microfilaments and microtubules in cell movement, endocytosis and exocytosis. *Adv. Cytopharmac.* **2**, 237–248

Allison, A. C. and Nunn, J. F. (1968). Effects of general anaesthetics on microtubules. *Lancet* ii, 1326–1329

Allison, A. C. and Young, M. R. (1969). Vital staining and fluorescence microscopy of lysosomes. In *Lysosomes in Biology and Pathology,* pp. 600–628. J. T. Dingle and H. B. Fell (ed.) Amsterdam: North Holland Press

Allison, A. C., Hulands, G. H., Nunn, J. F., Kitching, J. A. and Macdonald, A. C. (1970). The effect of inhalational anaesthetics on the microtubular system in *Actinosphaerium nucleofilum. J. Cell Sci.* **7**, 483–499

Armstrong, C. M. and Binstock, L. (1964). The effects of several alcohols on the properties of the squid giant axon. *J. gen. Physiol.* **48**, 265–277

Ashwell, M. and Work, T. S. (1970). The biogenesis of mitochondria. *A. Rev. Biochem.* **39**, 251–290

Baker, P. F. (1972). Transport and metabolism of calcium ions in nerve. *Progr. Biophys. molec. Biol.* **24**, 177–193

Barondes, S. H. (ed.) (1967). Axoplasmic transport. *Neurosci. Res. progr. Bull.* **5**, 307–419

Behnke, O. (1965). Further studies on microtubules: a marginal bundle in human and rat thrombocytes. *J. Ultrastruct. Res.* **13**, 469–477

Behnke, O. and Forer, A. (1967). Evidence for four classes of microtubules in individual cells. *J. Cell Sci.* **2**, 169–192

Bennet, M. V. L. (1966). Physiology of electronic junctions. *Ann. N. Y. Acad. Sci.* **137**, 509–542

Bennet, M. V. L., Nakajima, Y. and Pappas, G. D. (1967). Physiology and ultrastructure of electronic junctions. 1. Supramedullary neurons. *J. Neurophysiol.* **30**, 161–179

Bensch, G. and Malawista, E. (1969). Microtubular crystals in mammalian cells. *J. Cell Biol.* **40**, 95–107

Bernard, C. (1875). *Anesthésiques et l'asphyxie.* Paris: Ballière

Biebuyck, J. F., Dedrick, D. F. and Scherer, Y. D. (1975). Brain cyclic AMP and putative transmitter amino acids during anaesthesia. In *Molecular Mechanisms of Anesthesia,* pp. 451–470. B. R. Fink (ed.) New York: Raven Press

Blaustein, M. P. and Goldman, D. E. (1966). Action of anionic and cationic nerve blocking agents: experiment and interpretation. *Science, N.Y.* **153**, 429–432

Bretscher, M. S. (1972). Asymmetrical lipid bilayer structures for biological membranes. *Nature (New Biol.)* **236**, 11–13

Brinley, F. J. (1928). Effects of chemicals on viscosity of protoplasm of amoeba as indicated by brownian movement. *Protoplasma* **4**, 177–182

Bruce, D. L. (1966). Effect of halothane anesthesia on extravascular mobilization on neutrophils. *J. cell. Physiol.* **68**, 81–83

Bruce, D. L. (1967). Effect of halothane anesthesia on experimental salmonella peritonitis in mice. *J. surg. Res.* **7**, 180–185

Bruce, D. L. and Christiansen, R. (1965). Morphologic changes in the giant amoeba *Chaos chaos* induced by halothane and ether. *Expl Cell Res.* **40**, 544–553

Caro, L. G. and Palade, G. E. (1964). Protein synthesis, storage and discharge in the pancreatic exocrine cell. *J. Cell Biol.* **20**, 473–495

Cohen, P. J. and Marshall, B. E. (1968). Effects of halothane on respiratory control and oxygen consumption of rat liver mitochondria. In *Toxicity of Anesthetics,* pp. 24–36. B. R. Fink (ed.) Baltimore, Md: Williams & Wilkins

Crawley, J. C. W. (1966). Fine structure and cytoplasmic streaming in *Physarum polycephalum. Jl R. microsc. Soc.* **85**, 313–322

Dahlström, A. (1967). The transport of noradrenaline between two simultaneously performed ligations of the sciatic nerves of rat and cat. *Acta physiol. scand.* **69**, 158–166

Dingle, J. T. and Fell, H. B. (ed.) (1969). *Lysosomes in Biology and Pathology.* Amsterdam: North-Holland

Durham, A. C. H. (1974). A unified theory of the control of actin and myosin in nonmuscle movements. *Cell* **2**, 123–135

Eckert, R. (1972). Bioelectric control of ciliary activity. *Science* **176**, 473–476

Eldefrawi, M. E. and Eldefrawi, A. T. (1977). Acetylcholine receptors. *Recept. Recogn., A* **4**, 199–258

Fedorko, M. E. and Hirsch, J. G. (1966). Cytoplasmic granule formation in myelocytes. An electron microscope radioautographic study on the mechanism of formation of cytoplasmic granules in rabbit heterophilic myelocytes. *J. Cell Biol.* **29**, 307–316

Ferguson, F. C. Jr and Theodore, P. S. (1952). Colchicine. I. General pharmacology. *J. Pharmac. exp. Ther.* **106**, 261–270

Finean, J. B., Coleman, R., Green, W. G. and Limbrick, A. R. (1966). Low angle x-ray diffraction and electron microscopic studies of isolated membranes. *J. Cell Sci.* **1**, 287–298

Foreman, J. C., Mongar, J. L. and Gomperts, B. D. (1973). Calcium ionophores and movement of calcium ions following the physiological stimulus to a secretory process. *Nature, Lond.* **245**, 249–251

Furshpan, E. J. and Potter, D. D. (1959). Tramission of giant motor synapses in the crayfish. *J. Physiol., Lond.* **145**, 289–325

Gatfield, P. D., Lowry, O. H., Schulz, D. W. and Passanneau, J. V. (1966). Regional energy reserves in mouse brain and changes with ischaemia and anaesthesia. *J. Neurochem.* 13, 185–195

Gillespie, E., Levine, R. J. and Malawista, S. E. (1968). Histamine release from rat peritoneal mast cells: inhibition by colchicine and potentiation by deuterium oxide. *J. Pharmac. exp. Ther.* 164, 158–165

Goldacre, R. J. (1952). The action of general anaesthetics on amoebae and the mechanism of the response to touch. In *Structural Aspects of Cell Physiology*, pp. 128–143. Symposia of the Society for Experimental Biology, No. 6. Cambridge: University Press

Gomperts, B. (1976). Calcium and cell activation. In *Receptors and Recognition*, Vol. 2, pp. 43–102. P. Cuatrecasas and M. F. Greaves (ed.). London: Chapman and Hall

Graham, E. A. (1911). The influence of ether and ether anesthesia on bacteriolysis, agglutination and phagocytosis. *J. infect. Dis.* 8, 147–175

Gray, E. G. (1969). Electron microscopy of excitatory and inhibitory synapses: a brief review. *Progr. brain Res.* 31, 141–155

Gray, E. G. (1977). The synapse. In *Carolina Biology Readers*. J. J. Head (ed.). Burlington, N. Carolina: Carolina Biological Supply Co.

Halsey, M. J., Smith, E. B. and Wood, T. E. (1970). Effects of general anaesthetics on Na^+ transport in human red cells. *Nature, Lond.* 225, 1151–1152

Hamburger, H. J. (1916). Researches in phagocytosis. *Br. med. J.* 1, 37–41

Harrison, G. G., Saunders, S. J., Biebuyck, J. F., Hickman, R., Dent, D. M., Weaver, V. and Terblanche, J. (1969). Anaesthetic-induced malignant hyperpyrexia and a method for its prediction. *Br. J. Anaesth.* 41, 844–852

Hauser, H., Penkett, S. A. and Chapman, D. (1969). Nuclear magnetic resonance spectroscopic studies of procaine hydrochloride and tetracaine hydrochloride at lipid–water interfaces. *Biochim biophys. Acta* 183, 466–475

Heilbrunn, L. V. (1920). The physical effect of anesthetics upon living protoplasm. *Biol. Bull. mar. biol. Lab., Woods Hole* 39, 307–315

Heilbrunn, L. V. (1952). *An Outline of General Physiology*, 3rd edn. Philadelphia, Pa: W. B. Saunders

Hirsch, J. G. and Fedorko, M. E. (1968). Ultrastructure of human leukocytes after simultaneous fixation with glutaraldehyde and osmium tetroxide and 'postfixation' in uranyl acetate. *J. Cell Biol.* 38, 615–627

Inoue, F. and Frank, G. B. (1967). Effects of ethyl alcohol on excitability and on neuromuscular transmission in frog skeletal muscle. *Br. J. Pharmac. Chemother.* 30, 186–193

Ishikawa, H., Bischoff, R. and Holtzer, H. (1969). Formation of arrowhead complexes with heavy meromyosin in a variety of cell types. *J. Cell Biol.* 43, 312–328

Kalow, W., Britt, B. A., Terreau, M. E. and Haist, J. (1970). Metabolic error of muscle metabolism after recovery from malignant hyperthermia. *Lancet* ii, 895–898

Katz, B. (1966). *Nerve, Muscle and Synapse.* New York: McGraw-Hill

Kornberg, R. D. and McConnell, H. M. (1971). Lateral diffusion of phospholipids in a vesicle membrane. *Proc. Natn. Acad. Sci. U.S.A.* 195, 135

Lacy, P. E., Howell, S. L., Young, P. L. and Fink, C. J. (1968). A new hypothesis of insulin secretion. *Nature, Lond.* 219, 1177–1179

Lehninger, A. L. (1965). *The Mitochondrion.* New York: Benjamin

Llinas, R., Blinks, J. R. and Nicholson, C. (1972). Calcium transport in presynaptic terminal of squid giant synapse: detection with aequorin. *Science* 176, 1127–1128

McDowall, D. G. (1965). Effects of general anaesthesia on cerebral metabolism. *Br. J. Anaesth.* 37, 236–245

McIlwain, H. (1959). *Biochemistry and the Central Nervous System.* London: Churchill

McLaughlin, S. (1975). Local anesthetics and the electrical properties of phospholipid bilayer membranes. In *Molecular Mechanisms of Anesthesia*, pp. 193–200. B. R. Fink (ed.). *Progress in Anesthesiology*, Vol. 1. New York: Raven Press

Marsland, D. (1968). Cell division: enhancement of the anti-mitotic effects of colchicine by low temperature and high pressure in the cleaving eggs of *Lytechinus variegatus. Expl Cell Res.* 50, 369–376

Michenfelder, J. D., Van Dyke, R. A. and Theye, R. A. (1970). The effects of anesthetic agents and techniques on canine cerebral ATP and lactate levels. *Anesthesiology* 33, 315–321

Moore, J. W., Ulbricht, W. and Takata, M. (1964). Effect of ethanol in the sodium and potassium conductances of the squid axon membrane. *J. gen. Physiol.* 48, 279–295

Narahashi, T., Andersen, N. C. and Moore, J. W. (1967). Comparison of tetrodotoxin and procaine in internally perfused squid axons. *J. gen Physiol.* 50, 1413–1428

Narahashi, T., Frazier, D. and Yamada, M. (1970). The site of action and active forms of local anesthetics. 1. Theory and pH experiments with tertiary compounds. *J. Pharmac. exp. Ther.* 171, 32–44

Nass, S. (1969). The significance of the structural and functional similarities of bacteria and mitochondria. *Int. Rev. Cytol.* 25, 55–129

Neutra, M. and Leblond, C. P. (1966). Synthesis of the carbohydrate of mucus in the Golgi complex, as shown by electron microscope. *J. Cell Biol.* 30, 119–136

Nilsson, L. and Siesjö, B. K. (1970). The effect of anaesthetics upon labile phosphates and upon extra- and intracellular lactate, pyruvate and bicarbonate concentrations in the rat brain. *Acta physiol. scand.* 80, 235–248

Northcote, D. H. and Pickett-Heaps, J. D. (1966). A function of the Golgi apparatus in polysaccharide synthesis and transport in the root cap cells of wheat. *Biochem. J.* 98, 159–167

Nunn, J. F., Sharp, J. A. and Kimball, K. L. (1970). Reversible effect of an inhalational anaesthetic on lymphocyte motility. *Nature, Lond.* 226, 85–86

Östergren, G. (1944). Colchicine mitosis, chromosome contractions, narcosis, and protein chain folding. *Hereditas* 30, 429–467

Palay, S. L., Sotelo, C., Peters, A. and Orkland, P. M. (1968). The axon hillock and the initial segment. *J. Cell Biol.* 38, 193–201

Pierce, E. C. Jr, Lambertsen, C. J., Deutsch, S., Chase, P. E., Linde, H. W., Dripps, R. D. and Price, H. L. (1962). Cerebral circulation and metabolism during thiopental anesthesia and hyperventilation in man. *J. clin. Invest.* 41, 1664–1671

Pollard, B. J. and Millar, R. A. (1973). Potentiating and depressant effects of inhalational anaesthetics on the rat phrenic nerve–diaphragm preparation. *Br. J. Anaesth.* 45, 404–410

Porter, K. R. (1966). Cytoplasmic microtubules and their functions. In Ciba Symposium on *Principles of Biomolecular Organisation*, pp. 308–345. G. E. W. Wolstenholme and M. O'Connor (ed.). London: Churchill

Poste, G. and Allison, A. C. (1973). Membrane fusion. *Biochim. biophys. Acta* 300, 421–465

Quastel, J. H. and Wheatley, A. H. M. (1932). Narcosis and oxidations of the brain. *Proc. R. Soc. B.* 112, 60–79

Ritchie, J. M. and Greengard, P. (1966). On the mode of action of local anesthetics. *A. Rev. Pharmac.* 6, 405–430

Ritchie, J. M. and Ritchie, B. (1968). Local anesthetics: effect of pH on activity. *Science, N.Y.* 162, 1394–1395

Robertson, J. D. and Reid, D. D. (1952). Standards for the basal metabolism of normal people in Britain. *Lancet* i, 940–943

Satow, Y. and Kung, C. (1974). Genetic dissection of active electrogenesis in *Paramecium aurelia. Nature, Lond.* 247, 69–70

Saubermann, A. J. and Gallagher, M. L. (1973). Mechanisms of general anesthesia: failure of pentobarbital and halothane to depolymerize microtubules in mouse optic nerve. *Anesthesiology* 38, 25–35

Sax, M. and Pletcher, J. (1969). Local anesthetics: significance of hydrogen bonding in mechanism of action. *Science, N.Y.* 166, 1546–1548

Seeman, P. (1972). The membrane actions of anesthetics and tranquillizers. *Pharmac. Rev.* 24, 583–655

Seifriz, W. (1941). A theory of anesthesia based on protoplasmic behavior. *Anesthesiology* 2, 300–309

Singer, S. J. and Nicolson, G. L. (1972). The fluid mosaic model of the structure of cell membranes. *Science* 175, 720

Sjöstrand, J., Frizell, M. and Hasselgren, P. O. (1970). Effects of colchicine on axonal transport in peripheral nerves. *J. Neurochem.* 17, 1563–1570.

Slater, T. F. (1968). Aspects of cellular injury and recovery. In *The Biological Basis of Medicine*, Vol. 1, pp. 369–414. E. E. Bittar and N. Bittar (ed.). London: Academic Press

Smith, D. S., Järlfors, V. and Beránek, R. (1970). The organization of synaptic axoplasm in the lamprey (*Petromyzon marinus*) central nervous system. *J. Cell Biol.* 46, 199–219

Stephens, R. E. (1968). Reassociation of microtubule protein. *J. molec. Biol.* 33, 517–519

Strichartz, G. (1975). Inhibition of ionic currents in myelinated nerves by quaternary derivatives of lidocaine. In *Molecular Mechanisms of Anesthesia*, pp. 1–11. B. R. Fink (ed.). *Progress in Anesthesiology*, Vol. 1. New York: Raven Press

Strobel, G. E. and Bianchi, C. P. (1970). The effects of pH gradients on the action of procaine and lidocaine in intact and de-sheathed sciatic nerves. *J. Pharmac. exp. Ther.* 172, 1–17

Taylor, R. B., Duffus, P. H., Raff, M. C. and de Petris, S. (1971). Redistribution and pinocytosis of lymphocyte surface immunoglobin molecules induced by anti-immunoglobin antibody. *Nature (New Biol.)* 233, 225

Taylor, R. G. (1959). Effect of procaine on electrical properties of squid axon membrane. *Am. J. Physiol.* 196, 1071–1075

Tilney, L. G. (1968). Studies on the microtubules of *Heliozoa*. IV. The effect of colchicine on the formation and maintenance of the axopodia. *J. Cell Sci.* 3, 549–562

Uchizono, K. (1965). Characteristics of excitatory and inhibitory synapses in the central nervous system of the cat. *Nature, Lond.* 207, 642–643

Uy, Q. L., Moen, T. H., Johns, R. J. and Owens, A. H. Jr (1967). Vincristine neurotoxicity in rodents. *Johns Hopkins med. J.* 121, 349–360

Wardley-Smith, B. and Nunn, J. F. (1970). The effect of halothane on bacterial division rate. *Br. J. Anaesth.* 42, 89

Weber, A. and Murray, J. M. (1973). Molecular control mechanisms in muscle contraction. *Physiol. Rev.* 53, 612–621

Wiklund, R. A. and Allison, A. C. (1972). Effects of anaesthetics on the mobility of *Dictyostelium discoideum. Nature (Lond.)* 239, 221–222

Winterstein, H. (1919). *Die Narkose.* Berlin: Springer

2 Cellular metabolism in relation to anaesthesia
I. C. Geddes

Anaesthetists play a major role in life support. Cardiac arrest is no longer an inevitable lethal event and prolonged artificial respiration is now common practice. However, maintenance of the energy requirements of these patients still brings its problems. It behoves all anaesthetists to meet this challenge. Much remains to be discovered, especially concerning the essentials for brain survival and to prevent the onset of prolonged coma and the tragedy of patients surviving with irreversible coma. Many new laboratory techniques, currently in use, have created an explosion of knowledge but the clinical worker often does not have direct access to this literature. This chapter attempts a simplified approach to the modern concept of energy transfer and its importance in relation to anaesthesia.

ENERGY PRODUCTION IN THE CELL

The integrity of all living tissue revolves round its unique properties of utilization and storage of energy. A flame and a living cell both consume fuel and liberate energy. The flame achieves this in a one-stage reaction while the living cell requires a complicated series of steps with little loss of energy as heat. Most of the stored energy of foodstuffs in the cell is converted to a labile chemical energy store which is later converted, under rigidly controlled conditions, into such uses as mechanical energy in muscles, electrical energy in nerves and luminescence in certain special cells which are capable of releasing energy as light.

Thermodynamic laws state that energy must run 'downhill', as in a flame, and that equilibrium can only be reached when all atoms and molecules assume the most random configuration with the least energy content. For a cell to remain viable, continuous 'uphill' work is necessary and it is this ability to employ energy in an orderly manner that characterizes all living matter.

Physicochemical aspects

The chemical bond joining atoms is more than a physical link: it is an energy relationship. This can be measured in units of energy such as kilojoules of potential energy per mole of a compound. When this is done it is found that some chemical bonds contain more energy than others. Thus, if a carbon–hydrogen bond is ruptured, more energy is released than when a carbon–carbon bond is broken. All chemical change is associated with movement of energy and there is also a receiving or giving up of electrons. Atoms must be located close enough for their electron clouds to overlap and have sufficient kinetic energy to overcome forces of repulsion due to the negative charges of their electron clouds. Spatial orientation at an atomic level thus becomes critical and its study can explain many observed phenomena.

Structure orientation

When three or more atoms combine to form a molecule, the molecule takes on a specific configuration due to a geometric relationship between the atoms involved. The shape of the molecule can be predicted by measuring bond angles and polarity. These are important in explaining chemical reactions between molecules, the specificity of enzymes, construction of membranes and other repetitive patterns seen in living matter.

Oxidation and reduction

When electrons are lost the process is called oxidation and the atom which loses electrons is said to be oxidized. When electrons are gained the process is called reduction and the atom which gains the electrons is said to have been reduced.

Oxygen is not necessarily involved for oxidation to take place. Any loss of electrons in a chemical reaction is termed oxidation. The oxidizing agents then give electrons while the reducing agents accept electrons. In biological systems the removal of electrons from one substance and their transfer to another is the chief method of energy release.

Role of protons

Electron transport mechanisms situated in membranes are claimed by Mitchell (1976) to be there to pump protons across that membrane and thus set up an imbalance in proton distribution between its two sides, the proton gradient being generated across the inner wrinkled membrane. Protons carry positive charges, thus the proton gradient across the membrane creates an electrical potential difference. Since Nature abhors unequal distributions of this sort, protons flow back through the inner membrane of the mitochondrion, and Mitchell (1976) says that ATP is thus generated through activation of ATPase. This potential difference has been calculated to be of the order of 230 mV, which is sufficient to 'drive' the ATPase enzyme. The concept of energy by proticity is simple but effective. All that is required is a thin, topologically closed insulating lipid membrane between two aqueous proton-conducting phases. In addition, because of the relatively high reactivity and mobility of the proton, it is able to function at very low concentrations. This type of power transmission is unique in its ubiquitous occurrence in biology. Little is known concerning the role of anaesthetic agents on this form of energy transfer.

High energy bonds

One form of energy storage in living organisms is high energy phosphate bonds. These bonds contain more potential energy than ordinary or low

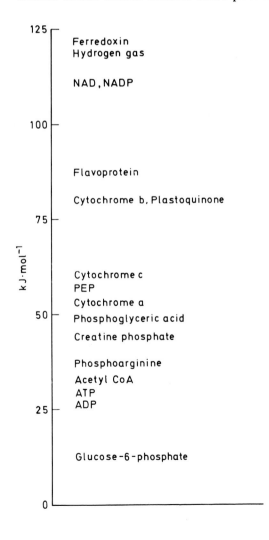

Figure 2.1
The relative energy levels of some common phosphoryl and electron carriers. The baseline for phosphoryl carriers is the transfer of phosphoryl to water (hydrolysis), whereas the baseline for electron carriers is the transfer of one electron to molecular oxygen. (Reproduced from Dupraw, 1968, by courtesy of the author and Academic Press Inc. ©)

energy phosphate bonds. Adenosine triphosphate (ATP) is of great importance in metabolism but there are many other chemical bonds in living
organisms that have greater potential energy than is associated with the
phosphate bonds. Thus the term energy is somewhat misleading and it is a
relative one (*Figure 2.1*).

A high energy bond results from the attachment of new groups to an
existing molecule (for example, adenosine diphosphate (ADP) + inorganic
phosphate $(PO_4) \rightarrow$ adenosine triphosphate (ATP)) so that there is a maximum amount of energy concentrated in bonding certain groups of atoms
together. The phosphate grouping is well suited to this purpose. The rate
of conversion is normally limited by the level of either ADP or PO_4.

In energy exchange it is necessary to capture the energy or else it is
lost for useful work in the cell. There are two advantages in having the
energy stored as high energy phosphate bonds. The first is that the energy
is readily available to the cell for immediate use, it being a one-step
reaction to release it. The second advantage is that the energy available
from such a high energy bond is generally that which is most useful for
producing biochemical reactions. There is thus little waste of energy.

ATP can release energy by detaching one phosphate group to give ADP.
The energy made available can move chemicals across cell membranes,
build molecules and perform other essential cellular functions. ADP can
further be broken down to adenosine monophosphate (AMP) and release
more energy, but usually it is returned to ATP using energy released from
fuel molecules (*Figure 2.2*). ATP is found in the cells of all living organisms
from bacteria to man, and without it life as known would not be possible.

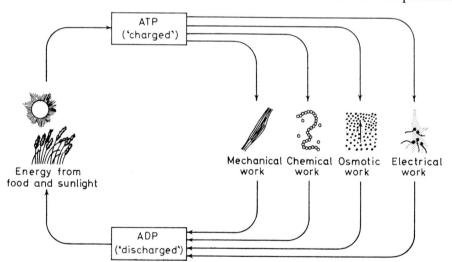

Figure 2.2
ADP, the common carrier of energy in animal and plant cells, is
formed in the mitochondria and chloroplasts. It supplies energy for
muscle contraction, protein synthesis, absorption or secretion against
an osmotic gradient and transfer of nerve impulses. 'Discharged'
ADP thus formed is 'charged' by solar or food energy. (Reproduced
from Lehninger, 1961, by courtesy of the author and the Editor of
Scientific American)

PHOSPHATE/OXYGEN RATIO

The P/O ratio is a measure of the yield of phosphate esterified per atom of oxygen consumed. This can be determined if the hydrolytic breakdown of ATP by ATPase is prevented. From the quantity of oxygen consumed and the ADP added, the P/O ratio can be calculated under different experimental conditions in isolated mitochondrial preparations (*Table 2.1*).

TABLE 2.1. Basic characteristics of oxidative phosphorylation

Substrate oxidized	P/O ratio
NAD^+-linked	3
Flavoprotein-linked: succinate glycerophosphate	2
Non-enzymatic reduction: cytochrome c	1

Phosphorylation sites

Site 1   Between NAD^+ and flavoprotein
Site 2   Between cytochrome b and cytochrome c
Site 3   Between cytochrome c and oxygen

Decoupling of oxidative phosphorylation

In the phenomenon of uncoupling, isolated mitochondria in the presence of certain agents become able to consume oxygen at maximal rate without the formation of ATP and regardless of whether or not inorganic phosphorus and ADP are available.

2,4-Dinitrophenol uncouples oxidative phosphorylation from cellular respiration. This has been compared to putting a car into neutral gear and leaving the engine running. If the respiratory activities are regarded as the engine and the phosphorylation as a process of making the car go, then dinitrophenol uncouples the engine from the transmission of the car. The engine continues to run but the car does not move; in the cell, respiration continues but no ATP is formed.

It has recently been demonstrated that certain unsaturated fatty acids such as oleic acid are also found to be active as uncoupling agents. The fact that an uncoupling agent can be produced *in vivo* suggests that the presence of such a substance in mitochondria might function as an agent regulating tissue respiration and oxygen consumption.

Weinbach and Garbus (1969) suggested that, during uncoupling of oxidative phosphorylation, this was achieved by interaction with proteins. It was found empirically that in damaged mitochondria bovine serum albumin improved the efficiency of oxidative phosphorylation by binding liberated fatty acids acting as endogenous uncouplers. Subsequently, albumin has been shown to counteract the action of many other uncoupling agents by binding to them. Protein in mitochondria can also bind uncoupling agents. This can take place at sites which do not interfere with oxidative phosphorylation. It is suggested that structural changes in lipoprotein complexes in the membrane may be responsible for an alteration in activity of the enzymes responsible for the coupling of phosphorylation to electron transport.

METABOLISM OF CARBOHYDRATES

The main source of energy for cell activities is carbohydrate metabolism. There are two types of metabolism: anaerobic and aerobic. Anaerobic metabolism occurs normally in muscle during exercise and results in the production of lactic acid. Muscle, however, has an abundant supply of blood, which can be greatly increased during muscle activity and a large amount of oxygen is thus made available to be utilized by muscle. However, despite this large blood supply, during strenuous work the tissue content of lactic acid can rise considerably and only returns slowly to normal. Carbohydrates are broken down anaerobically and lactic acid accumulates. During aerobic conditions lactic acid does not accumulate but pyruvate does. This latter, however, can be oxidized almost as rapidly as it is formed.

Lactate metabolism

Cohen and Simpson (1975) have reviewed the problems associated with accumulation of lactate in the body. Severe hypoxia causes rapid accumulation of lactic acid, which has a pK of 3.86. This is considerably lower than the pH range of the body fluids. Lactic acid is thus always virtually completely dissociated and, when buffer systems are overloaded, metabolic acidosis ensues. Cardiac muscle can utilize lactic acid for its energy requirements. Renal excretion is slow, and this builds up over 2—4 hours after onset of acidosis. If the pH falls below 7.1, lactate uptake by the liver ceases and death rapidly follows.

The conversion of pyruvate to lactic acid creates a serious loss of potential energy in the body. It has been shown by Selwyn and Walker (1977) that bicarbonate ions enter mitochondria by an electrogenic process under non-energized conditions. The bicarbonate ions may have a role in regulating mitochondrial metabolism in relation to the electrical potential and pH differences across mitochondrial membranes. Administration of sodium bicarbonate will correct the intracellular metabolic acidosis and allow normal metabolism to be re-established.

Chronic production of lactic acid may result from the administration of fructose, sorbitol or xylitol infusions used for parenteral nutrition. If ethanol is also included in infusion solutions containing fructose, this increases the lactic acidosis by lowering the redox state and elevating the lactate/pyruvate ratio. Sorbitol, which is converted to fructose, may also give rise to overproduction of lactic acid. Thus caution must be exercised when long-term use of these solutions for nutrition is contemplated, especially if hepatic dysfunction is present.

PHENFORMIN AND LACTIC ACIDOSIS

Lactic acidosis has followed the administration of phenformin to patients (Gong and Kato, 1975). It is thought that phenformin lowers blood sugar by potentiating the action of endogenous and exogenous insulin, particularly in its effect on adipose tissue. Oxidation in the citric acid cycle is also inhibited and anaerobic glycolysis is stimulated. The end-result of all these actions is an increased production of lactic acid and lactic acidosis. Gong and Kato (1975) reported that their patient was successfully treated by the intravenous administration of sodium bicarbonate.

Control mechanisms

There has recently been much interest in the mechanisms responsible for the control of metabolism, apart from the well known influence of hormones. One mechanism of control is associated with the accumulation of various metabolites which influence enzyme activity by 'feedback' mechanism. These can be small molecules such as citric acid which influences the activity of phosphofructokinase. This enzyme converts fructose-6-phosphate into fructose-1-6-diphosphate. This reaction takes place many steps away from the site of production of citrate in the Krebs citric acid cycle. These chemicals which influence enzyme activity many steps away from their production are known as allosteric effectors. They play a most important role in regulating metabolism.

The presence and absence of ADP also has an effect regulating the conversion of fructose-6-phosphate to fructose-1-6-diphosphate. As ATP is broken down to ADP, liberating energy, the accumulation of ADP stimulates metabolism and this continues until all the ADP has been reconverted to ATP.

Effect of anaesthesia

Almost 50 years ago Quastel and Wheatley (1932) demonstrated that barbiturates and other drugs affected the metabolism of isolated brain tissue. At the concentrations tested *in vitro*, there was a parallel between hypnotic activities and depression of brain respiration as measured by oxygen uptake in Warburg flasks. When the substrate was glucose, pyruvate or lactate, depression of respiration was seen, but this did not occur in the presence of succinate.

Succinate is an intermediate of the tricarboxylic acid cycle and is oxidized rapidly only to fumarate. This in turn is converted non-oxidatively to malate and only slowly further. Associated with the addition of succinate to medium containing brain and other tissues there is a rapid increase in oxygen uptake but this does not lead to any increase in the tissue content of phosphocreatine. This indicates that the rapid succinate oxidation is not productive of high energy phosphate. The concentrations of anaesthetics required to depress oxygen uptake were relatively high when compared with those needed to induce clinical anaesthesia.

In 1951 Webb and Elliott studied the effects of increasing concentrations of various narcotic drugs on the respiration of both aerobic and anaerobic glycolysis of brain suspensions (*Figure 2.3*). As the concentration of the narcotic was increased the respiration was progressively

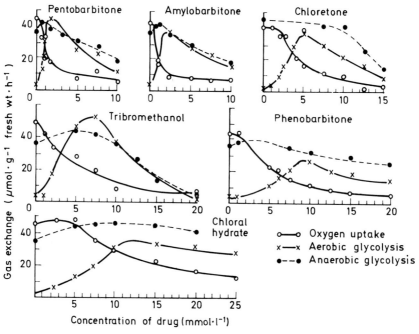

Figure 2.3
Effects of narcotics on oxygen uptake and aerobic and anaerobic glycolysis of rat brain suspensions in bicarbonate-buffered medium. (Reproduced from Webb and Elliott, 1951, by courtesy of the authors and Williams & Wilkins Co., Baltimore, Md. 21202 ©)

inhibited, but about 15–20% of the respiratory activity was resistant to the highest drug concentration. The rate of aerobic glycolysis first increased and reached a maximum when the respiration was about 50% inhibited and then it decreased. At low drug concentrations the rate of anaerobic glycolysis usually showed a slight increase but, at about the same concentration that caused aerobic glycolysis to fall, inhibition was observed to take place. The concentration at which these effects occurred varied widely from drug to drug but was consistent in repeated experiments with one drug. It was shown that following washout of phenobarbitone there was reversibility of the effect on oxygen uptake. However, when the drug concentration was raised beyond the level at which aerobic glycolysis was inhibited the effects on respiration and blood level rapidly became irreversible.

In the absence of oxygen and glucose, brain tissue rapidly and irreversibly loses metabolic activity. When convulsant agents such as nikethamide were added to brain suspensions, little effect was observed on metabolism except at relatively high concentrations. This suggests that convulsants may not enter or reach enzymes responsible for metabolism.

The turnover rate of 6-phosphogluconate was measured by Hakim and Moss (1974), using an isotope technique, in awake rats and those receiving ether. This allowed direct determination of the role of the pentose—phosphate shunt during anaesthesia. It was found that during ether anaesthesia there was a drastic fall in the total cerebral glucose oxidation while the pentose pathway was still able to function.

LIPOLYSIS

In rats, Mäkeläinen (1974) demonstrated the occurrence of lipolysis *in vivo* following anaesthesia and suggested that it was due to an indirect action involving catecholamines. Only slight hyperglycaemia was observed. Bennis, Olsson and Smith (1976) studied specimens of human adipose tissue exposed to varying concentrations of halothane and found that lipolysis was significantly increased by low concentrations of halothane. When higher concentrations were used, lipolysis was reduced. Yang *et al.* (1973) have demonstrated that halothane stimulates the adenyl cyclase as well as phosphodiesterase activities in rat uterine muscle. At the higher concentrations of halothane, increased phosphodiesterase activity may give an over-all effect of inhibition of the observed lipolysis.

When trifluoracetic acid, a known metabolite of halothane, was given to rats by Mäkeläinen and Rosenberg (1974) this was also found to stimulate lipolysis *in vivo,* as was sodium fluoride from methoxyflurane metabolism. It was suggested that elevated free fatty acids and glycerol seen after anaesthesia with halothane or methoxyflurane were due to these metabolites and not the agents themselves.

Carbon dioxide and brain metabolism

In cats, Granholm and Siesjo (1969) studied both hypercapnia and hypocapnia in relation to lactate/pyruvate ratios in cerebrospinal fluid and brain tissues. Hypercapnia leads to a decrease and hyperventilation an increase in tissue concentrations of these acids.

In rats, Carlsson, Nilsson and Siesjo (1974) found increases of lactate and pyruvate occurring within 2 minutes of hyperventilation to a Pa_{CO_2} of 1.3 kPa (10 mmHg). No changes were seen in phosphocreatine, ATP, ADP or AMP at 2–5 minutes. Lactic acidosis was unrelated to derangement of the energy state of the tissue. Activation of phosphofructokinase was observed but it was suggested that other enzymes may also be involved.

Alexander *et al.* (1968) have studied cerebral carbohydrate metabolism in man under conditions of normal acid—base balance, respiratory alkalosis and combined respiratory and metabolic alkalosis. When the $P_{a}CO_2$ was below 2.7 kPa (20 mmHg) there was an increase in glucose consumption by brain (compared with normocarbia), with lower oxygen consumption and an increase in conversion to lactate. The Bohr effect and decreased cerebral perfusion both played a part in these metabolic upsets. Following the administration of sodium bicarbonate, brain perfusion increased and counteracted the Bohr effect on brain metabolism.

Hypoxia, cerebral oedema and metabolism

It has been demonstrated in decapitated animals that a sequence of events is associated with increasing periods of hypoxia, as can be seen in *Figure 2.4*. Following the acute period of stagnant anoxia attendant on cardiac

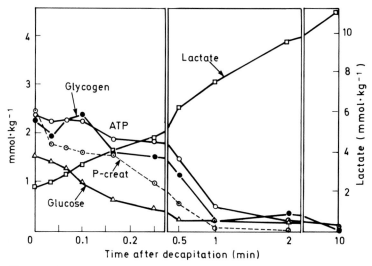

Figure 2.4
Concentration of phosphocreatine, ATP, glucose, glycogen and lactate in the brains of anaesthetized adult mice frozen quickly at different intervals after decapitation. Each point is the average of values from 2—4 mice, a total of 28 animals. (Reproduced from Lowry *et al.*, 1964, by courtesy of the authors and the American Society of Biological Chemists, Inc.)

arrest, nerve cells, astrocytes and oligodendroglia undergo destructive changes leading to irreversible death. This process has been called morphotropic necrobiosis by Lindenberg (1963) and is associated with the rapid accumulation of toxic cellular metabolites.

If, however, stagnant anoxia is preceded by a period of hypoxaemia during which circulation is maintained, toxic metabolites are carried away from the brain as they are produced. There is absence of oedema and histologically the cells remain structurally normal even if stagnant anoxia lasts for 24 hours or longer. This has been called morphostatic necrobiosis (*Figure 2.5*).

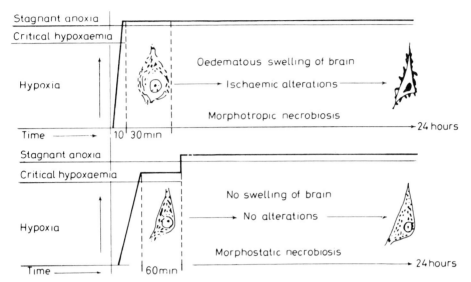

Figure 2.5
Two types of transition from hypoxaemia to stagnant anoxia and their significance for the development or absence of morphological changes. (Reproduced from Lindenberg, 1963, by courtesy of the author and Blackwell Scientific Publications)

Neurostenin and hypoxia

Actin and myosin are major protein components of vertebrate striated muscles. They are able to convert the chemical energy present in ATP to movement. Actin and myosin are also to be found in adult vertebrate brain, nerve cells in culture and in fragments such as synaptosomes (Bray, 1976). The amount of actin in nerve is surprisingly high while less myosin is present. To facilitate the differentiation between muscle and brain proteins, brain actomyosin has been designated as neurostenin, where brain actin is known as neurin and brain myosin as stenin. It has been proposed by Halsey (1975) that neurotransmitter release of neurons is linked to the contraction of neurostenin.

Following short intervals of cerebral ischaemia, neurostenin decreases to a greater extent than other enzymes apart from tyrosine hydroxylase. The exact role of depletion of neurostenin after cerebral hypoxia requires further study. It is, however, possible that, if this controller of transmitter release is destroyed, irreversible cerebral function must inevitably follow.

MITOCHONDRIA

The major site of aerobic respiration is in mitochondria (*Figure 2.6*). These are found in a wide variety of animal tissues and all possess the same basic morphology. There is an apparently structureless matrix bounded by two membranes. The inner of these is periodically invaginated

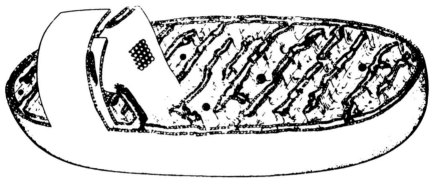

Figure 2.6
An interpretation of mitochondrial ultrastructure. The cristae are folds of an inner membrane composed of spheroid subunits; a relatively unfolded outer membrane encloses the inner membrane and matrix. Polyp-like particles line the cristae surfaces in regular arrays. (Reproduced from Dupraw, 1968, by courtesy of the author and Academic Press Inc. ©)

to form highly characteristic infoldings known as cristae. The function of this infolding of the inner membrane seems to be to provide access to the respiratory enzymes and to provide additional membrane surfaces to accommodate these enzymes. Mitochondria from tissues with high oxygen uptake have large numbers of tightly packed cristae.

Chance (1957) has assigned different states of metabolic balances such as those associated with starvation. Where this is present the cells have a high content of ADP, respiration rate is slow and here the rate-limiting factor is lack of substrate. During active metabolism the ADP level is high, there is also a high substrate content with fast respiration. Here the rate-limiting factor is associated with the passage of electrons down the respiratory chain. During resting conditions ADP is at a low concentration while the substrate level is high and respiration slow. The rate-limiting factor here is the absence of ADP. Under anaerobic conditions the ADP level is high and the substrate content is also high. There is no consumption of oxygen and the rate-limiting factor here is the lack of oxygen.

Halothane and respiratory control

Snodgrass and Piras (1966), using standard manometric techniques, showed that halothane was a true uncoupling agent of rat liver mitochondria *in vitro*. By using amylobarbitone, which is known to block electron transport in the first part of the respiratory chain (*Figure 2.7*), it could be shown that halothane did not act in a similar way. Halothane appeared to uncouple at all three phosphorylation sites along the electron transfer chain. It was also suggested that halothane impaired the function of the enzyme systems which generate NADH within the mitochondria.

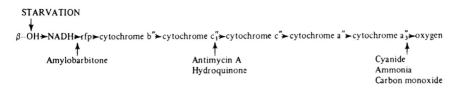

Figure 2.7
Components of cytochrome chain and site of action of inhibitors.
(rfp = reduced flavoprotein)

When mitochondria, in a resting state with low ADP or 'acceptorless' respiration, were equilibrated with halothane at a partial pressure of 4.5 kPa (34 mmHg), there was a loss of respiratory control. This may be associated with a breakdown in some high energy intermediate before the uptake of inorganic phosphate. The solubility of anaesthetics in the lipid of lipoprotein membranes found in mitochondria was thought to be an important factor.

Cohen and Marshall (1968) also studied the effect of halothane on liver mitochondria and found significant effects at concentrations of halothane used clinically. Instead of using manometric techniques, they used a rapidly responding oxygen electrode which was able to provide a more sensitive indication of altered mitochondrial oxygen consumption. They examined the mitochondria in both the active and resting states. It was observed that alteration in the function of the mitochondrial respiratory chain and loss of respiratory control occurred.

In the active state, with excess of substrate, oxygen, phosphate and phosphate acceptor, the rapid transfer of electrons from glutamate to oxygen by the respiratory chain was decreased in a dose-related manner (*Figure 2.8*). Cohen and McIntyre (1972) exposed rat liver mitochondria to a wide range of concentrations of halothane, methoxyflurane, enflurane and diethyl ether. It was found that all these volatile anaesthetics produced a dose-dependent diminution in state 3 respiration with ADP present, when glutamate or NADH was the substrate. However, when succinate was present, both halothane and enflurane failed to depress state 3 respiration. With methoxyflurane and diethyl ether a diminished rate of oxidation of succinate was observed but this was much less than when glutamate was present. All four agents acted at the same site of glutamate oxidation, namely that of NADH dehydrogenase. Since this effect is seen only in intact mitochondria, it has been suggested that the metabolic effect may be associated with interference of delivery of the substrate to the site of utilization.

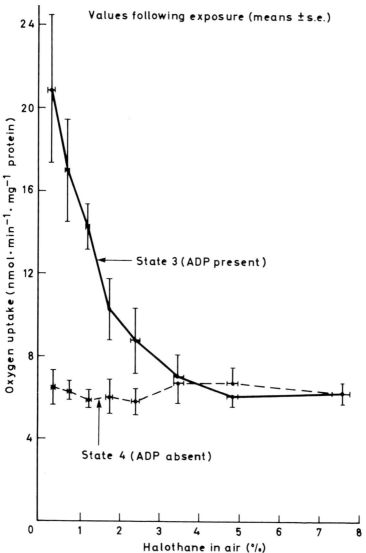

Figure 2.8
Effect of halothane on oxygen uptake by rat liver mitochondria in
the presence and absence of ADP; 2-ml cuvettes were used containing
0.187 mol mannitol, 0.062 mol sucrose, 0.010 mol Tris buffer,
0.010 mol KH_2PO_4 and 0.010 glutamate at a pH of 7.2. (Reproduced
from Cohen and Marshall, 1968, by courtesy of the authors and
Williams & Wilkins Co., Baltimore, Md. 21202 ©)

EFFECT ON LABILE PHOSPHATES

Volatile anaesthetics have been used by Nilsson and Siesjo (1970) and
Biebuyck and Hawkins (1972) to study their effect on labile phosphates
in brain tissue. Concentrations of phosphocreatine, ATP or AMP were
found not to be affected, and this indicates that the anaesthetics studied
did not inhibit electron transport or energy transfer in brain tissue.

LOW CONCENTRATIONS OF ANAESTHETICS AND CEREBRAL OXYGEN CONSUMPTION

Stullken *et al.* (1977), in dogs, studied the effect of low concentrations of anaesthetics and cerebral oxygen consumption. When concentrations of halothane, enflurane, isoflurane and thiopentone between 0 and 1 MAC* were administered a non-linear dose response curve was observed. Changes in the EEG to an 'anaesthetic' pattern which took place at concentrations well below MAC were accompanied by abrupt falls in metabolic rate. This was presumed to be linked to the onset of functional cerebral depression. The non-linear dose response curves seen at low anaesthetic concentrations are contrary to previous observations.

MICROSOMES

By means of centrifugation of liver cell homogenates at the highest speed of centrifugation, a range of microscopic particles is obtained. One fraction consists of microsomes containing a high concentration of ribonucleic acid. Under the electron microscope, small vesicles can be seen with ribonucleic acid granules attached to them. It has been established that, following homogenization of the liver, the endoplasmic reticulum is broken up into little vesicles and these are the source of the microsomes. It is now possible, by the use of sugar gradients, to separate two major fractions — one predominantly arising from smooth endoplasmic reticulum and the other from the ribonucleic-rich rough endoplasmic reticulum. These microsomes can be shown to be involved in the metabolism of drugs.

Metabolism of drugs

Located in hepatic microsomes are enzymes responsible for the metabolism of many drugs. These include esterases, amidases and glucuronyl transferases. There are also reduced nicotinamide adenine dinucleotide phosphate (NADPH) dependent enzymes which catalyse the breakdown of a variety of aromatic and aliphatic compounds. When used with appropriate co-factors, the enzymes in the microsomal fraction can metabolize a wide variety of drugs *in vitro*. Oxidations may be straightforward as aromatic or aliphatic hydroxylations but can also include oxidative N-, S- or O-de-ethylation, deamination, demethylation, desulphuration and certain dehalogenations. Thus there are a large number of biotransformations which can take place in the microsomes of the liver and probably some other organs as well.

    Cytochrome P450 describes a group of haemoproteins located in cell membranes, which are responsible for the metabolism of many chemicals foreign to the body. The label P450 is derived from the fact that these cytochromes have a strong absorption of light at a wavelength of 450 nm when reduced and coupled with carbon monoxide. They are the terminal

*MAC is defined on p. 45. *Ed.*

cytochrome of an electron transport chain, and many drugs and metabolic inhibitors have been shown to combine with the oxidized form of cytochrome P450.

Alvares *et al.* (1969) have demonstrated that cytochrome P450 and cytochrome b_5 are present in human liver. There is less cytochrome P450 in human than in rat and rabbit liver.

The duration and the intensity of action of many drugs and foreign chemicals depend upon the tissue content of oxidized cytochrome P450. Brain and skeletal muscle, being devoid of cytochrome P450, are unable to oxidize many foreign chemicals. An increase or decrease of cytochrome P450 content has been shown to parallel drug-induced changes in tissue hydroxylating activity.

Certain drugs, such as barbiturates, tend to accelerate the reduction of cytochrome P450 and are known as type 1 substrates; other drugs, known as type 2 substrates, such as pyridine tend to decrease the reduction rate. Cytochrome b_5 has also been thought to be responsible for some drug oxidations.

Ullrich and Schnabel (1973) describe a 'catalytic site' in cytochrome P450 where the oxygen molecule is bound to the ferrous iron, and an 'active site' of the enzymes where binding of the substrate takes place. These two sites are in close proximity to each other. When considering inhibition studies of cytochrome-P450-catalysed reactions there are two possibilities of action of inhibitors, given below.

(1) Binding to the active site and thus competition for the formation of the enzyme substrate complex. This is typical of lipophilic compounds such as anaesthetics.
(2) Binding to the catalytic site of the cytochrome or ferrous iron. Here competition takes place for oxygen binding and this has non-competitive characteristics. The best known is carbon monoxide, which competes effectively with the oxygen-binding reaction.

The most potent inhibitors of cytochrome P450 are those compounds which bind to both active sites. Typical examples are metapyranone and octylamine where the free electron pairs of the nitrogen atoms provide the necessary binding forces for complex formation. Chlorinated hydrocarbons such as carbon tetrachloride and halogenated volatile anaesthetics can all form an enzyme—substrate complex with cytochrome P450 of liver microsomes.

Pharmacological implications are that new routes of metabolism now become evident. If a free radical is unstable in the presence of oxygen, peroxides can be formed which are either reduced to alcohols or may result in destruction of auto-oxidizable cell components. It is possible that there are alternate pathways of metabolism during hypoxia. These have already been described for halothane (Van Dyke and Gandolfi, 1976; Widger, Gandolfi and Van Dyke, 1976).

Low concentrations of volatile anaesthetics have been shown to have a significant effect on the microsomal mixed function oxidase system in animals (Berman and Bochantin, 1970).

Enzyme induction

Many drugs that induce their own metabolic breakdown by hepatic microsomes also stimulate the metabolic destruction of other pharmacologically active agents (Conney, 1967).

During enzyme induction, hydroxylation is one of the detoxicating systems which is stimulated. Others affected are glucuronylating systems and increases in the activities of oxidation by mitochondrial enzymes. The glucuronyl pathway, using a readily available carbohydrate closely related to glucose, is possibly the most important route of drug detoxication. Many drugs are excreted in bile and urine in water-soluble forms as glucuronides after direct esterification or prior hydroxylation.

There is a direct relationship between the duration and intensity of action of many drugs and their speed of metabolism in the body. The microsomal enzymes in liver are mainly responsible for the disposal of many pharmacologically active agents. Dietary and nutritional factors, hormonal changes in the body and ingestion of foreign chemicals can alter the activities of these enzymes. An increase in activity appears to represent an increased concentration of enzyme protein and is referred to as 'enzyme induction'.

Spurious results from environmental factors have marred some experiments. These include the presence of cedar wood shavings in animal cages. These shavings may contain enzyme-inducing chemicals (Vessel, 1968). The use of fly-sprays containing fluorinated aerosols must be avoided in animal houses when studying enzyme induction.

Pretreatment of animals with drugs, such as phenobarbitone given daily to rats, results in maximal increase in enzyme activity in 3 days. Other inducers may take as long as 5—10 days before maximal increase in activity can be observed.

Associated with enzyme induction is an increase in the weight of the liver and the content of cytochrome P450 which can increase two- or threefold. Chronic treatment with the drug accelerates metabolism, lowers its blood level and decreases the pharmacological effects. Tolerance to several barbiturates is related to accelerated metabolism in the liver. However, whilst phenobarbitone stimulates its own metabolism when high doses are administered chronically to dogs, tolerance developed. In dogs and humans this is not related to enhanced metabolism but occurs presumably by an adaptation of the central nervous system. Enzyme induction, however, can seriously affect the measurement of metabolism and influences the acute or chronic toxicity of drugs.

Berman *et al.* (1976) suggest that enzyme induction, in man, is present when (1) the rate of clearance of a foreign chemical from plasma is increased, (2) its half-life in plasma is less, or (3) the excretion of its metabolites is increased. A non-invasive method of testing for enzyme induction is based on the observation that hydroxylation of steroid hormones is also increased in the presence of enzyme induction. This can be monitored by estimation of the urinary levels of a metabolite of cortisol, 6β-hydroxycortisol, relative to the total of 17-hydroxycorticosteroids (Conney, 1967).

Volatile anaesthetics and enzyme induction

HALOTHANE

Van Dyke, Chenoweth and Van Poznak (1964) described halothane biotransformation *in vitro* which occurred primarily in the hepatic microsomal fraction and was inducible by phenobarbitone. Thus halothane was metabolized by the classic mixed function oxygenase pathway.

Chronic administration of halothane (0.5%) to mice caused liver enlargement of 50% in 2 weeks, similar to that observed after administration of phenobarbitone (Schimassek, Kunz and Gallwitz, 1966). There was a decrease in trioses of the glycolytic pathway and an increase in the substrates of the citric acid cycle, which was maximal in the third week. Most of the observed actions of halothane concern the mitochondrial compartment with substrates of the citric acid cycle.

Malic enzyme which connects the cytoplasmic and mitochondrial compartments increased in activity and this was associated with a rise in glycerol-1-phosphate oxidase. This latter may be looked upon as a compensatory mechanism to allow transport of hydrogen from the glycolytic pathway to the respiratory chain.

Phenobarbitone administered prior to anaesthesia with ^{14}C–halothane in animals, was found by Reynolds and Moslen (1975) to increase the cytochrome P450 content of liver. In addition, the amount of ^{14}C exhaled was almost halved and the total urinary ^{14}C metabolites was doubled. This indicated that more halothane was being metabolized. However, no change was observed after enzyme induction in the binding of radioactivity to liver at either 2 or 24 hours following exposure to ^{14}C–halothane. This suggests that there is no alteration of normal metabolic pathways following induction with phenobarbitone.

Carbon tetrachloride pretreatment deactivated cytochrome P450 and injured the endoplasmic reticulum with the result that there was a decrease in the total ^{14}C metabolites excreted in urine. In the liver there was less total radioactivity but, once again, no alteration in the pattern of incorporation of ^{14}C into the metabolites in liver was observed.

Aroclor 1254, a polychlorinated biphenyl, is typical of a group of chemicals now widely distributed in the environment. Aroclor 1254 was used by Reynolds and Moslen (1977) as an inducer of enzyme activity 7 days prior to exposure to halothane. Damage to the rough endoplasmic reticulum and deactivation of cytochrome P450 was seen. In these experiments there was no increase in the protein-bound metabolites in liver, nor excretion of water-soluble metabolites in urine.

Sipes and Brown (1976) pretreated rats with a single dose of Aroclor 1254 before exposure to halothane anaesthesia. This was followed by pronounced centrilobular necrosis in 80% of the rats and these lesions resembled those seen in the reported halothane-induced hepatic lesions. The Aroclor 1254 pretreatment increased the covalent binding of reactive intermediates of halothane to microsomal lipids and proteins. The biotransformation of halothane was altered, and elevated levels of microsomal protein and cytochrome P450 associated with increased activity of NADP-cytochrome c reductase were seen. A P450 variant with a CO-binding absorption at 449 nm was also observed and thought to be responsible for these alterations in halothane metabolism.

The initial step in halothane metabolism has been postulated to be its conversion to a free radical by an electron-capture reaction displacing bromine, this being the least stable atom present in halothane due to its larger molecular weight and lowest bond energy (Atallah and Geddes, 1973).

Recent studies by Van Dyke and Gandolfi (1976) and Widger, Gandolfi and Van Dyke (1976) have shown that active cytochrome P450 and NADPH give rise to trifluoracetic acid, inorganic bromide and chloride as the main metabolites of halothane. In the presence of low oxygen tensions (7% oxygen) inorganic fluoride released was approximately 60% of the total bound material, assuming that one fluorine atom was released per halothane molecule defluorinated. Obese patients also have elevated serum fluoride levels after halothane anaesthesia (Young *et al.,* 1975).

METHOXYFLURANE

Pretreatment of rats with a subanaesthetic concentration of methoxy-flurane (0.13%) vapour for 7 hours a day was found by Berman and Bochantin (1970) to result in the following responses, different from a control group of rats. After 15 days' exposure to subanaesthetic concentration of methoxyflurane, hexobarbitone sleeping times were reduced by 79%. Aminopyrine demethylase activity was markedly increased in microsomes prepared from rats exposed for 10 days; after this same time of exposure a significant number of rats subsequently survived a lethal concentration of methoxyflurane as determined by LD_{50} experiments. The hepatic microsomal enzyme inhibitor SKF-525-A reversed all these effects of pretreatment with methoxyflurane.

In separate experiments, in rats, Berman *et al.* (1973) demonstrated that pretreatment with phenobarbitone for 3 days increased uptake of methoxyflurane by 36%, and the rate of elimination from a closed circuit was decreased by 21%. Metabolism of methoxyflurane, as determined by the content of inorganic fluoride in livers and kidneys, was markedly increased. These effects of phenobarbitone were partially blocked by SKF-525-A.

In these experiments induced rats were found to have significantly lower blood concentrations of methoxyflurane than seen in control rats on induction of anaesthesia. The induced rats took longer to be anaesthetized than the controls. Altered metabolic patterns can thus influence the clinical practice and behaviour of patients during anaesthesia if the results of these experiments in animals can be extrapolated to man.

ENFLURANE

Berman *et al.* (1976) measured the concentrations of 6β-hydroxycortisol and 17-hydroxycorticosteroids in urines of six male volunteers exposed to enflurane anaesthesia. The ratio of 6β-hydroxycortisol to 17-hydroxy-corticosteroids was increased markedly in five and decreased slightly in one volunteer after anaesthesia. These results indicate that enflurane can cause induction of hepatic microsomal enzymes.

Studies with individual cells

Progress has been made in analysis of individual enzymes, metabolic pathways and metabolic control mechanisms within the intact cell. Chance *et al.* (1962) have described a method to analyse reduced pyridine nucleotides in cells. NADH and NADPH have the property of fluorescence when they are excited by ultraviolet light of wavelength around 340 μm. This emitted fluorescence has a maximum wavelength around 450 μm. Since NAD^+ and $NADP^+$ do not fluoresce, it is possible, using a suitable microscopic system, to check for the presence and absence of these fluorescent compounds. Thus oxidation/reduction reactions can be followed in nerve tissue, when simultaneous recording of action potentials can yield valuable information.

Giacobini (1968) has reviewed chemical studies in individual neurons and discusses the practical aspects of microchemical techniques. It is possible that it will be in this field that the next major breakthrough in metabolism and anaesthesia will take place.

References

Alexander, S. C., Smith, T. C., Strobel, G., Stephen, G. W. and Wollman, H. (1968). Cerebral carbohydrate metabolism of man during respiratory and metabolic aklalosis. *J. appl. Physiol.* 24, 66–72

Alvares, A. P., Schilling, G., Levin, W., Kuntzman, R., Brand, L. and Mark, L. C. (1969). Cytochromes P450 and b$_5$ in human liver microsomes. *Clin. Pharmac. Ther.* 10, 655–659

Atallah, M. M. and Geddes, I. C. (1973). Metabolism of halothane during and after anaesthesia in man. *Br. J. Anaesth.* 45, 464–470

Bennis, J., Olsson, J. and Smith, U. (1976). Effects of halothane on the metabolism of human adipose tissue. *Acta anaesth. scand.* 20, 327–333

Berman, M. L. and Bochantin, J. F. (1970). Non specific stimulation of drug metabolism in rats by methoxyflurane. *Anesthesiology* 32, 500–506

Berman, M. L., Lowe, H. J., Bochantin, J. and Hagler, K. (1973). Uptake and elimination of methoxyflurane as influenced by enzyme induction in the rat. *Anesthesiology* 38, 352–357

Berman, M. L., Green, O. C., Calverley, R. K., Smith, N. T. and Eger, E. I. (1976). Enzyme induction by enflurane in man. *Anesthesiology* 44, 496–500

Biebuyck, J. F. and Hawkins, R. A. (1972). The effect of anaesthetic agents on brain tissue metabolite patterns. *Br. J. Anaesth.* 44, 226–227

Bray, D. (1976). Actin and myosin: their role in the growth of nerve cells. *Biochem. Soc. Trans.* 4, 543–544

Carlsson, C., Nilsson, L. and Siesjo, B. K. (1974). Cerebral metabolic changes in arterial hypocapnia of short duration. *Acta anaesth. scand.* 18, 104–113

Chance, B. (1957). Cellular oxygen requirements. *Fedn Proc.* 16, 671–680

Chance, B., Cohen, P., Jobsis, F. and Schoener, B. (1962). Intracellular oxidation-reduction states *in vivo. Science, N.Y.* 137, 499–508

Cohen, P. J. and McIntyre, R. (1972). The effects of general anesthesia on respiratory control and oxygen consumption of rat liver mitochondria. In *Cellular Biology and Toxicity of Anesthetics*, pp. 109–116. B. R. Fink (ed.). Baltimore, Md: Williams & Wilkins

Cohen, P. J. and Marshall, B. E. (1968). Effects of halothane on respiratory control and oxygen consumption of rat liver mitochondria. In *Toxicity of Anesthetics*, p. 24. B. R. Fink (ed.). Baltimore, Md: Williams & Wilkins

Cohen, R. S. and Simpson, R. (1975). Lactate metabolism. *Anesthesiology* 43, 661–673

Conney, A. H. (1967). Pharmacological implications of microsomal enzyme induction. *Pharmac. Rev.* 19, 317–366

Dupraw, E. J. (1968). *Cell and Molecular Biology.* New York: Academic Press

Giacobini, E. (1968). Chemical studies on individual neurons. I. Vertebral nerves. In *Neurosciences Research,* Vol. 1, p. 1. S. Ehrenpreis and O. C. Solnitzky (ed.). New York and London: Academic Press

Gong, W. C. and Kato, D. B. (1975). Phenformin-induced lactic acidosis. A case report and review of the literature. *Drug Intell. clin. Pharm.* 9, 236–240

Granholm, L. and Siesjo, B. K. (1969). The effects of hypercapnia and hypocapnia upon the cerebrospinal fluid lactate and pyruvate concentrations and upon the lactate, pyruvate, ATP, ADP, phosphocreatine and creatine concentrations of cat brain tissue. *Acta physiol. scand.* 75, 257–266

Hakim, A. M. and Moss, G. (1974). The effect of ether anesthesia on cerebral glucose metabolism – the pentose phosphate pathway. *Anesthesiology* 40, 261–267

Halsey, J. H. Jr (1975). Studies in cerebral metabolism. *Clin. Neurosurg.* 22, 67–75

Lindenberg, R. (1963). Patterns of CNS vulnerability in acute hypoxaemia, including anaesthesia accidents. In *Selective Vulnerability of the Brain in Hypoxaemia,* p. 189. A Symposium Organised by the Council for International Organisations of Medical Sciences. J. P. Schade and W. H. McMenemey (ed.). Oxford: Blackwell

Lowry, O. H., Passonneau, J. V., Hasselberger, F. X. and Schulz, D. W. (1964). Effect of ischaemia on known substrates and cofactors of the glycolytic pathway on brain. *J. Biol. Chem.* 239, 18–30

Mäkeläinen, A. (1974). Methoxyflurane and lipid carbohydrate metabolism in rate. *Acta anaesth. scand.* 18, 144–152

Mäkeläinen, A. and Rosenberg, P. (1974). The effect of halothane and methoxyflurane metabolites on lipolysis 'in vitro'. *Acta anaesth. scand.* 18, 153–160

Mitchell, P. (1976). Vectorial chemistry and the molecular mechanics of chemiosmotic coupling: power transmission by proticity. *Biochem. Soc. Trans.* 4, 399–430

Nilsson, L. and Siesjo, B. K. (1970). The effect of anesthetics upon labile phosphates and upon extra- and intracellular lactate, pyruvate and bicarbonate concentrations in the rat brain. *Acta physiol. scand.* 80, 235–248

Quastel, J. H. and Wheatley, A. H. M. (1932). Narcosis and oxidations of the brain. *Proc. R. Soc. B* 112, 60–79

Reynolds, E. S. and Moslen, M. T. (1975). Metabolism of halothane-^{14}C 'in vivo'. Effects of multiple halothane anesthesia phenobarbital and carbon tetrachloride pretreatment. *Biochem. Pharmac.* 24, 2075–2081

Reynolds, E. S. and Moslen, M. T. (1977). Halothane hepatoxicity: enhancement by polychlorinated biphenyl pretreatment. *Anesthesiology* 47, 19–27

Schimassek, H., Kunz, W. and Gallwitz, D. (1966). Differentiation of liver metabolism on the molecular level during chronic application of halothane. *Biochem. Pharmac.* 15, 1957–1964

Selwyn, M. J. and Walker, H. A. (1977). Permeability of the mitochondrial membranes to bicarbonate ions. *Biochem. J.* 166, 137–139

Sipes, I. G. and Brown, B. R. (1976). An animal model of hepatotoxicity associated with halothane anesthesia. *Anesthesiology* 45, 622–628

Snodgrass, P. J. and Piras, M. M. (1966). The effects of halothane on rat liver mitochondria. *Biochemistry* 5, 1140–1149

Stullken, E. H., Milde, J. H., Michenfelder, J. D. and Tinker, J. H. (1977). The non linear responses of cerebral metabolism to low concentrations of halothane, enflurane, isoflurane and thiopental. *Anesthesiology* 46, 28–34

Ullrich, V. and Schnabel, K. H. (1973). Formation and binding of carbanions by cytochrome P-450 of liver microsomes. *Drug Metab. Disposit.* 1, 176–182

Van Dyke, R. A. and Gandolfi, A. J. (1976). Anaerobic release of fluoride from halothane relationship to the binding of halothane metabolites to hepatic cellular constituents. *Drug Metab. Disposit.* 4, 40

Van Dyke, R. A., Chenoweth, M. B. and Van Poznak, A. (1964). Metabolism of volatile anesthetics. 1. Conversion 'in vivo' of several anesthetics to $^{14}CO_2$ and chloride. *Biochem. Pharmac.* 13, 1239–1247

Vessel, E. S. (1968). Genetic and environmental factors affecting hexobarbital metabolism in mice. *Ann. N.Y. Acad. Sci.* 151, 900–912

Webb, J. L. and Elliott, K. A. C. (1951). Effect of narcotics and convulsants on tissue glycolysis and respiration. *J. Pharmac. exp. Ther.* 103, 24–34

Weinbach, E. C. and Garbus, J. (1969). Mechanism of action of reagents that uncouple oxidative phosphorylation. *Nature, Lond.* 221, 1016–1018

Widger, L. A., Gandolfi, A. J. and Van Dyke, R. A. (1976). Hypoxia and halothane metabolism 'in vivo' release of inorganic fluoride and halothane metabolite binding to cellular constituents. *Anesthesiology* 44, 197–201

Yang, J. C., Triner, L., Vulliemoz, Y., Verosky, M. and Ngai, S. H. (1973). Effects of halothane on the cyclic 3', 5'-adenosine monophosphate (cyclic AMP) system in rat uterine muscle. *Anesthesiology* 38, 244–250

Young, S. R., Stoelting, R. K., Peterson, C. and Madura, J. A. (1975). Anesthetic biotransformation and renal function in obese patients during and after methoxyflurane or halothane anesthesia. *Anesthesiology* 42, 451–457

3 Physicochemical properties of inhalational anaesthetics

M. J. Halsey

The physicochemical properties of the inhalational general anaesthetics determine their potencies, modes of administration and rates of uptake, distribution and elimination. In addition, certain characteristics have been found to be of considerable importance in relation to possible mechanisms of anaesthetic action. The physical and chemical data in this chapter have been assembled from the references which are indicated in the legend of each table. In some cases it has been necessary to choose between discrepant values, and it is surprising how much the data have continued to be revised for many years after the release of the agent.

ANAESTHETIC POTENCY AND MAC

The agents in all the tables have been arranged in order of their anaesthetic potency. The *minimum alveolar concentration* (MAC) of an anaesthetic is defined as the concentration at 1 atmosphere that produces immobility in 50% of patients or animals exposed to a noxious stimulus (Eger, 1974). Clinical practice is, of course, more concerned with the *inspired* anaesthetizing concentration of an agent, but the required inspired concentration is a complex function of both the intrinsic potency of the agent (MAC), duration of anaesthesia and the uptake and distribution of the agent in that particular patient. MAC is determined by maintaining the alveolar (or end-tidal) concentration at a predetermined level for at least 10 minutes in order to allow for anaesthetic equilibration between the alveolar gas, arterial blood and the site of action in the central nervous system. Under these circumstances, the alveolar concentration at 1 atm is, in fact, the partial pressure throughout these regions. Partial pressure is a very useful concept in a multiphase system because, unlike concentration, it is the same in different compartments which are in equilibrium with each other. This overcomes the problem that the solubility characteristics of the site of action are not yet completely known.

It used to be thought that the clinical usefulness of the MAC concept would be limited because it was defined as the anaesthetizing dose for only half a group of patients. However, the dose response curve for surgical anaesthesia turned out to be relatively steep and it is only necessary to increase the dose by 10—15% to be sure of anaesthetizing the vast majority of patients (de Jong and Eger, 1975). The end-point chosen for the determination of MAC was surgical skin incision but there are many other clinical criteria for assessing the depth of anaesthesia. These are very useful when administering a particular agent but they do not necessarily apply to all agents.

GENERAL CHEMICAL AND PHYSICAL PROPERTIES

The structural formulae of the general anaesthetics in *Table 3.1* only indicate the relative positions of the atoms making up the molecule. For example, nitrous oxide is a linear molecule as illustrated, but the equilibrium bond length between the two nitrogen atoms is shorter than that between the nitrogen and oxygen atom. The relative Van der Waals radii of the different terminal atoms are of the order $Br > Cl > F > H$, and the over-all shape and size can only be seen satisfactorily in molecular models made up with 'space filling' atoms (e.g. the Corey—Pauling—Koltun atomic models).

The inhalational anaesthetics have diverse structures and do not act by forming covalent-ionic bonds with the site of action. Since the state of general anaesthesia is rapidly reversible, the type of bonding involved must be the weak Van der Waals type which is produced by the electrostatic attraction between opposite dipoles. Dipoles are electric charges formed by the unequal distribution of electrons between the atoms of the molecule. These forces are, however, sufficient for anaesthetics to be able to bind reversibly to various cell components, including internal sites of proteins (Schoenborn, 1968; Brown, Halsey and Richards, 1976).

The mole volume

The molecular weight and density are used in many calculations in anaes-thesia, particularly when it is necessary to convert from liquid to vapour volumes. A *mole* (the molecular weight in grams) of any substance contains the same number of molecules (6.022×10^{23} — Avogadro's number). *Avogadro's principle* states that equal volumes of gas under standard conditions of temperature and pressure contain equal numbers of molecules. Thus the volume of one mole of any gas should be the same, and for an *ideal* gas at $0°C$ and 1 atmosphere pressure the molar volume is 22.414 litres. In general, the molar volumes of gases, as calculated from their measured gas densities, are less than the theoretical value but, since the volatile anaesthetics are used at low partial pressures (when their behaviour

TABLE 3.1. Physical data of inhalational anaesthetics

Agent (Trade name)	Structure	Molecular weight	Boiling point at 1 atm (°C)	Vapour pressure at 20°C kPa (mmHg)		Latent heat of vaporization (kJ·mol⁻¹)	Liquid density at 20°C (g·ml⁻¹)	MAC (% vol/vol)	Antoine constants A (kPa)	B	C	ml of vapour/ ml of liquid (at 20°C)
Methoxy-flurane (Penthrane)	$CH_3-O-CF_2CHCl_2$	165.0	104.7	3.0	(22.5)	33.9	1.43	0.16	6.206	1336.58	213.5	208
Trichloro-ethylene (Trilene)	$CCl_2 = CHCl$	131.4	86.7	7.7	(58)	31.3	1.46	(0.6)	5.961	1198.48	216.4	267
Chloroform	$CHCl_3$	119.4	61.2	21.3	(160)	29.5	1.47	(0.77)	5.978	1125.05	222.0	296
Halothane (Fluothane)	$CF_3-CHClBr$	197.4	50.2	32.1	(241)	28.9	1.86	0.75	5.892	1043.70	218.3	227
Enflurane (Ethrane)	$CHF_2-O-CF_2-CHFCl$	184.5	56.5	23.3	(175)	32.3	1.52	1.68	6.112	1107.84	213.1	198
Diethyl ether	$CH_3-CH_2-O-CH_2-CH_3$	74.1	34.6	59.1	(442)	27.6	0.72	1.92	6.151	1109.58	233.2	233
Cyclo-propane	$H_2C \overset{CH_2}{\underset{}{\triangle}} CH_2$	42.1	−34.0	640	(4800)	20.1	—	9.2	5.769	723.32	225.7	—
Nitrous oxide	$N \equiv N \rightarrow O$	44.0	−88.0	5200	(39 000)	18.2	—	101	6.702	912.90	285.3	—

Physical data are from manufacturer' literature and/or Secher (1971). MAC values are for man (30—55-year-old age group) except where not available; i.e. trichloro-ethylene (rat), chloroform (dog). The references for the MAC values are (in order of agents): Saidman *et al.* (1967); Chand, Halsey and White (1978); Eger *et al.* (1969); Gregory, Eger and Munson (1969); Gion and Saidman (1971); Saidman *et al.* (1967); Stevens *et al.* (1975). Antoine constants are from Rodgers and Hill (1978).

is a better approximation of the 'ideal' situation), the value of 22.4 $l \cdot mol^{-1}$ is acceptable. Thus, for example:

$$1 \text{ ml of liquid halothane at } 20°C = 1 \times 1.86 \text{ g}$$

$$= \frac{1 \times 1.86}{197.4} \text{ mol}$$

$$= \frac{1 \times 1.86}{197.4} \times 22.4 \times \frac{293}{273} \text{ litres}$$

$$= 227 \text{ ml of gas at } 20°C$$

The equivalent figures for the other volatile agents are included in *Table 3.1*.
This type of calculation can be used to estimate the consumption of liquid anaesthetics in a vaporizer; e.g. 2% enflurane for 1 hour with a total output gas flow of 7 $l \cdot min^{-1}$ uses approximately 42.5 ml of liquid, whereas 0.5% trichloroethylene under the same conditions uses 7.8 ml. It is also the basis of determination of concentration attained with a liquid injection system of vaporization.

Vaporization

All the clinical inhalational anaesthetics are normally supplied as liquids. The same physical principles apply to those agents which are liquids at room temperature and pressure, and to the liquefied gases in cylinders at elevated pressures.

SATURATED VAPOUR PRESSURE AND TEMPERATURE

The essential feature of vaporization of liquids is that the saturated vapour pressures are effectively independent of the total atmospheric pressure but highly dependent on temperature. *Table 3.1* includes the saturated vapour pressure at 20°C as well as the boiling points of the liquids when their saturated vapour pressures are equal to atmospheric pressure. The variation of saturated vapour pressure with temperature is described theoretically by the *Clapeyron–Clausius equation*, of which one form is:

$$\log P_2/P_1 = - \frac{\Delta H}{19.14} \left[\frac{1}{T_2} - \frac{1}{T_1} \right]$$

where ΔH is the latent heat of vaporization in $J \cdot mol^{-1}$ and T is the temperature in K.

The derivation of this equation assumes that the latent heat of vaporization is independent of temperature and neglects the volume of the liquid in comparison with that of the vapour. It has been found that these assumptions hold good over narrow temperature ranges. However, an alternative empirical equation is the *Antoine equation* — proposed some

50 years later in 1888 — which describes the variation in saturated vapour pressure with temperature (°C) in the form:

$$\log (P) = A - \frac{B}{t + C}$$

where t is the temperature in °C.

If C is 273.15°C (i.e. conversion of °C → K), this equation is the same as the Clapeyron–Clausius but, by varying C as well as A and B, a better fit to the original data can usually be obtained. Rodgers and Hill (1978) have tabulated the Antoine constants from which the vapour pressure at any particular temperature can be calculated and the general graph relating these two functions is shown in *Figure 3.1*.

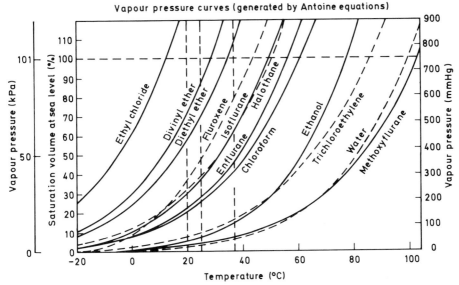

Figure 3.1
Vapour pressure as a function of temperature for water, ethanol and 10 different anaesthetic substances. Vertical dashed lines are at 20, 25 and 37°C. Horizontal dashed line intersects curves at their boiling points at sea level. (Adapted with permission from Rodgers and Hill, 1978)

The vapour pressure at 37°C is of theoretical interest in its relation to anaesthetic potency — as is discussed in the section on physicochemical theories. The vapour pressure at room temperature is used primarily in the calculation of the concentration of anaesthetic produced by passing carrier gas through an efficient vaporizer, as represented in *Figure 3.2*.

CALCULATION OF VAPORIZER ANAESTHETIC CONCENTRATIONS

The concentration produced by a vaporizer is not dependent on whether the carrier gas is oxygen or oxygen–nitrous oxide mixtures. In unit time a certain volume of carrier gas (V_{car}) passes through the vaporizing chamber

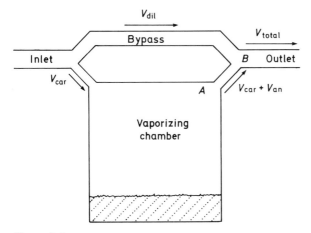

Figure 3.2
Theoretical model of a vaporizer to illustrate the method of calculating
the delivered concentrations

(*Figure 3.2*) and is mixed with a volume of anaesthetic vapour (V_{an}). If
the vaporizing chamber is efficient, the carrier gas passing through it
becomes completely saturated with vapour and the partial pressure of
anaesthetic in the chamber (P_{an}) is equal to the saturated vapour pressure
at that temperature. Now:

$$\% \text{ anaesthetic at } A = \frac{P_{an}}{P_{bar}} \times 100\% \tag{3.1}$$

$$= \frac{V_{an}}{V_{an} + V_{car}} \times 100\% \tag{3.2}$$

P_{bar} is the barometric pressure, assuming that there are no pressure gradients
between A and the external atmosphere. Equations (3.1) and (3.2) relate
the percentage of anaesthetic to either the volumes or the partial pressures
of the different components. They are derived from *Dalton's law of
partial pressures*, which states that the pressure of a mixture of gases is the
sum of the partial pressures of the component gases.

The percentage of anaesthetic at the outlet of the vaporizer B can now
be calculated:

$$\% \text{ of anaesthetic at } B = \frac{V_{an}}{V_{total}} \times 100\% \tag{3.3}$$

$$= \frac{V_{an}}{V_{dil} + V_{car} + V_{an}} \times 100\% \tag{3.4}$$

Where, in unit time, the total outflow volume (V_{total}) comprises the
diluent volume bypassing the vaporizer chamber (V_{dil}) plus the anaesthetic vapour and carrier gas volumes.

Since V_{an} is difficult to measure directly, it can be calculated from equations (3.1) and (3.2):

$$V_{an} = V_{car} \times \frac{P_{an}}{(P_{bar} - P_{an})} \tag{3.5}$$

Substituting equation (3.5) into equation (3.3):

$$\% \text{ of anaesthetic at } B = \frac{V_{car} \times P_{an}}{(P_{bar} - P_{an}) \times V_{total}} \times 100\% \tag{3.6}$$

Substituting equation (3.5) into equation (3.4) and then multiplying out and tidying up:

% of anaesthetic at B =

$$\frac{V_{car} \times P_{an} \times 100}{(P_{bar} - P_{an})(V_{dil} + V_{car}) + V_{car} \times P_{an}}\%$$

$$= \frac{V_{car} \times P_{an} \times 100}{P_{bar} \times V_{dil} + P_{bar} \times V_{car} - (P_{an} \times V_{dil}) - (P_{an} \times V_{car}) + (V_{car} \times P_{an})}\%$$

$$= \frac{V_{car} \times P_{an} \times 100}{V_{dil} \times (P_{bar} - P_{an}) + V_{car} \times P_{bar}}\% \tag{3.7}$$

The percentage of anaesthetic at the outflow point can thus be calculated from equations (3.3) or (3.6) or (3.7). For practical purposes, equation (3.7) is the most useful since it is usual to know the gas flow rates into vaporizing chamber and bypass rather than the total gas flow leaving the vaporizer.

This expression has direct application in the copper kettle type of vaporizer and also in the flow and temperature compensated vaporizer such as the Fluotec Mark 3, in which the ratio V_{car}/V_{dil} is controlled by the knob which is used to select the delivered concentration. The temperature compensation is achieved by increasing the carrier gas flow as the temperature, and hence P_{an}, decreases. The proportionality of the different terms is illustrated in equation (3.6).

Solubility

Probably the most important physical properties of an anaesthetic from a clinical point of view are the solubilities in different body tissues. As is described in Chapter 4, the partition coefficient between blood/gas, brain/blood, muscle/blood and fat/blood are the main factors determining the uptake, distribution and removal of the inhalational anaesthetics. A *partition coefficient* is the ratio of anaesthetic concentrations in the two phases when they are at equilibrium. When the second phase is gas, the partition coefficient is equal to the *Ostwald solubility coefficient*, which is the volume of gas absorbed per unit volume of solvent at the temperature of the measurement and at a pressure of 1 atm. The advantage in using partition coefficients is that they are generally independent of the absolute concentrations of the agent. This follows from *Henry's law*, which states that the number of molecules of gas dissolving in the solvent is directly proportional to the partial pressure of the gas at the surface of the liquid. It is easy to calculate partition coefficients (λ) between two liquids from the appropriate liquid/gas coefficients. For example, the muscle/blood λ is equal to the muscle/gas λ divided by the blood/gas λ.

TABLE 3.2. Partition coefficients

Agent	Water/Gas (37°C)	Blood/Gas (37°C)	Oil/Gas (37°C)	'Rubber'/Gas (20–25°C)
Methoxyflurane	4.5	13.0	950	630
Trichloroethylene	1.7	9.0	714	830
Chloroform	4.0	8.0	400	300
Halothane	0.8	2.4	220	120
Enflurane	0.8	1.9	98	74
Diethyl ether	13.0	12.0	65	58
Cyclopropane	0.21	0.55	11.5	6.6
Nitrous oxide	0.47	0.47	1.4	1.2

The majority of these data are taken from the 'preferred values' in the compilation by Steward *et al.* (1973), with the following exceptions: methoxyflurane blood/gas: Eger and Shargel (1963); trichloroethylene oil/gas: Sherwood (1976). The rubber/gas partition coefficients refer to 'conductive rubber used in standard anesthesia breathing tubes' and are taken from Titel and Lowe (1968), with the addition of that for enflurane which is a personal communication from H. J. Lowe.

The solubility data presented in *Table 3.2* illustrate some of the factors which influence anaesthetic solubility. First, not surprisingly, the agent itself has a profound effect. Thus, for the same solvent — oil — methoxyflurane is almost 700 times as soluble as nitrous oxide. The second factor is the solvent and, in general, anaesthetics are less soluble in water and more soluble in oil or lipids. Thus halothane is almost 300 times more soluble in oil than in water. Blood solubility is usually between those for the other two solvents as would be expected from its chemical composition. One of the problems with solubility in blood is that since it does not have a fixed composition, the partition coefficient can vary from individual to individual and with the nutritional and haematological status of any particular individual. Diethyl ether is the only exception to the usual water < blood ≪ oil ranking order of the solubilities of the clinical agents in that its blood solubility is slightly lower than its water solubility.

It is known that the electrolytes in the blood decrease the aqueous solubility of an agent (the 'salting out' effect). This is normally out-weighed by the increased solubility associated with the protein and lipid components. Indeed, to a first approximation:

$$\lambda_{blood/gas} = \lambda_{water/gas} + 0.01\ \lambda_{oil/gas}$$

However, diethyl ether, being a polar molecule, probably is particularly susceptible to the salting out effect and definitely has a relatively low $\lambda_{oil/gas}$ (65), and thus does not obey the above numerical approximation. The only other agent which is a serious exception to the approximation is cyclopropane which, as will be explained below, appears to have definite binding sites in haemoglobin.

The rubber/gas partition coefficients have been included in *Table 3.2* to indicate the relative solubility characteristics of a non-biological 'solvent'. These are approximately 0.7 $\lambda_{oil/gas}$ — with the exception of trichloroethy-lene (where the data are not certain). The rubber/gas partition coefficients also emphasize the importance of allowing for the substantial uptake of the more potent agents into any rubber components of anaesthetic delivery systems.

The third factor which influences anaesthetic solubility is temperature. Heat is usually liberated when gases dissolve, and the higher the temperature the lower is the solubility (*Table 3.3*). The temperature coefficients for a wide range of gases in both aqueous and oil media have been collated by Allott *et al.* (1973); it was found that there was a correlation with solubility

TABLE 3.3. Variation of partition coefficients with temperature

Agent	Water/Gas λ at 20°C	Aqueous temperature coefficient (% per °C)	Oil/Gas λ at 20°C	Oil temperature coefficient (% per °C)
Methoxyflurane	9.3	− 4.18	2108	− 4.58
Trichloroethylene	3.4	− 3.94	1570	− 4.53
Chloroform	7.7	− 3.76	881	− 4.54
Halothane	1.6	− 4.01	469	− 4.36
Enflurane	1.4	− 3.22	180	− 3.51
Diethyl ether	30.5	− 4.89	117	− 3.39
Cyclopropane	0.3	− 2.11	16.7	− 2.18
Nitrous oxide	0.7	− 2.33	1.7	−1.13

The temperature coefficients have been taken from a compilation by Allott *et al.* (1973). They are the mean of various published values, except those for enflurane and for nitrous oxide (oil/gas) which have been estimated from the observed correlation of temperature coefficient with solubility. The values of the water/gas and oil/gas partition coefficients at 20°C have been calculated from the data in *Tables 3.2 and 3.3*.

itself — the more soluble the agent, the greater the negative temperature coefficient. These data are relevant clinically because the increase in oil/gas partition coefficient with decreasing temperature means that the effective concentration at the hydrophobic site of action is increasing and hence the apparent potency of the agent increases; i.e. MAC decreases in hypothermia and increases in hyperthermia (Regan and Eger, 1967; Steffey and Eger, 1974). Temperature does not appear to affect consciousness directly until extremes of temperature are reached ($<30°$C or $>40°$C).

The final factor which sometimes affects partition coefficients is the concentration of the agent. For the majority of the agents the partition coefficients are independent of the anaesthetic partial pressure because, as already discussed, Henry's law is obeyed. However, in the case of cyclopropane the blood/gas partition coefficient decreases as the concentration increases above 1%. This has been found to be because the cyclopropane is binding to the haemoglobin which has only a limited capacity for the agent, and when it is effectively saturated the partition coefficient decreases towards that of the plasma (Eger, 1974). This is a good example of the potential complexity of the real situation when anaesthetics dissolve in

TABLE 3.4. Equilibrium partial pressures and concentrations of halothane

Units	Gas phase (37°C)	Water phase (37°C)	Blood phase (37°C)	Water phase (20°C)
Partial pressure:				
% of 1 atm	1	1	1	1
kPa	1.01	1.01	1.01	1.01
mmHg	7.6	7.6	7.6	7.6
Concentration:				
% (gas vol./phase vol.)	1	0.8	2.4	1.6
ml·dl^{-1}	1	0.8	2.4	1.6
ml·l^{-1}	10	8	24	16
mmol·l^{-1}	0.39	0.31	0.94	0.63
mg·l^{-1}	77.6	62.1	186.3	124.2
mg·dl^{-1}	7.8	6.2	18.6	12.4
ml (liquid at 20°C)·dl^{-1}	0.0042	0.0033	0.01	0.0067

All the equilibrium partial pressures and concentrations in various media and at different temperatures in this Table are equivalent to 1% halothane in the gas phase. All the units selected have appeared in the anaesthetics literature in the last ten years.

biological media which are not simply bulk solvents. Fortunately, Henry's law seems to be obeyed by the other agents at clinical concentrations. The opposite effect — an increase in solubility with an increase in partial pressure — has been found for very high concentrations of chloroform in oil (Nunn, 1960) but in this case so much anaesthetic is dissolving in the solvent that the characteristics of the solvent are changing and it is not surprising that the apparent solubility also changes.

The difficulty of understanding the quantitative aspects of partition coefficients arising from various methods of expressing partial pressure and concentration is illustrated in *Table 3.4*. A lot of confusion has arisen in the literature because of the different units used to express the anaesthetic concentration under loosely defined conditions in media which themselves may not have a consistent composition. This problem has particularly bedevilled many of the early cellular studies in which the halothane was sometimes added as a liquid.

In conclusion, the solubilities of the inhalational agents are of crucial importance in determining their kinetics of administration. The speed of induction and recovery is related to aqueous tissue solubility to a first approximation and correlates inversely with $\lambda_{blood/gas}$. The relevance of $\lambda_{oil/gas}$ to the potency and mode of action of the anaesthetic is discussed in the section on physicochemical theories.

Non-flammability

The concern with anaesthetic fires and explosions has diminished over the years with the introduction of 'non-flammable' volatile agents and the reduced clinical use of cyclopropane and diethyl ether. Nevertheless, the potential problem still exists and it contributes enormously to the cost of theatres. The problem has also recently come to the fore in connection with the hazards (real or otherwise) of alternative scavenging systems for reducing anaesthetic contamination of operating areas. The upper and lower limits of flammability (*Table 3.5*) give some indication of the situations when explosions may or may not occur, but it is important to realize that the data refer to laboratory experiments which have used different ignition conditions from each other and from those likely to occur in clinical practice. For example, many people would correctly classify halothane or enflurane as 'non-flammable' and the specific data for these agents referred to in the Table were obtained in a closed combustion tube with very high ignition energies.

The minimum flammable concentrations of different agents have been related previously to the minimum alveolar concentration (Leonard, 1975), but it is probably more appropriate to compare them with the maximum inspired concentrations which would be used during induction. The comparison is complicated by the concomitant or sequential addition of nitrous oxide, which reduces the amount of volatile agent required but increases the danger of flammability. Methoxyflurane is an interesting example of an agent which was developed despite its potential flammability because it was clear that the hazards in clinical practice were minimal. Thus the only agents in current clinical practice which present a serious hazard are ether and cyclopropane. Ether has the additional hazard that it reacts with air to form peroxides which are unstable compounds capable

TABLE 3.5. Flammability limits of anaesthetics (vols %)

Agent	In air	In oxygen	In nitrous oxide
Methoxyflurane	7.0–	5.4–	4.6–
Trichloroethylene	NI	NI	NI
Chloroform	NI	NI	NI
Halothane	NI	NI	4.75–
Enflurane	NI	NI	5.75–
Diethyl ether	1.9–48	2.0–82	1.5–24
Cyclopropane	2.4–10.3	2.5–60	1.6–30
Nitrous oxide	NI	NI	

The lower and (where available) upper flammability limits are taken from the manufacturers' data and/or, for halothane and enflurane, from Leonard (1975) and, for diethyl ether and cyclopropane, from Coward and Jones (1952). The nitrous oxide data are for 50% nitrous oxide–balance oxygen. NI, non-inflammable.

of exploding regardless of the flammability range; i.e. impure ether is far more likely to explode (see *Table 3.5*).

For further reading the second edition of *Physics for Anaesthetists* (Macintosh, Mushin and Epstein, 1958) contains four chapters on explosions which provide an excellent background to the subject. The recommendations of the Association of Anaesthetists on explosion hazards have been published (1971), and Walter (1966) has published an interesting 'case history' of an ether vaporizer explosion.

Chemical stability

The inhalational anaesthetics are normally regarded as chemically stable except in a few specific circumstances. The formation of peroxides of diethyl ether in air has been mentioned in the non-flammability section, above. In fact, all the volatile agents, with the exception of enflurane, can be slowly oxidized in air, and for this reason a variety of antioxidant chemical stabilizers are added to the liquid agents (*Table 3.6*).

The concern with stability in the presence of ultraviolet light is primarily because of the use of physical analysers which measure anaesthetic concentrations by the absorption of radiation in that range of wavelengths. There is, of course, a component of ultraviolet light in normal daylight but the intensity of this is relatively weak and the majority of the volatile agents are supplied in amber bottles. However, in the vapour phase the agents contain only trace amounts of the chemical stabilizers and are fully exposed to any potential photochemical decomposition. Fortunately, the

TABLE 3.6. Chemical stability

Agent	Chemical stabilizer	UV light	Soda lime and baralyme
Methoxyflurane	0.01% Butylated hydroxytoluene	Decomposes; products unknown	Stable
Trichloroethanol	0.01% Thymol 0.001% Vaxolin blue	Unknown	Decomposes to $CCl \equiv CCl$
Chloroform	0.6–1.0% Ethanol	Unknown	Forms phosgene $(COCl_2)$ when heated in air
Halothane	0.01% Thymol	Decomposes; products unknown	Slight decomposition to $CF_2 = CBrCl$
Enflurane	None	Stable	Stable
Diethyl ether	4% Ethanol 0.001% Diphenylamine	Peroxides in air	Stable

The data on chemical stabilizers are taken from manufacturers' data and/or Secher (1971). The decomposition data are also included in Vitcha (1971) and in Raventos and Lemon (1965) (for halothane).

extent of this decomposition appears to be insignificant in clinical practice. For example, halothane gas is decomposed to trace quantities of halides, free halogen and 2-chloro-2-dibromo-1,1,1-trifluoroethane (a solid at room temperature) by 17 hours of ultraviolet radiation (H. E. Hudson, 1964, unpublished observations). Further experiments circulating the halothane through an ultraviolet monitor demonstrated that the halides and halothane could be removed by soda lime. If, therefore, it is desired to recirculate halothane gases sampled through an ultraviolet monitor, it is desirable to include a soda lime trap on the outlet side of the monitor.

The interaction of the volatile agents with alkaline carbon dioxide absorbers is currently being reconsidered. Trichloroethylene is the classic example of an agent which forms a toxic compound, dichloroacetylene, under alkaline conditions:

$$CCl_2 = CHCl + OH^- \rightleftarrows CCl \equiv CCl + Cl^- + H_2O$$

Halothane also has been known to undergo a slight decomposition under the same conditions (Raventos and Lemon, 1965) but only traces of the products were detected in comparison with the toxic levels (250 p.p.m. in mice):

$$CF_3CHBrCl + OH^- \rightleftarrows CF_2 = CBrCl + F^- + H_2O$$

However, Sharp, Trudell and Cohen (1979) have detected up to 5 p.p.m. of the decomposition product in a closed circuit system used for one hour's clinical anaesthesia with two patients. These levels appear to stabilize out rather than continually increase, and their absolute magnitude is at least of an order of magnitude lower than the toxic levels. However, it is ironic that closed circuit anaesthesia, which has been advocated as one of the best methods for reducing the potential hazards of anaesthetic pollution, should itself be associated with a further possible toxic hazard to the patient.

THE MECHANISMS OF NARCOSIS

The mechanism by which anaesthetics cause loss of consciousness is unknown. Explanation of the phenomenon of anaesthesia will require elucidation of the mechanism of action at no less than four levels. The first level is the interaction of anaesthetics with receptor sites at the molecular level, and this aspect of the problem is considered below. The second level is the disorder of cellular functions, caused by exposure to anaesthetics; a number of such actions are considered in Chapters 1, 2 and 10. Many of these effects are unlikely to be related to the production of narcosis. Third, it is necessary to define the action of anaesthetics on the synapse, which is almost certainly the part of the neuron concerned in the production of anaesthesia; this problem is considered in Chapters 1 and 5. Finally, an understanding of anaesthesia will require definition of those parts of the central nervous system which are affected by anaesthetics, because it is already clear that there is not a uniform depression of the entire central nervous system. Chapter 6 reviews the present state of knowledge of the effects of anaesthetics on the central nervous system of the intact animal.

PHYSICOCHEMICAL THEORIES OF ANAESTHESIA

The physicochemical theories of anaesthesia consider interactions of anaesthetics with some part of the cell dependent on the physical properties of the anaesthetic agent. Some correlations have been proposed which involve the physical properties of the anaesthetics themselves. Thus correlations with boiling points, vapour pressure, parachor* and Van der Waals constants have all been noted (Wulf and Featherstone, 1957; Adamson, 1964). All these properties may be related more or less directly to the intermolecular forces exerted between the anaesthetic molecules themselves and are therefore not very informative about the interaction between the anaesthetic and its site of action.

Parachor is a measure of the molecular volume of a substance at a standard internal pressure. It is determined from the effect of temperature on surface tension of the liquid.

Thermodynamic activity

Ferguson (1939) noted that at equilibrium the thermodynamic activity of an anaesthetic is the same in all phases, and he proposed that equal thermodynamic activities ($P_{an} \div$ sat. vap. pressure, i.e. analogous to 'relative humidity') produce equal degrees of anaesthesia. Essentially, this is a correlation with the ideal solubility of a gas or vapour as calculated from Raoult's law when due allowance is made for the molecular forces between the gas molecules themselves (see Nunn, 1960). Emphasis is thus removed from the interaction of the anaesthetic with the system and concentrated on its interaction with itself. Although the correlation is quite good, both Carpenter (1954) and K. W. Miller, Paton and Smith (1965) have shown that other correlations are better.

Solubility theories

Recent work on the physicochemical theories of general anaesthesia has been concerned with distinguishing between two main groups of theories: those based on theories about aqueous media and those about non-aqueous media.

AQUEOUS THEORIES

These theories are derived from the apparent relationship between the anaesthetic partial pressure and the decomposition pressure of the gas hydrates (or clathrates) formed by the anaesthetics (*Figure 3.3*). The hydrate or 'iceberg' theory was proposed independently by Pauling (1961) and S. L. Miller (1961), and postulates that anaesthetic action occurs in the aqueous or hydrophilic protein areas of the central nervous system. Pauling considered that anaesthetic hydrate microcrystals, which do not exist at physiological temperatures and pressures, are stabilized by charged protein side chains and increase the impedance to impulse conduction in nerve fibres. Miller did not invoke the presence of actual hydrates in the body but considered the ordering effects which simple solutes are supposed, by some, to exert on neighbouring water molecules. It was suggested that this ordering of water molecules might lower the conductance of brain tissue, 'stiffening up' the lipid membrane or occlude pores in the membrane.

These theories of primary interaction with an aqueous phase are no longer accepted, for three main reasons. First, the correlations with potency failed for the fluorocarbons such as SF_6. Second, the theories did not predict the additivity of anaesthetic potencies which is observed with the common clinical agents. Third, some of the more potent volatile agents do not form clathrates under the conditions originally proposed ($0°C$ in pure water).

NON-AQUEOUS THEORIES

These theories stem from the Meyer–Overton fat solubility hypothesis (H. Meyer, 1899; Overton, 1901) which has been formulated by K. H. Meyer (1937):

> 'Narcosis commences when any chemically indifferent substance has attained a certain molar concentration in the lipids of the cell. This concentration depends on the nature of the animal or cell but is independent of the narcotic.'

This theory is not a mechanistic theory of narcosis but rather a recognition of the remarkable relationship between the anaesthetic pressure of a substance and its lipid solubility (*Figure 3.3*). The latter is usually represented by solubility in olive oil or oleyl alcohol.

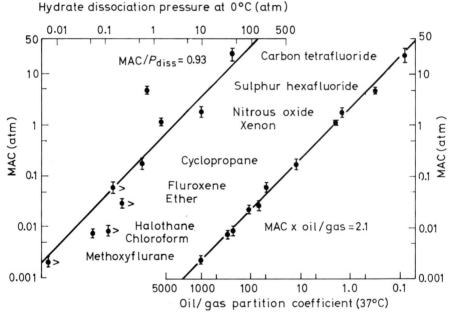

Figure 3.3
Correlation of anaesthetic potency (MAC) with either hydrate dissociation pressure or oil/gas partition coefficient. The solid lines have unit slope as predicted by the theory. (Adapted from Eger *et al.*, 1969)

In 1961 both the aqueous and the non-aqueous theories were supported by equally good correlations. These correlations were for the interaction of the anaesthetic with possible sites of action. However, the data were misleading because regular relationships are often found with forces between a homologous series of compounds and a third molecule or phase. It is known from studies on solutions that nearly all the gaseous anaesthetics roughly follow the same regular relationships even though they do not all belong to the same homologous series. It has been found that only fully fluorinated anaesthetics depart strongly from this behaviour (Hildebrand and Scott, 1962). This fact was used by K. W. Miller, Paton and Smith (1965), who included the fluorinated anaesthetics in a study of the relationship of the anaesthetic pressure and solubility of various agents in a variety of solvents having a range of solubility parameters (δ). The solubility parameter provides a measure of the cohesive energy density of the solvent, an indication of the strength of its intermolecular forces. This made it possible to determine the solubility parameter of the phase in which the anaesthetic action takes place. They concluded that a satisfactory correlation between anaesthetic pressures and solubilities is found only for solvents with $\delta = 8.5 \pm 1$ (cal $\frac{1}{2} \cdot$ cm$^{-3/2}$). This would eliminate both the aqueous phase ($\delta \triangleq 24$) and the protein membrane cover ($\delta \triangleq 14$) from serious consideration, and suggests that the search for a mechanism of anaesthesia should be concentrated on the lipid regions of the cell membrane or the hydrophobic region of protein molecules.

Mullins (1954) had suggested that anaesthetic potency should depend on molecular size as well as on solubility. Subsequent studies by the Oxford group (Miller *et al.*, 1972) demonstrated that inclusion of the molar volume of the agents in the hydrophobic correlation did not produce a lower coefficient of variation of the data but did suggest that the most appropriate solvent in this case would have a slightly higher solubility parameter (greater than 10).

The correlation of anaesthetic potency with hydrophobic solubility (*Figure 3.3*) is one of the most impressive correlations in biology, and has been demonstrated to hold for anaesthetics differing in potencies by a factor of 300 000. At one end are the clinical volatile agents which have been studied, particularly by Eger and his colleagues (1969). The correlation has been extended by an order of magnitude in the case of thiomethoxyflurane, which is the most lipid-soluble anaesthetic known, with an oil/gas partition coefficient of 7230 and a MAC value of 0.035% in dogs (Tanifuji, Eger and Terrell, 1977). There is controversy as to whether another highly lipid-soluble substance, *n*-decane, is an anaesthetic (Mullins, 1954). However, the work with thiomethoxyflurane suggests that an extremely high lipid solubility *per se* does not result in a deviation from the correlation.

At the other end of the scale, with agents of very low lipid solubility requiring high anaesthetic partial pressures, there is an apparent deviation from the predicted values. However, as will be seen in the section on pressure reversal, the observed anaesthetic potencies of these gases (hydrogen, neon and helium) are decreased by the effects of pressure *per se*, and when correlation is made for this, the calculated potencies are in agreement with their lipid solubilities (Halsey, 1974).

Within the extremes of lipid solubility there are remarkably few exceptions to the correlation. The physiological gases, oxygen and carbon dioxide, both have anaesthetic properties (Paton, 1967; Eisele, Eger and Muallem, 1967). However, oxygen appears to be twice as potent as predicted (Smith and Paton, 1976) although this is probably due to complications with distinguishing between anaesthesia and postconvulsant effects of the gas. Carbon dioxide is almost five times as potent as predicted but this is due to the fact that the special anaesthetic effect (CO_2 narcosis) is mediated via associated pH changes in the central nervous system, rather than simple solution in hydrophobic areas. Finally, one exception which at present is unexplained is the unexpectedly high potency of isoflurane (Forane) in mice — its ED_{50} only 30% of that predicted by its lipid solubility (Kent *et al.*, 1977). However, this anomaly appears to be restricted to mice, and the potencies of the same agent in other species are as predicted (Eger, 1974).

In conclusion, the correlation studies with anaesthetic potencies have identified hydrophobic areas of the body as the most probable site of anaesthetic action. These hydrophobic areas are most likely to be the lipids or internal hydrophobic sites of macromolecules which make up the nerve membrane. The correlation studies do not prove that these cellular regions are the anaesthetic sites but they are consistent with such a hypothesis.

The effects of anaesthetics on lipids is discussed further in Chapter 1. Anaesthetic perturbation of protein functions and conformations are illustrated by studies on glutamate dehydrogenase (Brammall, Beard and Hulands, 1974), luciferase (Halsey and Smith, 1970; White and Dundas, 1970) and haemoglobin (Barker *et al.*, 1975). The last-named is not altered functionally (Millar, Beard and Hulands, 1971) and has been used as a model protein to study the 'ground rules' for anaesthetic protein interactions (Halsey, Wardley-Smith and Green, 1978). The many potential links between protein perturbations and mechanisms of anaesthesia have been reviewed by Allison (1974).

Pressure reversal of anaesthesia

The interaction of high hydrostatic pressures with anaesthesia has proved to be of considerable importance in the development of the physical mechanisms of anaesthesia. The phenomenon can be demonstrated in mice, for example; they are first anaesthetized with halothane inside a pressure chamber and then, if helium is added to the chamber until the total pressure is 50 atm, the mice wake up, in spite of the fact that the partial pressures of halothane and oxygen are unaltered. This surprising effect is not due to some peculiarity of helium, because similar results have been obtained with newts where the pressure may also be applied by compressing the surrounding water (Lever *et al.*, 1971).

The phenomenon of pressure reversal of anaesthesia (as it has become known) should not be confused with inert gas narcosis, associated for example with increasing pressures of nitrogen used in diving. In the latter case, the partial pressure of the 'anaesthetic' gas (nitrogen) is increasing with pressure, and anaesthesia occurs at the pressure predicted by its relatively low lipid solubility. In the pressure reversal phenomenon the anaesthetic (halothane) partial pressure remains effectively constant, and any additional anaesthetic effect of the helium gas is too weak to have an appreciable effect at these pressures.

The modifications of drug responses by increased hydrostatic pressure have been studied intermittently since the 1940s. The initial work involved luminous bacteria (Johnson, Brown and Marsland, 1942) and the data on pressure-drug interactions were interpreted in terms of enzyme kinetics (Johnson, Eyring and Stover, 1974). Subsequently, aquatic and amphibious animals were used to study the molecular mechanisms of general anaesthesia produced by the inhalational agents (Lever *et al.*, 1971). These investigations led to the formulation of the critical volume hypothesis — a convenient theoretical model which postulated that a critical hydrophobic molecular site was expanded by anaesthetics and contracted by hydrostatic pressure; i.e. narcosis occurred with a fixed degree of expansion regardless of the type of anaesthetic or the actual level of pressure. The mathematical formulation of this hypothesis (Miller *et al.*, 1973) predicted that the percentage decrease in anaesthetic potency should be linearly related to the total pressure, with the slope being the same for all agents. The data obtained in newts (Miller, 1975) and in the early mammal experiments (Halsey *et al.*, 1975) were in agreement with this prediction, and the observed range of compressibilities of the molecular site was consistent with that calculated from its presumed solubility parameter. The critical volume hypothesis stimulated further research, particularly with mammals, and has provided a convenient framework for analysing the data. However, since it was first formulated in 1971, a number of discrepancies have become apparent. Although the qualitative pressure reversal phenomena appear to be common to all inhalational and intravenous anaesthetic agents so far studied (Halsey and Wardley-Smith, 1975), the quantitative data in mammals are not as simple as predicted by the critical volume hypothesis (Halsey, Wardley-Smith and Green, 1978).

It no longer appears that all anaesthetics behave in the same way at pressure and it is likely that the simple unitary hypothesis will have to be modified to allow for different types of molecular sites with a limit to their capacities for anaesthetics. In spite of such complications, high pressure studies in whole animals provide a framework into which fit the more detailed molecular, cellular and neurophysiological experiments with anaesthetics and high pressure such as are described in Chapter 5.

References

Adamson, R. H. (1964). Correlation of parachor with anaesthetic potency. *Life Sci.* 3, 1131–1134

Allison, A. C. (1974). The effects of inhalational anaesthetics on proteins. In *Molecular Mechanisms in General Anaesthesia*. M. J. Halsey, R. A. Millar and J. A. Sutton (ed.). Edinburgh: Churchill Livingstone

Allott, P. R., Steward, A., Flook, V. and Mapleson, W. W. (1973). Variation with temperature of the solubilities of inhaled anaesthetics in water, oil and biological media. *Br. J. Anaesth.* 45, 294–300

Association of Anaesthetists of Great Britain and Ireland (1971). Recommendations on explosion hazards. *Anaesthesia* 26, 155

Barker, R. W., Brown, F. F., Drake, R., Halsey, M. J. and Richards, R. E. (1975). Nuclear magnetic resonance studies of anaesthetic interactions with haemoglobin. *Br. J. Anaesth.* 47, 25–29

Brammall, A., Beard, D. J. and Hulands, G. H. (1974). Inhalational anaesthetics and their interaction *in vitro* with glutamate dehydrogenase and other enzymes. *Br. J. Anaesth.* 46, 643–652

Brown, F. F., Halsey, M. J. and Richards, R. E. (1976). Halothane interactions with haemoglobin. *Proc. R. Soc. Lond. B* 193, 387–411

Carpenter, F. G. (1954). Anesthetic action of inert and unreactive gases on intact animals and isolated tissues. *Am. J. Physiol.* 178, 505–509

Chand, S. C., Halsey, M. J. and White, D. C. (1978). Unpublished observations

Coward, H. F. and Jones, G. W. (1952). Limits of flammability of gases and vapors. *Bull. U.S. Bur. Mines* No. 503

De Jong, R. H. and Eger, E. I. (1975). MAC expanded: AD_{50} and AD_{95} values of common inhalation anesthetics in man. *Anesthesiology* 42, 384–389

Eger, E. I. (1974). *Anesthetic Uptake and Action.* Baltimore, Md: Williams & Wilkins

Eger, E. I. and Shargel, R. (1963). The solubility of methoxyflurane in human blood and tissue homogenates. *Anesthesiology* 24, 625–627

Eger, E. I., Lundgren, C., Miller, S. L. and Stevens, W. C. (1969). Anesthetic potencies of sulfur hexafluoride, carbon tetrafluoride, chloroform and Ethrane in dogs. *Anesthesiology* 30, 129–135

Eisele, J. H., Eger, E. I. and Muallem, M. (1967). Narcotic properties of carbon dioxide in the dog. *Anesthesiology* 28, 856–865

Ferguson, J. (1939). The use of chemical potentials as indices of toxicity. *Proc. R. Soc. Lond. B* 127, 387–404

Gion, H. and Saidman, C. J. (1971). The minimum alveolar concentration of enflurane in man. *Anesthesiology* 35, 361–364

Gregory, G. A., Eger, E. I. and Munson, E. S. (1969). The relationship between age and halothane requirements in man. *Anesthesiology* 30, 488–491

Halsey, M. J. (1974). Structure activity relationships of inhalational anaesthetics. In *Molecular Mechanisms in General Anaesthesia.* M. J. Halsey, R. A. Millar and J. A. Sutton (ed.). Edinburgh: Churchill Livingstone

Halsey, M. J. and Smith, E. B. (1970). Effects of anaesthetics on luminous bacteria. *Nature, Lond.* 227, 1363–1365

Halsey, M. J. and Wardley-Smith, B. (1975). Pressure reversal of narcosis produced by anaesthetics, narcotics and tranquillizers. *Nature, Lond.* 257, 811–813

Halsey, M. J., Wardley-Smith, B. and Green, C. J. (1978). The pressure reversal of general anaesthesia – a multi-site expansion hypothesis. *Br. J. Anaesth.* 50, 1091–1097

Halsey, M. J., Eger, E. I., Kent, D. W. and Warne, P. J. (1975). High pressure studies of anesthesia. *Progr. Anesthesiol.* 1, 353–361

Hildebrand, J. H. and Scott, R. L. (1962). *Regular Solutions.* Englewood Cliffs, NJ: Prentice-Hall

Hudson, H. E. (1964). Unpublished observations

Johnson, F. H., Brown, D. E. S. and Marsland, D. A. (1942). Pressure reversal of the actions of certain narcotics. *J. cell. Comp. Physiol.* 20, 269–276

Johnson, S. H., Eyring, H. and Stover, B. J. (1974). *The Theory of Rate Processes in Biology and Medicine.* New York: John Wiley

Kent, D. W., Halsey, M. J., Eger, E. I. and Kent, B. (1977). Isoflurane anesthesia and pressure antagonism in mice. *Anesth. Analg. curr. Res.* 56, 97–101

Leonard, P. F. (1975). The lower limits of flammability of halothane, enflurane and isoflurane. *Anesth. Analg. curr. Res.* 54, 238–240

Lever, M. J., Miller, K. W., Paton, W. D. M. and Smith, E. B. (1971). Pressure reversal of anaesthesia. *Nature, Lond.* 231, 368–371

Macintosh, R., Mushin, W. W. and Epstein, H. G. (1958). *Physics for the Anesthetist: including a section on explosions,* pp. 284–416. Philadelphia: Davis

Meyer, H. H. (1899). Zur theorie der alkoholnarcose. I. Mitt welche Eigenschaft der anasthetiken bedingt ihre narkotische Wirkung? *Archs exp. Path. Pharmak.* 42, 109–119

Meyer, K. H. (1937). Contributions to the theory of narcosis. *Trans. Faraday Soc.* 33, 1062–1068

Millar, R. A., Beard, D. J. and Hulands, G. H. (1971). Oxyhaemoglobin dissociation curves *in vitro* with and without the anaesthetics halothane and cyclopropane. *Br. J. Anaesth.* 43, 1003–1011

Miller, K. W. (1975). The pressure reversal of anesthesia and the critical volume hypothesis. *Progr. Anesthesiol.* 1, 341–351

Miller, K. W., Paton, W. D. M. and Smith, E. B. (1965). Site of action of general anaesthetics. *Nature, Lond.* 206, 574–577

Miller, K. W., Paton, W. D. M., Smith, E. B. and Smith, R. A. (1972). Physicochemical approaches to the mode of action of general anesthetics. *Anesthesiology* 36, 339–351

Miller, K. W., Paton, W. D. M., Smith, R. A. and Smith, E. B. (1973). The pressure reversal of general anesthesia and the critical volume hypothesis. *Molec. Pharmac.* 9, 131–143

Miller, S. L. (1961). A theory of gaseous anesthetics. *Proc. natn. Acad. Sci. U.S.A.* 47, 1515–1524

Mullins, L. J. (1954). Some physical mechanisms in narcosis. *Chem. Rev.* 54, 289–323

Nunn, J. F. (1960). The solubility of volatile anaesthetics in oil. *Br. J. Anaesth.* 32, 346–352

Overton, E. (1901). *Studien über die Narkose.* Jena: G. Fisher

Paton, W. D. M. (1967). Experiments on the convulsant and anaesthetic effects of oxygen. *Br. J. Pharmac. Chemother.* 29, 350–366

Pauling, L. (1961). A molecular theory of general anesthesia. *Science, N.Y.* 134, 15–21

Raventos, J. and Lemon, P. G. (1965). The impurities in fluothane: their biological properties. *Br. J. Anaesth.* 37, 716–737

Regan, M. J. and Eger, E. I. (1967). The effect of hypothermia in dogs on anesthetizing and apneic doses of inhalation agents. *Anesthesiology* 28, 689–700

Rodgers, R. C. and Hill, G. E. (1978). Equations for vapour pressure versus temperature. *Br. J. Anaesth.* 50, 415–423

Saidman, L. J., Eger, E. I., Munson, E. S., Babad, A. A. and Muallem, M. (1967). Minimum alveolar concentrations of methoxyflurane, halothane, ether and cyclopropane in man. *Anesthesiology* 28, 994–1002

Schoenborn, B. P. (1968). Binding of anesthetics to protein: an x-ray crystallographic investigation. *Fedn Proc.* 27, 888–894

Secher, O. (1971). Physical and chemical data on anaesthetics. *Acta anaesth. scand.* Suppl. 42

Sharp, J. H., Trudell, J. R. and Cohen, E. N. (1979). Volatile metabolites and decomposition products of halothane in man. *Anesthesiology* 50, 2–8

Sherwood, K. J. (1976). Ostwald solubility coefficients of some industrially important substances. *Br. J. ind. Med.* 33, 106–107

Smith, R. A. and Paton, W. D. M. (1976). The anesthetic effect of oxygen. *Anesth. Analg. curr. Res.* 55, 734–736

Steffey, E. P. and Eger, E. I. (1974). Hyperthermia and halothane MAC in the dog. *Anesthesiology* 41, 392–396

Stevens, W. C., Dolan, W. M., Gibbons, R. T., White, A., Eger, E. I., Miller, R. D., de Jong, R. H., Elashoff, R. M. (1975). Minimum alveolar concentrations of isoflurane with and without nitrous oxide in patients of various ages. *Anesthesiology* 42, 197–200

Steward, A., Allott, P. R., Cowles, A. L. and Mapleson, W. W. (1973). Solubility coefficients for inhaled anaesthetics for water, oil and biological media. *Br. J. Anaesth.* 45, 282–293

Tanifuji, Y., Eger, E. I. and Terrell, R. C. (1977). Some characteristics of an exceptionally potent inhaled anesthetic: thiomethoxyflurane. *Anesth. Analg. curr. Res.* 56, 387–390

Titel, J. H. and Lowe, H. J. (1968). Rubber–gas partition coefficients. *Anesthesiology* 29, 1215–1216

Vitcha, J. F. (1971). A history of Forane. *Anesthesiology* 35, 4–7

Walter, C. W. (1966). Explosion of an ether vaporizer. *Anesthesiology* 27, 681–686

White, D. C. and Dundas, C. R. (1970). Effects of anaesthetics on emission of light by luminous bacteria. *Nature, Lond.* 226, 456–458

Wulf, R. J. and Featherstone, R. M. (1957). A correlation of van der Waals' constants with anesthetic potency. *Anesthesiology* 18, 97–105

4 Inhalational anaesthesia: pharmacokinetics
Edmond I. Eger, II

Anaesthesia results from the development of an appropriate brain anaesthetic partial pressure. To achieve this brain partial pressure we administer a far higher pressure from the anaesthetic machine. Thus, between anaesthetic machine and brain exists a hierarchy of intervening partial pressure differences. A difference exists between machine and anaesthetic circuit, between circuit and lungs, between lungs and arterial blood and finally between blood and body tissues. The purpose of this chapter is to examine and explain these differences.

UPTAKE AND ALVEOLAR CONCENTRATION

Of greatest importance is the anaesthetic partial pressure difference between the anaesthetic circuit and that in the lungs. The partial pressure in the circuit may be directly and precisely controlled by the anaesthetist. The partial pressure in the lungs governs the partial pressure in arterial blood and hence, ultimately, the partial pressure in all tissues. Because of its pivotal role in anaesthetic uptake and distribution, the relationship between the inspired and alveolar anaesthetic concentrations will be examined first and in greatest detail.

For the moment, assume that the inspired concentration is constant and that the alveolar concentration rises towards it (in other words, we will examine what happens with a non-rebreathing system). Two factors cause the alveolar concentration to rise: (1) the inspired concentration itself and (2) alveolar ventilation. The effect of concentration is intuitively obvious although one aspect of it — the concentration effect — may not seem so: this is discussed later. Ventilation, if unaccompanied by uptake of anaesthetic agent, produces a rapid rise in the alveolar anaesthetic partial pressure. For example, in a normal lung with a functional residual capacity of 2 litres and an alveolar ventilation of 4 litres per minute, a 63% rise in the alveolar concentration toward the inspired concentration would occur in only 0.5 minute, an 86% change would occur in 1 minute and a 95% change in 1.5 minutes. However, uptake opposes the effect of ventilation to raise the alveolar concentration. Although ventilation brings anaesthetic into the lung, uptake of anaesthetic by lung tissue and the blood passing through the lung limits the alveolar concentration attained. The alveolar concentration results as a balance between ventilatory input and loss through uptake.

Three factors affect uptake at the lungs. These are: anaesthetic solubility in blood (and, to a minor extent, in lung tissue), cardiac output and the alveolar-to-venous anaesthetic partial pressure difference. Uptake equals the product of all three factors, divided by the barometric pressure. The implication of this fact is that if any one factor approaches zero then uptake becomes negligible. Thus if any one factor approaches zero, the effect of ventilation rapidly to narrow the difference between inspired and alveolar concentrations is unopposed.

SOLUBILITY

A greater solubility in blood and tissues produces a greater uptake. Solubility is defined as the ratio of anaesthetic (vapour or gas) concentrations existing in two phases when the two phases are in equilibrium (Eger and Larson, 1964). In *Figure 4.1* the concentration of anaesthetic in the

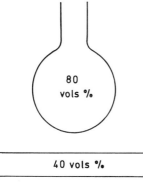

Figure 4.1
The equilibrium relationship described by a blood/gas partition coefficient of 0.5. The partial pressure produced by 80 vols % in the lung is the same as that produced by 40 vols % in the blood: that is, the capacity of the blood phase to hold anaesthetic is half the capacity of the gas phase

lungs is 80 vols % while that in the blood is 40 vols %, giving a blood/gas partition coefficient of 40/80 or 0.5. This describes the relative attraction to the gas compared with the blood phase. To describe solubility, the two phases and their ratio must be stated. In addition, since solubility varies with temperature, the temperature at which the determination of solubility was made must also be stated. Statement of a single solubility figure assumes that Henry's law is followed. Both Dr Harry Lowe (1971, personal communication) and Gregory (Gregory and Eger, 1968) have demonstrated that Henry's law may not always be followed for all anaesthetics. That is, the ratio of concentrations between the two phases may not be constant and may be a function of the partial pressure at which the ratio is determined (*Figure 4.2*). However, this deviation from Henry's law has only been found for cyclopropane and xenon, and for these agents appears to occur only when haemoglobin or myoglobin comprises one of the solvent phases (e.g. see *Figure 4.2*). The phenomenon is probably due to saturation of protein binding sites. We have not found deviations from Henry's law for nitrous oxide or halothane in blood. It is likely that other potent agents are similar to halothane.

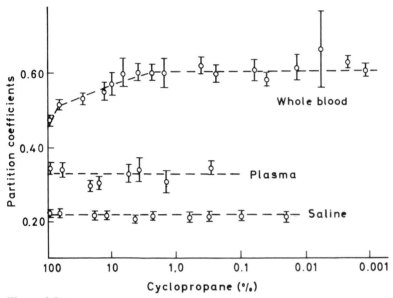

Figure 4.2
Relationship of cyclopropane partial pressure (100% cyclopropane equals 100 kPa or 750 mmHg) to saline/gas, plasma/gas and blood/gas partition coefficients. The saline/gas and plasma/gas partition coefficients are unaffected by an increase in partial pressure; that is, Henry's law is obeyed. However, the blood/gas partition coefficient decreases with increasing partial pressure; Henry's law is not obeyed. The disobedience probably results from saturation of the haemoglobin component. As saturation is approached, the haemoglobin can accept less and less additional cyclopropane with increase in cyclopropane partial pressure. (From unpublished data of G. A. Gregory and E. I. Eger, II)

Several terms describe solubility. Perhaps most descriptive is 'partition coefficient' since solubility is defined by the partition of a gas between two phases. The Ostwald solubility coefficient, or λ, refers to a special partition coefficient. When 100% of a gas is equilibrated with a liquid or tissue, the volume of gas dissolved per unit volume of liquid or tissue is called the Ostwald solubility coefficient. This is no different from a liquid or tissue to gas partition coefficient since it is the concentration in the liquid phase divided in this case by a fractional concentration of 1 (i.e. 100%). The Ostwald solubility coefficient is useful in that the phase ratio need not be stated. It is always a liquid or tissue to gas ratio. The Bunsen absorption coefficient equals the Ostwald solubility coefficient times 273 divided by absolute temperature at which the Ostwald coefficient was measured. That is, it is the Ostwald coefficient corrected to 0°C. The term 'blood solubility' means the blood/gas partition coefficient. 'Tissue solubility' means either a tissue/blood or tissue/gas partition coefficient.

Table 4.1 lists some common solubility data. The phases and ratios are stated. All determinations were made at $37\pm0.5°C$. The listings are in order of increasing blood/gas partition coefficients. For the same conditions, the anaesthetics at the top of the Table have the smallest uptake. Thus, the rise of the alveolar concentration towards the inspired concentration is more rapid with nitrous oxide than with enflurane; enflurane more rapid than with halothane; and halothane more rapid than with methoxyflurane. Speed of induction and recovery is inversely related to the blood/gas partition coefficient.

TABLE 4.1. Partition coefficients of some anaesthetic gases at 37°C

Anaesthetic gas	Blood/Gas	Brain/Blood	Muscle/Blood	Fat/Blood	Oil/Gas
Cyclopropane	0.4–0.6	0.76	1.2	13	12
Nitrous oxide	0.47	1.1	1.2	2.3	1.4
Isoflurane	1.4	2.6	4.0	45	98
Enflurane	1.8	1.4	1.7	36	98
Halothane	2.3	2.3	3.5	60	224
Chloroform	8.4	1.4	1.9	31	394
Trichloroethylene*	9	1.7	1.5	52	714
Diethyl ether	12	1.0	1.0	3.7	65
Methoxyflurane	12	1.7	1.3	49	970

Adapted from Eger, 1974*
* Values for trichloroethylene have been taken from Chapter 3. *Ed.*

CARDIAC OUTPUT

Cardiac output also influences anaesthetic uptake: a larger output increases uptake (Yamamura, 1968). This is most obvious at the extremes: if output were zero, there would be no uptake. If output were infinite, then all anaesthetic entering the lungs would immediately equilibrate with the entire body and uptake would be determined by the loss into this rather large capacity — the rise in alveolar concentration would be slow — at least during the early part of anaesthesia.

VENOUS ANAESTHETIC LEVELS

The last factor which determines uptake is the anaesthetic partial pressure difference between alveolus and returning venous blood: the larger this difference, the greater is uptake. The flow-weighted mean of anaesthetic partial pressures in the blood flowing from the tissues of the body determines the mixed venous partial pressure. When all tissues are equilibrated with the alveolar anaesthetic partial pressure, there is no difference between anaesthetic partial pressure in the alveoli and in the returning venous blood, and uptake is zero regardless of solubility or cardiac output. Complete equilibration occurs only after an infinitely long anaesthetic.

Tissue uptake

Each tissue removes anaesthetic from the blood coming to it. The amount removed determines the partial pressure reduction occurring on passage through that tissue. Three factors determine this uptake by the tissue: (1) the tissue anaesthetic solubility (the tissue/blood partition coefficient), (2) the tissue volume relative to blood flow and (3) the anaesthetic partial pressure difference between the arterial blood and the tissue. An increase in any of these factors increases removal of anaesthetic. As with uptake at the lung, tissue uptake is determined by the product of the above three factors. If any one factor approaches zero then uptake by that tissue approaches zero.

What is the combined effect of all the tissues on the partial pressure of an anaesthetic agent in the blood returning to the lungs? It would be difficult to examine each tissue and its contribution since the number of tissues is enormous and differences in blood flow between tissue parts within a single organ are sometimes considerable (for example, grey and white matter in brain). To simplify this problem, tissues having common flow per unit volume and solubility characteristics are combined. Mapleson (1963a) has shown that such groupings still permit a reasonable prediction of anaesthetic uptake provided at least three groups are used.

TISSUE GROUPS

We have chosen the groupings given in *Table 4.2* (Eger, 1963a). The vessel-rich group (VRG) includes those tissues having a high perfusion

TABLE 4.2. Tissue groups

	VRG (vessel-rich)	MG (muscle)	FG (fat)	VPG (vessel-poor)
Body mass	9	50	19	22
Volume (litres) in a 70 kg man	6	33	14.5	12.5
Cardiac output (%)	75	18.1	5.4	1.5
Perfusion ($l \cdot min^{-1}$) with 6 $l \cdot min^{-1}$ cardiac output	4.5	1.09	0.32	0.08

(After Eger, 1963a)

per unit volume such as brain, heart, kidneys, viscera and endocrine glands. Only a short time is required for these tissues to achieve equilibrium with the anaesthetic partial pressure in arterial blood. Muscle and skin make up the muscle group (MG), which differs from the VRG by a far lower rate of perfusion per volume of tissue and therefore has a far longer time to equilibration. The fat group (FG) is made up of fat and is separated from the muscle group, not on the basis of any significant difference in perfusion but on the basis of solubility. This difference in solubility varies considerably from one anaesthetic to another (see *Table 4.1*) ranging from a low fat/blood partition coefficient of 2.3 for nitrous oxide to a high of 60 for halothane. The longest time will be required for equilibration with the FG. The vessel-poor group (VPG) contains tissues such as bone, tendons, ligaments and cartilage, which have little or no perfusion but constitute a significant fraction of the body mass. Mapleson (1963a), in his analysis of uptake and distribution, ignored this tissue group and in fact this is what is done here by assigning it an extremely small perfusion per unit volume.

ALVEOLAR CONCENTRATION CURVES

Now let us examine the effects of solubility and the alveolar—venous partial pressure difference on the rate of rise of the alveolar concentration toward the inspired anaesthetic concentration (*Figure 4.3*). The rate of rise is inversely related to the solubility of the anaesthetic in blood and tissues. Therefore the alveolar ether concentration rises most slowly while the concentration of nitrous oxide rises rapidly. The height of each curve differs as a function of solubility but the shape of each curve is similar. Initially there is a rapid rise in alveolar concentration for all anaesthetics including the most soluble. Why is this? Because initially there is no anaesthetic in the alveoli and therefore the alveolar—venous anaesthetic partial pressure difference is zero. Uptake is consequently zero and the effect of ventilation to increase the alveolar concentration is unopposed. However, as the alveolar anaesthetic concentration rises, the alveolar—venous anaesthetic partial pressure difference increases and uptake increases. Within 0.5—1.5 minutes the alveolar—venous partial pressure difference is sufficient to produce an uptake counterbalancing the anaesthetic input by ventilation. The alveolar rate of rise then slows. This initial 'knee' is perhaps best seen with halothane or enflurane.

From 2 to 10 or 15 minutes there is a continuing, although slower, rise of the alveolar concentration. This results from a progressive decrease in uptake due to the rapid equilibration of the VRG with the arterial anaesthetic partial pressure. This decrease in uptake is considerable since three-quarters of the cardiac output flows through the VRG.

With final equilibration of the VRG a second 'knee' is seen at perhaps 10—15 minutes for halothane. Following the second knee there is a continuing but still slower rise in alveolar concentration. This slower rise results from the progressive but slow equilibration of muscle and fat anaesthetic partial pressure with that in the alveoli.

The curves in *Figure 4.3* suggest that induction of anaesthesia with a highly soluble anaesthetic is likely to be more prolonged than induction with a poorly soluble anaesthetic. This difficulty can be, and is, overcome

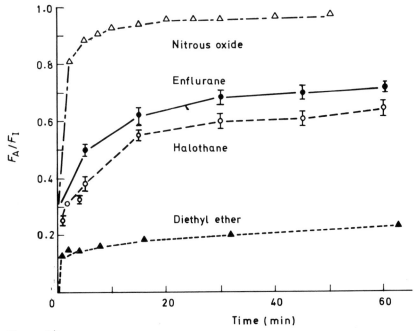

Figure 4.3
The rate of rise of alveolar (F_A) anaesthetic concentration toward the inspired (F_I) concentration is most rapid with the least soluble agent (nitrous oxide), and least rapid with the most soluble agent (diethyl ether). The data all are from studies in man: the nitrous oxide values are from Salanitre *et al.* (1962), the enflurane values from Torri *et al.* (1972) and the halothane and ether values are from Wahrenbrock *et al.* (1974)

by administering an inspired concentration far in excess of the alveolar concentration desired. Thus anaesthesia may be induced with 4 or 5% inspired halothane although the achievement of an alveolar concentration of 4% halothane would prove lethal. This process is sometimes called 'overpressure'.

THE CONCENTRATION EFFECT

The concentration effect augments the rate of rise of the alveolar nitrous oxide concentration toward the inspired nitrous oxide concentration (Eger, 1963b). The higher the inspired concentration, the more rapid is the alveolar rate of rise toward the inspired concentration. Note that this is not saying that the absolute alveolar concentration rises more rapidly when the inspired concentration is high: although this is true, it is not the point. The point is that the ratio of alveolar to inspired concentrations (F_A/F_I) rises more rapidly. Thus if a patient could breathe 80 or 8% of some imaginary anaesthetic, his alveolar/inspiratory concentration ratio would reach 40%/80% faster than 4%/8%. This is illustrated for nitrous oxide in *Figure 4.4*. In addition, the concentration effect results in the administration of 100% of any anaesthetic producing an equal rate of rise of alveolar concentration for all anaesthetics, a rate of rise which is dictated solely by ventilation relative to the functional residual capacity. That is, at 100% inspired concentration the effect of uptake on the alveolar concentration is nil. Part of the reason for this may be shown with a simple example. If a lung contains 100% of any gas and half the gas

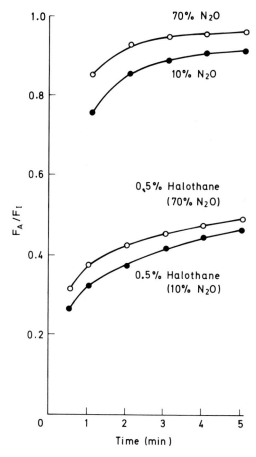

Figure 4.4
The concentration effect and the second gas effect alter the rate of rise of alveolar concentration. In the two upper curves the rate of nitrous oxide is greatest with administration of the higher nitrous oxide concentration (concentration effect). In the two lower curves the rate of halothane rise is different, not because of a difference in halothane concentration but because of the difference in the concentration of the concomitantly administered nitrous oxide (second gas effect). (Reproduced from Epstein *et al.*, 1964, by courtesy of the authors and the Editors of *Anesthesiology*)

is removed, then what remains is still 100%. The concentration effect exerts its influence in two ways. First there is a concentrating effect as illustrated with the lung filled with 100% of any anaesthetic. Second, a collapse of lung with absorption of anaesthetic does not occur; that is, if half the anaesthetic is taken up, this is replaced by more anaesthetic drawn down the trachea from the anaesthetic system. Thus the volume of gas inspired – the effective ventilation – is increased. The clinical significance of the concentration effect is that elevation of the inspired anaesthetic concentration disproportionately increases the rate of rise of the alveolar concentration.

Uptake of an appreciable volume of nitrous oxide accompanies induction with this anaesthetic. As noted above, such uptake results in a concentrating effect and an increase in the volume of gas inspired. Thus, any gas given concomitantly with nitrous oxide will be both concentrated (Stoelting and Eger, 1969a) and subjected to an increased ventilation (Epstein *et al.*, 1964). The alveolar rate of rise of such a concomitantly administered gas would therefore be more rapid. This augmentation in the alveolar rate of rise is shown in *Figure 4.4* and is called by Epstein *et al.* (1964) the second gas effect.

ENTRY OF ANAESTHETICS INTO GAS LOCULI

Now consider the movement of anaesthetic from blood or tissues to a gas phase. First, anaesthetic can move to a closed gas space surrounded by compliant walls. An example of this would be bowel gas or gas in an iatrogenically produced space such as a pneumothorax. If the gas is poorly soluble (such as nitrogen) and if the patient breathes a much more soluble gas (such as nitrous oxide) then the space volume will increase (Eger and Saidman, 1965; Hunter, 1955). The increase occurs because blood cannot carry away appreciable quantities of the poorly soluble gas (if the gas were completely insoluble, none could be carried by blood). On the other hand, blood can carry considerable quantities of the gas from the lungs to the space. The maximum theoretical increase in volume is determined by the concentration of the gas in the lungs. At equilibrium an identical concentration must exist in the closed gas space. If 50% nitrous oxide is in the lungs, then at equilibrium there must be 50% nitrous oxide in the closed gas space. Thus, a volume of nitrous oxide equal to the initial gas volume must enter and the space size doubles. If 80% nitrous oxide is in the lungs then 80% must be reached in the closed gas space, thereby increasing the space by a factor of 5. The volume increases disproportionately with the increase in concentration, approaching infinity at 100%. As seen in *Figures 4.5 and 4.6,* these theoretical limits are not achieved in practice. In the experiments illustrated 75–80% nitrous oxide was breathed while bowel or pneumothorax contained air. The gas volumes should show a four- or fivefold increase but the volumes increased only two- or threefold. In part this is because equilibrium is incomplete and in part because the theoretical analysis assumes that none of the gas originally contained within the closed gas space is lost. Although the solubility of nitrogen is one-thirtieth that of nitrous oxide, it is not totally insoluble and some must be lost with time.

These changes in volume have clinical implications. The use of nitrous oxide in the presence of intestinal distension may be contraindicated, particularly if concentrations of nitrous oxide exceeding 50% are used and if anaesthesia is prolonged. Anaesthesia of short duration may not be

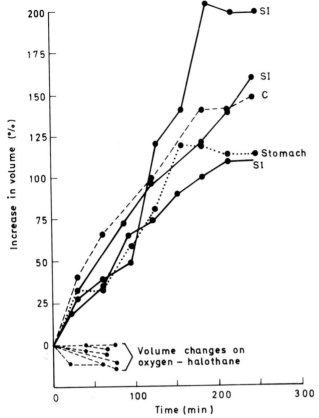

Figure 4.5
A loop of dog small intestine (SI), or colon (C) or stomach was
isolated and filled with air. At zero time the inspired halothane–
oxygen anaesthetic was either continued (lower curves, small circles)
or was changed to halothane, nitrous oxide (75–80%) and oxygen
(upper curves, large circles). (Reproduced from Eger and Saidman,
1965, by courtesy of the authors and the Editors of *Anesthesiology*)

contraindicated since the percentage change is small in the first half hour
to hour. Nitrous oxide is contraindicated in the presence of pneumothorax or non-communicating pulmonary blebs where increase in volume
occurs rapidly and is larger than seen in the bowel. These changes may
compromise ventilation or circulation (Hunter, 1955).

The expansion of one air space approaches the theoretical limit. Nunn
predicted (1959) and Munson demonstrated (Munson and Merrick, 1966)
that the volume of intravenously injected air required to produce death
was reduced by a factor of 3–4 during 75% nitrous oxide breathing.
Nitrous oxide apparently markedly increases the size of injected bubbles.
The use of nitrous oxide anaesthesia for procedures where air embolism
might occur (for example, posterior craniotomy in the upright position)
might be debatable. Use of nitrous oxide will allow a smaller bubble to
produce a significant effect. On the other hand, use of nitrous oxide will
allow a smaller bubble to produce earlier signs of embolism which may

be quickly reversed by elimination of nitrous oxide (and the air leak). In any case, if air embolism occurs during nitrous oxide anaesthesia, one of the most important parts of treatment is the immediate discontinuance of nitrous oxide.

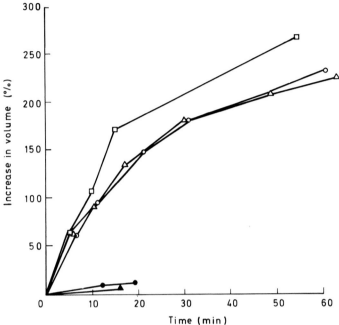

Figure 4.6
An artificial pneumothorax was produced in a dog with air. At zero time the halothane—oxygen anaesthetic was either continued (lower curves, black symbols) or changed to halothane, nitrous oxide (75—80%) and oxygen (upper curves, white symbols). (Reproduced from Eger and Saidman, 1965, by courtesy of the authors and the Editors of *Anesthesiology*)

The air injected into the endotracheal tube cuff also may be expanded by the presence of nitrous oxide (Stanley, Kawamura and Graves, 1974). Again, solubility may be important but in this case the importance lies in the greater diffusivity it confers on nitrous oxide. Nitrous oxide can diffuse through the rubber cuff more rapidly than the nitrogen or oxygen used to inflate the cuff. As a result, the gas space within the cuff expands and may exert an unwanted excess of pressure on the tracheal wall. This effect can be avoided by filling the cuff with gas from the anaesthetic circuit.

Gas spaces such as the sinus or middle ear or the space produced for pneumoencephalography are surrounded by poorly compliant walls. These spaces commonly contain air. On administration of a relatively soluble gas such as nitrous oxide, more gas enters than leaves. Since the volume cannot change, the pressure rises (Saidman and Eger, 1965; Matz, Rattenborg and Holaday, 1967). The theoretical limit to the pressure rise equals the partial pressure of the anaesthetic achieved in the arterial blood. In an experiment illustrating the pressures achieved, Saidman injected air into the cisternal space of dogs (Saidman and Eger, 1965). He then administered nitrous oxide, 70—80%, and recorded the change in pressure. The maximum increase in pressure of 5.3—9.3 kPa (40—70 mmHg) was rapidly reached in 3—5 minutes (*Figure 4.7*). Such pressures may exceed the mean cerebral arterial pressure and thereby impede blood flow. The pressure increase may be avoided either by not using nitrous oxide as the anaesthetic or by using nitrous oxide both as the anaesthetic and the contrast gas. Use of nitrous oxide as the contrast gas has an additional advantage. The ventricular nitrous oxide is rapidly eliminated on cessation of anaesthesia, thereby reducing the incidence of nausea and headache following pneumoencephalography.

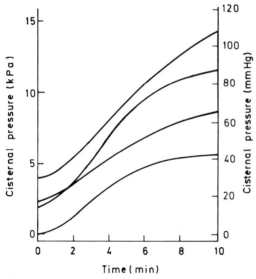

Figure 4.7
Air was placed in the cisternal space of four dogs anaesthetized with halothane in oxygen. At zero time the inhaled anaesthetic was changed to halothane plus 70—80% nitrous oxide (Reproduced from Saidman and Eger, 1965, by courtesy of the authors and the Editors of *Anesthesiology*)

The time for reabsorption of air from the cerebral ventricles is variable. Substantial amounts may remain for several days to a week. In a patient who had undergone pneumoencephalography some five days previous to craniotomy, we found a bulging brain at surgery (Artru, Sohn and Eger, 1978). Insertion of a cannula into the ventricle permitted the unexpected exit of gas and decompression of the brain. The anaesthetic included 60% nitrous oxide. Such experiences suggest the avoidance of nitrous oxide for a week following pneumoencephalography.

EFFECT OF CHANGES IN CARDIAC OUTPUT

Thus far, a constancy of body function has been assumed which may not be encountered in practice. For example, a normal cardiac output and distribution of blood flow have been assumed, as have a constant ventilation and an absence of ventilation/perfusion abnormalities. An assumption has also been made that an anaesthetic delivered to a tissue either remains within that tissue or leaves in the effluent blood. That anaesthetic may leave that tissue by transfer to adjacent tissues or, in the case of skin, by loss to air, has not been considered. There has been the further assumption that no degradation of an anaesthetic occurs. None of these assumptions is correct and in the succeeding sections it will be seen how these deviations may affect the alveolar and arterial anaesthetic partial pressure.

Cardiac output increases with excitement, hyperthermia and hyperthyroidism, while hypothermia, shock and hypothyroidism induce a decrease. An increased output increases uptake of anaesthetic and thereby hinders the rise in alveolar concentration. This is seen in *Figure 4.8* for nitrous oxide, halothane and ether at 2, 6 and 18 l·min^{-1} output (Eger,

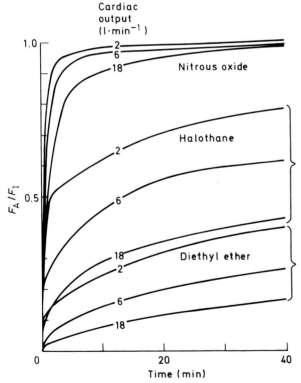

Figure 4.8
When ventilation is maintained at 4 l·min^{-1}, then an increase in cardiac output decreases the rate at which the alveolar concentration rises. The effect of changes in cardiac output on the anaesthetic dose is greatest with the most soluble agent and least with the poorly soluble nitrous oxide. (Reproduced from Eger, 1974)

1974). An increased output produces a slower rate of rise of alveolar concentration with all three anaesthetics, but the impact is greatest with the most soluble anaesthetic. The difference between the rate of rise associated with 2 versus 18 l·min^{-1} cardiac output is small with nitrous oxide. It becomes larger with halothane and is proportionately greatest with the most soluble agent, ether. Although the absolute spread between the 2 and 18 l·min^{-1} curves is approximately the same for both halothane and ether, examination of the curves at 10 minutes illustrates the proportionate difference. The 18 l·min^{-1} halothane curve rises to 30% of the inspired concentration, whereas at 2 l·min^{-1} it rises to 60% — a twofold increase. The alveolar ether concentrations are, respectively, 10 and 30% of the concentrations inspired — a threefold increase. Thus, changes in cardiac output most affect rate of induction of soluble anaesthetics. Excitement or hyperthermia may delay induction with a very soluble agent but shock accelerates induction. There is danger in the last since not only induction but also the achievement of lethal depths of anaesthesia may be rapid.

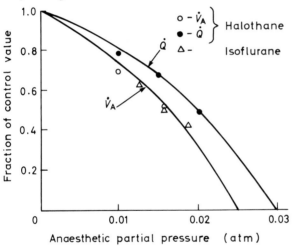

Figure 4.9
The $\dot{V}_A$ graph gives the decrease in ventilation produced by halothane (white circles) or isoflurane (triangles) in male volunteers. The $\dot{Q}$ graph gives the cardiac output decrease produced by halothane when ventilation is controlled to hold $Pa{CO_2}$ between 4.8 and 5.3 kPa (35 and 40 mmHg). (Reproduced from Munson, Eger and Bowers, 1973, by courtesy of the authors and the Editors of *Anesthesiology*)

The computation of the curves in *Figure 4.8* assumed that flow to all tissues changes proportionately with changes in total cardiac output. That is, as output increases from 2 to 18 l·min^{-1}, the VRG, muscle and fat all receive a ninefold inflow increase. Such is not the case. In shock, flow to the brain and heart is spared while flow to the viscera, muscle and fat is reduced. In excitement, flow to brain is unchanged while that to muscle increases. This differential change in flow alters the rate of rise of both alveolar and brain anaesthetic partial pressure (Munson and Eger, 1968).

The limitation of flow to muscle and fat in shock reduces still further the loss of anaesthetic to these tissues and thus reduces uptake. Therefore the alveolar rate of rise with differential reduction of blood flow is greater than with a proportional reduction. The impact is greatest with the most soluble anaesthetic. Not only is the alveolar rate of rise more rapid, but so is the brain rate of rise. The reverse effect may be seen when blood flow is increased to muscle alone, such as might occur during excitement. This results in a greater anaesthetic uptake and hence a slower rate of rise of alveolar anaesthetic concentration than predicted from a proportional change. Again, the impact of this effect parallels solubility.

Various anaesthetics may alter cardiac output and thereby may influence their own uptake. Enflurane and halothane each are potent circulatory depressants which decrease cardiac output in a dose-related fashion (*Figure 4.9*). As a result, anaesthetic uptake of these agents may be progressively reduced at increasing alveolar concentrations — thereby

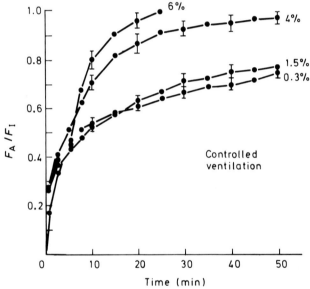

Figure 4.10
Using dogs whose ventilation was controlled, Gibbons and colleagues found that increasing the inspired concentration decreased cardiac output. The resulting decrease in uptake allowed the accelerated rise in the alveolar concentration. (Reproduced from Gibbons, Steffey and Eger, 1977, by courtesy of the authors and the Editors of *Anesthesia and Analgesia*)

permitting a progressively more rapid approach to the inspired concentration (Gibbons, Steffey and Eger, 1977) (*Figure 4.10*). That is, an increase in the inspired concentration may produce a disproportionate increase in the rate of rise of the alveolar concentration. This may lead to a positive feedback which may in turn culminate in anaesthetic overdose and cardiovascular collapse.

EFFECT OF CHANGES OF VENTILATION

Hyperventilation is more common than normal respiration in the patient about to be anaesthetized. Frequently excitement and occasionally hypermetabolic states occur, both of which increase ventilation. The patient in shock also may have increased ventilation. On the other hand, depressed ventilation is produced by excessive premedication or by impaired lung function. The impact of different ventilations is illustrated in *Figure 4.11*, again for three anaesthetics of widely different solubilities.

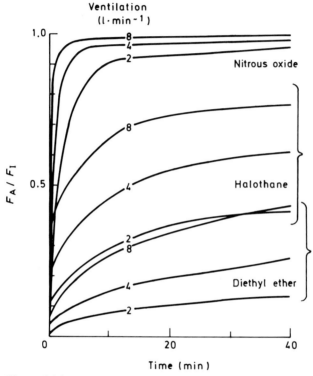

Figure 4.11
An increase in alveolar ventilation accelerates the increase in anaesthetic concentration. The effect on the anaesthetic dose is greatest
for the most soluble agent, ether, and least for the least soluble
agent, nitrous oxide. (Reproduced from Eger, 1974)

An increase in ventilation from 2 to 4 to 8 $l \cdot min^{-1}$ increases the rate at which the alveolar concentration rises. These results are confirmed by the work of Yamamura *et al.* (1963). As with changes induced by alteration of cardiac output, these changes are greatest with the most soluble agent, ether. The clinical implications also are similar to those of changes in cardiac output: the most predictable induction of anaesthesia in the face of variations in ventilation is achieved with the least soluble anaesthetic.

The above predictions ignore the decrease in cerebral blood flow that results from a decrease in Pa_{CO_2}. The lower cerebral blood flow due to

hyperventilation may decrease the cerebral anaesthetic partial pressure
rate of rise to or below normal (that is, the same as when ventilation is
normal) during induction with a poorly soluble agent. The effect is small
with a highly soluble agent (Munson and Bowers, 1967).

Anaesthetics may affect their rate of rise in the alveoli by depressing
ventilation. For halothane or isoflurane, alveolar ventilation is decreased
to half of normal at a concentration of 1.5% in the alveoli (see *Figure 4.9*).
A similar depression is produced by 2.5% enflurane. This depression
increases to apnoea at 2.5% halothane or isoflurane, and at 3% enflurane.
The progressive decrease in ventilation limits the rate at which the alveolar

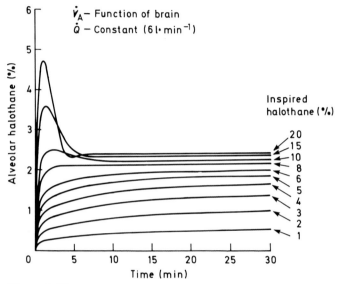

Figure 4.12
When ventilation is spontaneous, cardiac output is sustained despite
high inspired halothane concentrations. Ventilation itself is depressed
and thereby limits the alveolar anaesthetic concentration which can
be achieved. Since apnoea occurs at 2.5% alveolar halothane, this
level cannot be exceeded in the steady state regardless of the inspired
concentration. (Reproduced from Munson, Eger and Bowers, 1973,
by courtesy of the authors and the Editors of *Anesthesiology*)

concentration rises and the ultimate level of anaesthetic achieved in the
alveoli (*Figure 4.12*). Obviously in the steady state the alveolar concentration cannot exceed that concentration which produces apnoea. This
'negative feedback' increases the safety of anaesthesia when ventilation is
spontaneous since it lessens the danger of achieving an alveolar anaesthetic
partial pressure which might compromise myocardial function.

CONCOMITANT CHANGES IN VENTILATION AND CIRCULATION

Many conditions may affect ventilation and perfusion per kilogram of
body tissue. Fever, hyperthyroidism and hypercapnia each increase both

ventilation and circulation, while hypothermia and hypothyroidism may do the opposite. Since an increase in ventilation accelerates the alveolar rate of rise (see *Figure 4.11*) while an increase in cardiac output slows the rate of rise (see *Figure 4.8*), the effects of concomitant increases in ventilation and cardiac output should tend to cancel each other and the alveolar anaesthetic rate of rise should not differ greatly from normal. Indeed, if the distribution of blood flow remains constant (i.e. blood flow increases proportionally in all tissues) then the alveolar rate of rise is only slightly accelerated (Eger, Bahlman and Munson, 1971) (*Figure 4.13*).

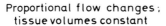

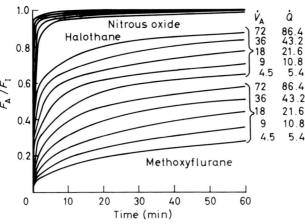

Figure 4.13
A concomitant doubling of ventilation and circulation accelerates the alveolar anaesthetic rate of rise. The simulation portrayed here assumed that each increase in cardiac output was distributed proportionally to all tissues (e.g. a doubling of flow meant that flow to each tissue was doubled). The effect on alveolar anaesthetic concentration is relatively small for cardiorespiratory changes that commonly are found (i.e. a doubling of cardiac output $-\dot{Q}-$ or alveolar ventilation $-\dot{V}_A$). (Adapted from Eger, Bahlman and Munson, 1971, by courtesy of the authors and the Editors of *Anesthesiology*)

The acceleration achieved results from the increased rate of equilibration of tissues with anaesthetic due to the higher blood flow. This increases the venous anaesthetic partial pressure, decreases the alveolar-to-venous difference in anaesthetic partial pressure and hence reduces anaesthetic uptake.

   Uptake in the young — particularly in the newborn — is affected by their higher ventilation and perfusion per kilogram of body tissue. However, unlike the situation described in the preceding paragraph, the perfusion per kilogram is not increased proportionally to all tissues. The vessel-rich group of tissues receives a disproportionately larger share than other tissues. Since the VRG equilibrates rapidly with the anaesthetic partial pressure delivered in arterial blood, an increase in perfusion would act to shunt anaesthetic back to the lung and hence decrease the alveolar-to-venous partial pressure difference. This effect significantly accelerates the alveolar rate of rise of anaesthetic concentration in the young (Salanitre and Rackow, 1969) (*Figure 4.14*), and in part explains the more rapid induction of anaesthesia in the young when an inhalational approach is used.

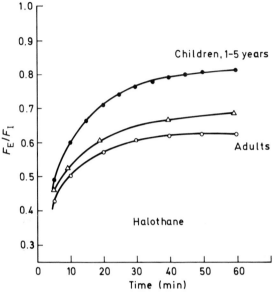

Figure 4.14
The alveolar rate of rise of halothane in infants or children is more rapid than in adults in part because of their greater ventilation and perfusion per kilogram of tissue and in part because of the diversion of most of the increase in blood flow to the vessel-rich group. (Adapted from Salanitre and Rackow, 1969, by courtesy of the authors and the Editors of *Anesthesiology*)

VENTILATION/PERFUSION ABNORMALITIES

Ventilation/perfusion abnormalities are the rule rather than the exception in patients undergoing anaesthesia. Anaesthetists are well aware that abnormalities are produced by emphysema, pneumonitis or atelectasis. The anaesthetist may cause them by endobronchial intubation or by anaesthesia itself. These abnormalities influence the rates of rise of both alveolar and arterial anaesthetic partial pressures: raising the former and lowering the latter. The impact of ventilation/perfusion abnormalities on the rate of induction of anaesthesia depends on the solubility of the anaesthetic (Eger and Severinghaus, 1964). The alveolar anaesthetic partial pressure rises more rapidly than usual with highly soluble anaesthetics, but the arterial anaesthetic partial pressure rise is scarcely affected. The converse is true with poorly soluble anaesthetics. The reason for this is illustrated in *Figure 4.15* (Saidman and Eger, 1967). The normal state is shown in *Figure 4.15a* where the anaesthetic partial pressure of 1.3 kPa (10 mmHg) is achieved equally in both alveoli and the blood leaving these alveoli. The inspired anaesthetic partial pressure required to achieve an alveolar partial pressure of 1.3 kPa (10 mmHg) depends on anaesthetic solubility. It might be 6.7 kPa (50 mmHg) for a highly soluble gas and 1.6 kPa (12 mmHg) for a slightly soluble gas. Imagine now that one bronchus is obstructed and that the ventilation normally directed through that bronchus is added to the ventilation to the unobstructed lung. The effects of such a change on the alveolar and arterial anaesthetic partial

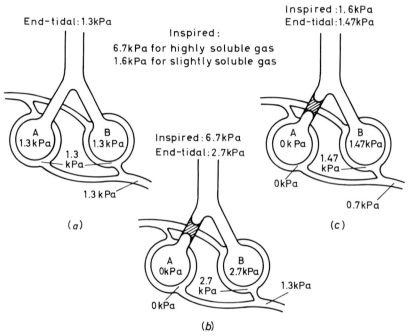

Figure 4.15
Anaesthetic partial pressure achieved normally (*a*) and during obstruction of one bronchus (*b* and *c*) in the case of a highly soluble anaesthetic (*b*) and a poorly soluble anaesthetic (*c*). See the text for a detailed explanation. (Reproduced from Saidman and Eger, 1967, by courtesy of the authors and the Editors of *Clinical Anesthesia*)

pressures for a highly and for a slightly soluble anaesthetic are illustrated in *Figure 4.15b and c*, respectively. Doubling ventilation nearly doubles the alveolar concentration of a highly soluble gas (see *Figure 4.11*) and thus the alveolar anaesthetic partial pressure in *Figure 4.15b* equals 2.7 kPa (20 mmHg). However, only half the pulmonary blood flow receives this increased partial pressure. Since half the blood has double the normal anaesthetic partial pressure while half has none, the mean arterial anaesthetic partial pressure is unchanged from normal (that is, it equals that in *Figure 4.15a*. The situation is reversed for a slightly soluble agent. Doubling ventilation scarcely affects the alveolar concentration of a slightly soluble anaesthetic such as nitrous oxide (*Figure*

4.15b) and therefore the alveolar anaesthetic partial pressure in *Figure 4.15c* is only raised to 1.5 kPa (11 mmHg) (the most it could rise is to the inspired partial pressure of 1.6 kPa; 12 mmHg). However, the arterial partial pressure is reduced to almost half normal (0.7 kPa; 5.5 mmHg) by the dilution of the blood from the unventilated lung. Since it is the arterial anaesthetic partial pressure with which the brain eventually achieves equilibrium, the rate of induction with highly soluble anaesthetics will scarcely be affected by ventilation/perfusion abnormalities, but may be delayed considerably with slightly soluble anaesthetics.

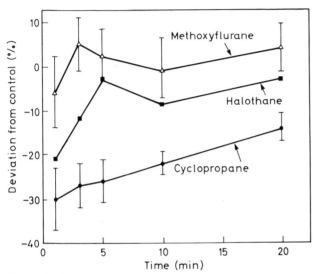

Figure 4.16
In dogs the introduction of an endobronchial blocker slows the arterial anaesthetic rate of rise of the poorly soluble cyclopropane but does not affect the arterial concentration of the very soluble methoxyflurane. (Reproduced from Stoelting and Longnecker, 1972, by courtesy of the authors and the Editors of *Anesthesiology*)

The impact of solubility on the effect of ventilation/perfusion abnormalities was studied in dogs by Stoelting and Longnecker (1972). They found that introduction of an endobronchial blocker delayed the rate of rise of cyclopropane in arterial blood but had no effect on methoxyflurane (*Figure 4.16*). Halothane was slightly delayed.

METABOLISM OF ANAESTHETICS

At one time it was thought that all inhaled anaesthetics (with the exception of trichloroethylene) were eventually excreted unchanged via the lungs. However, it is now known that a significant amount of potent inhaled anaesthetic is metabolized (Van Dyke and Chenoweth, 1965). The amount varies from agent to agent: as much as 50% of the methoxyflurane which is taken up is metabolized (Holaday, Rudofsky and Treuhaft, 1970), while as little as 2.5% of enflurane is degraded (Chase *et al.*, 1971). Halothane occupies an intermediate position, with the fraction metabolized equalling 10–25% of uptake (Rehder *et al.*, 1967). However, the impact of biodegradation on uptake is uncertain because a substantial fraction of the biodegradation takes place after the administration of anaesthetic. Furthermore, it appears that saturation of the enzymes responsible for metabolism occurs at anaesthetizing anaesthetic concentrations (Sawyer *et al.*, 1971). Nevertheless, at least with methoxyflurane there is evidence that an increase in biodegradation can significantly alter the rate at which anaesthetic blood levels rise (Berman *et al.*, 1973).

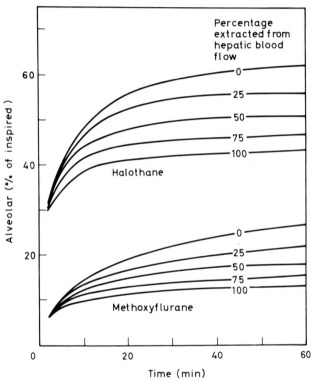

Figure 4.17
An increase in the percentage of halothane or methoxyflurane removed (metabolized) by the liver increases anaesthetic uptake and thereby decreases the rate of rise of alveolar anaesthetic. The effect on anaesthetic dose is greater with the more soluble agent, methoxyflurane. (Reproduced from Eger, 1974)

The ultimate effect of metabolism on the alveolar or arterial anaesthetic concentration will depend both on its rate of metabolism and on the solubility of the anaesthetic (*Figure 4.17*) (Eger, 1974). The alveolar concentration of a more soluble anaesthetic will be more affected by a given increase in its rate of metabolism. Metabolism of anaesthetics is considered further in Chapter 7.

PERCUTANEOUS LOSS OF ANAESTHETICS

In 1933 Orcutt and Waters demonstrated the passage of nitrous oxide and ethylene through skin. Stoelting (Stoelting and Eger, 1969b) confirmed these observations for nitrous oxide and extended them to cyclopropane, halothane and diethyl ether (*Figure 4.18*). Percutaneous loss of

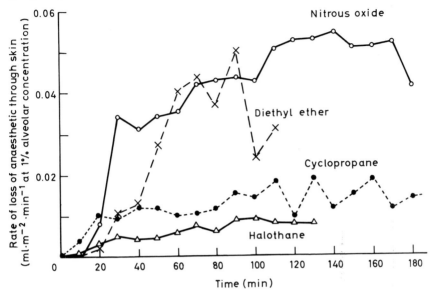

Figure 4.18
Rates of loss per minute through 1 m² of skin are shown for nitrous oxide, diethyl ether, cyclopropane and halothane when the alveolar concentration of each anaesthetic equals 1%. (Reproduced from Stoelting and Eger, 1969b), by courtesy of the authors and the Editors of *Anesthesiology*)

these anaesthetics is too small to influence uptake except after prolonged anaesthesia. However, the results are interesting for another reason. Loss of nitrous oxide at a given partial pressure is three times the cyclopropane loss, although these gases are similar in lean tissue solubility and molecular size. Another explanation is possible. The dermis is sandwiched between epidermis and subcutaneous fat. Anaesthetic in the dermis may move either to subcutaneous fat or through the epidermis. Loss to subcutaneous fat would reduce the dermal partial pressure of anaesthetic and thereby would reduce the pressure driving anaesthetic across the epidermis. Loss to subcutaneous fat should be greatest and reduction of dermal partial pressure most with cyclopropane because the cyclopropane fat/lean tissue partition coefficient is five to ten times that for nitrous oxide. The difference between cyclopropane and nitrous oxide percutaneous excretion therefore suggests that significant intertissue diffusion occurs. Intertissue diffusion might occur not only at the skin but also between all adjacent tissues. Perl (1963) suggested this possibility, and Rackow supported Perl's hypothesis by showing that the alveolar rate of rise of nitrous oxide significantly exceeded the rate of rise of cyclopropane (Rackow *et al.*, 1965). The most rational interpretation for the difference in the cyclopropane and nitrous oxide rates of rise appeared to be inter-tissue diffusion between well perfused tissues and adjacent lipid tissues. However, this interpretation assumed an identical solubility of cyclo-propane and nitrous oxide for all tissues except fat, and subsequent experiments demonstrated that cyclopropane blood solubility is signifi-cantly higher than nitrous oxide (Gregory and Eger, 1968). If other tissues show a higher affinity for cyclopropane, then Rackow's experiment may not support the intertissue diffusion hypothesis.

Cohen, Chow and Mathers (1972) have indirectly demonstrated inter-tissue diffusion of halothane in the monkey brain. They gave radioactive halothane intravenously and, using radioautography, demonstrated the following sequence. Initially the halothane was confined to the grey matter — that is, to a 3–4 mm thick surface band of tissue. This greater partial pressure of anaesthetic in grey matter caused the transfer of halothane to the adjacent white matter. Evidence for this transfer appears in the subsequent radioautographs. The high initial concentration of halothane in grey matter is markedly reduced by the level of perfusion accorded this tissue. A band of radioactivity remains in the white matter underlying the grey. The degree of radioactivity decreases progressively at greater depths in the white matter.

RECOVERY

Recovery occurs by anaesthetic loss from blood to the alveolar gas space. The factors controlling recovery are, with one exception, identical to the factors influencing induction. The rate of fall of alveolar concentration (that is, recovery) is proportional to ventilation: an increase in ventilation accelerates recovery. Output of agent from blood to lungs opposes this fall in alveolar concentration. Three factors determine output: blood solubility, cardiac output and the venous–alveolar anaesthetic partial pressure difference. An increase in any one of these increases output. Thus the rate at which the alveolar concentration falls is slower for methoxyflurane or ether than for halothane; slower for halothane than for enflurane; and slower for enflurane than for nitrous oxide (*Figure 4.19*).

After a long anaesthetic with saturation or near-saturation of most tissues, the decay of the alveolar concentration is similar to the rise in concentration seen on induction except that the curves are 'turned upside down'. Initially, there is a very rapid fall because output is zero and thus the effect of ventilation is unopposed. Output is initially zero because the venous–alveolar anaesthetic partial pressure difference is zero. As ven-tilation reduces the alveolar partial pressure, the venous–alveolar difference increases and output increases. Within the first minute of recovery the removal of anaesthetic by ventilation equals the output of anaesthetic from blood and the decline in alveolar concentration slows.

The anaesthetic partial pressure in the tissues next falls toward the reduced partial pressure in arterial blood. The rate of fall of tissue anaesthetic pressure is determined by the same factors which influenced the rate of rise on induction: tissue/blood partition coefficient, tissue volume relative to blood flow and the tissue–blood anaesthetic partial pressure difference. The most rapid reduction in anaesthetic partial pressure occurs in the most highly perfused tissues (the VRG). The rapid fall in the VRG anaesthetic partial pressure reduces the venous anaesthetic partial pressure

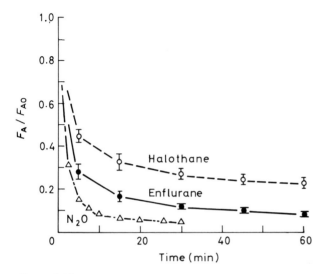

Figure 4.19
These graphs illustrate the fall in alveolar anaesthetic concentration (F_A) from the alveolar concentration achieved at the end of an hour of anaesthetic administration (F_{AO}) in man. The rate of fall is most rapid with the least soluble agent (nitrous oxide) and least rapid with the most soluble agent (halothane). The halothane and enflurane data are from Torri *et al.* (1972), while those for nitrous oxide are from Salanitre *et al.* (1962).

and thereby reduces the venous–alveolar partial pressure difference. This decreases output of anaesthetic and allows ventilation to further reduce the alveolar concentration (albeit at a slower rate than during the first minute) until the venous–alveolar anaesthetic partial pressure difference is restored and anaesthetic output balances removal by ventilation. The influence of the VRG disappears at 10–15 minutes as its anaesthetic partial pressure approaches the reduced partial pressure in the alveoli. After this time a still more gradual decline is seen resulting from the continuing desaturation of muscle and fat.

CONCENTRATION EFFECT

The concentration effect associated with nitrous oxide is prominent only on induction of anaesthesia. During recovery there is no infinite gaseous reservoir of anaesthetic: the anaesthetic contained by blood is finite and no more can be drawn from blood after that is lost. Further-more, the outpouring of nitrous oxide — which may equal $1-2$ $l \cdot min^{-1}$ initially — dilutes alveolar CO_2 and thereby depresses ventilation.

EFFECT OF DURATION OF ANAESTHESIA

In clinical practice, rarely are all tissues completely equilibrated with the alveolar anaesthetic partial pressure. The time for 95% equilibration of fat tissue with a constant arterial halothane partial pressure is 150 hours; 95% equilibration of halothane with muscle requires 5 hours. Therefore, the venous anaesthetic partial pressure during clinical anaesthesia is lower than the alveolar partial pressure, and the initial fall in the alveolar partial pressure necessary to develop a sufficient venous–alveolar difference to balance the ventilatory removal of anaesthetic will have to be greater than the fall after total equilibration. Since duration of anaesthesia determines

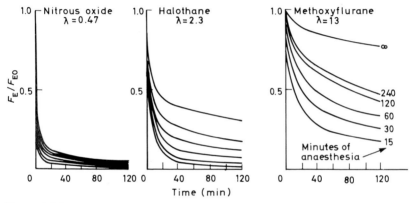

Figure 4.20
The fall in alveolar concentration (F_E) relative to the alveolar concentration immediately preceding cessation of anaesthetic administration for nitrous oxide, halothane and methoxyflurane. A constant alveolar anaesthetic concentration prior to recovery (F_{EO}) was of various durations: the curves from uppermost to lowest followed anaesthetics of infinite duration, 4 hours, 2 hours, 1 hour, 30 minutes and 15 minutes respectively. (Reproduced from Stoelting and Eger, 1969c, by courtesy of the authors and the Editors of *Anesthesiology*)

the venous anaesthetic partial pressure relative to the alveolar partial pressure, then duration of anaesthesia also determines the rate at which the alveolar concentration falls: the longer the anaesthetic, the slower the rate of fall (Mapleson, 1963b; Stoelting and Eger, 1969c). As shown in *Figure 4.20*, an increase in anaesthesia time from 15 to 60 to 240 minutes to an anaesthetic of infinite duration slows the rate of fall of alveolar concentration on recovery. However, anaesthetic solubility determines the impact of anaesthetic duration. With a poorly soluble anaesthetic such as nitrous oxide, there is a negligible difference between the percentage fall following a 15-minute anaesthetic and that which follows an anaesthetic of infinite duration. Recovery is rapid in either case. The difference in percentage fall is greatest with a highly soluble anaesthetic such as methoxyflurane. Recovery is prompt following a short methoxyflurane anaesthetic but is prolonged following a long anaesthetic.

Diffusion hypoxia

During recovery from nitrous oxide anaesthesia, large volumes of nitrous oxide may be lost via the lungs, producing a phenomenon described by Fink (1955) as 'diffusion anoxia'. The effect of this large volume transfer on oxygenation is illustrated in *Figure 4.21*. About 2—3 minutes after the

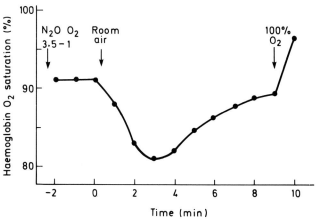

Figure 4.21
The change in arterial haemoglobin saturation occurring in a patient when the inspired gas was changed from nitrous oxide and oxygen to room air. The consequent decrease in saturation Fink called diffusion anoxia. (Reproduced from Fink, 1955, by courtesy of the author and the Editors of *Anesthesiology*)

respired gas mixture is changed from nitrous oxide and oxygen to air, the oxygen saturation falls from 91 to 81% and then gradually returns toward 91%. Fink explained this decreased saturation by the dilution of inspired oxygen with the outpouring nitrous oxide. This hypothesis is supported by the appearance of the maximum desaturation at a time when the outpouring of nitrous oxide is greatest (Sheffer, Steffenson and Birch, 1972). Rackow and coworkers (Rackow, Salanitre and Frumin, 1961) suggested that oxygen is not the only gas diluted by the outpouring of nitrous oxide; the partial pressure of carbon dioxide also is reduced. A lower alveolar CO_2 depresses ventilation and thereby aggravates the hypoxia induced by dilution of oxygen. Diffusion hypoxia is of little consequence to a normal patient, but may be important to the patient with impaired respiration or circulation. Administration of oxygen during the greatest outpouring of nitrous oxide (the first 5 minutes of recovery) prevents most of the decrease in oxygen saturation.

Effect of ventilatory changes

Changes in ventilation also influence recovery from anaesthesia (Stoelting and Eger, 1969c). An increase in ventilation from 2 to 4 to 8 $l \cdot min^{-1}$ increases the rate of fall (*Figure 4.22*). These curves, obtained after anaesthetic equilibration with all tissues, are essentially upside down images of those seen in *Figure 4.11* for the effect of different ventilations

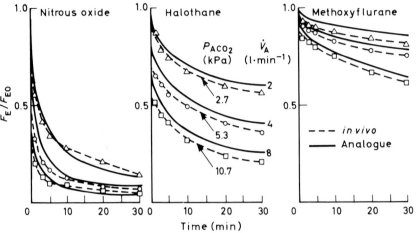

Figure 4.22
The effect of different alveolar ventilations on recovery from three anaesthetics. The *in vivo* data (dashed lines) at 2.7, 5.3 and 10.7 kPa (20, 40 and 80 mmHg $PACO_2$) are comparable to predicted rates of fall, assuming alveolar ventilations of 8, 4 and 2 $l \cdot min^{-1}$ respectively. Recovery in all cases follows total body equilibration. (Reproduced from Stoelting and Eger, 1969c, by courtesy of the authors and the Editors of *Anesthesiology*)

on induction. The implications of these curves, however, are different. During recovery it is not the proportionate change but the absolute change in alveolar anaesthetic partial pressure which is important. Recovery from the anaesthetic showing the greatest separation of curves will therefore be most influenced by changes in respiration. For the periods shown in *Figure 4.22*, this anaesthetic is halothane – an agent of intermediate solubility. With the poorly soluble agent, nitrous oxide, the alveolar anaesthetic partial pressure falls rapidly regardless of ventilation. With the highly soluble methoxyflurane, the partial pressure falls slowly regardless of ventilation. Thus, following total body equilibration, different ventilations most influence recovery during the first 30 minutes following halothane anaesthesia. However, after longer periods of time the separation of the halothane curves becomes smaller, while the separation of methoxyflurane curves increases.

Complete tissue equilibration is rarely accomplished since it requires an anaesthetic of infinite duration. As shown in *Figure 4.23*, shortening the duration of anaesthesia accelerates the fall in alveolar anaesthetic partial

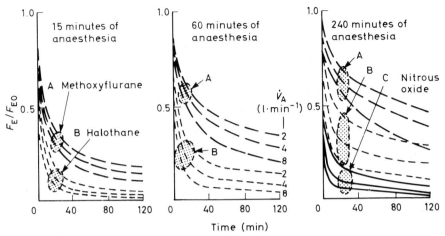

Figure 4.23
As illustrated for methoxyflurane (A), halothane (B) or nitrous
oxide (C), recovery is more rapid after 15 minutes of constant
alveolar anaesthetic concentration than after 60 minutes; recovery
after 60 minutes of anaesthesia is more rapid than after 240 minutes.
However, the impact of an increase in alveolar ventilation (from
2 to 4 to 8 l·min^{-1}) on the rate of recovery is progressively decreased
with decrease in time of anaesthesia. (Reproduced from Stoelting
and Eger, 1969c, by courtesy of the authors and the Editors of
Anesthesiology)

pressure and reduces the impact of changes in ventilation (Stoelting and
Eger, 1969c). In effect, shortening anaesthesia makes the anaesthetic
appear less and less soluble: for example, the halothane curves after
15 minutes of anaesthesia are similar to those seen with nitrous oxide
after total body equilibration.

EPILOGUE

The importance of anaesthetic pharmacokinetics is not always apparent.
Until 20 years ago anaesthesia was administered without this knowledge.
Nevertheless, the majority of patients survived and benefited. Why, then,
should we trouble ourselves with the effort required to assimilate the
concepts of 'uptake and distribution'? The same question might be
asked of a knowledge of the cardiovascular, respiratory or neuromuscular
effects of anaesthetics. An understanding of basic pharmacology is not
necessary to the administration of anaesthesia: anaesthesia can be administered by trial and error. But the time required to learn to give a satisfactory
anaesthetic is much less when the learning process is based on an understanding of the underlying principles, rather than on trial and error. The
safest use of anaesthetics does require this understanding. It does require
the ability to anticipate the impact of variations in patient physiology,
disease or surgery on the effect of these potentially lethal drugs we
administer.

References

Artru, A., Sohn, Y. J. and Eger, E. I. II (1978). When it is safe to administer nitrous oxide after pneumoencephalography? *Anesthesiology* 49, 136–137

Berman, M. L., Lowe, H. J., Hagler, K. J. and Bochantin, J. (1973). Uptake and elimination of methoxyflurane as influenced by enzyme induction in the rat. *Anesthesiology* 38, 352–357

Chase, R. E., Holaday, D. A., Fiserova-Bergerova, V., Saidman, L. J. and Mack, S. E. (1971). The biotransformation of Ethrane in man. *Anesthesiology* 35, 262–267

Cohen, E. N., Chow, K. L. and Mathers, L. (1972). Autoradiographic distribution of volatile anesthetics within the brain. *Anesthesiology* 37, 324–331

Eger, E. I. II (1963a). A mathematical model of uptake and distribution. In *Uptake and Distribution of Anesthetic Agents,* Chapter 7. E. M. Papper and R. Kitz (ed.). New York and Maidenhead: McGraw-Hill

Eger, E. I. II (1963b). Effect of inspired anesthetic concentration on the rate of rise of alveolar concentration. *Anesthesiology* 24, 153–157

Eger, E. I. II (1974). *Anesthetic Uptake and Action.* Baltimore, Md: Williams & Wilkins

Eger, E. I. II and Larson, C. P. Jr. (1964). Anaesthetic solubility in blood and tissues. *Br. J. Anaesth.* 36, 140–149

Eger, E. I. II and Saidman, L. J. (1965). Hazards of nitrous oxide anesthesia in bowel obstruction and pneumothorax. *Anesthesiology* 26, 61–66

Eger, E. I. II and Severinghaus, J. W. (1964). Effect of uneven pulmonary distribution of blood and gas on induction with inhalation anesthetics. *Anesthesiology* 25, 620–626

Eger, E. I. II, Bahlman, S. H. and Munson, E. S. (1971). Effect of age on the rate of increase of alveolar anesthetic concentration. *Anesthesiology* 35, 365–372

Epstein, R. M., Rackow, H., Salanitre, E. and Wolf, G. L. (1964). Influence of the concentration effect on the uptake of anesthetic mixtures; the second gas effect. *Anesthesiology* 25, 364–371

Fink, B. R. (1955). Diffusion anoxia. *Anesthesiology* 16, 511–519

Gibbons, R. T., Steffey, E. P. and Eger, E. I. II (1977). The effect of spontaneous versus controlled ventilation on the rate of rise of alveolar halothane concentration in dogs. *Anesth. Analg.* 56, 32–34

Gregory, G. A. and Eger, E. I. II (1968). Partition coefficients in blood and blood fractions at various concentrations of cyclopropane. *Fedn Proc.* 27, 705

Holaday, D. A., Rudofsky, S. and Treuhaft, P. S. (1970). Metabolic degradation of methoxyflurane in man. *Anesthesiology* 33, 579–593

Hunter, A. R. (1955). Problems of anaesthesia in artificial pneumothorax. *Proc. R. Soc. Med.* 48, 765–768

Mapleson, W. W. (1963a). An electric analogue for uptake and exchange of inert gases and other agents. *J. appl. Physiol.* 18, 197–204

Mapleson, W. W. (1963b). Quantitative prediction of anesthetic concentrations. In *Uptake and Distribution of Anesthetic Agents,* Chapter 9. E. M. Papper and R. Kitz (ed.). New York and Maidenhead: McGraw-Hill

Matz, G. J., Rattenborg, C. G. and Holaday, D. A. (1967). Effects of nitrous oxide on middle ear pressure. *Anesthesiology* 28, 948–950

Munson, E. S. and Bowers, D. L. (1967). Effects of hyperventilation on the rate of cerebral anesthetic equilibration. *Anesthesiology* 28, 377–381

Munson, E. S. and Eger, E. I. II (1968). The effects of changes in cardiac output and distribution on the rate of cerebral anesthetic equilibration. *Anesthesiology* 29, 533–537

Munson, E. S. and Merrick, H. C. (1966). Effect of nitrous oxide on venous air embolism. *Anesthesiology* 27, 783–787

Munson, E. S., Eger, E. I. II and Bowers, D. L. (1973). Effects of anesthetic-depressed ventilation and cardiac output on anesthetic uptake. *Anesthesiology* 38, 251–259

Nunn, J. F. (1959). Controlled respiration in neurosurgical anaesthesia. *Anaesthesia* 14, 413–414

Orcutt, F. S. and Waters, R. M. (1933). Diffusion of nitrous oxide, ethylene and carbon dioxide through human skin during anesthesia; including a new method of estimating nitrous oxide in low concentrations. *Curr. Res. Anesth. Analg.* 12, 45

Perl, W. (1963). Large-scale diffusion between body compartments. In *Uptake and Distribution of Anesthetic Agents,* p. 224. E. M. Papper and R. Kitz (ed.). New York and Maidenhead: McGraw-Hill

Rackow, H., Salanitre, E. and Frumin, M. J. (1961). Dilution of alveolar gases during nitrous oxide excretion in man. *J. appl. Physiol.* 16, 723–728

Rackow, H., Salanitre, E., Epstein, R. M., Wolf, G. L. and Perl, W. (1965). Simultaneous uptake of N$_2$O and cyclopropane in man as a test of compartment model. *J. appl. Physiol.* 20, 611–620

Rehder, K., Forbes, J., Alter, H., Hessler, O. and Stier, A. (1967). Halothane biotransformation in man: a quantitative study. *Anesthesiology* 28, 711–715

Saidman, L. J. and Eger, E. I. II (1965). Change in cerebrospinal fluid pressure during pneumoencephalography under nitrous oxide anesthesia. *Anesthesiology* 26, 67–72

Saidman, L. J. and Eger, E. I. II (1967). The influence of ventilation/perfusion abnormalities upon the uptake of inhalation anesthetics. *Clin. Anesth.* 1, 79–87

Salanitre, E. and Rackow, H. (1969). The pulmonary exchange of nitrous oxide and halothane in infants and children. *Anesthesiology* 30, 388–394

Salanitre, E. and Rackow, H., Greene, L. T., Klonymus, D. and Epstein, R. M. (1962). Uptake and excretion of subanesthetic concentrations of nitrous oxide in man. *Anesthesiology* 23, 814–822

Sawyer, D. C., Eger, E. I. II, Bahlman, S. H., Cullen, B. F. and Impelman, D. (1971). Concentration dependence of hepatic halothane metabolism. *Anesthesiology* 34, 230–235

Sheffer, L., Steffenson, J. L. and Birch, A. A. (1972). Nitrous oxide-induced diffusion hypoxia in patients breathing spontaneously. *Anesthesiology* 37, 436–439

Stanley, T. H., Kawamura, R. and Graves, C. (1974). Effects of nitrous oxide on volume and pressure of endotracheal tube cuffs. *Anesthesiology* 41, 256–262

Stoelting, R. K. and Eger, E. I. II (1969a). Additional explanation for the second gas gas effect: a concentrating effect. *Anesthesiology* 30, 273–277

Stoelting, R. K. and Eger, E. I. II (1969b). Percutaneous loss of nitrous oxide, cyclopropane, ether, and halothane in man. *Anesthesiology* 30, 278–283

Stoelting, R. K. and Eger, E. I. II (1969c). Effect of ventilation and solubility on recovery from anesthesia: an in vivo and analog analysis before and after equilibrium. *Anesthesiology* 30, 290–296

Stoelting, R. K. and Longnecker, D. E. (1972). Effect of right-to-left shunt on rate of increase in arterial anesthetic concentration. *Anesthesiology* 36, 352–356

Torri, G., Damia, G., Fabiani, M. L. and Frosa, Y. (1972). Uptake and elimination of enflurane in man. *Br. J. Anaesth.* 44, 789–794

Van Dyke, R. A. and Chenoweth, M. B. (1965). Metabolism of volatile anesthetics. *Anesthesiology* 26, 348–357

Wahrenbrock, E. A., Eger, E. I. II, Laravuso, R. B. and Maruschak, G. (1974). Anesthetic uptake – of mice and men (and whales). *Anesthesiology* 40, 19–23

Yamamura, H. (1968). The effect of ventilation and blood volume on the uptake or elimination of inhalation anaesthetic agents. In *Anaesthesiology,* Proc. 4th Wld Congr. of Anaesthesiologists; International Congress Series. Amsterdam and London: Excerpta Medica

Yamamura, H., Wakasugi, B., Okuma, Y. and Maki, K. (1963). The effects of ventilation on the absorption and elimination of inhalation anaesthetics. *Anaesthesia* 18, 427–438

5 Axon and synapse in relation to anaesthesia
Joan J. Kendig

The problem to be addressed in this chapter is the isolation and identification of the nerve cell functions, modification of which produces the state of anaesthesia. Except for comparative purposes, the discussion is limited to the inhalation agents, and to the inert gases and organic solvents thought to act in a fashion similar to them. The cellular structure to be primarily considered is the cell membrane.

It may be said very simplistically that nerve cells perform two different but related functions, employing membranes with distinct characteristics for each. The first is the conveying of digitally coded information in the form of action potentials, sometimes over long distances. The part of the nerve cell which is most associated with this function of impulse conduction is the axon. In this mode, as we have come to perceive it from studies on peripheral nerves, the nerve cell acts much like a telephone wire. The most important considerations for proper performance are that the signal should not be degraded nor information lost. To this end, the peripheral nerve axon does not operate upon the signal to transform it, and is highly resistant to environmental factors, including anaesthetics, which might degrade it. Conduction of the action potential in this type of axon has a high safety factor, and is difficult to disrupt. During clinical anaesthesia conduction in the peripheral nerve axon is relatively unimpaired; interference with the function of axons of this type therefore plays little part in general anaesthesia. The phenomenon of impulse conduction, however, may be more fragile elsewhere in the nervous system, and thus remains of interest with respect to anaesthesia.

The second function of nerve cells is to process or translate the information: to ignore a weak, possibly random or irrelevant signal, and to act on coherent patterns of impulses which 'make sense'. This translating function is carried out primarily at the synaptic structures where nerve cells contact each other, and is mediated by chemical neurotransmitters released by one cell to act on another. The synapse is thus a bicellular structure comprising the presynaptic terminal of one cell and the post-synaptic chemically sensitive membrane of another. The presynaptic terminal includes impulse-conducting membranes whose properties, as opposed to those of axonal membrane, are relatively little known; it also contains the machinery for synthesis, storage and release of neurotransmitter, as well as for reuptake of enzymatically degraded transmitter fragments. The postsynaptic membrane contains the receptor specific to the transmitter at that synapse, and has the capability of responding to the transmitter, most commonly by graded changes in electrical ion conductivity. Synaptic transmission is therefore not one process but a series of processes, including conduction.

The existence of two such separate regions of function, axonal and synaptic, prompted the question as to which was most implicated in the induction of unconsciousness by anaesthetic agents. The experiments reported in the classic paper by Larrabee and Posternak (1952) were designed to test whether in sympathetic ganglia anaesthetic agents blocked conduction or synaptic transmission first, i.e. at a lower concentration. This paper is often quoted as showing that anaesthetics block synaptic transmission at a lower concentration than conduction in the preganglionic axons, and therefore cited as evidence that synaptic transmission, rather than conduction of the action potential, is the process interfered with by anaesthetic agents. However, this is a misquotation of the findings, and moreover one which reduces the information to be gained from them. Larrabee and Posternak actually showed that different anaesthetics vary in the extent to which they selectively block synaptic transmission; and that the short-chain alcohols, often considered as models of anaesthetic agents, do not selectively block transmission at all. For these agents, conduction is blocked first. Furthermore, they found that as lipid solubility (and thus anaesthetic potency) increases with increasing chain length in the alcohols, so does the tendency to block synaptic transmission selectively. Methyl, ethyl and propyl alcohol all block conduction at lower concentrations than they block transmission. Butyl alcohol depresses both at the same concentration, while pentyl and octyl alcohol selectively depress transmission. These findings, that agents of differing lipid solubility may selectively act at different membrane sites, have important implications for the biophysical basis of anaesthesia. They suggest that the site of anaesthesia may vary with the lipid solubility of the agent. Taken together with considerations described below in the discussion of anaesthetic effects on axons, they demonstrate that the site of anaesthesia may not be exclusively axon or synapse, but both.

The rest of the chapter will consider the specific actions of anaesthetic agents on the processes of impulse conduction, transmitter release and postsynaptic response, and how these may be related to anaesthesia. Two themes will be emphasized. First, the preponderance of evidence demonstrates that selective depression of excitatory postsynaptic responses must be considered to play an important part in the central effects of most clinically useful anaesthetic agents. Second, the evidence does not permit the exclusion of other processes including depression of conduction, transmitter release and more subtle modulations of these properties as important to anaesthesia.

ANAESTHETIC ACTIONS ON AXONAL MEMBRANE

Membrane events underlying the action potential

It is beyond the scope of this chapter to treat in detail the basic neurophysiology of the nerve cell membrane. It is assumed that the reader is familiar with the relationship between active ion transport, membrane ion permeabilities and the electrical potential difference across the membrane, and with terms such as resting potential, depolarization, threshold, action potential and refractory period. These topics are covered in Chapter 15 of this text as well as in most neurophysiology textbooks. An excellent introduction is the now classic small book by Katz (1966), *Nerve, Muscle and Synapse*.

The membrane of the axon, and indeed of all excitable cells, is composed of a lipid bilayer matrix in which are embedded proteins. Some of these proteins (or shorter polypeptides) constitute channels which allow the passage of charged ions through the membrane (*Figure 5.1*). The channels of primary importance to the generation of the action potential are those which selectively pass sodium ions. The sodium channels are remarkably sparse in the membrane, their density being estimated at approximately ten channels per square micrometre (micron) of axon surface. Knowledge concerning their structure is therefore based on indirect evidence derived from studies of their function, of agents which block them, and of enzymes and toxins which selectively destroy parts of them. The sodium channels are presently considered to exist in three alternative states: resting, open and inactive (*Figure 5.1a*). In the resting state, the channels are closed and do not conduct sodium ions, but respond to depolarization of the membrane by opening. The opening corresponds to the Hodgkin—Huxley m^3h term in the equations describing the sodium current, and the channel is described in neurophysiological jargon as having both 'm' and 'h' gates open. In the open state, the channel is briefly permeable to sodium ions. The channel then enters the inactive state, in which it can neither conduct nor respond to a depolarization by opening. The 'h' or inactivation gate is said to have closed. This state corresponds to the refractory period of the nerve. Following the passage of an impulse, the channels slowly (over several milliseconds) revert to the resting state. The sodium channels in impulse-conducting membrane are therefore time- and voltage-sensitive, responding to a sudden membrane depolarization by first opening, then closing (inactivating). The production of a propagated action potential depends on a sufficient number of channels opening to conduct sodium ions (*Figure 5.1b*). An anaesthetic agent could conceivably block conduction by preventing channels from opening (blocking m gating), by altering the ability of open channels to pass sodium ions, or by favouring the inactive state (preventing the h gate from opening). The last action is now considered to be important in local anaesthetic block (Hille, 1977). In addition, any agent which chronically depolarizes the membrane will favour the inactive state and thus prevent channel opening.

The potassium channel is also active during the course of the action

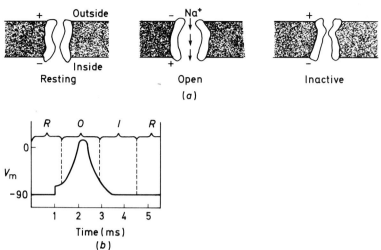

Figure 5.1
Function of the sodium channel in action potential generation.
(*a*) The three states of the sodium channel. In the resting state, the channel is not permeable to sodium ions. When the membrane potential undergoes a depolarizing change, the resting channel opens to conduct sodium ions. The increase in sodium permeability further depolarizes the membrane, as shown by the shift in the charge from inside negative to inside positive. The period of time spent in the open state is brief; channels in the depolarized membrane then enter the inactive state, in which they neither conduct sodium ions nor respond to a further depolarization by opening. The changes in channel state are represented as changes in the conformation of a protein which constitutes the channel. Although this is a reasonable model, it is not yet firmly established. (*b*) The state of a 'typical' sodium channel during various phases of the action potential. When the membrane is subjected to an abrupt depolarization (drop in V_m, membrane voltage), channels in the resting state (R) begin to open (O), further depolarizing the membrane. At the peak of the potential, the open channels begin to pass into the inactive state (I). As more and more channels inactivate, the membrane potential returns toward its previous level. While the inactive state exists, the channel will not respond by opening, and the nerve is in the refractory period. Anaesthetic molecules may block conduction either by preventing channels from opening or by changing the properties of open channels so that sodium ions cannot pass through

potential, providing the late outward current which aids in terminating the impulse and repolarizing the membrane. However, many nerves can generate action potentials, of more or less distorted shape, even when potassium channels have been completely blocked. Anaesthetic block of potassium channels alone would therefore not necessarily block conduction, but would prolong the falling phase of the action potential and depolarize the membrane by decreasing potassium conductance.

Anaesthetic actions on ion channels

Having considered what general anaesthetics might, in theory, do to sodium and potassium channels, let us consider what they in fact do. Unfortunately, here we are on stony ground, for few investigators have looked at the problem. First of all, most neurophysiologists, even those with a pharmacological bent, are at least as interested in the nature of the channels as they are in anaesthetic action. The small, structurally simple anaesthetic molecule, with its lack of well defined structure—activity relationships, holds little promise of revealing channel structure by its manner of blocking conduction. Second, there is considerable technical difficulty in working with volatile agents of limited aqueous solubility in *in vitro* preparations. This is compounded by the necessity of using the largest available axons to study ionic currents. These require exceedingly high anaesthetic concentrations for observable effects, since general anaesthetics block smaller axons more readily than larger. However, a few such experiments have been done. Trichloroethylene and halothane were found to depolarize the membrane of squid axon (Shrivastav *et al.,* 1976). In addition, trichloroethylene decreased the magnitude of the currents associated with both sodium and potassium channels. These findings are in accord with those of an earlier study, which showed that alcohols also decreased both sodium and potassium currents and depolarized the axon membrane (Armstrong and Binstock, 1964). Anaesthetics and alcohols may therefore act in part by depolarizing the membrane and thus (1) reducing the absolute magnitude of the action potential and (2) favouring the persistence of sodium channels in the inactive state. Both short- and long-chain alcohols, as well as trichloroethylene, probably also reduce the number of open conducting sodium channels by a poorly understood mechanism independent of depolarization.

A recently described property of local anaesthetics raises interesting possibilities concerning the modulation of nerve excitability by drugs. Many local anaesthetics prolong the refractory period of axons and thus produce a conduction block whose depth varies with the frequency of impulses in the nerve (Courtney, Kendig and Cohen, 1978). The basis for frequency-dependent block appears to consist in part of an effect of sodium channel state on drug-receptor affinity (Hille, 1977). Channels in the open or the inactive state bind drugs more strongly than those in the closed state. Since sodium channel state is determined by membrane potential, the latter has a very marked influence on the depth of conduction block by local anaesthetic agents. Whether sodium channel state also influences the interaction between general anaesthetics and their receptor has yet to be determined.

The role of conduction block in anaesthesia

Granted that anaesthetic agents block conduction, one must ask whether this action is relevant to anaesthesia. The report by Larrabee and Posternak

(1952), cited in the introduction to this chapter, suggested that the volatile anaesthetic agents act at synapses, and do not block conduction in the axons of presynaptic nerve cells. More recent studies have produced similar evidence in the central nervous system. Spinal cord motor neurons show depressed postsynaptic potentials in animals anaesthetized with diethyl ether and thiopentone, while the impulse in the presynaptic terminal appears unimpaired (Somjen, 1963, 1967; Somjen and Gill, 1963). Similarly, trans-synaptically evoked potentials in olfactory cortex are depressed by ether and methoxyflurane at concentrations which do not alter the compound action potential recorded from the presynaptic tract (Richards, Russell and Smaje, 1975). Also, in the hippocampus, the massed postsynaptic responses of granule cells are depressed at lower concentrations than the presynaptic compound action potential by four volatile anaesthetics: ether, halothane, methoxyflurane and trichloroethylene (Richards and White, 1975). This is certainly strong evidence that synaptic transmission is involved in anaesthesia; it is less than conclusive evidence, however, that conduction is not involved. The reasons for still considering block of conduction as possibly relevant to anaesthesia, in the face of this kind of evidence, may be summarized as follows.

(1) It is technically difficult to measure the amplitude of the conducted impulse near the nerve terminal and, thus, the extent to which the terminal is invaded by the action potential. Therefore, although the extracellularly monitored action potential does not appear to be modified at anaesthetic partial pressures in the main portion of the axon, it may be affected in the terminal segment, whose properties are much less well understood. In this regard the terminal of the axon is considered part of the synapse, since it usually cannot be measured separately; effects on the synapse then may be, in reality, effects on conduction in the presynaptic terminal.

(2) Conduction is usually studied in large diameter axons. Conduction block obeys a size principle wherein smaller diameter fibres are blocked more readily than larger. In the central nervous system there are many very small nerve fibres impossible to investigate experimentally. By size considerations alone, these would be predicted to be blocked during anaesthesia.

(3) Apart from questions of size, *per se,* conduction is strongly influenced by cellular geometry. Areas in which axon diameter changes or in which there is extensive branching may be more vulnerable to conduction block than the more usually studied uniform axon segment. Very little is known about the effects of anaesthetics on, for example, branching dendrites.

SYNAPTIC TRANSMISSION

Let us now turn to a consideration of how anaesthetics may influence events at the synapse. Of the several components of synaptic function outlined in the introduction, the discussion of anaesthetic effects will be confined to two: transmitter release at the presynaptic terminal, and the response of the postsynaptic membrane. There is little in the literature concerning the effects of volatile agents on reuptake or synthesis of transmitter. Some changes in brain transmitter levels have been reported, but their significance is unclear (Biebuyck, Dedrick and Scherer, 1975).

Release of transmitter

At synapses transmitter is constantly being released in small amounts from the presynaptic terminal. At excitatory synapses (and at the neuro-muscular junction, from which much of our understanding of transmission is derived), the constant leak of transmitter gives rise to small depolarizations of the postsynaptic membrane, called miniature synaptic potentials. The uniform height of the smallest miniatures and the size relationships between smallest and larger miniatures led to the hypothesis that the leaked transmitter is released in packets containing uniform numbers of transmitter molecules. The massive release of transmitter which occurs

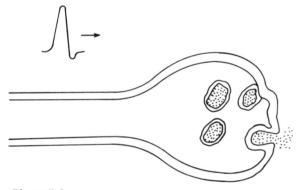

Figure 5.2
Release of transmitter from the presynaptic terminal. Transmitter molecules are contained in synaptic vesicles within the terminal. Depolarization of the terminal membrane by an arriving impulse leads to the fusion of numerous vesicles with the terminal membrane, and the release of their contents into the synaptic cleft. Anaesthetic agents may affect transmitter release either by interfering with conduction in the terminal or by altering one of the steps between depolarization and release of transmitter

at the terminal following the arrival of an action potential is triggered by depolarization of the terminal membrane. The coupling between depolarization and transmitter secretion, like the coupling between excitation and contraction in muscle, is mediated by a translocation of calcium — in this case across the presynaptic membrane. It is thought that the calcium then promotes the fusion of the vesicular membrane containing transmitter with the cell membrane of the presynaptic terminal, the transmitter molecules being extruded into the synaptic cleft by the process of exocytosis (*Figure 5.2*).

This sequence of events provides a number of points at which anaesthetic drugs might, in theory, intervene. A chronic depolarization of the nerve terminal, by reducing the amplitude of the action potential, would reduce the amount of transmitter released per impulse. Such an action would be similar to the mechanism of presynaptic inhibition. As cited above, anaesthetics may indeed depolarize nerve cell membrane. Also, any conduction-blocking effect of anaesthetics at the presynaptic terminal would inhibit transmitter release. Very little is yet known about calcium currents and specific calcium channels in presynaptic terminals, but this is presently an area of intense study. Specific effects of anaesthetics on calcium entry might be of considerable interest. Among other ways in which anaesthetics might disrupt transmitter release is the movement of vesicles toward the terminal membrane and their fusion with it. A role for microfilaments in this process has been proposed, and a disruptive effect of anaesthetics on microfilaments demonstrated (Hinckley and Telser, 1975). Interference with vesicle fusion through an effect on membrane lipids has also been proposed (Trudell, 1977).

Do volatile anaesthetic agents indeed depress transmitter release? Evidence on this is hard to collect. It is firmest for barbiturates, which have been shown in independent studies to depress the quantal transmitter content of evoked synaptic potentials (Weakly, 1969) and to reduce the amount of acetylcholine collected at cholinergic synapses (Matthews and Quilliam, 1964). For volatile agents there appear to be at least two different effects on transmitter release. Counts of miniature potential frequency suggest that both ethyl alcohol and anaesthetic agents enhance spontaneous transmitter release at the mouse phrenic nerve—diaphragm junction (Quastel, Hackett and Cooke, 1970). In this preparation the synchronous release of transmitter evoked by stimulating the nerve is depressed by ether and trichloroethanol, but not by alcohol. At the frog sartorius junction, however, methoxyflurane in low concentrations increases evoked potential amplitude by increasing the quantal content of the response (Richter, Landau and Cohen, 1977a). In this array of contradictory evidence, the most that can be said at the present time is that anaesthetic depression of synaptic transmission in the central nervous system is not inconsistent with a mechanism which includes anaesthetic inhibition of transmitter release (Richards, 1973; Richards and White, 1975).

Depression of the postsynaptic response

Here one is on firmer ground because a method is available to separate postsynaptic effects from effects on the entire synaptic chain of events. Whereas measurements of presynaptic events are difficult to perform with unequivocal results, the technique of directly applying the known or suspected transmitter to the postsynaptic membrane, combined with intracellular recording from the postsynaptic cell, allows a direct evaluation of anaesthetic effects on the postsynaptic chemically excitable membrane.

When this technique is employed, the results indicate that anaesthetic agents depress the postsynaptic response at excitatory synapses (Thesleff, 1956; Bloom, Costa and Salmoiraghi, 1965; Barker, 1975; Richter, Landau and Cohen, 1977a, b). In the arguments presented above, the conclusion has been drawn that one cannot exclude the processes of conduction or of transmitter release from participation in anaesthesia. In the case of chemically sensitive postsynaptic membrane, the conclusion is more positive. Whatever else is implicated in anaesthesia, it is highly likely that depression of the postsynaptic response occurs in the anaesthetized patient.

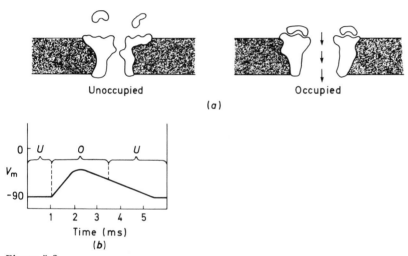

Figure 5.3
Response of the postsynaptic membrane. (*a*) When the postsynaptic receptors are unoccupied, the channel is closed. Binding of receptor to arriving transmitter opens the channels to the passage of ions, in a manner analogous to sodium channel opening in impulse-conducting membrane. In postsynaptic membrane, the stimulus is chemical rather than electrical. (*b*) At many excitatory synapses, occupancy (*O*) of unoccupied (*U*) receptors produces a depolarizing change in membrane potential (V_m). As transmitter leaves the receptor (to be broken up by specific enzymes), the channels close and the excitatory potential passively decays to the original level.
Anaesthetic agents may distort receptors so as to prevent transmitter-receptor binding. They may also, as in the case of electrically excitable membrane, prevent channel opening or block ion passage through open channels

In the consideration of how anaesthetics may diminish the postsynaptic response, the elements are much the same as in the case of conduction. The postsynaptic membrane of the most commonly studied synapses also is traversed by ion-selective pores, the 'opening' of which leads to changes in transmembrane potential due to transient increases in specific ion conductances (*Figure 5.3*). Instead of electrical depolarization, however, the key to the gates of postsynaptic ion channels is the arrival of the appropriate transmitter, thus the contrast between 'electrically excitable' and 'chemically excitable' membrane. The transmitter binds to its receptor at or near the ion channels, and in doing so opens the channel (*Figure 5.3*). Receptor-transmitter binding is the step blocked by specific transmitter antagonists such as the competitive neuromuscular blocking agents and adrenergic antagonists. The small, simple and diverse anaesthetic molecules are highly unlikely candidates for competitive binding. Instead they must block the ion permeability of postsynaptic channels either by diminishing the probability of their opening (blocking the 'gate') or by altering the ion permeability of the 'open' but blocked channel. It is also possible that they may alter the binding of transmitter to receptor in a non-competitive fashion. In addition to these possible mechanisms, it has been proposed that anaesthetics may depress the response by increasing the rate of decay of the postsynaptic current (Gage and Hamill, 1975).

Temporal modulation of synaptic efficacy

Every anaesthetist is familiar with the properties of fatigue, facilitation and post-tetanic potentiation as they are observed at the neuromuscular junction. The same properties are important at central synapses, only more so. At the neuromuscular junction they are, as normally observed in the clinical situation, artefacts of junctional block or of neuromuscular disease. In the central nervous system they are important elements of normal information coding. Indeed, many synapses will not transmit effectively until several impulses have arrived, each generating a larger postsynaptic potential than the one before it; others will respond with large potentials to the first few impulses, but with progressively diminishing ones to succeeding impulses (*Figure 5.4*). The mechanism of these short-term changes in synaptic efficacy is presynaptic; in the case of fatigue, it is due to depletion of 'available' transmitter; facilitation and post-tetanic potentiation, on the other hand, are due to poorly understood processes collectively called transmitter mobilization.

Little research has been undertaken to explore the possibility that anaesthetics might depress facilitation. However, a recent report suggests that anaesthetics may shorten the time course of post-tetanic potentiation, limiting the 'memory' of the synapse for preceding activity (Woodson *et al.*, 1976). The significance of this effect has yet to be evaluated, but it is an intriguing demonstration that not all the effects of anaesthetics can be revealed by the study of responses to single stimuli. Alterations in the pattern of impulses at a synapse are conceivably more relevant to anaesthesia than complete block of synaptic transmission.

Selectivity for specific types of synapse

The list of compounds which serve as chemical neurotransmitters is long and still growing; its most spectacular new additions are the endorphins and enkephalins, polypeptides occurring in mammalian brain, with pro-

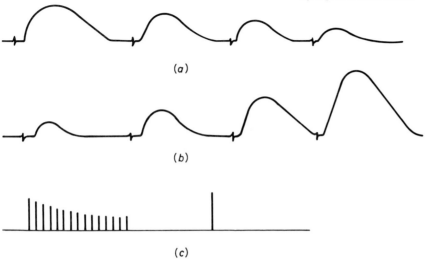

(a)

(b)

(c)

Figure 5.4
Temporal modulation of synaptic efficacy. (*a*) Excitatory postsynaptic potentials demonstrating fatigue. The first stimulus evokes a
relatively large response, the size of which diminishes with subsequent
stimuli. (*b*) Responses of a synapse where facilitation is prominent.
The first evoked synaptic potential is small, while subsequent ones
are markedly enhanced. Synapses differ in the extent to which
facilitation is present. (*c*) Post-tetanic potentiation. A series of
stimuli evokes a progressively diminishing response. After a pause,
a subsequent stimulus evokes a response larger than the first in the
train. The specific effects of anaesthetics on these changes with use
over time have been relatively little studied

perties similar to those of opiate narcotics. The oldest identified transmitter
on the list is, of course, acetylcholine. In between are a number of compounds more or less firmly established as transmitters: catecholamines
(adrenaline, noradrenaline, dopamine); indoleamines (serotonin); amino
acids (glycine, glutamine, γ-amino butyric acid (GABA)) and purines.

Postsynaptic responses may also be diverse, but the types best explored
are conductance increases to specific ions. An excitatory response of this
sort consists of an increase in membrane permeability to sodium and to
potassium, which depolarizes the postsynaptic membrane and thus brings
the postsynaptic cell nearer to the threshold for action potential initiation.
The best-known example is the neuromuscular junction, described in
Chapter 15. Transmitters known to produce this response at many sites
in the central nervous system are acetylcholine and glutamine. A different
specific conductance increase accounts for a common type of inhibition:
increases in permeability to potassium and chloride clamp the membrane
near the potassium equilibrium potential, far from threshold. These
inhibitory responses thus prevent the depolarization due to excitatory
inputs from initiating an action potential. Transmitters known to be
associated with inhibition of this type include glycine and GABA.

With respect to the role of specific kinds of synaptic transmission in
anaesthesia, there is now evidence in two invertebrate systems that volatile

depressant anaesthetic agents may preferentially depress excitatory transmission as opposed to inhibitory (Barker, 1975; Richter, Landau and Cohen, 1977b).

Of other types of synaptic response, a theory has been proposed that anaesthetics might plausibly oppose the potassium conductance decrease thought to be responsible for excitatory responses at some muscarinic cholinergic synapses (Krnjevic, 1975). Other forms of postsynaptic response have been less clearly defined. A mechanism involving modulation of active ion transport rather than ionic permeability changes has been proposed as the basis for inhibition at some adrenergic synapses (Siggins, Hoffer and Bloom, 1969). Anaesthetic agents, however, have been shown to exert no effects on the response of caudate neurons to iontophoresis of noradrenaline or dopamine (Bloom, Costa and Salmoiraghi, 1965).

For the sake of completeness, it is necessary to include a mention of presynaptic inhibition — the type of inhibition mediated by a synaptic connection between one neuron and the presynaptic terminal of a second. The ending on the presynaptic terminal depolarizes it and thus decreases the transmitter released from it to the third, postsynaptic, neuron. This is an important means of selective inhibition in the spinal cord. Barbiturates significantly enhance it (Larson and Major, 1970); there is evidence that nitrous oxide may do so as well (Chin, Crankshaw and Kendig, 1974). However, evidence for other inhalation agents is lacking.

The discovery of endorphins and enkephalins as endogenous regulators of pain perception has enormous implications for the future of anaesthesia. Although these are not yet clearly defined, it seems reasonable to propose that some of the analgesic properties of anaesthetics may be due to interactions with the endorphin system. That these interactions contribute to anaesthesia is strongly suggested by the demonstration that naloxone, a competitive inhibitor of endorphin binding, increases the responses to painful stimuli in rats anaesthetized with cyclopropane, halothane or enflurane (Finck, Ngai and Berkowitz, 1977). The implication of this finding is that anaesthetic agents may act to release endorphins.

The evidence concerning the specific effects of anaesthetics on synaptic transmission may be summarized as follows. Inhalation anaesthetics depress the postsynaptic depolarization at excitatory synapses. The sensitivity of inhibitory transmission to anaesthetics appears to be much less than that of excitatory. Depolarizing conductance changes at postsynaptic membranes therefore appear to be necessary entrants on the list of neuronal functions which are most probably altered during anaesthesia.

SELECTIVITY FOR CELLS ASSOCIATED WITH PARTICULAR FUNCTIONS: UNCONSCIOUSNESS, ANALGESIA, AMNESIA

Unconsciousness: reticular formation versus cortical neurons

The early finding that cortical evoked responses mediated through the reticular formation were depressed at lower anaesthetic concentrations than those evoked directly led to the long-held concept that depression of reticular formation might be the central action of anaesthetic agents basic to the production of unconsciousness (French, Verzeano and Magoun, 1953). This was an attractive concept in light of the then newly discovered relationship between reticular formation and consciousness. However, single-cell studies of cortical neurons by many investigators have repeatedly demonstrated that their responsiveness is directly modified at anaesthetic levels. Moreover, comparisons between cortical and reticular formation spontaneous activity have shown that effects of halothane on the cortex may be detected at lower concentrations than changes in reticular formation activity (Hosick *et al.,* 1971). The difficulty of systematic single-cell studies in reticular formation is a stumbling block to detailed comparisons of sensitivity between these two structures, both of undoubted importance to the conscious state. However, for the present it seems likely that the activity and responsiveness of cortical neurons are directly altered during anaesthesia, in addition to whatever indirect effects are mediated *via* the reticular formation.

A difference in sensitivity of synaptic transmission to anaesthetics between different central nervous system areas has been suggested by recent studies. Monosynaptic transmission in the cuneate nucleus appears to be depressed relatively slightly by anaesthetic agents, whereas transmission through the ventrobasal thalamic complex appears to be much more sensitive (Angel, 1977). The basis for such differences in sensitivity is not known with certainty. A high safety factor for transmission in the cuneate, similar to that at the neuromuscular junction, may account for its apparent stability during anaesthesia. 'High safety factor' corresponds to the number of postsynaptic receptors, and the amount of acetylcholine normally released, being much higher than the minimal requirements for successful transmission. Under these conditions, even a significant impairment of postsynaptic response will not result in failure to generate an action potential in the postsynaptic neuron.

Analgesia

Kitahata (1975) has demonstrated that cells in cat spinal cord laminae known to be related to transmission of nociceptive stimuli are more sensitive to anaesthetic agents than non-nociceptive cells. These findings are relevant not only to the analgesic properties of anaesthetics; it is also proposed that by reducing noxious stimulating input to the brain, depressant effects on the pain pathways may reduce anaesthetic requirement.

Amnesia

A significant retrograde amnesia follows exposure to anaesthetics at subanaesthetic doses. The sensitivity to anaesthetics of neurons in the hippocampus, an area of the central nervous system thought to be important in the consolidation of memory traces, has been suggested to be relevant to anaesthetic-related amnesia (Richards and White, 1975).

CONVULSANT–ANTICONVULSANT PROPERTIES OF ANAESTHETICS

It has long been a puzzle why some halogenated hydrocarbons are anaesthetics and others are convulsants. An example of the latter is hexafluorodiethyl ether (Indoklon), an agent used in convulsant therapy for depression. A commonly proposed explanation for convulsant responses to drugs has been that they may selectively depress inhibitory synaptic transmission. Such a selective action has now been satisfactorily demonstrated in the case of anaesthetic and convulsant inhalation agents. Whereas anaesthetic agents such as methoxyflurane depress postsynaptic responses to glutamate, an excitatory transmitter in crustaceans, hexafluorodiethyl ether does so only at higher concentrations. The opposite is true for the response to the inhibitory transmitter GABA, which is more readily depressed by hexafluorodiethyl ether than by methoxyflurane (Richter, Landau and Cohen, 1977b). These findings are consistent with earlier studies showing that anaesthetics depress excitatory, but not inhibitory, transmission in molluscan neurons (Barker, 1975).

BIOPHYSICAL CONSIDERATIONS

The above information shows a widespread effect of anaesthetic agents on events in the nerve cell membrane. How may these be related to the molecular actions of anaesthetics outlined in Chapter 3? It is widely conceded that the inhalation agents and inert gases act at a lipoid site: either hydrophobic regions of proteins or the structural lipid bilayer of the cell membrane. A connection between the first proposed site and impairment of function is easy to imagine. Effects on the lipid bilayer are intuitively less easy to relate to membrane functional changes, although the connection has been made in some experimental studies (Gage and Hamill, 1975; Traynor *et al.*, 1976; Woodson *et al.*, 1976) and a theory has been proposed to relate them (Trudell, 1977). The present discussion is confined to three phenomena which might shed light on the relationship between molecular action and cellular functional impairment: pressure–anaesthesia antagonism, tolerance and synaptic selectivity.

Pressure–anaesthesia antagonism

Pressure antagonizes anaesthesia in animals (pressure 'reversal' of anaesthesia), and anaesthetic agents antagonize the convulsant effects of high pressure. The mutual antagonism is not known with certainty to be due to a direct opposition between pressure and anaesthetic effects at an identical site. However, pressure and anaesthetics have been shown to oppose each other's effects on the fluid state of lipid bilayers (Trudell, Hubbell and Cohen, 1973), and in theory could do so on protein conformation (Eyring, Woodbury and D'Arrigo, 1973). At the cellular level the effects of pressure are as yet little known. There appears to be a limited pressure-related antagonism to anaesthetic conduction block (Spyropoulos, 1957; Kendig, Trudell and Cohen, 1975; Roth, Smith and Paton, 1976). High pressure also antagonizes local anaesthetic conduction block; local and general anaesthetics may therefore share a common pressure-sensitive site of action in the nerve cell membrane (Kendig and Cohen, 1977). Both anaesthetics and pressure, however, depress synaptic transmission. There seems to be no antagonism detectable in their effects on this process (Kendig, Trudell and Cohen, 1975; Kendig and Cohen, 1976). Thus, although at the molecular level there is a basis for a direct antagonism between pressure and anaesthetic agents, either the antagonism at the cellular level is indirect or conduction block is more relevant to anaesthesia and its reversal by pressure than synaptic transmission is.

The membrane events subject to pressure—anaesthesia antagonism are still unknown. A single study on sodium and potassium currents in the squid axon at high pressure has shown no obvious basis for antagonism in the effect of pressure alone (Henderson and Gilbert, 1975).

Tolerance and cross-tolerance

Tolerance and chronic anaesthetic exposure, followed by withdrawal, has recently been demonstrated to be similar in its behavioural manifestations to alcohol tolerance and withdrawal (Winter *et al.*, 1976). Cross-tolerance between alcohol and inhalation agents has long been suspected clinically. If cross-tolerance can be demonstrated, it will suggest a similar molecular basis for tolerance to both types of agents.

The basis for alcohol tolerance is not yet established. Recent evidence, however, has shown a decreased sensitivity to alcohol effects in nerve cell membrane lipids derived from alcohol-tolerant mice compared to lipids derived from normal controls (Chin and Goldstein, 1977a,b). The alteration responsible for tolerance may thus be a change in the lipid bilayer, perhaps a homoeostatic change in phospholipid composition so as to maintain a constant favourable membrane fluidity (Hill and Bangham, 1975). Such a concept links depressant action directly to tolerance and addiction. There is still little direct evidence for the relationship between functional changes and lipid changes in tolerance and withdrawal. However, membrane lipid fluidity has been invoked as a possible basis for alcohol-induced shortening of post-tetanic potentiation in *Aplysia* (Traynor *et al.*, 1976). This phenomenon displays tolerance in the form of decreased sensitivity to alcohol following chronic exposure.

Synaptic selectivity

The data of Larrabee and Posternak (1952) showed an increasing sensitivity of synaptic transmission to alcohol depression as chain length increased. The more lipid soluble an agent, the more readily did it block synaptic transmission. These findings were used by Mullins as a basis for the proposal that the sites involved in block of conduction and of synaptic transmission had different solubility parameters (Mullins, 1954). This hypothesis would account for selectivity among agents solely on the basis of their physical properties and those of their respective membrane sites. The same hypothesis, that hydrophobic receptor sites might have different solvent properties, might explain the findings of Richter, Landau and Cohen (1977a, b), namely that anaesthetic agents and related convulsants exert different effects on excitatory and inhibitory transmission. Although this hypothesis explains the different pharmacological characteristics of the simple small anaesthetic molecules, there is no direct evidence on the differences between, for example, axonal and postsynaptic membrane lipids, to confirm it.

CONCLUSIONS

At the present time the weight of evidence compels the consideration that the postsynaptic membrane at excitatory synapses is a crucial site with respect to anaesthesia. The evidence is strongest for the potent clinical agents of high lipid solubility and for those synapses at which a depolarizing conductance increase to sodium is the excitatory response. Membrane of this type may not be the sole important site either of anaesthesia or of the side effects peculiar to each agent. The necessity of continuing to consider other sites is based primarily on the experimental difficulty of obtaining satisfactory evidence to exclude them. Thus, it is impossible at present to weigh the relative importance to anaesthesia of conduction block or of alteration of events in presynaptic terminals, in comparison with anaesthetic blockade of the postsynaptic excitatory response. Until better evidence is forthcoming, it is necessary to consider all the many effects of anaesthetics on axon and synapse as potentially relevant to anaesthesia.

ACKNOWLEDGEMENTS

Discussions with many investigators helped to shape this review. In particular, the author would like to thank Dr Kenneth Courtney of the Stanford University Department of Anesthesia. Dr Jane Chin of the Department of Pharmacology and Dr James Trudell of the Department of Anesthesia, Stanford University, contributed many ideas concerning the effects of anaesthetics and alcohols on membrane lipids. Miss Erika Prince rendered valuable clerical assistance.

   This work was supported by Office of Naval Research and Naval Medical Research and Development Command Contract N00014-75-C-1021 and by National Institutes of Health Grants NS13108 and GM22113. Part of the work was carried out during the author's tenure of a Mellon Faculty Fellowship.

References

Angel, A. (1977). Processing of sensory information. *Progress in Neurobiology* 9, 1–122

Armstrong, C. M. and Binstock, L. (1964). The effects of several alcohols on the properties of the squid giant axon. *J. gen. Physiol.* 48, 265–277

Barker, J. L. (1975). C.N.S. depressants: effects on postsynaptic pharmacology. *Brain Res.* 92, 35–55

Biebuyck, J. F., Dedrick, D. F. and Scherer, Y. D. (1975). Brain cyclic AMP and putative transmitter amino acids during anesthesia. In *Progress in Anesthesiology.* Vol. 1, *Molecular Mechanisms of Anesthesia,* pp. 451–470. B. R. Fink (ed.). New York: Raven Press

Bloom, F. E., Costa, E. and Salmoiraghi, G. C. (1965). Anesthesia and the responsiveness of individual neurons of the caudate nucleus of the cat to acetylcholine, norepinephrine and dopamine administered by microelectrophoresis. *J. Pharmac. exp. Ther.* 150, 244–252

Chin, J. H. and Goldstein, D. B. (1977a). Effects of low concentrations of ethanol on the fluidity of spin-labeled erythrocyte and brain membranes. *Molec. Pharmac.* 13, 435–441

Chin, J. H. and Goldstein, D. B. (1977b). Drug tolerance in biomembranes: a spin label study of the effects of ethanol. *Science* 196, 684–685

Chin, J. H., Crankshaw, D. P. and Kendig, J. J. (1974). Changes in the dorsal root potential with diazepam and with the analgesics aspirin, nitrous oxide, morphine and meperidine. *Neuropharmacology* 13, 305–315

Courtney, K. R., Kendig, J. J. and Cohen, E. N. (1978). Frequency-dependent conduction block: the role of nerve impulse pattern in local anesthetic potency. *Anesthesiology* 48, 111–117

Eyring, H., Woodbury, J. W. and D'Arrigo, J. S. (1973). A molecular mechanism of general anesthesia. *Anesthesiology* 38, 415–424

Finck, A. D., Ngai, S. A. and Berkowitz, B. A. (1977). Antagonism of general anesthesia by naloxone in the rat. *Anesthesiology* 46, 241–245

French, J. D., Verzeano, M. and Magoun, H. W. (1953). A neural basis of the anesthetic state. *Archs Neurol. Psychiat.* 69, 519–529

Gage, P. W. and Hamill, O. (1975). General anesthetics: synaptic depression consistent with increased membrane fluidity. *Neurosci. Letters* 1, 61

Henderson, J. V. and Gilbert, D. L. (1975). Slowing of ionic currents in the voltage-clamped squid axon by helium pressure. *Nature, Lond.* 258, 351–352

Hill, M. W. and Bangham, A. D. (1975). General depressant drug dependency: a biophysical hypothesis. *Adv. exp. Med. Biol.* 59, 1–9

Hille, B. (1977). Local anesthetics: hydrophilic and hydrophobic pathways for the drug-receptor interaction. *J. gen. Physiol.* 69, 497–515

Hinckley, R. E. and Telser, A. G. (1975). The effects of halothane on microfilamentous systems in cultured neuroblastoma cells. In *Progress in Anesthesiology.* Vol. 1, *Molecular Mechanisms of Anesthesia,* pp. 103–118. B. R. Fink (ed.). New York: Raven Press

Hosick, E. C., Clark, D. L., Adam, N. and Rosner, B. S. (1971). Neurophysiological effects of different anesthetics in conscious man. *J. appl. Physiol.* 31, 892–898

Katz, B. (1966). *Nerve, Muscle and Synapse* New York: McGraw-Hill

Kendig, J. J. and Cohen, E. N. (1976). Neuromuscular function at hyperbaric pressures: pressure-anesthetic interactions. *Am. J. Physiol.* 230, 1244–1249

Kendig, J. J. and Cohen, E. N. (1977). Pressure antagonism to conduction block by anesthetic agents. *Anesthesiology* 47, 6–10

Kendig, J. J., Trudell, J. R. and Cohen, E. N. (1975). Effects of pressure and anesthetics on conduction and synaptic transmission. *J. Pharmac. exp. Ther.* 195, 216–224

Kitahata, L. M. (1975). Modes and sites of 'analgesic' action of anesthetics on the spinal cord. *Int. Anesthesiol. Clins* 13, 149–170

Krnjevic, K. (1975). Is general anesthesia induced by neuronal asphyxia? In *Progress in Anesthesiology.* Vol. 1, *Molecular Mechanisms of Anesthesia,* pp. 93–101. B. R. Fink (ed.). New York: Raven Press

Larrabee, M. G. and Posternak, J. M. (1952). Selective action of anesthetics on synapses and axons in mammalian sympathetic ganglia. *J. Neurophysiol.* 15, 91–114

Larson, M. D. and Major, M. A. (1970). The effect of hexobarbital on the duration of the recurrent IPSP in cat motor neurons. *Brain Res.* 21, 309–311

Matthews, E. K. and Quilliam, J. P. (1964). Effects of central depressant drugs upon acetylcholine release. *Br. J. Pharmac.* 22, 415–440

Mullins, L. J. (1954). Some physical mechanisms in narcosis. *Chem. Rev.* 54, 289–323

Quastel, D. M. J., Hackett, J. T. and Cooke, J. D. (1970). Calcium: is it necessary for transmitter secretion? *Science* 172, 1034–1036

Richards, C. D. (1973). On the mechanism of halothane anaesthesia. *J. Physiol., Lond.* 233, 439–456

Richards, C. D. and White, A. E. (1975). The actions of volatile anaesthetics on synaptic transmission in the dentate gyrus. *J. Physiol., Lond.* 252, 241–257

Richards, C. D., Russell, W. J. and Smaje, J. C. (1975). The action of ether and methoxyflurane on synaptic transmission in isolated preparations of the mammalian cortex. *J. Physiol., Lond.* 248, 121–142

Richter, J., Landau, E. M. and Cohen, S. (1977a). The action of volatile anesthetics and convulsants on synaptic transmission: a unified concept. *Molec. Pharmac.* 13, 548–559

Richter, J., Landau, E. M. and Cohen, S. (1977b). Anaesthetic and convulsant ethers act on different sites at the crab neuromuscular junction *in vitro. Nature., Lond.* 266, 70–71

Roth, S. H., Smith, R. A. and Paton, W. D. M. (1976). Pressure antagonism of anaesthetic-induced conduction failure in frog peripheral nerve. *Br. J. Anaesth.* 48, 621–628

Shrivastav, B. B., Narahashi, T., Kitz, R. J. and Roberts, J. D. (1976). Mode of action of trichloroethylene on squid axon membranes. *J. Pharmac. exp. Ther.* 199, 179–188

Siggins, G. R., Hoffer, B. J. and Bloom, F. E. (1969). Cyclic adenosine monophosphate: possible mediator for norepinephrine effects on cerebral Purkinje cells. *Science* 175, 720

Somjen, G. G. (1963). Effects of ether and thiopental on spinal presynaptic terminals. *J. Pharmac. exp. Ther.* 140, 396–402

Somjen, G. G. (1967). Effects of anesthetics on spinal cord of mammals. *Anesthesiology* 28, 135–143

Somjen, G. G. and Gill, M. (1963). The mechanism of the blockade of synaptic transmission in the mammalian spinal cord by diethyl ether and by thiopental. *J. Pharmac. exp. Ther.* 140, 19–30

Spyropoulos, C. S. (1957). The effects of hydrostatic pressure upon the normal and narcotized nerve. *J. gen. Physiol.* 40, 849–857

Thesleff, S. (1956). The effect of anesthetic agents on skeletal muscle membrane. *Acta physiol. scand.* 37, 335–349

Traynor, M. E., Woodson, P. B. J., Schlapfer, W. T. and Barondes, S. H. (1976). Sustained tolerance to a specific effect of ethanol on post-tetanic potentiation in *Aplysia. Science* 193, 510–511

Trudell, J. R. (1977). A unitary theory of anesthesia based on lateral phase separations in nerve membranes. *Anesthesiology* 46, 5–10

Trudell, J. R., Hubbell, W. L. and Cohen, E. N. (1973). Pressure reversal of inhalation anesthetic induced disorder in spin-labelled phospholipid vesicles. *Biochim. biophys. Acta* 291, 328–334

Weakly, J. N. (1969). Effect of barbiturates on 'quantal' synaptic transmission in spinal motor neurons. *J. Physiol., Lond.* 204, 63–77

Winter, P. M., Smith, R. A., Smith, M. and Eger, E. I. (1976). Tolerance to and dependence on some gaseous anesthetics. American Society of Anesthesiologists Annual Meeting, October 9–13, 1976. *Abstracts* pp. 315–316

Woodson, P. B. J., Traynor, M. E., Schlapfer, W. T. and Barondes, S. H. (1976). Increase of membrane fluidity implicated in acceleration of decay of post-tetanic potentiation by alcohols. *Nature, Lond.* 260, 797–799

6 Effect of anaesthetics on nervous pathways
A. Angel

It is better to light one small candle than
to curse the darkness.   *Confucius*

The effect of general anaesthetic agents is to disrupt the normal function
of many body systems. This may produce, for example, (1) a decrease
(partial or total) of skeletomotor responses to overtly or potentially
noxious stimuli, coupled with the absence of volitional movement and
muscle flaccidity; (2) a change in level of consciousness coupled with
obvious alterations in spontaneous electrocortical activity; and (3) a
complete loss of all sensory experience. Therefore, to explain the anaesthetic state one must either (1) propose a variety of different actions on
different systems, or (2) suggest that one system is affected which, by its
inter-relations with other systems, causes a general effect, or (3) assume
naively that general anaesthetic agents non-specifically decrease the
excitability of all nervous tissue. It is the second of these views which I
wish to expand in this chapter, concerning the over-all relations and
influences of the brain stem reticular formation and its thalamic extensions.

The implication that this structure serves a role in the co-ordination of
sensory and motor systems related to the level of arousal of an animal was
given by the researches of Magoun and his various collaborators. They
showed that the brain stem reticular formation could control the excitability of spinal motoneurons (Magoun and Rhines, 1946; Rhines and
Magoun, 1946), and that high frequency electrical stimulation of any part
of the reticular system, in brain stem and thalamus, could produce electrocortical arousal (Moruzzi and Magoun, 1949). These two observations
were brought together by Euler and Söderberg (1956, 1957) and Hongo,
Kubota and Shimazu (1963), who showed that during conditions of slow-
frequency high-voltage electrocortical activity, either induced by warming
the hypothalamus or occurring spontaneously, the peripheral drive via
muscle spindles to spinal motoneurons was decreased. These authors
proposed the existence of a neural system causing drowsiness coupled
with a diminution in muscle tone.

This chapter will therefore be devoted to the anatomy and physiology of the reticular system and its inter-relations with the sensory and motor systems. The original designation of the reticular formation as an area of diffuse cellular aggregation criss-crossed by a network of fibres has lost its meaning with the demonstration by Olszewski (1954) and Brodal (1957) that it consists of a complex of several fairly discrete cellular regions. Therefore, to remove the mental image of an arrow-bearing sausage placed in the brain, as is usually indicated in textbooks of physiology, it will be referred to as the sensorimotor modulation system.

ANATOMY OF THE SENSORIMOTOR MODULATION SYSTEM

Ascending system

The anatomical arrangement of this system is shown simplified in *Figure 6.1*. The separation of the medulla and pons into ascending and descending portions is based upon areas of maximal projection, and the indicated

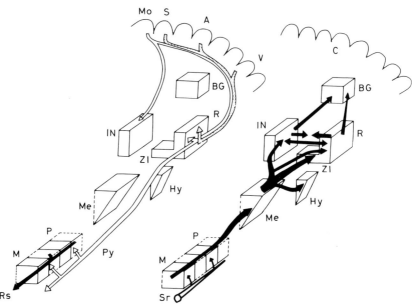

Figure 6.1
Summary diagrams for the structure of the ascending (right-hand side) and descending (left-hand side) components of the sensori-motor modulation system. Each diagram represents the right half of the brain and indicates areas of maximum termination and projection. Mo, motor cortex; S, somatosensory cortex; A, auditory cortex; V, visual cortex; C, cerebral cortex; BG, basal ganglia; R, thalamic reticular nucleus; IN, intralaminar nuclei; ZI, zona incerta; Hy, hypothalamus; Me, mesencephalon; P, pons; M, medulla; Py, pyramidal tract; Rs, reticulospinal tract; Sr, spinoreticular tract. In all cases the arrows represent both projection to and termination within the structure to which they point. (For further details, see text)

connections being to one side of the brain is again one of predominance (see Brodal, 1957, pp. 20, 26). The sensory input to the system is via the spinoreticular tract which ascends in the anterolateral white matter of the spinal cord. This tract terminates in medial 'reticular' nuclei in the caudal medulla and caudal pons. The cells in these two regions project upwards to the mesencephalon, with very few axons from the cells in the caudal part of the medulla ascending beyond the medulla (Nauta and Kuypers, 1958). Axons from cells in the caudal part of the pons join with those from cells in the mesencephalon to project into thalamic and subthalamic nuclei. At the caudal border of the ventral thalamus this projection divides into a main component, terminating in subthalamic structures (zona incerta, hypothalamus and the ventral part of the nucleus reticularis thalami); and a lesser but still considerable component, to the intralaminar nuclei and the dorsal and anterior parts of the nucleus reticularis thalami (Nauta and Kuypers, 1958; Fairén, 1973; Edwards and de Olmos, 1976). The intralaminar nuclei and nucleus reticularis thalami project mainly to the basal ganglia, the specific thalamic relay nuclei (tactile, visual, auditory and motor thalamic relay nuclei) and show reciprocal connections with each other (Cowan and Powell, 1955; Scheibel and Scheibel, 1958, 1966a, b; Minderhoud, 1971; Jones and Leavitt, 1974). There is a suggestion that the intralaminar nuclei are concerned with motor mechanisms (e.g. their projection to the caudate nucleus and thalamic cerebellocortical relay nuclei) whereas the nucleus reticularis thalami is concerned with sensory mechanisms (e.g. its projection into the sensory relay nuclei and the organized projection it receives from the various sensory cortical receiving areas).

Descending system

The motor cortex projects to the intralaminar nuclei, nucleus reticularis thalami and, via collaterals from the pyramidal tract, into the rostral part of the medial pons and rostral part of the medial medulla. Cells in these last two locations send long descending axons via the reticulospinal tract to influence both α and fusimotor spinal motoneurons. In contrast to other parts of the system, the nucleus reticularis thalami receives a well organized projection from all the primary sensory cortical areas. Noteworthy is the lack of a cortical projection to the mesencephalic portion of the modulatory system (Brodal, 1957; Rossi and Zanchetti, 1957).

General

The wealth of afferent and efferent connectivity would seem to indicate a correlational activity for this system. Reference to any textbook of physiology reveals the close anatomical localization for those brain stem areas involved in respiratory, circulatory and visceral control with the ascending and descending components of the sensorimotor modulation system. Whether this represents an intermingling of functionally dissimilar neurons or separate groups of neurons with reciprocal connections is not clear. Teleologically the latter would be preferable, but in any case the system considered as a whole could participate in a co-ordinated viscero-skeletomotor act of obvious advantage in 'arousing' reactions; for example, waking a person and changing him from a horizontal to a vertical posture without concomitant circulatory changes would not be desirable.

Lastly there are two other systems implicated in the modulation of brain and behavioural activity. These are the midline raphe nuclei (Taber, Brodal and Walberg, 1960) and the locus coeruleus (Swanson, 1976), both with a predominantly longitudinal efferent projection. The raphe nuclei receive afferents from the spinal cord and cerebral cortex and give rise to long descending and long ascending efferents (Brodal, Taber and Walberg, 1960; Brodal, Walberg and Taber, 1960). Raphe neurons contain 5-hydroxytryptamine and project, via the median forebrain bundle, to ipsilateral forebrain structures and the hypothalamus (Dahlstrom and Fuxe, 1964; Andén *et al.*, 1966; Ungerstedt, 1971). This system has been implicated in the sleep/waking cycle (Jouvet, 1967).

The noradrenergic locus coeruleus projects, also via the median forebrain bundle, to ipsilateral hypothalamic, limbic forebrain structures and to the neocortex (Dahlstrom and Fuxe, 1964; Andén *et al.*, 1966; Ungerstedt, 1971). These paired pontine nuclei have a possible role to play in the genesis of the paradoxical phase of sleep (REM sleep; see Jouvet, 1967).

PHYSIOLOGY OF THE SENSORIMOTOR MODULATION SYSTEM

Research into the physiology of the modulatory system has, in the main, been concerned with two techniques: ablation and stimulation. Both of these are crude and make no distinction between destruction or stimulation of cells, fibres terminating or fibres merely passing through the lesion or stimulation site. What is possibly more invidious is the common practice of concentrating exclusively on one system, the behaviour of which such experiments alter, or the use of preparations with total transections of the neuraxis and overinterpreting the results obtained from such animals to refer to the whole intact animal. Another confusing aspect is the interpretation of an electrocortical arousal as being synonymous with 'awakening'. Electrocortical arousal and behavioural arousal (awakening) are two different, though often inter-related, phenomena — the former under the control of the ascending modulatory system, the latter under hypothalamic control (see Feldman and Waller, 1962). Dissociation between electrocortical and behavioural activity can easily be demonstrated, either after atropine when an animal can be behaviourally awake but electrocortically asleep (Wikler, 1952; Bradley and Elkes, 1957) or electrocortically awake but behaviourally deeply asleep seen in the paradoxical phase of sleep (REM sleep; Jouvet, 1967).

Role of level of consciousness

The initial observation which implicated the modulatory system in determining the level of consciousness was that of Moruzzi and Magoun (1949),
that high frequency stimulation (50–300 Hz) anywhere within the system
gave an electrocortical desynchronization (i.e. a change from high-voltage
low-frequency to low-voltage higher frequency activity; see, for example,
Figure 6.2). This was followed by the observations that stimulation

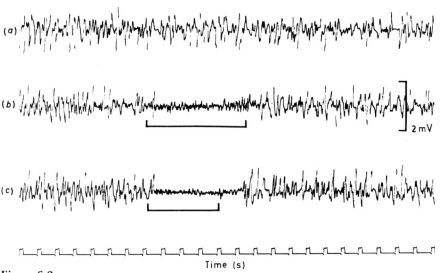

Time (s)

Figure 6.2
The electrocortical activity recorded from the primary sensory
cortical receiving area for the right forepaw in a rat surgically
anaesthetized with urethane. (*a*) Spontaneous activity. (*b*) The
effect of stimulating (indicated by the horizontal bar) within the
medullary compartment of the sensorimotor modulation system,
on the same side as the cortex, via a glass macroelectrode (tip
diameter, 80 μm; stimulus, 10 V; 0.5 ms pulse duration, 50 pulses
per second). (*c*) The effect of stimulating the skin at the right wrist
with potentially noxious electrical stimulation (100 V; 0.5 ms
pulses, 50 per second)

within the system could mimic behavioural arousal (Segundo, Arano-Iniguez
and French, 1955) and that lesions within the modulatory system — sparing
the direct sensory pathways — led to an inability of sensory stimulation to
alter electrocortical activity and also produced, postoperatively, a comatose
state (French and Magoun, 1952). This last was not prolonged if the
posterior hypothalamus was not involved in the lesion (Feldman and
Waller, 1962). These observations led to the postulate that the level of
consciousness was attributable to the level of activity within the system
(Moruzzi, 1964). That this view was too simplistic has been pointed out
repeatedly.
    First, Moruzzi and Magoun (1949) themselves showed that low frequency
stimulation of thalamic structures gave electrocortical patterns similar in

many respects to synchronized activity but that high frequency stimulation at the same site gave electrocortical desynchronization. Second, the work of Hess (1954) showed that behavioural sleep could occur as a result of thalamic stimulation. Third, the possible existence of structures in the lower brain stem concerned with the genesis of synchronized electrocortical activity was demonstrated: a complete transection of the neuraxis just rostral to the trigeminal nerve (the mid-pontine pretrigeminal preparation) in the cat produced an animal in which the time the cortex spent in desynchronized activity was almost twice that seen in the intact animal (Batini *et al.*, 1959; Cordeau and Mancia, 1959), implying the existence of a caudally located synchronizing structure. This was also implied by the observation of Magni *et al.* (1959) that, in *encéphale isolé* cats with internal carotid and intervertebral arterial communications ligated, intra-carotid injection of thiopentone (to midbrain, thalamus, forebrain and anterior cerebellum) gave electrocortical synchronization, whereas intra-vertebral arterial injection (to medulla, pons and posterior cerebellum) gave electrocortical desynchronization. Fourth, stimulation in the region of the solitary tract (Magnes, Moruzzi and Pompeiano, 1961) and in the pontine component of the system (Frederickson and Hobson, 1970; Monti, 1970) could cause electrocortical synchronization. Fifth, depletion of central nervous levels of 5-hydroxytryptamine can lead to insomnia, implying a sleep-generating role for the midline raphe nuclei (Jouvet, 1967). Sixth, at all levels of the modulatory system, three types of cell can be distinguished according to their level of spontaneous (i.e. without intentional stimulation) activity (see Angel, 1977c).

Figure 6.3
The change in pattern of the two major types of cell found in the nucleus reticularis thalami of the rat surgically anaesthetized with urethane when the electrocorticogram (ECoG) shows a spontaneous change in activity pattern from low-voltage high-frequency (DES) to high-voltage low-frequency (SYN). The graphs on the left are plots of each interimpulse interval (Int.) of the discharge of a single cell (ordinate) versus its succeeding interimpulse interval (abscissa) on a log scale. The top two are from a cell which increased its discharge frequency when the ECoG passed from a desynchronized (DES) to a synchronized (SYN) activity pattern; and the bottom two from the other type of cell which decreased its discharge frequency when the ECoG passed from DES to SYN. The graphs on the right show the number of impulses (ordinate) versus the log interimpulse interval (abscissa). A completely steady discharge would be represented as a spot (left-hand graphs) or a single vertical line (right-hand graphs). Thus the cellular discharges represented here show reciprocal changes from an orderly distribution of interimpulse intervals to a dis-orderly one. That at the top represents the type of cell firing steadily during SYN and with bursts of impulses at high frequency, followed by periods of silence with interspersed low-frequency steady discharge during DES. That at the bottom represents a steady discharge during DES and a pattern of steady discharge interspersed with periods of silence terminated with a burst of two to three impulses at high frequency, followed by a period of silence during SYN. (Angel, unpublished records)

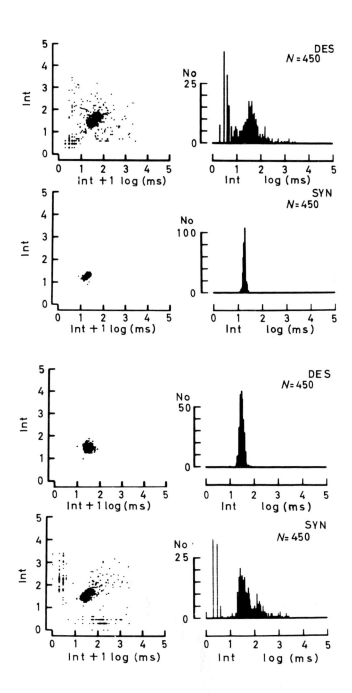

(1) Cells with a low irregular frequency of discharge, including those cells which show a pattern of high frequency activity with intervening periods of silence. This type of cell has been shown, with intracellular techniques, to discharge as a result of the summation of excitatory and inhibitory postsynaptic events (Limanskii, 1962; 1963; 1965; Segundo, Takenaka and Encabo, 1967; Waszak, 1974).

(2) Cells with a higher regular frequency of discharge showing, intracellularly, an increasing depolarization similar to that seen in the pacemaker potentials of cardiac tissue (Limanskii, 1965); Segundo, Takenaka and Encabo, 1967).

(3) Cells with no spontaneous activity, with an intracellular picture of subthreshold synaptic noise (Limanskii, 1963; Magni and Willis, 1964; Segundo, Takenaka and Encabo, 1967).

That the first two types of cell are functionally distinct is shown by the fact that, when isolated from the same compartment of the system, they show reciprocal changes in discharge frequency and pattern to various perturbations (see Angel, 1977b, c) (*Figure 6.3*). Seventh, in addition to the reciprocal activity of cells within one compartment there is also the possibility of antagonistic behaviour between different cell groups (see Hobson *et al.*, 1974; Hobson, McCarley and Wyzinski, 1975; Pompeiano and Hoshino, 1976).

Thus with both postulated synchronizing and desynchronizing components of the modulating system and two cell types showing reciprocal frequency changes within, and possibly between, compartments it is better to postulate that the level of consciousness is due *to a balance in synchronizing and desynchronizing activities within the system.*

That the system is undoubtedly organized to promote a change in level of behavioural and electrocortical arousal is shown by the response of its cells to sensory stimuli. For example, the cells show very large receptive fields to stimulation of the integument compared with those in the specific centripetal pathways (*Figure 6.4*). For the caudal medullary component of the system, Bowsher (1970) found that, for a population of isolated cells, 77% responded to stimulation of all four appendages, 5% to three, 15% to two and only 3% to one. They respond with longer latencies and much greater scatter in individual response latencies than do cells in the specific pathways. This is illustrated in *Figure 6.4*, which compares a cell from the cuneate nucleus with one some 300 μm distant in the nucleus reticularis ventralis. This behaviour can probably be accounted for in the possibly slower rise time of the excitatory postsynaptic potential (EPSP) when the postsynaptic current has to be integrated over a long dendrite with synaptic terminations remote from the cell soma (see Rall, 1967; Burke, 1967). Reticular cells have long dendrites with diffuse afferent synaptic termination compared with the shorter dendritic arborization and dense afferent synaptic terminations in the dorsal column nuclei. Therefore the longer latency will be given by the interpolation of a cell in the spinal cord between the reticular cell and the receptor as well as a slower EPSP rise time and thus time to depolarize to threshold, and

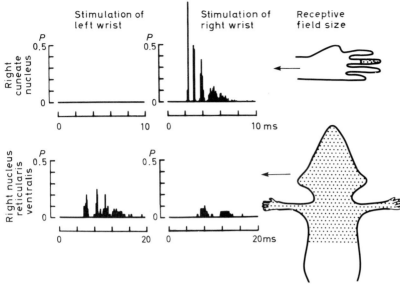

Figure 6.4
The difference in receptive field sizes (right-hand diagrams) and
cellular responsiveness (graphs) of a cell located in the right cuneate
nucleus (upper line) and another located some 300 μm deeper within
the nucleus reticularis ventralis (lower line) from a rat surgically
anaesthetized with urethane (1.25 g·kg^{-1}). Each graph represents
the responsiveness of the cell to 100 consecutive electrical stimuli
applied to the left wrist (left-hand graphs) or right wrist (right-hand
graphs). The graphs are expressed as probability (P) of response
(ordinate: with unit probability defined as 100 impulses to 100
consecutive stimuli) versus latency of response (ordinate). The
cuneate cell responded with a train of four to five impulses to
stimulation of the right wrist; and the reticular cell with four
impulses to stimulation of the left wrist and two to stimulation of
the right. Note the doubled time scale for the reticular cell. (Angel,
unpublished records)

the latter also will give a longer interspike interval if the cell is repeatedly
bombarded by a necessarily more temporally dispersed input. The relative
remoteness of the input and the diffuse nature of the terminations will
thus confer upon a reticular cell a lower degree of synaptic security (i.e.
ability of the input to discharge the cell) than for cells in the direct
pathways. It is less easy to explain the inability of reticular cells to follow
relatively low frequency (2—5 per second) iterative peripheral stimuli,
especially when a reticular cell ceases to follow stimuli along one channel
but immediately responds to stimuli along a new channel (see Angel,
1977c).

The type of sensory stimulus most often effective in exciting cells in
the ascending part of the modulatory system is overtly or potentially
noxious — i.e. pinching, cutting or heating the skin above 45°C. That this
is a response to an 'arousing' stimulus rather than any implied function of
the system in pain perception is the total lack of spatial resolution for
noxious stimuli shown by cells in the system (see Angel, 1977c). In

agreement with the diverse array of inputs to the system, the cells behaviourally display heterosensory convergence (i.e. are discharged by different sensory modalities). For cells in the caudal medulla, Bowsher (1970) showed that 47% responded only to somatic stimulation, 26% to somatic and auditory stimulation, 7.5% to somatic plus visual stimulation and 19.5% to all three.

Coupled with the obvious alterations in electrocortical activity consequent upon the administration of anaesthetic agents, both the responses of cells within the system and the electrocortical desynchronization given by electrical stimulation at sites in the system are also affected. The difficulty of obtaining an electrocortical arousal with electrical stimulation of the modulatory system during barbiturate anaesthesia was remarked upon by Moruzzi and Magoun (1949). Suppression of the ascending activation was shown to be dependent upon anaesthetic dose in the cat

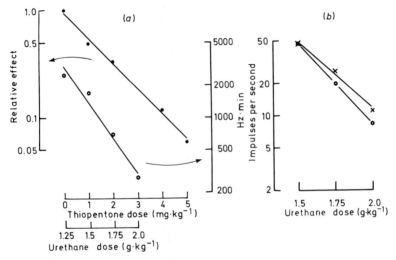

Figure 6.5
(a) The effect of intravenous pentobarbitone (upper abscissa) on electrocortical arousal in the feline *encéphale isolé* preparation. Each dot represents the relative effect (left-hand ordinate) of the electrical stimulation within the 'reticular formation' on electrocortical arousal (derived from Paul-David, Riehl and Unna, 1960). The circles represent the integrated electrical activity (Hz·min, right-hand ordinate) seen after intraperitoneal injection of a 'reticular excitant' chemical (catechol 60 mg·kg^{-1}) at various levels of urethane anaesthesia (bottom abscissa) in a rat with an intact neuraxis. (Angel and Fox, unpublished observations). (b) Shows the mean peak change (ordinate) in the frequency of discharge of two thalamic reticular cells to 20 consecutive trains of electrical stimuli applied to the left ankle (34 shocks, duration of 0.1 ms, separation 3 ms, of sufficient intensity to activate peripheral C-fibres, delivered once per 5 s) in an intact rat at various levels of urethane anaesthesia (abscissa). The crosses are from a cell which decreased its frequency of discharge; the circles from one which increased its frequency of discharge to each stimulus train. (Angel and Knox, unpublished observations)

by Bradley and Key (1958). This was seen for both behavioural and electrocortical arousal to afferent and brain stem stimulation. Using an integrating technique for measuring electrocortical desynchronization, Paul-David, Riehl and Unna (1960) showed in the cat *encéphale isolé* preparation a diminution in 'units of arousal' which was dose dependent such that, as the dose of pentobarbitone was increased, electrocortical arousal to stimulation within the system was both of shorter duration and less intense (*Figure 6.5a*). A similar effect in the intact rat on the frequency—time integrated electrocortical activity to chemical stimulation of the modulatory system can also be demonstrated with increasing anaesthetic depth (*Figure 6.5a*).

Using macroelectrodes and recording mass responses to peripheral stimulation from within the brain stem component of the modulatory system, French, Verzeano and Magoun (1953) and Arduini (1954) demonstrated that anaesthetic agents blocked the responses of 'cells' in the modulatory system at doses which left conduction over the direct peripherocortical pathways seemingly unimpaired. Unfortunately, such recording methods cannot adequately differentiate between presynaptic (input) or postsynaptic (output) components of the system and ignore responses of the cell type which is slowed by peripheral stimuli. From the decreased responses they obtained, French, Verzeano and Magoun (1953) offered the suggestion which nowadays must be totally refuted that conduction through the system was via long chains of short-axoned cells. Since these cells do not exist (see Cajal, 1911; Brodal, 1957), let us hope that people will forget the initial suggestion. Recording from single spontaneously active cells in the thalamic compartment of the system, it can be shown that both functional types of cell (either slowed or accelerated by peripheral stimulation) show a diminished responsiveness to peripheral stimulation on increasing depth of anaesthesia, with both the duration and the intensity of frequency change decreasing as anaesthetic depth is increased (*Figure 6.5b*).

Role in control of access of information to the cerebral cortex

The idea to be advanced in this part of the chapter is that, in addition to its capability to control states of behavioural and electrocortical 'arousal', the sensorimotor modulatory system is also capable of altering the excitability of cells in the sensory pathways from the periphery to the cerebral cortex (see *Figure 6.6*). Three important facets are examined. First, that the modulatory system exerts both excitation and inhibition on sensory relay cells. Second, that the ability of sensory relay cells to respond to their inputs may be profoundly affected by the modulation they receive, with cells in the thalamic sensory relay nuclei showing this modulation to the greatest extent. Third, evidence will be presented to show that anaesthetics block transmission of information through the thalamic relay nuclei by a combined effect of decreased excitatory and increased inhibitory drives from the modulatory system.

One peculiar property of all groups of sensory cells along the various major specific afferent pathways is the relatively small proportion (15–20%) of synaptic knobs which degenerate after the total severance of the afferent input (see, for example, Walberg, 1966). This means that the majority of synapses within a sensory nucleus come from axons either originating within the nucleus itself or from other sites in the nervous system. It is not surprising, therefore, to find that, as well as obvious changes in electrocortical or motor and behavioural activity seen after electrical stimulation of the modulatory system, such stimulation also modifies the transfer of information through various sensory nuclei.

Such modulation has been described in the spinal cord (Hagbarth and Kerr, 1954; Hagbarth and Fex, 1959; Tolle, Feldman and Clemente, 1959), dorsal column nuclei (Hernández-Péon, Scherrer and Velasco, 1956) and ventrobasal thalamus (Li, 1956; King, Naquet and Magoun, 1957) as well as along the auditory and visual pathways (Bremer and Stoupel, 1958, 1959a, b; Dumont and Dell, 1958). The results from low frequency stimulation of the thalamic nuclei in the modulatory system – i.e. recruiting responses (Dempsey and Morrison, 1942) – had clearly shown that there were potent, indirect functional connections between this compartment of the modulatory system and the cerebral cortex. For the recruiting responses obtained from the motor cortex to intra-laminar stimulation, Purpura and Cohen (1962) produced convincing evidence that this was consequent upon phasic activation of cells in the thalamic motor relay nucleus which, via its direct corticopetal projection, gave the phasic activation of motor cortical cells. With the lack, or paucity, of a direct cortical connection from the modulatory system, an alternative mechanism to influence cerebral cells would be to modulate the activity of the specific thalamic relay projecting onto it.

Evidence gained from a study of the mass responses at thalamic and cortical sites points to a facilitation of transfer of information across the thalamic relay nuclei in the direct peripherocortical paths (*Figure 6.6*) during electrocortical arousal (see Steriade, 1970). Koella and his associates were the first to remark upon the similar changes, in cortical mass responses to peripheral stimulation, to electrical stimulation of the posterior hypothalamus and noxious cutaneous stimulation (Gellhorn, Koella and Ballin, 1954, 1955; Nakao and Koella, 1956). This was followed by the observation that noxious stimulation of the skin prior to an electrical test stimulus to the forepaw, in the surgically anaesthetized rat, gave an increase in the amplitudes of the short latency components, coupled with a decrease in latency, of the cortical response evoked by the test stimulus, unaccompanied by any change in the mass response recorded from the cuneate nucleus (Dawson, Podachin and Schatz, 1959, 1963). However, noxious stimulation was shown to modulate the responsiveness of cells in the ventrobasal thalamic complex to electrical stimulation of the forepaw, and that this modulation showed a parallel time course to that of the increase in cortical mass response (Angel and Dawson, 1961, 1963). Next, a similar time course of change in frequency of discharge of cells in the thalamic reticular nucleus to noxious peripheral stimulation was shown,

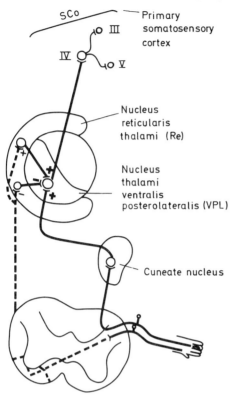

Figure 6.6
A diagrammatic representation of the
arrangement of the modulatory influence
of the nucleus reticularis thalami on
transmission through the somatosensory
pathway. (SCo, primary somatosensory
cortex and cells in layers III, IV and V.)
The terminations on the cells in VPL
and Re are shown as (+) for excitation
and (−) for inhibition. The dashed line
from the ventrolateral white matter to
the nucleus reticularis thalami indicates
relative ignorance of the knowledge of
the afferent path to this cellular mass

which paralleled both the increase in specific thalamic cellular response
and cortical evoked response under four different conditions.

(1) In the rat anaesthetized with trichloroethylene (ca 1%), where a
    train of 34 electrical shocks with a 3 ms separation and an intensity
    sufficient to excite C fibres (i.e. potentially noxious) gave changes in
    ventrobasal thalamic cell responsiveness, reticular thalamic cell dis-
    charge and cortical mass responses, with a peak change at 200 ms
    after the start of the train and a duration of 0.8—1.0 s (Angel, 1964).
(2) In the rat anaesthetized with urethane (1.3—1.5 g·kg^{-1}), where the
    changes were bimodal, with peaks at 300—500 ms and 1.0—1.5 s, and
    the effect lasted for 2.5—3.0 s (Angel, 1964).
(3) In the urethane-anaesthetized rat after intravenous 1,2-dihydroxy-
    benzene (a powerful reticular 'excitant' giving a pronounced electro-
    cortical arousal) at a dose of 4.0 mg·kg^{-1} where the peak change at all
    three sites was seen 30—45 s after injection and the effect lasted for
    8—12 min (Angel, 1969).
(4) In the urethane-anaesthetized rat during spontaneous electrocortical
    desynchronization (Angel, Dodd and Gray, 1976; Angel and Blake,
    1977).

Since two types of reticular cell were isolated in the above experiments,
one showing an increase in frequency of discharge (80%) and the other a

decrease (20%), it was postulated (Angel, 1964, 1977c) that the correlation between change in discharge frequency and increased ventrobasal thalamic responsiveness was due to both an increased excitatory and a decreased inhibitory influence of the thalamic extension of the modulatory system upon the ventrobasal thalamus complex, the anatomical basis for which has already been mentioned (see above).

If the effect of anaesthetic agents were to employ the same modulatory mechanism, transmission through the specific thalamic relay nuclei should be altered; indeed, these nuclei should also show an increased susceptibility to anaesthetic action compared to lesser order sensory relay cells in cochlear and dorsal column nuclei or retinal ganglion cell for the auditory, somaesthetic and visual paths, respectively. If we confine our attention to the somaesthetic pathway and examine the available evidence, it is apparent that such a modulation could indeed exist.

Dawson, Podachin and Schatz (1963) demonstrated that the mass response recorded from the cuneate nucleus (*Figure 6.6*) to electrical stimulation of the forepaw in the rat remained unaltered at anaesthetic (trichloroethylene) levels from very deep to light enough to just allow reflex withdrawal to a strong pinch. Galindo (1968, 1969), on the other hand, presented evidence which showed a depression of activity of feline cuneate neurons to systemic pentobarbitone and halothane given either by inhalation or by medullary superfusion. It is not merely a matter of author semantics if one points out that this was seen in the decerebrate animal in which preparation, with its drastically truncated neuraxis, it is difficult to determine whether one is investigating anaesthesia *per se* or action of anaesthetic agents. In the urethane-anaesthetized intact rat, cells in the cuneate nucleus, monosynaptically excited by a peripheral input, show little or no change. Thus they will discharge once with little increase in latency to each peripheral stimulus if the anaesthetic level is increased with a variety of anaesthetic agents, and only show a decrement in responsiveness at near-threshold stimulus levels or at suprathreshold stimulus levels if near-fatal anaesthetic levels are reached (Angel and Unwin, 1970; Angel, Berridge and Francis, 1976; Angel, 1977b). However, cells possibly activated multisynaptically show a much greater susceptibility to anaesthetic agents (Gordon and Paine, 1960; McComas, 1963; Gordon and Jukes, 1964), as do the later responses of cells which respond iteratively to a single peripheral stimulus (Angel, 1977b). Nevertheless, the evidence points to an unchanged monosynaptically discharged cuneothalamic volley as anaesthetic depth is increased.

At the level of the ventrobasal thalamus it had already been argued by King, Naquet and Magoun (1957) that the effects of pentobarbitone and thiopentone could be interpreted as being due to a heightened susceptibility of specific thalamic cells to anaesthetic agents. In a comparative study on the effect of ethyl carbamate anaesthesia on cellular responses in rat cuneate nucleus and ventrobasal thalamic complex, it was shown (Angel and Unwin, 1970) that thalamic cells with response latencies compatible with monosynaptic excitation to cuneothalamic volleys showed a clear-cut decrease in response probability and an increase in latency as anaesthesia was increased with no change in cuneate cell responses under the same experimental conditions. Further, the responses of cortical cells could be entirely explained by the anaesthetic acting solely at the thalamic relay level. This was subsequently shown to be a general observation for a variety of anaesthetic agents (Angel, 1977a, b). A marked reduction in the excitation of ventrobasal thalamic cells to iontophoretically applied acetylcholine or inhibition to noradrenaline has been shown after administration of pentobarbitone, nitrous oxide or halothane (Phillis and Tebēcis, 1967; McCance *et al.*, 1968).

Most authors report that deepening anaesthesia results in a diminution in amplitude and an increase in latency of the short latency components of the cerebral mass response evoked by peripheral stimulation (see Angel, 1977c). Unfortunately, using this response as the indicative parameter of anaesthetic action is subject to interpretive difficulties. First, considering the amplitude of the response, without regard to its sign or configuration, is not equatable as a sign of cortical cellular responsiveness (see Angel, 1977c; Darbinyan and Bogdanov, 1977). Second, in the primate and cat, the early part of the response to stimulation of the anterior limb is a composite of activity conveyed to the cerebral cortex over dorsal column, spinothalamic and spinocervical paths so that the question arises upon which of these paths the anaesthetic exerts its action. Third, increasing depth of anaesthesia gives a larger volume of cortex to which the afferent input can gain access (Angel, Berridge and Unwin, 1973) so that, unless one records from the centre of the projection area, an apparent increase in response may be recorded.

In the modulatory system, recording from diencephalic and mesencephalic sites, obvious changes are seen in the discharge of single cells when anaesthetics are administered, cells showing either an increase or decrease in frequency of discharge or a change in pattern of discharge (Schlag, 1956). In the mesencephalic compartment of the system, Shimoji and Bickford (1971) showed that, of 37 cells, 32 showed a decrease in discharge frequency and 5 an increase as the animals (paralysed, artificially ventilated cats) were anaesthetized with halothane, diethyl ether, thiopentone and nitrous oxide. Of 233 spontaneously active cells in the thalamic reticular nucleus of the rat surgically anaesthetized with ethyl carbamate, 178 were of the type showing an irregular low frequency discharge increased by noxious cutaneous stimulation and 45 were of the type showing a higher regular discharge which was decreased by noxious stimuli. The first type of cell showed a steady decrease in discharge frequency as anaesthetic depth was increased, regardless of the anaesthetic agent used, and the latter type a steady increase. These changes in frequency showed an exact correlation with the concomitant reduction in ventrobasal thalamic, primary sensory cortical cellular responses and evoked cortical potential changes (Angel and Knox, 1970; Angel, 1977b). Since the changes are the reverse of those seen after an arousing stimulus, one can forward the hypothesis that anaesthetic agents affect specific thalamic cell responsiveness via decreased excitatory and increased inhibitory inflow from the modulatory system. In common with other authors, it was seen that the most dramatic effect of anaesthetic agents on thalamic reticular cellular discharge was one of change in pattern. Those cells 'excited' by noxious stimulation tend to show periods of fairly regular discharge interspersed with irregular components, which latter are accentuated by increase in anaesthesia while those 'inhibited' by noxious stimuli tend to have their irregular components removed by increasing anaesthesia.

In summary (see *Figure 6.6*), one can say that the modulation of transmission of information from the periphery to the cerebral cortex is affected by anaesthetic agents in such a way that transmission across the various specific thalamic relay nuclei is decreased, proportionately more than at other relay sites, and that this action effectively and transiently (for the duration of anaesthetic action) denervates the specific sensory cortical receiving areas. This, combined with the observations of Andersson and Wolpow (1964) and Andersson, Norssell and Wolpow (1964) that the electrocortical activity recorded from the somatosensory cortex becomes synchronized after dorsal column section, may indicate that block of access of information to the cerebral cortex may play a part in the genesis of the anaesthetic state. A further link, albeit tenuous, between this and altered states of consciousness may be inferred from the observation of Strümpell (1877) that in a patient with progressive sensory loss exclusion of information from the remaining channels caused him to 'fall asleep'.

Its role in motor control

In a series of experiments, Magoun and his various collaborators produced a map of the sites, stimulation of which influenced extensor motoneurons. Some areas decreased the discharge of motoneurons to muscle stretch or cortical stimulation while other areas increased the discharge. The facilitatory area extended through the thalamus, hypothalamus, mesencephalon, pontile tegmentum and a large part of the lateral bulbar 'reticular' formation. The inhibitory area was located in the ventromedial part of the bulbar 'reticular' formation; this area appears to be incapable of intrinsic activity but requires an inflow from cerebral and cerebellar cortices as well as the basal ganglia to provide a drive to its cells (see Lindsley, Schreiner and Magoun, 1949). Both the facilitatory and the inhibitory areas were later shown to give reciprocal effects on extensors and flexors, such that extensor facilitation was accompanied by flexor inhibition and *vice versa* (Sprague and Chambers, 1954; Gernandt and Thulin, 1955). Reference to *Figure 6.7* will show that the spinal motoneurons supplying the direct drive to the skeletal muscles can be discharged by three mechanisms (see also Granit, 1970).

(1) Stretching the muscle will stretch the muscle spindle which will increase the firing rate of the spindle afferents, which in turn will increase the discharge of the α-motoneurons which will cause a reflex contraction (*Figure 6.7a*).

(2) Direct excitation of the α-motoneurons will cause the muscle to contract; its shortening will unload the muscle spindles and cause a decreased discharge of the spindle afferents proportional to the degree of muscular contraction (*Figure 6.7b*).

(3) Excitation of the γ-motoneurons will cause the polar ends of the spindle to contract, thus increasing the length of the non-contractile equatorial region which will be signalled by an increase in discharge rate of the spindle afferents and via their direct action on the α-motoneurons an increased α-motoneuronal discharge giving muscular contraction with a timing equal to the γ-to-α loop delay (*Figure 6.7c*).

That the effects of stimulation of the brain stem motor modulatory system could be via this latter mechanism was indicated by the experiments of Granit and Kaada (1952) who showed, using the discharge from spindle afferents as an indicator of fusimotor drive (i.e. state of spindle

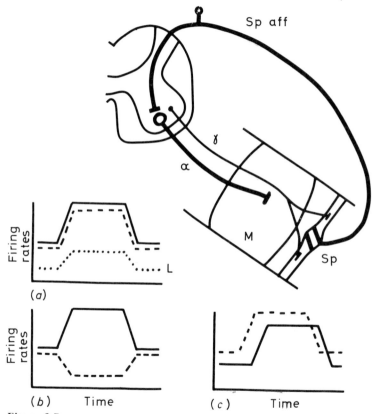

Figure 6.7
The monosynaptic arc from muscle spindles (Sp) via the group Ia spinal afferents (Sp aff) to the α-motoneurons which innervate the muscle (M) via the α-efferents (α). The spindle muscle fibres are innervated by the smaller γ-efferents (γ). The small graphs represent the change in α-motoneural (——) and muscle spindle (- - -) firing rates with (a) muscle stretch (muscle length indicated by . . . . . . L); (b) direct excitation of motoneurons; and (c) increased γ-motoneuronal discharge

muscle fibres), that stimulation of the extensor facilitatory/flexor inhibitory area gave an increase in spindle discharge from extensor muscles and, conversely, a decrease by stimulation within the extensor inhibitory/ flexor excitatory area. This was also seen by Shimazu, Hongo and Kubota (1962) and Hongo, Kubota and Shimazu (1963) but, perhaps more importantly, they also showed non-reciprocal effects with spindle discharge from both flexor and extensor muscles decreasing coincidentally with signs of electrocortical synchronization (see also Euler and Söderberg, 1956, 1957), pointing to a mechanism of generalized diminution of muscle tone correlated with drowsiness. A similar coexcitation of both flexor and extensor spindles can be shown to occur after administration of the modulatory system excitant 1,2-dihydroxybenzene. This chemical produces spontaneous muscle twitches accompanied by a powerful electrocortical desynchronization (Angel and Lemon, 1974). The muscular twitches are reduced by some 80—96% by deafferentation (Angel and Lemon, 1973), pointing to a powerful γ-motoneuronal excitation. Direct recordings from spindle afferents show this to be the case (Angel, Clarke and Taylor, 1976) and further, subconvulsive, doses of 1,2-dihydroxybenzene, can raise the excitability of the α-motoneurons, via the γ-to-α loop, such that a normally ineffective phasic excitatory volley from the motor cortex can cause them to discharge (Angel and Lemon, 1976).

It is pertinent to note here that, although quick phasic movements can be produced by direct α-motoneuronal excitation, precise, well controlled movements demand an additional form of control such that the length of the spindles can be altered to the required length by γ-motoneuronal action and the muscle automatically contracted to the required degree by titrating spindle afferent excitatory drive and α-motoneuronal discharge — the servo control idea formulated by Merton (1951, 1953). Thus an awakening animal needs both a general and a specific control of the γ-motoneuronal apparatus both to raise the general level of α-motoneuronal excitation and to control their discharge during specific motor acts. There is good evidence (see, for example, Granit, 1970) that control of posture and locomotion requires coactivation of both α- and γ-motoneuronal systems.

Very little has been reported on the effects of anaesthesia on the control of α-motoneuronal discharge. That the α-motoneurons are extremely sensitive to anaesthesia can be deduced from the complete suppression of their monosynaptic excitation at anaesthetic levels which leave the monosynaptic excitation of dorsal horn or dorsal column cells apparently little affected. Andrew (1961) showed that, recording from γ-afferents to hindlimb muscles in the urethane-anaesthetized rat, the lighter the anaesthetic level the greater the number of active γ-efferents, the more variable their discharge rate and the more easily they could be influenced by sensory stimulation. Increasing depth of anaesthesia with various anaesthetic agents gave two effects: either (1) an initial excitation coupled with transient behavioural arousal and limb movements followed by a tonic increase in γ-motoneuronal discharge with suppression of the reflex accessibility of these motoneurons to sensory stimulation — this was seen with ether, ethyl chloride, trichloroethylene and chloroform, with the tonic phase of excitation being via a central nervous mechanism (Diete-Spiff and Pascoe, 1959); or (2) a rapid suppression of γ-moto-neuronal discharge and their reflex accessibility to sensory stimuli — seen with urethane, halothane and nitrous oxide. The initial excitation seen with some anaesthetics could possibly explain the phase of hyper-excitability seen when inducing anaesthesia with these agents; the tonic excitation, if it occurs in γ-motoneurons to intercostal spindles, may play a role in maintaining an excitatory drive to respiratory motoneurons and may be used to explain in part the respiratory excitement seen with some anaesthetic agents (e.g. trichloroethylene and ethyl chloride). Preferential depression of intercostal muscles is a normal feature of deepening anaesthesia (Chapter 25).

In summary, the modulatory system does play a role in the control of the skeletal musculature, exerting both a general and a specific control on motor movements. The extent of the nervous system involved is rather loosely defined by the method of central stimulation and the resultant inability to determine whether the effects are from stimulation of cells near the stimulating electrode tip, or fibres projecting to or from this area or to fibres of passage.

CONCLUSIONS

We are now in a position to explain, in general terms, the disruption by anaesthetic agents of motor control, sensory experience (excluding that of pain) and consciousness. By their action on the sensorimotor modulation system to switch off excitation and turn on inhibition, messages from the periphery to the brain are blocked mainly at the thalamic level. A similar action on the fusimotor system could explain the loss of motor control. If the muscle spindles are temporarily paralysed, then the powerful spindle drive to the spinal motoneurons would be removed and their over-all excitability depressed. For the loss of consciousness we have to postulate a similar dis-excitation and increased inhibition of the system favouring the waking state and the reverse action on the system favouring the sleeping state giving an exaggerated 'sleep' state which could be reinforced by denying the cortex access to its normal sensory inflow.

Finally, one must negate the generally held belief that the depressive effect of anaesthetics is greater in pathways containing multiple synaptic links. This stemmed from the work of French, Verzeano and Magoun (1953) on responses evoked from the reticular formation by peripheral stimulation, a supposedly multisynaptic structure. However, we now know that the pathway from the periphery to the thalamic reticular nucleus is only trisynaptic (see above) and comparable with the specific somatosensory pathway from the skin to the cerebral cortex. Of much greater importance is the ability of the synapse to transfer its information, i.e. its synaptic security. Comparison of two monosynaptic transmission systems — that from muscle spindle afferents to α-motoneurons with that from dorsal column afferents to cuneate neurons — shows a marked difference, with the former blocked at relatively low anaesthetic levels and the latter showing minimal changes until fatal levels of anaesthesia are reached. Since synaptic security appears to depend upon the degree of supraspinal modulation of postsynaptic membrane excitability, we are again forced to look at the modulatory system for the prime site of anaesthetic action and to disregard the number of synapses along a pathway.

References

Andén, N. E., Dahlströhm, A., Fuxe, K., Larsson, K., Olson, L. and Ungerstedt, U. (1966). Ascending monoamine neurons to the telencephalon and diencephalon. *Acta physiol. scand.* 67, 313—326

Andersson, S. A. and Wolpow, E. R. (1964). Localized slow wave activity in the somatosensory cortex of the cat. *Acta physiol. scand.* 61, 130—140

Andersson, S. A., Norrsell, U. and Wolpow, E. R. (1964). Cortical synchronization and desynchronization via spinal pathways. *Acta physiol. scand.* 61, 144—158

Andrew, B. L. (1961). The effect of certain anaesthetics on the activity of small motor fibres serving the hind limb of the rat. *J. Physiol., Lond.* 155, 59—71

Angel, A. (1964). The effect of peripheral stimulation on units located in the thalamic reticular nuclei. *J. Physiol., Lond.* 171, 42—60

Angel, A. (1969). An analysis of the effect of 1-2,dihydroxybenzene on transmission through the dorsal column sensory pathway. *Electroenceph. clin. Neurophysiol.* 27, 392—403

Angel, A. (1977a). Theories of the mechanism of action of general anaesthetic agents. In *Anaesthesiology*, pp. 67—76. E. Hülsz, J. A. Sandrez-Hernandez, G. Vasconcelos and J. N. Lunn (ed.). Amsterdam and Oxford: Excerpta Medica

Angel, A. (1977b). Modulation of information transmission in the dorsal column—lemniscothalamic pathway by anaesthetic agents. In *Anaesthesiology*, pp. 82—89. E. Hülsz, J. A. Sandrez-Hernandez, G. Vasconcelos and J. N. Lunn (ed.). Amsterdam and Oxford: Excerpta Medica

Angel, A. (1977c). Processing of sensory information. *Progr. Neurobiol.* 9, 1—122

Angel, A. and Blake, K. (1977). The relation between changes in frequency of discharge of thalamic reticular cells and thalamic relay cell responses to afferent input during spontaneous fluctuations in 'anaesthetic depth' in the rat anaesthetized with urethane. *Br. J. Anaesth.* 49, 1169

Angel, A. and Dawson, G. D. (1961). Modification of thalamic transmission by sensory stimulation. *J. Physiol., Lond.* 156, 23—24P

Angel, A. and Dawson, G. D. (1963). The facilitation of thalamic and cortical responses in the dorsal column sensory pathway by strong peripheral stimulation. *J. Physiol., Lond.* 166, 587—604

Angel, A. and Knox, G. V. (1970). The effect of anaesthesia on units in the thalamic reticular formation. *J. Physiol., Lond.* 210, 167—168P

Angel, A. and Lemon, R. N. (1973). An analysis of the myoclonic jerks produced by 1,2-dihydroxybenzene in the rat. *Electroenceph. clin. Neurophysiol.* 35, 589—601

Angel, A. and Lemon, R. N. (1974). An experimental model of sensory myoclonus produced by 1,2-dihydroxybenzene in the anaesthetized rat. In *Epilepsy*, Proceedings of the Hans Berger Centenary Symposium, pp. 37—47. P. Harris and C. Mawdsley (ed.). Edinburgh, London and New York: Churchill Livingstone

Angel, A. and Lemon, R. N. (1976). Cortical and pyramidal influences on rat motoneurons. *J. Physiol., Lond.* 259, 14—15P

Angel, A. and Unwin, J. (1970). Effect of urethane on transmission along dorsal column sensory pathway in rat. *J. Physiol., Lond.* 208, 32P

Angel, A., Berridge, D. A. and Francis, H. (1976). The effect of anaesthetic agents on the response of cells in the cuneate nucleus of the rat. *J. Physiol., Lond.* 259, 15—17P

Angel, A., Berridge, D. A. and Unwin, J. (1973). The effect of anaesthetic agents on primary cortical evoked responses. *Br. J. Anaesth.* 45, 824—836

Angel, A., Clarke, K. A. and Taylor, C. (1976). Effect of catechol on the discharge of hind-limb muscle spindles in the anaesthetized rat. *J. Physiol., Lond.* 259, 12—14P

Angel, A., Dodd, J. and Gray, J. D. (1976). Fluctuating anaesthetic state in the rat anaesthetized with urethane. *J. Physiol., Lond.* 259, 11—12P

Arduini, A. and Arduini, M. G. (1954). Effects of drugs and metabolic alterations and brain stem arousal mechanism. *J. Pharmac. exp. Ther.* 110, 76—85

Batini, C., Moruzzi, G., Palestini, M., Rossi, G. F. and Zanchetti, G. (1959). Effects of complete pontine transections on the sleep–wakefulness rhythm: the mid-pontine pretrigeminal preparation. *Archs ital. Biol.* 96, 1–12

Bowsher, D. (1970). Place and modality analysis in caudal reticular formation. *J. Physiol., Lond.* 209, 473–486

Bradley, P. B. and Elkes, J. (1957). The effects of some drugs on the electrical activity of the brain. *Brain* 80, 77–117

Bradley, P. B. and Key, B. J. (1958). The effect of drugs on arousal responses produced by electrical stimulation of the reticular formation of the brain. *Electroenceph. clin. Neurophysiol.* 10, 97–110

Bremer, F. and Stoupel, N. (1958). De la modification des réponses sensorielles corticales dans l'éveil réticulaire. *Acta neurol. psychiat. belg.* 58, 401–403

Bremer, F. and Stoupel, N. (1959a). Facilitation et inhibition des potentiels évoqués corticaux dans l'éveil cérébral. *Archs int. Physiol.* 67, 240–275

Bremer, F. and Stoupel, N. (1959b). Etude pharmacologique de la facilitation des réponses corticales dans l'éveil réticulaire. *Archs int. Pharmacodyn.* 122, 234–238

Brodal, A. (1957). *The Reticular Formation of the Brain Stem: anatomical aspects and functional correlations*, p. 87. Edinburgh and London: Oliver and Boyd

Brodal, A., Taber, E. and Walberg, F. (1960). The raphe nuclei of the brain stem in the cat. II. Efferent connections. *J. comp. Neurol.* 114, 239–259

Brodal, A., Walberg, F. and Taber, E. (1960). The raphe nuclei of the brain stem in the cat. III. Afferent connections. *J. comp. Neurol.* 114, 261–279

Burke, R. E. (1967). Composite nature of the monosynaptic excitatory postsynaptic potential. *J. Neurophysiol.* 30, 1114–1137

Cajal, R. S. (1911). *Histologie du Système Nerveux de l'Homme et des Vertébrès.* Paris: Maloine

Cordeau, J. P. and Mancia, M. (1959). Evidence for the existence an electroencephalographic synchronization mechanism originating in the lower brain stem. *Electroenceph. clin. Neurophysiol.* 11, 551–564

Cowan, W. M. and Powell, T. P. S. (1955). The projection of the midline and intralaminar nuclei of the thalamus of the rabbit. *J. Neurol. Neurosurg. Psychiat.* 18, 266–279

Dahlström, A. and Fuxe, K. (1964). Evidence for the existence of monoamine neurons in the central nervous system. I. Demonstration of monoamines in the cell bodies of brain stem neurons. *Acta physiol. scand.* 62, Suppl. 232, 1–55

Darbinyan, T. M. and Bogdanov, K. Y. (1977). Comparative significance of evoked responses, high frequency EEG and mean frequency EEG during general anaesthesia. In *Anaesthesiology*, pp. 77–81. E. Hülsz, J. A. Sandrez-Hernandez, G. Vasconcelos and J. N. Lunn (ed.). Amsterdam and Oxford: Excerpta Medica

Dawson, G. D., Podachin, V. P. and Schatz, S. W. (1959). Facilitation of cortical responses by competing stimuli. *J. Physiol., Lond.* 148, 24–25P

Dawson, G. D., Podachin, V. P. and Schatz, S. W. (1963). Facilitation of cortical responses by competing stimuli. *J. Physiol., Lond.* 166, 363–381

Dempsey, E. W. and Morison, R. S. (1942). The production of rhythmically recurrent cortical potentials after localized thalamic stimulation. *Am. J. Physiol.* 135, 293–300

Diete-Spiff, K. and Pascoe, J. E. (1959). The spindle motor nerves to the gastrocnemius muscle of the rabbit. *J. Physiol., Lond.* 149, 120–134

Dumont, S. and Dell, P. (1958). Facilitations spécifiques et non spécifiques des réponses visuelles corticales. *J. Physiol., Paris* 50, 261–264

Edwards, S. B. and de Olmos, J. S. (1976). Autoradiographic studies of the projections of the midbrain reticular formation: ascending projections of nucleus cuneiformis. *J. comp. Neurol.* 165, 417–432

Euler, C. V. and Söderberg, U. (1956). The relation between gamma motor activity and the electroencephalogram. *Experientia* 12, 278

Euler, C. V. and Söderberg, U. (1957). The influence of hypothalamic thermoreceptive structures on the electroencephalogram. *Electroenceph. clin. Neurophysiol.* 9, 391–408

Fairén, A. (1973). Conexiones ascendentes del tegmento pontino caudal: un estudio experimental en la rata blanca. *An. de Anat.* 22, 463–508

Feldman, S. M. and Waller, H. J. (1962). Dissociation of electrocortical activation and behavioural arousal. *Nature, Lond.* 196, 1320–1322

Frederickson, C. J. and Hobson, J. A. (1970). Electrical stimulation of the brain stem and subsequent sleep. *Archs ital. Biol.* 108, 564–576

French, J. D. and Magoun, H. W. (1952). Effects of chronic lesions in central cephalic brain stem of monkeys. *Archs Neurol. Psychiat., Chicago* 68, 591–604

French, J. D., Verzeano, M. and Magoun, H. W. (1953). A neural basis of the anesthetic state. *Archs Neurol. Psychiat., Chicago* 69, 519–529

Galindo, A. (1968). Some observations on presynaptic action of drugs, including anaesthetic agents in the cuneate nucleus. *Fedn Proc.* 27, 756

Galindo, A. (1969). Effects of procaine, pentobarbital and halothane on synaptic transmission in the central nervous system. *J. Pharmac. exp. Ther.* 169, 185

Gellhorn, E., Koella, W. P. and Ballin, H. M. (1954). Interaction on cerebral cortex of acoustic or optic with nociceptive impulses: the problem of consciousness. *J. Neurophysiol.* 17, 14–21

Gellhorn, E., Koella, W. P. and Ballin, H. M. (1955). The influence of hypothalamic stimulation on evoked cortical potentials. *J. Psychol.* 39, 77–88

Gernandt, B. E. and Thulin, C. A. (1955). Reciprocal effects upon spinal motoneurons from stimulation of bulbar reticular formation. *J. Neurophysiol.* 18, 113–129

Gordon, G. and Jukes, M. G. M. (1964). Dual organization of the exteroceptive components of the cat's gracile nucleus. *J. Physiol., Lond.* 173, 263–290

Gordon, G. and Paine, C. H. (1960). Functional organization in nucleus gracilis of the cat. *J. Physiol., Lond.* 153, 331–349

Granit, R. (1970). *The Basis of Motor Control.* London and New York: Academic Press

Granit, R. and Kaada, B. (1952). Influence of stimulation of central nervous structures on muscle spindles in cat. *Acta physiol. scand.* 27, 130–160

Hagbarth, K. E. and Fex, J. (1959). Centrifugal influences on single units activity in spinal sensory paths. *J. Neurophysiol.* 22, 321–338

Hagbarth, K. E. and Kerr, D. I. B. (1954). Central influences on spindle afferent conduction. *J. Neurophysiol.* 17, 295–307

Hernández-Péon, R., Scherrer, H. and Velasco, M. (1956). Central influences on afferent conduction in the somatic and visual pathways. *Acta neurol. latinoam.* 2, 8–22

Hess, W. R. (1954). The diencephalic sleep centre. In *Brain Mechanisms and Consciousness*, p. 117. J. F. Delafresnaye (ed.). Oxford: Blackwell

Hobson, J. A., McCarley, R. W., Freedman, R. and Pivik, R. J. (1974). Time course of discharge rate changes by rat pontine brain stem neurons during sleep cycle. *J. Neurophysiol.* 37, 1297–1309

Hobson, J. A., McCarley, R. W. and Wyzinski, P. W. (1975). Sleep cycle oscillation, reciprocal discharge by two brainstem neuronal groups. *Science* 189, 55–58

Hongo, T., Kubota, K. and Shimazu, H. (1963). EEG spindle and depression of gamma motor activity. *J. Neurophysiol.* 26, 568–580

Jones, E. G. and Leavitt, R. Y. (1974). Retrograde axonal transport and the demonstration of non-specific projections to the cerebral cortex and striatum from thalamic intralaminar nuclei in the rat, cat and monkey. *J. comp. Neurol.* 154, 349–378

Jouvet, M. (1967). Neurophysiology of the states of sleep. *Physiol. Rev.* 47, 117–177

King, E. E., Naquet, R. and Magoun, H. W. (1957). Alterations in somatic afferent transmission through thalamus by central mechanisms and barbiturates. *J. Pharmac. exp. Ther.* 119, 48–63

Li, C. L. (1956). The facilitatory effect of stimulation of an unspecific thalamic nucleus on cortical sensory neuronal responses. *J. Physiol., Lond.* 131, 115–124

Limanskii, Y. P. (1962). Synaptic modifications of the resting potential of individual neurones in the medulla oblongata reticular formation. *Sechenov physiol. J.* 48, 126–133

Limanskii, Y. P. (1963). Characteristics of afferent convergence on neurons of the medullary reticular formation. *Fedn Proc. Transl. Suppl.* 22, 1090–1093T

Limanskii, Y. P. (1965). Slow and fast prepotentials in neurons of medullary reticular formation. *Fedn Proc. Transl. Suppl.* 24, 1008–1010T

Lindsley, D. B., Schreiner, L. H. and Magoun, H. W. (1949). An electromyographic study of spasticity. *J. Neurophysiol.* 12, 197–216

McCance, I., Phillis, I. W., Tebēcis, A. K. and Westerman, R. A. (1968). The pharmacology of ACh-excitation of thalamic neurones. *Br. J. Pharmac. Chemother.* 32, 652–662

McComas, A. J. (1963). Responses of the rat dorsal column system to mechanical stimulation of the hind paw. *J. Physiol., Lond.* 166, 435–448

Magnes, J., Moruzzi, G. and Pompeiano, O. (1961). Synchronization of the EEG produced by low-frequency electrical stimulation of the region of the solitary tract. *Archs ital. Biol.* 99, 33–67

Magni, F., Melzack, R., Moruzzi, G. and Smith, C. J. (1959). Direct pyramidal influences on the dorsal column nuclei. *Archs ital. Biol.* 97, 357–377

Magni, F. and Willis, W. D. (1964). Subcortical and peripheral control of brain stem reticular neurons. *Archs ital. Biol.* 102, 434–448

Magoun, H. W. and Rhines, R. (1946). An inhibitory mechanism in the bulbar reticular formation. *J. Neurophysiol.* 9, 165–171

Merton, P. A. (1951). The silent period in a muscle of the human hand. *J. Physiol., Lond.* 114, 183–198

Merton, P. A. (1953). Speculations on the servo-control of movement. In *The Spinal Cord*, Ciba Symposium, pp. 247–260. London: Churchill

Minderhoud, J. M. (1971). An anatomical study of the efferent connections of the thalamic reticular nucleus. *Expl Brain Res.* 12, 435–446

Monti, J. M. (1970). Effect of recurrent stimulation of the brain stem reticular formation on REM sleep in cats. *Exp. Neurol.* 28, 484–493

Moruzzi, G. (1964). Reticular influence on the EEG. *Electroenceph. clin. Neurophysiol.* 16, 2–17

Moruzzi, G. and Magoun, H. W. (1949). Brain stem reticular formation and activation of the EEG *Electroenceph. clin. Neurophysiol.* 1, 455–473

Nakao, H. and Koella, W. P. (1956). Influence of nociceptive stimuli on evoked subcortical and cortical potentials in cat. *J. Neurophysiol.* 19, 187–195

Nauta, W. J. H. and Kuypers, H. J. G. M. (1958). Some ascending pathways in the brain stem reticular formation. In *The Reticular Formation of the Brain,* Henry Ford Hospital International Symposium, pp. 3–30. L. D. Procter (ed.). Boston: Little, Brown

Olszewski, J. (1954). The cytoarchitecture of the human reticular formation. In *Brain Mechanisms and Consciousness,* pp. 54–76. E. D. Adrian, F. Bremer and H. H. Jasper (ed.). Oxford: Blackwell Scientific

Paul-David, J., Riehl. J-L. and Unna, K. R. (1960). Quantification of effects of depressant drugs on E.E.G. activation response. *J. Pharmac. exp. Ther.* 129, 69–74

Phillis, J. W. and Tebēcis, A. K. (1967). The effects of pentobarbitone, sodium on acetylcholine excitation and noradrenaline inhibition of thalamic neurones. *Life Sci.* 6, 1621

Pompeiano, O. and Hoshino, K. (1976). Central control of posture: reciprocal discharge by two pontine neuronal groups leading to suppression of decerebrate rigidity. *Brain Res.* 116, 131–138

Purpura, D. P. and Cohen, B. (1962). Intracellular recording from thalamic neurons during recruiting responses. *J. Neurophysiol.* 25, 621–635

Rall, W. (1967). Distinguishing theoretical synaptic potentials computed for different soma-dendritic distributions of synaptic inputs. *J. Neurophysiol.* 30, 1138–1168

Rhines, R. and Magoun, H. W. (1946). Brain stem facilitation of cortical motor response. *J. Neurophysiol.* 9, 219–229

Rossi, G. F. and Zanchetti, A. (1957). The brain stem reticular formation. *Archo ital. Biol.* 95, 199–435

Scheibel, M. E. and Scheibel, A. B. (1958). Structural substrates for integrative patterns in the brain stem reticular core. In *Reticular Formation of the Brain,* pp. 31–55. H. H. Jasper, L. D. Proctor, R. S. Knighton, W. C. Noshay and R. T. Costello (ed.). Boston, Mass: Little, Brown

Scheibel, M. E. and Scheibel, A. B. (1966a). Patterns of organization in specific and nonspecific thalamic fields. In *The Thalamus,* pp. 13–46. D. P. Purpura and M. D. Yahr (ed.). New York: Columbia University Press

Scheibel, M. E. and Scheibel, A. B. (1966b). The organization of the nucleus reticularis thalami: a Golgi study. *Brain Res.* 1, 43–62

Schlag, J. (1956). A study of the action of nembutal on diencephalic and mesencephalic unit activity. *Archs int. physiol. Biochim.* 44, 470–488

Segundo, J. P., Arano-Iniguez, R. and French, J. D. (1955). Behavioral arousal by stimulation of the brain in monkey. *J. Neurosurg.* 12, 601–613

Segundo, J. P., Takenaka, T. and Encabo, H. (1967). Electrophysiology of bulbar reticular neurons. *J. Neurophysiol.* 30, 1194–1220

Shimazu, H., Hongo, T. and Kubota, K. (1962). Two types of central influences on gamma motor system. *J. Neurophysiol.* 25, 309–323

Shimoji, K. and Bickford, R. G. (1971). Differential effects of anesthetics on mesencephalic reticular neurons. I. Spontaneous firing patterns. *Anesthesiology* 35, 68–75

Sprague, J. H. and Chambers, W. W. (1954). Control of posture by reticular formation and cerebellum in the intact anaesthetized and unanaesthetized and in the decerebrate cat. *Am. J. Physiol.* 176, 52–64

Steriade, M. (1970). Ascending control of thalamic and cortical responsiveness. *Int. Rev. Neurobiol.* 12, 87–144

Strümpell, A. (1877). Ein Beitrag zur Theorie des Schlafs. *Pflügers Arch. ges. Physiol.* 15, 573–574

Swanson, L. W. (1976). The locus coeruleus: a cytoarchitectonic Golgi and immunohistochemical study in the albino rat. *Brain Res.* 110, 39–56

Taber, E., Brodal, A. and Walberg, F. (1960). The raphe nuclei of the brain stem in the cat. I. Normal topography and cytoarchitecture and general discussion. *J. comp. Neurol.* 114, 161–183

Tolle, A., Feldman, S. and Clemente, C. D. (1959). Effects of bulbar stimulation and decerebration on visceral afferent responses in the spinal cord. *Am. J. Physiol.* 196, 674–680

Ungerstedt, U. (1971). Stereotaxic mapping of the monoamine pathways in the rat brain. *Acta physiol. scand.* Suppl. 367, 1–50

Walberg, F. (1966). The fine structure of the cuneate nucleus in normal cats and following interruption of afferent fibres – an electron microscopical study with particular reference to findings made in Glees and Nauta sections. *Expl Brain Res.* 2, 107–128

Waszak, M. (1974). Firing pattern of neurons in the rostal and ventral part of nucleus reticularis thalami during EEG spindles. *Exp. Neurol.* 43, 38–59

Wikler, A. (1952). Pharmacologic dissociation of behavior and EEG 'sleep patterns' in dogs: morphine, *n*-allylmorphine, and atropine. *Proc. Soc. exp. Biol. Med.* 79, 261–265

7 Biotransformation of anaesthetics in relation to toxicity
M. J. Halsey

Originally, the inhaled general anaesthetics were thought to be chemically inert *in vivo*, one of the advantages being that they could be easily removed from the body via the lungs. Although Barrett and Johnston (1939) reported the biotransformation of trichloroethylene only five years after its introduction as a clinical agent, this was regarded as an exception rather than the general rule. However, such ideas had to be revised when Van Dyke, Chenoweth and Van Poznak (1964) demonstrated the breakdown of all the common volatile agents during anaesthesia in animals. These studies were made possible by the development of radioactive labelling of different atoms of the anaesthetics, which allowed their biodegradation to be followed *in vivo*. Administration of ^{14}C-chloroform and diethyl ether, and ^{36}Cl-methoxyflurane, ^{36}Cl-halothane and ^{36}Cl-chloroform resulted in the production of ^{14}C- and ^{36}Cl-urinary metabolites and $^{14}CO_2$. However, in spite of continuing work both *in vivo* and *in vitro* (Van Dyke and Chenoweth, 1965; Van Dyke, 1966), including the qualitative demonstration of the metabolism of halothane in man (Stier *et al.*, 1964), the potential clinical relevance of this area of research was generally disregarded.

Since 1970, the metabolism of the volatile agents has been determined quantitatively in man, and the extent of the phenomenon is surprisingly large. The fraction of the anaesthetic recovered as metabolites also varies considerably between agents: 0.2% of isoflurane (Holaday *et al.*, 1975), 2.4% of enflurane (Chase *et al.*, 1971), 25% of halothane (Cascorbi, Blake and Helrich, 1970) and 44–47% of methoxyflurane (Holaday, Rudofsky and Treuhaft, 1970; Yoshimura, Holaday and Fizerova-Bergerova, 1976). These figures may be an underestimate of the total amount metabolized because careful balance studies have demonstrated that it was not possible to account for all the anaesthetic taken up in the body, and the fraction not recovered may represent non-volatile breakdown products bound intracellularly. For example, F^- is taken up by bone to approximately the same extent as renal excretion (Fiserova-Bergerova, 1973). (The fractions not recovered in the above studies were: 5% of the isoflurane, 15% of the enflurane, 38% of the halothane and 18—36% of the methoxyflurane.) The extent of the metabolism in man is also emphasized by relating it to the total amount of any agent absorbed into the body during an anaesthetic. The latter is, to a first approximation, independent of the agent and averages about 9 g·h^{-1}. Thus for a two-hour operation with methoxyflurane, almost 10 g of the agent is biotransformed by the patient. This contrasts dramatically with the more usual medical situation of the body biodegrading, say, 100 mg of a specific drug.

The primary clinical relevance of these observations is that in some cases the biotransformation intermediates or end-products are toxic if sufficiently high concentrations are attained intracellularly. The concentrations are dependent both on the rate of formation and on the rates of redistribution and elimination. Furthermore, the actual biodegradation pathway also appears to be dependent on a variety of environmental and genetic factors (illustrated in the discussion of the fluroxene studies). These facts have made the clinical and basic research in this area complicated and sometimes inconclusive.

There are now over 500 papers, published in approximately 100 journals, relevant to the subject; in an attempt to make the topic comprehensible, the present chapter is deliberately not divided into each anaesthetic, its breakdown products and its potential toxicity. Instead, the present position is summarized by considering first the site and mode of breakdown of the agents and then the relationships between biotransformation, postoperative toxicity and chronic toxicity. To illustrate these aspects, the biotransformation of all the current clinical volatile agents will be included (*Table 7.1*). The biotransformation of the gaseous agents such as cyclopropane and nitrous oxide have not yet been established unequivocally in animal or human studies. However, it is interesting to note that *in vitro* nitrous oxide reacts with vitamin B_{12}, oxidizing the cobalt (Blackburn, Kyaw and Swallow, 1977), and this type of reaction may also occur *in vivo*.

SITE AND MODE OF BIOTRANSFORMATION

The principal organ associated with anaesthetic biotransformation is the liver but it should not be forgotten that other areas also have this capability. For example, cerebral biotransformation may account for up to 5% of the total amount metabolized, and recently pulmonary biotransformation has been demonstrated (Blitt, Brown and Wright, 1977). The biotransformation enzymes in these extrahepatic sites appear to be equally efficient but the liver predominates because of both the high concentration of enzymes in its cells and its very large over-all size. In addition, the liver microsomal enzymes in particular are susceptible to enzyme induction.

TABLE 7.1. Summary of inhalational anaesthetics biotransformation

Agent	Breakdown intermediates	Final products
$CH_3OCF_2CHCl_2$ (methoxyflurane)		$\boxed{F^-}$
	CH_3OCF_2COOH (methoxydifluoroacetic acid) $CHCl_2COOH$ (dichloroacetic acid)	COOH | COOH (oxalic acid) Cl^-
	HCHO (formaldehyde) $\longrightarrow$	CO_2
$CCl_2 = CHCl$ (trichloroethylene)	$[CCl_2OHCHClOH]$ (chloral hydrate)	CCl_3COOH (trichloroacetic acid) $\boxed{CCl_3CH_2OH}$ (trichloroethanol)
$CHCl_3$ (chloroform)	$\boxed{\cdot CCl_3}$ $\boxed{: CCl_2}$ chloromethyl radicals	CO_2
CHF_2OCF_2CHFCl (enflurane)		F^-
$C_2H_5OC_2H_5$ (diethyl ether)	CH_3CH_2OH (ethanol) CH_3CHO (acetaldehyde) CH_3COOH (acetic acid)	CO_2
$CF_3CH_2OCH = CH_2$ (fluroxene)	$\boxed{CF_3CH_2OH}$ (trifluoroethanol)	CF_3COOH (trifluoroacetic acid) CO_2
$CF_3CHClBr$ (halothane)	Oxidation intermediates	$\left\{ \begin{array}{l} CF_3COOH \\ \text{(trifluoroacetic acid)} \\ Br^- + Cl^- \end{array} \right.$
	Reduction intermediates	$\left\{ \begin{array}{l} CF_3CH_2Cl \\ \text{(1,1,1-trifluoro-2-chloroethane)} \\ CF_2CHCl \\ \text{(1,1-difluoro-2-chloroethylene)} \end{array} \right.$
	$(CF_3C.^{\nearrow O})$	$CF_3CONHCH_2CH_2OH$ (trifluoroacetyl ethanolamide)
		N-Acetyl-cysteine-$CF_2CHBrCl$ (2-Bromo-2-chloro-1,1-difluoro ethyl-N-acetyl-L-cysteine)

Types of biotransformation

Within the cell, two types of transformation can take place (*Table 7.2*). Phase I involves an oxidation, reduction or hydrolysis of the drug. The volatile agents normally undergo oxidation although reduction has also been demonstrated in the case of halothane in particular (Van Dyke and Gandolfi, 1976). Phase II reactions are conjugations in which the products of phase I (or drugs not subject to phase I attack) are combined with a naturally occurring constituent such as glutathione. The results of these processes are that the products of phase I reactions have an increased water solubility and also an increased chemical reactivity for phase II conjugations which, in turn, produce end-products suitable for excretion via the kidneys.

TABLE 7.2. Biotransformation reactions
(those particularly important in inhaled anaesthetic reactions are in bold type)

Type of reaction		*Examples*
Phase I	**Oxidation**	Hydroxylation (aliphatic and aromatic)
		O-**Dealkylation** (ether cleavage)
		N-Dealkylation
		Dehalogenation
		Sulphoxidation
		Desulphuration
		Epoxidation
	Reduction	Nitro reduction
		Azo reduction
		Halothane reduction
	Hydrolysis	De-esterification
Phase II	**Conjugation**	**Glucuronic acid conjugation**
		Mercapturic acid conjugation
		Sulphate conjugation
		Amide synthesis

Intracellular site of biotransformation

The intracellular locations of the different enzymes for these processes are related to their functions and the physical properties of the substrates on which they act. The phase I oxidation and reduction enzymes are in the hydrophobic areas of the endoplasmic reticulum membranes while the phase I hydrolysis and phase II conjugation enzymes are associated with the more aqueous environment of the cell cytoplasm. The endoplasmic reticulum is a system of membranes which are either smooth or rough (i.e. studded with ribosomes) when observed with electron microscopy (Chapter 1). Both types of membrane are thought to be involved in the over-all process of assembling the enzymes and substrates in the appropriate locations for the various transformations. However, the endoplasmic reticulum cannot be separated from the cell intact and, when liver tissue is homogenized and centrifuged, the membrane breaks up and forms small spheres known as microsomes. The enzyme systems in these microsomes have been extensively studied *in vitro* and are known to be primarily concerned with metabolism of foreign compounds as well as of some endogeneous substrates such as steroid hormones and cholesterol.

Cytochrome P450

The enzyme system associated with the oxidation reaction — known as 'the microsomal mixed function oxidase system' — has a key enzyme, cytochrome P450, so called because it binds carbon monoxide when reduced and absorbs light at a wavelength of 450 nm. The intensity of this absorption can be used as an assay of the amount of enzyme present. More sophisticated biochemical experiments (e.g. Welton *et al.*, 1975) have demonstrated that this enzyme is not a single substance but probably

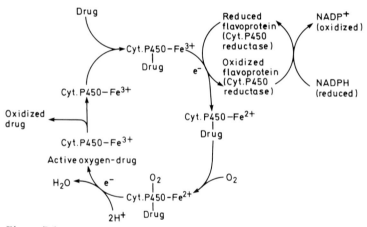

Figure 7.1
Part of the biochemical pathways for lipid-soluble drug
biotransformation

consists of an association of at least three haemoproteins. Furthermore, if the system is induced by pretreatment with polycylic hydrocarbons, another cytochrome absorption maximum occurs at 448 nm and this enzyme has been termed cytochrome P448. Some of the complexities of the biochemistry are illustrated in *Figure 7.1*. It will be seen that there is yet another enzyme termed NADPH-cytochrome c reductase, which has been demonstrated to increase specifically after both halothane and enflurane anaesthetic (Rietbrock, 1974). Further details of the biochemistry of biotransformation are included in Chapter 2.

The enzymes' capacities to biotransform anaesthetics are negligible in the mammalian fetus and the newborn infant but subsequently increase with age. However, genetic and environmental factors determine both the extent and the pattern of biochemical degradation for the different anaesthetics. For any specific anaesthetic the extent of biotransformation is determined not only by its chemical structure but also by its hydrophobic solubility. If it is very fat-soluble, the agent will be retained in the body for a long time and will continue to be biotransformed as it passes and repasses through the liver. In addition, increased hydrophobicity of the agent increases its access to the phase I enzymes located in hydrophobic areas. The biochemical pathway for the biotransformation of a particular anaesthetic is determined primarily by the chemical structure of the agent. For example, the initial steps in the oxidation reactions are favoured by electrons associated with bonding between the atoms being unequally distributed to particular parts of the molecule. It is possible to calculate these distributions using molecular orbital theory; on this basis Loew, Trudell and Motulsky (1973) predicted that the relative ease of defluorination of fluorinated methyl ethyl ethers would be methoxyflurane > enflurane > isoflurane. As will be seen in the next section, other features can modify these basic concepts.

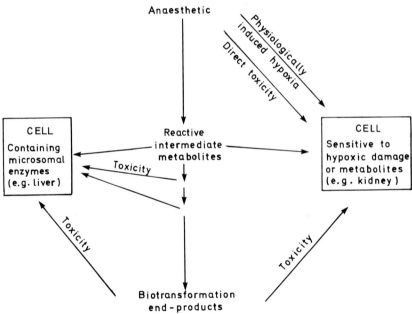

Figure 7.2
Possible routes of cellular toxicity for anaesthetics and/or biotransformation products

BIOTRANSFORMATION AND POSTOPERATIVE TOXICITY

Cellular damage associated with anaesthesia can be due either to direct toxicity or alteration of physiological variables producing tissue hypoxia, etc., or to the indirect effect of biotransformation producing toxic intermediates or end-products (*Figure 7.2*). It is sometimes difficult to distinguish between these alternatives, but the distinctions are important because the clinical solutions to the problems may be very different. In general, if it is direct or physiologically induced toxicity, the maximum concentration of the agent is critical, whereas if it is indirect biotransformation-induced toxicity, it is the total accumulated dose which is more important. In addition, the clinical implications of potential drug interactions are completely different in the two cases.

Chloroform and free radical formation

One example of distinguishing between alternative mechanisms of toxicity is provided by the studies on chloroform. In the 1960s there were two alternative hypotheses for its hepatotoxicity: vasoconstriction of the blood flow in liver lobules (Calvert and Brody, 1960) or toxic metabolites (Butler, 1961). One of the first applications of low temperature autoradiography to studies on anaesthetic metabolism demonstrated the accumulation of non-volatile metabolites of ^{14}C-labelled chloroform (Cohen and Hood, 1969), but it was not known if this was coincidental to the hepatotoxicity or its cause. Scholler (1970) then carried out the critical studies relating hepatotoxicity to biotransformation of the agent. He increased the activity of the microsomal enzymes which split up chloroform by pretreating rats with phenobarbitone (60 mg·kg^{-1} intramuscularly, daily for 11 days) and then found that the increased biotransformation of chloroform was associated with a statistically significant increase in hepatotoxicity, as measured by increasing both serum transaminases and the zone of liver cell necrosis. Furthermore, the preadministration of disulfiram, which inhibits the breakdown of many lipid-soluble drugs, was found to suppress the toxicity of chloroform completely.

This demonstration of increased toxicity with enzyme induction and decreased toxicity with enzyme inhibition is one of the classic tests for biotransformation-related effects. The other obvious test is to administer the presumed breakdown products and see if these produce the same pattern of toxicity. Although, as will be discussed later, this has been done for other agents, this was not possible in the case of chloroform because it is the short-lived reactive intermediates rather than the end-products which cause the toxicity. Chloroform is postulated to form the free radicals ·CCl$_3$ and :CCl$_2$ (Van Dyke, 1969). A free radical has an unpaired electron in the outer molecular orbital of the compound. It is thus highly reactive and can bind covalently to any other molecule which is close. This in turn may make the second molecule reactive and the induced chain of reactions may result in tissue damage. For example, the hepatic endoplasmic reticulum containing the biotransformation enzymes initiating this process can itself be attacked by free radicals. These decompose the unsaturated fatty acid components of the membranes by removing hydrogen from the α-methylene carbon and subsequent attack by oxygen results in lipoperoxidation. As it continues, lipoperoxidation produces severe functional and structural impairment to the adjacent lipids and ultimately the cell membrane is destroyed. Studies have now demonstrated this lipoperoxidation damage *in vitro* in hepatic microsomes prepared from rats anaesthetized with chloroform (and halothane) (Brown, 1972). Thus chloroform provides a clear example of an agent which is biotransformed, producing highly reactive intermediates which in turn cause tissue damage in the locality of the enzymes associated with the transformation.

Methoxyflurane and fluoride ion

The alternative type of biotransformation toxicity results from the end-products of the process which may then be redistributed throughout the body and cause toxicity in the most vulnerable tissues or organs. The best documented example is methoxyflurane. In summary, the polyuric renal insufficiency which can follow its administration has been correlated with total dose (rather than concentration) of the agent and with the concentrations of its breakdown products. The toxicity has been demonstrated to be enhanced by enzyme induction, attenuated by enzyme inhibition and produced by the administration of the presumed toxic metabolites on their own.

Methoxyflurane was administered to approximately 12 million patients before the link with postoperative renal tubular dysfunction was seriously considered (Committee on Anesthesia, NAS–NRC, 1971). Although there had been isolated case reports before, the coincidence of three separate studies in 1970 drew attention to the potential problem. Frascino and his colleagues (Frascino, Venemee and Rosen, 1970) reported finding a high degree of oxalate precipitation in the renal tubules of 11 patients in renal failure after methoxyflurane anaesthesia. As always in such clinical studies, many factors, including the fact that some of the operations were on the urinary tract, complicated the interpretation. Then two papers from Rochester, New York (Panner *et al.*, 1970; Taves *et al.*, 1970) reported the death of two obese patients within 24 hours of methoxyflurane anaesthesia for abdominal operations. They had polyuric renal failure, and autopsy revealed oxalate crystals in the renal tubules. In addition, the concentrations of fluoride ion in the serum of one of the patients had been measured. These increased postoperatively to levels ($275\ \mu\text{mol·l}^{-1}$) higher than those estimated to have been attained in the much earlier experiments of Goldemberg (1930) who produced polyuria in man by sodium fluoride administration.

The third study was carried out by Mazze and his colleagues at Stanford, who had had a long-standing interest in renal function following anaesthesia. In a prospective study they compared the renal functions of two groups of 12 patients who had received either methoxyflurane or halothane. Abnormalities were found in all cases with the former but none with the latter agent. They separated their methoxyflurane group of patients into those with serious clinical nephrotoxicity and those with only laboratory observable abnormalities in renal function. The daily serum inorganic fluoride concentration and oxalic acid excretions were found to reach a maximum approximately two days postoperatively and the levels in those patients with clinically evident nephrotoxicity were about twice those in patients with laboratory abnormalities only (Mazze, Trudell and Cousins, 1971). From the patterns of renal dysfunction (e.g. polyuria rather than classic anuric renal failure), it was argued that the primary nephrotoxin was probably the fluoride ion.

One problem in determining the general clinical significance of the Stanford study was that, in order to avoid difficulties in interpretation which are inherent when many drugs are involved, the methoxyflurane was administered without anaesthetic adjuvants (except *d*-tubocurarine).

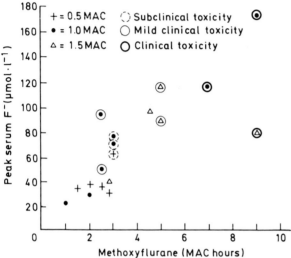

Figure 7.3
Peak serum inorganic fluoride concentration (F⁻) and degree of nephrotoxicity at increasing doses of methoxyflurane (MAC hours). Methoxyflurane dose correlated with both peak serum inorganic fluoride concentration and degree of nephrotoxicity. Patients with subclinical toxicity: 2.5–3 MAC hours; F^-, 50–80 $\mu mol \cdot l^{-1}$. Patients with mild clinical toxicity: 5 MAC hours; F^-, 90–120 $\mu mol \cdot l^{-1}$. Patients with clinical toxicity: 7–9 MAC hours; F^-, 80–175 $\mu mol \cdot l^{-1}$. (Reproduced with permission from Cousins and Mazze, 1973, *J. Am. med. Ass.*, **255**, 1611, © 1971 American Medical Association)

Thus the concentrations of methoxyflurane used were several times higher than those normally needed when administered with nitrous oxide and oxygen. A subsequent prospective clinical study of general surgical patients in which anaesthetic adjuvants were used cleared up this problem and defined the general dose range associated with nephrotoxicity (Cousins and Mazze, 1973). The patients were divided into groups receiving low, medium or high anaesthetic concentrations (i.e. 0.5, 1.0, 1.5 MAC)*

* The concept of MAC is defined in Chapter 3. *Ed.*

of methoxyflurane, and a control group receiving high concentrations (i.e. 1.0—1.5 MAC) of halothane. The serum fluoride concentrations were measured daily postoperatively and there was a reasonable correlation with the total methoxyflurane dose expressed as the average end-tidal concentration multiplied by the duration of anaesthesia (MAC hours) (*Figure 7.3*). This method of measuring dose is, of course, only an approximation, primarily because it does not include the long period of elimination of the agent. The resulting nephrotoxicity in the patients was classified into: (1) subclinical — delayed return to maximum preoperative urinary osmolality, unresponsiveness to vasopressin administration and elevated serum uric acid concentrations; (2) mild clinical — serum hyperosmolality, hypernatraemia, polyuria and low urine osmolality; (3) clinical toxicity — vasopressin-resistant polyuria, hypernatraemia, serum hyperosmolality, elevated blood urea and serum creatinine, and marked thirst. Although, as would be expected. the correlation between toxicity and MAC hours of methoxyflurane or peak serum fluoride (*Figure 7.3*) was not perfect, the clinical conclusions were clear. The onset of subclinical renal toxicity occurred at approximately 2.5 MAC hours, which corresponded to a serum inorganic fluoride level above 50 μmol$\cdot$l^{-1}. At 2.5—5.0 MAC hours corresponding to serum inorganic fluoride concentrations of 50—120 μmol$\cdot$l^{-1}, there was usually mild clinical toxicity while, at levels above 6 MAC hours (and above 80 μmol$\cdot$l^{-1} fluoride concentration), there was clinical toxicity. Allowing for the inaccuracies of determining anaesthetic dosage in clinical practice, it was suggested that surgical anaesthesia with methoxyflurane should be limited to two hours. This approach should ensure that some renal reserve would be present even if a patient were particularly sensitive to inorganic fluoride as a nephrotoxin, or metabolized methoxyflurane unexpectedly rapidly.

The threshold nephrotoxic serum concentration of inorganic fluoride indicated by the Stanford studies is of the order of 50 μmol$\cdot$l^{-1}. However, it should be noted that most of the patients in these studies needed prolonged intravenous feeding and there were frequent periods of dehydration. Holaday and his colleagues at Miami (1972) found that, following methoxyflurane anaesthesia in volunteers, careful maintenance of fluid balance prevented hypernatraemia and dehydration, and minimized the clinical signs and symptoms of nephrotoxicity. However, they found the urine-concentrating ability (as revealed by challenging with standard water deprivation and exogenous vasopressin) was depressed by over 50% on days 2 to 5 following methoxyflurane anaesthesia of only an hour's duration. It subsequently returned to preanaesthetic control values within a fortnight. More recently, a study at San Diego (Mazze, Calverley and Smith, 1977) indicated a 25% reversible depression of maximum urinary osmolality following nearly 10 MAC hours of enflurane anaesthesia which had resulted in a mean peak fluoride concentration of only 34 μmol$\cdot$l^{-1}. However, the urine-concentrating ability appears to be a very sensitive test of potential nephrotoxicity, and minor impairment, such as that in the enflurane study, probably has no serious clinical consequences provided there is sufficient renal reserve.

Halothane and the bromide ion

In both the Miami and the San Diego studies, volunteers exposed to halothane anaesthesia were used as control groups and their postanaesthetic urine-concentrating ability was actually slightly enhanced rather than depressed. Since halothane does not appear to form significant quantities of fluoride ion, the lack of any impairment is not surprising. However, halothane does form bromide ions, which is interesting for two reasons. First, the quantification of this effect (Tinker, Gandolfi and Van Dyke, 1976) is one of the best examples of the levels of a breakdown product being directly related to the anaesthetic concentration multiplied by the duration of exposure (i.e. MAC hours); this is probably because the removal of bromide from the blood is relatively slow (half-life 11.5 days) and so the kinetics of elimination do not complicate the issue. Second, the values of bromide following very long periods of anaesthesia (up to 10–14 MAC hours) can approach 3 $mmol \cdot l^{-1}$ (Tinker, Gandolfi and Van Dyke, 1976; Mazze, Calverley and Smith, 1977), which is high enough to produce postoperative sedation.

Trichloroethylene and trichloroethanol

The other agent whose metabolites may produce postoperative depression of the central nervous system is trichloroethylene. This agent is bio-transformed to trichloroethanol, which is also the pharmacologically active metabolite of chloral hydrate. One example of the clinical relevance of this was provided by an epileptic patient who had had chronic treatment with phenobarbitone and phenytoin for many years prior to an hour-long operation with trichloroethylene anaesthesia. He remained drowsy and barely rousable for 40 hours, with the plasma trichloroethanol levels ($7–13$ $mg \cdot l^{-1}$) sufficient to account for heavy sedation (A. M. Hewlett and M. J. Halsey, unpublished observations). In this case, the clinical consequences of toxicity related to biotransformation were not subtle or slowly developing but obvious to everybody concerned.

THE PROBLEM OF SPECIES DIFFERENCE

The majority of the data described in the previous section has been obtained in man but it is not always possible to define the extent of the clinical problem.

Methoxyflurane

One unanswered question is how far does enzyme induction by a variety of drugs affect the potential for biotransformation toxicity? It is unusual to find patients with as dramatic a case of enzyme induction as the trichloroethylene example cited above, and the majority of work in this area has been done in animals. For example, pretreatment of Fisher 344 rats with phenobarbitone prior to a low dose of methoxyflurane resulted in increased biotransformation producing more severe renal lesions and functional impairment (Cousins *et al.*, 1974). The same animal model has been used for demonstrating that combinations of gentamicin and methoxy-flurane resulted in higher serum fluoride levels and greater renal insufficiency than either drug used alone (Barr *et al.*, 1973). Not only are animal models necessary for drug interaction experiments which are not ethically possible to undertake in man, but also they provide essential complementary evidence about the putative toxicity of alternative metabolites. For example, methoxyflurane produces two metabolic end-products: fluoride ion and oxalic acid. Either might be expected to cause changes in renal function, but injection of F^- into rats produced changes in renal function and histology similar to those seen following methoxyflurane administration, whereas injection of the alternative toxic agent, oxalic acid, did not (Cousins *et al.*, 1974). However, it should not be forgotten that the data from animal models can be difficult to interpret, especially in biotransformation research. Five different rat strains were screened before it was found that only one, the Fisher 344, developed methoxyflurane nephrotoxicity (Mazze, Cousins and Kosek, 1973). There is also a sixfold variation in the amount of methoxyflurane defluorination in the mouse, rat, guinea-pig, rabbit, calf and monkey (Murray and Fleming, 1972).

Fluroxene

One of the most dramatic examples of misleading evidence from animal data is provided by the studies on fluroxene (Wardell, 1973). After more than a decade of apparently safe clinical use, the agent was demonstrated to be lethal if given in long or repeat exposures in the dog, cat and rabbit (Johnston *et al.*, 1973), mice (Cascorbi and Singh-Amaranath, 1972) and rats (Harrison and Smith, 1973). If these particular experiments had been carried out 20 years earlier, the agent would never have been released. There have been studies on the contributions of various component groups of the fluroxene molecule to its toxicity (Harrison *et al.*, 1976), and on the toxicity of trifluoroethanol, one of the end-products of biotransformation (Blake, Cascorbi and Rozman, 1969). These demonstrated that trifluoroethanol was the toxic metabolite. It is now thought that, although at least 10% of fluroxene is metabolized in man, the amount of trifluoroethanol produced is very small (Gion *et al.*, 1974). Subsequent studies in rhesus monkey are consistent with the data in man but have emphasized the potential dangers of fluroxene administration following enzyme induction with phenobarbitone (Munson, Malagodi and Shields, 1975). It now appears that 'enzyme induction' can change the pathway of biotransformation as well as the extent of the phenomenon.

Halothane and the liver

Animal studies are continuing, in spite of the difficulties of interpretation, in the area of halothane hepatotoxicity. Halothane hepatitis in man is a rare and unpredictable occurrence, which makes research in man virtually impossible. However, in view of its severity, research is important and it is therefore necessary to develop an animal model. The early attempts to do so were not successful because, although halothane was metabolized to a variety of metabolites (including trifluoroacetic acid, chloride and bromide), the hepatic injury was inconsistent except in long-term chronic exposures (which is discussed in the next section). Induction of the hepatic microsomal enzymes of rats with phenobarbitone slightly enhanced the binding of halothane metabolites to microsomes – suggesting the formation of reactive intermediates – but did not lead to massive centrilobular necrosis (Brown, Sipes and Sagalyn, 1974). Recently, however, hepatic necrosis has been induced in rats by a single exposure to 1% halothane in oxygen following pretreatment of an alternative enzyme inducer – Aroclor 1254, a polychlorinated biphenyl compound (Sipes and Brown, 1976). Within 2 hours of anaesthesia the serum transaminase levels were above normal, and 24 hours later centrilobular hepatocyte necrosis was prominent (Reynolds and Moslen, 1977). The mechanisms of this toxicity have not yet been defined but the toxic pathways for biotransformation of halothane may not involve increased protein binding or its oxidation to soluble excretable metabolites. An alternative set of circumstances which may lead to halothane hepatotoxicity is anaesthesia at reduced oxygen tensions. In the first experiments rats were exposed to halothane in 7% oxygen and the amount of defluorination increased (Widger, Gandolfi and Van Dyke, 1976). Subsequently, halothane anaesthesia following phenobarbitone pretreatment with only a moderate degree of hypoxia (14% inspired oxygen concentration) has been demonstrated to produce consistent hepatic necrosis and rises in transaminases in male (but not female) rats. Interestingly, blocking of oxidative phosphorylation by the common enzyme inhibitor, SKF-525-A, enhanced rather than inhibited the toxicity. It is possible that the inhibitor shunted more halothane to a reductive biotransformation path (McLain *et al.,* 1977). It must be emphasized that any clinical implications of these current animal studies are at present speculative, although few would disagree that even mild hypoxia during anaesthesia is potentially dangerous for more than one reason.

BIOTRANSFORMATION AND CHRONIC TOXICITY

There is an important distinction between toxicity produced directly by an administered compound and toxicity produced indirectly by its biotransformation to a toxic metabolite. Except in the case of a sensitivity reaction, the former is normally directly related to the concentration of the compound and decreasing the concentration reduces the toxicity proportionately. However, the latter has a more complicated dependence on concentration since the rates of formation, distribution and elimination of metabolites can vary independently of the rate of administration. Thus, reducing the concentration of an administered compound, say, tenfold might be expected to reduce the direct toxicity below its threshold but this is not necessarily the case for indirect toxicity. There is already good evidence for this anomaly in the concentration dependence of biotransformation.

Dependence of biotransformation on concentration of anaesthetics

In man, excretion of urinary metabolites of methoxyflurane is sustained at relatively constant levels for up to 40 hours post anaesthesia (Holaday, Rudofsky and Treuhaft, 1970). At first sight this is surprising since the methoxyflurane partial pressure decreases exponentially over this period while apparently the absolute rate of metabolism remains constant. The problem was investigated by Sawyer and his colleagues at San Francisco (1971, 1972). Most of the previous studies had used the appearance of metabolites as an indication of metabolism but this group studied the disappearance of anaesthetic from the hepatic circulation. They determined the fraction of anaesthetic removed by the livers of surgically prepared miniature swine. At high alveolar concentrations (i.e. at MAC) the liver extracted little of the anaesthetic passing through it but at one-hundredth of MAC the fraction extracted was 50% and at one-thousandth of MAC it approached 100%. The most reasonable explanation for the extraction was its metabolism by the liver. Subsequent studies (Halsey *et al.*, 1971), using the same animal model, demonstrated quantitatively that the amounts of metabolism of the agents halothane, methoxyflurane, enflurane and isoflurane correlated very well with those in man (the amount of isoflurane metabolism in man was not known until four years later – Holaday *et al.*, 1975). This phenomenon in miniature swine is also consistent with the fact that halothane anaesthesia in man decreases the metabolism of tracer amounts of radioactive halothane (Cascorbi, Blake and Helrich, 1970).

The mechanism of this concentration dependence is unknown. It appears that the biotransformation rate reaches a maximum at relatively low concentrations of anaesthetic, and thus as the concentration increases, the efficiency of the system (i.e. rate of biotransformation divided by rate of hepatic supply) decreases. The maximum or plateau in the biotransformation rate could be because the amount of enzyme becomes the rate-limiting factor or because the activity of the enzyme is depressed either by substrate (i.e. anaesthetic) or by product (i.e. metabolite) inhibition. However, regardless of the exact mechanism, the important implication for toxicity caused by products of biotransformation is that a greater quantity of metabolites may be produced by subanaesthetic concentration than by exposure to an anaesthetizing concentration when each is administered for the same number of MAC hours. Furthermore, it would be predicted that increasing the length of anaesthesia would not proportionately increase the quantity of metabolites.

Recent experiments by Anne White *et al.* (1975) have confirmed these predictions. Fluoride excretion was used as a measure of anaesthetic biotransformation of enflurane (*Figure 7.4*). It was found that sub-anaesthetic doses produced four to eight times the amount of metabolites produced by the comparable anaesthetizing doses. Increasing the sub-anaesthetic exposure increased the amount of metabolites whereas the

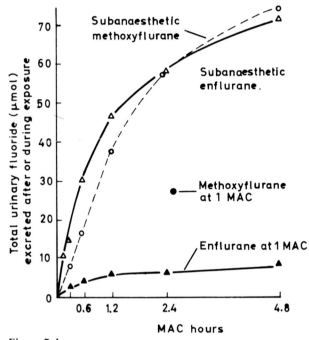

Figure 7.4
Comparison of urinary fluoride excreted after or during exposure to methoxyflurane or enflurane at subanaesthetic or 1 MAC doses. Points represent an average of data from 8 animals. (Reproduced from White *et al.*, 1975, by courtesy of the authors)

increase with anaesthetizing exposure came to a definite plateau. The clinical implication of these data is that breathing low concentrations for a prolonged period is at least as dangerous, if not more so, as breathing higher concentrations for a proportionately shorter period. This view is supported by the work of Atallah and Geddes (1973), who demonstrated that the levels of blood bromide were up to six times greater post anaesthesia (44 hours) than those measured during the actual anaesthetic period. Thus the generalized concept of MAC hours being directly related to toxicity is an oversimplification if the range of anaesthetic levels is very large.

Continuous exposure to anaesthetics

The toxic aspects of chronic exposure have been investigated in a series of experiments in San Francisco, where mice, rats and guinea-pigs were exposed to low doses of anaesthetics day and night for periods varying from 7 to 35 days. In the initial series there were dose-related hepatic injuries with halothane exposure but not with isoflurane or diethyl ether (Stevens *et al.*, 1975). This can be related to biotransformation because the agent which produced the toxicity (halothane) is known to be metabolized and some metabolites are toxic (see previous section). On the other hand, the two agents which were relatively innocuous were either minimally biotransformed (isoflurane) or biotransformed to compounds normally found in the body (diethyl ether).

In the second series (Stevens *et al.*, 1977), fluroxene was demonstrated to be toxic even in doses as low as 0.0005 MAC (30 p.p.m.), whereas enflurane at 0.1 MAC was toxic in mice only. Nitrous oxide appeared to be as relatively innocuous as isoflurane or ether. These experiments all featured continuous exposure day and night but the threshold concentration for halothane hepatotoxicity was in the range of 15–50 p.p.m., which contrasts with the much higher anaesthetizing concentration failing to produce injury under oxidative conditions. In conclusion, it should be noted that these hepatic effects in animals occur at very low concentrations of halothane which are orders of magnitude lower than those which may cause significant fetotoxicity. It has not proved possible to repeat many of the chronic exposure studies on pregnant animals but, for example, fetal growth retardation is now thought to occur in rats only if the chronic halothane concentration is above 1500 p.p.m. (Pope *et al.*, 1978).

The essential features of chronic exposure are that (1) the formation of the intermediate and end-products of biotransformation occurs continuously and at maximum efficiency; (2) there is a slow progressive accumulation of the products which are chemically stable and not immediately eliminated from the body — many of the non-volatile products have long half-lives; and (3) in the case of toxic products, the tissues or cell constituents are being attacked continuously and the repair processes of the cell are severely hampered.

CONCLUSION

The postoperative and chronic toxicity of the currently used clinical anaesthetics is often related to their biotransformation. This has led to the search for new anaesthetics which are not biotransformed at all, but this goal appears to be unattainable. In any case, it is clear that metabolism of an agent *per se* does not necessarily lead to toxicity (e.g. the diethyl ether chronic exposure studies). However, in view of the importance in understanding the underlying mechanisms of toxicity, there is very active research in this area and the subject is advancing rapidly. For example, after the first draft of this chapter was written, the first volatile halogenated metabolites of halothane were discovered (Mukai *et al.*, 1977) as well as the importance of the reductive biochemical pathways (see section 'Halothane and the liver'). For those who wish to read further about the background work and the state of the subject up to the beginning of 1977, the monograph by Cohen and Van Dyke (1977) is both comprehensible and comprehensive.

References

Atallah, M. M. and Geddes, I. C. (1973). Metabolism of halothane during and after anaesthesia in man. *Br. J. Anaesth.* 45, 464–469

Barr, G. A., Mazze, R. I., Cousins, M. J. and Kosek, J. C. (1973). An animal model for combined methoxyflurane and gentamicin nephrotoxicity. *Br. J. Anaesth.* 45, 306–312

Barrett, H. M. and Johnston, J. H. (1939). The fate of trichoroethylene in the organism. *J. Biol. Chem.* 127, 765

Blackburn, R., Kyaw, M. and Swallow, A. J. (1977). Reaction of cob(I)alamin with nitrous oxide and cob(III)alamin. *J. Chem. Soc.* 73, 250–255

Blake, D. A., Cascorbi, M. F. and Rozman, R. S. (1969). Animal toxicity of 2,2,2-trifluroethanol. *Toxic. appl. Pharmac.* 15, 83

Blitt, C. D., Brown, B. R. and Wright, B. J. (1977). Pulmonary biotransformation of halogenated inhalational anaesthetics. American Society of Anesthesiologists Annual Meeting, *Scientific Abstracts* pp. 489–490

Brown, B. R. (1972). Hepatic microsomal lipoperoxidation and inhalation anesthetics: a biochemical and morphologic study in the rat. *Anesthesiology* 36, 458–465

Brown, B. R., Sipes, I. G. and Sagalyn, A. M. (1974). Mechanisms of acute hepatic toxicity: chloroform, halothane and glutathione. *Anesthesiology* 41, 554–561

Butler, T. C. (1961). Reduction of carbon tetrachloride *in vivo* and reduction of carbon tetrachloride and chloroform *in vitro* by tissue and tissue constituents. *J. Pharmac. exp. Ther.* 134, 311

Calvert, D. N. and Brody, T. M. (1960). Role of the sympathetic nervous system in CCl_4 hepatotoxicity. *Am. J. Physiol.* 198, 669

Cascorbi, H. F. and Singh-Amaranath, A. V. (1972). Fluroxene toxicity in mice. *Anesthesiology* 37, 480–482

Cascorbi, H. F., Blake, D. A. and Helrich, M. (1970). Differences in the biotransformation of halothane in man. *Anesthesiology* 32, 119–123

Chase, R. E., Holaday, D. A., Fiserova-Bergerova, V., Saidman, L. J. and Mack, F. E. (1971). The biotransformation of Ethrane in man. *Anesthesiology* 35, 262–273

Cohen, E. N. and Hood, N. (1969). Application of low temperature autoradiography to studies of the uptake and metabolism of volatile anesthetics in the mouse. I. Chloroform. *Anesthesiology* 30, 306–314

Cohen, E. N. and Van Dyke, R. A. (1977). *Metabolism of Volatile Anesthetics.* Reading, Massachusetts: Addison-Wesley

Committee on Anesthesia, NAS–NRC (1971). Statement regarding the role of methoxyflurane in the production of renal dysfunction. *Anesthesiology* 34, 505–509

Cousins, M. J. and Mazze, R. I. (1973). Methoxyflurane nephrotoxicity; a study of dose response in man. *J. Am. med. Ass.* 225, 1611–1616

Cousins, M. J., Mazze, R. I., Kosek, J. C., Hitt, B. A. and Love, F. V. (1974). The etiology of methoxyflurane nephrotoxicity. *J. Pharmac. exp. Ther.* 190, 530–541

Fiserova-Bergerova, V. (1973). Changes of fluoride content in bone; an index of drug defluorination *in vivo. Anesthesiology* 38, 345–351

Frascino, J. A., Venemee, P. and Rosen, P. P. (1970). Renal oxalosis and azotemia after methoxyflurane anesthesia. *New Engl. J. Med.* 283, 676–679

Gion, H., Yoshimura, N., Holaday, D. A., Fiserova-Bergerova, V. and Chase, R. E. (1974). Biotransformation of fluroxene in man. *Anesthesiology* 40, 553–562

Goldemberg, L. (1930). Tratamiento de la enfermedad de Basedow: y del hipertiroidismo por fluor. *Revta Soc. Med. interna Soc. tisiol.* 6, 217–242

Halsey, M. J., Sawyer, D. C., Eger, E. I., Bahlman, S. H. and Impelman, D. M. (1971). Hepatic metabolism of halothane, methoxyflurane, cyclopropane, Ethrane and Forane in miniature swine. *Anesthesiology* 35, 43–47

Harrison, G. G. and Smith, J. S. (1973). Massive lethal hepatic necrosis in rats anesthetized with fluroxene, after microsomal enzyme induction. *Anesthesiology* 39, 619

Harrison, G. G., Ivanetich, K. M., Kaminsky, L. and Halsey, M. J. (1976). Fluroxene (2,2,2-trifluoroethyl vinyl ether) toxicity: a chemical aspect. *Anesth. Analg.* 55, 529–533

Holaday, D. A., Rudofsky, S. and Truehaft, P. S. (1970). The metabolic degradation of methoxyflurane in man. *Anesthesiology* 33, 579–593

Holaday, P. A., Yoshimura, N., Fiserova-Bergerova, V., Hotchkiss, J. L. and Vaamonde, C. A. (1972). Relationship between methoxyflurane and renal concentrating ability. American Society of Anesthesiologists Annual Meeting, *Scientific Abstracts* pp. 41–42

Holaday, D. A., Fiserova-Bergerova, V., Latto, I. P. and Zumbiel, M. A. (1975). Resistance of isoflurane to biotransformation in man. *Anesthesiology* 43, 325–332

Johnston, R. R., Cromwell, T. H., Eger, E. I., Cullen, D., Stevens, W. C. and Joas, T. (1973). The toxicity of fluroxene in animals and man. *Anesthesiology* 38, 313–319

Loew, G., Trudell, J. and Motulsky, H. (1973). Quantum chemical studies of the metabolism of a series of chlorinated Ethane anesthetics. *Molec. Pharmac.* 9, 152–162

McLain, G. E., Sipes, I. G., Brown, B. R. and Thompson, M. F. (1977). An animal model of halothane hepatotoxicity on reductive biotransformation. American Society of Anesthesiologists Annual Meeting, *Scientific Abstracts* pp. 481—482

Mazze, R. I., Calverley, R. K. and Smith, N. T. (1977). Inorganic fluoride nephrotoxicity: prolonged enflurane and halothane anesthesia in volunteers. *Anesthesiology* 46, 265—271

Mazze, R. I., Cousins, M. J. and Kosek, J. C. (1973). Strain differences in metabolism and susceptibility to the nephrotoxic effects of methoxyflurane in rats. *J. Pharmac. exp. Ther.* 184, 481

Mazze, R. I., Trudell, J. R. and Cousins, M. J. (1971). Methoxyflurane metabolism and renal dysfunction: clinical correlations in man. *Anesthesiology* 35, 247—252

Mukai, S., Morio, M., Fujii, K. and Hanaki, C. (1977). Volatile metabolites of halothane in the rabbit. *Anesthesiology* 47, 248—251

Munson, E. S., Malagodi, M. H. and Shields, R. P. (1975). Fluroxene toxicity induced by phenobarbital. *Clin. Pharmac. Ther.* 18, 687

Murray, W. J. and Fleming, P. J. (1972). Defluorination of methoxyflurane during anesthesia: comparison of man with other species. *Anesthesiology* 37, 620—625

Panner, B. J., Freeman, R. B., Roth-Mayo, L. A. and Markowitch, W. (1970). Toxicity following methoxyflurane anesthesia. I. Clinical and pathological observations in two fatal cases. *J. Am. med. Ass.* 214, 86—90

Pope, W. D. B., Halsey, M. J., Lansdown, A. B. G., Simmonds, A. and Bateman, P. E. (1978). Fetotoxicity in rats following chronic exposure to halothane, nitrous oxide, or methoxyflurane. *Anesthesiology* 48, 11—16

Reynolds, E. S. and Moslen, M. T. (1977). Halothane hepatotoxicity enhancement by polychlorinated biphenyl pretreatment. *Anesthesiology* 47, 19—27

Rietbrock, I. (1974). Tierexperimentelle untersuchungen der leberfunktion unter Ethrane und halothan. In *Ethrane,* Proceedings of the First European Symposium on Modern Anesthetic Agents, pp. 42—58. P. Lawin and R. Beer (ed.). Berlin: Springer Verlag

Sawyer, D. C., Eger, E. I., Bahlman, S. H., Cullen, B. F. and Impelman, D. (1971). Concentration dependence of hepatic halothane metabolism. *Anesthesiology* 34, 230—235

Sawyer, D. C., Eger, E. I., Bahlman, S. H., Halsey, M. J., Cullen, B. F. and Impelman, D. M. (1972). Metabolism of inhalation anesthetics. In *Cellular Biology and Toxicity of Anesthetics,* pp. 238—244. B. R. Fink (ed.). Baltimore: Williams and Wilkins

Scholler, K. L. (1970). Modification of the effects of chloroform on the rat liver. *Br. J. Anaesth.* 42, 603—605

Sipes, I. G. and Brown, B. R. Jr. (1976). An animal model of hepatotoxicity associated with halothane anesthesia. *Anesthesiology* 45, 622—628

Stevens, W. C., Eger, E. I., White, A., Halsey, M. J., Munger, W., Gibbons, R. D., Dolan, W. D. and Shargel, R. (1975). Comparative toxicity of halothane, isoflurane, and diethyl ether at subanesthetic concentrations in laboratory animals. *Anesthesiology* 42, 408—419

Stevens, W. C., Eger, E. I., White, A., Biava, C. G., Gibbons, R. D. and Shargel, R. (1977). Comparative toxicities of enflurane, fluroxene and nitrous oxide at subanaesthetic concentrations in laboratory animals. *Can. Anaesth. Soc. J.* 24, 479—490

Stier, A., Alter, H., Hessler, O. and Rehder, K. (1964). Urinary excretion of bromide in halothane anesthesia. *Anesth. Analg.* 47, 723—728

Taves, D. R., Fry, B. W., Freeman, R. B. and Gillies, A. J. (1970). Toxicity following methoxyflurane anesthesia. II. Fluoride concentrations in nephrotoxicity. *J. Am. med. Ass.* 214, 91—95

Tinker, J. H., Gandolfi, A. J. and Van Dyke, R. A. (1976). Elevation of plasma bromide levels in patients given halothane anesthesia: time correlation with total halothane dosage. *Anesthesiology* 44, 194—196

Van Dyke, R. A. (1966). Metabolism of volatile anesthetics. III. Induction of microsomal dechlorinating and ether-cleaving enzymes. *J. Pharmac. exp. Ther.* 154, 364—369

Van Dyke, R. A. (1969). On the fate of chloroform. *Anesthesiology* 30, 257—258

Van Dyke, R. A. and Chenoweth, M. B. (1965). The metabolism of volatile anesthetics. *Anesthesiology* 26, 348—357

Van Dyke, R. A. and Gandolfi, A. J. (1976). Anaerobic release of fluoride from halothane. *Drug Metab. Disposit.* 4, 40—44

Van Dyke, R. A., Chenoweth, M. B. and Van Poznak, A. (1964). Metabolism of volatile anaesthetics. I. Conversion *in vivo* of several anaesthetics to $^{14}CO_2$ and chloride. *Biochem. Pharmac.* 13, 1239—1247

Wardell, W. M. (1973). Fluroxene and the penicillin lesson. *Anesthesiology* 38, 309—312

Welton, A. F., O'Neal, F. O., Chaney, L. C. and Aust, S. D. (1975). Multiplicity of cytochrome P-450 hemoproteins in rat liver microsomes. *J. Biol. Chem.* 256, 5631—5639

White, A. E., Stevens, W. C., Eger, E. I., Mazze, R. I. and Hitt, B. A. (1975). Enflurane and methoxyflurane metabolism of anesthetic versus sub-anesthetic concentrations. American Society of Anesthesiologists Annual Meeting, *Scientific Abstracts* pp. 135—136

Widger, L. A., Gandolfi, A. J. and Van Dyke, R. A. (1976). Hypoxia and halothane metabolism *in vivo;* release of inorganic fluoride and halothane metabolite binding to cellular constituents. *Anesthesiology* 44, 197—210

Yoshimura, N., Holaday, D. A. and Fiserova-Bergerova, V. (1976). Metabolism of methoxyflurane in man. *Anesthesiology* 44, 372—379

8 Cardiovascular, respiratory and hepatic effects of inhalational anaesthetics
Gerald W. Black

It is now more than 40 years since cyclopropane was introduced into clinical practice, and it was not long before the new agent rivalled ether in popularity — smooth and rapid induction of anaesthesia and maintenance of arterial pressure at all levels of narcosis being desirable features of its use.

In the early 1950s, however, there was increasing use of cautery, diathermy and x-ray equipment in the operating room area, and ether and cyclopropane became progressively less popular because of their inflammable and explosive nature. The limitations of the non-inflammable compounds available at that time — chloroform and trichloroethylene — stimulated the search for better and more versatile anaesthetics, particularly those with a halogen structure since these agents are generally non-inflammable. This chapter reviews the cardiovascular, respiratory and hepatic effects of the general anaesthetic agents. Renal effects are discussed in Chapter 39.

HALOTHANE AND METHOXYFLURANE

Halothane, a halogenated hydrocarbon first investigated by Raventos in 1956, has been the most widely used inhalational anaesthetic during the last 20 years. It has been popular because it is a potent, non-explosive agent producing a level of anaesthesia which is readily controllable. However, it has become apparent that halothane possesses some undesirable features such as the precipitation of arrhythmias and incompatibility with adrenaline.

Methoxyflurane has had some success as an inhalational anaesthetic during the past decade, the great advantage of this halogenated ether being that it produces only minimal sensitization of the myocardium to the effects of catecholamines. Although superior to halothane in this respect, it has a high blood/gas partition coefficient and, unless low concentrations are administered, there may be undesirable sequelae such as prolonged recovery and drowsiness.

Until recently it was assumed that halothane and methoxyflurane were inert substances eliminated from the body in an unchanged state. It is now known, however, that some metabolic breakdown of these agents occurs, and concern has been expressed that biotransformation products may exert toxic effects on the liver and kidney.

The occasional occurrence of postoperative hepatic dysfunction has led to curtailment of the use of halothane and, to a lesser extent, of methoxy-flurane, even though a definitive causal relationship has not been verified (see below). There is now a widely held view that, because of medicolegal and other considerations, administration of these volatile anaesthetics should be restricted. On the other hand, many believe that this is a trend which should be regarded with concern when the excellent safety record of halothane is considered. Alternative methods of anaesthesia, relying upon the use of narcotics and muscle relaxants, may be accompanied by such problems as postoperative respiratory depression and awareness. In addition, they are often unsuitable for short procedures and there is, in fact, no guarantee that an increased use of these methods will not increase morbidity and even mortality. The move to abandon halothane in the absence of clear incriminatory evidence should be resisted.

A dose-related nephrotoxicity associated with the inhalation of methoxy-flurane may be due to the toxic effects of metabolic breakdown products, and Mazze, Trudell and Cousins (1971) found elevations of serum and urinary inorganic fluoride levels in patients with clinical signs of renal dysfunction (see Chapter 39).

OUTLINE PHARMACOLOGY OF NEWER AGENTS

Evidence is now forthcoming that personnel in operating and recovery rooms may be exposed to an occupational hazard because of atmospheric contamination with subanaesthetic concentrations of inhalational agents — another reason for seeking more stable compounds.

For these reasons much interest is being shown in newer and more inert volatile anaesthetics. Halogenated ethers have proved more promising compounds than hydrocarbons (Vitcha, 1971); they produce better muscular relaxation, cause less cardiovascular depression and tend to maintain normal cardiac rhythm in the presence of raised concentrations of circulating catecholamines. The methyl ethyl ethers constitute the group giving most encouraging results, and two new compounds at present receiving most attention — enflurane (Ethrane) and its isomer, isoflurane (Forane) — are both members of this series.

Enflurane

Enflurane is a potent, non-inflammable inhalational anaesthetic widely used in Europe and North America, which has recently undergone clinical trial in the UK (Black, Johnston and Scott, 1977) and is now generally available.

Although it resembles methoxyflurane in chemical structure, the physical properties of enflurane are more closely related to halothane (*Figure 8.1*). Because it has a low blood/gas partition coefficient, enflurane produces a level of anaesthesia which is readily controllable and both induction and recovery phases are rapid. Induction of anaesthesia may be accomplished by using 3–5% inspired enflurane vaporized either in oxygen or nitrous oxide–oxygen mixture. Unconsciousness may be produced with an intravenous thiobarbiturate which will facilitate the

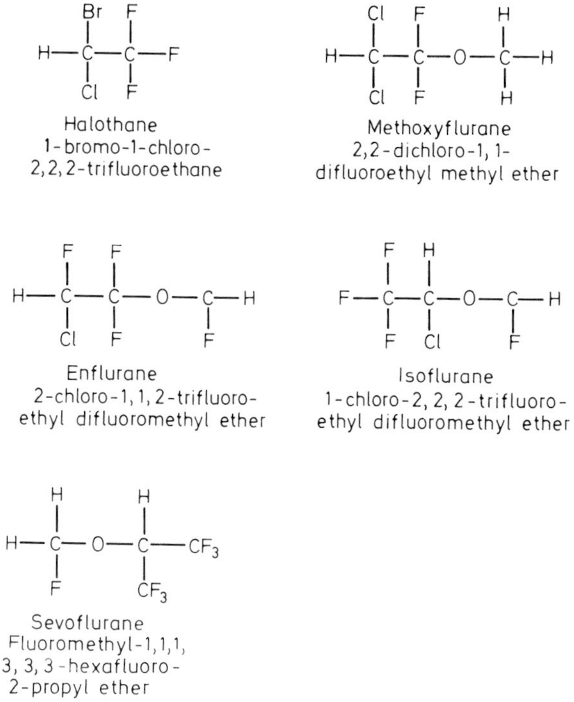

Halothane
1-bromo-1-chloro-
2,2,2-trifluoroethane

Methoxyflurane
2,2-dichloro-1, 1-
difluoroethyl methyl ether

Enflurane
2-chloro-1, 1, 2-trifluoro-
ethyl difluoromethyl ether

Isoflurane
1-chloro-2, 2, 2-trifluoro-
ethyl difluoromethyl ether

Sevoflurane
Fluoromethyl-1,1,1,
3, 3, 3-hexafluoro-
2-propyl ether

Figure 8.1
Chemical structure of halothane, methoxyflurane, enflurane, isoflurane and sevoflurane

establishment of enflurane anaesthesia and eliminate any element of excitement. In general, 1–3% vapour strength is adequate for the maintenance of anaesthesia. As with all potent agents, a vaporizer capable of accurately delivering concentrations of anaesthetic vapour should be used for the administration of enflurane. This precaution lessens the likelihood of overdosage with the attendant risks of hypotension and respiratory depression.

A drawback to the use of enflurane is the occurrence of muscular tonic–clonic twitchings of the face and limbs which may develop during deep anaesthesia when passive pulmonary hyperventilation is used. Clark, Hosick and Rosner (1971) have shown that the neural effects of enflurane in man include electroencephalographic changes indicating nervous irritability and spike–dome complexes following ulnar nerve stimulation.

These responses, which are exacerbated by hypocarbia and suppressed by hypercarbia, can readily be terminated by lightening the level of anaesthesia and increasing the minute volume ventilation. Investigations of cerebral blood flow (CBF) and metabolism indicate that the stimulation of the central nervous system caused by enflurane is not accompanied by any evidence of impaired cerebral oxygenation.

Although there is some muscular relaxation when clinical concentrations of enflurane are inhaled, muscle relaxant drugs should be used rather than resort being made to higher concentrations of anaesthetic vapour to provide muscle relaxation. All the commonly used neuromuscular-blocking drugs are compatible with enflurane but the actions of the non-depolarizing group may be markedly potentiated so that a smaller than normal dose will usually suffice. High concentrations of enflurane may themselves cause depression of twitch height (Lebowitz, Blitt and Walts, 1970), in which case muscular relaxation may not be reversed completely by neostigmine.

Investigations in animals (Halsey *et al.*, 1971) and in man (Chase *et al.*, 1971), show that the degree of enflurane biotransformation is much less than with many other inhalational agents. The metabolism of enflurane to inorganic fluoride is not usually sufficient to produce renal dysfunction in subjects with normal renal activity (Cousins *et al.*, 1976).

Although spontaneous skeletal muscular activity and the potential hazard to the kidney from fluoride toxicity are disadvantages of enflurane anaesthesia, they are unlikely to occur if high vapour strengths are avoided. It is not certain if enflurane is a suitable alternative to halothane, especially when anaesthesia has to be repeated. However, no case has yet been reported which could be unreservedly called 'enflurane hepatitis' and some 15 million patients have received the agent.

Isoflurane

When isoflurane was introduced in 1971 it showed considerable promise and seemed to merit further comprehensive investigation. Chemical and pharmacological properties are comparable to those of halothane and enflurane (*Figure 8.1, Table 8.1*). As with other inhalational agents, isoflurane may be administered either in oxygen or in nitrous oxide—oxygen mixtures in concentrations comparable to enflurane, and again it is advisable to use a thermocompensated vaporizer. Induction of anaesthesia may be associated with some breath-holding and coughing because of the slightly pungent odour of isoflurane, but this may be avoided by putting the patient to sleep with an intravenous anaesthetic agent. Clinical signs of anaesthesia are like those seen with halothane, the skin being warm, pink and dry, and the pupils usually fixed and constricted.

As with enflurane, there is considerable potentiation of the action of non-depolarizing muscle relaxants and it has been shown that isoflurane enhances the effect of *d*-tubocurarine three times as much as halothane (Miller *et al.*, 1971).

Isoflurane, like most inhalational anaesthetics, undergoes some bio-chemical degradation in the body, the main metabolites being trifluoroacetic acid and inorganic fluoride ion. However, the degree of biotransformation appears to be minimal, being less than with enflurane and considerably less than with halothane. Indeed, the peak serum inorganic fluoride level after prolonged isoflurane anaesthesia was found to be only 4.4 μmol/l, a concentration which renders the possibility of nephrotoxicity very remote

TABLE 8.1. Some physical properties of fluorinated inhalational anaesthetics

	Boiling point (°C)	*Molecular weight*	*Partition coefficients at 37°C*		*Vapour pressure at 20°C*	*Minimal alveolar concentration (MAC)* (vols %)
			Blood/Gas	*Oil/Gas*		
Halothane	50.2	197	2.3	236	243	0.8
Methoxyflurane	104.7	164	13	825	22	0.2
Enflurane	56.5	184	1.9	99	180	1.7
Isoflurane	48.5	184	1.4	99	250	1.2
Sevoflurane	58.5	200	0.6	99	160	2.5

(Mazze, Trudell and Cousins, 1971). At comparable anaesthetic exposures there was approximately ten times more production of fluoride ion with methoxyflurane, an agent known to produce toxic changes in the kidney. These workers also found that the production of trifluoroacetic acid was ten times less during isoflurane anaesthesia than during the administration of halothane.

Isoflurane was due to be released for general clinical use in 1975 but a report by Corbett of the University of Michigan suggested that the agent had carcinogenic properties in mice (Kramer, 1975). The data, however, were disputed and the future of isoflurane is still awaiting the outcome of the extensive toxicity studies now in progress.

Sevoflurane

Clinical studies are about to begin on yet another halogenated ether, sevoflurane. It has lower distribution coefficients than other agents (*Table 8.1*), and if clinical trials are satisfactory it may prove ideal for outpatient anaesthesia. Animal experiments with repeated administrations have not uncovered any adverse reactions or toxicity (Wallin *et al.*, 1975).

HAEMODYNAMIC EFFECTS OF INHALATIONAL ANAESTHETICS

Anaesthetic agents may exert effects both on the central nervous system and on the periphery. Thus there may be vasomotor depression with accompanying diminution of sympathetic activity, while possible peripheral effects include alterations of myocardial function and actions on the baroreceptors and chemoreceptors, vascular smooth muscle and autonomic ganglia.

There is a correlation between the pharmacological actions of anaesthetics and the nature of the sympathetic responses they provoke. For example, there is a close relationship between the level of circulating noradrenaline on the one hand and peripheral vascular changes and cardiac rate and rhythm on the other, while respiration and metabolism are influenced by prevailing catecholamine concentrations. Many of the cardiovascular signs of anaesthesia appear to be the expression of the balance between sympathetic stimulation and the direct depressant effects of the inhalational anaesthetic (Cullen *et al.*, 1972).

Most general anaesthetics cause depression of heart—lung preparations. Measurements made in these circumstances, however, do not take into account the compensatory reflexes of the sympathoadrenal system on the circulation and are not comparable with those made in the intact animal. For these reasons, particular consideration is given in this section to the sympathoadrenal responses elicited by the different anaesthetic agents.

Halothane, methoxyflurane and enflurane produce central nervous inhibition of the sympathoadrenal system with reduction in catecholamine production; in contrast, diethyl ether causes central nervous stimulation with increased adrenaline and noradrenaline liberation.

Nitrous oxide

This is not a potent anaesthetic and it is not surprising that its effects on the cardiovascular system were overlooked until recent years.

Marked falls in arterial pressure have been reported when nitrous oxide is administered during deep halothane anaesthesia and these are reversed when its use is discontinued (Bloch, 1963). The so-called 'second gas effect' (see Chapter 4) has been postulated as a possible explanation for such responses, the addition of high concentrations of a relatively insoluble gas to a second gas in lower concentrations increasing the uptake of the latter (Epstein *et al.*, 1964).

In studies of volunteers inhaling 40% nitrous oxide, Eisele and Smith (1972) found reductions in ballistocardiographic measurements of cardiac output suggestive of cardiac depression; also noted were falls in heart rate, decreases in limb blood flow and evidence of some rise in plasma noradrenaline concentration. It may be that nitrous oxide has negative inotropic and chronotropic effects on the heart and at the same time produces α-adrenoreceptor stimulation of the peripheral circulation. In spite of the cardiac depression, normal arterial pressure appears to be maintained because of the increased peripheral resistance. It is of interest that only peripheral circulatory effects of nitrous oxide are manifest in the presence of inhalational anaesthetics, and it is suggested that its depressant effects on the heart are masked by the depressant actions of the other anaesthetics.

Diethyl ether

Many of the features of ether anaesthesia are manifestations of increased sympathetic activity. There is usually an increase in arterial pressure, heart rate and cardiac output during light anaesthesia, although hypotension and diminished output may occur when higher concentrations are inhaled.

Diethyl ether depresses myocardial contractility in the heart—lung preparation but this is not readily seen in the intact animal and, indeed, increases in cardiac output have been reported under clinical conditions. This difference is probably due to the fact that a properly functioning sympathetic nervous system is required for the maintenance of circulatory homoeostasis during ether anaesthesia, and corresponding increases in plasma noradrenaline concentrations have been reported (Black *et al.*, 1969).

The cardiovascular effects of ether are thus complex and can alter with the depth and duration of anaesthesia. Compare, for example, accounts by McArdle, Black and Unni (1968), Skovsted and Price (1970) and Gregory *et al.* (1971).

Cyclopropane

This differs from other general anaesthetics in possessing the quality of maintaining the arterial blood pressure; indeed, this may even be elevated due to the presence of hypercarbia resulting from inadequate ventilation.

The reductions in cardiac output which anaesthetic concentrations of cyclopropane produce in the isolated heart—lung preparation are not readily demonstrable in the intact human subject. As in the case of ether, this difference is in all probability due to an increased discharge at sympathetic nerve endings, the homoeostatic role of the sympathetic nervous system being reflected by increases in circulating plasma catecholamines.

The positive inotropic activity caused by cyclopropane anaesthesia produces the marked increases in stroke volume and cardiac output which occur in man, although these return to normal, and may decrease, when the concentrations of inhaled gas exceeds 20% (Jones *et al.*, 1960); even when this happens, however, there is little change in arterial pressure because of the increases in peripheral vascular resistance which accompany the reductions in cardiac output associated with the inhalation of high concentrations.

The compensatory mechanisms of the circulation remain largely intact during cyclopropane anaesthesia; there is only slight blockade of sympathetic ganglia, interference with the pressor response to carotid occlusion is minimal and baroreceptor functions are unhindered.

It was for these reasons that, in the past, cyclopropane was often regarded as the anaesthetic of choice for the 'shocked' patient. However, during the inhalation of cyclopropane the maintenance of arterial pressure is brought about by an increased vascular resistance throughout the body and this may lead to impaired tissue perfusion, especially in the patient who is hypovolaemic.

Studies of regional blood flow indicate that cyclopropane causes vasoconstriction in the main sites of peripheral vascular resistance. There is a substantial reduction in splanchnic blood flow (Price *et al.*, 1965) and in renal blood flow (Deutsch *et al.*, 1966), changes consistent with raised sympathetic activity. Vasoconstriction also occurs in the limbs, and since it persists in the nerve-blocked forearm it cannot be nervously mediated and must be due to the direct action of cyclopropane on vascular smooth muscle or to the presence of catecholamines in the circulating blood (McArdle and Black, 1963). Cyclopropane is known to have a direct action on smooth muscle contractility and has been shown to potentiate the contractile response of strips of rabbit aorta to adrenaline (Price and Price, 1962). The nature of the effect on smooth muscle has recently been clarified by Sprague and Ngai (1974), whose work suggests that it is due to decreased formation of intracellular cyclic AMP.

It seems reasonable to assume that the enhanced responsiveness of smooth muscle to noradrenaline is mainly responsible for the moderate vasoconstriction of light anaesthesia, sympathoadrenal activity being largely within normal limits. It is probable, however, that the progressive increase in limb vascular resistance which occurs during the administration of higher concentrations of cyclopropane is initiated chiefly by the concomitant rise in circulating noradrenaline. There has been continuing debate regarding the manner in which increased sympathetic nervous activity is produced during cyclopropane anaesthesia. Price *et al.* (1969) suggested it was due to a central stimulant effect from selective depression of certain medullary-inhibiting neurons as well as direct stimulation of excitatory 'pressor' neurons. However, it now seems more likely that baroreceptor reflexes are responsible and that the central effects of cyclopropane are purely depressant (Fukunaga and Epstein, 1974).

Trichloroethylene

This resembles two other halogenated anaesthetics — methoxyflurane and halothane — in that it does not induce rises in plasma catecholamine concentrations (Unni, McArdle and Black, 1970). However, arterial hypotension which may occur with other agents is not usually seen during trichloroethylene anaesthesia. Clinical concentrations of trichloroethylene cause little alteration in either cardiac output or peripheral vascular resistance, and this probably accounts for the circulatory stability which is a feature of anaesthesia with this agent. The preservation of circulatory homoeostasis without any compensatory increase in sympathetic activity may be due to the low vapour concentrations which are often sufficient to produce anaesthesia but it also suggests that trichloroethylene exerts only a minimal depressant effect on the cardiovascular system.

Halothane

The main circulatory effect of halothane is to cause a fall in arterial pressure, the extent of the hypotension being related to the concentration of inhaled vapour. The cause is debated: possible explanations include central sympathetic depression (Price, Price and Morse, 1965), ganglionic blockade (Raventos, 1956), myocardial depression (Severinghaus and Cullen, 1958) and a direct action on vascular smooth muscle (Black and McArdle, 1962).

EFFECT ON THE MYOCARDIUM

Halothane causes a reduction in the cardiac output of the dog heart—lung preparation and is about 70% as potent as chloroform in this respect. Studies made in the isolated cat papillary muscle indicate that it has negative inotropic effects on the heart, causing decreased maximal velocity of shortening and decreased maximal isometric force (Sugai, Shimosato and Etsten, 1968). In other animal studies, Prys-Roberts *et al.* (1972) concluded that the major cause of arterial hypotension is a fall in cardiac output, due to depression of myocardial contractility.

THE PERIPHERAL CIRCULATION

During halothane anaesthesia the limbs are warm and dry with prominent superficial veins, suggesting vasodilatation. Though an early study (using a water-filled plethysmograph) suggested that halothane caused substantial reductions in limb vascular resistance (Black and McArdle, 1962), more recent work (using a mercury-in-rubber strain gauge) has shown reductions in flow during the inhalation of halothane (Scott, McArdle and Black, 1978). This latter finding is in keeping with animal work (Ngai and Bolme, 1966; Westermark, 1969; Amory, Steffenson and Forsyth, 1971).

Plasma catecholamine levels are not raised during halothane anaesthesia (see below) and, consequently, increases in peripheral vascular resistance would not be anticipated. Millar and Biscoe (1966), however, found that halothane produced increased postganglionic sympathetic discharge in the rabbit, a factor which may partly account for a raised vascular resistance. On the other hand, Cristoforo and Brody (1968) reported that halothane induced vasoconstriction in isolated dog muscle and, since this response persisted in spite of complete α-adrenergic blockade, concluded that the vasoconstriction resulted from the liberation of antidiuretic hormone (ADH), vasopressin. There is evidence that halothane interferes with the ability of noradrenaline to cause vasoconstriction; therefore, if this postulate with regard to ADH is correct, the action of the ADH must oppose and overcome the direct depressant action on vascular smooth muscle. It can thus be seen that the mode of action of halothane on the peripheral vasculature is confusing and controversial.

There is no evidence to indicate that halothane produces vasoconstriction in other parts of the body. It causes an increase in cerebral blood flow (CBF), although it is not clear if this is due to a direct effect on the cerebral vessels or to alterations in cerebral metabolism; thus in studies made in animals, Smith (1973) found that the arterial halothane content correlated poorly with changes in CBF but well with changes in cerebral oxygen consumption.

Domenech *et al.* (1977) found marked reductions in coronary vascular resistance in both the intact and the isolated heart of the dog during the inhalation of halothane, which was probably due to vasodilatation produced by a direct action of the agent.

Halothane causes a reduction in splanchnic perfusion pressure with a parallel fall in splanchnic blood flow and no significant change in splanchnic vascular resistance (Epstein *et al.*, 1966). This suggests that hypotension rather than increased vasomotor tone may be responsible for the reductions in splanchnic blood flow.

CATECHOLAMINE PRODUCTION

Using a newly developed and extremely sensitive radiometric assay, Roizen *et al.* (1974) have been able to show that in rats the total plasma catecholamine concentration during 1% halothane anaesthesia is only about 12% of that in awake animals. As the concentration of inhaled halothane was increased the titre of plasma catecholamines fell further, *pari passu* with the drop in arterial pressure. The decreases in catecholamine levels appear to be due to diminished release of adrenaline from the adrenal medulla as well as noradrenaline from the sympathetic nerve endings.

These findings, and those of Perry, Van Dyke and Theye (1974) who demonstrated comparable decreases in plasma catecholamines in the dog, may well help to explain the reductions in mean arterial pressure, cardiac output and myocardial contractility which occur during halothane anaesthesia. Although it seems that sympathetic suppression is largely responsible for the circulatory depression observed during halothane anaesthesia, the site (or sites) at which this inhibiting effect may be exerted has not been clearly defined.

Methoxyflurane

Although methoxyflurane is an ether, it is a halogenated compound and its effects on the cardiovascular system resemble those of halothane rather than diethyl ether. Arterial pressure falls in proportion to the concentration of inhaled vapour but, in spite of the fact that the reductions in ventricular force are not significantly different from halothane, hypotension appears to be less pronounced during methoxyflurane anaesthesia. The fall in arterial pressure may result solely from the reduction in cardiac output because it has been shown that vascular resistance is unchanged and the normal vasoconstrictor ability of noradrenaline is unaffected by methoxyflurane (Black and McArdle, 1965). In baroreceptor-denervated animals, methoxyflurane produces a slight reduction in sympathetic activity, believed to be due to a depressant action on the medullary pressor neurons, an action which in normal animals is counteracted by the reflex response to arterial hypotension (Skovsted and Price, 1969). Catecholamine concentrations from the adrenal vein of the dog were found to decrease during methoxyflurane anaesthesia in proportion to the strength of inhaled vapour (Li, Shaul and Etsten, 1968) — a decrease due, at least in part, to a direct effect of methoxyflurane on the chromaffin cell (Dreyer, Bischoff and Gothert, 1974). When consideration is given to the circulatory effects of methoxyflurane, this absence of sympathoadrenal activity is not unexpected.

Enflurane

As with other halogenated compounds, there is a fall in arterial pressure which is commensurate with the concentration of vapour inhaled. In general, enflurane produces comparable effects to halothane on the cardiovascular system, both agents producing a negative inotropic effect on the heart of the intact dog, which is accompanied by equivalent decreases in cardiac oxygen demand. Assessments of the inotropic effect of enflurane on the intrinsic contractile state of the cat papillary muscle suggest that it may produce less depression of myocardial contractility than halothane (Shimosato *et al.,* 1969). Studies made by Marshall *et al.* (1971) indicate that normal circulatory responses may persist during enflurane anaesthesia. They found that in the presence of hypocarbia, normocarbia and hypercarbia cardiac output and arterial pressure were better maintained with the newer agent than with halothane.

However, marked dose-dependent impairment of cardiac function has been observed during prolonged enflurane anaesthesia in fit volunteers (Calverley *et al.,* 1975). Comparable findings in dogs are reported by Horan *et al.* (1977a), who noted that in equipotent concentrations enflurane caused slightly greater impairment of left ventricular function than halothane. Hypotension is often a conspicuous feature of the clinical use of enflurane although it tends to be counterbalanced by the stimulation of the surgical procedure. *In vivo* investigations show that there is inhibition of adrenal medullary catecholamine secretion during enflurane anaesthesia (Gothert and Wendt, 1977).

Isoflurane

Stevens *et al.* (1971) found that isoflurane caused little impairment of cardiovascular function in human volunteers in whom the arterial carbon dioxide tension was kept constant. Hypotension was only minimal in spite of a dose-related decrease in peripheral vascular resistance. There was little reduction in cardiac output because of an increase in heart rate which compensated for a diminished stroke volume.

During spontaneous ventilation there are further increases in heart rate and cardiac output, changes which are probably due to a raised Pa_{CO_2} associated with the respiratory depressant effect of isoflurane. Several workers (Cromwell *et al.*, 1971; Graves, McDermott and Bidwai, 1974) have also found that decreases in stroke volume are counteracted by increases in pulse rate and systemic resistance. It has been pointed out that although isoflurane depresses the contractile properties of the isolated myocardial preparation, apparently this does not occur in the intact human subject; it has therefore been suggested that the β-adrenergic effects seen during deep isoflurane anaesthesia may be the result of sympathetic responses to arterial hypotension.

Studies made in dogs confirm that equipotent concentrations of isoflurane cause less myocardial impairment than either enflurane or halothane (Horan *et al.*, 1977b), and there can be little doubt that minimal cardiovascular depression is one of several advantages of this halogenated ether, the future of which has yet to be determined.

EFFECTS ON HEART RATE AND RHYTHM

Most of the changes in cardiac rate and rhythm which occur during anaesthesia may be explained on the basis of altered autonomic balance, a preponderance of vagal or sympathetic activity producing characteristic changes.

Vagal stimulation causes slowing of the sinus rate with decrease or disappearance of the P-wave in the electrocardiogram. If the SA node is sufficiently depressed, the role of the pacemaker may be taken over by the AV node, so that often the stimulus passes backwards over the atria. This is seen on the electrocardiogram as nodal rhythm. There may be independent activation of the atria and ventricles (atrioventricular dissociation), while intense vagal stimulation leads to partial or complete heart block, or even asystole.

Sympathetic stimulation induces sinus tachycardia with, perhaps, occasional ventricular extrasystoles. These become more frequent and arise from an increasing number of foci in the ventricle as sympathetic activation becomes more profound, and multifocal ventricular extrasystoles and ventricular tachycardia may be followed by ventricular fibrillation.

Vagal inhibition has long been cited as a cause of sudden death during induction of anaesthesia with chloroform, and it is believed that the mechanism largely responsible for this is sensitization of the sinus and aortic baroreceptors.

It has long been known that general anaesthetics which have a hydrocarbon structure in some way sensitize to the effects of catecholamines. The manner in which chloroform, cyclopropane and halothane produce this effect is not clear but it would seem that reduction of heart rate and depression of ventricular automaticity play an important role (Vick, 1966; Reynolds, Chiz and Pasquet, 1970; Hashimoto and Hashimoto, 1972).

Halothane

There is frequently some degree of cardiac slowing during halothane anaesthesia. This becomes more pronounced in deeper levels of anaesthesia and may be accompanied by a shift of pacemaker and nodal rhythm. It is probable that these changes are mainly due to increased vagal activity since they can often be counterbalanced by the action of atropine (see below). They are more likely to occur when high concentrations of anaesthetic vapour are being inhaled, and both halothane and methoxyflurane have been shown to produce a dose-dependent increase in the functional refractory period of the AV conducting system (Morrow, Haley and Logic, 1972).

The effects of halothane were recently studied in intact and isolated heart preparations in which the papillary muscle and sinoatrial node of a recipient dog were separately infused with arterial blood from a donor animal (Hashimoto *et al.*, 1975). The inhalation of 1% halothane by the donor dog decreased arterial pressure and heart rate and sensitized the ventricle to the effects of noradrenaline in the same animal. Halothane did not cause irregularities of rhythm in the papillary muscle preparation, and the maximum rate produced by noradrenaline in this preparation was much less than the sinoatrial rate. The authors concluded that it is unlikely that halothane causes changes in ventricular automaticity and they believe that some form of 're-entry' mechanism is a likely cause for production of hydrocarbon—catecholamine-induced arrhythmia.

In common with other hydrocarbons, halothane 'sensitizes' the myocardium to the effects of catecholamines, and respiratory depression and retention of carbon dioxide may give rise to bigeminal rhythm, multifocal ventricular extrasystoles and ventricular tachycardia. In contrast to cyclopropane, arrhythmias are not commonly encountered during uncomplicated halothane anaesthesia in man in the presence of normal arterial $P\text{CO}_2$ levels (Black, 1965). Also, a higher degree of hypercarbia is required to provoke ventricular extrasystoles and their incidence is not related to the concentration of inspired halothane. The correction of respiratory acidosis will often abolish ventricular irregularities even though the concentration of halothane is unaltered.

It is essential that changes in heart rate and rhythm during halothane anaesthesia should not be treated indiscriminately with atropine since the abolition of any restraining vagal tone may accentuate their severity and even induce ventricular fibrillation.

Although tachyarrhythmia usually results from a source of increased adrenergic discharge such as hypercarbia, the use of adrenaline for haemostatic purposes during halothane anaesthesia may also cause irregularities of heart action. It has been suggested that, provided ventilation is adequate and that the concentration and total dose of adrenaline are kept within prescribed limits, subcutaneous injection of adrenaline may safely be given during halothane anaesthesia. However, endogenous amines are an important factor in the causation of arrhythmia and, at the time of injection, their concentration may be already elevated by light anaesthesia or surgical stimulation. In such circumstances the absorption of even small amounts of injected adrenaline may have serious consequences. It is therefore best to avoid the use of adrenaline during halothane anaesthesia.

Cyclopropane

During cyclopropane anaesthesia the heart rate is usually within normal limits in spite of a pronounced increase in sympathetic nervous activity. This may be because a high degree of vagal tone is present during the inhalation of cyclopropane — a theory which is supported by the finding that when atropine is given unduly rapid heart rates are noted, presumably because of the unmasking of excess sympathetic activity.

It would appear that two factors are necessary to cause appearance of ventricular arrhythmias during anaesthesia. The myocardium should be sensitized and there should be a source of increased catecholamine production. Cyclopropane is the sole anaesthetic to possess both these properties, so arrhythmias are an extremely common occurrence. Ether causes increased sympathoadrenal activity but not myocardial sensitization, while the reverse situation pertains during uncomplicated halothane anaesthesia. Other adrenergic influences which may give rise to ventricular irregularities are preoperative apprehension, light anaesthesia and surgical stimulation, hypoxaemia, retention of carbon dioxide and the injection or infusion of adrenaline, noradrenaline or other catecholamine.

Cyclopropane is the only gaseous anaesthetic which causes serious tachyarrhythmias and adequate ventilation is of prime importance in their prevention. However, when high concentrations of cyclopropane are inhaled (over 20 vols %), ventricular extrasystoles may appear even though the end-tidal P_{CO_2} is within normal limits (Lurie *et al.*, 1958). Also, the higher the concentration of inspired cyclopropane, the lower is the alveolar P_{CO_2} level at which arrhythmias appear.

An intravenous infusion of adrenaline or noradrenaline will produce ventricular arrhythmia in man during cyclopropane anaesthesia. When ventricular extrasystoles are associated with hypercarbia during cyclopropane anaesthesia, the level of plasma noradrenaline concentration at which they appear is significantly less than ·when they are initiated by noradrenaline infusion. This suggests that the cause of the arrhythmias is not an increase in circulating catecholamines but rather that they may be due to the local release of noradrenaline from the cardiac β-adrenoreceptors where the liberated amine is in close contact with the sensitized myocardium. The use of adrenaline or noradrenaline during cyclopropane anaesthesia is highly dangerous and should be avoided.

Methoxyflurane

Methoxyflurane is a halogenated ether, not a hydrocarbon, and the evidence suggests that it causes only minimal myocardial sensitization. Normal sinus rhythm is a feature of anaesthesia with this agent and ventricular arrhythmias do not appear even in the presence of intense hypercarbia (Black, 1967). On this basis it is suggested that adrenaline may be used for haemostatic purposes during methoxyflurane anaesthesia, provided care is taken to minimize other adrenergic influences. The agent has been used successfully for the management of patients requiring surgical removal of phaeochrome tumours, normal heart action persisting in the presence of high concentrations of circulating catecholamines.

Trichloroethylene

Trichloroethylene does not give rise to an increase in circulating catecholamines and, although it causes myocardial sensitization, arrhythmia is infrequent in the absence of excessive adrenergic activity.

It was previously suggested that the use of trichloroethylene was associated with a high incidence of ventricular irregularities but accurately calibrated vaporizers were not available at that time and unnecessarily high concentrations of gas were probably inhaled. If the inspired vapour strength does not exceed 0.5%, adequate ventilation will be maintained and cardiac arrhythmia will rarely occur.

Enflurane

Earlier studies carried out in dogs suggested that enflurane sensitized the myocardium to the effects of catecholamines and that the incidence of severe arrhythmia following adrenaline challenge was similar to that associated with halothane (McDowell, Hall and Stephen, 1968). However, a recent comparison made in dogs of the dose of adrenaline required to produce arrhythmia when given by constant rate intravenous infusion provides evidence that enflurane, like methoxyflurane, is less likely to induce cardiac arrhythmia than halothane (Munson and Tucker, 1975).

Clinical work, too, suggests that subcutaneous injections of adrenaline do not cause serious cardiac irregularities during enflurane anaesthesia, provided precautions are taken regarding the amount and concentration of the amine (Reisner and Lippmann, 1975). Enflurane is a halogenated ether and it would not be surprising if arrhythmias were less common than with halothane.

Isoflurane

It has also been shown, both in animal (Tucker, Rackstein and Munson, 1974) and in clinical investigations (Pauca and Dripps, 1973), that the incidence of adrenaline-induced arrhythmias is considerably less with the other new halogenated ether, isoflurane, than with halothane. As is the case with enflurane, this should prove to be a major advantage over halothane because of the unsuitability of the latter in such fields as plastic surgery where there is widespread use of adrenaline to reduce operative bleeding.

Effects of β-blocking drugs

Since there is good evidence that β-adrenergic stimulation is primarily responsible for the causation of ventricular irregularities, it is not surprising that β-adrenoreceptor-blocking drugs can be of considerable value in their prevention and abolition. However, drugs such as propranolol and practolol may cause hypotension and bradycardia and should be used with care, particularly in the presence of hypovolaemia and metabolic acidosis.

Methoxyflurane and practolol appear to have an additive depressant action on the myocardium because their combination causes reductions in contractility indices and cardiac output (Saner *et al.*, 1975); in contrast, no such depression is observed during halothane anaesthesia (Roberts *et al.*, 1973). Since neither of these inhalational anaesthetics evokes sympathetic activation, β-adrenoreceptor blockade is unlikely and some central or peripheral vascular effect may be the cause of the adverse interaction of methoxyflurane and practolol.

The vast majority of disorders of ventricular rhythm usually disappear when the concentration of inspired anaesthetic is reduced and ventilation improves, and the use of these drugs is rarely necessary for this purpose. Beta-adrenoreceptor-blocking compounds should be reserved for the intractable tachyarrhythmia which is liable to progress to ventricular fibrillation. These drugs are contraindicated in the management of disorders of heart action arising because of excessive vagal activity.

EFFECTS ON RESPIRATION

Inhalational anaesthetics may influence respiration in various ways. The plasma pH, Pao_2 and $Paco_2$ play an important homoeostatic role in the control of the level of ventilation, and anaesthetic agents may alter respiratory function by means of the responses to hypoxaemia and acidaemia.

Some controversy exists regarding the nature of the respiratory response to a raised $Paco_2$; since this is not abolished by denervation of the chemoreceptors, there is reason to believe that the response is controlled by receptors in the central nervous system. These central chemoreceptors are probably situated close to the ventrolateral aspect of the medulla in the vicinity of the respiratory centre. Their function is to respond to pH changes in the CSF/brain/ECF compartment. Depression of central regulatory mechanisms, alterations in the pH of the blood, sensitization of chemoreceptor and pulmonary stretch receptors, and the release of catecholamines are factors which may produce ventilatory changes during anaesthesia. The respiratory effects of several of the inhalational anaesthetics have been comprehensively reviewed by Ngai (1967).

Diethyl ether

The vapour of ether is irritating and may cause coughing, salivation, laryngeal spasm and apnoea if a high concentration is introduced rapidly. Ether differs from other inhalational anaesthetics in that pulmonary ventilation is well sustained provided deep planes of narcosis are avoided. Although there may be some reduction in amplitude, the respiratory rate and minute volume are increased so that Paco$_2$ levels usually remain unaltered or are even reduced except in very deep anaesthesia. The increased respiratory rate may be partly due to sensitization of pulmonary stretch receptors but, because tachypnoea may persist after bilateral vagotomy, it cannot be completely responsible.

Studies made in animals reveal that an increase in respiratory rate may be produced by respiratory acidosis and that tachypnoea does not occur if hypercarbia is avoided. However, increases in respiratory rate were found in a clinical study of ether in which neither respiratory nor metabolic acidosis was present, suggesting that alterations in the pH of the blood cannot be held responsible (Black *et al.*, 1969).

It may be that some of the respiratory changes which occur when ether is inhaled are due to increases in circulating catecholamine levels. Studies of the ventilatory response to inhaled carbon dioxide provide evidence of respiratory depression, and it may be that this response and the reduction in amplitude which occurs during ether anaesthesia result from central depression. The important clinical implication is that with ether, in contrast to other agents, Paco$_2$ levels usually do not rise and ventilation may be maintained without recourse to assisted or controlled ventilation.

Cyclopropane

There is a progressive decrease of alveolar ventilation as the concentration of inspired gas is increased. The accompanying retention of carbon dioxide results mainly from a diminished tidal volume secondary to ineffective action of the intercostal muscles.

There is usually an increased respiratory rate and, because of this, the alveolar ventilation is reduced by only about half as much as the tidal volume. This may be due to a central response to the raised Paco$_2$ or it may be the result of sensitization of the pulmonary stretch receptors by cyclopropane. It is of interest that subjects who receive morphine prior to cyclopropane do not respond with a raised respiratory rate as anaesthesia deepens, with the result that respiratory acidosis is more severe.

The inhalation of higher concentrations of cyclopropane may induce laryngospasm and bronchospasm. These manifestations of parasympathetic activity are more liable to occur when vagal tone is augmented by respiratory acidosis.

Trichloroethylene

The concentrations of trichloroethylene normally used in clinical practice cause little irritation of the respiratory tract and do not produce any significant depression of respiration. There is usually a fall in tidal volume but this is more than compensated for by a raised respiratory rate, with the result that the minute volume may also be increased. However, when concentrations of trichloroethylene greater than 1% are inhaled, tachypnoea becomes pronounced and the resulting hypercarbia may initiate the appearance of cardiac irregularities.

Stimulation of pulmonary stretch receptors probably accounts for the marked increase in respiratory rate and this increase can usually be eliminated by reducing the concentration of trichloroethylene. The use of a narcotic (such as pethidine) has been advocated to control excessive respiratory rate but since tachypnoea is a sign of overdosage, such drugs can usually be avoided if a calibrated vaporizer is employed.

Halothane

This agent is also non-irritant to the respiratory tract so that it is possible to induce surgical anaesthesia smoothly and rapidly. There is depression of the pharyngeal and laryngeal reflexes, which may facilitate endotracheal intubation without the use of muscle relaxants. There is little increase in salivary and bronchial secretions even in subjects who have not received atropine.

The inhalation of concentrations of halothane used in clinical practice produces bronchodilatation and this is probably mediated largely through β-adrenoreceptor stimulation since it is decreased by drugs which block these receptors (Aviado, 1975). Halothane is especially suitable for patients suffering from respiratory disabilities such as chronic bronchitis and emphysema.

Tachypnoea often occurs during anaesthesia and this may be pronounced when high concentrations of halothane are being administered, with the result that there are substantial reductions in tidal volume; there may then also be decreases in minute volume and in effective alveolar ventilation. The cause of the increase in respiratory rate has been attributed to the sensitization of pulmonary stretch receptors (Coleridge *et al.*, 1968), but it has been shown to persist following bilateral vagotomy (Ngai, Katz and Farhie, 1965).

Methoxyflurane

Respiratory features of methoxyflurane anaesthesia are very similar to those of halothane, although this agent has a slightly more potent depressant action. An increased respiratory rate with depression of amplitude of ventilation and minute volume produce hypercarbia when methoxyflurane is inhaled. For this reason it is often necessary to assist or control ventilation in order to avoid respiratory acidosis.

Using the concept of minimal (alveolar) anaesthetic concentration (MAC), comparative studies have been made on the effects of commonly used inhalational anaesthetics on ventilation (Larson *et al.*, 1969). These show that with diethyl ether, cyclopropane, halothane and methoxyflurane the ventilatory response to carbon dioxide progressively decreases with increasing depth of anaesthesia. It has also been found that at equipotent anaesthetic concentrations halothane and methoxyflurane produce the most profound depression of respiration, while ether causes only minimal reduction of ventilation.

Enflurane

Smooth and rapid induction of anaesthesia is a feature of this newer agent, probably because it is non-irritant and has a low blood/gas partition coefficient. It is possible to increase the strength of the inhaled vapour progressively with little risk of laryngospasm or bronchospasm.

In common with other halogenated anaesthetics, enflurane causes depression of respiration. This effect becomes pronounced when the patient is spontaneously breathing concentrations of vapour greater than 2%. Although respiratory depression becomes more marked as anaesthesia is deepened, the respiratory rate remains largely unaltered. Tidal volumes, however, are greatly reduced and, as a result, arterial carbon dioxide tension rises. Control of ventilation is recommended in the presence of decreasing alveolar ventilation in order to maintain normal acid–base equilibrium.

Isoflurane

This is a more powerful respiratory depressant than halothane and it has been suggested that the reason for this is a lack of increase in respiratory rate when higher concentrations of vapour are inhaled (Fourcade *et al.*, 1971). The studies showing this, however, were carried out in human volunteers and the workers concerned believe that lack of surgical stimulation may have accounted for the ventilatory insufficiency. That this is probably a correct assumption is shown by observations made during surgery, which indicate that the respiratory response to isoflurane is characterized by a raised respiratory rate, although in spite of this there is often a marked decrease in tidal volume with some elevations of Pa_{CO_2} (Pauca and Dripps, 1973).

EFFECTS ON THE LIVER

In this section consideration is given to the potential hepatotoxic effects of inhalational anaesthetics. It must be emphasized, however, that factors such as surgery, coincidental viral hepatitis, hypotension, changes in hepatic blood flow and concomitant drug therapy often play a more important role in the causation of postoperative liver dysfunction. Although chloroform and halothane are most frequently reported as being associated with hepatic malfunction, several other agents have also been incriminated. Many of the reports deal with one or more isolated cases of postoperative hepatic damage and such data are of little value in determining the causation and incidence of this complication (Dykes, 1970).

Chloroform

Although Orth, Pohle and Sims (quoted by Waters, 1951) found a 52% incidence of hepatic dysfunction associated with the use of chloroform, it is unlikely to cause damage to the liver provided only minimal concentrations are inhaled and hypoxaemia and hypercarbia are avoided. The dangers of deep anaesthesia and respiratory depression are greatly reduced by the use of muscle relaxants and mechanical ventilation.

Delayed chloroform poisoning is a major hazard of the use of the drug in obstetric practice. Little or no damage will follow the administration of chloroform in a patient with a normal nutritional state, but prolonged vomiting during labour may produce injury to the liver characterized by central lobular necrosis.

Cyclopropane

This anaesthetic has long been regarded as less hepatotoxic than other agents, although in the past decade there have been isolated case reports linking hepatic dysfunction following surgery with the administration of cyclopropane. It is of interest that the USA National Halothane Study (1966) in which other anaesthetics in addition to halothane were examined, revealed a higher incidence of massive hepatic necrosis following the use of cyclopropane than with other agents. However, a probable explanation for this may be related to the selective use of this anaesthetic in the shocked patient. Other possible factors may be the high circulating catecholamine levels and the intense splanchnic vasoconstriction associated with the use of cyclopropane.

Halothane

Halothane has a chemical structure similar to chloroform and, though it was initially thought that it might have toxic effects on the liver, studies in the experimental animal suggested that liver function was affected no more frequently with halothane than with other agents and that, when used in clinical practice, the incidence of adverse effects of halothane on the liver was no higher than with ether and cyclopropane.

However, by 1963 a number of cases of jaundice, presumed to be due to halothane, had been described. Concern that halothane might cause damage to the liver was again being expressed — mainly in the USA, probably because six of the first nine reports came from there (Little, 1968).

NATIONAL HALOTHANE STUDY

Isolated case reports can contribute little to an evaluation of the problem and several clinical studies, mostly of a retrospective nature, were therefore undertaken. The National Halothane Study (1966) in the USA was a retrospective study of over 800 000 administrations of anaesthesia, covering the years 1959—62, and its object was to compare halothane with other anaesthetics in respect of the frequency of fatal hepatic necrosis occurring within six weeks of surgery. The over-all incidence of hepatic necrosis was found to be less than 1 in 10 000 and in the vast majority of these cases a cause other than anaesthesia, such as circulatory shock, sepsis, previous hepatic disease or prolonged major surgery, could be incriminated (Mc-Caughey, 1972). Other findings were that hepatic necrosis did not occur more commonly with halothane than with other agents and that the mortality rate was higher if two or three surgical procedures were undertaken within one or two months. This, however, was not more likely to occur with repeated administration of halothane than with other anaesthetic agents.

Although no consistent histological pattern emerged in the National Halothane Study, it appeared that cases associated with the use of halothane exhibited a lesion simulating that encountered in fatal viral and some drug-induced forms of hepatitis more often than those associated with the administration of other anaesthetics.

REPEATED EXPOSURES

An increased incidence of jaundice and death occurs after all multiple anaesthetics given within one month, irrespective of the agent used and regardless of whether or not the cause of the jaundice can be explained (Strunin and Simpson, 1972). Nevertheless, although the incidence of liver dysfunction following halothane anaesthesia is low, there is continuing anxiety regarding the advisability of exposing a patient to this agent on more than one occasion within a short period of time. Inman and Mushin (1974) analysed 130 case reports of jaundice attributed to halothane received by the Committee on Safety of Medicines. Their main conclusion was that the interval between the last of a series of administrations of halothane and the appearance of jaundice is significantly shorter than the corresponding interval following a single exposure, a finding which suggests that the underlying mechanism may be some form of hypersensitivity. However, it has been pointed out (McPeek and Gilbert, 1974) that the scrutiny of data from the National Halothane Study (1966) and that reported by Simpson, Strunin and Walton (1971) fails to show any relationship between previous exposure to halothane and the rapidity with which jaundice develops.

At the beginning of 1974 the Medical Assessor to the Committee on Safety of Medicines issued a controversial circular to all anaesthetists ('Jaundice following repeated exposure to halothane') in which it was stated that repeated administration of the agent within a few weeks carried a greater risk of jaundice than a single exposure (Mansell-Jones, 1974). The Assessor may have subscribed to the view taken by Williams (1971) and others who feel that, in spite of the lack of absolute proof, 'halothane hepatitis' should be accepted as a definite clinical entity because of strong circumstantial evidence. Such recommendations place the anaesthetist in a clinical dilemma and make it difficult for clear guidelines to be given regarding the use of halothane. Medicolegal and other implications may force him to use intravenous and other inhalational agents which may be unsuitable and less safe than halothane. When this choice is being made, however, the outstanding safety record of halothane should not be forgotten.

'HALOTHANE HEPATITIS'

The jaundice which may occur in the postoperative period after halothane anaesthesia is often indistinguishable from viral hepatitis, and it may be that this latter disorder accounts for many cases of liver damage erroneously thought to be due to 'halothane hepatitis'. Antimitochondrial antibodies and positive lymphocytic stimulation tests have been found in cases of alleged 'halothane hepatitis' (suggesting autoimmune response) but they are probably not sufficiently reliable to be of value. Hepatitis-associated antigen is not detectable in all cases of viral hepatitis, and in addition it is often difficult to differentiate liver changes of the two disorders by electron microscopy. It may therefore be unreasonable to make a presumptive diagnosis of 'halothane hepatitis' in a patient suffering from otherwise unexplained hepatitis who has been exposed to halothane; it may not be possible to exclude the possibility of viral hepatitis with confidence.

A single case report of a recurrence of hepatitis after a challenge with the suspected drug, however, strongly incriminates the drug as a cause of hepatitis (Babior and Davidson, 1966). It has been suggested that only two true instances of a positive halothane challenge have appeared in the literature (Belfrage, Ahlgren and Axelson, 1966; Klatskin and Kimberg, 1969). In both instances the patients were anaesthetists chronically exposed to low concentrations of halothane, who showed evidence of severe liver injury following a challenging dose of the agent. Although these clinical records have some equivocal features, they provide reasonable evidence of the existence of the clinical entity of 'halothane hepatitis', and it may not be justifiable to insist that cases of hepatitis associated with the use of halothane must always be due to factors such as viral hepatitis, other hepatotoxic drugs or the influence of surgery.

THE IMPORTANCE OF METABOLIC PRODUCTS

When speculating upon the possible pathogenesis of halothane hepatitis oᵢe must consider the effects of its breakdown products in the body. Up to 20% of inhaled halothane is normally metabolized to bromide, chloride and trifluoroacetic acid, the major metabolite which has been detected in the urine many days after anaesthesia (Blake, Barry and Cascorbi, 1972). There is at present, however, no clear evidence that these breakdown products are toxic to the liver.

Obesity and the administration of several anaesthetics within a short period of time are factors which may tend to cause accumulation of halothane in the body. Slow release of large amounts of halothane taken up by fat depots during anaesthesia may mean that in the obese subject there are excessive metabolic demands made upon the liver. Since the metabolism and excretion of halothane may be protracted, repeated administrations at short intervals could, in theory, lead to the production of greater amounts of intermediate metabolites than can be managed by the available liver microsomal enzyme systems (Carney and Van Dyke, 1972).

ENZYME INDUCTION

Induction of the microsomal enzyme systems of the liver by an appropriate inducing agent (e.g. barbiturates) can result in increased rates of halothane metabolism. Initial work by Cascorbi, Blake and Helrich (1970) led them to believe that anaesthetists metabolized halothane to a greater extent than a control group of pharmacists because they excreted more breakdown products in the urine. These workers later formed the opinion that their own results were questionable because of the considerable individual variation in drug metabolism. It is, of course, difficult to know whether it is beneficial or harmful to have an increased ability to metabolize halothane.

IMMUNOLOGICAL ASPECTS

It may be that a pathogenic mechanism involving an immunological response to a complex of halothane metabolism and liver protein is responsible for hepatic injury associated with halothane anaesthesia (Reed and Williams, 1972). Accumulations of large amounts of non-volatile metabolites have been found in the liver of the mouse following injection of C-labelled halothane (Cohen and Hood, 1969). Although these metabolites accumulate rapidly, they leave the liver slowly and residual concentrations are present for at least 12 days. Their exact nature is not known with certainty and consequently the possibility of determining toxicity in relation to liver disease cannot be established. With regard to a hypersensitivity type of response, Cohen (1971) is of the opinion that the responsible haptene is unlikely to be the small halothane molecule and he has demonstrated the formation of large antigenic molecules, the result of the combination of halothane metabolites with protein. Van Dyke and Gandolfi (1974) have also produced evidence that one or more metabolites of halothane may combine with proteins in the liver. The findings of antimitochondrial antibodies and sensitization of lymphocytes to a halothane—protein complex in patients suspected of having 'halothane hepatitis' also suggest a hypersensitivity type of response (Paronetto and Popper, 1970), but these findings have not been confirmed by other workers.

PREDICTION AND PROGNOSIS

On reviewing the literature of the subject it is difficult to disagree with the thesis that, by suitable arrangement of the data, almost any theory relating postoperative jaundice to halothane can be supported or denigrated (Editorial, 1974).

Although the exact pathogenesis of the hepatitis which may follow halothane anaesthesia is still obscure, it is essential to know the absolute contraindications to its clinical use. It is generally advised that it should be avoided if there is a history of liver disease and especially if there has been unexplained pyrexia and jaundice following a previous halothane administration. Postoperative temperature elevations frequently follow surgery, however, and often no explanation can be given for them (Dykes, 1971).

In two recent studies, confined to women with carcinoma of the uterus requiring repeated anaesthesia for radium insertions, serum aspartate and alanine aminotransferase determinations were found to be elevated in those patients receiving halothane but not in the control groups (Trowell, Peto and Smith, 1975; Wright *et al.*, 1975). These findings suggest that obese, middle-aged women receiving radiotherapy for carcinoma are especially prone to hepatic dysfunction after halothane anaesthesia, and are a group in whom repeated administrations of the agent should be avoided. They do not provide sufficient evidence, however, that such considerations apply to the whole of the patient population.

In a study of 76 patients with unexplained hepatitis following halothane anaesthesia, Walton *et al.* (1976) found that rapid onset of jaundice after anaesthesia, male sex and obesity were poor prognostic signs. Those studied had a higher incidence of liver or kidney microsomal and autoimmune complement fixation. This suggests that obese patients with a tendency to organ-specific autoimmunity may be more at risk, although (as the authors point out) the comparative risks of halothane and non-halothane anaesthesia cannot be determined from their data. Further evidence that halothane may be immunogenic is contained in a case report of a patient who developed immune complexes in association with a metabolite of the anaesthetic (Williams *et al.*, 1977).

In a well documented clinical study of 26 cases of halothane-related hepatitis, Moult and Sherlock (1975) found that 24 (92%) had multiple exposures and that 11 (48%) died. Obesity, early onset of jaundice after anaesthesia and a low thrombotest were associated with a fatal outcome. The authors believe that unexplained jaundice or delayed pyrexia after a previous administration of halothane are contraindications to its further use.

It is disappointing to realize that, although halothane has now been in clinical service for some 20 years, the problem of 'halothane hepatitis' remains unsolved. Comprehensive prospective clinical studies appear to offer the only chance of obtaining satisfactory answers.

Methoxyflurane

This is also a halogenated compound and so it was natural that it should be suspected of being able to cause adverse effects on the liver. In spite of several isolated case reports, there is no firm evidence to indicate a causal relationship between the use of methoxyflurane and postoperative liver disturbance. It has been postulated, however, that 'cross-sensitization' may occur with halothane and in the present state of knowledge it would seem best to avoid its use in a patient who for any reason is considered unsuitable for halothane anaesthesia. It would also appear prudent not to use methoxy-flurane when surgery of the liver or gall bladder is contemplated.

Other factors

It has already been emphasized that factors other than the anaesthetic agent should be considered when evaluating the possible causes of post-operative liver dysfunction. Hypoxaemia and respiratory and metabolic acidosis may contribute to hepatic changes, while alterations in hepatic blood flow during anaesthesia and surgery may cause a diminution in venous oxygen saturation. It is thus apparent that the influence of surgery and respiratory and circulatory factors may induce changes in liver function in addition to the effects of the anaesthetic agent.

References

Amory, D. W., Steffenson, J. L. and Forsyth, R. P. (1971). Systemic and regional blood flow changes during halothane anesthesia in the rhesus monkey. *Anesthesiology* 35, 81–90

Aviado, D. M. (1975). Regulation of broncho-motor tone during anesthesia. *Anesthesiology* 42, 68–80

Babior, B. M. and Davidson, C. S. (1966). Hepatitis. Drug or viral? *Am. J. Med.* 41, 491–496

Belfrage, S., Ahlgren, I. and Axelson, S. (1966). Halothane hepatitis in an anaesthetist. *Lancet* ii, 1466–1467

Black, G. W. (1965). Review of the pharmacology of halothane. Br. J. Anaesth. 37, 688–705

Black, G. W. (1967). A comparison of cardiac rhythm during halothane and methoxyflurane anaesthesia at normal and elevated levels of $PaCO_2$. Acta anaesth. scand. 11, 103–108

Black, G. W. and McArdle, L. (1962). The effects of halothane on peripheral circulation in man. Br. J. Anaesth. 34, 2–9

Black, G. W. and McArdle, L. (1965). The effect of methoxyflurane (Penthrane) on the peripheral circulation in man. Br. J. Anaesth. 37, 947–951

Black, G. W., Johnston, H. M. L. and Scott, M. G. (1977). Clinical impressions of enflurane. Br. J. Anaesth. 49, 875–880

Black, G. W., McArdle, L., McCullough, Helen and Unni, V. K. N. (1969). Circulating catecholamines and some cardiovascular, respiratory, metabolic and pupillary responses during diethyl ether anaesthesia. Anaesthesia 24, 168–178

Blake, D. A., Barry, J. Q. and Cascorbi, H. F. (1972). Qualitative analysis of halothane metabolites in man. Anaesthesia 36, 152–154

Bloch, M. (1963). Some systemic effects of nitrous oxide. Br. J. Anaesth. 35, 631–639

Calverley, R. K., Smith, N. T., Prys-Roberts, C., Eger, E. I. II, Jones, C. W. and Ramme, F. B. (1975). Cardiovascular effects of prolonged enflurane anaesthesia in man. Abstracts of Scientific Papers, American Society of Anesthesiologists Annual Meeting, p. 57

Carney, F. M. T. and Van Dyke, R. A. (1972). Halothane hepatitis: a critical review. Anesth. Analg. curr. Res. 51, 135–160

Cascorbi, H. F., Blake, D. A. and Helrich, M. (1970). Differences in the biotransformation of halothane in man. Anesthesiology 32, 119–123

Chase, R. E., Holaday, D. A., Fiserova-Bergerova, V., Saidman, L. J. and Mack, F. E. (1971). The biotransformation of Ethrane in man. Anesthesiology 35, 262–267

Clark, D. L., Hosick, E. C. and Rosner, B. D. (1971). Neurophysiological effects of different anesthetics in unconscious man. J. appl. Physiol. 31, 884–891

Cohen, E. N. (1971). Metabolism of volatile anesthetics. Anesthesiology 35, 193–202

Cohen, E. N. and Hood, Nancy (1969). Application of low-temperature and autoradiography to studies of the uptake and metabolism of volatile anesthetics in the mouse. Anesthesiology 31, 553–559

Coleridge, H. M., Coleridge, J. C. G., Luck, J. C. and Norman, J. (1968). The effect of four volatile anaesthetic agents on the impulse activity of two types of pulmonary receptors. Br. J. Anaesth. 40, 484–492

Cousins, M. J., Greenstein, L. R., Hitt, B. A. and Mazze, R. I. (1976). Metabolism and renal effects of enflurane in man. Anesthesiology 44, 44–53

Cristoforo, M. D. and Brody, M. J. (1968). Non-adrenergic vasoconstriction produced by halothane and cyclopropane anesthesia. Anesthesiology 29, 44–56

Cromwell, T. H., Stevens, W. C., Eger, E. I., Shakespeare, T. F., Halsey, M. J., Bahlman, S. H. and Fourcade, H. E. (1971). The cardiovascular effects of compound 469 (Forane) during spontaneous ventilation and CO_2 challenge in man. Anesthesiology 35, 17–25

Cullen, D. J., Eger, E. I., Stevens, W. C., Smith, N. Ty., Cromwell, T. H., Cullen, B. F., Gregory, G. A., Bahlman, S. H., Dolan, W. M., Stoelting, R. K. and Fourcade, H. E. (1972). Clinical signs of anesthesia. Anesthesiology 36, 21–36

Deutsch, S., Goldberg, M., Stephen, G. W. and Wen-Hsien, W. (1966). Effects of halothane anesthesia on renal function in normal man. Anesthesiology 27, 793–803

Domenech, R. J., Macho, P., Valdes, J. and Penna, M. (1977). Coronary vascular resistance during halothane anesthesia. Anesthesiology 46, 236–240

Dreyer, C., Bischoff, D. and Gothert, M. (1974). Effects of methoxyflurane anesthesia on adrenal medullary catecholamine secretion: inhibition of spontaneous secretion and secretion evoked by splanchnic-nerve stimulation. Anesthesiology 41, 18–26

Dykes, M. H. M. (1970). Anesthesia and the liver. Int. Anesthesiol. Clins 8, 241

Dykes, M. H. (1971). Unexplained post-operative fever. Its value as a sign of halothane sensitization. J. Am. med. Ass. 216, 641–644

Editorial (1974). Jaundice and repeated exposure to halothane. Br. J. Anaesth. 46, 1–2

Eisele, J. H. and Smith, N. Ty. (1972). Cardiovascular effects of 40 per cent nitrous oxide in man. Anesth. Analg. curr. Res. 51, 956–961

Epstein, R. M., Rackow, H., Salanitre, E. and Wolf, G. (1964). Influence of the concentration effect on the uptake of anesthetic mixtures: the second gas effect. Anesthesiology 25, 364–371

Epstein, R. M., Deutsch, S., Cooperman, L. H., Clement, A. J. and Price, H. L. (1966). Splanchnic circulation during halothane anesthesia and hypercapnia in normal man. Anesthesiology 27, 654–661

Fourcade, H. E., Stevens, W. C., Larson, C. P., Cromwell, T. H., Bahlman, S. H., Hickey, R. F., Halsey, M. J. and Eger, E. I. (1971). The ventilatory effects of Forane, a new inhaled anesthetic. Anesthesiology 35, 26–31

Fukunaga, A. F. and Epstein, R. M. (1974). Effects of cyclopropane on the sympathetic nervous system and on neural regulation of circulation in the cat. *Anesthesiology* 40, 323–335

Gothert, M. and Wendt, J. (1977). Inhibition of adrenal medullary catecholamine secretion by enflurane: I. Investigations in vivo. *Anesthesiology* 46, 400–403

Graves, C. L., McDermott, R. W. and Bidwai, Arun (1974). Cardiovascular effects of isoflurane in surgical patients. *Anesthesiology* 41, 486–489

Gregory, G. A., Eger, E. I., Smith, N. Ty., Cullen, B. F. and Cullen, D. J. (1971). The cardiovascular effects of diethyl ether in man. *Anesthesiology* 34, 19–24; 35–41

Halsey, M. J., Sawyer, D. C., Eger, E. I., Bahlman, S. H. and Impelman, Dianne M. K. (1971). Hepatic metabolism of halothane, methoxyflurane, cyclopropane, Ethrane and Forane in miniature swine. *Anesthesiology* 35, 43–47

Hashimoto, K. and Hashimoto, K. (1972). The mechanism of sensitization of the ventricle to epinephrine by halothane. *Am. Heart J.* 83, 652–658

Hashimoto, K., Endoh, M., Kimura, T. and Hashimoto, K. (1975). Effects of halothane on automaticity and contractile force of isolated blood-perfused canine ventricular tissue. *Anesthesiology* 42, 15–25

Horan, B. F., Prys-Roberts, C., Roberts, J. G., Bennett, M. J. and Foex, P. (1977a). Haemodynamic responses to isoflurane anaesthesia and hypovolaemia in the dog, and their modification by propranolol. *Br. J. Anaesth.* 49, 1179–1187

Horan, B. F., Prys-Roberts, C., Hamilton, W. K. and Roberts, J. G. (1977b). Haemodynamic responses to enflurane anaesthesia and hypovolaemia in the dog and their modification by propranolol. *Br. J. Anaesth.* 49, 1189–1197

Inman, W. H. W. and Mushin, W. W. (1974). Jaundice after repeated exposure to halothane: an analysis of reports to the Committee on Safety of Medicines. *Br. med. J.* 1, 5–10

Jones, R. E., Guldmann, N., Linde, H. W., Dripps, R. D. and Price, H. L. (1960). Cyclopropane anesthesia. III. Effects of cyclopropane on respiration and circulation in normal man. *Anesthesiology* 21, 380–393

Klatskin, G. and Kimberg, D. V. (1969). Recurrent hepatitis attributable to halothane sensitization in an anesthetist. *New Engl. J. Med.* 280, 515–522

Kramer, B. (1975). Possible cancer link in new anesthetic is reported in Michigan study on mice. *Wall Street Journal,* March 20

Larson, C. P., Eger, E. I., Muallem, M., Buechel, D. R., Munson, M. D. and Eisele, J. H. (1969). The effects of diethyl ether and methoxyflurane on ventilation. 2. A comparative study in man. *Anesthesiology* 30, 174–184

Lebowitz, M. H., Blitt, C. D. and Walts, L. F. (1970). Depression of twitch response to stimulation of the ulnar nerve during Ethrane anesthesia in man. *Anesthesiology* 33, 52–57

Li, T. H., Shaul, M. S. and Etsten, B. E. (1968). Decreased adrenal venous catecholamine concentrations during methoxyflurane anesthesia. *Anesthesiology* 29, 1145–1152

Little, D. M. (1968). The effects of halothane on hepatic function. In *Halothane.* N. M. Greene (ed.). Philadelphia: F. A. Davis

Lurie, A. A., Jones, R. E., Linde, H. W., Price, M. L., Dripps, R. D. and Price, H. L. (1958). Cyclopropane anesthesia: cardiac rate and rhythm during steady levels of cyclopropane anesthesia in man at normal and elevated end-expiratory carbon dioxide tensions. *Anesthesiology* 19, 457–472

McArdle, L. and Black, G. W. (1963). Effects of cyclopropane on the peripheral circulation in man. *Br. J. Anaesth.* 35, 352–357

McArdle, L., Black, G. W. and Unni, V. K. N. (1968). Peripheral vascular changes during diethyl ether anaesthesia. *Anaesthesia* 23, 203–210

McCaughey, W. (1972). A summary of the National Halothane Study. *Br. J. Anaesth.* 44, 918

McDowell, S. A., Hall, K. D. and Stephen, C. R. (1968). Difluoromethyl 1,1,2-trifluoro-2-chloroethyl ether: experiments on dogs with a new inhalational anaesthetic agent. *Br. J. Anaesth.* 40, 511–516

McPeek, B. and Gilbert, J. P. (1974). Onset of post-operative jaundice related to anaesthesia history (halothane). *Br. med. J.* 3, 615–617

Mansell-Jones, D. (1974). Circular letter from the Committee on Safety of Medicines. CSM/S/121 3 January

Marshall, B. E., Cohen, P. J., Klingenmaier, C. H., Neigh, J. L. and Pender, J. W. (1971). Some pulmonary and cardiovascular effects of enflurane (Ethrane) anaesthesia with varying $PaCO_2$ in man. *Br. J. Anaesth.* 43, 996–1002

Mazze, R. I., Trudell, J. R. and Cousins, M. J. (1971). Methoxyflurane metabolism and renal dysfunction: clinical correlation in man. *Anesthesiology* 35, 247–252

Millar, R. A. and Biscoe, T. J. (1966). Post-ganglionic sympathetic discharge and the effect of inhalational anaesthetics. *Br. J. Anaesth.* 38, 92–114

Miller, R. D., Eger, E. I., Way, W. L., Stevens, W. C. and Dolan, W. M. (1971). Comparative neuromuscular effects of Forane and halothane along and in combination with d-tubocurarine in man. *Anesthesiology* 35, 38–42

Morrow, R. D. H., Haley, J. V. and Logic, J. R. (1972). Anesthesia and digitalis. VII. The effect of pentobarbital, halothane and methoxyflurane on the A-V conduction and inotropic responses to ouabain. *Anesth. Analg. curr. Res.* 51, 430–438

Moult, P. J. A. and Sherlock, S. (1975).
Halothane-related hepatitis. A clinical study
of twenty-six cases. *Q. Jl Med.* New Series,
44, 99–114

Munson, E. S. and Tucker, W. K. (1975) Doses
of epinephrine causing arrhythmia during
enflurane, methoxyflurane and halothane
anaesthesia in dogs. *Can. Anaesth. Soc. J.*
22, 495–501

National Halothane Study (1966). Possible
association between halothane anesthesia
and post-operative hepatic necrosis. Report
by Subcommittee on the National Halothane
Study of the Committee on Anesthesia,
National Academy of Science. *J. Am. med.
Ass.* 197, 775–788

Ngai, S. H. (1967). Pharmacological aspects of
the control of respiration. In *Modern Trends
in Anaesthesia – 3. Aspects of Metabolism
and Pulmonary Ventilation*, pp. 162–184.
F. T. Evans and T. C. Gray (ed.). London:
Butterworths

Ngai, S. H. and Bolme, P. (1966). Effects of
anesthetics on circulatory mechanisms in the
dog. *J. Pharmac. exp. Ther.* 153, 495–504

Ngai, S. H., Katz, R. L. and Farhie, S. E. (1965).
Respiratory effects of trichloroethylene,
halothane and methoxyflurane in the cat.
J. Pharmac. exp. Ther. 148, 123–130

Paronetto, F. and Popper, H. (1970). Lymphocyte stimulation induced by halothane in
patients with hepatitis following exposure to
halothane. *New Engl. J. Med.* 283, 277–280

Pauca, A. L. and Dripps, R. D. (1973). Clinical
experience with isoflurane (Forane). *Br. J.
Anaesth.* 45, 697–703

Perry, L. B., Van Dyke, R. A. and Theye, R. A.
(1974). Sympathoadrenal and hemodynamic
effects of isoflurane, halothane and cyclopropane in dogs. *Anesthesiology* 40, 465–470

Price, M. L. and Price, H. L. (1962). Effects of
general anesthetics on contractile response of
rabbit aortic strips. *Anesthesiology* 23, 16–20

Price, H. L., Price, M. L. and Morse, H. T.
(1965). Effects of cyclopropane, halothane
and procaine on the vasomotor 'center' of
the dog. *Anesthesiology* 26, 55–60

Price, H. L., Warden, J. C., Cooperman, L. H.
and Millar, R. A. (1969). Central sympathetic
excitation caused by cyclopropane. *Anesthesiology* 30, 426–438

Price, H. L., Deutsch, S., Cooperman, L. H.,
Clement, A. J. and Epstein, R. M. (1965).
Splanchnic circulation during cyclopropane
anesthesia in normal man. *Anesthesiology* 26,
312–319

Prys-Roberts, C., Gersh, B. J., Baker, A. B. and
Reuben, S. R. (1972). The effects of halothane
on the interactions between myocardial
contractility, aortic impedance, and left
ventricular performance. *Br. J. Anaesth.* 44,
634–649

Raventos, J. (1956). The action of Fluothane –
a new volatile anaesthetic. *Br. J. Pharmac.* 11,
394–410

Reed, W. D. and Williams, R. (1972). Halothane
hepatitis as seen by the physician. *Br. J.
Anaesth.* 44, 935–940

Reisner, L. S. and Lippmann, M. (1975).
Ventricular arrhythmias after epinephrine
injection in enflurane and halothane anesthesia. *Anesth. Analg. curr. Res.* 54,
468–470

Reynolds, A. K., Chiz, J. F. and Pasquet, A. F.
(1970). Halothane and methoxyflurane – a
comparison of their effects on cardiac pacemaker fibers. *Anesthesiology* 33, 602–610

Roberts, J. G., Prys-Roberts, C., Foex, P.,
Clarke, T. N. S. and Bennett, M. J. (1973).
A comparison of the effects of practolol and
propranolol on the response to haemorrhage
in anaesthetized dogs after myocardial infarction. *Br. J. Anaesth.* 45, 1230

Roizen, M. D., Moss, J., Henry, D. P. and
Kopin, I. J. (1974). Effects of halothane on
plasma catecholamines. *Anesthesiology* 41,
432–439

Saner, C. A., Foex, P., Roberts, J. G. and
Bennett, M. J. (1975). Methoxyflurane and
practolol: a dangerous combination. (Proc.
Anaesth. Res. Soc.) *Br. J. Anaesth.* 47, 1025

Scott, M. G., McArdle, L. and Black, G. W.
(1978). A critical appraisal of venous occlusion
plethysmography as a method of assessing
limb blood flow during halothane anaesthesia.
(Proc. Anaesth. Res. Soc.) *Br. J. Anaesth.* 50,
630

Severinghaus, J. W. and Cullen, S. C. (1958).
Depression of myocardium and body oxygen
consumption with fluothane. *Anesthesiology*
19, 165–177

Shimosato, S., Sugai, N., Iwatsuki, N. and
Etsten, B. E. (1969). The effect of Ethrane
on cardiac muscle mechanics. *Anesthesiology*
30, 513–518

Simpson, B. R., Strunin, L. and Walton, B.
(1971). The halothane dilemma: a case for
the defence. *Br. med. J.* 4, 96–100

Skovsted, P. and Price, H. L. (1969). The
effects of methoxyflurane on arterial pressure,
preganglionic sympathetic activity and
barostatic reflexes. *Anesthesiology* 31,
515–521

Skovsted, P. and Price, H. L. (1970). Central
sympathetic excitation caused by diethyl
ether. *Anesthesiology* 32, 202–209

Skovsted, P., Price, Mary L. and Price, H. L.
(1969). The effects of halothane on arterial
pressure, preganglionic sympathetic activity
and barostatic reflexes. *Anesthesiology* 31,
507–514

Smith, A. L. (1973). The mechanism of cerebral
vasodilatation by halothane. *Anesthesiology*
39, 581–587

Sprague, D. H. and Ngai, S. H. (1974). Effects
of cyclopropane on contractility and the
cyclic 3'5'-adenosine monophosphate system
in the rat aorta. *Anesthesiology* 40, 336–339

Stevens, W. C., Cromwell, T. H., Halsey, M. J., Eger, E. I., Shakespeare, T. F. and Bahlman, S. H. (1971). The cardiovascular effects of a new inhalation anesthetic, Forane, in human volunteers at constant arterial carbon dioxide tension. *Anesthesiology* 35, 8−16

Strunin, L. and Simpson, B. R. (1972). Halothane in Britain today. *Br. J. Anaesth.* 44, 919−924

Sugai, N., Shimosato, S. and Etsten, B. E. (1968). Effect of halothane on force-velocity relations and dynamic stiffness of isolated heart muscle. *Anesthesiology* 29, 267−274

Trowell, J., Peto, R. and Smith, A. C. (1975). Controlled trial of repeated halothane anaesthetics in patients with carcinoma of the uterine cervix treated with radium. *Lancet* i, 821−823

Tucker, W. K., Rackstein, A. D. and Munson, E. S. (1974). Comparison of arrhythmic doses of adrenaline, metaraminol, ephedrine and phenylephrine during isoflurane and halothane anaesthesia in dogs. *Br. J. Anaesth.* 46, 392−396

Unni, V. K. N., McArdle, L. and Black, G. W. (1970). Sympatho-adrenal, respiratory and metabolic changes during trichloroethylene anaesthesia. *Br. J. Anaesth.* 42, 429−433

Van Dyke, R. A. and Gandolfi, A. J. (1974). Studies on irreversible binding of radioactivity from halothane to rat hepatic microsomal lipids and protein. *Drug Metab. Disposit.* 2, 469−476

Vick, R. L. (1966). Effects of altered heart rate on chloroform−epinephrine cardiac arrhythmia. *Circulation Res.* 18, 316−322

Vitcha, J. F. (1971). A history of Forane (Editorial). *Anesthesiology* 35, 4−7

Wallin, R. F., Regan, B. M., Napoli, M. D. and Stern, I. J. (1975). Sevoflurane: a new inhalational anesthetic agent. *Anesth. Analg., Cleve.* 54, 758−766

Walton, B., Simpson, B. R., Strunin, L., Doniach, D., Perrin, J. and Appleyard, A. J. (1976). Unexplained hepatitis following halothane. *Br. med. J.* 1, 1171−1176

Waters, R. M. (ed.) (1951). *Chloroform: a study after 100 years.* Madison: University of Wisconsin Press; London: Clair

Westermark, L. (1969). Haemodynamics during halothane anaesthesia in the cat. *Acta anaesth. scand.* 35, Suppl., 20−25

Williams, R. (1971). Halothane hepatitis. *Br. med. J.* 3, 110

Williams, B. D., White, N., Amlot, P. L., Slaney, J. and Toseland, P. A. (1977). Circulating immune complexes after repeated halothane anaesthesia. *Br. med. J.* 2, 159−162

Wright, R., Chisholm, M., Lloyd, B., Edwards, J. C., Eade, O. E., Hawksley, M., Moles, T. M. and Gardner, M. J. (1975). Controlled prospective study of the effect on liver function of multiple exposures to halothane. *Lancet* i, 817−820

9 Chronic exposure to trace concentrations of anaesthetics

Alastair A. Spence

The use of gaseous anaesthetics is always associated with contamination of the ambient air of the operating room, recovery room or labour room. Sources of contaminants include the exhaust outlet of and leaks from a breathing system, the patient following disconnection of the breathing system, filling of vaporizers without the use of a locked safety system, and the use of volatile anaesthetics, such as diethyl ether, for cleansing equipment. Personnel working in these environments carry the contaminants in the alveolar gas, blood and other body tissues. It should be remembered that anaesthetics are not the only contaminants of operating rooms; Halliday and Carter (1978) found that ethanol and isopropanol were the most concentrated contaminants of an operating room in which the exhaust anaesthetic gases were scavenged.

For more than 50 years, but particularly in the last ten years, it has been suggested that occupational exposure to trace concentrations of anaesthetics may be a cause of ill health or of impaired psychomotor performance, or both. There have been several epidemiological, volunteer and small animal studies to determine if this is so. There is still no firm evidence of a risk of any type but we may be reasonably satisfied that some of the early anxieties, about an effect on mental performance for example, are not justified. At present, the greatest credence is given to reports of an increased risk of spontaneous abortion associated with operating room work during a pregnancy.

If there is a danger to health associated with anaesthetic contamination, it is important to realize that many people are at risk; in the USA alone, it has been estimated that 250 000 persons work regularly in places where anaesthetics are given.

LEVELS OF CONTAMINATION

There have been many reports of methods for measuring operating room contamination. The most popular techniques are based on gas chromatography, infrared analysis and mass spectrometry. The lowest concentration that can be detected varies between studies, even for the same type of apparatus. Halsey (reported by Barton and Nunn, 1975) achieved 0.01 p.p.m. (v/v) in the measurement of halothane. The value of 0.1 p.p.m. is more typical. Robinson *et al.* (1976) have drawn attention to the need for precision in both measuring and reporting the levels of contamination. The unqualified use of the unit 'parts per million' (p.p.m.), for example, is particularly ambiguous unless we know whether a volume (v/v) or weight (w/w) ratio is intended (halothane 100 μg·l^{-1} = 11.3 p.p.m. [v/v] = 83.0 p.p.m. [w/w]). In the ten years since Linde and Bruce (1969) reported on the concentrations of halothane and nitrous oxide in operating theatre air, there have been more than 50 similar or more detailed studies.

TABLE 9.1. Measurement of air contamination [p.p.m. (v/v)] in areas in which anaesthetic gases occur, showing the improvements which result from scavenging of breathing systems

	Highest value reported	Average or typical range of averages	
		Unscavenged	Scavenged
Operating room:			
Halothane	199	3—12	0.8—2
Nitrous oxide	9700	130—929	14—135
Dental surgery:			
Halothane	36	18—25	—
Nitrous oxide	6767	—	7—14
Recovery room:			
Halothane	8.2	3.0	—
Nitrous oxide	500	169	—

Data based principally on NIOSH report (1977) table 13, pp. 168—169, and Pfäffli, Nikki and Ahlman (1972).

Table 9.1 shows the wide range of values for the anaesthetic contaminants which occur commonly. Often, but not always, the use of scavenging devices is associated with lesser concentrations.

It should be appreciated, however, that the value of such measurements is limited since it is generally assumed that any deleterious effects of operating theatre contamination (pollution) would be related to the concentration of the anaesthetics in the tissues of theatre workers. It is well established that even random simultaneous sampling of operating room air can reveal widely differing concentrations from one part of the room to another (Langley and Steward, 1974). Thus the doctor or nurse who is positioned within a few centimetres of an unscavenged exhaust valve or who fills a vaporizer from an open bottle may be exposed to concentrations of anaesthetics of a different order of magnitude from those reported as being 'representative' of the working environment.

Not surprisingly, there have been several demonstrations of both nitrous oxide and halothane in the expired gas of operating room personnel; concentrations of halothane as great as 12 p.p.m. have been noted by Nikki, Pfäffli and Ahlman (1972) who were able to demonstrate the presence of halothane in venous blood. The elimination of trace concentrations of anaesthetics to the point at which they are no longer detectable in expired gas continues for a period of as much as 64 hours for halothane and 7 hours for nitrous oxide (Corbett, 1973).

EPIDEMIOLOGICAL STUDIES

Eight retrospective surveys have sought to determine if there is a relationship between working in an operating room ('exposure') and obstetric mishap, notably spontaneous abortion. The first suggestion of a link between spontaneous abortion and anaesthetic practice came from Vaisman (1967), although her enquiry was not designed specifically for this purpose. Several of these studies have considered the possibility of an effect on the wife of an exposed male (*Table 9.2*). Vessey (1978) and Spence and Knill-Jones (1978) have discussed the problems of interpretation of such retrospective enquiries. Every one of the eight surveys is open to serious scientific criticism on a variety of grounds. For example, the Danish survey (Askrog and Harvald, 1970) compared the obstetric history of respondents before and after commencing the practice of anaesthesia, thus appearing to ignore the important effects of age on child bearing. The chief positive finding was an increase in the frequency of spontaneous abortion in the wives of male anaesthetists, but the data were not sufficient to allow conclusions about the risk to a pregnant woman from working in an operating room. Knill-Jones *et al.* (1972) were unable to derive more than mean values for the abortion rate in the exposed and non-exposed groups. Thus, important factors such as smoking habit, parity and maternal age could not be allowed for; the mean ages in the two groups were comparable but there were significantly fewer children born to anaesthetists, suggesting that they may become pregnant for the first time at a relatively older age.

Even more serious objections can be levelled at the fact that all the enquiries were retrospective, covering (except in the case of the US studies) the entire reproductive history of each respondent. Studies after 1970 could not guarantee a lack of bias on the part of responding anaesthetists, most of whom were fully aware of the possibility of the risks about which they were questioned, and, perhaps most serious of all, reply rates in the large enquiries were never better than about 80% (Knill-Jones *et al.*, 1972) while some yielded rates of less than 50% (Cohen *et al.*, 1974). Reporting bias is a serious possibility with such low response rates.

These objections are not just theoretical, for it is accepted widely that personal recollection of spontaneous abortion is notoriously unreliable. At the very least, it would be desirable to have clinical and laboratory confirmation of the fact that a pregnancy had become established, while

TABLE 9.2. Summary of nine reports relating anaesthetic or operating theatre work and problems of child bearing, notably spontaneous abortion

	Country of origin	Groups studied		Apparent risk associated with exposure	Comment
		Test	Control		
(1) Vaisman (1967)	USSR	An. (M & F)	—	Inc. Abtn	No controls
(2) Askrog and Harvald (1970)	Denmark	An. (M & F)	Same respondents before commencing anaesthesia	Inc. Abtn ? Inc. CA Fewer males	No controls
(3) Cohen, Bellville and Brown (1971)	USA	An. (F) An. nur. (F)	Paediatricians (F) Paed. nur. (F)	Inc. Abtn	Careful study. Small numbers
(4) Knill-Jones et al. (1972)	UK	An. (F)	Doctors (F)	Inc. Abtn ? Inc. CA Inc. infertility	First large study. Data superficial
(5) Rosenberg and Kirves (1973)	Sweden	An. nur. (F) Scrub nur. (F) ITU nur. (F)	Casualty nur. (F)	Inc. Abtn	ITU nurses had greatest frequency of Abtn
(6) Cohen et al. (1974)	USA	An. (M & F) An. nur. (M & F)	Paediatricians (M & F)	Inc. Abtn (F only) Inc. CA	Largest survey
(7) Cohen et al. (1975)	USA	Dentists (M) GA	Dentists (M)	Inc. Abtn	Males only; cf. (6) and (8)
(8) Knill-Jones, Newman and Spence (1975)	UK	An. (M & F)	Doctors (M & F)	Inc. Abtn ? Inc CA } F only	Detailed study with matching of respondents
(9) Pharaoh et al. (1977)	UK	An. (F)	Doctors (F)	None	Presumably included respondents to (4) and (8)

Abtn, spontaneous abortion; An, anaesthetist; CA, congenital abnormality; F, female; GA, general anaesthesia; Inc, increased; M, Male; Nur, nurse some authorities believe that histological examination of the products of conception is the only true confirmation. Neither verification has been sought in any of the epidemiological surveys. Finally, it is practically impossible to relate data on morbidity to the degree of exposure, which is usually unknown, and there are many obvious factors, such as levels of contamination and differences in working hours, which can be expected to vary widely among individuals in one job category (operating room nurse or anaesthetist).

Similar confusion or uncertainty surrounds reports of congenital abnormality in liveborn children. Cohen *et al.* (1974) found a statistically significant increase in the rate of abnormalities in children born to women who had been exposed to anaesthetics during the pregnancy. Moreover, there was a parallel increase in the frequency of multifactorial abnormalities which they held to be specially indicative of a drug-induced effect. Knill-Jones *et al.* (1972) and Knill-Jones, Newman and Spence (1975) also found that the children of both male and female anaesthetists appeared to have a greater risk of abnormality, but they stressed that the increase was not attributable to an increased involvement of any one system (neural groove defects are likely in the case of a drug-induced effect). When they classified the defects as major (life threatening) and minor, they found that much of the increased reporting by anaesthetists was in the latter category, so that again the possibility of bias in reporting cannot be excluded.

Knill-Jones *et al.* (1972) found that female anaesthetists in the UK reported involuntary infertility at twice the frequency of the control group. They considered that this might be regarded as complementing their data on spontaneous abortion; that is, early shedding of a fetus might present as apparent infertility whereas the factors causing such an effect might be the same as those responsible for the increased rate of spontaneous abortion in other women. Unfortunately, data on infertility have not been obtained in studies outside the UK. The marriages of UK male anaesthetists were not obviously less fertile than those of other doctors.

The data from anaesthetists for the two UK studies and the 1974 US study (*Table 9.2*) have been compared formally (Spence *et al.*, 1978). There is a striking agreement between the two countries in the estimated increased risk of spontaneous abortion in women who are exposed to anaesthetic contaminants (about 50%). However, this is based on averages for the populations studied. Knill-Jones, Newman and Spence (1975) were able to match exposed and non-exposed mothers in respect of age, parity and smoking habit (a technique which epidemiologists regard as more acceptable than the use of group averages) and estimated the increased risk for exposed women at between 100 and 200%. However, confidence in the UK figures must be tempered by the fact that Pharoah *et al.* (1977) found that a small increase in the frequency of spontaneous abortion in British women anaesthetists was not significantly greater than that of a substantial control group. This finding is all the more surprising when it is realized that there must have been considerable overlap between their respondents and those of Knill-Jones and his colleagues in 1972 and 1975. Pharoah's study found an increase in the reporting of congenital abnormalities by women anaesthetists, although the difference from the control group was not statistically significant. They suggested that defects of the heart and great vessels were commoner in infants born to anaesthetists.

ANIMAL STUDIES

At the time of the initial concern about the risk to pregnancy of operating theatre work, in the early 1970s, there existed a considerable amount of information to suggest that anaesthetic concentrations of several inhalation agents could cause various types of fetal damage in small animals. This included evidence of death, decreased growth and defects of the neural tube in chick embryos in response to halothane and nitrous oxide (B. E. Smith, Gaub and Moya, 1965a, b), and frank teratogenicity in the rat following nitrous oxide (Fink, Shepard and Blandau, 1967) and halothane (Basford and Fink, 1968). Shepard and Fink (1968) described resorption of the rat fetus (a process analogous to spontaneous abortion in humans) following prolonged nitrous oxide anaesthesia. It is fair to state that, except for these studies, there would have seemed little purpose in con-ducting the early epidemiological studies of anaesthetists or, at least, no one would have given credibility to the suggestion that the findings in humans might be attributable to operating room pollution. At best, however, the link was tenuous. Quite apart from the difficulties of extra-polating from one species to another, the doses of anaesthetics adminis-tered in these animal studies were of a different order of magnitude from those likely to contaminate an operating room.

The more appropriate animal data — chiefly studies of the rat — did not appear until 1973 and later (*Table 9.3*). In each of the studies an un-desirable effect on the fetus was demonstrated but, with the possible exception of one study (Schwetz, Leong and Gehring, 1974), there was no clear evidence of fetal abnormality such as had been presumed to occur in anaesthetists. In a study on pregnant mice, Bruce (1973) found that trace concentrations of halothane (16 p.p.m.) had no deleterious effect on the pregnancy. Kripke *et al.* (1976) have demonstrated a reversible inhibition of spermatogenesis induced by subanaesthetic concentrations of nitrous oxide.

Pope *et al.* (1978) considered that the decrease in rat fetal weight which they observed might be a result of stress in the mother because of increased handling. This aspect of the animal experiments had received little mention previously, although its importance was emphasized by Fink and Cullen (1976), who argued that the existing literature on the effects of stress on pregnant animals was sufficient to justify advancing 'occupational stress' as an alternative to environmental pollution in explaining the obstetric data from the epidemiological studies.

In view of the report by Sturrock and Nunn (1976), of a synergistic effect of halothane and nitrous oxide in the production of nuclear

Table 9.3. Experimental exposure of pregnant rats to subanaesthetic concentrations of anaesthetic gases. Summary of published reports

Authors	Species	Exposure		Effect on fetus
		Time	Gas	
Pope et al. (1978)	Rat	8 h/day 21 days	Hal. 0.16–0.32% N₂O 1–50% N₂O 10% Hal. 0.16% Methox. 0.01–0.08%	Decreased fetal weight No significant fetal loss No fetal abnormality
Pope et al. (1975)	Rat	8 h/day 8–12 days	Hal. 50–3200 p.p.m.	Small decrease of weight No fetal loss, fetal abnormality or growth effect
Lansdown et al. (1976)	Rat	8–12 days 1–21 days	Hal. 50–3200 p.p.m. Hal. 1600 p.p.m.	Decreased fetal weight No fetal abnormality
Chang et al. (1974)	Rat	8 h/day 5 days/week	Hal. 10 p.p.m.	Damage to brain cell ultrastructure
Chang et al. (1975a)	Rat	8 h/day 5 days/week	Hal. 10 p.p.m.	Damage to kidney cell ultrastructure
Chang et al. (1975b)	Rat	8 h/day 5 days/week	Hal. 10 p.p.m.	Damage to liver cell ultrastructure
Schwetz, Leong, Gehring (1974)	Rat	7 h/day days 16–15	Chloroform 30, 100, 300 p.p.m.	Increased frequency of fetal abnormalities with 100 and 300 p.p.m.
Corbett et al. (1973a)	Rat	8 or 24 h/day	N₂O 100, 1000, 15 000 p.p.m.	Greater death rate with 1000 and 15 000 p.p.m.
Healy and Wilcox (1977)	Rat	4 h/day from day 6	Trichloroethylene 100 p.p.m.	Decreased fetal weight Increased fetal resorption

Hal., halothane; Methox., methoxyflurane; N₂O, nitrous oxide. Concentrations are v/v.

abnormalities in dividing fibroblasts, it is particularly noteworthy that there was no additional harm to the rat fetus from a combination of these agents in the study of Pope *et al.* (1978).

STUDIES OF OTHER DISEASE IN OPERATING ROOM PERSONNEL

Background

Studies in a variety of small animals have shown that chronic exposure to both anaesthetic and trace concentrations of several inhalation anaesthetics can cause disorders ranging from leucopenia and lesions of the liver, kidney and brain to general retardation of growth. For a detailed summary of these effects, the reader is referred to NIOSH (1977, pp. 184–185).

Vaisman (1967) listed many disorders in theatre workers, including headache, malaise, and gastrointestinal and respiratory upset. From time to time, the anaesthetic literature has carried individual case reports of liver disease, laryngitis, myasthenia, ophthalmic hypersensitivity, migraine, atrial fibrillation and exacerbations of asthma – all attributed to anaesthetic contamination (see review by Smith, 1976).

Carcinogenicity

Some anaesthetics may be capable of inducing or influencing the course of cancer in experimental animals (Eschenbrenner, 1945; Corbett, 1976a), although the total doses required to produce the effect are very large.

Corbett (1976b) has presented reasons for considering that carcinogenicity may occur in man also.

(1) Most inhalation anaesthetics are halogenated hydrocarbons or halogenated ethers. A number of closely related chemicals are known carcinogens in man or animals.
(2) In animals, the carcinogenicity of chloroform has been demonstrated with repeated oral administration of large doses, while trichloroethylene and isoflurane are 'highly suspect'.
(3) Tissue binding of metabolites of halothane, methoxyflurane, enflurane and isoflurane have been demonstrated in man. It is argued that some of the intermediates are highly reactive and may interfere with DNA or other macromolecules to initiate a carcinogenic process.

It should, however, be noted that the anaesthetics in common use are not mutagenic (see Chapter 10).

There is extensive literature on the suppression of various aspects of the immune response by anaesthetics in man and animals, although Salo and Vapaaruori (1976) concluded that there was no demonstrable effect which might be attributed to trace concentrations of anaesthetics in operating room personnel.

Mortality

Bruce *et al.* (1968) surveyed retrospectively the causes of death among members of the American Society of Anesthesiologists, with the statistics of an insurance company for comparison. There were no statistically significant differences between the groups, although tumours of the lymphoid and reticuloendothelial system and suicide were more common and lung cancer and coronary artery disease less common in anaesthetists than would have been expected. A follow-up prospective enquiry (Bruce *et al.*, 1974) failed to confirm these trends. Doll and Peto (1977), in a careful prospective study of mortality among doctors in the UK, conducted over 20 years, found no outstanding differences between anaesthetists and others, although the former had a greater than expected frequency of carcinoma of the pancreas.

Studies of health patterns

Cohen *et al.* (1974) and Knill-Jones, Newman and Spence (1975) sought information about serious illness in the respondents (in addition to the obstetric history). The enquiry related to men and women in the USA but only to men in the UK. Specific questioning was confined to disease of the liver and kidneys and to cancer, although many respondents volunteered additional information. In neither country was there any suggestion that male anaesthetists were specially susceptible to cancer or heart disease. Significant increases in the reporting of peptic ulcer, gall bladder disease, arterial hypertension and lumbar disc problems by anaesthetists in the UK, and of colitis and migraine in the USA were not reflected in the other country. In both countries, hepatitis was more common in anaesthetists, and a similar observation was made in US dentists (Cohen *et al.*, 1975).

Female operating room personnel in the USA were found to have an increased frequency of various types of cancer as compared with the control groups (Cohen *et al.*, 1974), and a similar pattern was suggested by Corbett *et al.* (1973b) in a study of Michigan nurse-anaesthetists. Vessey (1978) has criticized the methods and conclusions of these enquiries and considers the evidence for regarding cancer as an occupational hazard of anaesthesia to be unconvincing.

EFFECTS ON PERFORMANCE

Some anaesthetists believe that exposure to pollution by anaesthetics may exacerbate feelings of fatigue (Wilkinson, Tyler and Varey, 1975). Bruce, Bach and Arbit (1974) found that 6 of the 20 volunteers whom they exposed to trace concentrations of halothane and nitrous oxide fell asleep, but this was not noted in several similar studies.

It is clearly important to ensure that operating room workers are not impaired in their psychomotor performance as a result of anaesthetic contaminants. However, this is a difficult matter to assess. Nearly all the published reports have considered the artificial situation of laboratory exposure of volunteers to measured low concentrations of anaesthetics, associated with a variety of tests of psychomotor function. G. Smith and Shirley (1978) have reviewed these reports in detail. Early studies in which volunteers breathed trichloroethylene had sometimes, but not always, yielded positive findings in respect of impaired visual perception, memory and manual dexterity, but the concentrations used (often in excess of 100 p.p.m.) were greater than those to be expected in an operating room.

Bruce, Bach and Arbit (1974) in Chicago examined the effects of 500 p.p.m. of nitrous oxide and found a small decrement in performance; the addition of halothane 15 p.p.m. caused a more marked effect. Bruce and Bach (1975) noted impairment of performance with a similar mixture of nitrous oxide and enflurane. In 1976, the same authors, in attempting to derive a dose—response relationship, found a measurable effect with as little as 50 p.p.m. of nitrous oxide. However, at least four similar studies have failed to demonstrate the findings of the Chicago workers even at higher concentrations than those which they used. Smith and Shirley (1978) cite evidence to suggest that the threshold for an effect on psycho-motor performance may be as much as 5—10% of MAC* for nitrous oxide, enflurane and halothane.

CONCLUSION ON HEALTH HAZARDS OF CONTAMINATION

Many of the fears about occupational hazards associated with the operating room have not been sustained by the best, if limited, attempts to submit them to objective scrutiny. The writer is in agreement with the conclusion of Vessey (1978):

> '[there is] . . . reasonably convincing evidence of a moderate increase in the risk of spontaneous abortion among exposed females, although it is possible that even this result is attributable to reporting bias. There is no convincing evidence of any other hazard.'

In spite of this view based on the facts, there remains the problem of deciding what further action, if any, should be taken. Should we take no action about reducing the levels of contaminants, for example, on the grounds that we cannot be sure of its worth? Given that exhaust gas scavenging systems are easy and inexpensive to install and use, such a view would appear to lack common sense. Certainly, it has never been suggested that environmental contamination is beneficial. At the same time, it is reasonable to suggest that an effective system for monitoring

* The concept of MAC is defined in Chapter 3. *Ed.*

the health of women who work in operating rooms should be followed, at least in the advanced industrial countries. Such a scheme is already in operation in the USA and the UK.

Measures to reduce and monitor levels of operating theatre contamination

In spite of the uncertainties which have been mentioned, various authorities have taken the view that there is sufficient cause for anxiety to justify recommendations for reducing the levels of contamination. In the UK, the Departments of Health (1976) have advised health authorities that reasonable measures should be taken to reduce the levels of contamination and to remind operating theatre staff of the possible risks associated with a contaminated environment. Scavenging devices should be provided for anaesthetic breathing systems and a nurse who is or who plans to become pregnant should have the opportunity of working in an area of the hospital in which anaesthetic gases are not employed (there is no guidance about women doctors). Similar, but more elaborate, recommendations have been published in the USA (NIOSH, 1977) and apparently arbitrary upper limits of acceptable contamination have been suggested. Detailed descriptions of scavenging techniques are given by Whitcher *et al.* (1975) and W. D. A. Smith (1978). Whitcher (1978) has discussed the difficult question of the extent to which surveillance of the effectiveness of scavenging should be pursued. A comprehensive programme would require:

(1) regular tests of anaesthetic equipment for gas leaks;
(2) effective scavenging;
(3) avoidance of accidental gas leaks and spillage of volatile agents;
(4) monitoring of operating room air.

A comprehensive programme for monitoring operating theatre air is expensive of both manpower and equipment. Whitcher favours the detection of nitrous oxide only, using an infrared analyser, and his sophisticated arrangements in Stanford appear to work well, although it is recognized that they are not easily reproducible in all types of hospital. However, the limitations of this type of monitoring have been discussed earlier in this chapter and it is the writer's opinion that this approach to the problem is of questionable value. A preferable method of monitoring would be the use of one of the personal monitors or samplers such as those described by Davenport *et al.* (1976) and Piziali and others (cited by Whitcher, 1978). These devices allow continuous sampling and collection of air near the breathing zone of the individual. Subsequent analysis by gas chromatography provides a time-averaged value for exposure to contaminants. Even in the absence of clear guidelines as to the 'safe' level of exposure, personal sampling might be expected to encourage a more disciplined approach to the handling of the gaseous anaesthetics. Of course, a comprehensive programme of personal monitoring would be expensive and, as yet, no field trials of its feasibility have been attempted.

References

Askrog, V. and Harvald, B. (1970). Teratogen effekt af inhalations anaestetika. *Nord. Med.* 83, 498—504

Barton, F. and Nunn, J. F. (1975). Totally closed circuit nitrous oxide—oxygen anaesthesia. *Br. J. Anaesth.* 47, 350—357

Basford, A. B. and Fink, B. R. (1968). The teratogenicity of halothane in the rat. *Anesthesiology* 29, 1167—1173

Bruce, D. L. (1973). Murine fertility unaffected by traces of halothane. *Anesthesiology* 38, 473

Bruce, D. L. and Bach, M. J. (1975). Psychological studies of human performance as affected by traces of enflurane and nitrous oxide. *Anesthesiology* 42, 194—196

Bruce, D. L. and Bach, M. J. (1976). Effect of trace anaesthetic gases on behavioural performance in volunteers. *Br. J. Anaesth.* 48, 871—876

Bruce, D. L., Bach, M. J. and Arbit, J. (1974). Trace anesthetic effects on perceptual cognitive and motor skills. *Anesthesiology* 40, 453—458

Bruce, D. L., Eide, K. A., Linde, H. W. and Eckenhoff, J. E. (1968). Causes of death among anesthesiologists: a 20 year survey. *Anesthesiology* 29, 565—569

Bruce, D. L., Eide, K. A., Smith, N. J., Seltzer, F. and Dykes, M. H. M. (1974). A prospective survey of anesthesiologist mortality 1967—1971. *Anesthesiology* 41, 71—74

Chang, L. W., Dudley, A. W. Jr., Katz, J. and Martin, A. H. (1974). Nervous system development following in utero exposure to trace amounts of halothane. *Teratology* 9, A-15

Chang, L. W., Dudley, A. W. Jr., Lee, Y. K. and Katz, J. (1975a). Ultrastructural studies on the pathological changes in the neonatal kidney following in-utero exposure to halothane. *Environ. Res.* 10, 174—189

Chang, L. W., Lee, Y. K., Dudley, A. W. Jr. and Katz, J. (1975b). Ultrastructural evidence of the hepatotoxic effect of halothane in rats following in-utero exposure. *Can. Anaesth. Soc. J.* 22, 330—337

Cohen, E. N., Bellville, J. W. and Brown, B. W. (1971). Anesthesia, pregnancy and miscarriage. A study of operating room nurses and anesthetists. *Anesthesiology* 35, 343—347

Cohen, E. N., Brown, B. W., Bruce, D. L., Cascorbi, H. F., Corbett, T. H., Jones, T. W. and Whitcher, C. E. (1974). Occupational disease among operating room personnel: a national study. *Anesthesiology* 41, 321—340

Cohen, E. N., Brown, B. W., Bruce, D. L., Cascorbi, H. F., Corbett, T. H., Jones, T. W. and Whitcher, C. E. (1975). A survey of anesthetic health hazards among dentists. *J. Am. dent. Ass.* 90, 1291—1296

Corbett, T. H. (1973). Retention of anesthetic agents following occupational exposure. *Anesth. Analg., Cleve.* 52, 614—617

Corbett, T. H. (1976a). Cancer and congenital anomalies associated with anesthetics. *Ann. N.Y. Acad. Sci.* 271, 56—66

Corbett, T. H. (1976b). Anesthetics: are they carcinogens? American Society of Anesthesiologists. *Abstracts.* Refresher Course 1976, San Francisco. Paper 211

Corbett, T. H., Cornell, R. G., Endres, J. L. and Millard, R. I. (1973a). Effects of low concentrations of nitrous oxide on rat pregnancy. *Anesthesiology* 39, 299—301

Corbett, T. H., Cornell, R. G., Leiding, K. and Endres, J. L. (1973b). Incidence of cancer among Michigan nurse anesthetists. *Anesthesiology* 38, 260—263

Davenport, H. T., Halsey, M. J., Wardley-Smith, B. and Wright, B. M. (1976). Measurement and reduction of occupational exposure to inhaled anesthetics. *Br. med. J.* 2, 1219—1221

Department of Health (1976). Pollution of operating theatres, etc. by anaesthetic gases. HC (76) 38 or SHHD/DS (76) 65. London: DHSS

Doll, R. and Peto, R. (1977). Mortality among doctors in different occupations. *Br. med. J.* 1, 1433—1436

Eschenbrenner, A. B. (1945). Induction of hamartomas in mice by repeated oral administration of chloroform with observations on sex differences. *J. natn. Cancer Inst.* 5, 251—255

Fink, B. R. and Cullen, B. F. (1976). Anesthetic pollution: what is happening to us? *Anesthesiology* 45, 79—83

Fink, B. R., Shepard, T. H. and Blandau, R. J. (1967). Teratogenic activity of nitrous oxide. *Nature, Lond.* 214, 146—147

Halliday, M. M. and Carter, K. (1978). A chemical adsorption system for the sampling of gaseous organic pollutants in operating theatre atmospheres. *Br. J. Anaesth.* 50, 1013—1018

Healy, T. E. J. and Wilcox, A. (1977). Chronic exposure of rats to inhalational anaesthetic agents. *J. Physiol., Lond.* 276, 24—25P

Knill-Jones, R. P., Newman, B. J. and Spence, A. A. (1975). Anaesthetic practice and pregnancy: controlled survey of male anaesthetists in the UK. *Lancet* ii, 807—809

Knill-Jones, R. P., Moir, D. D., Rodrigues, L. V. and Spence, A. A. (1972). Anaesthetic practice and pregnancy: controlled survey of women anaesthetists in the United Kingdom. *Lancet* i, 1326—1328

Kripke, B. J., Kelman, A. D., Shah, N. K., Balogh, K. and Handler, A. H. (1976). Testicular reaction to prolonged exposure to nitrous oxide. *Anesthesiology* 44, 104—113

Langley, D. R. and Steward, A. (1974). The effect of ventilation system design on air contamination with halothane in operating theatres. *Br. J. Anaesth.* 46, 736—741

Lansdown, A. B. G., Pope, W. D. B., Halsey, M. J. and Bateman, P. E. (1976). Analysis of fetal development in rats following maternal exposure to subanesthetic concentrations of halothane. *Teratology* 13, 299—304

Linde, H. W. and Bruce, D. L. (1969). Occupational exposure of anesthetists to halothane, nitrous oxide and radiation. *Anesthesiology* 30, 363—368

Nikki, P., Pfäffli, P. and Ahlman, K. (1972). End-tidal and blood halothane and nitrous oxide in surgical personnel. *Lancet* ii, 490—491

NIOSH (1977). Criteria for a recommended standard . . . occupational exposure to waste anesthetic gases and vapors. DHEW Publication No. 77—140. Washington DC: US Government Printing Office

Pfäffli, P., Nikki, P. and Ahlman, K. (1972). Concentrations of anaesthetic gases in recovery rooms. *Br. J. Anaesth.* 44, 230

Pharoah, P. O. D., Alberman, E., Doyle, P. and Chamberlain, G. (1977). Outcome of pregnancy among women in anaesthetic practice. *Lancet* i, 34—36

Pope, W. D. B., Halsey, M. J., Lansdown, A. B. G. and Bateman, P. E. (1975). Lack of teratogenic dangers with halothane. *Acta anaesth. belg.* 26, Suppl., 169—173

Pope, W. D. B., Halsey, M. J., Lansdown, A. B. G., Simmonds, A. and Bateman, P. E. (1978). Fetotoxicity in rats following chronic exposure to halothane, nitrous oxide, or methoxyflurane. *Anesthesiology* 48, 11—16

Robinson, J. S., Thompson, R. S., Barratt, R. S., Belcher, R. and Stephen, W. I. (1976). Pertinence and precision in pollution measurements. *Br. J. Anaesth.* 48, 167—177

Rosenberg, P. and Kirves, A. (1973). Miscarriages among operating theatre staff. *Acta anaesth. scand.* Suppl. 53, 37—41

Salo, M. and Vapaaruori, M. (1976). Peripheral blood T- and B-lymphocytes in operating theatre personnel. *Br. J. Anaesth.* 48, 877—880

Schwetz, B. A., Leong, B. K. J. and Gehring, P. J. (1974). Embryo and fetotoxicity of inhaled chloroform in rats. *Toxic appl. Pharmac.* 28, 442—451

Shepard, T. H. and Fink, B. R. (ed.). (1968). Teratogenic activity of nitrous oxide in rats. In *Toxicity of Anesthetics*, pp. 308—321. Baltimore: Williams & Wilkins

Smith, B. E., Gaub, M. L. and Moya, F. (1965a). Investigation into the teratogenic effects of anesthetic agents — the fluorinated agents. *Anesthesiology* 26, 260—261

Smith, B. E., Gaub, M. L. and Moya, F. (1965b). Teratogenic effects of anesthetic agents — nitrous oxide. *Anesth. Analg., Cleve.* 44, 726—732

Smith, G. and Shirley, A. W. (1978). A review of the effects of trace concentrations of anaesthetics on performance. *Br. J. Anaesth.* 50, 701—712

Smith, W. D. A. (1976). Pollution and the anaesthetist. In *Recent Advances in Anaesthesia and Analgesia — 12*, pp. 131—173. C. L. Hewer and R. S. Atkinson (ed.). Edinburgh: Churchill Livingstone

Smith, W. D. A. (1978). Atmospheric pollution and contamination with anaesthetics. *Br. J. clin. Equipment* 3, 49—53

Spence, A. A. and Knill-Jones, R. P. (1978). Is there a health hazard in anaesthetic practice? *Br. J. Anaesth.* 50, 713—719

Spence, A. A., Cohen, E. N., Brown, B. W., Knill-Jones, R. P. and Himmelberger, D. U. (1978). Occupational hazards in operating room personnel. A comparison of studies in the United States and United Kingdom. *J. Am. med. Ass.* 238, 955—959

Sturrock, J. M. and Nunn, J. F. (1976). Effect of mixtures of nitrous oxide and halothane on the nuclei of dividing fibroblasts. *Br. J. Anaesth.* 46, 267—268 (Abstract)

Vaisman, A. I. (1967). Work in operating theatres and its effect on the health of anesthesiologists. *Eksp. Khir. Anestesiol.* 12, 44—49

Vessey, M. P. (1978). Epidemiological studies of the occupational hazards of anaesthesia — a review. *Anaesthesia* 33, 430—438

Whitcher, C. E. (1978). Monitoring occupational exposure to the inhalation anesthetics. In *Monitoring in Anesthesia*, pp. 205—220. L. J. Saidman and W. T. Smith (ed.). New York: John Wiley

Whitcher, C. E., Piziali, R., Sher, R. and Moffat, R. J. (1975). *Development and evaluation of methods for the elimination of waste anesthetic gases and vapors in hospitals.* DHEW publication (NIOSH) 75, 137. Washington DC: US Government Printing Office

Wilkinson, R. T., Tyler, P. D. and Varey, C. A. (1975). Duty hours of young hospital doctors: effects on the quality of work. *J. occup. Psychol.* 48, 219—229

10 Cytotoxic effects of inhalational anaesthetics
Jean Sturrock

The inhalational anaesthetics produce various dose-dependent toxic side-effects in many types of cells. These side-effects include depression of cell multiplication rate, mitotic abnormalities in the nucleus, reduction in the synthesis of DNA and other macromolecules, and reduction in cell viability. There have also been some investigations into the possible mutagenic (and therefore potentially carcinogenic) effects of anaesthetics on cells in culture, but so far all results, with one exception, have been negative. Finally there are some rather contradictory effects on bacteria. Some toxic effects of anaesthetics are caused by biotransformation products which may be present after metabolism of the primary agent in the body or tissue, and this aspect is discussed in Chapter 3. This latter effect may not be detected with experimental cell lines, since such cells may not contain the necessary enzymes after years of culture under artificial conditions.

Effects of anaesthetics on microtubules and reduction in cell motility are described in Chapter 1.

INHIBITION OF CELL MULTIPLICATION

It has been known for a number of years that exposure of cultured cells to anaesthetics causes a dose-related depression of cell multiplication, and quantitative results have been obtained *in vitro* for various cell lines.

Mouse heteroploid cells were exposed by Fink and Kenny (1968) to six different inhalational anaesthetics, at clinical dose levels, for four days. Growth rate was reduced in a dose-related manner, methoxyflurane being the most potent in this respect, followed by trichloroethylene, halothane and chloroform equal, then fluroxene and finally diethyl ether. They also found that the yield of mouse sarcoma 1 cells was lower when grown for four days in 77.5% nitrous oxide than when exposed to the same tension of nitrogen. Mouse sarcoma 1 cells were more sensitive during four days' exposure to halothane than were mouse heteroploid cells when the growth rates of the two cell lines were compared.

Sturrock and Nunn (1975) exposed Chinese hamster lung fibroblast cells, for 24 hours, to five of the same volatile anaesthetics that were tested by Fink and Kenny. Dose response curves for inhibition of cell multiplication (*Figure 10.1*) were comparable with the results of Fink and Kenny, but fluroxene was not included in this study.

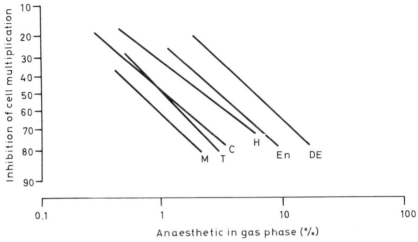

Figure 10.1
Regression lines for inhibition of cell multiplication, caused by exposure of Chinese hamster cells to various concentrations of six different inhalational anaesthetics. Log scale on the abscissa and probit scale on the ordinate. M, methoxyflurane; T, trichloroethylene; C, chloroform; H, halothane; En, enflurane; DE, diethyl ether. (Adapted from Sturrock, 1975)

Jackson (1972) exposed rat hepatoma cells to graded doses of halothane for 24 hours. Inhibition of cell replication was at levels comparable to the results of Fink and of Sturrock and Nunn, but Jackson reported that the viability of these cells was not reduced by exposure to as much as 5% halothane for 24 hours. However, measurement of cell viability in this study was based only on growth rate during recovery, after removal of the halothane. A more reliable assessment of cell survival can be obtained by measuring colony-forming ability as mentioned below. Jackson and Epstein (1971) also grew rat hepatoma cells in suspension culture and exposed them to various concentrations of lignocaine HCl or to prilocaine HCl. From their results they calculated the dose necessary to cause 50% inhibition of growth rate (I_{50}) in the treated cells, compared with control cells. The I_{50} for lignocaine was found to be 1.2×10^{-3} mol·l^{-1} (0.035%) and the value for prilocaine was 9.1×10^{-4} mol·l^{-1} (0.023%).

Telser and Hinkley (1977) grew mouse neuroblastoma cells for up to 72 hours in various concentrations of halothane. They found that growth rate was inhibited in a dose-dependent manner, and that exposure to halothane at 2% for 24 hours caused complete cessation of growth.

Effects of nitrous oxide on cell multiplication*

In 1957, Kieler showed that the treatment of explants of fetal mouse heart muscle with various gas mixtures containing nitrous oxide and oxygen caused a reduction in growth rate and some cell death. The toxic effect of nitrous oxide was greatest in cultures suffering from a lack of oxygen, but high oxygen tensions alone also resulted in cell death. Kieler found that nitrous oxide was a mitotic poison that caused destruction of the mitotic spindle, which structure is essential for normal movement of chromosomes during metaphase.

The effect of nitrous oxide on the growth of two forms of mouse ascites tumour cells *in vivo* was tested by Parbrook (1967). Mice were injected with tumour cells intraperitoneally and then maintained in an atmosphere of air or 25% or 40% nitrous oxide. After a set time each mouse was killed and the total number of tumour cells in the ascites fluid was calculated. Parbrook found that treatment with nitrous oxide significantly lowered the number of cells which had grown from the Ehrlich ascites tumour but it did not affect the growth rate of the 2146 ascites tumour cells. In contrast, Cullen and Sundsmo (1974) reported that halothane did not affect the growth rate of ascites sarcoma cells which had been injected into mice intraperitoneally. Green and Eastwood (1963) investigated the effect on haemopoiesis in rats, of exposure to 80% nitrous oxide with 20% oxygen for 2–6 days. They found that the production of leucocytes was reduced and that there was extensive destruction of bone marrow; only the platelets had a normal appearance. Subsequently, in a study of the comparative sensitivity of five distinct strains of laboratory rats and one cross-bred variety, Green (1968) found that a significant increase in sensitivity to nitrous oxide exposure in some rat strains was associated with a high initial white blood cell count, probably resulting from high activity in bone marrow and thymus in the sensitive rats. However, there were no significant differences in the analgesic effects of nitrous oxide between different rat strains.

In a later study, Kripke *et al.* (1977) exposed rats to either 20% or 40% nitrous oxide for a maximum of 35 days. This caused a decrease in cellularity in the bone marrow, but megakaryocytes were not affected. In the peripheral blood, lymphocytes were reduced in number, but polymorphs were not significantly affected and lymphoid tissues appeared to be normal. After a return to breathing air, bone marrow and peripheral blood became normal within three days.

Nunn, Sturrock and Howell (1976) found that halothane, alone or combined with nitrous oxide, caused a dose-related depression of growth rate in mouse bone-marrow cells grown in semisolid agar. These cells were not particularly sensitive when exposed to nitrous oxide; in fact, 75% nitrous oxide caused a slight insignificant depression in growth rate

---

* *Note added at proof.* Since this chapter was written, it has been demonstrated that prolonged administration of nitrous oxide will inactivate vitamin B_{12} and interfere with DNA synthesis. References are cited by Nunn (1978) *Br. J. Anaesth.* **50**, 1089–1090. *Ed.*

similar to the effect of 0.5% halothane, but 2% halothane stopped cell multiplication completely and there was very little recovery after this latter treatment. However, droperidol with fentanyl, at doses two to ten times those at clinical levels, was not found by Stamenkovic *et al.* (1977) to reduce the rate of colony formation by human bone-marrow cells in somewhat similar agar cultures, and these authors confirmed the minimal depression with nitrous oxide.

Sturrock and Nunn (1976a) also found that there was synergism between halothane and 75% nitrous oxide in the production of nuclear abnormalities in Chinese hamster cells (see below), although the combined effect of these two anaesthetics on growth rate was merely additive and nitrous oxide alone had very little effect in either case.

In summary, the *in vitro* data suggest that nitrous oxide has approximately the depressant effect on leucocyte precursors that would be predicted from its anaesthetic potency. It is therefore difficult to explain the occasional dramatic examples of leucopenia which have followed the prolonged use of nitrous oxide in the treatment of patients with tetanus (Ablett, 1956; Lassen *et al.*, 1956; Wilson, Martin and Last, 1956; Eastwood *et al.*, 1963). Ablett's review shows that leucopenia is not an inevitable sequel to the prolonged use of nitrous oxide, and in most cases the clinical picture is complicated by exposure to other drugs and by the effects of a severe illness. It should also be stressed that there is normally a large extravascular pool of leucocytes, release of which should mask the effects of short periods of suppression of haemopoiesis.

Nevertheless, there is ample evidence for inhibition of multiplication of all cell lines yet tested by a wide range of anaesthetics at clinical concentrations. However, there is no evidence of any effect at the trace concentrations which may contaminate operating theatres.

Nuclear abnormalities

In 1953, Howard and Pelc published a scheme for dividing up the cell growth cycle into four parts, as shown in *Figure 10.2*. These four phases were called G_1, S, G_2 and M. G_1, or gap 1, is the phase directly prior to S, which is the DNA synthetic phase. G_2, or gap 2, is the postsynthetic phase. M, or mitosis, is subdivided into prophase, metaphase, anaphase and telophase. During metaphase the chromosomes become attached to a structure called the spindle, which is largely composed of microtubules. At anaphase the two longitudinal halves of each chromosome separate and travel to opposite poles of the cell; in this way, two new daughter nuclei are formed at telophase. The whole process is completed by division of the cytoplasm so that two separate daughter cells are produced.

By means of microcinephotography, Sturrock and Nunn (1975) showed that 2% halothane caused an increase of cell cycle time in Chinese hamster cells from a duration of about 10 hours to nearly 21 hours, but prolongation of the actual duration of mitosis was only from 26 to 36 minutes.

Anaesthetics have been found to cause an abnormality of metaphase, known as C or colchicine metaphase, in which the chromosomes are scattered at random in the nucleus, with a similar appearance to the effect of treatment with colchicine. This effect is usually seen in plant cells when exposed to anaesthetics (Östergren, 1944; Nunn, Lovis and Kimball, 1971), but C mitosis is not seen so often in mammalian cells after exposure to anaesthetics. However, Sturrock and Nunn (1975, 1976a) saw numerous other abnormalities among Chinese hamster fibroblasts after exposure to halothane or to a mixture of halothane with

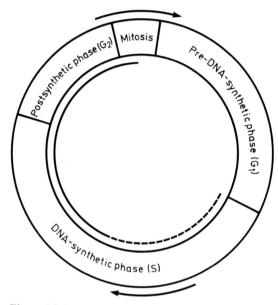

Figure 10.2
Diagrammatic representation of the cell cycle. The double inner line in the circle shows that the chromosomes split into two chromatids at the end of the G$_1$ phase and continue in this condition until anaphase, during mitosis, when one chromatid from every chromosome in a cell goes to each of its two daughter nuclei

nitrous oxide. There were many tripolar and tetrapolar metaphase and anaphase nuclei (*Figure 10.3*) and these abnormal mitoses resulted in binucleate and multinucleate cells and in the production of micronuclei, as seen in *Figure 10.4*.

Kusyk and Hsu (1976) also found abnormalities in the metaphase arrangement of chromosomes during division, after treatment of cells from a human lymphoid line, a mouse fibroblast line and chick embryos with halothane, enflurane or methoxyflurane, but owing to their experimental method the final concentrations of these agents in their cell cultures were uncertain.

It is known that various inhalational anaesthetics cause a reversible dispersal of the microtubules in the axonemes of the heliozoan *Actinosphaerium nucleofilum* (Allison *et al.*, 1970). Halothane at 2% has been seen to abolish the birefringence of the mitotic spindle in the fertilized

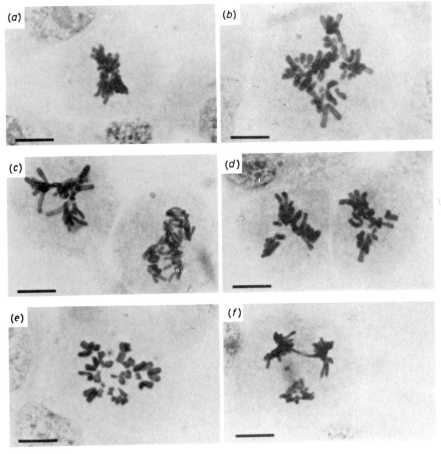

Figure 10.3
Mitotic figures stained with acetic orcein to show the chromosomes.
(*a*) Normal metaphase. (*b*) Tetrapolar metaphase after exposure to
3% halothane for 24 hours. (*c*) The right-hand nucleus shows a
tetrapolar division in early anaphase and the left-hand nucleus is a
tripolar metaphase; 1% halothane for 24 hours. (*d*) Tripolar meta-
phases in two adjacent sister cells after 1% halothane for 24 hours.
(*e*) C-metaphase after 0.75% halothane in 75% nitrous oxide for
24 hours. (*f*) Tripolar anaphase with a chromosome bridge between
two parts of the nucleus after 1.5% halothane in 75% nitrous oxide
for 24 hours. Black lines represent 10μm. (Reproduced from Sturrock
and Nunn, 1976a, by courtesy of the Editor of *Anesthesiology*)

sea-urchin egg (Nunn and Allison, 1972), but these agents have not been
found to disperse the microtubules in the mitotic spindle of dividing
mammalian cells.

Hinkley and Telser (1974) and Telser and Hinkley (1977) have reported
that halothane concentrations, even as low as 0.3%, caused complete but
reversible disruption of microfilaments in mouse neuroblastoma cells.
These authors suggest that the dose-dependent inhibition of cell growth
by halothane may be due to disruption of actin-like microfilaments in the

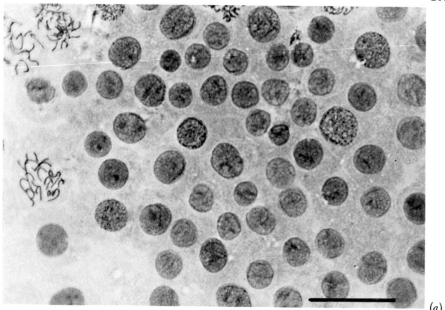

(a)

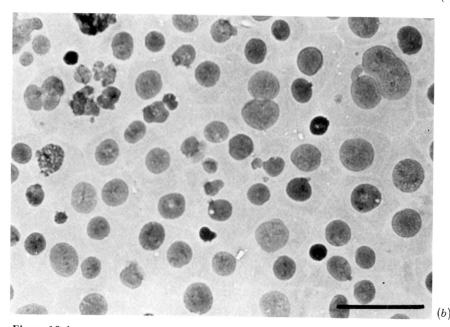

(b)

Figure 10.4
(a) Normal cells expanded by a short treatment with hypotonic
saline and stained with acetic orcein. Phase-contrast illumination.
(b) Cells treated as in (a) but exposed to 0.55% halothane in 75%
nitrous oxide for 24 hours. A multinucleate cell in the upper right
part of the picture also contains two micronuclei. Two multinucleate
and one binucleate cell can be seen in the upper left corner, and
several other binucleate cells are scattered throughout the picture.
The black lines represent 50 μm. (Reproduced from Sturrock and
Nunn, 1976a, by courtesy of the Editor of *Anesthesiology*)

mitotic apparatus, but Telser and Hinkley found no evidence to support the view that halothane disrupted the spindle microtubules. By means of fluorescent microscopy of labelled heavy meromyosin, which binds to actin in microfilaments, Sanger (1975a, b) demonstrated localization of actin in the spindle region during cell division and also in the cleavage furrow during cell separation at the end of mitosis. It therefore seems most likely that halothane interferes with mitosis by disrupting the microfilaments in the mitotic apparatus of dividing cells, thereby increasing cell cycle time and this effect is additional to the disturbance of events in interphase (see below).

DEOXYRIBONUCLEIC ACID (DNA) SYNTHESIS

DNA synthesis by cells in culture or in tissues *in vivo* can be estimated by observing the amount of radioactive tracer substance, such as tritiated thymidine (^{3}HTdR), which has been taken up by the cells from the medium and incorporated into the newly formed DNA during the S phase. The rate of uptake of a DNA precursor, such as ^{3}HTdR, depends on several factors, such as its ready availability in the medium, the permeability of the cell membrane and the concentration and competitive ability of unlabelled thymidine or of other DNA precursors which may be present in precursor pools within the cells. Nevertheless, its uptake into treated cells, as compared with control cells, forms a valid measure of the comparative amount of DNA synthesis in these cells.

Jackson (1973) with rat hepatoma cells, and Sturrock and Nunn (1976b) using Chinese hamster cells, tested the effect of halothane on uptake of labelled thymidine by cultured cells for incorporation into DNA. At low doses of anaesthetic, in short pulse treatments, there was only a small inhibition of DNA synthesis, which was insufficient to constitute the rate-limiting effect of anaesthetics on the prolongation of the cell cycle. Sturrock and Nunn also treated cultures of cells in synchronous growth with 1%, 2% or 3% halothane and examined the uptake of tritiated thymidine into the cells during a whole cell cycle: 1% halothane had little effect but 2% or 3% halothane for 3 or 5 hours, or a mixture of 1.3% halothane with 75% nitrous oxide for 5 hours, caused a marked delay in the onset of S phase (roughly equal to the duration of treatment) and a reduction in height of the S peak, combined with a prolongation of S phase. In all the treated cultures, cell cycle time was increased when compared with control cycle times.

Telser and Hinkley (1977) grew mouse neuroblastoma cells in 1% halothane, but found no significant effect on the biosynthesis of protein and RNA in these cells. Bruce and Traurig in 1969 injected rats with tritiated thymidine, then immediately exposed them to 0.1% or 0.5% halothane for from 1 to 24 hours. At stated intervals the rats were killed and sections of small intestinal wall, containing crypt cells, were processed and later examined to count those cells in mitosis which also showed uptake of labelled thymidine. From these data, curves for the duration of the phases of the cell cycle were plotted. Bruce and Traurig concluded that the S phase in the rat crypt cells was lengthened by 1.8 hours as a result of exposure to 0.1% halothane and by 4.1 hours by exposure to 0.5% halothane. Cell cycle time in treated cells was similarly increased.

Kuramoto and Takahashi (1977), in a similar but more extensive study of crypt cells from both duodenum and jejunum in mice, have confirmed the results of Bruce and Traurig. Kuramoto and Takahashi found that exposure to 0.45% halothane lengthened the G_1, S and M phases in the crypt cells, as shown in *Table 10.1*. The greatest increase in

TABLE 10.1. Duration of cell cycle phases (hours) in cells of the duodenum and jejunum of mice injected with ^{3}H-thymidine and immediately exposed to halothane at 0.45%, or N_2O at 64%

Groups	G_1	S	G_2	M	Cycle time
Duodenum:					
Air	5.67	6.47	1.17	0.82	14.13
Halothane (0.45%)	9.09	7.82	1.27	1.09	19.28
Nitrous oxide (64%)	4.46	6.63	1.06	0.77	12.92
Jejunum:					
Air	4.68	7.07	0.96	0.79	13.49
Halothane (0.45%)	7.41	9.19	0.37	1.15	18.12
Nitrous oxide (64%)	4.18	7.12	1.00	0.78	13.08

From Kuramoto and Takahashi, 1977, by courtesy of the authors and the Editor of *British Journal of Anaesthesia.*

the duration of any phase was found to be in G_1, so that there was corresponding delay in entry into the synthetic phase (S), as found by Sturrock and Nunn (1976b). Nitrous oxide at 64% had no effect on the cell cycle.

Evenwel, Keizer and van Putten in 1976 exposed mice to 0.8% halothane for 6 hours or for 24 hours and measured the uptake in various tissues of labelled iodo-deoxyuridine. Treatment for 6 hours had little effect, but exposure for 24 hours caused a significant depression of DNA synthesis in cells from the spleen, femoral bone marrow and, in some instances, also from the small intestine. However, no effect was observed for skin, muscle, or cells from a mammary carcinoma which had been implanted subcutaneously.

Resting small lymphocytes in the blood do not normally divide, but they can be stimulated to synthesize DNA, RNA and protein, thus becoming enlarged and ultimately dividing. This transformation process occurs in the body after stimulation by specific antigens, but lymphocytes can also be transformed experimentally *in vitro* by stimulation with a non-specific mitogen such as phytohaemagglutinin (PHA). Several authors have shown that *in vitro* exposure of human lymphocytes to halothane caused inhibition of PHA-induced transformation (Bruce, 1972a; Cullen, Sample and Chretien, 1972). It was also demonstrated by Bruce (1972b) that the halothane exposure did not prevent the actual uptake of tritiated thymidine by the human lymphocytes, but only affected some later event during the process of DNA synthesis.

From all this evidence we may conclude that halothane at clinical concentrations and for a duration of at least one cell cycle time causes a delay in onset and mild inhibition of DNA synthesis in various types of cells both *in vitro* and in the intact animal.

CELL SURVIVAL AS MEASURED BY COLONY-FORMING ABILITY

Contrary to expectations, very high doses of inhalational anaesthetics, such as 8% halothane, do not appear to kill mammalian cells in culture for many hours. It is impossible to discover by microscopic examination whether or not any particular cell will continue to live and to divide after an injury. However, long-term cell survival after exposure to anaesthetics can be quantified by the ability of the cells to form colonies. In this system, known as Puck plating (Puck and Marcus, 1955), the cultured cells are first exposed to an anaesthetic, then suitable dilutions of a suspension of single cells are transferred to petri dishes containing growth medium. The cells become attached to the bottom of the dishes and each viable cell will divide to form one colony. After six or seven days the colonies can be stained and counted, and cell survival may be calculated relative to untreated cells in control dishes. Injured cells will die, or fail to attach, or make small abortive colonies; it is known that abnormalities

TABLE 10.2. Comparison between concentrations of agents required for anaesthesia and those required for 50% inhibition of colony-forming ability (CFA) for 3 hours' or for 24 hours' exposure and for 50% inhibition of growth rate after 24 hours' exposure.

	MAC* (dog)	50% inhibition of CFA		50% inhibition of growth rate, 24 h exposure
		3 h exp.	24 h exp.	
Methoxyflurane	0.23	2.15	1.05	0.67
Trichloroethylene	0.6	4.0	2.7	1.05
Chloroform	0.77	3.6	2.1	1.06
Halothane	0.87	4.1	2.5	2.17
Diethyl ether	3.0	19.0	11.0	5.97
Enflurane	2.2	–	12.0	2.8

* From Eger *et al.* (1969), except trichloroethylene MAC for rat from M. J. Halsey (unpublished).

which prevent successful cell division ultimately lead to cell death during mitosis, although abnormal cells may survive in interphase until they come into mitosis.

The colony-forming ability (CFA) for Chinese hamster lung fibroblasts showed a dose-dependent inhibition following exposure to several different inhalational anaesthetics (Sturrock, 1975, 1977a, b). The median effective dose (ED_{50}) for the hamster cells was in relative proportion to dog MAC* values for all the agents tested, except trichloroethylene for which the MAC value is uncertain. *Table 10.2* shows ED_{50} values for inhibition of CFA in the hamster cells after 3 hours' or 24 hours' exposure to six different inhalational anaesthetics. It also shows ED_{50} values for inhibition of growth rate in these same cells after 24 hours' exposure to the same anaesthetics. It is evident from *Table 10.2* that cell growth rate is more easily inhibited than is CFA; however, it must be remembered that these figures show only the effect on growth rate at the end of 24 hours' exposure to anaesthetics and that (except at high doses) there will be recovery of cell growth soon after removal of the anaesthetics, whereas the cell survival figures show inhibition of the ability to form colonies during six or seven days after removal of the anaesthetic and, in fact, the cells that have failed to form a colony are dead.

MUTAGENESIS

Substances which produce chromosome breaks and other microscopic damage might be suspected of causing mutagenesis, perhaps leading to carcinogenesis. However, cells which had been exposed to anaesthetics were examined many times by Sturrock and Nunn (1975) in stained slide preparations, but no damage to the actual chromosomes was seen although there were many metaphase cells in which the arrangement of the chromosomes was abnormal.

In a series of papers from 1973 onwards, Ames and his co-workers described an experimental method which can be used for testing the mutagenicity, not only of many carcinogens and suspected carcinogens but also of their metabolites. Ames used rat liver cells to metabolize the substances to be tested. Any mutagens which were present caused changes in various *Salmonella* test strains. Ames *et al.* found that 90% of the known carcinogens they tested were also mutagenic and very few of the non-carcinogens were found to be mutagenic.

Baden and his group of workers (1976a) have tested the mutagenicity of halothane, using *Salmonella typhimurium*, with rat liver cell microsomes as a metabolic activation system, in the Ames test. Halothane was not found to be mutagenic in this system and, at a later date, Baden *et al.* (1976b) stated that enflurane, isoflurane and methoxyflurane were not mutagenic, but that fluroxene was mutagenic and was suspected of also being carcinogenic.

* The concept of MAC is defined in Chapter 3. *Ed.*

Halothane (with or without nitrous oxide) chloroform and, later, enflurane were tested by Sturrock (1977a, b) for mutagenicity, using the azaguanine system as specified by Chu and Malling (1968), on cultured Chinese hamster cells, but none of these four anaesthetics gave positive results in the tests. Therefore it may be concluded that several frequently used inhalational anaesthetics, as mentioned above, are not mutagenic when tested on *Salmonella typhimurium* or on Chinese hamster cells *in vitro* and are unlikely to have any carcinogenic effects at the concentrations tested.

THE EFFECT OF ANAESTHETICS ON BACTERIA

The antibacterial effect of five different inhalational anaesthetics was investigated by Horton, Sussman and Mushin (1970). They found that high doses of halothane, chloroform, trichloroethylene, methoxyflurane or diethyl ether caused a dose-related reduction in cell survival in cultures of *Escherichia coli* grown on cellulose acetate membranes. Wardley-Smith and Nunn (1971) tested 1–10% halothane on four different species of non-pathogenic bacteria grown in nutrient broth, and found that growth rate was inhibited only at high concentrations of the anaesthetic, the ED_{50} being between 7% and 8% halothane. Bacteria were also exposed to 5% or 10% halothane while growing on agar plates, and were slightly affected only by the higher concentration. There was no effect on growth rate when using halothane at clinical concentrations.

Mehta, Behr and Kenyon (1973) tested the effect of halothane, trichloroethylene and methoxyflurane on *Staphylococcus aureus* and *E. coli* cultures growing on blood agar or on cellulose acetate membranes, in petri dishes. Growth on blood agar plates was not affected by clinical concentrations of the three anaesthetics, but when the bacteria growing on membranes were exposed to the same anaesthetics, inhibition of cell multiplication relative to control was found to be highly significant, but was not dose-dependent except in the case of exposure to trichloroethylene. In a further study, Mehta, Behr and Kenyon (1974) exposed two species of respiratory pathogens, namely *Streptococcus pneumoniae* and *Haemophilus influenzae,* to clinical concentrations of halothane, trichloroethylene and methoxyflurane for 2, 3 or 4 hours. The bacteria were growing either on chocolate agar in plates or on cellulose acetate membranes resting on the agar surface in similar plates. In all cases they found a significant reduction in bacterial growth, which was dose-related, but the reduction was greater for cultures growing on membranes than for those exposed on the surface of chocolate agar plates.

These rather contradictory results may be explained by the suggestion of Mehta, Behr and Kenyon that the bacteria growing on blood agar plates were protected from the anaesthetic vapour by the serum proteins in the medium and this system was regarded as resembling conditions within the body; on the other hand, cultures growing on membranes were thought to present a model for bacterial contamination of anaesthetic equipment.

References

Ablett, J. J. L. (1956). Tetanus and the anaesthetist. *Br. J. Anaesth.* 28, 258–273

Allison, A. C., Hulands, G. H., Nunn, J. F., Kitching, J. A. and Macdonald, A. C. (1970). The effect of inhalational anaesthetics on the microtubular system of *Actinosphaerium nucleofilum. J. Cell Sci.* 7, 483–499

Ames, B. N., Lee, F. D. and Durston, W. E. (1973). An improved bacterial test system for the detection and classification of mutagens and carcinogens. *Proc. natn. Acad. Sci. U.S.A.* 70, 782–786

Ames, B. N., Durston, W. E., Yamasaki, E. and Lee, F. D. (1973). Carcinogens are mutagens: a simple test system combining liver homogenates for activation and bacteria for detection. *Proc. natn. Acad. Sci. U.S.A.* 70, 2281–2285

Baden, J. M., Brinkenhoff, M., Wharton, R. S., Hitt, B. A., Simmon, V. F. and Mazze, R. I. (1976a). Mutagenicity of volatile anesthetics: halothane. *Anesthesiology* 45, 311–318

Baden, J. M., Kelly, M., Wharton, R. S., Hitt, B. A., Mazze, R. I. and Simmon, V. F. (1976b). Mutagenicity of fluroxene. *Anesthesiology* 45, 695

Bruce, D. L. (1972a). Halothane inhibition of phytohemagglutinin-induced transformation of lymphocytes. *Anesthesiology* 36, 201–205

Bruce, D. L. (1972b). Normal thymidine entry into halothane-treated lymphocytes. *Anesthesiology* 37, 588–591

Bruce, D. L. and Traurig, H. H. (1969). The effect of halothane on the cell cycle in rat small intestine. *Anesthesiology* 30, 401–405

Chu, E. H. Y. and Malling, H. V. (1968). Chemical induction of specific locus mutations in Chinese hamster cells *in vitro. Proc. natn. Acad. Sci. U.S.A.* 61, 1306–1312

Cullen, B. F., Sample, W. F. and Chretien, P. B. (1972). The effect of halothane on phytohemagglutinin-induced transformation of human lymphocytes *in vitro. Anesthesiology* 36, 206–212

Cullen, B. F. and Sundsmo, J. S. (1974). Failure of halothane anesthesia to alter growth of sarcoma in mice. *Anesthesiology* 41, 580–584

Eastwood, D. W., Green, C. D., Lambdin, M. A. and Gardner, R. (1963). Effect of nitrous oxide on the white-cell count in leukemia. *New Engl. J. Med.* 268, 297–299

Eger, E. I., Lundgren, C., Miller, S. L. and Stevens, W. C. (1969). Anesthetic potencies of sulfur hexafluoride, carbon tetrafluoride, chloroform and ethrane in dogs. *Anesthesiology* 30, 129–135

Evenwel, R. F., Keizer, H. J. and van Putten, L. M. (1976). Preferential inhibition of DNA synthesis in mouse hemopoietic cells by halothane. *Cancer Res.* 36, 3156–3159

Fink, B. R. and Kenny, G. E. (1968). Metabolic effects of volatile anesthetics in cell cultures. *Anesthesiology* 29, 505–516

Green, C. D. (1968). Strain sensitivity of rats to nitrous oxide. *Anesth. Analg.* 47, 509–514

Green, C. D. and Eastwood, D. W. (1963). Effects of nitrous oxide inhalation on hemopoiesis in rats. *Anesthesiology* 24, 341–345

Hinkley, R. E. and Telser, A. G. (1974). The effects of halothane on cultured mouse neuroblastoma cells. 1. Inhibition of morphological differentiation. *J. Cell Biol.* 63, 531–540

Horton, H. N., Sussman, M. and Mushin, W. W. (1970). The anti-bacterial action of anaesthetic vapours. *Br. J. Anaesth.* 42, 483–486

Howard, A. and Pelc, S. R. (1953). Synthesis of deoxyribonucleic acid in normal and irradiated cells and its relation to chromosome breakage. *Heredity* Suppl. 6, 261–273

Jackson, S. H. (1972). The metabolic effects of halothane on mammalian hepatoma cells *in vitro.* 1. Inhibition of cell replication. *Anesthesiology* 37, 489–492

Jackson, S. H. (1973). The metabolic effects of halothane on mammalian hepatoma cells *in vitro.* II. Inhibition of DNA synthesis. *Anesthesiology* 39, 405–409

Jackson, S. H. and Epstein, R. A. (1971). The metabolic effects of nonvolatile anesthetics on mammalian hepatoma cells *in vitro.* I. Inhibition of cell replication. *Anesthesiology* 34, 409–414

Kieler, J. (1957). The cytotoxic effect of nitrous oxide at different oxygen tensions. *Acta pharmac. tox.* 13, 301–308

Kripke, B. J., Talarico, L., Shah, N. K. and Kelman, A. D. (1977). Hematologic reaction to prolonged exposure to nitrous oxide. *Anesthesiology* 47, 342–348

Kuramoto, T. and Takahashi, M. (1977). Cell cycle in mouse intestinal crypts during halothane or nitrous oxide anaesthesia. *Br. J. Anaesth.* 49, 1075–1080

Kusyk, C. J. and Hsu, T. C. (1976). Mitotic anomalies induced by three inhalation halogenated anesthetics. *Environ. Res.* 12, 366–370

Lassen, H. C. A., Henriksen, E., Neukirch, F. and Kristensen, H. S. (1956). Treatment of tetanus. Severe bone-marrow depression after prolonged nitrous-oxide anaesthesia. *Lancet* i, 527–530

Mehta, S., Behr, G. and Kenyon, D. (1973). The effect of volatile anaesthetics on bacterial growth. *Can. Anaesth. Soc. J.* 20, 230–240

Mehta, S., Behr, G. and Kenyon, D. (1974). The effect of volatile anaesthetics on common respiratory pathogens. *Anaesthesia* 29, 280–289

Nunn, J. F. and Allison, A. C. (1972). Effects of anesthetics on microtubular systems. In *Cellular Biology and Toxicity of Anesthetics*, pp. 138–146. B. R. Fink (ed.). Baltimore: Williams and Wilkins

Nunn, J. F., Lovis, J. D. and Kimball, K. L. (1971). Arrest of mitosis by halothane. *Br. J. Anaesth.* 43, 524–530

Nunn, J. F., Sturrock, J. E. and Howell, A. (1976). Effect of inhalational anaesthetics on division of bone-marrow cells *in vitro*. *Br. J. Anaesth.* 48, 75–81

Östergren, G. (1944). Colchicine mitosis, chromosome contractions, narcosis and protein chain folding. *Hereditas* 30, 429–467

Parbrook, G. D. (1967). Experimental studies into the effect of nitrous oxide on tumour cell growth. *Br. J. Anaesth.* 39, 549–553

Puck, T. T. and Marcus, P. I. (1955). A rapid method for viable cell titration and clone production with HeLa cells in tissue culture. *Proc. natn. Acad. Sci. U.S.A.* 41, 432–437

Sanger, J. W. (1975a). Changing patterns of actin localization during cell division. *Proc. natn. Acad. Sci. U.S.A.* 72, 1913–1916

Sanger, J. W. (1975b). Presence of actin during chromosomal movement. *Proc. natn. Acad. Sci. U.S.A.* 72, 2451–2455

Stamenkovic, L., van Leersum, R. H., Dicke, K. A. and Spierdijk, J. (1977). Effects of droperidol and fentanyl on human bone marrow cultures. *Anaesthesia* 32, 328–332

Sturrock, J. E. (1975). Effect of volatile anaesthetics on cell survival as measured by colony forming ability. *Br. J. Anaesth.* 47, 831–835

Sturrock, J. E. (1977a). Lack of mutagenic effect of halothane or chloroform on cultured cells using the azaguanine test system. *Br. J. Anaesth.* 49, 207–210

Sturrock, J. E. (1977b). No mutagenic effect of enflurane on cultured cells. *Br. J. Anaesth.* 49, 777–779

Sturrock, J. E. and Nunn, J. F. (1975). Mitosis in mammalian cells during exposure to anesthetics. *Anesthesiology* 43, 21–33

Sturrock, J. E. and Nunn, J. F. (1976a). Synergism between halothane and nitrous oxide in the production of nuclear abnormalities in the dividing fibroblast. *Anesthesiology* 44, 461–471

Sturrock, J. E. and Nunn, J. F. (1976b). Effects of halothane on DNA synthesis and the presynthetic phase (G1) in dividing fibroblasts. *Anesthesiology* 45, 413–420

Telser, A. and Hinkley, R. E. (1977). Cultured neuroblastoma cells and halothane: effects on cell growth and macromolecular synthesis. *Anesthesiology* 46, 102–110

Wardley-Smith, B. and Nunn, J. F. (1971). The effect of halothane on bacterial growth rate. *Br. J. Anaesth.* 43, 919–925

Wilson, P., Martin, F. I. R. and Last, P. M. (1956). Bone-marrow depression in tetanus. *Lancet* ii, 442–443

11 Non-inhalational anaesthetics
John W. Dundee and R. S. J. Clarke

The first effective rapidly acting intravenous anaesthetic agent was hexo-barbitone (Evipal, Evipan), introduced in Germany in 1932 (Weese and Scharpff, 1932). This was quickly followed by the much improved thio-pentone (thionembutal) which was first studied by Lundy and Waters in North America in 1935.

When the intravenous barbiturates were substituted as sole agents for ether and chloroform, some of the initial results were disastrous. Their continuing use has been due to an appreciation of the poor tolerance of ill patients and the use of small doses; perhaps more important, though, has been the development of 'balanced techniques' in which the barbiturate is combined with nitrous oxide—oxygen and latterly employed only in the induction of anaesthesia.

Thiopentone is still by far the most popular induction agent. It has been challenged by other barbiturates, some of which (thiamylal, thialbarbitone, thiobutobarbitone) have an almost identical action. The non-sulphur-containing methohexitone, introduced about 20 years ago, is the only drug in this chemical series which offers an alternative action to thiopentone.

The supremacy of the barbiturates as intravenous anaesthetics remained virtually unchallenged until comparatively recently when a clinically acceptable eugenol was introduced. The eugenols are related to oil of cloves, which has been used for many years as an anodyne in dental practice. The first eugenol, G 29 505, was abandoned because of its deleterious action on veins. Continuing systematic research at the labora-tories of Bayer in West Germany produced propanidid, which became available in Britain in 1967; it was popular for a few years but has fallen into disuse because of toxicity and, in particular, because of its cardio-vascular effects.

Hydroxydione, an early steroid anaesthetic in use mainly between 1955 and 1962, has been abandoned because of the delay in the onset of its action and the high incidence of venous sequelae. In the early 1970s, Glaxo Laboratories produced a mixture of two steroids in Cremophor EL — Althesin; it has never been given an official BP name. This has many admirable properties and seemed likely to challenge other barbiturates, but cases of hypersensitivity have been reported in increasing numbers. Its future is therefore uncertain.

Ketamine, a drug similar to the earlier phencyclidine, was introduced into clinical practice in 1966. Its early reception in Britain in 1970 was unsatisfactory, but gradually there has been the development of clear indications for its use and ketamine is probably now assured of a definite, although limited, place.

Continental European workers have recently studied etomidate, another non-barbiturate anaesthetic. Early British reports are not very encouraging and it is difficult to assess its ultimate place in intravenous anaesthesia.

The benzodiazepine tranquillizer, diazepam (Valium), has an effect very different from that of the barbiturates or eugenols, with some delay in onset of its soporific action. It is not a competitor with the barbiturates as a routine induction agent, but is of particular value as a safe basal narcotic. Other newer benzodiazepines are now being investigated as alternatives.

CLASSIFICATION

It is desirable that induction agents be rapidly acting and, in adequate doses, produce loss of consciousness in one arm—brain circulation time. This allows the dosage to be titrated against the patient's requirements. Other drugs with a slower onset of action are essentially basal hypnotics. In general, drugs with a rapid onset have a shorter duration of action than is the case with slower acting compounds. The primary induction agents (rapidly acting) also produce fewer side-effects — excluding immediate cardiovascular and respiratory depression — than the slower acting drugs. These latter should be used only when specifically indicated because of their unique properties. The following is a helpful classification as it embraces both the rate of onset and chemical constituents of each group:

Rapidly acting
Induction agents: thiobarbiturates, methylbarbiturates
      eugenols
      Althesin
      etomidate

Slower acting
Basal hypnotics: phencyclidines (ketamine)
      tranquillizers (diazepam, etc.)
      neuroleptic drug combinations and intravenous analgesics
      others: sodium oxybate (Gamma-OH), chlormethiazole
       edisylate (Heminevrin), barbiturates

It should be noted that the barbiturates, such as pentobarbitone, which are generally employed as oral hypnotics, have a slower onset of action than the thiobarbiturates when given intravenously.

The terms 'ultra-short' acting and 'short' acting are often applied to many intravenous anaesthetics and are not only confusing but may be misleading. These should be reserved for drugs which are rapidly broken down in the body and from which rapid recovery is not dependent on redistribution to non-nervous tissues. The only applicable drugs are:

ultra-short acting: propanidid
short-acting: Althesin, etomidate

In contrast with these, return of consciousness following an intravenous barbiturate (thiobarbiturate or methylbarbiturate) occurs with a large amount of active drug remaining in the body; there is a tendency for patients to lapse back to sleep if left undisturbed and drugs given in the early postoperative period can lead to reinduction of anaesthesia.

BARBITURATES

The terminology of the barbiturates varies between North America and Britain, the former using the ending *al* and the latter *one*. The group title 'barbiturates' is used to include the thiobarbiturates in this chapter.

Chemistry

Barbituric acid is usually regarded as the cyclic ureide of malonic acid (i.e. malonyl urea), and the chemical reaction for its synthesis is as follows:

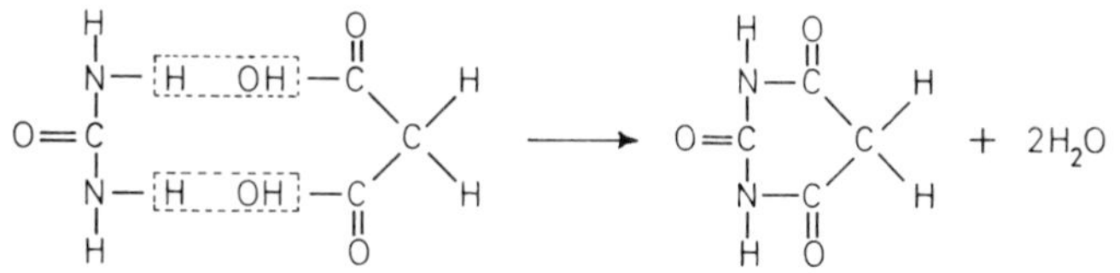

Urea and malonic acid → barbituric acid and water

Although it is more correct to regard barbituric acid as a pyrimidine derivative, it is usually depicted in either the keto or enol form shown below. The acidity is due to the hydrogen ion which migrates from the nitrogen in the 1 position. In aqueous solution it dissociates into hydrogen ion and barbiturate ion. The sodium salts (in the 3 position) are water soluble and can be administered parenterally.

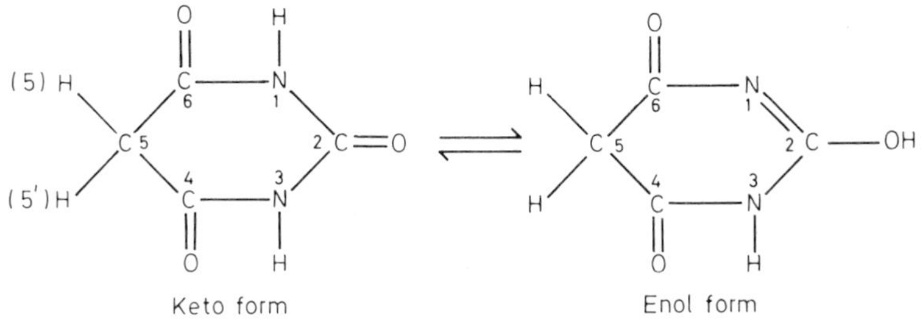

Keto form   Enol form

The many variations are all derived by alterations in the 1,2 and 5,5' positions. Varying substitutions in the 5 and 5' positions determine the degree and duration of narcosis, but apart from these the drugs fall into four distinct groups as follows:

(1) Barbiturates (or oxybarbiturates)   1 = H   2 = O
(2) Methylated oxybarbiturates   1 = CH$_3$ 2 = O
(3) Thiobarbiturates   1 = H   2 = S
(4) Methylated thiobarbiturates   1 = CH$_3$ 2 = S

The relationship of action to structure

Although one is inclined to consider changes in the 5 position as being of prime importance in determining the action of different compounds, it must be stressed that each of the four groups possesses a distinctive action by which it can be recognized clinically.

Sleep cannot be produced in one arm—brain circulation time after the intravenous injection of an effective hypnotic dose of any (unmodified) *barbiturate.* These have a very limited use in clinical anaesthesia and are mainly employed as hypnotics or sedatives.

Methylated barbiturates frequently, but not invariably, cause sleep in one arm—brain circulation time. The methyl radical confers convulsive activity, of which tremor, involuntary muscle movement and hypertonicity are manifestations. Their main use is as intravenous anaesthetics. Some undergo rapid demethylation in the body to form active, long-lasting compounds and hence are unsuitable in this field.

Sleep occurs in one arm—brain circulation time after intravenous injection of an effective dose of *thiobarbiturate,* and return to consciousness is more rapid than after the same dose of the comparable oxybarbiturate. These are used as anaesthetics or anticonvulsants, usually given by the intravenous route but on occasions by rectal or even intramuscular administration.

Methylated thiobarbiturates combine a similar rapidity of onset which is accompanied by convulsive activity, of such severity as to preclude their use in clinical anaesthesia.

Only the thiobarbiturates and the rapidly acting methylated barbiturates are used in anaesthetic practice. Before considering individual drugs, attention is drawn to the (5) (5') substitutions which determine the relative intensity and duration of action of the many possible compounds in these groups. Both hydrogen ions on the carbon must be replaced by alkyl or aryl groups in order to confer hypnotic properties on the barbiturate. In some circumstances substitution can lead to convulsant and other toxic properties.

There is good evidence to show that alterations in the (5) side chains will produce a comparable change in the action of drugs in each of the four groups of compounds mentioned above. Thus the net effect of substitutions at four possible sites may be predicted with a reasonable degree of certainty. This is illustrated in *Figure 11.1* which shows a barbiturate (pentobarbitone) with a slow onset of action when injected intravenously, two thiobarbiturates which are in widespread clinical use and a methylthiobarbiturate which causes an unacceptably high incidence of muscle movements.

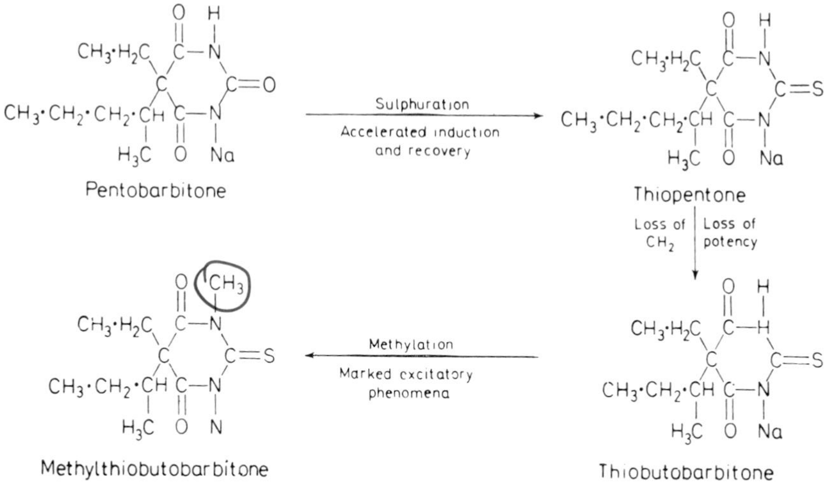

Figure 11.1
Chemical relationship between four compounds and the effects produced by various structural alterations. (Reproduced from Dundee and Barron, 1962, by courtesy of the Editor of *British Journal of Anaesthesia*)

The intravenous barbiturates of clinical importance are listed, together with their commonly used proprietary names, in *Table 11.1*. The authors have had an appreciable experience with the intravenous barbiturates and these are classified below according to their clinical usefulness:

Equally acceptable: thiopentone, thiobutobarbitone, thiamylal, thialbarbitone

Side-effects outweigh merits: hexobarbitone, buthalitone, methitural, all methylthiobarbiturates

Advantages more than outweigh side-effects: enibomal, methohexitone

Physical properties

All drugs are prepared for clinical use as sodium salts and, with the exception of enibomal, are available in powder form to be dissolved in water or saline before use. The sodium salt of thiopentone is a pale yellow hygroscopic powder with a bitter taste, and a melting point of 158–159°C. It is readily soluble in water. Commercial preparations of most barbiturates contain a mixture of 6 parts anhydrous sodium carbonate

TABLE 11.1. Intravenous barbiturates of clinical importance

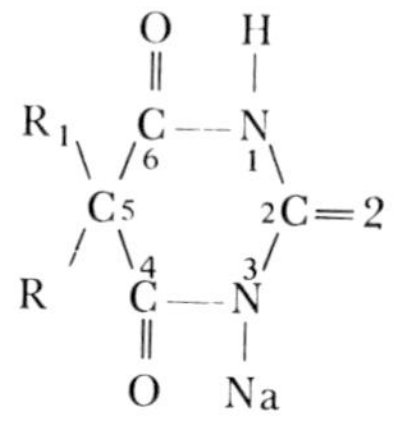

Cyclic ureide of malonic acid

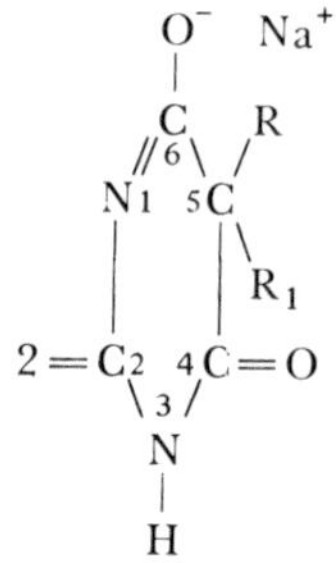

$$R_1 \begin{array}{c} O \ \ H \\ \| \ \ \ \| \\ C\text{---}N \\ /6 \ \ 1\backslash \\ C_5 \ \ \ \ 2C{=}2 \\ / \ \backslash_4 \ \ 3/ \\ R \ \ C\text{---}N \\ \| \ \ \ \| \\ O \ \ Na \end{array}$$

Pyrimidine derivative

$$\begin{array}{c} O^- \ \ Na^+ \\ | \\ C \ \ R \\ /\!/6\backslash / \\ N_1 \ {}_5C \\ | \ \ \ \backslash \\ | \ \ \ \ R_1 \\ 2{=}C_2 \ {}_4C{=}O \\ \backslash 3/ \\ N \\ | \\ H \end{array}$$

Preparation	1	2	5 R	$5'\ R_1$
Hexobarbitone (Evipan, Evipal)	CH_3	O	CH_3-	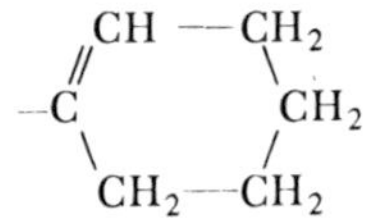 $-C\!\!\begin{array}{c}{}^{CH}\!\!=\!\!{}^{CH_2}\\ \big\backslash \ \ \ \ CH_2 \\ CH_2\!-\!CH_2 \end{array}$ (cyclohexenyl)
Thiopentone (Pentothal, Intraval, Nesdonal, Trapanal)	H	S	CH_3-CH_2-	$-CH-CH_2-CH_2-CH_3$ $\quad\ \|$ $\quad\ CH_3$
Thiobutobarbitone (Inactin)	H	S	CH_3-CH_2-	$-CH-CH_2-CH_3$ $\quad\ \|$ $\quad\ CH_3$
Thialbarbitone (Kemithal, Kemithene)	H	S	$CH_2{=}CH-CH_2-$	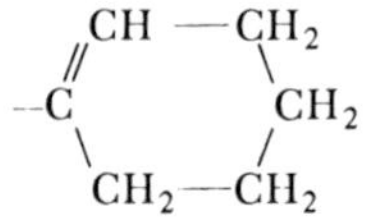 $-C\!\!\begin{array}{c}{}^{CH}\!\!=\!\!{}^{CH_2}\\ \big\backslash \ \ \ \ CH_2 \\ CH_2\!-\!CH_2 \end{array}$ (cyclohexenyl)
Thiamylal (Surital)	H	S	$CH_2{=}CH-CH_2-$	$-CH-CH_2-CH_2-CH_3$ $\quad\ \|$ $\quad\ CH_2$
Methohexitone (Brietal, Brevital)	CH_3	O	$CH_2{=}CH-CH_2-$	$CH-C{\equiv}C-C_2H_5$ $\ \|$ $\ CH_3$
Enibomal (Narcodorm, Narkotal, Eunarcon, narcobarbital)	CH_3	O	$\begin{array}{c}CH_3\\ {>}\,CH\\ CH_3\end{array}$	$-CH_2-CB_r{=}CH_2$

Hexobarbitone	sodium 1-methyl-5-methyl-5'-cyclohexenyl-2-barbiturate
Thiopentone	sodium 5-ethyl-5'-(1-methylbutyl)-2-thiobarbiturate
Thiobutobarbitone	sodium 5-ethyl-5'-(1-methylpropyl)-2-thiobarbiturate
Thialbarbitone	sodium 5-allyl-5'-cyclohexenyl-2-thiobarbiturate
Thiamylal	sodium 5-allyl-5'-(1-methylbutyl)-2-thiobarbiturate
Methohexitone	sodium 1-methyl-5-allyl-5'-(1-methyl-2-pentynyl)-2-barbiturate
Enibomal	sodium 1-methyl-5-isopropyl-5'-2(2-bromallyl)-barbiturate

and 100 parts (w/w) of the barbiturate to prevent participation of the insoluble free acid by atmospheric carbon dioxide. Aqueous solutions are strongly alkaline and the pH of 2.5% thiopentone is about 10.5. The solutions are incompatible with acids which include most of the analgesics, the phenothiazine derivatives, adrenaline and noradrenaline and some preparations of tubocurarine chloride. Although the precipitate which forms when thiopentone and suxamethonium are mixed dissolves in excess barbiturate if the mixture is allowed to stand, almost half of the relaxant will be hydrolysed in 1 hour.

Hexobarbitone and methohexitone are colourless compounds whose solutions are readily distinguishable from the thiobarbiturates.

Clinical preparations

Thiopentone and thiamylal are usually prepared for clinical use in a 2.5% solution, although some anaesthetists use the less safe 5%; to avoid the use of excessive volumes, thialbarbitone and hexobarbitone both require 5–10% solutions. Methohexitone is used in a 1 or 2% solution. Solutions of thiobarbiturates may remain stable at room temperature for up to two weeks after preparation but should not be used if they have become cloudy, while methohexitone can often be used for up to six weeks after preparation. Solutions will remain clearer for a longer period of time if stored at 4°C.

Relative potency

The approximate potency of the available compounds relative to thiopentone (1.0) is:

thiamylal	1.1	methohexitone	2.5–3.0
thialbarbitone	0.5	enibomal	1.0
thiobutobarbitone	0.7	hexobarbitone	0.5

Distribution and fate in the body

Most of the work in this field has been done with thiopentone, and its distribution and fate in the body are described in detail.

PROTEIN BINDING

Immediately on injection a large proportion of the barbiturate is rendered pharmacologically inactive by being bound to the non-diffusible constituents of the plasma. Thiobarbiturates are bound to a greater extent than their oxygen analogues, thiopentone being 65–70%. The degree of binding varies with the pH, passing through a maximum at about pH 8.0.

With increasing barbiturate concentration, the percentage of the bound drug diminishes, although the total amount inactivated by this means increases.

Methylation and sulphuration increase the lipoid solubility of un-ionized forms, and the rate at which barbiturates penetrate the central nervous system can be correlated with the lipoid solubility of the un-ionized molecules. For example, the onset of hypnotic action following intravenous pentobarbitone (oxybarbiturate) is slower than that following comparable doses of thiopentone (thiobarbiturate): that this is due to the differences in partition coefficients of the two drugs has been shown by analyses of their rate of passage into brain (Mark *et al.,* 1958). In practice one finds that the 'blood—brain barrier' is non-existent as far as rate of transfer of clinically used intravenous anaesthetics is concerned. Thus, factors which influence the arm—brain circulation time are important in determining the rate of onset of action.

Drugs which quickly penetrate into brain will also diffuse out rapidly and soon be distributed to skeletal muscle and other tissues. Thus, not only will the onset of action of thiopentone be quicker than that of pentobarbitone, but the duration of its hypnotic effect will be correspondingly shorter.

Barbiturates are weak acids and, at a pH near 1, as in the stomach, they are practically un-ionized. The rate of absorption through gastric mucosa will be related to their lipoid solubility. Thus, the methylated or thio-compounds are very rapidly absorbed by mouth and cause a brief period of intense hypnosis.

The effects of thiopentone on the electroencephalogram can usually be detected in 8—12 seconds after injection, and after one deep inspiration consciousness is lost. The temporal relationship of this respiratory effect to the onset of anaesthesia suggests that it is mediated via the chemoreceptors in the carotid body. The brain continues to take up thiopentone for a further 15—30 seconds or so, and thereafter the concentration of the drug in the efferent venous blood slightly exceeds the afferent arterial level and the brain concentration falls.

The immediate uptake of thiopentone by the brain is accompanied by a similar rapid uptake in other important vessel-rich tissues such as the liver and kidneys, and the plasma level falls quickly. The concentration of drug reaching the brain is thus lowered and the gradient is reversed; as the brain content falls, anaesthesia lightens. The cerebrospinal fluid concentration reaches a level almost as high as that of the unbound drug in the plasma, and thereafter it declines at a rate similar to that of other tissues.

The maximum tissue concentration of thiopentone in well perfused tissues is reached within 1 minute of a single intravenous injection and it is this rapid redistribution which is responsible for the short action of small doses (*Figure 11.2*). Equilibrium with the muscles is not attained until a quarter of an hour after injection and, thereafter, its concentration declines at a rate parallel to that of plasma. With a fat/blood partition coefficient in the region of 11:1, thiopentone will move from blood to fat as long as the concentration in the latter is less than 11 times that in

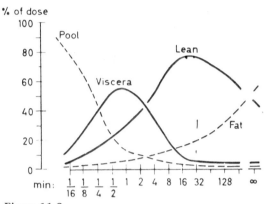

Figure 11.2
Distribution of thiopentone in different bodily tissues and organs at various times after its intravenous injection. (Reproduced from Price *et al.*, 1960, by courtesy of the Editor of *Clinical Pharmacology and Therapeutics*)

blood. Despite this affinity for fat, because of the poor blood supply, uptake of the drug in adipose tissues is slow and maximum deposition only occurs after approximately 2½ hours. By this time the thiopentone content of fat greatly exceeds that of other tissues, and body fat content may be a factor in determining the duration of action of large doses of thiopentone.

DETOXICATION AND BIOTRANSFORMATION

Very little attention has been paid to the role of detoxication in reducing the plasma thiopentone concentrations. Brodie (1952) calculated that 10–15% of the drug was broken down per hour. Animal experiments and observations in humans show prolongation of the action of large doses of thiopentone in the presence of hepatic dysfunction, pointing to the positive role of the liver in its breakdown and its importance in recovery from doses in excess of those rapidly removed from the brain by redistribution. Metabolic reactions (oxidation and reduction) which occur with highly lipophilic drugs such as thiopentone are due to the cytochrome P450 in the endoplasmic reticulum. The liver has the largest amount of endoplasmic reticulum and will carry out most of the oxidation. *In vivo* studies by Mark *et al.* (1965) showed that the liver removes up to 50% of the thiopentone from the hepatic blood flow and plays a definite role in the short duration of the action of the drug. The latest work in this field is that of Saidman and Eger (1966), who found that metabolism plays a not insignificant role in the early awakening seen with this anaesthetic. Uptake in muscle is mainly responsible for the early fall of the arterial concentration, with a modest but imprecisely defined contribution by metabolism and uptake in fat.

The reserve capacity of the liver is such that functional impairment must be great before the effect is manifest clinically and before one should consider withholding the administration of moderate doses. Side chain oxidation is the major mechanism of inactivation *in vivo*, but 5 demethylation plays some part.

Methohexitone is metabolized at a slightly faster rate than thiopentone (Breimer, 1976) and has the relatively short half-life of 70–125 minutes.

RECOVERY

This occurs when a large amount of thiopentone remains unchanged in the body and a cumulative effect is observed after repeated doses. Increments necessary to maintain sleep become gradually less as tissue equilibrium occurs until after 2–3 hours only small doses are required at long intervals. These not only replace the drug which has been detoxicated but compensate for the increasing tolerance which the brain shows to the depressant effects of thiopentone. As intermittent administration proceeds, the blood concentration at which various signs of anaesthesia are elicited increases and the blood level of the drug at recovery becomes higher.

Recovery from thiopentone is affected by the phenomenon of acute tolerance. Within certain limits, the higher the initial dose of thiopentone the greater will be the increments needed to maintain a constant degree of cerebral depression. The peak concentration of the drug attained in the brain, whether at induction or during intermittent administration, seems to determine in part the blood level at which consciousness is regained. There is little correlation between the blood thiopentone level and the depth of anaesthesia, as recorded on the electroencephalogram.

TIME COURSE OF DISTRIBUTION IN TISSUES

Price (1960) presented a mathematical analysis of the kinetics of thiopentone distribution and validated his conclusions by direct measurement of drug concentration in human tissue (Price *et al.*, 1960). His findings following a single injection of the drug (*Figure 11.2*) reveal that the course of anaesthesia depends passively upon competition between nervous and non-nervous tissues for the drug. The solution is injected into a central 'pool' of blood and within 1 minute after injection the blood has given up 90% of the injected dose, principally to the central nervous system, heart, liver and other rapidly perfused viscera. During the subsequent half hour these are in turn depleted as the result of further redistribution. About 80% of the thiopentone given up by the rapidly perfused viscera is distributed to the other aqueous tissues of the body ('lean') while the remainder enters fat. The blood supply of the latter is so low relative to other tissues that it cannot begin to store thiopentone to any significant degree until the central nervous system has lost over 90% of its peak content. Price did not allow for detoxication in his calculations, which show that fat should contain 55–60% of the injected dose 8–10 hours after its administration.

EFFECT OF pH ON LIPOID SOLUBILITY

Thiopentone has a pK value of 7.6 and the degree of ionization of such a drug can change considerably with physiological variations in blood pH. The effects of such changes can be best understood by regarding thiopentone as being distributed *in vivo* between two immiscible phases: one (mainly a water phase) consists of blood and parenchymatous tissues, and the other (the organic phase) is fat. The concentration of undissociated acid relative to that which is ionized largely determines the distribution of a weak organic acid, such as barbituric acid, between an aqueous buffer and an immiscible organic solvent. The lower the pH, the more drug will be in the organic phase, while at a higher pH the opposite is true. Brodie *et al.* (1950) found that decreasing the pH of plasma of dogs to 6.8, by the inhalation of 10% carbon dioxide, reduced the concentration of thiopentone in the plasma by about 40%. On stopping the inhalation, the blood pH returned to near the control level and the plasma level of the drug rose rapidly.

The degree of ionization also affects the renal excretion of barbiturates. The un-ionized drug which appears in the glomerular filtrate diffuses back into the circulation through the renal tubules. This diffusion will be less if the drug is ionized and, being weak organic acids, ionization will be maximal at an alkaline pH. This renal excretion of thiopentone is negligible.

As one would expect from the passage of highly lipoid-soluble agents across membranes, a barrier such as the placenta offers no barrier to thiopentone. The maximum concentration in fetal blood occurs about 3 minutes after injection, at which time there is equilibrium between maternal and fetal concentrations.

PERSISTENCE OF ACTION

The clinical implications of the redistribution, rather than rapid detoxication, of thiopentone are demonstrated by the well planned human electroencephalographic studies carried out by Doenicke and his coworkers (Doenicke *et al.*, 1966; Doenicke, Kugler and Laub, 1967) from Munich. This work is concerned with a comparison of propanidid with thiobutobarbitone and methohexitone, and it clearly shows that EEG changes could be detected for up to 24 hours after clinical doses of the two barbiturates but not after the rapidly detoxicated eugenol (*Figure 11.3*). Doses of alcohol which had little effect on the normal subject produced drunkenness when given up to 11 hours after either barbiturate. More important was the fact that at the time of taking alcohol the subjects showed little or no clinical evidence of persistence of the hypnotic effect of the barbiturate. In contrast, propanidid was a truly short-acting drug with rapid recovery and no potentiation of alcohol 2 hours after return of consciousness. It is now obvious that no modification of the side chains in the barbiturate nucleus is likely to produce a truly short-acting rapidly detoxicated drug, with no hangover effect.

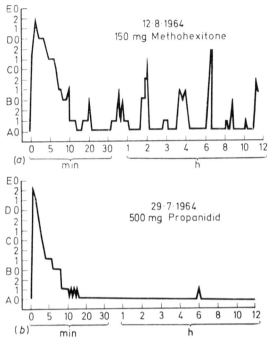

Figure 11.3
'Sleep depth curves' (from the integrated electroencephalogram) during and following approximately equivalent doses of (*a*) methohexitone and (*b*) propanidid. (Reproduced from Doenicke, Kugler and Laub, 1967, by courtesy of the author and the Editor of *Canadian Anaesthetists' Society Journal*)

There are other clinical implications of the slow detoxication of the barbiturates. Care is needed should a further anaesthetic be required within a short time of a previous one. Moderate doses of opiates can 'reinduce' anaesthesia if given in the early postoperative period, particularly if large amounts of barbiturate were given during operation and if the opiates are administered intravenously. This also occurs with other sedatives, particularly diazepam.

Return of mental faculties to normal following barbiturates does not coincide with apparent return of full consciousness. Hypnotic doses of oral barbiturate may impair over-all driving efficiency for up to 14 hours after administration while there is a significant impairment of visual perception, attention and arithmetic performance for between 5 and 8½ hours after the oral administration of 100 mg pentobarbitone. On recovering from intravenous barbiturates many patients complain of fatigue or grogginess, and the probability of some degree of mental impairment is such that, under no circumstances, should patients who have recently received these drugs be allowed to leave for home unaccompanied. It is recommended that, particularly with barbiturate anaesthesia, outpatients be warned not to drive a car and to restrict activities especially those involving the use of machinery until the following day.

Obesity, although it will not markedly influence the induction dose or the duration of action of normal doses, may increase requirements with intermittent injection and delay recovery after very large doses.

Non-drug factors influencing onset

With adequate doses the all-important factor is the forearm blood flow, which depends on the cardiac output and the state of the peripheral circulation. When cardiac output is decreased in disease, as in circulatory failure, the onset of action of thiopentone is slower than normal. Cardiac output is increased in thyrotoxicosis and severe anaemia, as well as after exercise, but this is not likely to affect noticeably the rate of onset of intravenous drugs. Inadvertent partial occlusion of blood flow by tight clothing or an improperly released tourniquet can occur. In clinical practice the effect of the environmental temperature is of great importance, and the vasoconstriction which occurs at lower temperatures will delay the drug effect.

Effects on the body

Before discussing the actions of intravenous barbiturates on the body, mention must be made of some of the effects which are related to the mode of administration.

The mechanism of transport of intravenous anaesthetics from vein to brain, as compared with inhalation agents, leads to a high concentration suddenly coming into contact with the heart, vasomotor and respiratory centres. Thus, in clinical practice, hypotension and respiratory depression occur frequently during the induction of intravenous anaesthesia. These phenomena are usually only transient because of rapid diffusion of the drugs throughout the body, but in patients with a decreased cardiovascular reserve hypotension leads to decreased venous return, which in turn causes a further fall in cardiac output and resulting decreased coronary blood flow. This vicious circle can be easily established and have disastrous results. For this reason, intravenous anaesthesia is more frequently contra-indicated because of its effect on the cardiovascular system than are the inhalation techniques, in which the depressant effects occur more gradually and can be more rapidly reversed.

The rapid onset of anaesthesia with intravenous agents leads to a more complete and sudden relaxation of the cardiac sphincter and loss of the protective reflexes. The dangers of regurgitation and aspiration of intestinal contents are thus greater than with conventional inhalation techniques and any intravenous injection carries the hazard of transmitting virus hepatitis unless proper sterilization is carried out. Haematomas and broken needles are two other dangers which are an inherent part of any intravenous injection.

CENTRAL NERVOUS SYSTEM

The rapid injection of doses of thiopentone in excess of 3.5 mg·kg^{-1} will normally produce loss of consciousness in one arm—brain circulation time, although there is a wide variation in the required dosage of intravenous agents, even in normal persons. The onset of anaesthesia is usually smooth and unaccompanied by any movement or respiratory upset, but these do occur on occasions with methohexitone.

Subnarcotic doses increase sensitivity to somatic pain and this state of antanalgesia, which is associated with a low brain barbiturate concentration, also occurs during recovery from large doses. This applies only to deep pain, such as that produced experimentally by pressure on the tibia, and small doses actually reduce the ability to appreciate a painful stimulus applied to the skin. Perhaps the term 'hyperalgesia' would better describe the increased appreciation of a painful stimulus which occurs with sub-anaesthetic doses of the intravenous barbiturates. Minute doses of thiopentone will antagonize the analgesia produced by nitrous oxide or pethidine and prolonged hyperalgesia has been produced by 100 mg phenobarbitone, an observation which is in keeping with the slower redistribution of this barbiturate in the body. Antanalgesia may result from the effect of the barbiturate on some inhibitory system in the brain.

The maximum depressant action of thiopentone on the nervous system does not occur until several seconds after its initial effect. The classic signs and stages of anaesthesia as described for the induction of ether anaesthesia are usually not seen with thiopentone, but hypersensitivity to stimuli can often be demonstrated after small doses if the patient is disturbed too soon. The high amplitude, fast, spiky activity of mixed frequencies, which is the first electroencephalographic evidence of the effects of the drug, is rapidly replaced by a complex pattern of mixed frequencies, with predominantly slower waveforms of very irregular contour and random occurrence. Depending on the dosage administered, there is a progressive suppression of cortical activity with short periods of relative quiescence separating groups or bursts of activity. The larger the dose, the greater will be the duration of the periods of cortical inactivity.

Although the basic action of the barbiturates on the nervous system is similar to that of the volatile and gaseous agents, because of the route of administration and the lack of analgesia, the signs and stages of anaesthesia differ somewhat from those observed with ether. Its irritant action on the tracheobronchial tree causes stimulation of respiration and this, together with irregularities of rhythm and depth of respiration, is rarely seen with thiopentone. In the absence of surgical or other stimuli, the degree of respiratory depression is a poor guide to the depth of anaesthesia with the barbiturates. Low concentrations of ether have a marked analgesic action in contrast to the hypersensitivity to touch or painful stimuli with thiopentone and a dangerous degree of cerebral depression may be required to abolish this latter completely. Muscular relaxation is also poor with a moderate depth of barbiturate anaesthesia.

With the barbiturates — more so than with any other drug used in anaesthesia — the clinical level of anaesthesia is related to the intensity of the surgical stimulus as well as to the degree of cerebral depression. An undisturbed patient, with depressed respiration and abdominal and masseteric relaxation, gives a picture of moderately deep surgical anaesthesia but on application of a surgical stimulus the respiration may be stimulated, relaxation lost and there may be a reflex movement of a limb. If this patient is now given sufficient thiopentone to produce surgical anaesthesia in the presence of strong stimulation, when the stimulation ceases a dangerous degree of respiratory depression may ensue and prolonged unconsciousness can be expected. While analgesic drugs will reduce the dose of thiopentone required to produce surgical anaesthesia, these also depress respiration and are long acting; a similar state of affairs can be produced if a large dose is given too near the end of the operation. With the use of nitrous oxide—oxygen to supplement thiopentone it is possible to produce a pattern of anaesthesia somewhat similar to that observed with other drugs without excessive dosage and without causing dangerous and prolonged periods of depression of vital functions.

Brain metabolism and oxygen consumption are reduced in proportion to the degree of cerebral depression. Carbon dioxide retention, the sequel of respiratory depression, will reduce cerebrovascular resistance and may lead to increased blood flow to the brain and an increase in cerebrospinal fluid pressure. At low arterial pressures cerebral blood flow will be reduced.

CARDIOVASCULAR SYSTEM

Thiopentone is a direct myocardial depressant, the degree of depression being proportional to the concentration of the drug but less than that of equivalent concentrations of ether, cyclopropane or nitrous oxide. A fall in the blood pH increases the cardiovascular toxicity of the barbiturates.

A variable degree of hypotension is the usual sequel to the injection of thiopentone. Its severity depends on the dose, rate of injection and the condition of the patient. A direct relationship exists between blood thiopentone concentration and the degree of arterial hypotension, which also varies with the electroencephalographic depth of anaesthesia. The maximum fall may occur within 10 seconds of injection of a single dose; hypertensive and hypovolaemic persons are more sensitive than fit adults, and any degree of cardiac inefficiency is an indication for the use of caution.

There is a consistent fall in cardiac index after induction of anaesthesia but, since venous pressure does not rise, it is unlikely that myocardial insufficiency is a major cause of this. The hypotension probably results from the vasodilatation produced by the thiopentone, with pooling of the blood in the periphery and a decreased venous return. Lightening of the depth of barbiturate anaesthesia is not necessarily accompanied by a return of blood pressure to normal. Hypotension can persist for long periods after the return of consciousness, and, if this is accompanied by any respiratory depression, the combined effects of a stagnant and anoxic hypoxia may affect the chances of complete recovery.

In the normal person, slow pulse rates are usually quickened, and fast rates slowed, by the induction of anaesthesia. In poor-risk patients or following excessive doses in normal persons, tachycardia is the usual response to injection of these drugs. Premedicant drugs such as the phenothiazines, which cause vasodilatation, increase the incidence, severity and duration of hypotension and tachycardia following the injection of thiopentone. Even opiate premedication may increase its hypotensive action.

Severe hypotension, with or without bronchospasm, occurs in the rare event of a hypersensitivity reaction. This is discussed later.

Thiopentone modifies the vasomotor response to positive pressure inflation of the lungs. Too vigorous controlled respiration (such as the Valsalva manoeuvre) increases the intrathoracic pressure and there is a temporary fall in the blood pressure from which recovery occurs as the result of compensatory vasoconstriction. This compensatory mechanism is reduced by the barbiturates and persistent hypotension may result.

RESPIRATORY SYSTEM

Although the barbiturates are among the most potent respiratory depressants used in modern anaesthesia, the effect of moderate single induction doses is of no great significance. The use of opiate premedication enhances the depressant action. Repeated doses do not have the same safety. As with all anaesthetic agents, the sensitivity of the respiratory centre to carbon dioxide is depressed in proportion to the depth of narcosis. In deep anaesthesia, the effect of hypoxia on the carotid body plays an important part in the maintenance of respiration but this shift to hypoxia control is accompanied by a decrease in the minute volume and hypoxaemia. In contrast with the opiates, respiratory tidal volume rather than frequency is affected by the barbiturates and there may even be a slight increase in respiratory rate.

Carbon dioxide retention is difficult to detect during the intermittent use of barbiturates, since the blood pressure rise in response to endogenous carbon dioxide may be depressed by the anaesthetic. When combined with nitrous oxide—oxygen, the use of a mixture containing more than 25 vols % of oxygen is recommended.

The respiratory pattern produced by thiopentone is modified markedly by surgical stimuli and an increase in the respiratory volume in response to tactile stimulation persists until a dangerously deep level of thiopentone narcosis is reached. Eckenhoff and Helrich (1958) have shown that the degree of respiratory depression is increased and the response to endogenous carbon dioxide is reduced when thiopentone is given following a moderate dose of morphine or pethidine, as compared with the effect of a similar dose of thiopentone alone. A 50% nitrous oxide—oxygen mixture slightly increases the depressant effects of the barbiturate, although not nearly as much as an opiate. Fetal respiration is particularly sensitive to the depressant effects of the barbiturates. Poor-risk subjects, with impaired cardiovascular or respiratory function, are also particularly prone to dangerous degrees of respiratory depression.

The irritative phenomena (coughing, hiccup) and laryngospasm are rare with thiopentone but not uncommon after methohexitone; their incidence and severity increase with dosage and rapid injection and decrease after vagolytic premedication. Coughing, sneezing and even bronchospasm may occur in the lightly anaesthetized patient, or even before consciousness is lost. They are more common in chronic bronchitics, asthmatics and vagotonic subjects.

The once feared danger of laryngospasm after thiopentone is now of little importance since the advent of suxamethonium. Barbiturates cause an apparent increase in sensitivity of the laryngeal reflexes, compared with the inhalational agents, but this is probably due more to their inability to depress the laryngeal reflexes than to any stimulant action. The presence of excess mucus or foreign bodies in the upper respiratory tract is a predisposing cause, while an effective dose of atropine or hyoscine and the avoidance of insertion of artificial airways or too light a level of anaesthesia are worthwhile prophylactic measures. Bronchospasm, which may be severe, is a manifestation of hypersensitivity to thiopentone and is discussed later.

MISCELLANEOUS

While the effects of thiopentone on blood sugar are insignificant, in large doses it interferes with the deposition of glycogen in the liver but this is of no clinical importance in routine anaesthesia. Liver function is impaired for several days after the use of large doses of thiopentone but therapeutic doses have no deleterious effects in normal persons. Renal blood flow varies with the mean arterial blood pressure and temporary oliguria can follow prolonged periods of hypotension after thiopentone.

Intravenous barbiturates do not have the curariform action of ether, and do not effectively block motor impulses. Muscular relaxation can be provided only through excessive central depression. Shivering is a common phenomenon on recovery from anaesthesia and may be due to the prolonged vasodilatation in contact with the cold surroundings. Its frequency, as compared with that following other agents, is probably a reflection of the lack of analgesic action of this group of drugs because it is readily controlled by postoperative analgesics.

Thiopentone and methohexitone cause a small, but consistent, fall in serum potassium concentration, with a peak effect occurring at about 2–3 minutes and returning to normal within 10 minutes. Thiopentone reduces the degree of hyperkalaemia caused by suxamethonium and in this respect it has a greater protective action than methohexitone.

Some degree of histamine release follows injection of thiopentone (and propanidid), but this has no special significance in normal patients. It is likely that, as with propanidid, massive histamine release can occur with anaphylactoid reaction to this drug, although this has not been confirmed by actual data.

Local irritant effects

Some detectable degree of venous damage occurs in a small percentage of patients following intravenous barbiturates. *Table 11.2* lists the incidence of thrombosis, phlebitis and thrombophlebitis found in a survey of over

TABLE 11.2. Incidence of thrombosis, phlebitis and thrombophlebitis following clinical doses of thiopentone and methohexitone

	Thiopentone		Methohexitone	
Percentage concentration	5.0	2.5	2.0	1.0
Percentage incidence of all sequelae	5.8	2.0	6.3	3.0

2000 patients on the second or third day after clinical doses of thiopentone and methohexitone. Extended thrombophlebitis or thrombosis is very rare with these two drugs, and with Althesin, but is a troublesome complication of propanidid.

PERIVENOUS INJECTION

Local irritation following perivenous injection of thiopentone is more likely to occur after a 5% solution than when 2.5% has been used. Sequelae vary from slight pain to extensive necrosis, depending on the amount of the drug injected outside the vein and, equally important, the condition of the skin at the site of the injection. Such effects are extremely uncommon following methohexitone. Both drugs can be given by deep intramuscular injection as premedication without any serious sequelae.

INTRA-ARTERIAL INJECTION

The sequelae to intra-arterial injection of thiopentone cannot be treated in adequate detail in this chapter, and the reader is referred to the publications of Cohen (1948), Forrester and Saunders (1955), Dundee (1956), Stone and Donnelly (1961) and Dundee and Wyant (1974). The immediate clinical signs are usually an agonizing pain shooting down the forearm and movement of the arm in an attempt to remove the needle and syringe. Unfortunately, in an occasional patient pain may not follow the injection and there is then no warning that the needle point is misplaced.

Severe arterial spasm, with blanching of the limb and disappearance of the radial pulse, usually follows and the onset of unconsciousness may be delayed. Vasomotor collapse may also occur. The end-result in untreated cases varies from loss of part of a limb to a small area of gangrene or loss of sensation.

Figures for the incidence of sequelae following intra-arterial injection of different barbiturates can only be approximate. In one survey there was an 82% incidence following a 10% solution, a 31% incidence with a 5% solution and only 7% when the solution was 2.5% or less. The severity of sequelae was also less after the more dilute solutions. There appear to be no reports of sequelae following the accidental intra-arterial injection of 1–2% methohexitone.

Many theories have been put forward to explain the sequelae following intra-arterial barbiturates. Burn and Hobbs (1959) and Burn (1960) have shown that the intra-arterial injection of thiopentone releases noradrenaline from the vessel walls and this is probably the cause of the intense vascular spasm which occurs and which may be followed by thrombosis and permanent damage to the limb. This does not occur with hexobarbitone, and the hypothesis of Burn is supported by the absence of reported cases of permanent damage resulting from the intra-arterial injection of this drug. Biopsy has shown that thrombosis occurs in all cases where there is permanent tissue damage.

When thiopentone is injected into blood with a pH of 7.4, crystals of insoluble acid form in the blood stream and block small vessels. The greater the concentration of the solution used, the greater will be the production of crystals. It is difficult, however, to explain the connection between barbituric acid crystals and thrombosis on the basis of mechanical blockage alone. Red blood cell haemolysis and platelet aggregation also occur and both these effects are accentuated by the acid crystals. These have been found with the barbiturate concentrations expected after accidental intra-arterial injection, assuming a normal forearm blood flow of $0.5–1$ ml·s^{-1} and rate of injection of 1 ml·s^{-1}. A study of the crystal-forming ability of aqueous solutions of clinically used drugs (Brown, Lyons and Dundee, 1968) showed that this was less likely to occur with dilute solutions. Release of adenosine triphosphate (ATP) from damaged red blood cells or platelets and an area of endothelial damage at the puncture site are adequate reasons for the initiation of thrombosis.

Although oxybarbiturates appear to be less likely to form crystals than are thiobarbiturates, dilution is the main factor in preventing crystal formation and maximum safety can best be achieved by the use of dilute solutions. This is particularly important with the thiobarbiturates. Metho-hexitone is safer in this respect since it need never be used in concentrations exceeding 2% and there may be the additional safety factor of the absence of a sulphur atom. Crystal formation also occurs in veins but it is unimportant because of the ever-increasing diameter of the vessels and subsequent resolution of the crystals. In developing new barbiturates, the above evidence points to a preference for the more potent drugs which can be used in dilute solutions.

To be effective, treatment must be carried out immediately. If the needle is still in the vessel, procaine, papaverine or tolazoline should be injected. A brachial plexus and stellate block will open up the collateral circulation and, where possible, either papaverine (40–80 mg in 10–20 ml of saline solution) or tolazoline (25–50 mg) should be injected into the vessel above the injection site and infiltrated around the segment which is in spasm. The operation should be postponed where possible and the patient immediately given heparin, but if surgery is absolutely essential, anaesthesia can be continued with a vasodilator such as halothane. For a fuller description of treatment, consult Dundee and Wyant (1974).

Factors influencing induction characteristics

A number of important factors can influence induction characteristics to the extent that, under certain circumstances, a quite acceptable drug can cause a very stormy induction with troublesome complications. These are summarized in *Table 11.3*.

TABLE 11.3. **Some factors known to influence side-effects of barbiturates**

Factor	Excitatory phenomena	Respiratory upset	Hypotension
Premedication	Reduced by analgesics	Reduced by atropine and hyoscine	Increased by opiates and phenothiazines
Dose related	++ (worst with methylated compounds)	++	+++ (Related to rate of injection)
Rate of injection	++ (worst with methylated compounds)	++	+++ (Related to dose administered)

Tremor, spontaneous involuntary muscle movements or hypertonus are more likely to occur with methylated compounds. At any given dosage, premedication with a potent analgesic (opiate) reduces the frequency and severity of these, while certain 'antanalgesic' drugs, which increase sensitivity to somatic pain (for example, promethazine, cyclizine, hyoscine), have the opposite effect and may increase them to a troublesome degree. This effect is more marked with methohexitone than with thiopentone (Dundee, 1965); promethazine–hyoscine can result in 50–70% excitatory phenomena after 1.6 mg·kg^{-1} methohexitone.

Other factors being equal, the larger the dose of any drug injected the greater will be the likelihood of excitatory phenomena occurring although, with any given dose, the incidence of these increases with the increasing speed of injection, especially with methylated compounds. Small changes in rate have no appreciable effect on the frequency of this complication with thiopentone.

RESPIRATORY UPSET AND HYPOTENSION

The occurrence of cough and hiccup is not reduced by opiate premedication. However, the preoperative use of 0.4 mg hyoscine, and to a lesser extent 0.6 mg atropine, reduces the incidence of either complication. This suggests that these complications may be of vagal origin. Like excitatory phenomena, the incidence of respiratory upset increases as the dose and rate of injection are increased, but in clinical practice these two factors are important only with methohexitone.

There is some evidence to suggest that hypotension is more common with the less potent drugs, where larger doses have to be given, and least common with methohexitone. The dosage and rate of administration are both important and inter-related in affecting the occurrence of hypotension, while premedication with phenothiazines and opiates increases this tendency. Methohexitone is particularly likely to cause tachycardia.

Contraindications

Absolute contraindications to the barbiturates are few and can be considered under the following headings.

CONTRAINDICATIONS TO ANY FORM OF GENERAL ANAESTHESIA

(1) Inadequate airway before induction, including where, even in the conscious state, adequate oxygenation is dependent on the use of the accessory muscles of respiration.
(2) Risk of loss of airway during anaesthesia; ensuring a free airway during the procedure removes this contraindication.
(3) Untreated adrenocortical insufficiency, due to the inability of such patients to respond to any form of stress.
(4) Unavailability of apparatus to inflate the lungs or perform suction.
(5) Outpatients who have to leave hospital alone.

SPECIFIC CONTRAINDICATIONS TO THE BARBITURATES WHERE, IF ADEQUATE CARE IS TAKEN, OTHER AGENTS CAN SAFELY BE USED

(1) Severe cardiac decompensation or peripheral circulatory failure. The depressant action and the peripheral vasodilatation precludes the safe use of even a small dose of barbiturate.
(2) Severe uraemia, where even a small dose of barbiturate may cause a prolonged effect.

TABLE 11.4. Comparison of the important properties of propanidid and Althesin with those of thiopentone and methohexitone

	Thiopentone	Methohexitone	Propanidid	Althesin
Introduced	1935	1957	1965	1971
Group	Thiobarbiturate	Methylbarbiturate	Eugenol	Steroid
Water solubility	high	high	low	low
Available as	powder	powder	viscid solution	viscid solution
Induction	smooth	frequent upset	smooth	smooth
CVS depression	moderate	tachycardia	marked with high doses	moderate
Respiratory effects	moderate depression	hiccup	stimulation	moderate depression
Complete recovery	slow	rapid	very rapid	rapid
Recovery due to	redistribution	redistribution and detoxication	detoxication	redistribution and detoxication
Hangover	marked	moderate	nil	moderate
Idiosyncrasy	infrequent	infrequent	frequent	not uncommon

(3) Porphyria — in the latent stage of this disease any barbiturate may cause an acute exacerbation, with porphyrinuria, paralysis and frequently death.
(4) History of hypersensitivity to barbiturates.
(5) Status asthmaticus.

WHERE A SMALL DOSE OF BARBITURATE CAN BE GIVEN WITH CARE, BUT THEIR USE MUST BE LIMITED TO THE INDUCTION OF ANAESTHESIA

(1) Hypovolaemia.
(2) Where the hypnotic effect may be prolonged, as in the presence of a raised blood urea or severe anaemia, or where an overdose of pre-operative medication has been given.
(3) Myocardial weakness.
(4) Raised intracranial pressure.
(5) Slight respiratory obstruction.
(6) Where prolonged periods of muscular relaxation are required.
(7) Asthma.
(8) Myasthenia gravis.
(9) Severe electrolyte imbalance, especially potassium intoxication.
(10) Untreated myxoedema.
(11) Very severe diabetes mellitus.
(12) Patients with arteriosclerosis, hypertension or a history of cerebral thrombosis.
(13) Obstetrics.
(14) Dystrophia myotonia.

RAPIDLY ACTING NON-BARBITURATES

Table 11.4 summarizes the important properties of propanidid and Althesin and compares these with thiopentone and methohexitone. The action of these is briefly compared.

EUGENOLS

Propanidid is the only one of these in current clinical use, G 29 505 and Propinal having been abandoned.

Propanidid is a yellowish oil, only sparingly soluble in water. It can, however, be solubilized by Cremophor EL or the closely related Micellophor, which consist of 16% glycerin–polyglycol ethers and polyglycolin (hydrophilic part) and about 84% of a hydrophobic part (mainly esters of ricinoleic and glycerin–polyglycol ethers). The commercial preparation (Epontol) contains 16 g of hydrophobic part of Cremophor EL, 5 g of propanidid and 0.7 g of sodium chloride in 100 ml. This hydrophobic part, known as Tensid, takes the form of aggregates or micelles, and the molecules of propanidid are incorporated into them as a colloidal solution.

Epontol remains stable for two years at normal room temperature. It can be diluted with water or normal saline solution before use to reduce the viscosity, but such solutions must be freshly prepared. It is also compatible with most anaesthetic adjuvants (pethidine, suxamethonium, tubocurarine, gallamine, atropine). The pH of a 5% solution of propanidid is 5.15.

Fate in the body

About half of the injected propanidid is rapidly bound to plasma protein, particularly albumin, and this reduces its anaesthetic activity. A low level of plasma protein could render debilitated patients more sensitive to the agent. It is rapidly broken down by the plasma cholinesterase, the resulting compound being anaesthetically inactive as well as of low toxicity. Where thiopentone is taken up from the plasma into non-nervous tissues and therefore slowly metabolized in the liver, this process of redistribution is not normally of importance for the eugenols, but in conditions where the plasma protein level is low or there is a deficiency of the enzymes responsible for its breakdown, propanidid has a longer anaesthetic action which is terminated by redistribution. In such circumstances, the drug behaves like the barbiturates and crosses the placental barrier freely.

Propanidid is approximately equipotent with thiopentone. Doses of $2-3$ mg·kg^{-1} will produce loss of consciousness but this is too transient and too light to be of value in inducing clinical anaesthesia; $4-6$ mg·kg^{-1} propanidid is satisfactory for induction and if more than 8 mg·kg^{-1} is given in a single dose, the toxicity is increased greatly.

Central nervous system

Propanidid produces sleep in one arm—brain circulation time but this is accompanied by various excitatory effects and there may be major convulsive activity in certain circumstances. The incidence of excitatory effects is related to dosage and increasing this to 12 mg·kg^{-1} or a very rapid administration of a smaller dose leads to frequent and violent movements. With any premedicant the incidence of these effects is intermediate between that following thiopentone and that with methohexitone, and the factors influencing them are similar to those known to affect induction with methohexitone. Hiccup occurs after propanidid with high dosage, rapid injection or phenothiazine premedication. Hyoscine and atropine diminish its frequency.

Electroencephalography during induction of anaesthesia, both in animals and man, shows the same type of change as with the barbiturates (Doenicke, Kugler and Laub, 1967). The resting α rhythm ($8-13$ cycles·s^{-1}) is replaced by the slow broad β rhythm of surgical anaesthesia ($1-4$ cycles·s^{-1}). However, prolonged EEG studies in the postanaesthetic phase have shown that, once the patient recovers from propanidid anaesthesia, the EEG returns to normal and shows no relapses during the first 24 hours. After thiopentone or even methohexitone anaesthesia, on the other hand, there is a tendency for all subjects to develop sleep patterns at various times (*Figure 11.3*).

In contrast with the barbiturates, propanidid does not have an antanalgesic action. It produces local anaesthesia whether applied topically or injected subcutaneously, and this may protect the patient from pain when the solution is accidentally injected outside a vein.

Other effects

The rapid recovery and minimal cumulative action are the main features of propanidid, particularly in relation to the barbiturates. In view of its almost complete eclipse in clinical practice it is not proposed to discuss its other actions in detail.

In normal induction doses propanidid has an action on the cardiovascular system which is similar to that of thiopentone. However, once the dose is raised to 8 mg·kg^{-1}, the incidence and severity of hypotension rise more rapidly than with thiopentone. Hypotension with propanidid is of short duration even when it is profound, but the drug should be used with caution for bad-risk patients. Induction with propanidid is accompanied by a sinus tachycardia which is greater than that with barbiturate induction and is probably secondary to the hypotension. Sudden severe

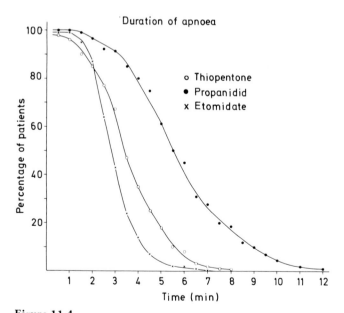

Figure 11.4
Distribution of duration of apnoea following 50 mg suxamethonium given to patients infused with thiopentone (o), propanidid (•) or etomidate (x). (Thiopentone and propanidid data taken from Clarke, Dundee and Hamilton, 1967.)

falls in blood pressure after normal doses of propanidid are probably a manifestation of hypersensitivity, discussed later.

Respiratory stimulation is the striking feature of the clinical use of propanidid, and the more rapidly the drug is given the greater is the intensity of the phenomenon. It is followed by hypoventilation or, in some cases, by apnoea. Opiate premedication diminishes the intensity of the hyperventilation and prolongs the apnoea.

Patients in whom anaesthesia is induced with propanidid will, on the average, have a longer period of apnoea and respiratory depression following suxamethonium than those induced with thiopentone. This prolongation usually amounts to an increase of 50% over the expected duration after thiopentone, but even with a single induction agent there is a wide variation in individual response to suxamethonium (*Figure 11.4*). The suxamethonium—propanidid interaction may be due to the fact that both are broken down by plasma cholinesterase. It appears to have a protective action against muscle pains induced by suxamethonium, both the incidence and severity being lower than after a thiopentone induction.

Propanidid causes more sickness than other induction agents and this cannot be explained solely on the basis of a more rapid recovery. In general, while slightly more irritant to veins than thiopentone, the incidence of venous thrombosis after propanidid is clinically acceptable.

Propanidid has proved to be a useful anaesthetic for short procedures where a rapid recovery is desired. It may be used as sole agent but it is preferable to give nitrous oxide and oxygen with or without halothane to achieve greater control of the duration of anaesthesia. The initial dose should be 4–6 mg·kg^{-1}, or less for those with cardiovascular disease or hypovolaemia. If this dosage is exceeded, muscle movements and hypotension become undesirably frequent. The viscosity of the preparation and the occurrence of postoperative sickness are minor disadvantages.

ALTHESIN

Despite its many clinical advantages, hydroxydione, the first steroid anaesthetic, had a high therapeutic index and continuing research in the field of steroids produced a number of hypnotic compounds of which alphaxalone was the most promising. This is virtually insoluble in water but can be injected in Cremophor; the addition of the weaker hypnotic alphadolone acetate increases the solubility of alphaxalone in Cremophor more than threefold. It has the highest therapeutic index (*Table 11.5*) of six compounds studied by Child *et al.* (1971).

Althesin is a mixture of these two steroids, the formulation of the commercially available preparation being:

alphaxalone	0.90 g
alphadolone acetate	0.30 g
polyoxyethylated castor oil	20.00 g
sodium chloride	0.25 g
water for injection BP	to 100 ml

Thus each millilitre of Althesin contains 9 mg of alphaxalone and 3 mg of alphadolone acetate. The ready-to-use solution is slightly viscid, has a pH of about 7 and is isotonic with blood. As with all solutions made up in Cremophor, it has a tendency to be frothy when drawn into the syringe.

TABLE 11.5. Anaesthetic (AD_{50}) and lethal (LD_{50}) doses of six intravenous anaesthetics given to male mice of the Charles River CDI strain (Child *et al.*, 1971)

	AD_{50} (mg·kg^{-1})	LD_{50} (mg·kg^{-1})	*Therapeutic index*
Thiopentone	13.2	90.5	6.9
Methohexitone	5.3	39.4	7.4
Propanidid	22.9	184.7	8.1
Ketamine	12.7	108.7	8.5
Hydroxydione	18.0	311.0	17.3
Althesin	1.8	54.7	30.6

Like propanidid, solutions are miscible with water. Some of its properties have been compared with those of other intravenous agents in *Table 11.4*.

Low water solubility is undoubtedly a disadvantage of Althesin and for many years it was believed that water solubility (as with hydroxydione) and rapidity of onset (as with alphaxalone—alphadolone) could not be achieved together in a steroid anaesthetic, but recent work suggests that this may eventually be possible.

Effects on the body

One may get the impression that there is a slight delay in the onset of action of Althesin as compared with thiopentone, but this is not so and the apparent delay may be due to the slower rate of injection due to viscosity of the solution. Anaesthesia will consistently be produced by doses of 50—60 μl·kg^{-1}. The electroencephalographic pattern of cerebral depression is similar to that produced by other anaesthetics. There is some evidence that Althesin selectively depresses cerebral oxygen consumption to an extent greater than can be attributed to a reduction in cerebral blood flow.

Induction is not as smooth as with thiopentone, but the small amount of muscle movement which occurs is of little clinical significance. It is less than from the equivalent dose of methohexitone. The excitatory effects are increased by hyoscine premedication and reduced by the opiates; a fast rate of injection also increases their incidence. Cough, hiccup and laryngospasm are rare after Althesin.

Excluding the not uncommon hypersensitivity reactions (q.v.), Althesin does not cause more cardiovascular depression than equivalent doses of other induction agents. It does not predispose to adrenaline-induced arrhythmias and is a satisfactory drug for induction in patients with limited cardiovascular reserve.

Recovery from Althesin is due to both rapid redistribution and breakdown in the body. It occurs sooner than following equivalent doses of thiopentone but not more rapidly than after methohexitone. Excitement in the early postoperative period is uncommon after Althesin, as is postoperative vomiting. Venous thrombosis is not a problem.

The high incidence of immediate hypersensitivity reactions to even very small doses of Althesin has affected its clinical use and many feel that it is no longer an acceptable alternative to thiopentone. As a guide to its continuing use, it is worth emphasizing the desirable properties of this agent which very nearly approaches the ideal intravenous anaesthetic.

(1) It is *stable in solution*, with only 3—5 ml being required for induction of anaesthesia in adults.
(2) It has a *shorter duration of action* than equivalent doses of thiopentone and a more rapid clear-headed recovery can be achieved in adults.
(3) It possesses a higher *safety margin*, demonstrated in both animals and man. This is of particular value in relation to its use in poor-risk patients.

It has properties which suggest that it may be a suitable drug for continous administration in dilute solutions as originally suggested by du Cailar (1972) and du Cailar *et al.* (1974):

(1) Reduction in cerebral blood flow, brain size and cerebral metabolism; it may have a place in head injuries and neurosurgery.
(2) Its lack of antanalgesic action and less cumulation than with thiopentone.
(3) Ability to produce 'light sleep' with almost instantaneous recovery, even after prolonged infusion.

Ramsay *et al.* (1974) and Savege *et al.* (1975) — both from The London Hospital — have investigated the potential use of infusions both in the intensive care and in the operative fields. In the former, 4.37 litres of Althesin was given over 20 days with no evidence of tachyphylaxis or delay in recovery. Concern has been expressed over the potential dangers of the large amount of solubilizing agent and also on the effects on liver function. Both these aspects need further investigation. Du Cailar *et al.* (1975) and Laurent and du Cailar (1977) have reported its use as an infusion combined with narcotic analgesia. This seems worthy of further study.

It would appear that Althesin can be given safely to patients with a personal or family history of malignant hyperpyrexia, when it may even have some protective effect. It should, however, be avoided in porphyrics.

ETOMIDATE

This is the latest addition to the field of intravenous anaesthetics; originally known as R 26490, etomidate is an intravenous hypnotic which was synthesized in the Belgian laboratories of Janssen Pharmaceutica at Beerse. It is a completely new type of anaesthetic belonging to the imidazole chemical group and chemically unrelated to any other hypnotic agent. Animal studies showed it to have the remarkably high therapeutic index of 26.4 as compared with 6.7 for propanidid and 9.5 for methohexitone. It was also shown to have minimal toxicity on repeated administration and to be free from teratogenic effects (Janssen, Niemegeers and Marsboom, 1975). These claims led to its investigation in man.

Etomidate is a white crystalline powder with a molecular weight of 342.4. The salt is very soluble in water, but unstable in aqueous solution. The base is very soluble in propylene glycol and ethanol, freely soluble in polyethylene glycol and chloroform, sparingly soluble in acetone and water and practically insoluble in ether and *n*-hexane. Although freely soluble in water, because of pain on injection two preparations in organic solvents (polyethylene glycol and propylene glycol) have been studied. It is not yet clear which will be made available for clinical use.

Once constituted, the aqueous solution (1.5 mg$\cdot$l^{-1}) should be used within 24 hours as it may lose its potency. The polyethylene glycol formulation is dispensed in 0.2% solution and is stable at room temperature. It may be immunologically active and is also a possible cause of haemolysis. There is no problem with the stability of the propylene glycol formulation (0.2% solution), which can be left at room temperature for over two years.

The normal induction dose of etomidate is around 0.3 mg$\cdot$kg^{-1}. In effective doses it causes sleep in one arm—brain circulation time. On a w/w basis it is approximately four times more potent than methohexitone and twelve times more potent than thiopentone.

Its pharmacokinetics have not been reported in detail. It is 78% bound to albumin. Like thiopentone, it quickly enters the brain and leaves it rapidly due to redistribution in the body. The fast component of the plasma decay curve has a half-life of 1.2 minutes. Etomidate is quickly broken down, being mainly hydrolysed by esterases, both in the liver and plasma. Blood levels decrease rapidly over the first half hour, less so over the next 3½ hours and more slowly thereafter. As with thiopentone, disappearance from the plasma occurs in three phases and detectable amounts of etomidate persist in plasma for at least 6 hours (Doenicke *et al.*, 1973a; Heykants *et al.*, 1975; Lewi, Heykants and Janssen, 1976). Of the total administered drug, 87% is excreted in the urine (3% of which is in an unchanged form) and 13% in the bile.

Pain on injection is a distinct disadvantage of etomidate. This is most troublesome with the aqueous solution. Its incidence is increased with slow injection (around 1 mg$\cdot$s^{-1}). Pain occurs most frequently when injections are given into small veins in the wrist or back of the hand.

The most important clinical problem with etomidate is spontaneous involuntary muscle movement, tremor and hypertonus following injection. The incidence is much higher than with methohexitone. It is reduced by premedication with diazepam and to a greater degree by pethidine. The frequency of cough and hiccup is similar to that with methohexitone. Respiratory depression is not a problem with clinical doses.

Lack of cardiovascular toxicity is claimed to be one of the outstanding features of etomidate and there have been many clinical studies which confirm this (Zindler, 1975). In fit patients, Bruckner *et al.* (1974) found that 0.3 mg·kg^{-1} produced a slight increase in cardiac index, accompanied by a slight fall in heart rate, a slight fall in arterial pressure (14%) and peripheral resistance (17%); dp/dt_{max} rose (9%) with maximum effects occurring about 3 minutes after injection. They considered changes to be small in comparison with the effects of other intravenous anaesthetics.

In a comprehensive comparative study, Kettler and Sonntag (1974) investigated coronary blood flow and myocardial oxygen consumption (MV_{O_2}) in healthy patients. Increases in heart rate are, in the main, responsible for the increases in MV_{O_2} which were found with propanidid (+82%), ketamine (+78%), Althesin (+63%), thiopentone (+55%) and methohexitone (+44%). In contrast, etomidate did not produce significant changes in MV_{O_2}. Coronary arteriovenous difference was not significantly altered by any of the other agents and etomidate alone seemed to have a true, but weak, coronary vasodilator effect. In another study, the same group of workers (Kettler *et al.*, 1974) gave an induction dose of 0.3 mg·kg^{-1} etomidate followed by an infusion of 0.12 mg·kg^{-1}·min^{-1} and found that coronary blood flow was increased by 19% and coronary resistance decreased 19%, leaving a constant coronary perfusion pressure. In clinical doses, etomidate reduces peripheral resistance with an increase of as much as 60% in blood flow.

Unlike other intravenous anaesthetics, etomidate does not release significant amounts of histamine (Doenicke *et al.*, 1973b).

Although the findings may not be of great clinical significance, our studies (Dundee and Zacharias, 1978) suggest that etomidate induction causes a slight decrease in the duration of action of 50 mg suxamethonium as compared with a barbiturate induction (*Figure 11.4*).

There would appear to be a significantly higher incidence of vomiting and nausea in the first 6 hours after operation in unpremedicated patients anaesthetized with etomidate—nitrous oxide—oxygen compared with patients in whom anaesthesia is induced with methohexitone or thiopentone. The propylene glycol preparation is followed by a very high incidence of venous sequelae and all preparations cause a slightly higher incidence than thiopentone or methohexitone. There is some evidence to suggest that rapid injection may slightly increase this; dosage is also important since the over-all incidence of 13% sequelae with 0.3 mg·kg^{-1} rose to 37% with doses in excess of 0.9 mg·kg^{-1} (Dundee and Zacharias, 1978).

At this stage in its development it would be unwise to comment on the place of etomidate in clinical anaesthesia. Pooling the available data from many thousands of administrations, in *Table 11.6* is given the relative incidence of the quality of induction compared with thiopentone and methohexitone.

TABLE 11.6. Relative quality of induction with etomidate, thiopentone and metho-hexitone

	Etomidate	*Thiopentone*	*Methohexitone*
Uneventful	26	78	51
Slight upset	46	18	32
Marked upset	17	4	13
Very troublesome	11	0	4

The thiopentone and methohexitone data were obtained in unpremedicated patients and these figures speak for themselves.

KETAMINE

This phenyl cyclohexylamine derivative differs markedly, both in its chemistry and physical properties and in its clinical effects from the non-inhalation agents already described.

Chemically ketamine (Ketalar, Ketaject) is *dl*-2-(*o*-chlorophenyl)-2-(methylamino)cyclohexanone hydrochloride. It is an acidic solution (pH 3.5–5.5) available in 10, 50 and 100 mg·ml^{-1} strengths and is suitable for intravenous or intramuscular injection. It contains 1:10 000 benzethonium chloride as a preservative but this is not included in the dilute solutions marketed in Britain. The 10 mg·ml^{-1} solution has been made isotonic with sodium chloride.

This drug is unique in being effective when given by both the intravenous and the intramuscular routes. When given intravenously, the time of onset is between 30 and 60 seconds and is slower than after thiopentone. The adult induction dose is 1–2 mg·kg^{-1}. With intramuscular injections the induction doses are 5–10 mg·kg^{-1}- and consciousness usually is lost in 2–4 minutes, but the onset may be delayed for 6–8 minutes. Subcutaneous administration is not satisfactory.

Ketamine has been described as having a 'cataleptic, analgesic and anaesthetic action, but without hypnotic properties' (Chen, 1965). Catalepsy is defined as 'a characteristic akinetic state with a loss of orthostatic reflexes but without impairment of consciousness in which the extremities appear to be paralysed by motor and sensory failure'. Another definition of the state produced by ketamine is 'dissociative anaesthesia' which is characterized by complete analgesia combined with only superficial sleep (Corssen, 1969). These descriptions point to a state which is clinically very different from anaesthesia produced by other induction agents. Spontaneous involuntary muscle movement and hypertonus are not uncommon during induction, and purposeless and tonic–clonic movements of the extremities may occur during anaesthesia. These latter may be taken to indicate a light plane of anaesthesia and the need for additional doses, and unless this possibility is recognized one can readily give an overdose. Instances of failure to produce anaesthesia with ketamine have been reported in patients where there is an absence of the appropriate cerebral development; likewise it may be ineffective in neonates and very young children.

In anaesthetic doses in man, ketamine depresses the α rhythm and produces fairly continuous θ waves and, rarely, δ wave bursts on the electroencephalogram. It also causes depression of late portions of the auditory evoked response. Detailed studies of the electroencephalogram show a functional dissociation between the thalamoneocortical and limbic systems, the former being depressed before there is a significant obtunding of the reticular activating and the limbic systems (Corssen, Miyasaka and Domino, 1968). The site of action of minimal anaesthetic doses of ketamine thus appears to be on the non-specific thalamoneocortical system.

This difference from the action of other non-inhalational anaesthetics is manifested by the state of the patient. Hypertonus and movement have already been mentioned; in addition, patients may remain with their eyes open, jaw tone is maintained or even increased, sometimes to the extent of obstructing the airway. Analgesia is extremely good, even with small doses. Ketamine increases both cerebral blood flow and oxygen consumption; cerebrospinal fluid pressure parallels changes in cerebral blood flow.

Cardiovascular effects

In contrast with the action of other intravenous induction agents, some degree of cardiovascular stimulation occurs almost invariably with ketamine, affecting both blood pressure and heart rate. In the absence of depressant premedication, the rise in systolic pressure in adults receiving clinical doses of ketamine is in the region of 20—40 mmHg, with a slightly lower rise in diastolic pressure. In the majority of patients the blood pressure rises steadily over the 3—5 minutes following injection and then declines to normal limits over the next 10—20 minutes. There is often a slight delay in the rise in diastolic pressure, which may still be rising when the systolic has begun to drop. In most patients the peak rises occur between the second and fourth minute after injection, but this is a highly individual response and on occasions the pressure rise may be alarming. The heart rate almost invariably increases following intravenous anaesthesia in man.

A number of factors are claimed to influence the extent of the cardiostimulatory response.

(1) Dose: with doses in excess of $1 \text{ mg} \cdot \text{kg}^{-1}$ there is very little variation in the hypertensive action of ketamine which has even been noted with subhypnotic doses.

(2) Rate of injection: this is not an important factor.

(3) Route: intramuscular administration results in no less hypertension than with the intravenous route.
(4) Preanaesthetic medication: large doses of opiate or normal doses of droperidol minimize the pressure rise.
(5) The subsequent use of halothane will prevent marked hypertension.
(6) Pancuronium, probably by virtue of its positive chronotropic action, increases the stimulatory effects of ketamine and this combination should not be used.
(7) Initial pressure does not influence the degree of hypertension produced by ketamine.

The picture is one of cardiostimulation, produced by an agent which has a direct depressant action on the isolated myocardium. Central and peripheral mechanisms have been suggested as possible explanations and the only consistent positive finding is an increase in circulating noradrenaline. Perhaps ketamine may interfere with its reuptake by adrenergic nerve terminals. Cardiac arrhythmias are uncommon with ketamine.

Despite the increase of blood pressure and heart rate in adults following ketamine, there are many well documented series of many thousands of administrations in which no untoward effects were produced by the hypertension.

Other effects

Respiratory depression is minimal and transient after clinical doses, and cough, laryngospasm and hiccup occur very rarely. Laryngeal reflexes are not markedly depressed with normal adult doses in the absence of opiate or benzodiazepine premedication but the degree of protection of the upper airway is less than was once thought.

Ketamine prolongs the action of suxamethonium to a significant degree (Bovill *et al.*, 1971) but appears to have no effect on other myoneural blockers.

Hepatic and renal function are unaffected by low doses but there is some doubt about the safety of continuous infusions in patients undergoing intermediate-type operations.

A slight increase in intraocular pressure may occur following the intravenous administration of ketamine. There is a tendency toward an increased uterine tone and, although its placental transmission has not been studied, there is some evidence of increased muscle tone in infants when ketamine is given to the mothers.

From the practical point of view, it is important to note that salivation may be profuse after either route of administration of ketamine, particularly in children.

Sequelae

Emergence sequelae produce major problems in adults. There is great discrepancy in reports of the incidence, severity and significance of the sequelae which occur on emergence. The psychological manifestations vary in severity from pleasant dream-like states, a floating feeling, vivid imagery to hallucinations and emergence delirium. These may be accompanied by delirium or irrational behaviour and may or may not be remembered. There are three related aspects of this problem: (1) emergence reactions, (2) dreams and hallucinations and (3) longer term psychotomimetic effects.

(1) Emergence delirium or excitement occurs in the immediate postoperative period and the patient becomes disorientated and extremely restless and agitated. It is often accompanied by irrational talking or uncontrolled crying or moaning.
(2) Vivid dreams or hallucinations can occur up to 24 hours after ketamine; frequently they have morbid content and are often experienced in vivid technicolour.
(3) Despite the theoretical possibility of these occurring, there have been no well authenticated reports of undesirable long-term effects of ketamine.

Emergence delirium or excitement does not upset the patients themselves as they are unaware of its occurrence. However, it does upset nurses and other attendants and is very undesirable in a situation where patients waiting to come to operation may hear the disturbance. In contrast, the vivid dreams or hallucinations do upset the patients, particularly when they have unpleasant content. The attendants may be unaware of these and they can be of such severity as to deter patients from having subsequent anaesthetics. Perhaps they are most important in patients who have had previous anaesthetics with orthodox drugs and who have not had this occurrence.

Factors which are thought to influence the incidence and severity of emergence delirium and dreams include the following.

(1) Age: they are uncommon in the elderly and children. It is generally assumed that these do not occur in children, particularly in the very young but one can never be sure of this. Perhaps failure to record them indicates inability to communicate rather than the fact that they have not occurred.
(2) Females are more prone than males.
(3) Absence of premedication increases the incidence and severity of both types of sequelae.
(4) Nature of operation and duration of anaesthesia are inter-related. A number of workers have found that sequelae occur less frequently after body surface operations of 30—40 minutes' duration than after minor procedures lasting 5—10 minutes. They are uncommon after prolonged surgery.
(5) Disturbance during arousal: it has been suggested that disturbing the patient during the arousal period is likely to cause emergence delirium but this is far from proven.

(6) Sequelae occur less frequently when ketamine is used repeatedly. It is rare to have any emergence delirium or dreams after the third administration.

It is difficult to comment on the incidence of dreaming because many patients, particularly those given nitrous oxide, have postoperative dreams and this only causes an upset when the content of the dreams is unpleasant. As an example of this, children often have postoperative dreams and although these may occur more frequently after ketamine they do not seem to upset the children nor do they appear to have a morbid content. Visual disturbances can lead to both delirium and hallucinations. Their severity varies from patient to patient but the 'sensory and perceptual' misinterpretations which occur obviously are of importance.

Heavy premedication such as opiate–hyoscine or opiate–hyoscine–droperidol is effective in reducing emergence delirium but has less effect in preventing unpleasant dreams. Intravenous droperidol, given near the end of the operation, is also effective against emergence delirium but, likewise, is ineffective in preventing the occurrence of dreams. In contrast, intravenous diazepam, although ineffective against emergence delirium, reduces the incidence of unpleasant dreams. An oral mixture of 10 mg nitrazepam and 20 mg droperidol has been recommended for patients undergoing abdominal operations with ketamine as the main anaesthetic (Johnstone, 1972) and this is reported to reduce all sequelae. Lorazepam premedication has proved particularly effective in reducing the incidence of both emergence delirium and unpleasant dreams and increases the patient's acceptance of ketamine. Large doses (4 mg) are required by adults to give full protection, and this may prolong recovery.

Postoperative nausea and vomiting are not uncommon after ketamine.

Clinical uses and present status

This aspect must, of necessity, reflect the personal view of the authors. Ketamine is a useful drug in children, particularly for repeat minor procedures (burn dressings, radiotherapy, marrow sampling, etc). Care should be taken with it for neurological investigations. It is suitable for cardiac catheterization in infants and children. Its place is less clear in adults but it may have a place in poor-risk geriatric patients and for repeat burn dressings, for mass casualties and in the asthmatic.

Among the contraindications one would include patients with hypertension, those with increased intracranial or intraocular pressure and patients who give a history of psychiatric disorders. Furthermore, the pressor effect of the drug contraindicates its use where there is cardiac decompensation. Operations on pharynx, larynx or tracheobronchial tree cannot be carried out satisfactorily under ketamine alone because of the active reflexes in this area. Alcoholics and thyrotoxic patients also react badly to ketamine and, in the light of its known effects on the cerebrum, one might question the wisdom of using it in known or suspected drug addicts.

In assessing the present status, the list of advantages and disadvantages given in *Table 11.7* is helpful (Dundee and Lilburn, 1978).

TABLE 11.7. Advantages and disadvantages of ketamine (Dundee and Lilburn, 1979)

Advantages	Disadvantages	
Soluble in water	Anaesthesia:	slow onset
Effective by i.m. and i.v. routes		hypertonus
Non-irritant		hypertension
Good analgesia	Recovery:	slow
Non-hypotensive		emergence delirium
Minimum organ toxicity		unpleasant 'dreams'
Suitable for repeat administration		vomiting

It is remarkable that a drug which has so many disadvantages is still used 10 years after its introduction. Perhaps we have underestimated its advantages and the fact that no case of hypersensitivity to it has been described.

HYPERSENSITIVITY REACTIONS

Isolated cases of generalized reactions following administration of an intravenous anaesthetic have been occurring for over 25 years but for most of this time they were viewed as manifestations of bad technique, overdosage or simply as an unexplained anaesthetic death. However, now that they have been described following all the commonly used drugs, we can see that they fall into a general pattern, varying in incidence and severity with the particular drug.

The clinical features include generalized erythema, hypotension, oedema, bronchospasm and, rarely, abdominal symptoms. These closely resemble features of histamine release; indeed, plasma histamine levels correlate with the severity of the reaction in those cases where it has been measured (Lorenz *et al.*, 1972). Possible mechanisms of the histamine release fall into two groups: (1) direct release from basophils caused by the drug in amounts varying with the sensitivity of the subject, dose and rate of injection and (2) secondary to complement C3 conversion with liberation of a polypeptide which in turn liberates histamine from granules in the leucocytes (Watkins *et al.*, 1976b). This can occur by the so-called 'alternate pathway' without involvement of immune recognition. Alternatively, a patient who has been previously exposed to the drug may have built up IgE antibodies which are bound to the basophils. Subsequent challenge with the specific antigen results in immediate histamine release from these cells, which in turn may be trivial or constitute a typical anaphylactic attack.

The first reactions described were to thiopentone and there are now 55 published reports of fairly convincing reactions to the barbiturates (Clarke, 1979). This is, of course, a very small number compared with the very widespread use of this group of compounds. They cannot, however, be disregarded considering the number of published and un-published reports in recent years and the number of deaths (six) among them. Propanidid is responsible for very many more reactions, probably as many as 1 in 1000 administrations, and this has led to its almost complete abandonment as an anaesthetic. Most of these consisted in moderate erythema with flushing and hypotension, and despite this there are only two recorded deaths.

The largest number of published or unpublished reports of reactions has occurred with Althesin. They have been mainly cardiovascular in type but half have included bronchospasm. The fatality rate has been very low and while this may have been partly due to efficient treatment, it does suggest a less severe type of clinical course. Estimates of incidence in anaesthetic practice have ranged from 1 in 10 000 (Clarke *et al.*, 1975) to about 1 in 1000 (Fisher, 1976) and the true incidence must lie somewhere between these, depending on the exact criteria for definition of an adverse reaction.

Factors predisposing to an adverse reaction that have been specifically investigated include history of atopy (asthma, hay fever or eczema), allergy and previous exposure to the same anaesthetic. Dundee *et al.* (1978) found an 8% incidence of atopic history in an unselected surgical popu-lation which is very similar to that in the published reports (Clarke, 1978). However, there is a higher incidence of allergy to various substances in the reactors than in surgical patients and this can be incriminated as a predisposing factor. Likewise, previous exposure to propanidid (Doenicke, 1975) and Althesin (Clarke, 1978) can predispose to an adverse reaction to these drugs. Absolute prevention of reactions would not appear to be possible though an antihistamine in the premedication may be of some value (Lorenz *et al.*, 1972) and disodium cromoglycate appears to block signs of immune recognition *in vitro* (Watkins *et al.*, 1976a).

Treatment of an established reaction consists first in the replacement of fluid lost to the circulation as oedema, by some form of balanced salt solution or, preferably, by plasma protein. A vasoconstrictor may be given for hypotension and a bronchodilator for bronchospasm. Tracheal intubation and inflation with oxygen will probably be essential. Other remedies such as antihistamines and steroids take longer to produce any effect but the latter would appear to be of value in counteracting both the bronchospasm and the hypotension. The main point to be stressed is that intravenous anaesthetics should be given only where one is equipped for treatment along these lines, as it is too late to send for resuscitation apparatus when a disaster actually happens.

References

Bovill, J. G., Coppel, D. L., Dundee, J. W. and Moore, J. (1971). Current status of ketamine anaesthesia. *Lancet* i, 1285–1288

Breimer, D. D. (1976). Pharmokinetics of methohexitone following intravenous infusion in humans. *Br. J. Anaesth.* 48, 643–649

Brodie, B. B. (1952). Physiological disposition and chemical fate of thiobarbiturates in the body. *Fedn Proc.* 11, 632–639

Brodie, B. B., Mark, L. C., Papper, E. M., Lief, P. A., Bernstein, E. and Rovenstine, E. A. (1950). Fate of thiopental in man and method for its estimation in biological material. *J. Pharmac. exp. Ther.* 98, 85–96

Brown, S. S., Lyons, S. M. and Dundee, J. W. (1968). Intra-arterial barbiturates: a study of some factors leading to intravascular thrombosis. *Br. J. Anaesth.* 40, 13–19

Bruckner, J. B., Gethmann, J. W., Patschke, D., Tarnow, J. and Weymar, A. (1974). Investigations into the effect of etomidate on the human circulation. *Anaesthetist* 23, 322–330

Burn, J. H. (1960). Why thiopentone injected into an artery may cause gangrene. *Br. med. J.* 2, 414–416

Burn, J. H. and Hobbs, R. (1959). Mechanism of arterial spasm following intra-arterial injection of thiopentone. *Lancet* i, 1112–1115

Chen, G. (1965). Evaluation of phencyclidine-type cataleptic activity. *Archs int. pharmacodyn. thér.* 157, 193–201

Child, K. J., Currie, J. P., Davis, B., Dodds, M. G., Pearce, D. R. and Twissell, D. J. (1971). The pharmacological properties in animals of CT 1341 – a new steroid anaesthetic agent. *Br. J. Anaesth.* 43, 2–13

Clarke, R. S. J. (1979). Hypersensitivity reactions to intravenous anaesthetics. In *Intravenous Anaesthetic Agents.* J. W. Dundee (ed.). Current Topics in Anaesthesia series. London: Edward Arnold

Clarke, R. S. J., Dundee, J. W. and Hamilton, R. C. (1967). Interactions between induction agents and muscle relaxants. *Anaesthesia* 22, 235–248

Clarke, R. S. J., Dundee, J. W., Garrett, R. T., McArdle, G. K. and Sutton, J. A. (1975). Adverse reactions to intravenous anaesthetics. A survey of 100 reports. *Br. J. Anaesth.* 47, 575–585

Cohen, S. M. (1948). Accidental intra-arterial injection of drugs. *Lancet* ii, 361–371; 409–416

Corssen, G. (1969). Allgemeine klinische erfahrungen mit ketamine bei mehr als 1500 fällen. *Anaesthetist* 18, 25

Corssen, G., Miyasaka, M. and Domino, E. F. (1968). Changing concepts in pain control during surgery: dissociative anesthesia with CI-581: a progress report. *Anesth. Analg. curr. Res.* 47, 746–759

Doenicke, A. (1975). Propanidid. In *Recent Progress in Anaesthesiology and Resuscitation,* pp. 107–113. A. Arias, R. Llaurado, M. A. Nalda and J. N. Lunn (ed.). Proceedings of the IVth European Congress of Anaesthesiology, Madrid, 5–11 September 1974. Amsterdam: Excerpta Medica

Doenicke, A., Kugler, J. and Laub, M. (1967). Evaluation of recovery and 'street fitness' by EEG and psychodiagnostic tests after anaesthesia. *Can. Anaesth. Soc. J.* 14, 567–583

Doenicke, A., Kugler, J., Schellenberger, A. and Gurtner, T. (1966). The use of electroencephalography to measure recovery time after intravenous anaesthesia. *Br. J. Anaesth.* 38, 580–590

Doenicke, A., Kugler, J., Penzel, G., Laub, M., Kalmar, L., Killian, I. and Bezecny, H. (1973a). Hirnfunktion and Toleranzbreite nach Etomidate einem neuen barbituratfreien i.v. applizierbaren Hypnoticum. *Anaesthesist* 22, 357

Doenicke, A., Lorenz, W., Beigl, R., Bezecny, H., Uhlig, G., Kalmar, L., Praetorius, B. and Mann, G. (1973b). Histamine release after intravenous application of short-acting hypnotics. A comparison of etomidate, Althesin (CT 1341) and propanidid. *Br. J. Anaesth.* 45, 1097–1104

du Cailar, J. (1972). The effects in man of infusions of Althesin with particular regard to the cardiovascular system. *Postgrad. med. J.* 48, Suppl. 2, 72–79

du Cailar, J., Evrard, O., Peguret, C. and Deschodt, J. (1974). Anesthésie a l'Alfatésine par perfusion a la seringue automatique a débit constant. *Annls anesthésiol. fr.* 15, 661–670

du Cailar, J., Deschodt, J., Bessou, D. and Cabanel, Ph. (1975). Anesthésie a debit constant par l'association Alfatésine–fentanyl. *Annls anesthésiol. fr.* 16, 331–340

Dundee, J. W. (1956). *Thiopentone and Other Thiobarbiturates.* Edinburgh: Churchill Livingstone

Dundee, J. W. (1965). Some effects of premedication on the induction characteristics of intravenous anaesthetics. *Anaesthesia* 20, 299–314

Dundee, J. W. and Barron, D. W. (1962). The barbiturates. *Br. J. Anaesth.* 34, 240–246

Dundee, J. W. and Lilburn, J. K. (1979). Pros and cons of ketamine. In *Intravenous Anaesthetic Agents.* J. W. Dundee (ed.). Current Topics in Anaesthesia series. London: Edward Arnold

Dundee, J. W. and Wyant, G. M. (1974). *Intravenous Anaesthesia.* Edinburgh: Churchill Livingstone

Dundee, J. W. and Zacharias, M. (1979). Etomidate. In *Intravenous Anaesthetic Agents*. J. W. Dundee (ed.). Current Topics in Anaesthesia series. London: Edward Arnold

Dundee, J. W., Fee, J. P. H., McDonald, J. R. and Clarke, R. S. J. (1978). Incidence of atopy and allergy in an anaesthetic patient population. *Br. J. Anaesth.* 50, 793–798

Eckenhoff, J. E. and Helrich, M. (1958). The effect of narcotics, thiopental and nitrous oxide upon respiration and respiratory response to hypercapnia. *Anesthesiology* 19, 240

Fisher, M. M. (1976). Severe histamine mediated reactions to Althesin. *Anaesth. Intens. Care* 4, 33–35

Forrester, A. C. and Saunders, R. C. O. (1955). Intra-arterial thiopentone. *Br. J. Anaesth.* 27, 594

Heykants, J. J. P., Meuldermauf, W. E. G., Michiels, L. J. M., Lewi, P. J. and Janssen, P. A. J. (1975). Distribution, metabolism and excretion of etomidate, a short-acting hypnotic drug, in the rat. Comparative study of (R)–(+) and (S)–(–) etomidate. *Archs int. Pharmacodyn. Thér.* 216, 113–129

Janssen, P. A. J., Niemegeers, C. J. E. and Marsboom, R. P. H. (1975). Etomidate, a potent non-barbiturate hypnotic. Intravenous etomidate in mice, rats, guinea-pigs, rabbits and dogs. *Archs int. Pharmacodyn. Thér.* 214, 96–132

Johnstone, M. (1972). The prevention of ketamine dreams. *Anaesth. Intens. Care* 1, 70–74

Kettler, D. and Sonntag, H. (1974). Intravenous anesthetics: coronary blood flow and myocardial oxygen consumption (with special reference to Althesine). *Acta anaesth. belg.* 25, 384–399

Kettler, D., Sonntag, H., Donath, U., Regensburger, D. and Schenk, H. D. (1974). Haemodynamics, myocardial function, oxygen requirement and oxygen supply of the human heart after the administration of etomidate. *Anaesthesist* 23, 116–121

Laurent, S. and du Cailar, J. (1977). Anesthésie a débit constant a l'Alfatésine-phénopéridine. Applications a l'anesthésie du sujet agé en chirurgie viscérale. *Annls anesthésiol. fr.* 18, 265–272

Lewi, P. J., Heykants, J. J. P. and Janssen, P. A. J. (1976). Intravenous pharmacokinetic profile in rats of etomidate, a short-acting drug. *Archs int. Pharmacodyn. Thér.* 220, 72–85

Lorenz, W., Doenicke, A., Meyer, R., Reimann, J., Barth, H., Geesing, H., Hutzel, M. and Weissenbacher, B. (1972). Histamine release in man by propanidid and thiopentone: pharmacological effects and clinical consequences. *Br. J. Anaesth.* 44, 355–369

Mark, L. C., Burns, J. J., Brand, L., Campomanes, C. I., Trousof, N., Papper, E. M. and Brodie, B. B. (1958). The passage of thiobarbiturates and their oxygen analogs into brain. *J. Pharmac. exp. Ther.* 123, 70–73

Mark, L. C., Brand, L., Kamvyssi, S., Britton, R. C., Perel, J. M., Landrau, M. A. and Dayton, P. G. (1965). Thiopental metabolism by human liver *in vivo* and *in vitro*. *Nature, Lond.* 206, 1117–1119

Price, H. L. (1960). A dynamic concept of the distribution of thiopental in the human body. *Anesthesiology* 21, 40–45

Price, H. L., Kovnat, P. J., Safer, J. N., Conner, E. H. and Price, M. L. (1960). The uptake of thiopental by body tissues and its relation to the duration of narcosis. *Clin. Pharmac. Ther.* 1, 16–22

Ramsay, M. A. E., Savege, T. M., Simpson, B. R. J. and Goodwin, R. (1974). Controlled sedation with alphaxalone–alphadolone. *Br. med. J.* 2, 656–659

Saidman, L. J. and Eger, E. I. II (1966). The effect of thiopental metabolism on duration of anesthesia. *Anesthesiology* 27, 118–126

Savege, T. M., Ramsay, M. A. E., Curran, J. P. J., Cotter, J., Walling, P. T. and Simpson, B. R. (1975). Intravenous anaesthesia by infusion: a technique using alphaxalone/alphadolone (Althesin). *Anaesthesia* 30, 757–764

Stone, H. H. and Donnelly, C. C. (1961). The accidental intra-arterial injection of thiopental. *Anesthesiology* 22, 995–1006

Watkins, J., Clark, A., Appleyard, T. N. and Padfield, A. (1976a). Immune-mediated reactions to Althesin (alphaxalone). *Br. J. Anaesth.* 48, 881–886

Watkins, J., Udnoon, S., Appleyard, T. N. and Thornton, J. A. (1976b). Identification and quantitation of hypersensitivity reactions to intravenous anaesthetic agents. *Br. J. Anaesth.* 48, 457–461

Weese, H. and Scharpff, W. (1932). Evipan, ein neuartiges Einschlaffmittel. *Dt. med. Wschr.* 58, 1205–1207

Zindler, M. (1975). Cardiovascular effects of etomidate. In *Recent Progress in Anaesthesiology and Resuscitation,* pp. 118–121. A. Arias, R. Llaurado, M. A. Nalda and J. N. Lunn (ed.). Proceedings of the IVth Congress of Anaesthesiology, Madrid, 5–11 September 1974. Amsterdam: Excerpta Medica

12 Opiate analgesics
R. S. J. Clarke

The analgesics which are of particular value to the anaesthetist are those known as strong analgesics, narcotics or opiates. These drugs originate in the age-old use of opium and its extracts as a pain killer, but it was only during the last century that individual alkaloids were identified — for example, morphine by Sertürner in 1806. An extract of opium contains many narcotic alkaloids, the most important of which are morphine and codeine. A purified extract, known as papaveretum and standardized to contain 50% of morphine base, is still very widely used.

MORPHINE

Chemistry

Morphine represents between 3 and 23% of the total alkaloids in crude opium. It is a phenanthrene derivative as shown in *Figure 12.1*, having an

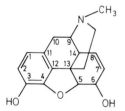

Figure 12.1
Formula of morphine

ethylene amine chain $-CH_2CH_2N(CH_3)-$ bridging the 9 and 13 positions. Alterations in the structure produce changes in properties which have been clinically useful.

(1) Alteration in the hydroxyl group at C_3 decreases the analgesic and respiratory depressant actions but increases the central stimulant effects (e.g. codeine).
(2) Changing the hydroxyl group at C_6 also increases central excitation but increases analgesic potency (with shorter duration).

(3) When the ether bridge is broken, oral absorption is improved (e.g. levorphanol).

(4) Substitution of an allyl group on the methyl radical attached to the nitrogen produces a substance with opiate antagonist and dysphoric actions (e.g. nalorphine).

Absorption and distribution

Morphine is well absorbed following intramuscular administration, with an onset of effect in 15–30 minutes and peak effect in 45–90 minutes. However, Laitinen *et al.* (1975) found a sevenfold range of concentration between individuals, in 1 hour, and there was no over-all correlation between plasma level and analgesia. Absorption from the gastrointestinal route is even less reliable. The onset following intravenous administration is in 1–2 minutes, reaching a maximum effect in 3–6 minutes. Morphine rapidly leaves the blood stream, lodging in nearly all body tissues. It is then detoxicated by oxidation and conjugation with glucuronic acid in the liver and excreted mainly in the urine, though some is found in bile and faeces.

Action on the central nervous system

Morphine, even in low doses, raises the threshold to pain and modifies the painful sensation so that it is no longer experienced as pain. There is also a modification in the reaction to pain, which is a most important aspect of clinical analgesia.

As the dose is raised, more widespread depression of the central nervous system usually follows in man, though stimulation occurs in other species. In man sedation progresses to sleep, but not to satisfactory anaesthesia unless another type of cerebral depressant is added. However, small doses can lead to excitement or delirium, particularly in women and older patients. A tendency to convulsions from other causes is enhanced. Euphoria is often reported where pain has been relieved, but it is not a feature of administration of the drug in routine preanaesthetic medication. Likewise, anxiety is not well relieved though powers of concentration and tendency to worry about a problem are reduced.

The site of action of morphine is widespread through the brain and spinal cord. It produces an effect on the electroencephalogram like that of sleep or anaesthesia; that is, the rapid α waves are replaced by slower δ waves. At still higher doses, spike waves begin to appear. In general not only do the cortical association areas seem to be depressed but also parts of the limbic system and thalamus.

The polysynaptic pathways of the spinal cord are also inhibited, though the increased activity of monosynaptic circuits may lead to muscular hypertonia occurring sometimes after large doses of the drug. Narcotics administered intrathecally in animals have been shown to be bound to the substantia gelatinosa and can exert a true analgesia at this level.

The exact mode of action of opiates and the nature of the opiate receptors is being increasingly studied (Hughes and Kosterlitz, 1977). It has been shown that various encephalins (pentapeptides) have a distribution in the CNS similar to that of the opiate receptors. When applied to certain mammalian brain areas they have an inhibitory effect and this in turn can be antagonized by naloxone. They may therefore act as an inhibitory neurotransmitter in particular brain regions and have the property of being rapidly destroyed, which is necessary for this role. However, it has not been shown that they are found naturally in nerve terminals or that they are released on stimulation.

A peptide has been found in human blood which produces long-lasting analgesia in rats — an effect reversed by naloxone. This substance appears to be produced in the pituitary under surgical stress and acts on various parts of the brain, leading to analgesia, sedation and euphoria. An endorphin is a larger peptide with opioid activity which can be extracted from brain tissue, particularly the pituitary. Kosterlitz (1977) has suggested that these endorphins could be involved in the fight and flight reactions, as well as making the individual insensitive to severe pain.

The inter-relation between morphine and the anticholinesterases (e.g. neostigmine) has been known for many years, and the latter group certainly potentiates morphine analgesia. While it is possible that morphine and the anticholinergics act by depressing central cholinergic synapses, this is still not proven.

Morphine increases cerebral blood flow but this is probably secondary to a rise in arterial $P\text{CO}_2$. There is a concomitant increase in intracranial and CSF pressure.

Cardiovascular actions

Morphine in low dosage, especially by the intramuscular route, has little effect on the cardiovascular system but, as the dosage is raised to the point where the analgesic response curve becomes flat (*Figure 12.2*), all side-effects become more evident. This is particularly important when the drug is used intravenously for postoperative analgesia or as a major part of the anaesthetic technique. Morphine (10 mg intravenously) does not appear to have any direct depressant action on the normal heart though the rate is slowed. The bradycardia has been attributed to both vagal stimulation and a depressant action on the sinoatrial node. The stroke volume is maintained but there is a fall in arterial pressure associated with peripheral vasodilatation. The exact mechanism of this is not clear and both release of sympathetic tone and a direct vasodilator action on smooth muscle appear to be involved. The latter action has been confirmed by intra-arterial infusion. The release of histamine which is a frequent accompaniment is not the cause of this increase in peripheral blood flow (Samuel, Clarke and Dundee, 1977; Samuel, Unni and Dundee, 1977).

Patients who have impaired circulatory function following cardiac surgery appear to have both a fall in blood pressure and a decrease in cardiac index when given morphine 10 mg intravenously. The most likely explanation for this is that morphine depresses the myocardium which has suffered from the physiological stress and trauma of cardiac surgery (Samuel, Clarke and Dundee, 1977). It also causes peripheral vasodilatation in these patients, so that the dose should be titrated to the effect.

This vasodilatory property is probably of value in patients with acute myocardial infarction, for Lee *et al.* (1976) have shown that neither morphine nor pethidine affects the heart rate or systemic blood pressure though they raise the pulmonary arterial pressure. The absence of hazardous haemodynamic effects was in contrast to pentazocine which

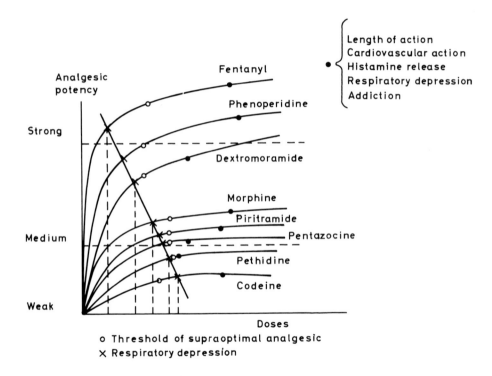

Figure 12.2
Diagrammatic representation of the occurrence, according to the doses used, of analgesia, respiratory depression and cardiovascular effects induced by the main central analgesics used in clinical practice

caused peripheral vasoconstriction and increased myocardial oxygen demand.

The use of potent analgesics as part of a neurolept technique is discussed later, but mention must be made here of the use of morphine in high dosage in 'analgesic anaesthesia'. The dose range studied has been 0.5–3.0 $mg \cdot kg^{-1}$ and detailed cardiovascular studies with special reference to cardiac surgery were carried out by Lowenstein *et al.* (1969). In patients with no obvious cardiorespiratory disease, doses of 0.5–1.0 $mg \cdot kg^{-1}$ had no effect on systemic or pulmonary blood pressure, central venous pressure or cardiac index. In a group about to undergo aortic valve replacement, the cardiac index rose by 30% after morphine 0.5 mg·kg⁻¹ and 49% after 1.0 mg·kg⁻¹. Lowenstein (1971) has postulated that morphine maintains the blood pressure by release of catecholamines but this has still not been fully investigated nor has the hypotension which sometimes occurs.

Action on respiration

Morphine causes a dose-related depression of respiration, which progresses to the point of apnoea. In addition, morphine depresses the sensitivity of the respiratory centre to carbon dioxide or other stimuli. It stimulates the stretch receptors in the lungs, inhibiting the inspiratory centres as well as facilitating vagal expiratory reflexes to cause slowing of respiration. Tidal volume is little affected or even increased, through compensation to maintain a normal $P\text{CO}_2$. The cough reflex is depressed and this property can be turned to advantage in patients subjected to positive pressure pulmonary ventilation.

Other cerebral depressants (as well as normal sleep) potentiate the respiratory depression of morphine, particularly in the newborn and the elderly. Analeptics antagonize this respiratory depression to some extent but narcotic antagonists have their main place in reversing this action of morphine.

Action on the gastrointestinal tract

Morphine stimulates the 'chemoreceptor trigger zone' (see Chapter 14) and, although it depresses the vomiting centre, it frequently causes nausea and vomiting by the former effect. In addition, it has a direct irritant action on the stomach. Like other undesirable effects of morphine, sickness is dose-related and its severity continues to increase when analgesia has reached its maximum. Its likelihood is accentuated by movements of the patient, particularly sitting up and attempting to take oral fluids. It is therefore a particular problem when narcotics are used for relief of chronic pain in ambulant patients. It is antagonized by all the principal varieties of antiemetics.

Morphine induces marked constipation by depression of the longitudinal muscle and prolonged stimulation of the circular muscle of the intestine. These effects are due to parasympathetic stimulation and a direct papaverine-like action on the smooth muscle fibres.

Another important action of morphine is in contracting the muscles of the pancreatic and biliary ducts and the sphincter of Oddi. This raises the back pressure in the biliary tree and may well be harmful in patients with partial biliary obstruction. It is not antagonized by atropine but is relieved by aminophylline and amyl nitrite.

Other actions of morphine

URINE OUTPUT

Morphine stimulates the hypothalamus to increase the output of antidiuretic hormone, leading to a fall in urine output. It also increases the tone of the lower part of the ureter and the detrusor muscle and sphincter of the bladder. This combination may lead to urgency and retention.

EYE

Morphine constricts the pupil by a central action on the Edinger—Westphal nucleus of the oculomotor nerve. This effect is antagonized by atropine and ganglion-blocking drugs.

HISTAMINE LIBERATION

This is a cause of several troublesome side-effects of morphine. It causes bronchoconstriction, and morphine is contraindicated in patients having an attack of bronchial asthma. It can also lead to flushing of the skin, itching, vasodilatation and tachycardia.

Clinical use of morphine

PREMEDICATION

The idea of opiate premedication was advocated as long ago as 1875 by Claude Bernard on the basis that it reduced the requirement of anaesthetic or increased the depth of anaesthesia. More recently, particularly in the USA, this view has been rejected and the use of narcotic premedication was restricted to patients actually suffering pain. However, there are definite advantages in including a narcotic, and morphine in particular, in a 'balanced' premedication. Morphine is not a good anxiolytic, as was pointed out above, but its analgesic properties are an advantage when preoperative infusions and monitoring lines are being set up and there is a more smooth onset of anaesthesia even when such a satisfactory drug as thiopentone is being used. These advantages are, of course, much more evident when the newer anaesthetic induction agents such as methohexitone, Althesin or etomidate are being given, though at the cost of a delayed recovery. It is probably unjustifiable to give morphine without the slightly antiemetic atropine or preferably hyoscine, the anti-emetic action of the latter being added to some useful sedation and powerful antisialogogue action. The combination of pentobarbitone, morphine and hyoscine has been recommended for major cardiac surgery for many years and could be applied to any major surgery where rapid recovery is not required. Its safety has been demonstrated even for severely ill patients by Lyons, Clarke and Vulgaraki (1975).

ANAESTHESIA

Morphine has only come into prominence in anaesthesia during the last ten years (Lowenstein *et al.*, 1969) because its prolonged action renders it inappropriate for most forms of surgery and it had been regarded as too depressant. Since it has been shown that in large doses it preserves cardiovascular stability, its use as main anaesthetic agent for coronary artery bypass surgery has increased. Detailed comparisons of the analgesics in this respect have still to be made but for prolonged surgery, where postoperative ventilation is an established routine, its long duration of action is an advantage.

The dose range is 1.5–2.5 mg·kg^{-1} infused over 10–15 minutes. The patient is encouraged to breathe deeply as long as he can but when he ceases to respond, ventilation is assisted and a muscle relaxant is administered. Even this does not always produce full anaesthesia and memory can be retained – hence the addition of diazepam (0.5 mg·kg^{-1}) to the infusate by many workers. This produces a cloudy mixture but appears to be satisfactory when freshly made up. Oxygen is inhaled from the onset of the infusion. It would appear that administration of 60% nitrous oxide in oxygen nullifies the cardiovascular advantages of morphine (Hasbrouck, 1970; Stoelting and Gibbs, 1973).

Morphine is less satisfactory for patients having short operations and where a rapid return to spontaneous respiration is required. Fentanyl is certainly the drug of choice here and is discussed later. In reversal of the action of morphine, the dose of naloxone will need to be repeated because of morphine's prolonged action (Evans *et al.*, 1974).

SUPPRESSION OF RESPIRATION AND COUGH REFLEX

This can be achieved in patients on artificial ventilation by any of the narcotics. There would seem to be little advantage in giving the shorter-acting, more potent drugs, and morphine 0.1 mg·kg^{-1} given intravenously is usually safe and effective. The dose may need to be reduced if there is additional hypovolaemia and increased if the patient is in particularly good general health or becomes tolerant to the drug.

POSTOPERATIVE ANALGESIA

There has been little change in this field for many years and, except where prolonged regional block renders analgesics unnecessary, morphine is still one of the most useful drugs. The standard practice is to give 5–10 mg by the intramuscular route when the patient has recovered consciousness and complains of pain, repeating the dose 4–6 hourly as required. With this regimen respiratory depression is rare, though it can occur if the same timing is applied to some of the longer-acting analgesics such as methadone or levorphanol. Sickness, too, occurs only rarely in patients lying prone after major surgery and routine use of combinations with antiemetics would seem to be undesirable. The action of cyclizine is shorter than that of morphine, and that of perphenazine, particularly its extrapyramidal effects, is much more prolonged. The practical problem in postoperative analgesia is not so much what drugs to give as to ensure that they are given in adequate dosage as soon as required.

Intravenous administration of morphine in small increments (2 mg for an adult) has the advantage of rapid action and reliable effect but it requires continuous intensive supervision of the patient and is probably only suitable for patients following major surgery. The advantages of the intravenous route have led to the technique of self-administration but this is most satisfactory with shorter-acting drugs such as pethidine or fentanyl.

Contraindications and restrictions on dosage

Morphine dosage can be calculated on a milligrams per kilogram body weight basis, but it must be remembered that infants are unduly sensitive to it. This is partly because the central nervous system in infants is immature and metabolism by the liver is also less efficient. The fetus is therefore very sensitive to morphine given during labour, since it readily crosses the placental barrier.

As has been stated earlier, cardiovascular depression occurs mainly in patients with heart disease. Morphine should be given with extreme caution in patients with severe respiratory disease or respiratory failure may be precipitated. This is particularly true where there is upper airway obstruction and this condition may be regarded as an absolute contraindication to its use until a safe airway has been provided.

Morphine is also contraindicated in all patients with head injury or any space-occupying lesion of the brain. In fact, it should probably be reserved for the time when a diagnosis has been established and the patient is being treated with pulmonary ventilation.

Hepatic failure due to widespread cirrhosis or viral hepatitis is another reason for extreme caution in dosage. A moderate dose given on a weight-for-weight basis can be followed by hepatic coma lasting for several days or from which the patient does not recover.

Myxoedema, adrenal hypofunction and mental deficiency are associated with sensitivity. Thyrotoxicosis leads to resistance to morphine. The interactions between morphine and other drugs are too widespread for description here apart from the obvious potentiation of its depressant effects by other depressants. However, particular watch should be kept for the severe cardiovascular and respiratory collapse which can occur with any opiate in patients who have recently had monoamine oxidase inhibitors, though pethidine was the opiate associated with collapse in most of the reported cases.

OTHER OPIATE ANALGESICS—AGONISTS

Drugs which are clinically available in the UK are listed in *Table 12.1*, classified according to their chemical derivation, into naturally occurring, semisynthetic and synthetic opiates. The synthetic compounds fall into

TABLE 12.1. Potent analgesics

Generic name and classification according to origin	Trade or other name	Relative potency	Dose range (mg)	Approximate duration (h)	Comments
Natural alkaloids of opium					
Morphine	–	100	8–16	4–6	Poor oral efficacy
Codeine	–	8–15	30–60 (O)	3–4	Very weak analgesic
Papaveretum	Omnopon	–	15–30	4–6	Regard 20 mg as equivalent to 13 mg morphine sulphate
Semisynthetic opium alkaloids					
Dihydrocodeine	DF 118	30	30–60 (O)	–	Good oral absorption; mild analgesic
Diamorphine	Heroin	200–300	4–8	2	Terminal malignancy. Unstable solution
Nalorphine hydrobromide*	Lethidrone	–	2–5	2–3	Used as an analgesic antagonist
Naloxone*	Narcan	–	0.4–0.8	–	Only available pure antagonist
Buprenorphine*	Temgesic	3000	0.3–0.6	8	Slow onset, cumulative
Synthetic compounds					
Morphinans and benzmorphinans:					
Levorphanol	Dromoran	330–500	2–4	4–6	Good oral absorption
Phenazocine	Narphen	500	2–4	4–6	As toxic as morphine. Sublingual use
Pentazocine hydrochloride*	Fortral	50	20–40	2–4	Low dependence liability
Levallorphan*	Lorfan	–	1–2	4–6	
Piperidine derivatives:					
Pethidine	–	10	75–125	2–3	High toxicity; rapid onset; short action
Phenoperidine	Operidine	500	2–3	2–3	Use in NLA
Fentanyl	Sublimaze	5000	0.2–0.3	1–2	Very short acting. Use in NLA
Piritramide	Dipidolar	90	15–20	6–8	More soporific than morphine
Diphenylheptane derivatives:					
Methadone	Physeptone	100–130	5–15	6–8	Good oral absorption
Dipipanone	Pipadone	40	10–25	5–6	Diconal = dipipanone + cyclizine
Dextromoramide	Palfium	200	5–8	2–3	Probably as toxic as morphine
Dextropropoxyphene	Doloxene	–	65–130 (O)	–	Mild analgesic

* Antagonist and partial agonist; also opiate antagonists.
Potency is given relative to morphine = 100. The dose range is for adults by intramuscular administration or oral (O) where more appropriate.

three groups — the morphinans and benzmorphinans, the piperidine derivatives and the diphenylheptane derivatives. These are not discussed in detail but their human pharmacology and therapeutic uses which concern the anaesthetist are mentioned. *Figure 12.2* illustrates the dose response curves of the principal opiates, classifying them according to their potential analgesic efficacy.

Codeine

Codeine is the weakest of these analgesics, its dose response curve flattening off at 60 mg. It is well absorbed by the oral route but overdosage leads to all the effects of other opiates in high dosage. However, a 15 mg dose by mouth has a definite antitussive effect.

Dihydrocodeine

This is a derivative of codeine which also has good oral absorption. It is a weak analgesic and its main side-effect is constipation.

Diamorphine

Diamorphine is an effective analgesic of about twice the potency of morphine, into which it is rapidly converted in the body. It is more lipid soluble and, because it crosses the blood—brain barrier rapidly, is more attractive to addicts using the intravenous route than morphine. Because of its instability in solution, it is preferable to use ampoules of dry powder which are dissolved immediately before administration.

Levorphanol

Levorphanol is very similar in structure and pharmacology to morphine, with about four times the potency. It has the advantage of better oral absorption than morphine with less tendency to produce nausea and vomiting.

Phenazocine

Phenazocine appears to have no advantages over morphine for clinical use.

Pethidine

This is probably the most widely used opiate analgesic after morphine and codeine. It has a totally different structure and, as well as having a lower potency weight for weight, is less analgesic in any dose that can be safely given. The onset is more rapid than that of morphine and its duration is only about half, but in equianalgesic doses its effects are very similar. For instance, pethidine 100 mg produces nausea or vomiting in about 65% of gynaecological patients compared with 61% in the case of morphine 10 mg, but the sickness comes on earlier and passes off more rapidly (Dundee, Clarke and Loan, 1965). It causes peripheral vasodilatation and a fall in arterial blood pressure when doses of 100—200 mg are given intravenously, similar in its action to morphine in equipotent doses, but higher doses lead to tachycardia and hypotension, which render it unsuitable for analgesic anaesthesia. It does not cause the constipation or spasm of the sphincter of Oddi associated with morphine and has a better spasmolytic effect on the ureter in colic. It is absorbed by the oral route, reaching its peak effect in about 90 minutes. Patients who are receiving monoamine oxidase inhibitors may experience a severe reaction on receiving pethidine, consisting in excitation, delirium, hyperpyrexia, respiratory depression and cyanosis, usually without hypotension.

Phenoperidine

Phenoperidine is about five times as potent as morphine but of shorter duration of action. It has a similar respiratory depressant effect but is less sedative, which may or may not be an advantage. If respiration is controlled, relatively high doses can produce a greater degree of analgesia than is possible with morphine. For this reason it was used in neurolept analgesic techniques. It has, however, been replaced by the shorter-acting fentanyl and its use is virtually confined to producing respiratory depression in ventilated patients.

Fentanyl

This is the most potent opiate so far to reach clinical use, both in terms of effect for weight and in considering the absolute degree of analgesia obtainable. Its use is almost confined to the intravenous route, mainly in neurolept analgesia, the effect of 0.1 mg beginning within 1 minute and lasting about 30 minutes. However, since the technique was introduced about 20 years ago fentanyl has been increasingly used as an intravenous analgesic without neuroleptics. It has the respiratory depressant and vasodilator effects associated with other opiates. The drug has been used in high doses in 'analgesic anaesthesia' but outside the 0.05—0.1 mg dose range it cannot be regarded as short-acting and patients will certainly need to be ventilated after its use, or the analgesia reversed, with the hazards of recurrent respiratory and cardiovascular depression. It may occasionally produce muscular rigidity which, by affecting the thoracic wall, renders respiration impossible and can only be managed by neuromuscular block.

Piritramide

Piritramide is very similar to morphine in dosage and properties but it appears to be less sedative and causes less sickness.

Methadone

Methadone is also very similar to morphine in many respects but has less addictive properties. Its main value is therefore in weaning patients off morphine dependence and reducing the withdrawal symptoms. It is, however, of value as a less hypnotic analgesic than morphine though its duration of action is longer and after repeated doses marked respiratory depression may occur. It is also very effective by the oral route.

Dipipanone

Dipipanone is well absorbed by the oral route and is useful in treating patients at home. Because of the frequency of sickness when used in this way, it is made up in a tablet in conjunction with cyclizine (Diconal).

Dextromoramide

Dextromoramide has about twice the potency of morphine but similar properties. Like phenoperidine, it has been used in neurolept analgesia (being the first of the potent analgesics to be introduced by Janssen) but its main advantages now would appear to be good oral absorption with less sedation than occurs with morphine or pethidine.

Dextropropoxyphene

Dextropropoxyphene is a weak analgesic usually taken orally. Its main interest to anaesthetists is that it is a common cause of opiate poisoning alone or in the mixture with paracetamol (Distalgesic).

OPIATE ANTAGONISTS AND PARTIAL AGONISTS

In 1915 it was observed that N-allyl-norcodeine prevented or abolished morphine-induced respiratory depression. It was another 25 years before the same properties were observed in N-allyl-normorphine or nalorphine. The clinical significance of this antagonistic effect was not explored until 1951 when Eckenhoff, Elder and King reported the use of nalorphine as an antidote to morphine poisoning in man. The next stage was the demonstration that nalorphine would precipitate acute withdrawal symptoms in addicts to morphine or other narcotics and in fact on its own produced dysphoria and anxiety rather than euphoria. The final step in the evolution of narcotic antagonists to our present ideas was Lasagna and Beecher's (1954) demonstration that, although nalorphine antagonized the analgesic effects of morphine, it was nevertheless an effective analgesic when given to patients in pain. It only remained to find a narcotic antagonist which was less dysphoric than nalorphine.

This group of drugs illustrates very well the structure–function relationships seen in barbiturates, steroids and other pharmacological groups. Four pairs need to be considered:

morphine→	nalorphine
levorphanol→	levallorphan
phenazocine→	pentazocine
oxymorphone→	naloxone

In each of these pairs the replacement of the *N*-methyl group by an *N*-allyl linkage (or similar double bond) alters the properties from mainly agonist to mainly antagonist. However, there are differences in the relationship of agonist to antagonist properties in each drug.

Nalorphine

This is the first antagonist to be used clinically but it has been largely replaced by the newer antagonists. The great objection to this drug is that about 20% of patients have psychotomimetic reactions. Some of these are very distressing — more hallucinatory and unpleasant than the dissociative feelings with ketamine. Although reports vary, many workers have found nalorphine to be as potent an analgesic as morphine, but its clinical use is precluded because of side-effects.

Nalorphine given to patients who have developed a drug dependence to morphine precipitates a withdrawal reaction characterized by sweating, nausea, weakness, tremor, anxiety and insomnia. In severe instances there may be epileptic fits and delirium. Nalorphine does *not* produce withdrawal symptoms in chronic users of pentazocine, in clear distinction to naloxone. That is, it is not a pure antagonist.

Levallorphan

This is the *N*-allyl analogue of levorphanol and came into clinical use after nalorphine. Its properties are very similar to those of nalorphine in that it is an agonist–antagonist with similar sedative and respiratory depressant actions and lack of analgesia and a similar ability to reverse opiate-induced respiratory depression. It also produces withdrawal symptoms in morphine addicts. Like nalorphine, levallorphan is an analgesic but antagonizes the analgesic action of pethidine.

Pentazocine

This drug emerged from a pharmaceutical attempt to produce an analgesic rather than an opiate antagonist and it is in fact a weak antagonist. The comparable dose to morphine 10 mg appears to be between 40 and 60 mg but it is not as good at relieving anxiety. It has marked emetic effects in the 60 mg dose range. Psychotomimetic effects are less marked than with nalorphine but with the 40 and 60 mg doses many patients do complain of feelings of impending death and other bizarre thought patterns.

It is possible to demonstrate experimentally an analgesic action with pentazocine 20–60 mg when given intramuscularly but the drug is not as good an analgesic as morphine. On the other hand, it does not antagonize the analgesic effects of opiates so it is more of an agonist than antagonist. It is not well absorbed from the gastrointestinal tract, since about three times the intramuscular dose is required for the same effect.

With regard to addiction, its position is intermediate also. Tolerance and dependence do develop especially to the parenteral preparation and addicts will accept the drug as a poor alternative to morphine. However, it can precipitate some withdrawal symptoms in such individuals.

Naloxone

This is the *N*-allyl analogue of oxymorphone but, being the newest antagonist, its general effects have not been fully studied. It appears to produce little drowsiness in doses up to 10 mg and indeed few subjective effects of any kind in clinical doses. It is not an analgesic.

As a pure antagonist, small doses (0.5–1.0 mg intramuscularly or intravenously) reverse the respiratory depressant action of opioid drugs and in higher doses it reverses the psychotomimetic actions of nalorphine. It also reverses the analgesia produced by pethidine. All the available evidence suggests that naloxone is a pure antagonist, with no addiction potential of its own and producing acute withdrawal symptoms in addicts. This drug should replace others for treatment of respiratory depression caused by opiates (though it must be remembered that repeated doses may be necessary) and it is the *only* antagonist to pentazocine overdosage.

Buprenorphine

This is an antagonist derived from thebaine, and animal studies suggested that it was a long-acting analgesic with a low physical dependence liability. A number of clinical studies have now been published (Orwin, 1977; Ward, 1977) and indicate that 0.3 mg is approximately equivalent to morphine 10 mg but doses of up to 0.6 mg appear to be safe by the parenteral routes.

Its onset of action following intramuscular administration is in about 30 minutes, the peak effect in 3 hours and duration at least 8 hours with some effects persisting for 24 hours. The prolonged action leads to the possibility of cumulation of side-effects so that users should be particularly aware of this aspect. Because of the slow onset of action the intravenous route of administration is preferred and onset time is reduced to 15 minutes.

Effects other than analgesia are similar to those of other opiates, the most prominent being sedation, respiratory depression and sickness. Major psychotomimetic effects have not been noted and physical dependence liability is low but not excluded.

Reversal of respiratory depression with naloxone has been demonstrated though the doses required are larger than in the reversal of a pure agonist. However, because of the inevitable reversal of its analgesic action at the same time, doxapram has been studied in this context and proved to be clinically more useful.

References

Dundee, J. W., Clarke, R. S. J. and Loan, W. B. (1965). Comparison of the sedative and toxic effects of morphine and pethidine. *Lancet* ii, 1262

Eckenhoff, J. E., Elder, J. O. and King, B. D. (1951). Effect of N-allyl normorphine in treatment of opiate overdosage. *Am. J. med. Sci.* 222, 115

Evans, J. M., Hogg, M. I. J., Lunn, J. N. and Rosen, M. (1974). Degree and duration of reversal by naloxone of effects of morphine in conscious subjects. *Br. med. J.* 2, 589

Hasbrouck, J. D. (1970). Morphine anaesthesia for open heart surgery. *Ann. thorac. Surg.* 10, 364

Hughes, J. and Kosterlitz, H. W. (1977). Opioid peptides. *Br. med. Bull.* 33, 157

Kosterlitz, H. W. (1977). Pharmacological advances in analgesics. In *Pain — New Perspectives in Measurement and Management*, p. 63. A. W. Harcus, R. B. Smith and B. A. Whittle (ed.). Edinburgh: Churchill Livingstone

Laitinen, L., Kanto, J., Vapaavuori, M. and Viljanen, M. K. (1975). Morphine concentrations in plasma after intramuscular administration. *Br. J. Anaesth.* 47, 1265

Lasagna, L. and Beecher, H. K. (1954). The analgesic effectiveness of nalorphine and nalorphine—morphine combinations in man. *J. Pharmac. exp. Ther.* 112, 356

Lee, G., De Maria, A. N., Amsterdam E. A., Realyvasquez, F., Angel, J., Morrison, S. and Mason, D. T. (1976). Comparative effects of morphine, meperidine and pentazocine on cardiocirculatory dynamics in patients with acute myocardial infarction. *Am. J. Med.* 60, 949

Lowenstein, E. (1971). Morphine anaesthesia — a perspective. *Anesthesiology* 35, 563

Lowenstein, E., Hallowell, P., Levine, F. H., Daggett, W. M., Austen, W. G. and Laver, M. B. (1969). Cardiovascular response to large doses of intravenous morphine in man. *New Engl. J. Med.* 281, 1389

Lyons, S. M., Clarke, R. S. J. and Vulgaraki, K. (1975). The premedication of cardiac surgical patients — a clinical comparison of four regimes. *Anaesthesia* 30, 459

Orwin, J. M. (1977). Buprenorphine — pharmacological aspects in man. In *Pain — New Perspectives in Measurement and Management*, p. 141. A. W. Harcus, R. B. Smith and B. A. Whittle (ed.). Edinburgh: Churchill Livingstone

Samuel, I. O., Clarke, R. S. J. and Dundee, J. W. (1977). Some circulatory and respiratory effects of morphine in patients without pre-existing cardiac disease. *Br. J. Anaesth.* 49, 927

Samuel, I. O., Unni, V. K. N. and Dundee, J. W. (1977). Peripheral vascular effects of morphine in patients without pre-existing cardiac disease. *Br. J. Anaesth.* 49, 935

Stoelting, R. K. and Gibbs, P. S. (1973). Hemodynamic effects of morphine and morphine nitrous oxide in valvular heart disease and coronary artery disease. *Anesthesiology* 38, 45

Ward, A. E. (1977). Buprenorphine — a summary of clinical experience in the United Kingdom. In *Pain — New Perspectives in Measurement and Management*, p. 160. A. W. Harcus, R. B. Smith and B. A. Whittle (ed.). Edinburgh: Churchill Livingstone

13 Sedatives, tranquillizers and hypnotics
John W. Dundee

Sedatives and tranquillizers are referred to under a number of names, including neuroleptics. As will be seen later, the differentiation between a tranquillizer, a sedative and a hypnotic is often one of degree of action related to dosage. In the past few years the tranquillizers have become very popular as preanaesthetic medication, often replacing the opiate—antisialogogue combination. This may be partly due to their efficacy by oral administration and the lower incidence of postoperative sickness following their use.

The tranquillizers are usually divided into major (including the phenothiazines and butyrophenones) and minor (including the benzodiazepines) although the clinical importance of this in relation to anaesthetic practice is not clear. According to the original classification only drugs which share the following characteristics (Delay, Deniker and Harl, 1952) can be classed as neuroleptics.

(1) A powerful central sedating action, without inducing sleep, but with marked potentiation of the effect of hypnotics and general anaesthesia.
(2) Reduction of psychomotor agitation, curiosity and aggression in animals.
(3) Capability of overcoming effectively some psychotic disorders.
(4) Main impact on the subcortical structures, with a diffuse inhibition of the reticular formation.
(5) Induction, as side actions, of diencephalic manifestations and a marked extrapyramidal syndrome.

It has been pointed out (Vourc'h and Viars, 1971) that this definition clearly distinguishes between the neuroleptics and tranquillizers and the latter 'can be considered on the whole as imperfect neuroleptics, devoid as a rule of at least one of the actions mentioned'. This division is not pursued further in this chapter.

DEFINITIONS

Although there are no agreed definitions of the different types of drugs or drug-induced states, the following is a useful clinical guide.

Hypnotics (hypnosis = drug-induced sleep)

These are depressants of central nervous system which enable patients to go to sleep more easily or which intensify the depth of sleep. Many drugs which are not primarily hypnotics have a hypnotic action as a side-effect. In general, hypnotics have no analgesic action and will not induce sleep in the presence of severe pain, although many analgesics have some hypnotic effect. Most hypnotics cause a concomitant depression of the medullary vasomotor and respiratory centres.

Sedatives

These are drugs which relieve tension and anxiety and, as the result of producing calmness, may make it easier for a patient to go to sleep. In practice one usually associates sedatives with drowsiness, but this is not necessary.

Tranquillizers

These are drugs which it is claimed have a predominant action in relieving anxiety without an undue sedative action.

While it is difficult to distinguish between sedatives and tranquillizers (ataractics), in practice the latter are usually given to ambulant patients who can continue their normal work. The same drug in a larger dose will be a sedative and this term is here reserved for hospitalized patients (thus one speaks of preoperative sedation, not preoperative tranquillization). The degree to which a preoperative drug will reduce anxiety without producing drowsiness will determine into which class it is included and will also determine its clinical use.

Neurolept anaesthesia/analgesia

These topics have not been included in detail in Chapter 11 and, although neurolept states will not be discussed, since the sedatives and tranquillizers described here are used in its production, the following definition (Foldes, 1973) is given. 'The term *neuroleptanalgesia* describes a state of indifference and immobilisation (mineralisation produced by the combination of . . . neuroleptic . . . and narcotic analgesic (de Castro and Mundeleer, 1959).

It can be modified by the use of intravenous induction agents or nitrous oxide—oxygen to produce unconsciousness and *neuroleptanaesthesia*. In contrast, neuroleptanalgesic patients, under the influence of neuroleptic and narcotic analgesia become analgesic, deeply sedated and partially or wholly amnesic, but yet remain capable of obeying commands and answering simple questions.'

Amnesia

Amnesia is total or complete inability to recall events occurring during a period when the subject was considered to be sufficiently awake to be aware of their happening. Drug-induced anterograde amnesia refers to memory loss *following* its administration, while retrograde implies impairment of recall prior to its administration.

BENZODIAZEPINES

The benzodiazepines are drugs with a dose-related tranquillizing—sedative—hypnotic action and with muscle relaxant and anticonvulsant properties. The latter two may be inter-related. In contrast with the barbiturates, they selectively inhibit activity in the limbic system, particularly the hippocampus. Their muscle relaxant effects are independent of their sedative actions and are due to an action on the spinal cord and brain stem.

There is no real evidence of qualitative differences between the sedative actions of equivalent doses of the individual benzodiazepines. Apart from the possibility that some may have a greater anticonvulsant action than others, there is little to differentiate between the pharmacological properties

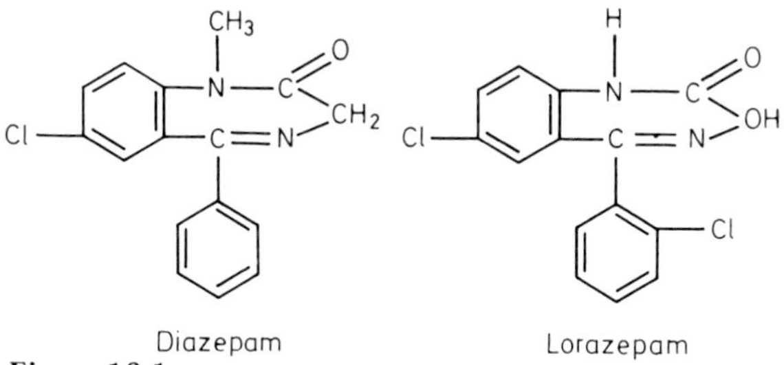

Diazepam   Lorazepam

Figure 13.1
Formulae of diazepam and lorazepam

of the many available drugs. Structurally they are very similar and share many active metabolites. The currently available compounds are either insoluble in water or unstable in solution. The commercially available injections are prepared in inorganic solvents.

Despite their widespread use, there is a paucity of controlled comparative data on the action of many of the available benzodiazepines. This survey discusses their action in general and concentrates on two compounds which differ markedly in their time-course of action – diazepam and lorazepam (*Figure 13.1*). These represent the extremes of duration of action, and if one has available a short-acting and a long-acting compound it should be possible to meet all clinical situations.

Diazepam was popularized as an oral tranquillizer which was followed by its use as an anticonvulsant (intravenous) and premedicant (intramuscular); the latter is now largely replaced by its oral administration. There have been several studies of its use as an intravenous anaesthetic but, generally speaking, it is not now used for this purpose except in the occasional patient with a known hypersensitivity to the other available agents. However, its intravenous use in subhypnotic doses is firmly established as a means of producing a light level of sedation. It is not intended here to describe fully the clinical pharmacology of diazepam, and interested readers are referred to the comprehensive review of Garattini, Mussini and Randall (1973), Brücke, Hornykiewicz and Sigg (1970) and Randall *et al.* (1961).

Preparations

Diazepam is insoluble in water, the commercially available preparation (Valium) containing several organic solvents. It is also readily soluble in Cremophor, but a commerical preparation with this as solubilizing agent has been withdrawn from use because of hypersensitivity reactions. Organic solvents are also used in the commercially available preparations of lorazepam (Ativan), which can be mixed with equal volumes of saline or water. Lorazepam causes venous thrombosis in fewer patients than diazepam.

Metabolism

Contrary to clinical impressions, the action of all benzodiazepines is prolonged and uncertain. This is supported by plasma levels which, like the clinical effects, show great individual person-to-person variation (Mandelli, Tognoni and Garattini, 1978). The major metabolic products of diazepam, desmethyldiazepam and oxazepam have a soporific effect and may contribute to its prolonged action. The elimination half-life of diazepam is 24–48 hours, which is similar to that of lorazepam. With both drugs the slow decline in plasma levels often shows a secondary 'peak' at 6–8 hours after administration, and this is accompanied by an intensification of the soporific action. This has been attributed to either enterohepatic recirculation or excretion into and reabsorption from the stomach, the latter being supported by the finding of a similar transient increase in diazepam levels following a carbohydrate meal (Korttila and Kangas, 1977). As evidence of the slow elimination we have found average plasma levels of 90 and 68 $ng \cdot ml^{-1}$ at 24 and 48 hours after 10 mg diazepam, the equivalent figures following 2.5 mg lorazepam being 17 and 10 $ng \cdot ml^{-1}$.

When given intravenously at 4—6-hourly intervals, as in an intensive therapy unit, the plasma levels of both drugs rose for 6—8 days and appeared to plateau after this. *Figure 13.2* is a typical finding when 4 mg diazepam is given 4-hourly for ⹂8 days: note the high concentrate of metabolite. The fall in plasma levels takes 8—10 days with both diazepam and lorazepam which do not seem to differ in this respect.

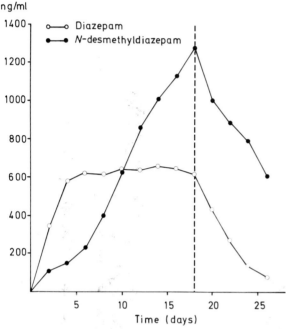

Figure 13.2
Plasma diazepam o-o and *N*-desmethyldiazepam •-• levels following 10 mg diazepam given 4-hourly for 18 days. (Reproduced from Gamble, Dundee and Gray, 1976, by courtesy of the authors and the Editor of *British Journal of Anaesthesia*)

Amnesic action

Both benzodiazepines have a calming effect in man, accompanied by a soporific action which increases with dosage. Large doses will cause loss of consciousness, although for a while patients may be capable of being roused. In adequate tranquillizing doses both cause a high incidence of anterograde (but not retrograde) amnesia. With the intravenous preparation the memory loss can occur independent of clouding of consciousness. *Figure 13.3* shows the frequency and duration of amnesia following the intravenous injection of 10 mg diazepam and 4 mg lorazepam. This is typical of the differences between these drugs. The findings of *Figure 13.3* apply to non-emotive stimuli, and in the absence of a definite soporific effect most patients premedicated with benzodiazepines will recall the actual journey to the operating room and the induction of anaesthesia. When taken by mouth it is not possible to demonstrate an amnesic action in the absence of drowsiness and the usual small tranquillizing doses (diazepam 5 mg and lorazepam 1 mg) produce no amnesia.

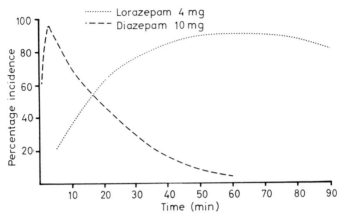

Figure 13.3
The incidence of amnesia, as assessed by the ability of patients to recall cards shown to them, after the intravenous injection of 10 mg diazepam (- - -) and 4 mg lorazepam (. . .). (Reproduced from George and Dundee, 1977, by courtesy of the authors and the Editor of *British Journal of Clinical Pharmacology*)

Their use to produce amnesia during labour has met with a mixed reception from the mothers, some of whom prefer to remember childbirth. When they are combined with other sedatives, amnesia is often complete, although patients remain co-operative. Diazepam, but not lorazepam, cumulates in the fetus; this is important to remember when they are given for their anticonvulsant action in eclampsia.

Preoperative use

The soporific and amnesic actions are the basis for the use of the benzo-diazepines in preanaesthetic medication. Small doses (10 mg diazepam and 2.5 mg lorazepam) have a predominantly calming action and, while an appreciable number of patients will fall asleep, 15 mg diazepam or 3.5 mg lorazepam are usually required for a consistent soporific action. Their simultaneous administration with hyoscine might seem an attractive proposition, but with lorazepam this causes a high frequency of restlessness (Pagano *et al.*, 1978). The oral route is recommended for both drugs, particularly as the intramuscular injection of diazepam is unpredictable in its effect. The prolonged action of lorazepam must be borne in mind and this makes it unsuitable for outpatients. However, its prolonged effect makes it a dependable means of minimizing the sequelae after the use of ketamine in adults. This can be achieved by the intravenous injection of diazepam near the end of the operation but not by its premedicant use. To be effective lorazepam has to be given in doses of 3.5—4 mg by mouth or 2.5 mg intravenously, and this may delay complete recovery from anaesthesia. Lilburn *et al.* (1978) found a 45% incidence of emergence delirium with a 20% incidence of unpleasant dreams following ketamine in adults premedicated with diazepam 15 mg compared with no sequelae in similar cases premedicated with lorazepam 4 mg. Perhaps more important was the fact that all those given lorazepam would have the same anaesthetic again as compared with only 70% of those premedicated with diazepam.

Effect on circulation and respiration

Clinical doses of both benzodiazepines have an insignificant effect on the cardiovascular and respiratory systems. Diazepam has been investigated in depth in this respect and has been shown to alter the respiratory response to hypoxia and to have a slight tendency to cause postural hypotension. In clinical doses neither drug has a significant effect on cardiac output.

Duration of action

It will be apparent that the time-course of action of diazepam and lorazepam to some extent determines their respective clinical uses. The comparison shown in *Table 13.1* is based on the effects of diazepam 10 mg and

TABLE 13.1. Duration of action of diazepam 10 mg and lorazepam 2—2.5 mg

	Diazepam	*Lorazepam*
Intravenous		
Peak effect	2—5 min	30—40 min
Duration of sedation	20—50 min	3—6 h
Amnesia	3—30 min	½—4 h
Oral		
Onset after administration	20—40 min	40—50 min
Route differences	Oral more rapid than intramuscular	Intramuscular more rapid than oral

lorazepam 2—2.5 mg, which are approximately equivalent as regards their depressant action on the central nervous system.

By all routes the onset of action of diazepam is more rapid than that of lorazepam. It will be obvious that lorazepam is not suitable for use as an intravenous induction agent, or even as a sedative during local anaesthesia or dental operations, whereas diazepam is valuable in this field.

Anticonvulsant action

While the benzodiazepines have a mild relaxant effect by virtue of their action on the spinal cord, they do not produce adequate relaxation for surgical procedures. Neither does their use during operations affect the requirements of myoneural blocking drugs. However, they are useful as anticonvulsants and diazepam is widely used for this purpose. It would seem that the slow rate of onset of lorazepam would make it unsuitable — even with intravenous use — for the control of status epilepticus, but it could be given as an anticonvulsant. Clonazepam, another benzodiazepine, is recommended as a more specific therapy for the control or prevention of convulsions. Animal experiments have shown that, in addition to its muscle-relaxing action, it has a central effect, raising the convulsion threshold. It is more potent on a weight for weight basis than either diazepam or lorazepam and the rate of action is at least as fast as that of diazepam.

Table 13.2 summarizes the important clinical differences between the two benzodiazepines which have been reviewed above.

TABLE 13.2. Comparison of some actions of diazepam and lorazepam

	Diazepam	*Lorazepam*
Equivalent dosage	10 mg	2–2.5 mg
Onset	Fairly rapid	Slow
Preparations		
Tablets	2, 5, 10 mg	1, 2.5 mg
Solution	5 mg·ml^{-1}	4 mg·ml^{-1}
Dilution	Not recommended	Recommended
Premedicant use	Oral preferred; i.m. too painful	Hospitalized patients only; before ketamine
Night before operation	Effective	Very effective
Intravenous anaesthesia	Can be used	Unsuitable
Anticonvulsant	Effective	Too slow onset for status epilepticus
Venous thrombosis	Very frequent	Infrequent
Placental transfer	Yes	Yes
Fetal : maternal ratio	1.4 : 1	1 : 1

PHENOTHIAZINES

These major tranquillizers are now second to the benzodiazepines as far as their use in anaesthesia is concerned, although they are still popular as antiemetics. Chlorpromazine and related drugs are employed primarily in the treatment of psychiatric patients. Since the phenothiazines have been in clinical use for over 30 years, it is not unexpected that a large number have been studied, but the differences in action between some of these is very slight indeed. To simplify matters only three are discussed in detail here and these are drawn from separate chemical subgroups. Their actions are, to some extent, qualitative representations of that of others in the same group.

Chemically the phenothiazines in clinical use are amino compounds with the basic general formula shown in *Figure 13.4*. They are soluble in

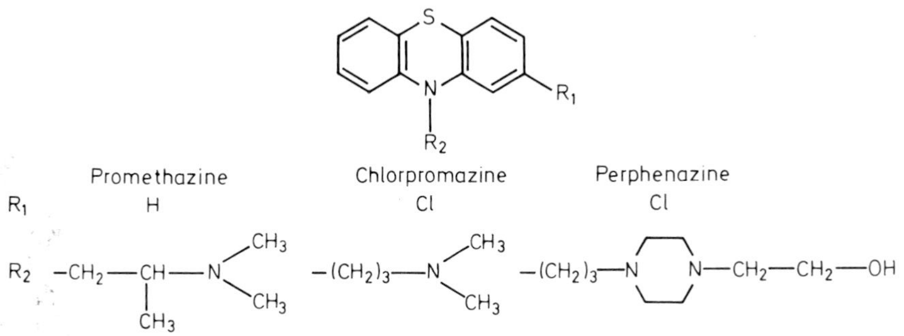

Figure 13.4
Formulae of three phenothiazines

water and available in injectable and oral forms. R_1 may be a methyl or methoxyl group or a halogen. R_2 is usually an X-N-Y group, the latter being a single heterocyclic ring or two similar alkyl groups. The X group may be a two- or three-carbon chain, sometimes (as in promethazine) with an additional methyl substitution.

The phenothiazines are often classified as belonging to either the dimethylamino group or piperazine group, promethazine and chlorpromazine being examples of the former and perphenazine of the latter (*Figure 13.4*). This is of some clinical importance as those with the ring structure are, generally speaking, the most useful antiemetics and also more likely to cause extrapyramidal side-effects. (This group also includes prochlorperazine, trifluoperazine, fluphenazine and thiopropazate.) The dimethylamino compounds are usually more soporific and affect the response to pain (these include promazine, triflupromazine, trimeprazine and methotrimeprazine).

The multiplicity of actions of the phenothiazines can be gauged from the trade name of chlorpromazine — Largactil. Not all of these are therapeutic as they cause a number of serious side-effects. Their various actions are discussed at length in reviews such as that of Forrest, Carr and Usdin (1974), and only those relating to anaesthesia are mentioned here.

The main action on the central nervous system is on behaviour, which is greatly modified in both man and animals. Therapeutic doses cause marked sedation with indifference to surroundings and loss of anxiety and emotions. Although patients become sleepy they can respond to questions, although perhaps somewhat slower than normal. In the absence of a soporific action they do not cause anterograde amnesia. Phenothiazines have a potent antiemetic action due to depression of the chemoreceptor trigger zone which occurs with even small doses. This means that they will be more effective against opiate-induced than motion sickness.

An anticonvulsant action is ascribed to the phenothiazines but the cause of this is not clear. They have insignificant direct depressant action on the spinal cord, but some cause hypotonia due to an action on the muscle fibre or motor-end plate.

The cardiovascular effects are complex, but basically all produce peripheral vasodilatation and postural hypotension with accompanying tachycardia. This may, in part, be due to a depression of the central regulatory mechanism, but antagonism of the peripheral effects of adrenaline and noradrenaline is a contributory factor. Theoretically, phenothiazine-induced hypotension should not respond to conventional sympathomimetic amines but this is not a problem in practice.

The peripheral vasodilation may contribute to the lowering of body temperature which occurs with the phenothiazines, but the direct depressant action on muscle, with reduced ability to generate heat by shivering, is an additional factor.

Other effects of phenothiazines include a local analgesic action, which is of no clinical significance. They can all induce extrapyramidal side-effects, which vary from drug to drug and also with the dose given. They potentiate or summate the action of hypnotics, general anaesthetics and analgesics to a degree which differs from compound to compound, and this and their other toxic effects are discussed in relation to the three drugs chosen for detailed documentation.

Promethazine

The hydrochloride is one of the older phenothiazines and was used initially for its antihistamine action. Doses which have an effective antihistamine action are probably too soporific for routine use and it is mostly employed as a sedative–tranquillizer. Its hypnotic, antiemetic action and drying actions make it useful as a premedicant, but when given alone it often induces akathisia (motor restlessness) which may be upsetting to patients. Paradoxically, the intravenous injection of promethazine will immediately abolish dyskinesia after piperazine-ring phenothiazines. The soporific action of other depressants is enhanced but it does not potentiate, and may even antagonize, analgesics with respect to this action on somatic pain. However, this is a complicated situation with respect to the types of pain — clinically it enhances the action of pethidine as an analgesic in labour, but this may be due to the production drowsiness and indifference to surroundings.

In clinical doses it has minimal depressant effects on the cardiovascular system, but there may be a slight fall in arterial pressure accompanied by tachycardia. It may produce a slight stimulation of respiration and it relaxes bronchial musculature, making it a suitable drug in asthmatics. It has not a potent antiemetic action, and it would not be the phenothiazine of choice for this effect alone.

Promethazine premedication will adversely affect the course of barbiturate anaesthesia, particularly methohexitone. It increases the incidence and severity of excitatory effects and this is particularly marked when it is combined with hyoscine. It is available in tablet, elixir and injection forms, the last causing some pain unless given by deep intramuscular injection. The administration of 25 mg tablets on the night before operation is very helpful for the asthmatic or bronchitic patient. Promethazine is also available premixed with pethidine, with and without atropine, and this is a potent hypnotic combination. Promethazine reduces the nausea and vomiting produced by pethidine and enhances its soporific action.

Promethazine theoclate is also available, and has very similar properties to the hydrochloride, although it may be less soporific. It is used as an oral antiemetic in early pregnancy and in travel sickness.

Chlorpromazine

This is the most widely used phenothiazine in anaesthetic practice; with promethazine and pethidine, it formed the lytic 'cocktail' used in the 'artificial hibernation' techniques of Laborit and Huguenard (1954). Some of its initial reputation was undoubtedly based on the effects of the combination of all three drugs, but more recently it has been possible to clarify the action of chlorpromazine alone. It produces indifference, lethargy and tranquillity without the accompanying motor restlessness of promethazine and is preferable as a premedicant. In contrast to promethazine, it does not antagonize the analgesic action of pethidine, but may rather enhance this by producing indifference to pain. Clinically it is a very useful adjunct in the treatment of chronic pain. It has a potent antiemetic effect, but this is only produced by soporific doses. Its actions appear to last longer than those of promethazine.

Cardiovascular depression, characterized by hypotension and tachycardia, is more marked after chlorpromazine than following an equivalent soporific dose of promethazine. This is due entirely to peripheral vasodilation and it should be avoided in hypovolaemic or hypertensive subjects. Clinical doses have like effects on respiration.

Hypotonia and muscle weakness occur with single premedicant doses of chlorpromazine and smooth muscle tone is depressed. Given with an analgesic it is useful as an adjunct in the production of hypothermia by surface cooling. Its antihistamine action is mild and of little clinical importance.

Although very large doses cause extrapyramidal side-effects, this is not a problem with a premedicant dose. Indeed, even when chlorpromazine is given intermittently in doses of 20—25 mg 4-hourly as a sedative—hypnotic to long-term intensive therapy patients this problem does not arise. Jaundice is a not infrequent complication of long-term chlorpromazine therapy (although its occurrence has been reported after just a single 50 mg dose). This is of the cholestatic type and its diagnosis may be confused with viral hepatitis or other cause of mechanical obstruction. The jaundice usually subsides within a few days of stopping therapy, although on occasions it has been followed by biliary cirrhosis. It is better to avoid chlorpromazine (even for premedication) in patients with a previous history of jaundice.

Like promethazine, the intramuscular administration of chlorpromazine may be painful unless injected deeply. It is recommended that the standard preparation of 25 mg·ml^{-1} be diluted for intravenous injection to reduce the incidence of venous thrombosis.

Perphenazine

This is a member of the group of phenothiazines which are potent anti-emetics and it is primarily used for this purpose. Doses of 2.5–5.0 mg will minimize opiate-induced vomiting and it is useful in the postoperative period, in uraemic or other metabolic disturbances but not in travel sickness.

Its sedative and soporific action is similar to that of promethazine. It may cause motor restlessness if given alone, although it is less likely to do so than promethazine. However, severe dystonic reactions, culminating in oculogyric crises, occur even after single doses of perphenazine and their onset may take 4–6 hours after administration, so that a causal relationship to the drug administration is not always obvious. They are very unlikely to occur when it is given with an opiate. They will respond immediately to antiParkinsonism treatment, but in anaesthetic practice it is often simpler to use promethazine which is equally effective in this respect. An initial dose of 12.5 mg i.v. and 12.5 mg i.m. is recommended and it may be necessary to repeat the former.

BUTYROPHENONES

This group includes droperidol, which is used as part of the 'neurolept' sequence and as a premedicant and antiemetic, and also haloperidol the use of which is now limited to psychiatric practice.

Droperidol cannot be classified as a sedative because, although it causes some drowsiness and 'dissociation', patients may be very apprehensive and restless. Many feel that it should never be given without an analgesic, which appears to reduce this complication, particularly preoperatively. Analgesics also seem to prevent dystonic reactions which are unacceptably common after droperidol alone. Droperidol has no analgesic action, nor does it increase the analgesic action of fentanyl or phenoperidine with which it is often combined in the neurolept sequence. The soporific action of the narcotics may be enhanced by droperidol.

In addition, droperidol has mild α-adrenergic-blocking properties, causing slight peripheral vasodilation, some fall in blood pressure and sometimes a compensatory tachycardia. These are only a problem when it is given intravenously. In fact, there is evidence to show that the droperidol—fentanyl mixture may have fewer deleterious effects on the cardiovascular system than any other agents which could be used to induce anaesthesia.

It is difficult to rationalize the administration of the rather long-acting droperidol concomitantly with the shorter-acting fentanyl, yet this combination has acquired some popularity. Whether this is due to the lack of cardiovascular depression of the fentanyl or the mild α-adrenergic-blocking agent of the droperidol is not clear. Perhaps the potent antiemetic action of the butyrophenone makes possible the intravenous use of the analgesic. Certainly in practice the combination behaves very differently from that of the individual drugs and one must hesitate in equating the action of droperidol with that of the mixture. Without an analgesic, droperidol can cause very unpleasant effects, including hallucinations, loss of body image and restlessness, and should be used cautiously in anaesthetic practice. In view of these complications, one cannot recommend it as an antiemetic.

HYPNOTICS

Here one is referring specifically to drugs used to facilitate the occurrence of sleep. Classically, the barbiturates have been most used in this field, but it is generally agreed that their prolonged use leads to dependence, and CURB (Campaign for Use and Restriction of Barbiturates) has campaigned for their abandonment. Nevertheless, they still form a useful standby in the hospitalized patient, provided it is appreciated that they are devoid of analgesic activity.

Barbiturates

The structural activity relationship of the barbiturates has been studied in detail (Dundee, 1974), but in practice the differences between those claimed as long acting and the slow-acting group is not as marked as once thought. For this chapter, pentobarbitone sodium is taken as the standard drug; the differences between its action and that of the other available drugs is really only one of potency.

Pentobarbitone sodium is the oxygen analogue of thiopentone, with substitution of O for S in the 2 position. The formula can be readily remembered from the trade name, Nembutal:

Na Ethyl MethylBUTyl barbiturate (barbit AL)

It is readily soluble in water, but the resulting solution is too unstable for storage. There is available a form for veterinary use, made up in organic solvents to BP standards of purity and very suitable for intramuscular and intravenous use. This contains 60 mg·ml^{-1} and the equivalent USP injection contains 50 mg·ml^{-1}. Tablets and capsules are available for oral administration.

When injected intravenously, pentobarbitone sodium takes 20–40 seconds to reach its full effect, the oral preparation takes 20–30 minutes to act and its hypnotic action lasts 4–6 hours. However, there is a persistent 'hangover' effect which, even if the patient is unaware of this, will impair performance for 12–24 hours. There is a dangerous degree of synergism between barbiturates and alcohol, and even social drinking may be dangerous in persons who have taken pentobarbitone sodium as a night time hypnotic. Administration on the night before operation will theoretically influence the dose of the subsequent anaesthetic, but this is not a problem in practice. More important is the restlessness which occurs postoperatively in patients in pain when they have been prescribed a barbiturate preoperatively.

Pentobarbitone sodium in clinical doses has little effect on vital functions but it may impair the sensitivity of the respiratory centre to carbon dioxide. Although it is broken down in the liver, prolonged hypnosis does not occur from normal doses in patients with liver disease. Like all barbiturates, it should be avoided in patients with a known or suspected history of acute intermittent porphyria and in those with a history of sensitivity to this group of drugs. Quinalbarbitone is slightly more powerful (on a weight basis) than pentobarbitone, while amylobarbitone has only half its potency.

With their reduced usage, overdosage of the barbiturates should become less frequent and in practice one is now encountering an increasing number of patients who have taken multiple drugs. A blood barbiturate analysis is little guide to the depth of hypnosis and to the treatment, which should be aimed at maintaining vital functions. With a small amount excreted unchanged in the urine, forced alkaline diuresis is not likely to help, although haemoperfusion may be of value (Vale *et al.*, 1975). Without condoning the use of analeptics, the author has found doxapram to be particularly useful in those patients with a marginal depth of respiratory depression when one does not want to institute artificial respiration.

In prescribing barbiturate hypnotics one must be aware of their possible interaction with other drugs. Pentobarbitone sodium is a potent inducer of liver enzymes, but the importance of this in a single administration is not known. The danger can arise when one changes to another hypnotic such as chloral which, by displacement from its binding sites, may increase the action and also the elimination of anticoagulants.

Benzodiazepines

Those who are most opposed to the barbiturates usually recommend the use of one or other of the benzodiazepines as hypnotics. This may be a sensible approach as the removal of anxiety will often induce sleep. There have been some suggestions that they can cause physical dependence, but a survey in Drug and Therapeutics Bulletin (1977) has commented that 'despite the fact that the benzodiazepines have been in use for 20 years their potential for producing dependence is still controversial'. This is of little importance in their use as hypnotics and here one is concerned with their efficacy, duration of action and the hypnotic action of metabolic products. Diazepam and flurazepam both have hypnotically active metabolites. Perhaps these should be used only as preoperative hypnotics on the night before operation when the residual effect may be desirable.

Nitrazepam is very popular as a night time hypnotic, probably because a hangover is not a feature of the drug. It has a half-life of 24—48 hours. However, the newer hypnotic, temazepam (which, like nitrazepam, has no active metabolite) has a half-life of only 8 hours and may eventually prove to be a safer hypnotic, but controlled clinical trials have not been reported.

Chloral derivatives

These include the well established but very unpalatable chloral hydrate, and triclofos which is the phosphoric ester of trichlorethanol. Both drugs are converted to trichlorethanol in the body and this appears to be the active hypnotic. Triclofos is available in tablet form, is not unpleasant to take and does not cause gastric irritation.

This group of drugs has a long tradition of safety, but their pharmacokinetics have not been studied in detail. They may have a longer action than was originally thought, as there is often some degree of drowsiness and confusion on awakening. Alternatively, this may result from their predominant use in the elderly who are prone to such problems. Certainly they are still preferred to the barbiturates in such patients.

Chlormethiazole

This is an interesting compound which is part of the vitamin B molecule and was once evaluated as an intravenous anaesthetic. It is basically an anticonvulsant and infusions are used in obstetrics to control the convulsions of eclampsia. It is effective by mouth and is available in tablet and syrup form. The latter is not pleasant to take.

Chlormethiazole is used as a safe hypnotic in the elderly, when it appears to be free from the tendency to produce confusion which characterizes some of the other hypnotics. Its main field of use is, however, in the treatment of acute alcoholism and in controlling delirium tremors. Here the treatment may start with its intravenous administration, but can be continued with the oral drug. This regimen is also used in the management of eclampsia and status epilepticus, and some recommend the infusion as a safe means of maintaining unconsciousness during treatment on a pulmonary ventilator.

References

Brücke, F. Th. v., Hornykiewicz, O. and Sigg, E. B. (1970). *The Pharmacology of Psychotherapeutic Drugs.* Berlin: Springer-Verlag

de Castro, G. and Mundeleer, P. (1959). Anesthésie sans sommeil 'La neuroleptanalgesie'. *Acta chir. belg.* 58, 689

Delay, J., Deniker, P. and Harl, M. (1952). Utilisation en thérapeutique psychiatrique d'une phenothiazine d'action central elective (4560 R.P.). *Ann. méd-psychol.* 100, 112

Drug and Therapeutics Bulletin (1977). Physical dependence on benzodiazepines? *Drug Ther. Bull.* 15, 85

Dundee, J. W. (1974). Molecular structure—activity relationships of barbiturates. In *Molecular Mechanisms in General Anaesthesia,* pp. 16–31. M. J. Halsey, R. A. Millar and J. A. Sutton (ed.). Edinburgh: Churchill Livingstone

Foldes, F. F. (1973). Neuroleptanesthesia for general surgery. In *Neuroleptanesthesia.* T. Oyama (ed.). *Int. Anesthesiol. Clins* 11, 1–35

Forrest, Irene S., Carr, C. J. and Usdin, E. (1974). Phenothiazines and structurally related drugs. in *Advances in Biochemical Psychopharmacology,* Vol. 9. New York: Raven Press

Gamble, J. A. S., Dundee, J. W. and Gray, R. C. (1976). Plasma diazepam concentrations following prolonged administration. *Br. J. Anaesth.* 48, 1087

Garattini, S., Mussini, E. and Randall, L. O. (ed.) (1973). *The Benzodiazepines.* New York: Raven Press

George, K. A. and Dundee, J. W. (1977). Relative amnesic actions of diazepam, flunitrazepam and lorazepam in man. *Br. J. clin. Pharmac.* 4, 45

Korttila, K. and Kangas, L. (1977). Unchanged protein binding and the increase of serum diazepam levels after food intake. *Acta pharmac. Tox.* 40, 241

Laborit, H. and Huguenard, P. (1954). *Pratique de L'hibernothérapie en chirurgie et en medicine.* Paris: Masson

Lilburn, J. K., Dundee, J. W., Nair, S. G., Fee, J. P. H. and Johnston, H. M. L. (1978). Ketamine sequelae. Evaluation of the ability of various premedicants to attenuate its psychic actions. *Anaesthesia* 33, 307

Mandelli, M., Tognoni, G. and Garattini, S. (1978). Clinical pharmacokinetics of diazepam. *Clin. Pharmacokin.* 3, 72

Pagano, R. R., Conner, J. T., Bellville, J. W., Graham, C. W., Schehl, D. and Katz, R. L. (1978). Lorazepam, hyoscine and atropine as i.v. surgical premedicants. *Br. J. Anaesth.* 50, 471

Randall, L. O., Heise, G. A., Schallek, W., Bagdon, R. E., Banziger, R., Boris, A., Moe, R. A. and Abrams, A. B. (1961). Pharmacological and clinical studies on Valium, a new psychotherapeutic agent of the benzodiazepine class. *Curr. Ther. Res.* 3, 404

Vale, J. A., Rees, A. J., Widdop, B. and Goulding, R. (1975). Use of charcoal haemoperfusion in the management of severely poisoned patients. *Br. med. J.* 1, 5–9

Vourc'h, G. and Viars, P. (1971). Neuroleptics. In *General Anaesthesia,* 3rd edn, Vol. 1, pp. 553–572. T. C. Gray and J. F. Nunn (ed.). London: Butterworths

14 Antiemetic Drugs
John W. Dundee

Antiemetics are used for the symptomatic control of nausea and vomiting, and it is desirable first to look at the causes of nausea and vomiting and the occasions where such drugs might be used. It need hardly be mentioned that antiemetics should be used only when the cause of vomiting cannot readily be removed.

CLINICAL CAUSES OF NAUSEA, VOMITING AND RETCHING

(1) Morphine, pethidine and similar drugs are among the most potent emetic compounds in clinical use although there is great individual variation in response to these.
(2) Certain other drugs, particularly when given in relative overdose (e.g. digitalis and some antibiotics), may lead to vomiting, and their importance as a possible cause of unexplained vomiting must be remembered.
(3) Reaction to disease, inflammation, injury or irritation of various abdominal organs.
(4) Metabolic disturbances or intoxications associated with emesis (e.g. hyperemesis gravidarum, radiation therapy, hyper- or hypoglycaemia).
(5) Vestibular disturbances.
(6) Psychogenic stimuli, including fear, anxiety and offensive sights, especially seeing other patients being sick.
(7) The local irritant effect of drugs on the gastrointestinal tract and changes in intraluminal pressure due to tumours, infection, ulcers, etc.
(8) Some inhalational anaesthetics.
(9) Raised intracranial pressure.

PHYSIOLOGY

The classical concept is of a vomiting centre anatomically located in the dorsal portion of the lateral reticular formation in the midst of other centres concerned with various motor activities which are affected during the act of vomiting (salivation, vasomotor control, etc.). More important is its action in the integration of the act of vomiting and of stimuli from both central and peripheral receptor sites. These may be from higher centres (including psychogenic stimuli), vestibular apparatus, the local irritant action of drugs on the gastrointestinal tract or from the chemo-receptor trigger zone (CTZ). This last lies superficially in the medulla on the floor of the fourth ventricle but it is not an integral part of the vomiting centre. Many drugs, such as apomorphine, act on the CTZ, as do certain antiemetics.

Different stimuli appear to cause vomiting by different mechanisms but there is often a summation of effects; thus opiates (which act on the CTZ) are more likely to cause sickness in the ambulant patient (because of additional labyrinthine function), and sickness is more likely to follow an emetic stimulus if the patient can see and hear another patient who is actually vomiting.

STUDY OF ANTIEMETICS

The organization of reliable clinical trials of antiemetics is particularly difficult. Not only has one to establish their efficacy which must be related to the emetic stimulus, but one must consider the time-course of action of the drugs and their route of administration. One must also evaluate their toxicity, particularly in relation to clinical situations in which they will be used. In addition, certain patient-factors have to be considered, including the sex of the patient (for example, women are more prone to vomit than men) and the individual tendency to sickness. This latter necessitates large numbers of patients in each series.

A 'standard' emetic stimulus is desirable and this may be motion sickness, drugs (e.g. opiates), certain pathological states (hyperemesis, uraemia, radiation therapy) or surgery and anaesthesia. The author and

TABLE 14.1. Standardization in an antiemetic study in which opiate-induced post-operative sickness is the emetic incident

Controllable factors	
Sex of patient	Female
Age of patient	Adult, reproductive years
Hospital unit	Standard, fixed visiting times and ward routine
Operation	D & C, 50% having cervical dilatation
Time of operation	Morning
Duration of operation	5—7 minutes
Anaesthetic	Methohexitone, nitrous oxide—oxygen
Postoperative analgesic	Nil
Observations standardized	Vomiting, nausea and retching noted preoperatively and 0—1 and 1—6 hours after operation

colleagues have used a combination of postoperative vomiting and opiate premedication, and *Table 14.1* is an example of the degree of standardization which is aimed at in these studies.

Preanaesthetic medication varies according to the study and is normally given by deep intramuscular injection about 90 minutes before operation. If studying the relative emetic effects of different agents, these are given alone as preanaesthetic medication or together with the appropriate emetic opiate (usually morphine 10 or 15 mg or pethidine 100 mg). Pethidine has an earlier onset and shorter duration of action than morphine and this also applies to its emetic action. This difference can be utilized in a study of the duration of action of antiemetics. Short-acting drugs may prevent the 'early' sickness which follows pethidine but be relatively ineffective against morphine. This type of study needs very rigorous control of variables and requires large numbers of patients.

DRUGS USED AS ANTIEMETICS

The drugs which are therapeutically useful for the control of nausea or vomiting can be grouped as follows.

(1) Parasympatholytic agents (belladonna alkaloids)
(2) Phenothiazines
(3) Butyrophenones
(4) Antihistamines
(5) Metoclopramide
(6) General sedatives and tranquillizers
(7) Miscellaneous

Parasympatholytic (vagolytic) drugs – the belladonna alkaloids

These drugs may act partially through their antimuscarinic (antispasmodic) action on the gastrointestinal tract but there is some evidence to suggest that the action of hyoscine on the vestibular mechanism plays a part in its efficacy in motion sickness.

Hyoscine is a well proven remedy for motion sickness. It is given in the form of the hydrobromide (scopolamine), 1 mg of which contains 0.7 mg of *l*-hyoscine base. Commercially available seasickness tablets usually contain 0.3 mg, and two are recommended as a single dose for protection for short journeys. Side-effects (drowsiness, blurred vision and dry mouth) preclude the long-term use of hyoscine for travel sickness. Atropine does not appear to have been used for this purpose.

Clinically used premedicant doses of atropine (0.6 mg) and hyoscine (0.4 mg) will suppress the emetic effects of 100 mg pethidine and 10 mg morphine. Although both vagolytic agents give good protection in the early postoperative period, the emetic action of 10 mg morphine lasts longer than the antiemetic action of either atropine or hyoscine (Dundee,

Moore and Clarke, 1964, Clarke, Dundee and Love, 1965). Hyoscine is a better antiemetic than atropine but neither has any notable effect on the incidence of nausea.

Phenothiazines

Chlorpromazine was one of the first drugs to be used specifically for the symptomatic control of vomiting and nausea. It appeared to be particularly effective against drugs which act on the CTZ, while larger doses may also depress the vomiting centre. Although chlorpromazine is now seldom used primarily as an antiemetic, other phenothiazines are justifiably popular in this field.

The piperazine—ring phenothiazines which are used for their antiemetic action are listed below, together with recommended doses.

perphenazine   2—5 mg
prochlorperazine   5—25 mg
thiethylperazine   10 mg
trifluoperazine   1—2 mg

All of these carry the very real risk of causing restlessness and dyskinesia with oculogyric crisis following large doses or repeated use.

PERPHENAZINE

This is probably the most widely used of the antiemetic phenothiazines and when one considers both efficacy and toxicity this popularity appears to be justified. Dundee *et al.* (1975) have studied the efficacy of perphenazine 2.5 and 5.0 mg against the emetic action of pethidine 100 mg and morphine 10 and 15 mg, and found that perphenazine has a rapid onset of action but its antiemetic activity does not last as long as the emetic effect of morphine. Perphenazine 5 mg may be needed to control effectively the emetic sequelae from morphine or pethidine but a dose of 2.5 mg, which is less toxic, has an appreciable antiemetic activity as well. Oral doses of 2—4 mg are useful for prophylaxis against nausea and vomiting in patients having radiation or chemotherapy, but they may have to be repeated in 4—6 hours. Perphenazine is a potent tranquillizer and may enhance the soporific action of opiates or other sedatives.

PROCHLORPERAZINE

Although prochlorperazine is less potent than perphenazine on a weight basis, the antiemetic and other effects of these two drugs are very similar. Prochlorperazine may have a slightly less soporific action than the effective antiemetic doses of other drugs in this group but the difference is negligible.

THIETHYLPERAZINE

This is a good antiemetic in doses of 10 mg. Like prochlorperazine, it is claimed to be less soporific than equivalent doses of perphenazine and, while this concurs with clinical impression, it is by no means proven. Its main clinical use is in the relief of vertigo associated with labyrinthine disturbances or surgery.

TRIFLUOPERAZINE

The main use of this potent antiemetic is in psychiatric practice and anxiety states, possible senile agitation and confusion. It appears to have all the advantages and disadvantages of the other related compounds.

These four useful phenothiazine antiemetics vary mainly in their absolute potency. Their action is principally on the CTZ and they are most effective against opiate-induced emesis and least effective in the prevention of travel sickness. Each carries the risk of extrapyramidal side-effects (q.v.), particularly after repeated use or when given in the absence of an opiate. Perphenazine is probably the most investigated of these but the less soporific prochlorperazine or thiethylperazine may be preferred on occasions.

Butyrophenones

Droperidol is a powerful antiemetic in clinical doses (Wheeler and Campman, 1971; Patton, Moon and Dannemiller, 1974). In view of the disturbing incidence of motor restlessness and anxiety found when 5 or 10 mg were given alone, its antiemetic use should be limited to patients who have been given opiates — particularly since these effects may outlast its antiemetic action. Droperidol enhances the soporific effect of opiate narcotics (Morrison, 1970). The antiemetic dose of droperidol for adults varies from 2.5 mg to 10 mg, which can be given intramuscularly or intravenously. Both droperidol and haloperidol can cause oculogyric crises and this precludes their repeated parenteral administration in antiemetic doses.

Antihistamines

A number of seemingly chemically unrelated compounds — most of which contain an ethylamine chain — have been shown to possess useful antiemetic properties and are most effective in the suppression of motion sickness. Drugs active in this respect may also relieve the emetic complications of labyrinthinic disturbances and are of value in controlling vomiting from other causes.

The antiemetic antihistamines fall into the following chemical groups.

Ethanolamines   Diphenhydramine hydrochloride
                     Dimenhydrinate theoclate

Piperazines   Cyclizine hydrochloride or lactate
                     Meclozine
                     Buclizine
                     Cinnarizine

Phenothiazines   Promethazine

The last has been discussed under the phenothiazines.

DIPHENHYDRAMINE AND DIMENHYDRINATE

These are potent and effective antihistamines. In clinical doses they possess significant atropine-like activity and both have a marked soporific effect. Dimenhydrinate was initially used in the control of vertigo. Reports on its efficacy as an antiemetic mainly refer to its use in controlling the nausea and vomiting of early pregnancy. There is no evidence to suggest that it has any teratogenic effects. Radiation and postoperative sickness are other fields in which it has been proved useful. Its popularity is now mainly limited to control of travel sickness in which it appears to be very effective, but the recommended 50 mg dose is probably more soporific than the equivalent dose of cyclizine.

CYCLIZINE

Cyclizine is a competitive antihistamine which is used primarily for its antiemetic action. It is available in tablet form as the hydrochloride and in injectable form as the lactate, and is well tolerated by both intramuscular and intravenous injection. It may be diluted and given slowly by the latter route. It is rapidly absorbed from the gastrointestinal tract and its effects start within 15—30 minutes of administration, persisting for about 3—6 hours.

Cyclizine is justifiably popular as an antiemetic for travel sickness. Many workers have studied its efficacy (usually doses of 50 mg given to adults) in postoperative vomiting (Dent, Ramachandra and Stephen, 1955; Moore *et al.*, 1956; Davis and Gallagher, 1957). In a comprehensive study, Dundee *et al.* (1975) found that cyclizine 50 mg reduced vomiting and nausea associated with morphine and pethidine premedication to about the same extent as did perphenazine 5 mg. It was noticeable that its efficacy against sickness induced by pethidine was maximal in the first 90 minutes after administration, emphasizing the short action of the drug.

The main side-effect of cyclizine is drowsiness. It also has an atropine-like action and clinical doses cause dryness of the mouth. It may also cause a slight rise in blood pressure when given by rapid intravenous injection. Although oculogyric crises have not been reported following cyclizine, patients may become restless and agitated after high or repeated doses.

It has been suggested that cyclizine may be teratogenic in man. Morphogenetic lesions were seen in groups of rats, mice and rabbits receiving $50-75$ mg·kg^{-1} as compared with the recommended clinical dose of about 1 mg·kg^{-1} three times daily. An extensive survey of congenital abnormalities in children was carried out by McBride (1963), one of the two investigators who first detected the teratogenic effect of thalidomide. In the latter years of his survey about 100 patients per month had been given cyclizine for morning sickness, yet this widespread use revealed no suggestion of a teratogenic action (Stalsberg, 1965). Five other large epidemiological series, each involving over 200 patients on meclozine or cyclizine, have shown that 'although it cannot be ruled out, they can give a reasonable assurance that these drugs are not teratogenic' (Midwinter, 1971).

Metoclopramide

This is chemically related to the procaine derivative, orthoclopramide, and its actions in animals include an ability to inhibit emesis due to locally acting emetics such as copper sulphate and also to prevent apomorphine-induced sickness. It has no antihistaminic effects.

Metoclopramide hastens emptying of the stomach and aids propulsion through the upper gastrointestinal tract, as well as abolishing irregular peristaltic activity. It is not surprising that it has been used in radiology of the gastrointestinal tract, to aid emptying of the stomach prior to operation in obstetrical and surgical emergency patients and as an antiemetic. It is not a very toxic drug but extrapyramidal symptoms, including oculogyric crises, have occurred after its prolonged use. Intravenous injection of normal doses can cause restlessness.

Despite its widespread popularity, there is considerable doubt as to the direct antiemetic efficacy of metoclopramide, particularly in relation to postoperative sickness. Handley (1967) and Lind and Breivik (1970) have demonstrated the effectiveness of metoclopramide 10 and 20 mg doses when given at the end of minor gynaecological procedures, but Dundee and Clarke (1973) found that it did not significantly reduce the incidence of postoperative sickness below that which occurred in patients following 100 mg pethidine. Its limited efficacy against morphine-induced sickness has been confirmed by Assaf *et al.* (1974) who have shown that this is due, at least in part, to its brevity of action. It may be of value in nausea and vomiting due to gastrointestinal disorders but a longer acting drug may be preferred in drug intolerance, malignant disease or after radiation therapy. A single dose may be recommended postoperatively, but if ineffective, another antiemetic should be used.

Sedatives and tranquillizers

These may reduce emetic symptoms when there is a large psychogenic element in their causation. They also reduce postoperative sickness by reducing the mobility of the patient. It is difficult to be sure whether some sedatives have a specific antiemetic action but this may be true of diazepam.

Others

BENZQUINAMIDE

This is a non-amine-depleting benzquinoline derivative chemically unrelated to other antiemetics. It has recently been introduced into clinical practice in North America (mostly in anaesthesia) but is not available in Europe. Using the apomorphine-induced vomiting as a stimulus, Pitts (1969) demonstrated the antiemetic action of benzquinamide 50 mg in human adult volunteers. Results with it were reproducible, and there was rapid and reliable absorption following both oral and rectal administration which compared favourably with the parenteral route. Klein *et al.* (1970), who reproduced these findings, also found the antiemetic activity of benzquinamide 50 mg was greater than that of prochlorperazine 10 mg but its duration of action was shorter. It is too soon to be certain of the efficacy of benzquinamide under clinical conditions.

One promising aspect of this new drug is its lack of toxicity. In contrast with the phenothiazines, it may have some pressor activity and it is also claimed to have some respiratory stimulant action.

To date there have been no reports of extrapyramidal side-effects associated with the antiemetic use of benzquinamide. Since this drug has been used as a minor tranquillizer, one would have expected such complications to have been reported had they occurred with any great frequency.

GROUP PHARMACOLOGY OF ANTIEMETIC DRUGS

Route and details of administration

Not all antiemetics are available in forms which are suitable for oral, intramuscular and intravenous administration, and the pharmaceutic presentation may, on occasions, affect the choice of drug. For patients already nauseated or actually vomiting, a parenteral preparation is obviously desired. Several antiemetic drugs can be given intravenously but some of these, such as the phenothiazines, carry a distinct risk if injected too rapidly. Intramuscular injections should be given deep into the buttock or outer aspect of the thigh to ensure good absorption. Oral preparations are desirable for long-term use, particularly when taken outside hospital, and are naturally the drugs of choice for motion sickness.

For effective self-medication, patients must be made aware that prophylaxis is often easier than cure and that the appropriate drugs should be taken well in advance of the emetic stimulus. This applies not only to travel sickness but also to opiate administration, cancer therapy or radio-therapy. In these circumstances it should be appreciated that the duration of the emetic stimulus may outlast the effective period of action of the antiemetic, which should be repeated towards the end of the period of its expected duration of action. It must be appreciated that many drugs can cumulate in the body with repeated administration and side-effects occurring 4–5 days after starting treatment may not be readily associated with the antiemetic.

It is easier to control vomiting than nausea and in some circumstances these two manifestations of the problem may occur independently. Persistent nausea is very unpleasant and is associated with dizziness, anorexia and listlessness and often with a 'drugged' feeling. Where possible, bed rest may be the most appropriate therapy for this distressing symptom.

Side-effects

The relative merits of antiemetic drugs cannot be divorced from their side-effects. If the patient is required to be mobile and ambulant (as in air or sea crew or travellers suffering from motion sickness) a drug with a soporific action or one which will produce postural hypotension is unacceptable. This also applies to many patients on opiates, although here postural hypotension may be less of a problem since they can lie down. In contrast, some bedridden patients may benefit from the soporific action of an antiemetic and this may be of value when sickness results from radiotherapy or chemotherapy. Patients quickly become tolerant to the soporific effect of antiemetics and this is not a problem of long-term therapy.

Akathisia (motor restlessness) and other extrapyramidal side-effects are undesirable and generally unacceptable complications of antiemetic therapy. Akathisia, which literally means 'the inability to sit down', is aptly termed 'the jitters' by patients who feel this compulsion to move about and, in addition, may be very apprehensive. Drug-induced dystonic extrapyramidal side-effects may not occur until 6–24 hours after administration and the relationship of these to the antiemetic may be missed (Ayd, 1961). Acute dystonia is characterized by painless spasmodic contractions of one or more muscle groups. Trismus, torticollis and opisthotonos indicate muscular spasms of the jaw, neck and spine respectively. The best-known dystonic condition is the oculogyric crisis, during which the eyes, after being fixed in a stare, later move to one side, while the head tilts uncomfortably and alarmingly backward and toward the same side (Dundee, Clarke and Carruthers, 1975).

Oculogyric crises or other severe dystonic reactions can be quickly controlled by the intravenous injection of promethazine 10–25 mg. Because of its antiemetic properties, this is preferred to antiParkinsonism drugs such as benztropine, biperiden or procyclidine. A similar dose of promethazine should be given subcutaneously or intramuscularly since the extrapyramidal dyskinesia may last longer than the action of a single intravenous dose of promethazine. Because of its prolonged action, the oral administration of diphenhydramine 50 mg also can be of benefit in preventing the recurrence of dyskinesia. The risk of extrapyramidal effects precludes the prophylactic use of 'depot' preparations of antiemetics which can cause this side-effect.

Use of antiemetic drugs in early pregnancy

Since morning sickness occurs in between 50 and 80% of pregnancies (mostly between the 6th and 14th weeks of gestation) and about 40% of patients are still vomiting, although less persistently, at 14 weeks, this aspect of the use of antiemetics is very important.

The effect of medication on the embryo during early pregnancy has caused much concern and this naturally involves antiemetic drugs which may be presented for morning sickness or hyperemesis gravidarum. The teratogenic effect of most of these is not known but, by virtue of their long-term consumption in 458 mothers who gave birth to infants with congenital abnormalities, out of a total of 11 369, Nelson and Forfar (1971) found only 48 who had taken antiemetics during the first trimester. Compared with controls, significantly fewer mothers of infants with major abnormalities consumed antiemetics during the first trimester. Perhaps mothers of abnormal infants may be less likely to suffer from morning sickness than those of normal infants. Wade and Dundee (1969) have suggested a compromise view on the importance of teratogenicity of antiemetics: 'while it is undesirable to give any drug during the first trimester of pregnancy for fear of causing fetal abnormality, occasionally a pregnant woman is so nauseated and anorexic that it is considered justifiable to use antiemetics such as cyclizine, meclozine or promethazine'. This view is supported by an obstetrician (Midwinter, 1971). In her review of vomiting in pregnancy, she lists the available antiemetics and comments: 'All these have been used widely for many years in early pregnancy in large series of patients. . . suggesting with reasonable assurance that they are not teratogenic'.

CHOICE OF ANTIEMETIC

It is obvious that there are large numbers of safe and effective antiemetics available for clinical use. In deciding which drug to use in a particular situation one should consider the cause of the symptoms and, where possible, use these as the basis for the choice of type of drug.

TABLE 14.2. Choice of antiemetic

Psychogenic stimuli: fear	Diazepam: sedatives
Motion sickness	Hyoscine, cyclizine
CTZ stimulation	Perphenazine, prochlorperazine, thiethylperazine, trifluoperazine
Gastrointestinal upset	Metoclopramide

While *Table 14.2* does not include all available antiemetics, it is recommended as a useful working hypothesis for the rational use of these drugs. Within each of these groups one can choose the drug which is not only most effective but which also produces the lowest incidence of side-effects in the particular patients.

References

Assaf, R. A. E., Clarke, R. S. J., Dundee, J. W. and Samuel, I. O. (1974). Studies of drugs given before anaesthesia. XXIV: Metoclopramide with morphine and pethidine. *Br. J. Anaesth.* **46**, 514

Ayd, F. J. Jr. (1961). A survey of drug-induced extrapyramidal reactions. *J. Am. med. Ass.* **175**, 1054

Clarke, R. S. J., Dundee, J. W. and Love, W. J. (1965). Studies of drugs given before anaesthesia. VIII: Morphine alone and with atropine or hyoscine. *Br. J. Anaesth.* **37**, 772

Davies, R. and Gallagher, E. (1957). Post-anaesthetic vomiting: a trial of cyclizine tartrate. *J. Ir. med. Ass.* **40**, 237

Dent, S. J., Ramachandra, V. and Stephen, C. R. (1955). Postoperative vomiting: incidence, analysis and therapeutic measures in 3,000 patients. *Anesthesiology* **16**, 564

Dundee, J. W. and Clarke, R. S. J. (1973). The premedicant and anti-emetic action of metoclopramide. *Postgrad. med. J.* **48**, Suppl. 4, 34

Dundee, J. W., Clarke, R. S. J. and Carruthers, S. G. (1975). Drug-induced extrapyramidal disorders. *Prescribers J.* **15**, 26

Dundee, J. W., Moore, J. and Clarke, R. S. J. (1964). Studies of drugs given before anaesthesia. V: Pethidine 100 mg alone and with atropine or hyoscine. *Br. J. Anaesth.* **36**, 703

Dundee, J. W., Assaf, R. A. E., Loan, W. B. and Morrison, J. D. (1975). A comparison of the efficacy of cyclizine and perphenazine in reducing the emetic effects of morphine and pethidine. *Br. J. clin. Pharmac.* **2**, 81

Handley, A. J. (1967). Metoclopramide in the prevention of postoperative nausea and vomiting. *Br. J. clin. Pract.* **21**, 460

Klein, R. L., Graves, Constance L., Yong, I. K. and Blatnick, R. (1970). Inhibition of apomorphine-induced vomiting by benzquinamide. *Clin. Pharmac. Ther.* **11**, 530

Lind, B. and Breivik, H. (1970). Metoclopramide and perphenazine in the prevention of postoperative nausea and vomiting. *Br. J. Anaesth.* **42**, 614

McBride, W. (1963). Cyclizine and congenital abnormalities. *Br. med. J.* **1**, 1157

Midwinter, A. (1971). Vomiting in pregnancy. *Practitioner* **206**, 743

Moore, D. C., Bridenbaugh, L. D., Piccioni, V. F., Adams, P. A. and Lindstrom, C. A. (1956). Control of postoperative vomiting with Merazine: a double blind study. *Anesthesiology* **17**, 690

Morrison, J. D. (1970). Studies of drugs given before anaesthesia. XXII: Phenoperidine and fentanyl, alone and in combination with droperidol. *Br. J. Anaesth.* **42**, 1119

Nelson, M. M. and Forfar, J. O. (1971). Associations between drugs administered during pregnancy and congenital abnormalities of the fetus. *Br. med. J.* **1**, 523

Patton, C. M., Moon, M. R. and Dannemiller, F. J. (1974). The prophylactic antiemetic effect of droperidol. *Anesth. Analg. curr. Res.* **53**, 361

Pitts, N. E. (1969). A clinical pharmacological evaluation of benzquinamide, a new antiemetic agent. *Curr. ther. Res.* **11**, 325

Stalsberg, H. (1965). Antiemetics and congenital deformities − meclozine, cyclizine and chlorcyclizine. *Norweg. Med. J.* **85**, 1840

Wade, O. L. and Dundee, J. W. (1969). Antiemetic drugs. *Prescribers J.* **9**, 69

Wheeler, M. W. and Campman, K. L. (1971). A comparative study of droperidol versus hydroxyzine hydrochloride as premedication. *J. Am. Ass. Nurse Anesth.* 401

15 Neuromuscular transmission and neuromuscular block

D. V. Roberts and T. C. Gray

This chapter is concerned with the physiological principles underlying neuromuscular transmission and the various ways in which this function may be blocked. The field to be covered includes events in the motor-nerve terminals, at the motor end-plate and in the muscle membrane; the links between electrical and mechanical activity in skeletal muscles will be described. In order for this account of neuromuscular transmission to be concise, many details have been omitted and the reader is advised to consult the works listed at the end of the chapter for a fuller account.

Transmission from nerve to skeletal muscle is a process which begins with the synthesis and storage of acetylcholine (ACh) inside motor-nerve terminals, from which the transmitter is released by nerve impulses. On arrival at the postjunctional (muscle) membrane, acetylcholine combines reversibly with receptor molecules; as a result, an increase in membrane permeability brings about a transient depolarization at the end-plate (the end-plate potential or EPP). Under normal circumstances the resulting ionic currents flowing across the adjacent muscle membrane are sufficiently intense to depolarize beyond the threshold and so initiate an action potential; this in turn rapidly invades the whole of the muscle membrane and activates the contractile mechanism. Various physiological and pharmacological factors may modify the several stages of neuromuscular transmission and use has been made of some of these factors to produce and overcome neuromuscular block.

IONIC CONCENTRATION, MEMBRANE PERMEABILITY AND ELECTRICAL POTENTIAL

Resting membrane potential

Many of the stages of neuromuscular transmission depend upon the relation between the concentration of various ions about the nerve and muscle membrane, the permeability of these membranes to the ions present and the resting and active membrane potentials. At rest, nerve and muscle membrane are relatively more permeable to K^+ ions than to Na^+ ions, and the resting membrane potential is proportional to the ratio $\ln [K]_o/[K]_i \times P_K$, where $[K]_o$ and $[K]_i$ are the concentrations of potassium outside and inside the cell membrane, and P_K is the permeability of the membrane to potassium. Values of the negative resting potentials calculated on this basis agree closely with those measured in various tissues. Changes in membrane potential from its resting value may be brought about by alterations in the concentration of potassium or permeability of the membrane to this ion, or by an increase in the membrane permeability to sodium. Thus, if the membrane is made permeable to sodium and not to potassium, the membrane potential becomes positive on the inside (because of the higher concentration of sodium in the fluid outside the fibre) with a value proportional to $\ln [Na]_o/[Na]_i \times P_{Na}$. When the membrane is permeable to both ions, the potential will assume a value and polarity in accordance with the ion concentrations and relative permeabilities. Such permeability changes form the basis for the action potential of nerve and skeletal muscle fibres, and the reduction in membrane potential produced by acetylcholine acting on the chemosensitive area of muscle membrane at the end-plate (the end-plate potential or EPP).

Action potential

In excitable membranes such as those of nerve and muscle, there is also an inverse relation between membrane potential and permeability to sodium, so that as the potential is reduced (for example, by action currents from an adjacent active region), permeability to sodium increases and supplements the depolarization already present. Once a threshold depolarization has been reached, the action is self-regenerative and results in a further rapid increase in permeability of sodium and reversal of membrane potential. Recovery of membrane potential to its resting negative value is brought about by inactivation of the sodium-permeability mechanism and by a transient increase in potassium permeability. During the action potential, there is also an increase in the membrane permeability to calcium, a change which is important for release of acetylcholine from motor-nerve terminals and for activation of the contractile mechanism in skeletal muscle.

End-plate potential

The muscle membrane at the end-plate does not possess the inverse relation between potential and sodium permeability and so it is electrically non-excitable. The potential change produced by acetylcholine when applied to this region is due to a simultaneous increase in permeability to sodium and potassium, so that the membrane depolarizes to a value of -10 to -15 mV, the equilibrium potential for the concentrations of these two ions. This change in potential serves as a source of ion current by which the adjacent electrically excitable muscle membrane is activated.

The magnitude of the EPP and of the currents it produces are proportional to the difference between the resting membrane potential and the equilibrium potential for sodium and potassium. When the end-plate is depolarized, EPP amplitude is reduced and this must be taken into account when the mechanisms of action of depolarization block are considered.

ACh receptors and ion permeability

The molecular effects responsible for permeability changes have not been elucidated, but one possibility is that when acetylcholine is joined to the receptor group in the end-plate membrane, the receptor molecule or perhaps an adjacent molecule (an ionophore) is induced to change its configuration and/or electrical charge, so that sodium and potassium ions can move more easily through the membrane. Acetylcholine agonists have a similar action, whereas the non-depolarizing blocking agents, while occupying the same receptors, do not induce the permeability changes.

Sodium/potassium pump

As a result of these changes in permeability, there is increased movement of ions across nerve and muscle membranes and a corresponding change in the concentrations of these ions on each side of the membranes, which, if unchecked, would lead to a decrease in membrane potential and loss of excitability. The unequal distribution of ions, which forms the basis for the resting membrane potential, is maintained by an active sodium/potassium pump which operates at particular sites within nerve and muscle membranes, at a rate which increases with the internal concentration of sodium. The sodium/potassium pump is a separate entity from the ion-permeability mechanism which is responsible for the resting and action potentials, and each function may be blocked selectively without affecting the other.

NEUROMUSCULAR TRANSMISSION: PREJUNCTIONAL ASPECTS

ACh synthesis

Most of the acetylcholine concerned with neuromuscular transmission is synthesized within the motor-nerve terminals, only a small amount being formed in the axon and moved to the terminal by axoplasmic transport. Synthesis is effected by acetylation of choline (actively transported across the nerve terminal membrane) by acetyl coenzyme A (from mitochondria), with choline-o-acetyltransferase as a catalyst. While the ultimate source of choline is the plasma, up to 50% of that which is actively transported into the nerve terminal is derived from the hydrolysis of previously released acetylcholine; moreover, the rate of uptake is increased by nerve stimulation, thus enabling synthesis of acetylcholine to keep pace with release. The importance of the choline-uptake mechanism is demonstrated when it is inhibited by hemicholinium-3; released acetylcholine is then not replaced by synthesis and eventually a block of transmission occurs due to the inadequate amount of acetylcholine released by each nerve impulse.

ACh storage

After synthesis, acetylcholine is stored within the nerve terminal in various ways. Part is stored in some molecular form in the cytoplasm and part is in multimolecular packets or quanta contained in the vesicles which are characteristic of prejunctional nerve terminals. Of the vesicular fraction, a small part (15—20%) is readily available for release by nerve impulses, while the rest acts as a depot from which the smaller (readily available) vesicular store of acetylcholine is replenished. The amount of acetylcholine present in each store at any moment depends on the rates of synthesis, hydrolysis by cytoplasmic cholinesterases and release from the nerve ending. Inhibition of these enzymes by anticholinesterase compounds such as eserine, which is able to penetrate the nerve membrane, results in a doubling of the total amount of acetylcholine in nerve—muscle preparations and better maintenance of acetylcholine release during prolonged nerve stimulation. The reader is reminded that cytoplasmic cholinesterase is not to be confused with the cholinesterase on the post-junctional membrane.

ACh release

Acetylcholine is released from the readily available store by each nerve impulse; the mechanism of release includes the fusion of vesicle and nerve membranes, an action which is facilitated by the inflow of calcium

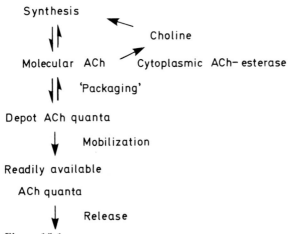

Figure 15.1
Diagrammatic representation of synthesis and various forms of storage of ACh. Note that a state of equilibrium exists between synthesis, molecular store and depot 'quantal' store of ACh and that excess ACh is hydrolysed by cytoplasmic ACh-esterase

during the nerve action potential. The most recent estimate of the number of acetylcholine molecules per vesicle is 6250 but, since all are released at the same time and act together on the postjunctional membrane, it is convenient to use the content of one vesicle as the unit or quantum of acetylcholine release. Estimates have been made of the number of acetylcholine quanta released by each nerve impulse, and the values obtained range up to several hundred. The size of the readily available store has been estimated at several thousand quanta. The arrival of an impulse in the nerve terminal releases a proportion of the quanta available and hence, if nerve stimulation continues, the number of quanta available and therefore the number released will be reduced (because of depletion of the readily available store) until the rate of release of quanta is just balanced by the rate of mobilization from the larger depot (*Figure 15.1*).

Calcium and ACh release

The actual number of quanta released per nerve impulse depends on several factors. For example, reduced calcium or increased magnesium concentrations in the immediate vicinity of the nerve terminal may reduce output to a few quanta per impulse and may abolish it completely. In these circumstances the impulse still reaches the nerve terminal which still contains acetylcholine quanta available for release but, for lack of calcium, fusion of vesicle and nerve membrane does not take place. Thus calcium determines the proportion of the available store which is released by controlling the probability of release of individual vesicles.

Frequency of stimulation and ACh release

Among the other factors affecting the number of quanta released per nerve impulse is the rate at which these impulses arrive at the motor-nerve terminal. Thus if the frequency of nerve stimulation increases, the quantal output per impulse decreases as depletion of the store of readily available vesicles takes place. However, the output of quanta per second (frequency of stimulation × quantal release per impulse) and the rate of mobilization of acetylcholine quanta increase. The effect is proportional to the frequency of stimulation and is particularly apparent when the quantal output per nerve impulse has been reduced by withdrawal of calcium. It forms the basis for the recovery of neuromuscular transmission after tetanization, and should be taken into account when neuromuscular transmission is measured by myographic or electromyographic (EMG) methods, using high frequency repetitive stimulation (*Figure 15.2*).

Prejunctional receptors

Release of acetylcholine quanta is also subject to modification by a mechanism which involves receptors in the membrane of the motor-nerve

terminal. When these receptors are occupied, the acetylcholine quantum
output per nerve impulse is decreased; substances which are active in this
way include acetylcholine and tubocurarine, although the neuromuscular
blocking action of the latter substance is principally due to its postjunctional action and only to a minor degree to its prejunctional action.
The same receptors may be involved in the generation of repetitive activity
in motor-nerve terminals by some anticholinesterase compounds.

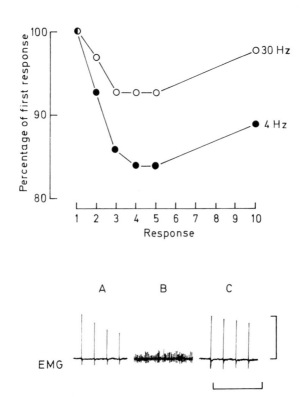

Figure 15.2
Effect of frequency of stimulation and voluntary activity on neuromuscular transmission. The graph shows the amplitude of the EMG
responses of the adductor pollicis muscle to trains of ten stimuli at
4 and 30 Hz applied to the ulnar nerve of a myasthenic patient.
Note (1) maximum decrease in EMG amplitude is attained after
three or four stimuli and that continued stimulation increases EMG
amplitude, and (2) greater facilitation of neuromuscular transmission
at 30 Hz results in a smaller initial decrease and a fuller recovery of
EMG amplitude. (Graph constructed from data of Roberts and
Wilson, 1969; similar results obtained in curarized subjects have
been reported by Lee and Katz, 1977.)
    The EMG records in the lower part of the figure show the response
to trains of four stimuli at 4 Hz (A) before and (C) after a 10-second
period of maximal voluntary activity in the tested muscle (B). Note
the decreased 'fade', indicating increased neuromuscular transmission
after voluntary activity. Calibration bars: 10 mV and 1 second. The
records have been retouched for publication

Cyclic AMP* and ACh release

In addition, it should be noted that the amount of acetylcholine released varies with the concentration of cyclic AMP within the nerve terminal. The mechanism of action is not known but it may involve the rate at which acetylcholine is mobilized into the store from which release takes place, with calcium playing an intermediary role. The increased amount of acetylcholine produced by adrenaline and ephedrine acting on motor-nerve terminals is attributed to an increase in cyclic AMP formation, whereas the similar effect of theophylline on acetylcholine output is thought to be due to its inhibitory effect on phosphodiesterase, so reducing the rate of inactivation of cyclic AMP.

NEUROMUSCULAR TRANSMISSION: POSTJUNCTIONAL ASPECTS

Postjunctional receptors

Once acetylcholine has been released from a motor-nerve terminal, it diffuses rapidly across the synaptic gap to combine with either of two receptor molecules incorporated into the postjunctional muscle membrane. Occupation of the cholinoreceptor molecules results in an increase in membrane permeability to sodium and potassium ions, and therefore in depolarization of the end-plate membrane, by an amount which is normally sufficient to generate an action potential in the adjacent membrane. Acetylcholine which is received by the acetylcholinesterase which is also present in the postjunctional membrane, side by side but separate from the cholinoreceptor molecules, undergoes hydrolysis and the products either move by diffusion into the plasma or, in the case of choline, are taken up by the nerve terminal and resynthesized to form new transmitter substance.

EPP amplitude and receptor activity

Just as the two receptors are in competition for acetylcholine, so are the end-results of their occupation by acetylcholine antagonistic in their actions. Thus, the depolarizing effect of acetylcholine is proportional to the number of occupied cholinoreceptors, which is in turn limited by the rate of hydrolysis of acetylcholine by acetylcholinesterase. Under normal circumstances, enzymatic hydrolysis restricts the duration of the active phase of the EPP to less than 1 ms, after which the membrane is re-polarized along a time course which is largely determined by the electrical characteristics of the end-plate region. Anticholinesterase compounds, by inhibiting the enzyme, prolong the active life of acetylcholine in the vicinity of cholinoreceptors, and so allow more of these receptors to be

* AMP is adenosine monophosphate. *Ed.*

successively occupied by acetylcholine before diffusion takes the transmitter away from the site of action. In this way, administration of an anticholinesterase agent increases the amplitude and duration of the end-plate potential.

Other factors related to EPP amplitude

In addition to the action of acetylcholinesterase, other factors influence the amplitude of the end-plate potential. Prejunctionally, variation in the number of acetylcholine quanta released by each nerve impulse will result in corresponding changes in EPP amplitude. For example, facilitation of release of transmitter by high frequency nerve activity will increase EPP amplitude, whereas depletion of the store of acetylcholine quanta (as occurs during a train of stimuli applied to the motor nerve at a frequency of 4 Hz) reduces EPP amplitude. Postjunctionally, the amplitude of end-plate potentials varies with the number of receptors available for combination with acetylcholine, a factor of importance in relation to neuromuscular block produced not only by non-depolarizing agents such as tubocurarine but also by the desensitization form of block which results from prolonged exposure to depolarizing agents, including acetylcholine itself. EPP amplitude also varies with the input impedance of the end-plate which is proportional to the diameter of the muscle fibre, so that, although acetylcholine quanta may contain similar numbers of molecules, their depolarizing effect is greater in small than in large muscle fibres.

Muscle action potential

The final stage of transmission from motor nerve to skeletal muscle is the initiation of an action potential in the muscle fibre by ionic currents originating in the depolarized end-plate region. The polarity of these currents is such as to depolarize the adjacent muscle membrane to a value at which, under normal circumstances, the resulting increased permeability to sodium is sufficient to allow an action potential to occur. Once this threshold depolarization has been reached, the muscle action potential is independent of the end-plate potential and rapidly spreads to involve all the muscle fibre membrane. During this process it is no longer sensitive to the effects of neuromuscular junctional blocking agents but it may be modified by other agents active against excitable membranes (e.g. tetrodotoxin, which selectively blocks the channels in the membranes which are the basis of the increased permeability to sodium essential for action potential formation).

ANALYSIS OF NEUROMUSCULAR TRANSMISSION

With the foregoing points in mind, an analysis of neuromuscular transmission may be made in terms of four principal factors, viz. the amount of

$$\text{Neuromuscular transmission} = \frac{\begin{array}{c} \text{Quantity} \\ \text{of ACh} \\ \text{released} \end{array} + \begin{array}{c} \text{No. of} \\ \text{receptors} \\ \text{available} \end{array} + \begin{array}{c} \text{Muscle} \\ \text{excitability} \end{array}}{\text{Hydrolysis by ACh-esterase}}$$

Figure 15.3
Principal factors in neuromuscular transmission

acetylcholine released, the availability of postjunctional acetylcholine receptors, the activity of acetylcholinesterase and the threshold for excitation in the muscle fibre membrane around the end-plate (*Figure 15.3*).

Factors affecting release of ACh

Two factors govern the amount of acetylcholine released: the number of acetylcholine molecules associated with each quantum, and the number of quanta released by each nerve impulse. The acetylcholine content of each quantum is remarkably constant under physiological conditions but may be reduced when synthesis of acetylcholine is depressed, for example, by inhibition of choline uptake into motor-nerve terminals by hemicholinium compounds. In contrast, the number of quanta released by a nerve impulse is subject to variation by many factors; for example, the number and frequency of nerve impulses, calcium/magnesium concentrations in the vicinity of the end-plate and presynaptically acting 'chemical' compounds.

Availability of ACh receptors

If output of acetylcholine from motor nerve terminals is constant, EPP amplitude is proportional to the number of acetylcholine receptors with which the transmitter can combine. This number may be reduced, for example, when some are occupied by tubocurarine and other non-depolarizing relaxants. An effective loss of receptors occurs when they temporarily lose their sensitivity to acetylcholine as a result of prolonged exposure to this or other depolarizing agents (such as suxamethonium).

Activity of acetylcholinesterase

Inhibition of this enzyme (for example, by neostigmine) effectively increases the number of receptors activated by acetylcholine because the transmitter is able to combine with several receptors before diffusion takes it away from the receptor area.

Action potential threshold and safety margin

The remaining factor of neuromuscular transmission is the amount of depolarization — the threshold — required to initiate an action potential. It should be noted that this factor is a function, not of the end-plate membrane which is not electrically excitable, but of the muscle membrane immediately around the end-plate. An increase in the threshold for excitation occurs as a response to prolonged depolarization and this factor may play a part in the neuromuscular blockade produced by depolarizing agents. Depolarization of the end-plate by an amount sufficient to exceed the threshold for excitation is a function of pre- and post-synaptic mechanisms and under normal circumstances the EPP exceeds the threshold by a factor of 5; this safety margin ensures full transmission from nerve to muscle and its elimination results in neuromuscular block.

MECHANISMS OF NEUROMUSCULAR BLOCK

From the foregoing account of the physiology of neuromuscular transmission, it is clear that a neuromuscular block may be produced at any one of the several stages in the process of transmission from nerve to muscle. In practice, however, neuromuscular block is usually achieved by modifying the activity of the postjunctional (muscle) membrane in one of two ways.

Non-depolarizing block

This form of block is produced when the postjunctional receptors are occupied by, for example, tubocurarine. This substance, while possessing sufficient affinity for the receptors to combine reversibly with them, does not bring about the changes in membrane permeability which underlie the end-plate potential. Thus, when acetylcholine is released from a motor-nerve ending it competes with tubocurarine for occupancy of receptor sites; the more sites that are occupied by tubocurarine, the fewer that are available for acetylcholine and so the smaller is the end-plate potential. Neuromuscular block occurs when the EPP amplitude fails to reach the threshold value, and it lasts as long as the tubocurarine concentration at the end-plate region is high enough to allow it to compete effectively with acetylcholine. While the rate of dissociation of tubocurarine molecules from the receptors is slower than that of acetylcholine, it is still a matter of seconds rather than minutes. The time course of a non-depolarizing block mainly reflects the removal of the blocking agent by distribution in body water, plasma protein binding, metabolism and excretion.

Depolarizing block

This mode of block is brought about by rapid application of a depolarizing agent such as acetylcholine or, in practice, suxamethonium (succinylcholine). The initial effect of the depolarization so produced is a short-lasting burst of repetitive activity in the affected muscle. Then follows a period of block due to the reduction in membrane potential of the electrically excitable muscle membrane around the end-plate. This reduction in membrane potential is due to persistent current flow from the end-plate region and it prevents the development of further electrical activity in muscle fibres by inactivating the normal relation between membrane potential and sodium permeability, which is the basis of the all-or-none potential mechanism. This period of block due to persistent end-plate depolarization has been termed phase 1; it is followed by phase 2, in which the block persists in spite of a recovery of end-plate resting potential. The mode of action of a phase 2 block is best described as a loss of sensitivity by acetylcholine receptors which have been occupied for too long a time by a depolarizing agent. In such circumstances the receptor assumes a more stable form or a more stable bond is formed between receptor and depolarizing agent. The receptor remains unavailable for acetylcholine released by motor-nerve activity, and the link between receptor and membrane permeability is broken so that the membrane potential of the end-plate is able to return toward the normal value. The adjacent muscle membrane regains electrical excitability but transmission is now blocked by receptor desensitization. It should be noted that there is no clear demarcation between phase 1 and phase 2 but rather a continuous transition from one to the other; the rate of transition depends on the degree of depolarization produced by the initial administration of the depolarizing agent and, in all probability, at any one time different end-plates in the same muscle may exhibit the two forms of block in different degrees. When the depolarizing agent is applied slowly, desensitization block may be produced with little or no evidence of prior depolarization.

Depolarization block in neonates and in myasthenia gravis

For any given concentration of depolarizing agent, the effect will be proportional to the number of available acetylcholine receptors. Where this is reduced, as in the neonate and in patients with myasthenia gravis, depolarizing agents may be expected to exert a smaller effect and the onset of phase 2 block will be more rapid. Such effects have been observed in practice.

Mechanism of presynaptic (low output) block

Both of the above-mentioned forms of block are due to postsynaptic changes; presynaptic block, while not used in anaesthetic practice, may occur and complicate the action of postsynaptic blocking agents. A notable although rare example is the block found in the Eaton–Lambert syndrome in which failure of transmission from nerve to muscle occurs because the number of acetylcholine quanta released by each nerve impulse is very much less than normal. Neomycin and other antibiotics also produce neuromuscular block by a presynaptic action, as do botulinum and black-widow spider toxins. This form of block may be described as 'low output' to distinguish it from the 'high output' depolarizing and non-depolarizing forms of block.

Reversal of neuromuscular block

This may be brought about either by removal of the blocking agent or by producing other changes in neuromuscular transmission which compensate for the blocking action. In practice, both mechanisms are likely to operate at the same time.

Reversal with anticholinesterase agents

The use of neostigmine to reverse a tubocurarine block is effective because the inhibition of acetylcholinesterase at the neuromuscular junction permits acetylcholine to interact with more receptors and so increase its depolarizing action. It should be noted, however, that the reversing action of neostigmine and other anticholinesterase compounds is limited; once the enzyme is fully inhibited, addition of more neostigmine cannot reduce the block any further and is more likely to increase the block by combining with acetylcholine receptors in a curare-like manner. In practice, owing to the sigmoid nature of the neostigmine dose/enzyme inhibition relation, maximal but not necessarily complete reversal of a neuromuscular block is obtained over a limited dose range; additional doses of neo-stigmine will be ineffective until the enzyme has recovered from the inhibition produced by previous doses (*Figure 15.4*).

Reversal of presynaptic block

In the case of low-output neuromuscular block, enzyme inhibition may not increase the effectiveness of the reduced quantities of acetylcholine released from motor-nerve endings to a level at which transmission is restored. In such cases, the effective method of reversing the block is to increase acetylcholine output by increasing plasma calcium concentration or by giving presynaptically acting drugs such as germine diacetate. Both procedures increase the number of acetylcholine quanta released by each nerve impulse; however, if acetylcholine synthesis is impaired, the stores of transmitter are likely to be further depleted by the increase in output and so any benefit may be short-lived.

Depolarizing block

There is no way of overcoming a pure depolarizing block because any agent which antagonizes the action of the depolarizing substance will also antagonize the action of acetylcholine. When a degree of desensitization

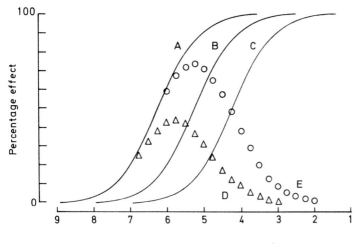

Negative   log. concentration

Figure 15.4
Illustration of the combined effect on neuromuscular transmission
of the anticholinesterase and curare-like action of neostigmine. The
percentage effect is plotted against the negative logarithm of the
concentration of neostigmine, curve A referring to anticholinesterase
activity, and curves B and C referring to curare-like activity, displaced
laterally by amounts equivalent to 10- and 100-fold increases in
concentration above those of curve A. The combined effect of these
antagonistic actions is obtained by subtracting from curve A, curve B
(triangles, D) and curve C (circles, E).

The following points should be noted. (1). The limited dose range
over which ACh-esterase inhibition (A) is linearly related to dose.
Above this range, large increases in dose result in little additional
increase in inhibition. (2). When, as with neostigmine, a curare-like
effect is produced at a concentration ten times that required to
inhibit significantly the ACh-esterase (B), the beneficial effect of
neostigmine on neuromuscular transmission is limited to less than
50% (D). (3). With a 100-fold difference in dose levels needed to
produce anti-ACh-esterase and curare-like action (C), the beneficial
effect of neostigmine is still no greater than 75% of the maximum (E)

of receptors has occurred, however, and the block is of the phase 2 type,
neostigmine may enhance the effect of released acetylcholine and so compensate for the reduced postjunctional sensitivity. This action is limited in
extent and excess neostigmine will increase the block by occupying those
postjunctional receptors which remain sensitive to acetylcholine.

Multiple actions on neuromuscular transmission

While it is customary to characterize neuromuscular agents in terms of
their main effect, it should be recognized that most, if not all, of these
compounds have more than one effect and that the relative importance of
these effects may alter with the state of neuromuscular transmission and
in the presence of other active compounds. Reference has already been

made to the anticholinesterase and curare-like actions of neostigmine and, in addition, this compound can also act presynaptically to increase acetylcholine output temporarily. Another example of a compound with multiple actions is procaine. This substance has been used to prolong the effect of suxamethonium by inhibiting plasma cholinesterase but it may itself produce neuromuscular block by reducing the amount of acetylcholine released, by decreasing the sensitivity of the end-plate muscle membrane to acetylcholine and by depressing the electrical excitability of the muscle membrane. Also of interest in the context of multiple actions is ether which, while used principally for its anaesthetic property, also has its own neuromuscular blocking action by reducing the sensitivity of the end-plate to acetylcholine. The precise mode of action of ether in this respect is not known but its relevance is clear.

RELATION BETWEEN ELECTRICAL AND MECHANICAL EVENTS

While neuromuscular transmission is a process confined to motor-nerve endings and muscle end-plates, in practice its end-product and the effects of neuromuscular blocking agents are seen in terms of contraction or tension of the whole muscle. When neuromuscular transmission is normal, each nerve action potential results in one muscle action potential which rapidly travels over the surface of the muscle fibre to activate the actin/myosin contractile system by a mechanism which includes the release of calcium from the sarcoplasmic reticular system. Thus, while there is a relation between neuromuscular transmission and muscle contraction, it is subject to modification by non-junctional factors.

Calcium and mechanical activity

One such non-junctional factor is the amount of calcium available to activate the interaction between actin and myosin filaments, which is the basis for muscle shortening and/or tension development. During each contraction/relaxation cycle, calcium is released from and then reabsorbed by the sarcoplasmic reticulum. When this movement of calcium is reduced, contraction and relaxation are impaired and muscle power is reduced. The ways in which such effects may occur are typified by three examples. First, the calcium content of the sarcoplasmic reticulum reflects the calcium concentration in the extracellular environment and so muscle power is reduced by a fall in plasma and interstitial fluid calcium. Second, a substance such as dantrolene sodium, which blocks the uptake and release of calcium by sarcoplasmic tubules, may be used to produce muscle relaxation at an intracellular level without impairing neuromuscular transmission. Third, experimental rupture of the transverse tubules prevents action or electrotonic potentials from reaching a point within the muscle fibre at which they can initiate the release of calcium from the longitudinal sarcoplasmic tubules. In all three instances, electrical activity of muscle continues in a normal manner but there is no resultant mechanical activity; substances which act on the neuromuscular junction are ineffective as antagonists to such a block.

Active state of skeletal muscle

Physiological changes in the strength of muscle contraction may occur as a result of variations in the active state of the contractile system. Not only is the energy of contraction proportional, within limits, to the length of muscle fibres before activation but it also depends on the frequency of stimulation and on previous activity. It is increased by adrenaline, an effect probably mediated via cyclic AMP and calcium.

Evaluation of twitch tension amplitude

Measurement of neuromuscular transmission is frequently carried out by recording the mechanical response to motor-nerve stimulation, using single shocks, trains of four at 2 Hz or tetanic stimulation (50 Hz). Changes in the amplitude of the contractions so produced are then interpreted in terms of events at the neuromuscular junction but, because of the many factors which influence the mechanical activity of muscle directly, this interpretation should be made with care. For example, the amplitude of single muscle twitches, recorded *in vivo,* may vary during the course of an experiment or clinical investigation as a result of changes in the catechol-amine level in plasma, or perhaps because of a change in the resting length or tension of the muscle under test. When trains of four stimuli are used, care is needed to make sure that the amplitudes of the second, third and fourth twitches are not influenced by previous twitches, either by simple summation or by increased contractility. In the case of tetanic stimulation, changes due to summation, increased contractility and mechanical fatigue may all be present at the same time. Finally, when evaluating the results of 'twitch' recordings, account should be taken of the possibility of action by some chemical compounds directly on the muscle as well as on the neuromuscular junction (e.g. calcium).

SUMMARY OF NEUROMUSCULAR TRANSMISSION AND NEUROMUSCULAR BLOCK (*Figure 15.5*)

Neuromuscular transmission consists of three principal components: the release of acetylcholine from motor-nerve endings, its reception by cholinoreceptors and the termination of its action by enzymatic hydrolysis and diffusion. All three are subject to modification, either pre- or post-junctionally, but when operating normally they combine to produce a transient depolarization of the muscle membrane, sufficient to initiate

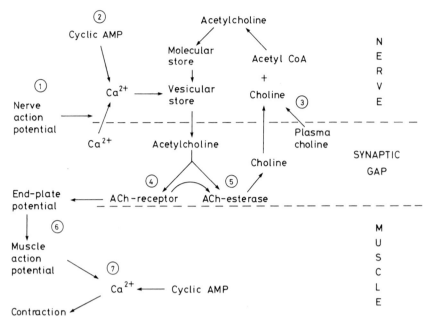

Figure 15.5

Diagrammatic representation of the main features of neuromuscular transmission, with examples of some factors which affect synaptic function.

(1) Anaesthetic and other agents may prevent the arrival of nerve action potentials at the motor terminals.

(2) Acetylcholine output is increased by substances which increase cyclic-AMP synthesis in the nerve terminals (e.g. adrenaline, ephedrine) or inhibit its hydrolysis by phosphodiesterase (e.g. theophylline).

(3) Hemicholinium compounds inhibit the active transport of choline into the nerve terminals so that synthesis of acetylcholine ceases and neuromuscular block occurs when the store of acetylcholine is depleted.

(4) Neuromuscular block also results when the ACh-receptors are occupied by non-depolarizing (e.g. tubocurarine) or depolarizing (e.g. suxamethonium) blocking agents.

(5) Neuromuscular block may be relieved when the ACh-esterase is inhibited by, for example, neostigmine. Note that this will reduce the amount of choline available for uptake, which in the long-term may affect synthesis and storage of acetylcholine.

(6) Neuromuscular block may occur if the EPP is too small to activate the action potential mechanism in the muscle fibre, or when this mechanism has been inactivated by previous depolarization.

(7) Electromechanical coupling in muscle fibres is blocked by lack of calcium. Irrespective of changes in electrical activity, mechanical activity will be modified by changes in the intracellular level of calcium, for example, by previous activity or by agents acting via cyclic AMP

an all-or-nothing, self-propagating action potential. The subsequent contraction depends on the successful activation of the contractile system and is subject to modification by factors operating on the muscle membrane and on its intracellular apparatus. Neuromuscular block occurs when the safety margin in transmission which is normally present is reduced by changes in the amount of acetylcholine released or in the sensitivity of postjunctional receptors, and relief of the block may be obtained by appropriate modification of the other principal component of neuromuscular transmission, acetylcholinesterase.

References

Lee, C. and Katz, R. L. (1977). Fade of neurally evoked compound electromyogram during neuromuscular block by *d*-tubocurarine. *Anesth. Analg., Cleve.* **56**, 271–275

Roberts, D. V. and Wilson, A. (1969). Electromyography in diagnosis and treatment. In *Myasthenia Gravis*. Raymond Green (ed.). London: Heinemann Medical

Further reading

Barnard, E. A., Dolly, J. O., Porter, C. W. and Albuquerque, E. X. (1975). The acetylcholine receptor and the ionic conductance modulation system of skeletal muscle. *Exp. Neurol.* **48**, 1–28

Csillik, B. (1965). *Functional Structure of the Post-synaptic Membrane in the Myoneural Junction*. Budapest: Publishing House of the Hungarian Academy of Sciences

Gage, P. W. (1976). Generation of end-plate potentials. *Physiol. Rev.* **56**, 177–247

Hebb, C. (1972). Biosynthesis of acetylcholine in nervous tissue. *Physiol. Rev.* **52**, 918–957

Hodgkin, A. L. (1964). *The Conduction of the Nervous Impulse*. Liverpool: Liverpool University Press

Hubbard, J. I. (1973). Microphysiology of vertebrate neuromuscular transmission. *Physiol. Rev.* **53**, 674–723

Hubbard, J. I. and Quastel, D. M. J. (1973). Micropharmacology of vertebrate neuromuscular transmission. *A. Rev. Pharmac.* **13**, 199–216

Hubbard, J. I., Llinas, R. and Quastel, D. M. J. (1969). *Electrophysiological Analysis of Synaptic Transmission*. London: Edward Arnold

Katz, B. (1962). The transmission of impulses from nerve to muscle, and the subcellular unit of synaptic action. The Croonian Lecture. *Proc. R. Soc. B.* **155**, 455–477

Katz, B. (1966). *Nerve, Muscle and Synapse*. New York: McGraw-Hill

Katz, B. (1969). *The Release of Neural Transmitter Substances*. Liverpool: Liverpool University Press

Kuffler, S. W. and Nicholls, J. G. (1976). *From Neuron to Brain*. Sunderland, Mass: Sinauer Associates

Martin, A. R. (1966). Quantal nature of synaptic transmission. *Physiol Rev.* **46**, 51–66

Singer, J. J. and Goldberg, A. L. (1970). Cyclic AMP and transmission at the neuromuscular junction. In *Role of Cyclic AMP in Cell Function*. P. Greengard and E. Costa (ed.). *Advances in Biochemical Psychopharmacology*, Vol. 3. New York: Raven Press

Thesleff, S. (ed.) (1976). *Motor Innervation of Muscle*. London: Academic Press

Whittaker, V. P. (1973). The biochemistry of synaptic transmission. *Naturwissenschaften* **60**, 281–289

16 Muscle relaxant drugs and their antagonists
T. N. Calvey and H. Wilson

In this chapter, various aspects of the pharmacology of muscle relaxants and their antagonists are considered.

RELATION OF CHEMICAL AND MOLECULAR STRUCTURE TO NEUROMUSCULAR BLOCK

The molecular requirements of depolarizing muscle relaxants have been clearly defined for many years. Both decamethonium and suxamethonium are slender, elongated and flexible molecules ('leptocurares'): they possess two quaternary centres separated by a distance of 1.2—1.4 nm. Comparable concepts relating to competitive muscle relaxants have been modified recently. Until 1970, all competitive agents used in clinical anaesthesia were believed to possess at least two quaternary groups; the interquaternary distance associated with optimal neuromuscular block appeared to be similar in both competitive and depolarizing muscle relaxants. This view is no longer accepted, as it is known that some competitive drugs (e.g. tubocurarine) are monoquaternary rather than *bis*-quaternary compounds. The interquaternary distance is not of crucial importance in the production of neuromuscular block, since it ranges from 0.75 nm (fazadinium) to 1.11 nm (pancuronium). Other molecular features — for instance, steric interactions and the number of functional asymmetric centres — play an important part in determining the potency and receptor affinity of relaxant drugs.

The chemical formulae of the muscle relaxants currently used in clinical anaesthesia in Great Britain are shown in *Figure 16.1*.

KINETICS OF MUSCLE RELAXANTS

After intravenous administration, suxamethonium is rapidly hydrolysed by plasma cholinesterase. The plasma concentration falls exponentially and is consistent with a one-compartment pharmacokinetic model. All

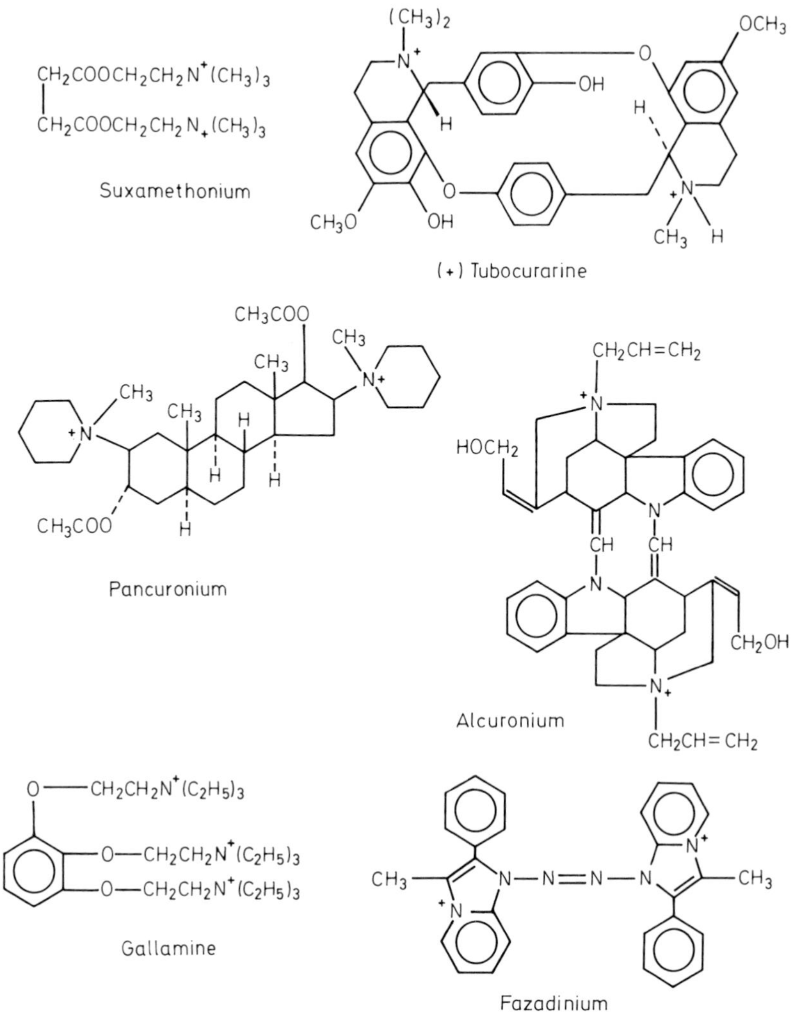

Figure 16.1
Chemical structure of muscle relaxants in current use. The associated
anion has been omitted

other muscle relaxants are eliminated from plasma in a multiexponential
manner. There is an initial rapid fall in plasma concentration during the
first 2–10 minutes, followed by one or more slower phases of exponential
decline. The initial fall in plasma concentration is mainly due to rapid
distribution in extracellular fluid, although uptake by certain organs may
be involved. Distribution studies in experimental animals suggest that
most muscle relaxants can readily enter hepatic and renal cells; small
but significant amounts are bound by end-plate receptors and anionic
groups associated with mucopolysaccharides. The final phase of exponential decline, characterized by the elimination half-life, reflects the
removal of the muscle relaxant from the body by renal or biliary excretion,
or by metabolism.

The pharmacokinetics of tubocurarine and pancuronium have been most widely studied. Until 5 years ago, measurement of tubocurarine was dependent on relatively insensitive methods; for instance, bioassay, spectrophotometry and spectrofluorimetry. The recent advent of more specific and sensitive techniques (i.e. radioimmunoassay and radiometric assay) have modified current concepts of the kinetics of tubocurarine. In patients with normal renal function, estimates of the elimination half-life range from 152 to 231 minutes, and traces of the drug are still detectable in plasma for more than 24 hours after intravenous administration. Approximately 38–44% of the dose is eliminated in urine during this time. In renal failure, the terminal half-life is prolonged to 256–330 minutes, and only 13–15% is excreted unchanged in urine within 24 hours. There is a significant correlation between the plasma concentration of tubocurarine and the degree of neuromuscular block; recovery from paralysis begins at a plasma concentration of 0.7 μg·ml^{-1}, and is complete when the concentration falls to 0.2 μg·ml^{-1}.

Pancuronium is eliminated from plasma in a comparable manner. After intravenous administration, there is an immediate decline in plasma concentration, followed by a relatively slow phase of elimination. In patients with normal renal function, the elimination half-life of pancuronium is 108–147 minutes, and the plasma clearance of the drug is similar to the glomerular filtration rate. By contrast, the clearance of pancuronium is decreased in renal disease, and the elimination half-life is two to five times longer than normal. Clearly, renal excretion of unchanged pancuronium is the most important route of drug elimination; most of the evidence suggests that tubocurarine is preferable to pancuronium in patients with renal failure.

The decline in the plasma concentration of tubocurarine or pancuronium has been interpreted in terms of two- or three-compartment kinetic models. A three-compartment open model has generally been used. The site of action of both drugs is in the central compartment or in a specific compartment, and the amount of drug in this compartment at the time of recovery from neuromuscular block is constant irrespective of the dose. These models have been used to predict the effect of renal failure on the duration of action of muscle relaxants in man. Computer simulation suggests that the effect of small, single doses of tubocurarine will not be modified by renal failure, although the action of large or multiple doses will be prolonged. These predictions are generally consistent with clinical observations.

The kinetics of alcuronium have been studied by radioisotopic methods. After intravenous administration of labelled alcuronium, there is a (slow) initial phase of distribution lasting 1–2 hours, followed by the slow elimination of the drug from plasma. In patients with normal renal function, the elimination half-life of the drug is 3.3 hours (range, 2.0–4.3 hours). By contrast, in a single anuric patient the half-life was 16 hours.

Fazadinium is removed more rapidly from plasma after intravenous administration. The elimination half-life is approximately 76 minutes, although traces of the drug are still detectable after 24 hours. The duration of action of fazadinium may be unrelated to its plasma concentration, and appears to be primarily determined by the rate of drug—receptor dissociation.

Metabolism and elimination of muscle relaxants

Suxamethonium is rapidly hydrolysed by plasma cholinesterase, and is completely removed from blood within 3—5 minutes of intravenous injection. Metabolism of the drug occurs in two distinct stages. Initially, suxamethonium is rapidly converted to succinylmonocholine; this compound, which is much less potent than suxamethonium, is then broken down to choline and succinic acid. Genetic variants in plasma cholinesterase have a profound effect on the duration of action of suxamethonium. In general terms, about 96% of the population have plasma cholinesterase activity within the normal range. Some 3—4% of individuals possess a genotype that produces slower than normal hydrolysis of suxamethonium, resulting in a prolonged action of the drug. Rarely, plasma cholinesterase is entirely absent; in these conditions, neuromuscular block may persist for several hours and the removal of the drug is entirely dependent on adequate renal function.

Low levels of plasma cholinesterase may be caused by liver disease and malnutrition; certain drugs have anticholinesterase actions, while some cytotoxic drugs may inhibit enzyme synthesis. In all these instances, the action of suxamethonium may be prolonged.

Tubocurarine, alcuronium and gallamine are not significantly metabolized, either in experimental animals or in man. Although earlier work suggested that tubocurarine was demethylated or oxidized in certain species, this has not been substantiated. Gallamine is entirely eliminated unchanged in urine, and the drug cannot be identified in bile. Tubocurarine is predominantly eliminated in urine, although 10—12% of the dose is normally present in bile, and is actively secreted from the liver cell into the biliary canaliculus. Minor amounts of alcuronium (10—15%) may also be eliminated in bile. The biliary elimination of muscle relaxants is of considerable clinical significance in patients with reduced or absent renal function. In these conditions, gallamine is excreted to a negligible extent, and prolonged neuromuscular block not antagonized by anticholinesterase drugs ('neostigmine-resistant curarization') may occur. By contrast, in renal failure tubocurarine is eliminated in increased amounts in bile, and its plasma half-life is prolonged by only 40—50%. The potential hazards of gallamine in patients with reduced or absent renal function have restricted its use in current anaesthetic practice.

Both pancuronium and fazadinium are partially metabolized in man. Approximately 20% of pancuronium is eliminated in urine and bile as a hydroxylated metabolite (3-hydroxypancuronium). Two additional metabolites (17-hydroxypancuronium and 3,17-dihydroxypancuronium) have been identified in experimental animals. Approximately 37—44% of pancuronium and its 3-hydroxy metabolite is eliminated in urine and 11%

in bile, although there are large interindividual differences in renal and hepatic elimination. Fazadinium is also mainly excreted unchanged in urine (60–80% within 48 hours). Some 10% or less is metabolized to at least three different products, including a hydroxylated derivative and its glucuronide conjugate. Minor amounts of fazadinium are eliminated in bile.

Binding of muscle relaxants to plasma protein

A variety of *in vitro* techniques (e.g. electrophoresis, equilibrium dialysis and ultrafiltration) have been used to assess the binding of drugs by plasma proteins. Unfortunately, values for the degree of protein binding of muscle relaxants vary widely and appear to be critically dependent on the particular technique employed. Recent evidence suggests that only minor amounts of gallamine and fazadinium (less than 20%) are bound by plasma proteins. By contrast, 30–50% of tubocurarine and 70–80% of pancuronium in plasma may be bound by gammaglobulin (IgG) and by albumin. In consequence, the concentration of these drugs at the motor end-plate may be one-half to one-fifth of their plasma concentration.

Protein binding of muscle relaxants may account for the classical observation that patients with liver disease, bilharziasis, burns or dehydration (in whom IgG levels are raised) may be resistant to tubocurarine. Nevertheless, in these conditions it should be recognized that the bound drug will be gradually released from plasma proteins, and that its duration of action may be prolonged and present problems in reversal. A number of attempts have been made to correlate the dosage requirements of muscle relaxants with the concentration of different plasma proteins. In general, there was a positive correlation between tubocurarine dosage and IgG and between gallamine and alcuronium dosage and albumin. The requirements of pancuronium were not correlated with any fraction. The clinical significance of these results is a matter of conjecture.

Placental transfer of muscle relaxants

Extremely small concentrations of most muscle relaxants (approximately 1–5% of the level in maternal plasma) can be detected in fetal plasma or cord blood after administration to the mother. Fetal apnoea is rarely, if ever, due to transplacental transport of muscle relaxants during caesarian section. Nevertheless, when these drugs are used for prolonged periods in pregnancy (e.g. in the control of status epilepticus or tetanus, or to adapt patients to a pulmonary ventilator), fetal paralysis may occur. Gallamine and alcuronium may be more liable to cross the placental barrier than other relaxants, and their use is best avoided during caesarian section.

INDIVIDUAL MUSCLE RELAXANTS

Suxamethonium

Suxamethonium is a widely used muscle relaxant with a short duration of action which usually lasts 4–6 minutes after an intravenous dose of 50 mg to a 70 kg adult.

Muscle paralysis is due to depolarization of the motor end-plate region. There is no direct evidence that depolarizing drugs impair prejunctional function or reduce transmitter release in man.

If suxamethonium is given repetitively or in an infusion, the nature of the neuromuscular block changes with time and resembles that produced by competitive inhibitors such as tubocurarine. This change in response has been referred to as desensitization, phase II or dual block. The term 'dual block', introduced by Zaimis in 1952 to describe the biphasic response of different species to decamethonium, is perhaps the most appropriate.

Inhibitors of plasma cholinesterase such as neostigmine, pyridostigmine, organophosphorus insecticides, tetrahydroaminacrine (tactrine), hexa-fluorenium and ecothiopate increase and prolong the action of suxa-methonium by delaying its hydrolysis. Some of these drugs have been used to prolong the muscular paralysis produced by suxamethonium but, because such procedures can produce difficulties in clinical practice, it is more reasonable to use a longer acting relaxant of the competitive type.

Procaine prolongs the action of suxamethonium. When the dose of procaine is increased, a greater prolongation of the action of suxamethonium occurs. Higher doses of procaine prevent the hydrolysis of suxamethonium by plasma cholinesterase by displacing it from the enzymatic sites.

Propanidid also prolongs considerably the action of suxamethonium. This is partially due to its anticholinesterase activity. Other mechanisms have been suggested such as a depolarization of the muscle cell membrane which would potentiate the depolarization produced by suxamethonium in the vicinity of the end-plate.

FASCICULATIONS

The intravenous injection of depolarizing agents may give rise to muscle fasciculations and to a transitory increase in height of the muscle twitch elicited by motor-nerve stimulation. These phenomena are well marked with suxamethonium in human patients. Many explanations have been suggested for this preliminary facilitatory effect. They include an anti-dromic response to stimulation of the motor-nerve terminal, and excitation of the first node of Ranvier in the nerve propagating an impulse to the several terminals of the motor nerve. They may also be produced by an increased random motoneuron discharge through partially blocked end-plates due to the increase in afferent discharge from muscle spindles induced by suxamethonium. A postsynaptic action may also be involved because depolarizing drugs are known to produce a contracture of chronically denervated muscle.

Muscle fasciculations may also cause an increase in intragastric pressure.

POSTSUXAMETHONIUM MUSCLE PAINS

Postsuxamethonium muscle pains remain the greatest drawback to the use of this relaxant.

The pains occur chiefly in the subcostal region, shoulder girdle and back, and may be of considerable intensity and indeed disabling. They last for periods ranging from hours to days and in one case they were reported to be present for weeks. The incidence of nearly 70% in ambulant patients is reduced to about 14% in those kept at bed rest for 24 hours. The incidence is approximately seven times greater in subjects unaccustomed to exercise than in those who are used to strenuous physical activity. The pains are more frequent in women and are rare in the first decade of life, but increase in frequency thereafter, reaching the adult incidence at 14 years of age.

The increase in serum creatine phosphokinase following the use of suxamethonium during anaesthesia and the occasional occurrence of myoglobinuria indicate that suxamethonium pains are probably due to muscle damage caused by drug-induced fasciculations, although some investigators have failed to find any correlation between the degree of fasciculation and pain.

A small preceding dose of a muscle relaxant of the competitive type reduces the muscle fasciculations but there remains a small incidence of muscle pains in ambulatory patients.

CARDIAC EFFECTS: THE PATIENT WITH SEVERE BURNS AND NEUROLOGICAL INJURIES

Suxamethonium has muscarinic effects, the most obvious being bradycardia which may be severe after a large single dose or repeated doses or in children. Bradycardia has been reported in over 33% of patients and atrioventricular nodal rhythm in 7% of cases. Caution should therefore be exercised in administering this drug to patients already receiving β-adrenoreceptor blocking agents. Other strong vagal stimulation during the bradycardia caused by high concentrations of irritant vapours and anaesthetic agents such as halothane could also lead to cardiac arrest. Atropine is, to an extent, protective and should always be given, preferably intravenously.

There have been numerous accounts of cardiac arrest following the use of suxamethonium in patients with severe burns. This has been ascribed to vagal overactivity, toxaemia, acidosis and hypovolaemia but evidence has been found of hyperkalaemia in severely burned patients prior to cardiac arrest. Similar findings have been reported in patients with neurological injury. Depolarization produced by suxamethonium is known to liberate potassium from striated muscle but, because hyperkalaemia and the abnormal response to suxamethonium occur only several weeks after injury, it has been suggested that a greater area of muscle membrane is probably being depolarized. Although this could arise during the development of depolarization supersensitivity following denervation, it may not be the entire explanation because some cases of burns lack definite evidence of denervation changes. The hyperkalaemia produced by suxamethonium is antagonized by pretreatment with tubocurarine. As no hyperkalaemia is produced by tubocurarine or gallamine alone, these neuromuscular blocking agents would appear to be the most suitable for use in such patients.

OCULAR EFFECTS

Multiply innervated muscle fibres occur in the extraocular muscles of man. These slow fibres have many discrete end-plates which are probably innervated by one axon. In contrast to fast muscle fibres with a single end-plate which respond to a single impulse with a propagated action potential and twitch, slow fibres cannot propagate action potentials and need a number of impulses to cause contraction. The contraction is slow and maintained; it is in fact a contracture. The development of tension and relaxation is slower than in the fast fibres.

Slow muscle fibres respond to depolarizing drugs such as suxamethonium with a contracture, and the rise in intraocular tension long recognized clinically may be attributed to this. The effect is transient and it is in fact reasonable to use the drug in patients undergoing intraocular procedures. It can be dangerous, however, to use suxamethonium where there is a damaged sclera as in penetrating injuries (see Chapter 63).

In contrast, tubocurarine reduces intraocular tension. The rise in intraocular pressure produced by suxamethonium is antagonized by a previous dose of competitive-type neuromuscular blocking drugs, by an increase in depth of anaesthesia and by hexafluorenium.

Tubocurarine chloride

Tubocurarine chloride, the active alkaloid of *Chondodendron tomentosum*, was the first relaxant to be used clinically and remains the standard by which others are assessed.

This relaxant produces muscle paralysis by competing with receptors on the muscle end-plate for acetylcholine. The drug is therefore best described as a competitive neuromuscular blocking drug rather than a non-depolarizer which relies upon the absence of a pharmacological action to describe a substance, or as an antidepolarizer.

In recent years it has been reported that tubocurarine produces its effect by a presynaptic action. This view has been challenged by many. There is, however, no direct evidence that tubocurarine produces its effect on man other than by a postsynaptic action — that is, by a process of competition for acetylcholine at the motor end-plate.

The elimination and recovery from neuromuscular block produced by tubocurarine are favoured by a low Pa_{CO_2} and, as most anaesthetists overventilate the lungs to some extent, this tends to produce more complete reversal.

The disadvantages of this muscle relaxant clinically are its histamine-releasing properties, ganglion block and, in relation to the other relaxants, its slow onset of action.

The dose used for full curarization is of the order of 0.6 mg·kg^{-1} body weight. In the obese a reduction should be made and in the adult it is seldom necessary to exceed an induction dose of 45 mg. A reduction must also be made in the neonate up to the third or fourth week of life. A dose of 0.25 mg should be given and increments added until the desired effect is achieved. These doses are suitable only if no potentiating inhalational agents are being used, and it is wise to reduce them by one-third if tubocurarine is preceded by suxamethonium during induction. This applies to other drugs which act in the same way as tubocurarine (see Chapter 79).

Gallamine triethiodide

Gallamine triethiodide was the first synthetic competitive inhibitor type of neuromuscular blocking agent to be introduced as a substitute for tubocurarine. It is no longer widely used by clinicians because of its main side-effect of tachycardia, the mechanism of which is unclear. It is also hazardous to use in patients with renal disease or renal failure. Some anaesthetists find it useful with inhalation anaesthetics such as halothane.

The dose of gallamine for induction comparable to that quoted for tubocurarine is 2 mg·kg^{-1} body weight with a reduction to 0.6 mg·kg^{-1} for the neonate. Its speed of onset is greater than that of tubocurarine and its duration shorter. Recovery from the block is delayed in hypocarbia and difficulties in its reversal reported from time to time may be due to this effect.

An advantage of the drug is that it is relatively cheap.

Alcuronium

Tubocurarine is the active principle of that brand of the native arrow poison, curare, stored in hollowed-out bamboo tubes — tube curare. Among the tribes of Amazonian South America are other varieties of curare, which are stored in earthenware pots and calabashes or gourds. It is from the latter that the extremely potent alkaloid 'toxiferene' was extracted. Toxiferene was found to be six to eight times as potent as tubocurarine, lasting two to three times longer. It is reversed by anticholinesterases but because its long action makes recurarization after reversal likely, it has fallen into disfavour.

Diallylnortoxiferene (alcuronium), a synthetic derivative of toxiferene, has a duration similar to tubocurarine but, like toxiferene, it has little histamine-releasing and ganglion-blocking activity. It has been claimed to be more readily and completely reversible than tubocurarine but this remains doubtful. It has been reported that variations in the Pa_{CO_2} of the blood do not affect the duration of the block, but this is difficult to understand as the drug is eliminated through the kidneys and conditions varying renal blood flow should have an effect.

Alcuronium is an acceptable substitute for tubocurarine, although perhaps more work is required to confirm the claims made for it with regard to the absence of side-effects and the effectiveness of anticholinesterases in reversing the action. It occasionally produces the same degree of hypotension as tubocurarine.

Pancuronium

Pancuronium bromide is a *bis*-quaternary ammonium steroid with potent neuromuscular blocking activity of the competitive inhibitor type. It is used to produce muscular relaxation of rapid onset and medium duration in clinical anaesthesia. Although it is a steroid, it is free from hormonal activity. The exact site and mode of action of pancuronium at the neuro-muscular junction are not yet fully elucidated. Experimental studies in animals indicate that it produces neuromuscular block by a pre- and postsynaptic action, but clinical evidence suggests that its main action is postjunctional because of a greater affinity for muscle receptors.

Clinically, pancuronium is about five times as potent as tubocurarine. It has a more rapid onset of action than tubocurarine but the duration of action of both relaxants is similar.

A dose of 0.15 mg·kg^{-1} is recommended for endotracheal intubation. A similar initial dose (0.1 mg·kg^{-1}) would seem to be required, however, if intubation is carried out with suxamethonium and the anaesthesia supplemented with halothane or narcotic agents.

Hypotension following pancuronium is not common because of its low ganglion-blocking activity and the absence of histamine-releasing property. Occasional increases in pulse rate and arterial blood pressure have been reported which are dose-dependent. Although no such changes were found with doses of 0.04 mg·kg^{-1}, a significant increase in pulse rate, arterial blood pressure, stroke volume and cardiac output have been reported to occur after 0.07 mg·kg^{-1}. This may be due to the drug releasing adrenaline and noradrenaline from the adrenal medulla.

There is experimental evidence that halothane—adrenaline arrhythmias in the dog are reduced in severity and duration by pancuronium, but this requires further study.

The absence of hypotension following the use of pancuronium is a particular advantage in cardiac surgery, and the absence of histamine release makes it justifiable for use in asthmatic patients.

Fazadinium

Fazadinium bromide is a potent member of a series of azopyridinium compounds.

This relaxant has the characteristic features of a competitive neuro-muscular-blocking drug such as tubocurarine but with an onset of action nearly as rapid as suxamethonium. The duration of action is shorter than that of pancuronium and tubocurarine. Fazadinium has approximately only one-half of the neuromuscular-blocking potency of tubocurarine.

The termination of the neuromuscular-blocking action of fazadinium is largely independent of the plasma concentration and depends on the rate of dissociation of the drug from cholinergic receptor sites at the motor end-plate.

Muscular paralysis after fazadinium is reversed with neostigmine approximately as fast as that following tubocurarine.

Fazadinium may cause a mild tachycardia and hypotension although some cases of hypertension have also been reported after its use. The hypotension is probably due to the mild ganglion-blocking activity of the drug.

There is little clinical evidence that fazadinium causes histamine release in man, although care should be exercised when considering its use in asthmatics. Local irritation, possibly due to histamine release, has been reported after the intravenous use of fazadinium, particularly in children.

FACTORS AFFECTING THE ACTIVITY OF MUSCLE RELAXANTS IN MAN

Many factors (e.g. age, the concurrent administration of other drugs, body temperature, extracellular pH, genetic abnormalities and neuro-muscular disease) may influence the response to muscle relaxants in man. Some of these factors are considered in detail in other chapters.

Age

Neonatal infants are generally resistant to depolarizing drugs and more sensitive to competitive neuromuscular block (particularly during the first few days of life). In early life, suxamethonium may induce some characteristics of competitive antagonism; for instance, children rarely fasciculate before the age of 10. The explanation for this phenomenon is obscure; both changes in end-plate sensitivity and altered drug kinetics may be involved. There is no evidence that the response to muscle relaxants is affected by advancing age.

Administration of other drugs

Many other drugs may affect the response to muscle relaxants in man. Any compound with anticholinesterase properties will prolong the effect of suxamethonium and tend to antagonize competitive neuromuscular block. Drugs that modify acid—base balance may affect neuromuscular block; in particular, compounds that induce metabolic or respiratory acidosis will intensify the effect of tubocurarine (as discussed below). Many drugs (e.g. steroids, antacids, chelating agents and most diuretics) may modify the plasma concentration of potassium, calcium or magnesium; in these conditions, altered reactions to muscle relaxants have been reported. Several antibiotics (in particular, neomycin and the amino-glycosides) may produce or enhance competitive block in susceptible patients, possibly by inducing hypocalcaemia or by influencing the binding of calcium at presynaptic sites. However, antibiotic-induced block is not invariably reversed by calcium salts or by anticholinesterase drugs. Most local anaesthetic drugs and drugs with local anaesthetic properties (e.g. quinidine, phenothiazines, propranolol and diphenylhydantoin) may also enhance competitive block.

General anaesthetics may profoundly influence the degree of competitive neuromuscular block. Ether has long been known to potentiate non-depolarizing relaxants, and halothane (1—2%) potentiates the action of tubocurarine and pancuronium on the motor end-plate. Similar effects are produced by other halogenated anaesthetics (viz. fluroxene, methoxyflurane and isoflurane). The mechanism responsible for this interaction is obscure, although indirect evidence suggests that presynaptic and haemodynamic effects may be involved.

Body temperature

The effect of muscle and body temperature on the potency and duration of action of muscle relaxants is a matter of controversy. Approximately 20 years ago, it was shown that hypothermia increased the magnitude and duration of depolarization block but diminished the response to competitive block. More recent evidence has not confirmed these results. Indeed, any effect of body temperature on either depolarizing or competitive block may be mediated by changes in regional blood flow induced by hypothermia. Reduction in body temperature decreases the renal, hepatic and biliary elimination of competitive muscle relaxants; in these conditions, reduced doses may be required to produce a given degree of neuromuscular block. Clinical evidence is consistent with the view that the requirements of competitive muscle relaxants are decreased during moderate hypothermia.

Plasma and extracellular pH

Alterations in plasma and extracellular pH may modify the potency and duration of action of muscle relaxants. In particular, hypoventilation and respiratory acidosis undoubtedly augment and enhance tubocurarine block and oppose its reversal by neostigmine. The effects of metabolic acidosis and alkalosis are inconsistent and difficult to evaluate; both increased and decreased potency have been reported. Changes in plasma pH affect the activity of other muscle relaxants in a different manner. The effect of gallamine is potentiated and prolonged by alkalosis although its plasma concentration is not significantly altered. Alcuronium and pancuronium block is usually unaffected by variations in Pa_{CO_2}, although suxamethonium may be potentiated by acidosis.

A great deal of accurate and careful investigation is needed to confirm these findings, which are difficult to explain by any one hypothesis. A number of explanations have been advanced to account for the variation in tubocurarine block produced by acid—base disturbances; the effects of pH on (1) protein binding, (2) the ionization of the tertiary group ($pK_a = 8.0$) and the two hydroxyl groups ($pK_a = 8.0$ and 9.3) (*Figure 16.1*) and (3) receptor ionization may be important factors. Changes in the ionization of acetylcholinesterase and the reduction of renal blood flow by low Pa_{CO_2} levels have also been incriminated.

Genetic factors

The effect of genetic abnormalities in plasma cholinesterase on the duration of action of suxamethonium is considered in detail in Chapter 46.

Neuromuscular disease

Patients with myasthenia gravis are extremely sensitive to competitive neuromuscular-blocking agents, but resistant to depolarizing drugs. Both phenomena have been used as diagnostic tests in myasthenic patients. The differential effects of competitive and depolarizing drugs in myasthenia are partially due to the presence of antibodies to acetylcholine receptors at the motor end-plate; in these conditions, the end-plate potential induced by acetylcholine release is diminished, so that the effects of competitive agents are enhanced. In myasthenia gravis, different muscle groups are affected to a varying extent, and the reaction to muscle relaxants may be extremely variable. Nevertheless, the use of all muscle relaxants should be avoided in all myasthenic patients undergoing surgery (including thymectomy). In these circumstances, competitive agents may induce prolonged postoperative curarization. Large doses of suxamethonium may be required to produce muscle relaxation, and the elimination of the drug may be retarded by concurrent anticholinesterase therapy.

In some myopathies (e.g. dystrophia myotonica and myotonia congenita), suxamethonium produces prolonged muscle contraction. Abnormal responses to muscle relaxants may occur in the Eaton—Lambert syndrome, but are unusual in other neurological or muscle disorders.

The action of muscle relaxants on the motor end-plate and neuromuscular transmission is discussed in Chapter 15. Nevertheless, some muscle relaxants may produce additional effects (particularly on the cardiovascular system).

OTHER PHARMACOLOGICAL EFFECTS

Histamine release

Certain drugs (particularly those containing tertiary amine groups) release histamine from mast cells in tissues into the circulation, and it has been recognized for over 40 years that tubocurarine is particularly potent in this respect. In the past, insufficient attention has been paid to the marked species difference shown by animals in their sensitivity to histamine, and evidence adduced from dog or guinea-pig experiments is likely to be fallacious when applied to man. In clinical practice the problem has been investigated by measuring wealing of the skin when different relaxants are injected intradermally, and by measuring plasma histamine levels after intra-arterial injection of tubocurarine. After intravenous administration of the drug during clinical anaesthesia, local vasodilatation and wealing, a slight increase in airway resistance and some degree of hypotension are not uncommon. Occasionally, severe anaphylactoid responses are observed.

Histamine release is much less common with other relaxant drugs. It is occasionally observed with gallamine, and isolated cases of broncho-constriction have been reported with alcuronium and pancuronium.

Many experienced anaesthetists do not consider histamine liberation a hazard, even when tubocurarine is given to asthmatic patients; nevertheless, when significant asthma is present, and certainly in status asthmaticus, tubocurarine should not be used when such acceptable alternative relaxants are available.

Actions at autonomic ganglia

Since muscle relaxants are quaternary amines, their affinity for cholinergic receptors may produce effects on autonomic ganglia where acetylcholine is the transmitter. Tubocurarine is the most active and induces a moderate degree of ganglionic block; similar but less marked effects are evoked by alcuronium. Minor effects are produced by other muscle relaxants. Gallamine and fazadinium may induce slight ganglionic blockade of no clinical significance.

Actions on the cardiovascular system

Relaxant doses of tubocurarine (45 mg) produce moderate hypotension, and both systolic and diastolic blood pressure usually fall by 20—30 mmHg. Hypotension is probably due to both histamine release and sympathetic ganglion blockade. Reflex tachycardia is extremely rare, suggesting that ganglion blockade may be the important factor.

Pancuronium and alcuronium usually have little effect on either heart rate or blood pressure. Severe hypotensive responses to both drugs are extremely uncommon, although they have been recorded. Pancuronium may cause a slight rise in pulse rate and blood pressure (possibly due to ganglionic stimulation).

Gallamine and, to a lesser extent, fazadinium characteristically induce tachycardia (usually 90—100 beats per minute). Pulse rates higher than 120 beats per minute are extremely uncommon, even after large doses of these relaxants. Gallamine-induced tachycardia has been attributed to the atropine-like action of the drug (although intravenous atropine invariably causes a further increase in heart rate). Recent experimental evidence suggests that gallamine and fazadinium may reduce the affinity of the sinoatrial node to acetylcholine, thus accounting for the atropine-sensitive tachycardia induced by these two relaxants. Gallamine and fazadinium have little or no effect on blood pressure. Due to their action on heart rate, both drugs are best avoided in cardiac surgery and in patients with hypertension or ischaemic heart disease.

Suxamethonium usually produces a minor increase in blood pressure and some degree of bradycardia, particularly in children. Cardiac arrhythmias (e.g. atrioventricular nodal rhythm) may also be induced. It is unclear whether these effects are due to a direct action on the SA node, to hyperkalaemia or to other factors.

REVERSAL OF NEUROMUSCULAR BLOCK

Neostigmine and atropine are most usually employed to antagonize competitive neuromuscular block. In these conditions, the muscarinic effects of neostigmine are adequately controlled and its duration of action is usually sufficiently long to avoid recurarization with relaxants in common use (except, perhaps, in renal failure). Although anaesthetic practice varies, most anaesthetists use neostigmine methylsulphate $(0.07 \text{ mg·kg}^{-1}$; maximum dose, 5.0 mg) and atropine sulphate $(0.02 \text{ mg·kg}^{-1}$; maximum dose, 1.5 mg) to antagonize standard doses of tubocurarine (0.6 mg·kg^{-1}), pancuronium $(0.12 \text{ mg·kg}^{-1})$ or other relaxants.

Both drugs are usually mixed in the same syringe and administered simultaneously; in these circumstances, significant bradycardia or tachycardia is unusual and maximal reversal occurs within 5–10 minutes. The effect of atropine on the heart usually precedes the muscarinic effects of neostigmine by 1–2 minutes. Titration of atropine against neostigmine, by observing the effects of the drugs on pulse rate, is usually unnecessary, but may be prudent in patients with a previous history of cardiovascular disease. Some anaesthetists prefer to give half the dose of atropine some minutes before the remaining dose of atropine and neostigmine in order to reduce the salivation and gut contraction which follow neostigmine administration. During the injection of these potentially dangerous drugs it is important to ensure that pulmonary ventilation is sufficient to ensure full oxygenation and to avoid hypercarbia.

To ensure good reversal there must be some return of muscle tone before neostigmine is given; indeed, it should not be administered less than half an hour after full doses of any of the commonly used muscle relaxants, unless there is pronounced muscle activity. If necessary, reversal should be delayed and pulmonary ventilation continued until there are signs of returning muscle tone; for instance, decreasing total chest compliance in the presence of a clear airway, attempts at spontaneous breathing or movement in response to sensory stimuli.

In the USA, pyridostigmine has been used as an alternative to neostigmine for the reversal of neuromuscular block. It has a longer latency and duration of action than neostigmine, and generally produces less marked muscarinic effects. It has no significant advantages over neostigmine except in certain specialized circumstances (e.g. reversal in atropine-sensitive patients and possibly in renal failure).

Assessment of adequate reversal

The clinical signs of residual curarization are facial weakness (ptosis, lack of expression and loss of tone in the masseters), inability to raise the head and hold it up for 5 seconds, inability to protrude the tongue and loss of a firm, sustained handgrip. However, these cannot be observed unless the patient has recovered from the anaesthetic. Tracheal tug and any paradoxical indrawing of the intercostal muscles during inspiration in the presence of a clear airway and in the absence of any central nervous, cardiac or pulmonary cause very strongly suggest residual curarization and should always be treated as such.

The use of a peripheral nerve stimulator may be helpful, although the signs elicited in the semiconscious patient are often equivocal. The use of these stimulators to distinguish between depolarizing and competitive block by the elicitation of tetanic fade and post-tetanic decurarization is largely of theoretical interest, as persistent block is almost always competitive.

More sophisticated means of detecting minor degrees of myoneural block entail the use of a square wave stimulator and some method of recording the evoked isometric muscle twitch or electromyogram. The twitch or the compound muscle action potential evoked in the adductor pollicis by supramaximal stimulation of the ulnar nerve is usually recorded. These two parameters of neuromuscular function are not strictly comparable; in expert hands, measurement of the compound action potential by electromyography is probably the best method of assessing the effects of muscle relaxants and their antagonists. In partially curarized patients, a train of stimuli (0.1–0.2 ms duration) should be given at a frequency of 2–5 Hz; in these conditions, the maximum depression is observed at the fourth stimulus. The ratio of the amplitude of the last response to the train of four stimuli expressed as a percentage of that of the first is a useful method of measuring objectively the degree of curarization. Comparative measurements have shown that head lifting for 5 seconds is possible when there is 80% recovery of neuromuscular block, as assessed by the ratio of the fourth to the first twitch evoked by the train of four stimuli. At this stage adequate respiratory function is restored.

Actions and kinetics of neostigmine

Neostigmine probably reverses the effects of competitive muscle relaxants by inhibiting junctional acetylcholinesterase. After an initial phase of reversible inhibition, the enzyme is converted to a carbamylated derivative which is slowly hydrolysed; the half-life of recovery of the inhibited enzyme is 37 minutes. Most of the available evidence suggests that the antagonism of neuromuscular block is primarily due to the action of acetylcholine at postsynaptic receptor sites. Thus, when acetylcholinesterase is inhibited, acetylcholine released from the motor-nerve ending accumulates in the synaptic cleft and displaces competitive muscle relaxants from their site of action on the postsynaptic membrane. The role of prejunctional receptors associated with the motor-nerve terminal in the reversal of neuromuscular block is controversial. Undoubtedly, receptors for acetylcholine are present at the motor-nerve ending and at the first node of Ranvier, and they are responsive to both competitive and depolarizing drugs. Acetylcholinesterase is also present at presynaptic sites. Although some authors consider that the nerve terminal is the main site of action of both neuromuscular blocking drugs and their antagonists, this view has not been generally accepted.

After intravenous injection in man, the plasma concentration of neostigmine falls in a bi-exponential manner. There is a rapid fall between 2 and 5 minutes, when the concentration of the drug is only 8% of its initial value. The level then declines more slowly, and traces of neostigmine can be detected in plasma for at least an hour. In consequence, the distribution half-life of the drug is less than 1 minute, while the elimination half-life is 15–30 minutes. When the data are interpreted in terms of a two-compartment kinetic model, the drug does not appear to act in either the central or the peripheral compartment. The time of maximal reversal in man (5–10 minutes after intravenous administration) may reflect the relatively slow access of neostigmine to a small subcompartment that cannot be distinguished kinetically from either the central or the peripheral compartment. Its relatively long duration of action, which far outlasts its clearance from plasma and usually prevents residual curarization, probably reflects the slow hydrolysis of the inhibited enzyme within the synaptic space.

Further reading

Ali, H. H. and Savarese, J. J. (1976). Monitoring of neuromuscular function. *Anesthesiology* 45, 216–249

Ali, H. H., Utting, J. E. and Gray, T. C. (1971). Quantitative assessment of residual anti-depolarising block (Part I). *Br. J. Anaesth.* 43, 473–477

Buckett, W. R. (1975). Steroidal neuromuscular blocking drugs in man. *Adv. Drug Res.* 10, 53–92

Buzello, W. and Agoston, S. (1978). Kinetics of intercompartmental disposition and excretion of tubocurarine, gallamine, alcuronium and pancuronium in patients with normal and impaired renal function. *Anaesthesist* 27, 319–321

Feldman, S. A. (1973). *Muscle Relaxants*, pp. 1–190. London: W. B. Saunders

Galindo, A. (1972). The role of prejunctional effects in myoneural transmission. *Anesthesiology* 36, 598–608

Katz, R. L. (1973). Electromyographic and mechanical effects of suxamethonium and tubocurarine on twitch, tetanic and post-tetanic responses. *Br. J. Anaesth.* 45, 849–859

Katz, R. L. and Ryan, J. F. (1969). The neuromuscular effects of suxamethonium in man. *Br. J. Anaesth.* 41, 381–390

MacLagan, J. (1976). Competitive neuro-muscular blocking drugs. *Handbuch der Experimentellen Pharmakologie*, Vol. 42, pp. 421–486. Berlin: Springer-Verlag

Miller, R. D. (1976). Antagonism of neuro-muscular blockade. *Anesthesiology* 44, 318–329

Smith, S. E. (1976). Neuromuscular blocking drugs in man. *Handbuch der Experimentellen Pharmakologie*, Vol. 42, pp. 593–660. Berlin: Springer-Verlag

Speight, T. M. and Avery, G. S. (1972). Pancuronium bromide: a review of its pharmacological properties and clinical application. *Drugs* 4, 163–226

II Principles of conduction anaesthesia

17 Pharmacology and toxicity of local anaesthetics
I.C. Geddes

General anaesthesia had been in clinical use for 38 years before local anaesthesia was shown to be possible. Carl Koller in 1884 was working with Sigmund Freud in Vienna. At that time cocaine was being used to treat a physician for morphine addiction. Cocaine is an alkaloid obtained from the leaves of a shrub, *Ethythroxylum coca,* cultivated for centuries by Indians high in the Andes of Peru. The prepared leaves were chewed with the addition of alkali for the cerebral stimulating properties of the active principle erythroxylon. It was well known that the application of cocaine to the tongue produced numbness, but it was Koller who followed this observation by experiments on animals to show that this loss of sensation could be of value for surgery on the eye. These findings were announced at an ophthalmological meeting in Heidelberg. Within a year of the topical use of cocaine, it had been used in over 1000 surgical operations by Halstead (1885) and many other surgeons. Unfortunately, the toxicity of cocaine was not appreciated and by 1890 Falk had collected 176 cases of acute intoxication from cocaine, of which 10 were fatal. Addiction was also another problem associated with the use of cocaine. Olch (1975) gives an account of Halstead's personal difficulties with cocaine.

CHEMICAL STRUCTURE (*Figure 17.1*)

Esters

Cocaine is the benzyl derivative of the methyl ester of ecgonine. It was found that the tropane ring was not essential for local anaesthetic activity and this encouraged the synthesis of simpler compounds.

The ester procaine was introduced by Einhorn in 1905 (Einhorn and Uhlfelder, 1909) and became the most widely used local anaesthetic for well over half a century. Its principal attributes were high water solubility, reasonable stability in solution, compatibility with adrenaline, acceptable margin of safety for clinical use and lack of irritation on injection.

Agent	Chemical configuration			Physicochemical properties			
	Aromatic (lipophilic)	Intermediate chain	Amine (hydrophilic)	Partition coefficient	Protein binding (%)	pK$_a$	Relative potency
Esters							
Procaine	H_2N–(ring)	COO CH$_2$ CH$_2$	–N(C$_2$H$_5$)(C$_2$H$_5$)	0.6	5.8	8.9	1
Amethocaine	H_9C_4–N(H)–(ring)	COO CH$_2$ CH$_2$	–N(CH$_3$)(CH$_3$)	80.0	75.0	8.5	4
Amides							
Mepivacaine (Carbocaine)	(ring with CH$_3$, CH$_3$)	NHCO	piperidine N–CH$_3$	12.0	65.0	7.69	1
Bupivacaine (Marcain)	(ring with CH$_3$, CH$_3$)	NHCO	piperidine N–C$_4$H$_9$	130.0	84.0	8.05	4
Lignocaine (Xylocaine)	(ring with CH$_3$, CH$_3$)	NHCO CH$_2$	–N(C$_2$H$_5$)(C$_2$H$_5$)	3.6	55.0	7.87	1
Prilocaine (Citanest)	(ring with CH$_3$)	NHCOCH–CH$_3$	–N(H)(C$_3$H$_7$)		66.0	7.89	1
Etidocaine (Duranest)	(ring with CH$_3$, CH$_3$)	NHCOCH–C$_2$H$_5$	–N(C$_2$H$_5$)(C$_3$H$_7$)	191.0	94.0	7.74	4

Amides

LIGNOCAINE

In 1943, in Sweden, Lofgren w⸱s investigating the substance responsible for causing a haemorrhagic disease in animals fed spoilt hay during the long northern winters. Lofgren tasted one of the suspected compounds and observed that his tongue was anaesthetized. After considerable work involving the synthesis of allied compounds and testing them for local anaesthetic activity, lignocaine was made available to clinicians. A full report of these studies was presented by Lofgren (1948). Lignocaine was the prototype of a whole series of amides with local anaesthetic activity.

Lignocaine is now the most extensively used local anaesthetic. Apart from procaine and amethocaine, the local anaesthetics in common use are all of the amide type: lignocaine, mepivacaine, prilocaine, bupivacaine and etidocaine.

Guanidines

Naturally occurring substances containing guanidine have potent local anaesthetic properties.

Tetrodotoxin originates in the pufferfish found in the seas surrounding Japan, and saxitoxin comes from dinoflagellates which are found in excess numbers in sea water at certain times of the year. They contaminate shellfish and, if these are then eaten, cause paralysis and death in man. Both these toxins are strong bases due to the presence of guanidine, and are extremely potent as local anaesthetics.

Structure activity relationships

A common chemical pattern present in clinically useful local anaesthetics is: aromatic group — intermediate chain — amine group. The aromatic group gives lipophilic properties and the amine group is hydrophilic. The intermediate chain is usually either an ester or an amide. The ester linkage can be hydrolysed by esterases, while the amide group is resistant and can only be broken down by enzymes found in the liver.

Modification of chemical structure alters the local anaesthetic activity and physical properties of the molecule. Lengthening of the intermediate chain or addition to the number of carbon atoms on the aromatic or amine group results in an increase in potency up to a maximum, when any futher increase in molecular weight is followed by a loss of local anaesthetic activity.

Procaine and amethocaine are both esters of para-aminobenzoic acid. The addition of a butyl group to the aromatic end of the procaine molecule increases lipid solubility markedly and also gives a tenfold increase in protein binding. There is also increased duration of local anaesthetic activity and systemic toxicity which is typically seen in amethocaine. Similarly, the substitution of a butyl group for the methyl group on the amine of mepivacaine gives bupivacaine greater anaesthetic potency and a prolonged duration of anaesthesia. There is also an increase in lipid solubility and a significantly greater degree of protein binding when compared with mepivacaine.

Etidocaine bears a similar relationship with lignocaine. Here a propyl group has been substituted for an ethyl group at the amine end, with the addition of an ethyl group on the α carbon of the intermediate chain of lignocaine. There is a 50-fold increase in the lipid solubility of etidocaine and much greater protein binding. The duration of anaesthesia and of anaesthetic potency are also significantly increased.

The chemical structure of local anaesthetics influences their rate of degradation and subsequent toxicity. The ester group derived from benzoic acid are all hydrolysed in plasma by the enzyme cholinesterase (Brodie, Lief and Poet, 1948). However, since the liver is also rich in esterases it, too, plays a significant role in the breakdown of these local anaesthetics. White, Dearborn and Swiss (1955) demonstrated in dogs that half or more of a dose of procaine was destroyed in the liver, which also had the ability to bind procaine and thus remove it from the general circulation.

Allergy to local anaesthetics

Aldrete and Johnson (1969), using intracutaneous injections, showed that there was a cross-reaction between local anaesthetics derived from para-aminobenzoic acid. That this was due to the presence of the metabolite para-aminobenzoic acid was confirmed by observations made by Gaul (1955), who reported cross-sensitization from para-aminobenzoic acid used to absorb the damaging rays from the sun in sunburn lotions. It is now accepted that the amide group of local anaesthetics are not associated with allergic reactions. However, when some multidose ampoules of lignocaine have been used, allergic reactions have been reported. Aldrete and Johnson (1969) have shown that this was associated with the presence of methyl hydroxybenzoate (methylparaben), related to para-aminobenzoic acid, used as a preservative in these solutions.

STRUCTURE OF NERVES

Peripheral nerves are made up of myelinated and non-myelinated fibres which belong to the nerve cell and its processes, the dendrites and the axon or axis cylinder. The axon is dependent upon its connection with the nerve cell for nutrition and contains mitochondria, microtubules and neurofilaments. Non-myelinated fibres are surrounded by a single wrapping of a Schwann cell sheath which is shared by groups of axons.

Myelinated nerves are enclosed in spirally wrapped layers of lipoprotein, the myelin sheath, derived from specialized Schwann cells. The outermost layer of myelin is composed of the Schwann cell and its nucleus. The myelinated nerves are insulated by the myelin sheath, which is impermeable to local anaesthetics. The events accompanying an impulse only take place at the nodes of Ranvier, which are spaced at regular intervals along the nerve. The internodal distance is proportional to the diameter of the fibre. The exposed myelin-free parts of the membrane surface have a width of approximately 0.5 μm and a surface area of approximately 4 μm². At the nodes, extracellular fluid is in contact with the membrane surrounding the area. The myelin sheath effectively prevents migration of ions except at the nodes. Since conduction in a nerve is dependent upon an action potential with its associated ionic flux, this can take place only in myelinated nerves across the membrane at the node.

When dyes are applied to myelinated nerves, it is only at the nodes that they enter and diffuse along the fibres. Using methylene blue, it is possible to demonstrate that nodes are also present in the central nervous system.

The size of the individual Schwann cell fixes the distance separating nodes in a myelinated nerve. The larger the nerve, the greater the distance between nodes, and this can be up to 2 mm in the largest nerves.

Since extracellular fluid is in contact with the axon membrane at the nodes, the current in myelinated nerves can flow from one node to the next, or may jump the distance equal to two or even three nodes. This jumping from node to node is called saltatory conduction. Its function is to permit an extremely efficient fast conduction of the electrical impulse with the expenditure of much less energy than would otherwise be required.

Tasaki (1953) demonstrated with single medullated nerve fibres that, if one node was blocked by local anaesthetic, the impulse could jump this node and thus no block in conduction was seen. For a nerve to be completely blocked, it was necessary to expose at least two and preferably three successive nodes in a myelinated fibre. There is thus a minimal length of nerve which must be exposed to local anaesthetic solution at a concentration above the minimal effective concentration before complete block occurs. Smaller nerves have short internodal distances while larger nerves with longer distances between nodes may, in the largest nerves, have to be exposed to a local anaesthetic for up to 5—6 mm. Franz and Perry (1974) confirmed these observations.

In non-myelinated nerves there is a similar state for potential changes required to cause depolarization, and passage of an impulse can be observed to occur some 3—5 mm ahead of the action potential.

When a nerve is stimulated and an action potential recorded by means of a cathode ray oscilloscope, the recording is the sum of the action potentials of all the individual neurons and is known as a 'compound action potential'. A full analysis of electrophysiology of nerve conduction and local anaesthesia is given by de Jong and Wagman (1963).

An action potential is dependent on there being a separation in time between the activation of the sodium and the potassium conductances (Jack, 1975). When the action potential rises rapidly, the sodium conductance is about ten times larger than for potassium conductance. When a decrease in the action potential occurs, this is associated with a slowing of sodium conductance and there is then less difference between it and the potassium conductance, which ultimately leads to insufficient 'local circuit' current and the action potential is not propagated.

Differential nerve fibre block (*Table 17.1*)

Franz and Perry (1974) examined single nerve fibres in nerves exposed to local anaesthetic solution over different lengths. If the nerve was exposed for 4 mm or more, all fibres were blocked by 0.2% procaine. If, however, the nerve was exposed for only 2 mm, Aδ fibres could be blocked completely without any block of Aα fibres. Here most of the Aδ fibres with a 0.3–0.7 mm internodal length will have at least three nodes blocked but few of the Aα fibres (0.8–1.4 mm internodal length) will have more than one node blocked. This concept can also explain the differential rate

TABLE 17.1. Classification of nerve fibres

Group	Fibre diameter (μm)	Conduction velocity (m·s^{-1})	Resistance to block by local anaesthetics	Function	
A (myelinated)					
α	12.22	95*(62.5)†	Highest	Motor:	Efferent muscle movement
β	‡	19*		Motor:	Afferent proprioception light touch
γ	‡	‡		Motor:	Efferent only to muscle spindles
δ	1–12	10–20	Intermediate	Sensory:	Afferent pain, temperature, touch
B (thinly myelinated)	<3	10–20	Intermediate	Autonomic:	Efferent preganglionic
C (non-myelinated)	0.2–1.5	0.5–2.0	Lowest	Sensory:	Dorsal roots Peripheral nerves Pain, temperature, touch
				Autonomic:	Postganglionic Sympathetic

Conduction velocity in metres per second is approximately equal to six times the over-all fibre diameter including the myelin sheath. *cat; †man; ‡no data given (de Jong and Wagman, 1963).

All group A fibres are further characterized by the similarity of their action potential, length of refractory period, and nature and duration of their after potentials. These are all different in group B and C fibres. The after potentials are relatively small, slow electrical changes of the nerve membrane, which may be either positive or negative, occurring after an action potential. In both A and certain C fibres the after potentials are negative for a period and then display a longer lasting positive potential. The B fibres have only positive after potentials. These after potentials are probably related to membrane metabolic activity after conduction. A negative after potential is associated with increased excitability and a positive one with lowered excitability (Bernhard, 1958).

of blocking of nerves. As the anaesthetic diffuses through the nerve bundle, a minimal effective concentration not only penetrates inwards to block the smaller axons first but also diffuses laterally to involve the nodes in the larger myelinated nerves.

It is harder to explain differential block for the non-myelinated nerves, but once again there is separation of potential changes and the area of depolarization of these nerves. This means that the potential changes precede depolarization by some 3—5 mm and thus it is necessary for the local anaesthetic to blanket the non-myelinated nerve for at least this minimal length to prevent depolarization.

The clinical importance of differential block is that, when low concentrations of local anaesthetics are used, C fibres and small and medium sized A fibres are blocked with loss of sensation for pain and temperature. However, since touch, proprioception and motor function are still present, the patient may feel the surgeon's knife but not experience actual pain. In an anxious patient, any sensation may be expected to be misinterpreted as pain and the local anaesthetic could be claimed to have failed. Complete block, including motor nerves, requires twice the minimal analgesic concentration of local anaesthetic.

MECHANISMS OF NERVE BLOCK

Conduction in nerves is dependent on ionic flow through selective 'channels' in nerve membranes. At rest the electrical potential inside the nerve membrane is negative relative to that outside. Sodium ions are at a higher concentration in the extracellular fluid outside the nerve membrane. The passage of a nerve impulse is associated with an alteration in the permeability of the membrane. Sodium ions enter the axon through sodium selective channels which open and close as the electrical potential alters. These sodium channels are linked to the distribution of lipoprotein in the membrane. Potassium channels also exist and these play an important role during repolarization of the nerves but, unlike the sodium channels, are not affected by local anaesthetics.

The radius of hydrated K^+ and Cl^- ions is approximately 0.2 nm while the hydrated Na^+ ion is larger, being 0.34 nm.

Membranes and local anaesthetic agents

To fulfil its vital functions, a biologically active membrane must operate differentially on the two compartments it separates. It must be asymmetrical and the outer surface must differ from the inner one. The nerve membrane surrounding the axon is about 10 nm thick. Whilst a lot of detailed information is available concerning the major phospholipid classes (Meymaris, 1975), less is known of the proteins present.

Proteolytic enzymes, such as pronase, have been used to study the role of proteins in nerve membranes. Tetrodotoxin binds at the outer openings of the sodium channels whether they are open or shut. If, however, the nerves are previously exposed to proteolytic enzymes this binding is inhibited. This suggests that the binding takes place with proteins which form the outer openings of the sodium channels.

Fluorescent probes

Fluorescent probes are chemicals which fluoresce when they come into contact with proteins. Their value in studying the dynamics of excitable membranes has been reviewed by Waggoner (1976). These fluorescent probes have been used to identify the binding sites for the different compounds which possess local anaesthetic activity. Tasaki, Watanabe and Hallet (1972) studied the effect of tetrodotoxin in the presence of fluorescent chemicals and found that there was suppression of the initial component of the fluorescent signal when depolarizing clamping pulses were applied to the nerves. Here is a non-invasive method of following the interaction of local anaesthetic agents and nerve protein, which is a powerful research tool. Using similar techniques, Wagner and Ulbricht (1976) demonstrated on single myelinated frog nerves that saxitoxin and procaine blocked the sodium channel by binding to separate and independent protein receptor sites. From their data they eliminated any possibility of competitive block being present. They concluded that the saxitoxin site of action was most likely situated near the external mouth of the sodium channel, while the procaine site was located on the internal aspect of the channel near the axon.

Model membranes

Papahadjopoulous (1972) used phospholipid membranes to study the mechanism of action of local anaesthetics. These model membranes have the advantage of having known chemical composition, but their very simplicity is also a handicap. Skou (1954a, b, c) used monomolecular layers of lipids and observed increases in the surface pressure from local anaesthetics which appeared to depend on the uncharged form of the molecule since they were more effective in alkaline conditions.

Effect of pH

Trevan and Booch (1927) drew attention to the importance of pH on the molecular form of local anaesthetics. Since they are tertiary amines, they can exist in a charged or uncharged form.

$$
\begin{array}{ccc}
\quad \text{R} & \qquad\qquad & \text{R} \\
\quad | & & | \\
\text{R} - \text{N}^+ - \text{H} & \qquad\qquad & \text{R} - \text{N} \quad + \text{H}^+ \\
\quad | & & | \\
\quad \text{R} & & \text{R}
\end{array}
$$

The greater the alkalinity of the solution, the more uncharged or free base is present. The pK_a is defined as being equal to the pH at which the solution contains equal proportions of charged and uncharged molecules.

The pK_a of currently used local anaesthetics lies between 7.7 and 8.5. The more alkaline the pH of the solution, the greater is the proportion of the uncharged form present. Alkaline solutions of local anaesthetics go cloudy due to the presence of free base which is insoluble in water. Commercial solutions of local anaesthetics are always acid. This is important if adrenaline is present, for it is unstable at alkaline pH.

Skou (1958) found that local anaesthetics were more effective in alkaline solutions and this conclusion was generally accepted up till the 1960s. The un-ionized form of the local anaesthetic is essential for penetration of membranes to reach the site of local anaesthetic action, since the ionized form is unable to penetrate tissue barriers. However, when experiments were carried out with desheathed nerve preparations (Ritchie, Ritchie and Greengard, 1965a, b), a less alkaline local anaesthetic solution, which contained a greater amount of charged cation (BH^+), was found to have an increased local anaesthetic activity. It was thus suggested that both the un-ionized base (B) and the ionized cationic form (BH^+) are important for local anaesthetic activity.

Effect of carbon dioxide

It has been known for many years that carbon dioxide can increase the speed of onset of nerve block. Catchlove (1972) has suggested that since carbon dioxide can rapidly cross membranes, the pH is lowered at the axoplasmic surface. The receptor located here is thus exposed to a higher concentration of local anaesthetic in the cationic form. Bromage (1965) found confirmation of this in epidural anaesthesia where latency of action and the quality of block were much improved when carbonated salts of lignocaine and prilocaine were used.

Membrane expansion theory and local anaesthetics

During anaesthesia the components of the membrane are expanded and disordered due to the presence of volatile anaesthetics. Johnson and Miller (1970) and Halsey and Wardley-Smith (1975) were able to demonstrate reversal with recovery from general anaesthesia by compression to pressures over 100 atm absolute. It has been suggested by Seeman (1972) that a similar mechanism might be responsible for local anaesthetic action where the presence of local anaesthetic drug in the membrane would distort the sodium pore, giving rise to nerve block. Kendig and Cohen (1977) performed experiments with the preganglionic sympathetic nerve of the superior cervical ganglion of the rat exposed to high atmospheric pressure. This was found to reverse local anaesthesia with benzocaine and lignocaine but not procaine. The studies were carried out at pH 7.4. At this pH, benzocaine is completely uncharged, lignocaine has 25% uncharged base while procaine has only 3% uncharged base. High pressure thus reversed the uncharged lipid-soluble component of local anaesthetic action.

Quaternary ammonium compounds

Further support for the concept that it is the cation which is essential for anaesthesia comes from the use of quaternary analogues of lignocaine (*Figure 17.2*). These can exist only as charged cations and not as uncharged bases at physiological pH. When these drugs are applied to the outside of myelinated nerves they have no local anaesthetic activity but, if applied to the inside of the axon sheath, they are as active as their tertiary analogues (Stritchartz, 1973).

In myelinated nerves, quaternary derivatives of lignocaine were observed to have two binding sites within the membrane pore. The first binding site

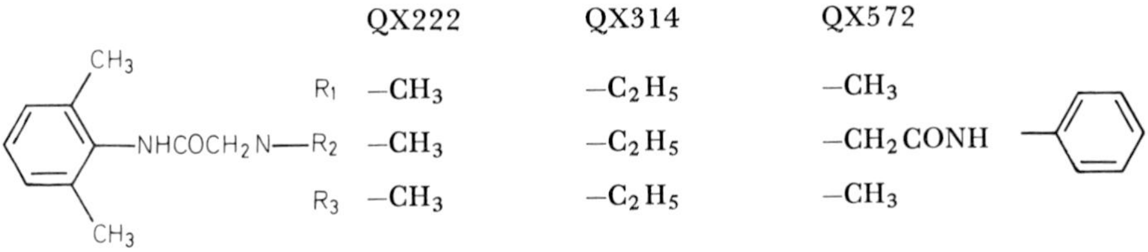

		QX222	QX314	QX572	
R_1		$-CH_3$	$-C_2H_5$	$-CH_3$	
R_2		$-CH_3$	$-C_2H_5$	$-CH_2CONH$	
R_3		$-CH_3$	$-C_2H_5$	$-CH_3$	

$-NHCOCH_2N-$

Figure 17.2
These quaternary ammonium compounds are analogues of lignocaine and have local anaesthetic properties (see text)

had a much higher affinity for the quaternary compounds and was located near the axoplasmic opening of the channel but outside the region in the channel which could support an electric potential gradient. The second site for binding was located well within the channel and binding here was less strong.

Sites of action of local anaesthetics

Takman (1975) classified local anaesthetics according to their sites of action (*Figure 17.3*). At the external surface of the sodium channel, tetrodotoxin and saxitoxin act as charged agents. Benzocaine, which is uncharged, acts in a non-specific manner inside the sodium channel. The quaternary analogues of lignocaine act in a charged form both on the internal axoplasmic channel and inside the sodium channel. The clinically acceptable agents are characterized by being in both charged and uncharged

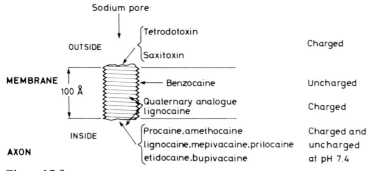

Figure 17.3
Sites of action of local anaesthetics

forms. They all act at specific receptor sites at the internal opening of the sodium channel. The differing characteristics of these local anaesthetics are related to variations in their pK_a, binding to proteins and lipid solubility.

Local anaesthetics and the axon

There is slow somatofugal flow of axoplasm of some 1–2 mm per day (Weiss and Hiscoe, 1948). In addition, rapid transport of some 100 mm per day takes place, presumably with the aid of axonal microtubules.

Kerkut, Shapira and Walker (1967) observed that 0.01% lignocaine had a marked effect on the rapid transport in a snail brain–muscle preparation. Fink *et al.* (1972) used the rabbit vagus nerve to study the effect of lignocaine on the transport of ^{3}H-leucine. It was found that lignocaine at concentrations below 0.1% had no consistent effect on the migration of the radioactive label. At concentrations above 0.1%, the distance travelled by the ^{3}H-leucine was decreased in proportion to the local anaesthetic concentration. The inhibition of axoplasmic transport by 0.6% lignocaine could be reversed by washing the nerves, but only if the lignocaine had been in contact with the nerve for less than 60 minutes. Nerves were examined by electron microscopy and, in control nerves, microtubules were well preserved in both axons and Schwann cells. Neurofilaments, mitochondria and smooth endoplasmic reticulum were also normal. However, marked changes were observed in nerves incubated in 0.6% lignocaine for 90 minutes. In both myelinated and non-myelinated axons there was almost complete loss of microtubules with no increase in cytoplasmic filaments. There was dissociation of neurofilament bundles while the individual neurofilaments appeared unchanged. Disruption of many cell and cytoplasmic membranes, including those of mitochondria, was present. The Schwann cells also lost microtubules, being more affected than the axons in this respect. Microtubules were lost in both myelinated and non-myelinated axons, but the latter suffered most damage. In experiments where reversal of blockage of rapid axonal transport by 0.6% lignocaine was studied, it was noted that conduction of an action potential was not present unless rapid axonal transport recovered as well.

Fink and Kish (1976) presented further evidence, from *in vivo* studies with rat trigeminal nerve, that lignocaine inhibits at least some of the elements of rapid axonal transport. It was suggested that there was interference with oxidative energy production. Ochs and Hollingsworth (1971) have previously demonstrated that high energy phosphate is an essential requirement for rapid axonal transport, and lignocaine was shown by Haschke and Fink (1975) to be a potent depressant of mitochondrial oxidative metabolism.

OTHER PHARMACOLOGICAL ACTIONS

Cardiovascular effects of local anaesthetics

Although most local anaesthetics are generally regarded as vasodilators, when they are injected their systemic effects are different in that peripheral resistance may be increased, cardiac output and heart rate can vary and many of the depressant effects can be counterbalanced by the sympathetic system (Blair, 1975).

ACTION ON THE HEART

In experiments on isolated cardiac tissue with concentrations of lignocaine which control arrhythmias but are not toxic, Bigger and Mandel (1970) showed that automaticity was strongly suppressed. The duration of the action potential was shortened, as was the effective refractory period in both Purkinje fibres and ventricular muscle. It was suggested that these effects were responsible for the stabilizing effect of lignocaine on cardiac irregularities. Toxic concentrations of lignocaine were associated with a decrease in the maximum rate of depolarization of Purkinje fibres and ventricular muscle, a reduction in amplitude of the action potential and a marked decrease in conduction velocity. These changes resemble the action of lignocaine on nerve tissue. With increasing doses of lignocaine there is prolongation of conduction time of impulses through various parts of the heart as well as an increase in diastolic threshold. On the electrocardiogram these can be observed as an increase in the P–R interval and in the duration of QRS. Clinically, sinus bradycardia is present and this may proceed to cardiac arrest at high concentrations of lignocaine. Sugimoto *et al.* (1969) confirmed these findings in awake dogs.

At concentrations of lignocaine which were sufficient to control arrhythmias, no interference with myocardial contractility and cardiac output was observed. However, as the concentration in the blood rose, failure of the myocardial contraction, increased diastolic volume, decreased intraventricular pressure and decreased cardiac output followed due to pump failure (Binnion *et al.*, 1969). Klein, Sutherland and Morch (1968) reported similar findings to animal studies in man. When lignocaine is used for regional anaesthesia, under normal circumstances, the concentrations in the blood do not reach levels that can affect the heart. Accidental intravenous administration of excessive doses may, however, reach concentrations which result in circulatory collapse.

Lignocaine is particularly useful in the control of ventricular arrhythmias. Kabela (1973) used ^{42}K in isolated cardiac tissue exposed to lignocaine, which was found to enhance the efflux of potassium from ventricular muscle strips and Purkinje fibres but not from atrial tissue.

PERIPHERAL VASCULAR EFFECTS

Cocaine is the only local anaesthetic which produces vasoconstriction. This is due to inhibition of uptake of catecholamines into tissue-binding sites (Iversen, 1965).

Mepivacaine and bupivacaine were shown by Åberg and Wahlstrom (1972) to have a biphasic action on isolated smooth muscle. At low concentrations the muscle tension and the frequency of contractions were increased, while at higher concentrations relaxation was present. Prilocaine was found to produce the greatest effect on smooth muscle contraction while etidocaine had the least effect. Basal tone was increased most by procaine, prilocaine and mepivacaine. Lignocaine, amethocaine, bupivacaine and etidocaine were associated with only minimal effects.

In man, a decrease in forearm blood flow followed the intra-arterial injection of mepivacaine in the absence of any alteration in arterial pressure, thus indicating that there was a rise in peripheral resistance (Jörfeldt *et al.*, 1970). It has been suggested that this biphasic peripheral vascular effect may be related to changes in smooth muscle concentrations of Ca^{2+} which is displaced from membrane-binding sites and thus results in vasoconstriction followed by vasodilatation as cytoplasmic Ca^{2+} decreases (Åberg and Andersson, 1972).

Covino and Vassallo (1976) have summarized the effects of increasing dosage of local anaesthetics on the cardiovascular system. At doses where non-toxic blood levels are present, there may be a slight rise in blood pressure due to an increase in either cardiac output or heart rate. This is believed to be due to sympathetic activity and a direct action causing vasoconstriction of certain peripheral vascular beds. At concentrations approaching toxicity there is hypotension from peripheral vasodilatation due to a direct action on peripheral smooth muscle. At higher concentrations there is a direct action on cardiac muscle which gives a fall in cardiac output. Profound hypotension then results from a combination of reduced peripheral vascular resistance and decreased cardiac output. At lethal concentrations there is cardiovascular collapse with marked bradycardia and finally cardiac arrest.

Indirect effects of local anaesthetics

Secondary effects independent of the direct actions of local anaesthetic agents can occur due to the regional procedures used. Hypotension takes place in 38—45% of patients receiving spinal or epidural anaesthesia (Moore *et al.*, 1968). In spinal anaesthesia, sympathetic blockade is responsible for hypotension rather than any direct effect of the small dose of local anaesthetic drug. In epidural anaesthesia, there are not only vasomotor alterations which resemble those of spinal anaesthesia but also a complex interplay of other factors. These include the type and concentration of the local anaesthetic drug, the level of anaesthesia, presence of vasoconstrictor and the state of the patient. Much larger quantities of local anaesthetics are used in epidural than spinal anaesthesia.

For the heart to be able to compensate for falls in blood pressure, the presence of the upper two cardioaccelerator nerves T1 and T2 are necessary. At this level of block there is also a significant increase in both upper and lower limb blood flow and a fall in total peripheral resistance. This is due to widespread sympathetic blockade and peripheral vasodilatation. If the block goes to T4, there is an increase in lower limb blood flow but, since the sympathetic nerves to the upper limb are unaffected, there is compensatory vasoconstriction in the upper half of the body.

Central effects of local anaesthetics absorbed into the blood stream include increases of cardiac output associated with stimulation of the vasomotor centre in the central nervous system, while excessive amounts can result in central depression aggravating hypotension from sympathetic blockade.

A decrease in renal plasma flow and hepatic blood flow can also result from central neural blockade. This will result in a decrease in both renal excretion and liver metabolism of the local anaesthetics belonging to the amide group (Kennedy *et al.*, 1969, 1971).

Central nervous system effects

Since local anaesthetics readily cross the blood—brain barrier, the brain is very sensitive to the presence of local anaesthetics circulating in arterial blood. At low concentrations, minimal symptoms are present such as numbness of the tongue and circumoral tissues. These are most likely the result of concentrations of local anaesthetics reaching these highly vascular areas. Light-headedness and dizziness with visual and auditory disturbances are evidence of an effect on the central nervous system. Drowsiness and sleep are typically associated with lignocaine overdosage.

In rhesus monkeys, Munson *et al.* (1975) observed that, with constant-rate infusions of lignocaine or bupivacaine, there was a period of drowsiness prior to the onset of convulsions. Malagodi, Munson and Embro (1977) observed that, with etidocaine, there was no tendency to sleep before the onset of convulsions. In clinical work this may be associated with some hazard, as no warning signs of impending toxicity may be associated with the use of etidocaine. In general, it was found that amide-type local anaesthetic drugs affected the central nervous system before depressing either ventilation or circulation.

In animals with implanted electrodes, Wagman, de Jong and Prince (1968) found that the earliest and most prominent changes in spontaneous cerebral activity after the administration of intravenous lignocaine were in the amygdaloid nuclear complex. There was a dose-related sequence of changes. Low doses associated with sedation gave an exaggeration of normal spindle discharges which were related to respiration. At convulsant doses of lignocaine, focal amygdaloid epileptiform spiking was seen and this was independent of respiration. When the amygdala was completely destroyed, Eidelberg, Lesse and Gault (1961) reported that, following the administration of a convulsive dose of cocaine, no seizure was observed. Munson *et al.* (1975), however, were unable to find any specific seizure focus in the amygdala of monkeys for either lignocaine or etidocaine. Robinson and Jenkins (1975), in cats, observed rhythmic activity in the amygdala during bupivacaine infusion. This also occurred in the hippocampus. These subcortical changes are similar to those seen with lignocaine in the cat.

Variations in the central nervous effects of local anaesthetics can be explained by differences in potency, speed of passage through the blood–brain barrier and their rate of breakdown. Each factor is also dependent upon the speed of injection and rapidity of build-up of a toxic concentration in the blood stream. If there is a slow administration or absorption is slowed, by the presence of adrenaline, detoxication mechanisms have time to act. However, if there is rapid absorption, the rate of passage through the blood–brain barrier is faster and then the intrinsic potency of the individual drug becomes important. Procaine can be broken down in circulating blood by cholinesterase and is less potent than the amide, lignocaine. This latter requires liver enzymes for metabolism and thus, following injection of toxic amounts, there is a greater risk of convulsions, which will last for a longer time than if the drug could be metabolized locally. Procaine is thus a safer drug as regards the action on the central nervous system.

ANTICONVULSANT ACTION

Bernhard, Bohm and Hojeberg (1955) used intravenous injections of lignocaine to control status epilepticus in humans. In general, the dose required is less than that associated with convulsions and a marked antiepileptic effect is observed. Berry, Sanner and Keasling (1961) found mepivacaine to be equally effective in animal experiments. The mode of action of local anaesthetics in epilepsy is due to depression of the hyperexcitable cortical neurons.

EFFECT OF VARIATION IN Pa_{CO_2}

In acute experiments in animals it was found that at a high Pa_{CO_2} convulsions took place, while at low Pa_{CO_2} the same dose of lignocaine was without effect. At elevated Pa_{CO_2} cerebral blood flow is higher than at low Pa_{CO_2}. This increased blood flow may be responsible for bringing more local anaesthetic to the brain. A fall in intracellular pH associated with a high Pa_{CO_2} will mean that there is an increase in the intraneuronal level of the active cationic form of the local anaesthetic.

Sakabe *et al.* (1974), in dogs, reported that at doses of lignocaine which did not cause seizures, cerebral respiration (as measured by oxygen consumption) was depressed. At concentrations giving rise to convulsions there was a preliminary period of depressed cerebral metabolic uptake for oxygen before onset of seizures. After convulsions, the oxygen consumption was markedly increased. Further administration of local anaesthetic drug resulted in flattening of brain waves and generalized depression of the central nervous system, including respiratory depression leading to respiratory arrest.

The explanation for the period of cerebral excitement is that local anaesthetics stabilize plasma membranes even at low concentrations; they are thus depressant from the start. The majority of the cells in the central nervous system are inhibitory. These inhibitory pathways are initially blocked, releasing the facilitatory neurons to act unopposed, thus giving rise to excitation and convulsions. Then, as the concentration of local anaesthetic rises, depression of both facilitatory and inhibitory pathways occurs, with over-all depression of the central nervous system.

EFFECT ON SPINAL CORD

Following intravenous injection of lignocaine $5-25$ mg·kg^{-1} in cats, de Jong, Robles and Corbin (1969) measured its effect on spinal synaptic transmission. It was found that lignocaine markedly facilitated monosynaptic transmission and inhibited polysynaptic transmission. The central seizure discharges associated with convulsant doses of local anaesthetics would find greatly facilitated spinal motoneurons and thus increase the likelihood of generalized motor activity.

TREATMENT OF CONVULSIONS

Barbiturates are effective in controlling convulsions. Maykut and Kalow (1955) demonstrated in guinea-pigs that, when barbiturates are injected, they augment the over-all depression of the brain. It is thus important to use only the minimum dose required to control convulsions. An alternative approach is the use of a neuromuscular blocking agent. Usubiaga *et al.* (1966) observed in human volunteers that, though muscle activity is controlled by suxamethonium, electroencephalographic evidence for convulsions continued and consciousness was not always lost.

de Jong and Heavner (1974) demonstrated in cats that a single intramuscular injection of diazepam gave rapid and prolonged protection from convulsions induced by local anaesthetics. Diazepam has been shown to enter the brain quickly. Van der Kleijn and Wijffels (1971) reported high concentrations of diazepam to be present in the spinal cord, brain stem and nuclei of the medulla oblongata and cerebellum ten minutes after the intravenous injection of ^{14}C-diazepam in newborn monkeys. The protection of diazepam exceeded the intravascular half-life of a few hours, and de Jong and Heavner (1974) suggested that a metabolite might be present with anticonvulsant properties. This may be oxazepam, which is nearly as potent an anticonvulsant as diazepam. This long duration of protection is important during continuous administration of lignocaine or, if topping-up doses are being administered, for the management of cardiac irregularities, since the monoethylglycine metabolite of lignocaine also possess convulsant properties in its own right (Blumer, Strong and Atkinson, 1973).

Ausinsch, Malagodi and Munson (1976) measured the arterial plasma concentrations of lignocaine in rhesus monkeys at the onset of convulsions during constant rate infusion of 4 mg·kg^{-1} min^{-1}. Pretreatment with diazepam raised the lignocaine seizure dose of lignocaine 24–34% above control values. Previous studies by de Jong and Heavner (1971, 1973) were complicated by the cardiovascular depression and resultant hypotension associated with the bolus administration of lignocaine. Ausinsch, Malagodi and Munson (1976) observed an increased threshold for local anaesthetic seizures but the prodromal signs of an impending convulsion were masked by diazepam. Following treatment with diazepam, prolonged depression was noted after the end of convulsions.

Maintenance of a patent airway, full oxygenation, use of diazepam or minimal doses of barbiturates to control seizures, and administration of vasopressor drugs to support circulation should hypotension be present are all important in the treatment of overdosage of local anaesthetic drugs.

Local anaesthetics and the placenta

Local anaesthetics can cross the placenta and may affect the fetus. Finster *et al.* (1972), working with animals, were able to detect fetal blood levels of lignocaine as early as 1–2 minutes after maternal administration. Relatively high concentrations were found in the fetal liver, heart and brain but it was only in fetal liver that the concentration was higher than in the mother's liver. Little lignocaine was present in the placenta itself.

Thomas *et al.* (1976) measured the transplacental distribution of bupivacaine and found that the umbilical venous plasma concentration was lower than the maternal venous plasma concentration. Binding of bupivacaine was greater with maternal than fetal plasma protein. Poppers (1975) gives data concerning the protein-binding capacity for various local anaesthetics as follows: prilocaine < lignocaine < mepivacaine < bupivacaine = etidocaine. The drugs with high protein binding in the mother's blood leave less available to cross the placenta. Thus, provided the mother does not receive a gross overdose of local anaesthetic, bupivacaine and etidocaine are safest for management of labour since less will reach the fetus.

METABOLISM

Ester group

Cocaine, procaine and many other early synthetic local anaesthetics have an ester linkage being derived from benzoic acid. Their safety in clinical use was related to the speed of their metabolism following injection and absorption into the systemic circulation.

PROCAINE

Cholinesterase is the enzyme responsible for hydrolysis of the ester group (Brodie, Lief and Poet, 1948). Procaine splits into para-aminobenzoic acid, which is excreted unchanged in the urine, and diethylaminoethanol, which is further metabolized since only 30% is found in urine. Para-aminobenzoic acid has been infused in humans by Foldes *et al.* (1960) and found to give rise to no symptoms of toxicity.

Cholinesterase activity is low in debilitated patients and in those with liver disease. In uraemic patients, procaine is also hydrolysed more slowly than in the healthy. Reidenberg, James and Dring (1972) found a negative correlation between the speed of hydrolysis of procaine and the patient's blood urea nitrogen. Since the safety of procaine depends upon its rapid metabolism, a reduced dosage is indicated in these patients. In patients with atypical forms of cholinesterase, prolongation of systemic toxic effects has resulted from failure of hydrolysis of procaine (Foldes *et al.*, 1963).

COCAINE

Until now, little has been known of the metabolism and distribution of cocaine. Nayak, Miska and Mulé (1976) used randomly labelled ^{3}H-cocaine for tissue distribution studies in rats. The main site of detoxication of cocaine was the liver. Only minor quantities of cocaine (1—1.5%) were excreted free in urine and faeces, while metabolites continued to be excreted for several days. In the rat, ecgonine is not metabolized and benzoylecgonine was converted mainly to ecgonine.

It is suggested that, on repeated administration of cocaine, the *in vivo* oxidation of norcocaine to a highly reactive nitroxide free radical may account for the systemic toxicity of cocaine. It is accepted that nitroxide free radicals reduce to norcompounds with membrane SH groups. Another factor responsible for the toxicity of cocaine on a chronic basis is its prolonged sequestration in fat.

In dogs, Miska *et al.* (1976) studied the metabolism of ^{3}H-cocaine on both acute and chronic administration. After intravenous dosage, cocaine was found to have disappeared from all areas of the central nervous system in 12—14 hours. Significant amounts of tritiated compounds were, however, still present in the brain even one week afterwards. In both acutely and chronically cocaine-treated dogs this radioactivity was identified as being due to metabolites of cocaine. These were identified as norcocaine, benzoylnorecgonine, benzoylecgonine and ecgonine. In chronically treated dogs there was accumulation of norcocaine and benzoylnorecgonine. When given intracisternally, benzoylnorecgonine and benzoylecgonine were associated with a stimulant action on the brain. These two metabolites are both polar compounds which could interfere with neuronal bound Ca^{2+}. This action was suggested to cause conformational changes in the membrane proteins, resulting in excitatory effects on the brain.

Amide group

Replacement of an ester linkage by a stable amide group gives rise to more complex metabolic patterns. Enzymes, which are capable of breaking this bond, are, however, present in the liver. The nature of the aminoacyl moiety exerts a profound influence on the different metabolic profiles seen in this group of local anaesthetics.

PRILOCAINE

Prilocaine (see *Figure 17.1*), which lacks one methyl group on the aromatic portion of the molecule, is the most rapidly metabolized amide. Its principal metabolites are *o*-toluidine and L-*N*-*n*-propylamine. Prilocaine is metabolized not only in liver but also *in vitro* in kidney (Geddes, 1965) and in lung (Åkerman *et al.*, 1966). The release of *o*-toluidine causes methaemoglobinaemia which is maximal some six hours after the administration of prilocaine and gives rise to undesirable clinical cyanosis.

LIGNOCAINE

Lignocaine is not only used for local anaesthesia but is of value in the control of cardiac arrhythmias. There has thus been considerable interest in its metabolites. In man, 72.6% of the dose administered is excreted in urine as 4,hydroxy-2,6-xylidine.

The first step in the metabolism of lignocaine is oxidative de-ethylation with the formation of monoethylglycinexylidide and acetaldehyde (*Figure 17.4*). Further de-ethylation takes place to give glycinexylidide (Hollunger, 1960). Splitting of the amide linkage gives *N*,*N*-diethylglycine which may also come direct from lignocaine. The major pathway, however, is thought to proceed through monoethylglycinexylidide to give *N*-ethylglycine and 2,6-xylidine. This latter is then hydroxylated in position 4 to give the major metabolite excreted in the urine. Conjugated metabolites excreted in rat bile were found to undergo enterohepatic recirculation prior to their excretion in the urine.

Another pathway for metabolism involves hydroxylation in position 3 to give 3-hydroxylignocaine and 3-hydroxymonoethylglycinexylidide. In addition, 2-amino,3-methylbenzoic acid is also thought to be present in urine (Keenaghan and Boyes, 1972).

Strong, Parker and Atkinson (1973) identified glycinexylidide in the urine of patients given intravenous infusions of lignocaine. When glycine-xylidide was administered by Strong *et al.* (1975) to humans, 50% of the dose was excreted unchanged in the urine while a further 15% was excreted as conjugates of 2,6-xylidine and 4-hydroxy-2,6-xylidine. Glycinexylidide possesses local anaesthetic activity when injected intracutaneously. Whilst glycinexylidide does not itself cause convulsions, it was found to potentiate seizures associated with lignocaine and another metabolite, mono-ethylglycinexylidide. This latter was shown by Blumer, Strong and Atkinson (1973), in animals, to have near equipotency with lignocaine in

358

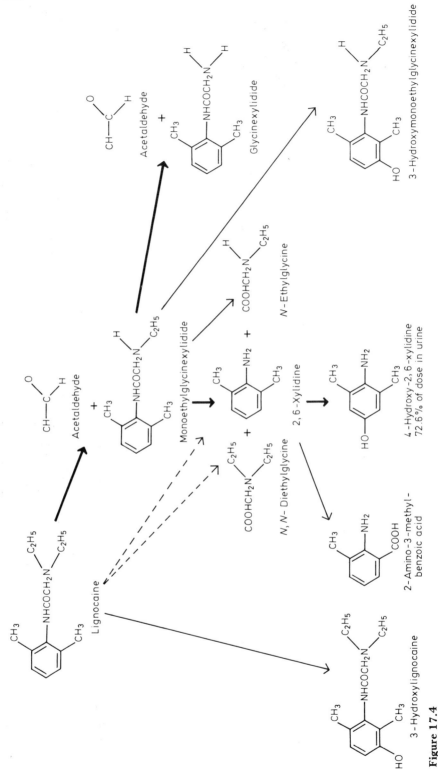

Figure 17.4
Metabolic pathways for lignocaine

causing convulsions. When blood levels of lignocaine are used to control infusions of lignocaine, it is advisable to sum these with monoethylglycine-xylidide levels, and those for glycinexylidide, when evaluating the risk of convulsions. Monoethylglycinexylidide has been reported by Smith and Duce (1971) to have emetic and antiarrhythmic properties.

In four uraemic patients on dialysis, given continuous infusion of lignocaine, the kinetics of distribution and elimination of monoethyl-glycinexylidide and glycinexylidide were studied by Collinsworth *et al.* (1975). No abnormal accumulation of lignocaine or monoethylglycine-xylidide was observed. Blood levels of glycinexylidide, however, increased progressively for as long as 1.5–2.5 days. Glycinexylidide, in man, has been shown by Strong *et al.* (1975) to be responsible for symptoms of headache and impaired concentration, especially if plasma levels exceeded 2–5 μg·ml^{-1}. The long half-life of glycinexylidide is also important when lignocaine is used to control cardiac irregularities. These patients should continue to be monitored with the electrocardiogram until all the glycine-xylidide has been eliminated from the body, as it may continue to be effective in controlling arrhythmias in the period after stopping lignocaine.

MEPIVACAINE

Mepivacaine (see *Figure 17.1*) is rapidly metabolized in the body since only a small percentage of the drug is excreted unchanged in the urine. It is rapidly *n*-demethylated in the liver (Hansson, Hoffman and Kristerson, 1965). Meffin *et al.* (1973) identified three neutral metabolites of mepivacaine, which accounted for 10% of the oral dose in humans. Hydroxylation of mepivacaine also takes place in rats and man so that up to 60% of the administered dose is excreted in urine as 3-hydroxy or 4-hydroxy derivatives (Meffin and Thomas, 1973). Initially, more of the 3-hydroxy metabolite was excreted at a higher concentration in urine but after 24 hours there was a greater proportion of the 4-hydroxy metabolite present in urine.

BUPIVACAINE

Reynolds (1971) found that, in humans, after the administration of bupivacaine (see *Figure 17.1*) approximately 5% was excreted as the *N*-dealkylated metabolite, pipecolylxylidide. This debutylation took place in the liver. When pipecolylxylidide was administered to humans, approximately half the dose was excreted unchanged in the urine. This suggested that further metabolism was taking place. Goehl, Davenport and Stanley (1973) found that, in monkeys, over 50% of bupivacaine was excreted as pipecolic acid while, in rats, an aromatic hydroxy metabolite was recovered from urine.

ETIDOCAINE

Etidocaine (see *Figure 17.1*) is very closely related to lignocaine but its metabolic pathways have been shown to be different by Thomas, Morgan and Vine (1976). Following administration of etidocaine to man, the proportion excreted unchanged was somewhat less than that for lignocaine. Only 31% of the total dose of etidocaine was recovered as metabolites which could be identified. These included 2,amino-2-butyroxylidide, 2-*N*-ethylamino-2-butyroxylidide, 2-*N*-propylamino-2-butyroxylidide,2,6-xylidine and 4-hydroxy-2,6-xylidine. In contrast to lignocaine, only trace amounts of 4-hydroxy-2,6-xylidine were found in urine after administration of etidocaine.

Heart failure and metabolism

In the presence of heart failure, Thomson, Rowland and Melmon (1971) observed decreased metabolism of lignocaine. They recommended markedly decreased dosage requirements in patients with either heart failure or liver disease such as advanced alcoholic cirrhosis. Halkin *et al.* (1975) measured the blood concentrations of lignocaine and monoethylglycine in patients receiving lignocaine for the treatment of cardiac arrhythmias. In three patients with heart failure, the concentration of monoethylglycine was equal to that of lignocaine and indicated failure of plasma clearance of lignocaine. Decreased liver blood flow is a positive indication for slowing the speed of administration of lignocaine.

SUMMARY

Local anaesthetic agents exert widespread actions on the body in addition to the desired effect at their site of injection. Recent advances are linked to the development of chemical groupings which confer stability, high lipid solubility and binding to proteins. Whilst there are many advantages associated with these properties, local anaesthetic agents must be treated with respect. There is no substitute for accurate placement of minimal effective amounts of local anaesthetics in clinical practice.

References

Åberg, G. and Andersson, R. (1972). Studies on mechanical actions of mepivacaine (Carbocaine) and its optically active isomers on isolated smooth muscle, role Ca⁺⁺ and cyclic AMP. *Acta pharmac. tox.* 31, 321–336

Åberg, G. and Wahlstrom, B. (1972). Mechanical electrophysiological effects of some local anaesthetic agents and their isomers on the rat portal vein. *Acta pharmac. tox.* 31, 255–266

Åkerman, B., Åström, A., Ross, S. and Telč, A. (1966). Studies on the absorption distribution and metabolism of labelled prilocaine and lidocaine in some animal species. *Acta pharmac. tox.* 24, 389–403

Aldrete, J. A. and Johnson, D. A. (1969). Allergy to local anesthetics. *J. Am. med. Ass.* 207, 356–357

Ausinsch, D., Malagodi, M. K. and Munson, E. S. (1976). Diazepam in the prophylaxis of lignocaine seizures. *Br. J. Anaesth.* 48, 309–313

Bernhard, C. G. (1958). On undifferentiated neuronal spread of excitation. *Expl Cell Res.* Suppl. 5, 201–220

Bernhard, C. G., Bohm, E. and Hojeberg, S. (1955). A new treatment of status epilepticus. *Archs Neurol. Psychiat.* 74, 208–214

Berry, C. A., Sanner, J. H. and Keasling, H. H. (1961). A comparison of the anticonvulsant activity of mepivacaine and lidocaine. *J. Pharmac. exp. Ther.* 133, 357–363

Bigger, J. T. and Mandel, W. J. (1970). Effect of lidocaine on the electrophysiological properties of ventricular muscle and Purkinje fibers. *J. clin. Invest.* 49, 63–77

Binnion, P. F., Murtagh, G., Pollock, A. M. and Fletcher, E. (1969). Relation between plasma lignocaine levels and induced haemodynamic changes. *Br. med. J.* 3, 390–392

Blair, M. R. (1975). Cardiovascular pharmacology of local anaesthetics. *Br. J. Anaesth.* 47, 247–252

Blumer, J. B., Strong, J. M. and Atkinson, A. J. (1973). The convulsant potency of lidocaine and its N-dealkylated metabolites. *J. Pharmac. exp. Ther.* 186, 31–36

Brodie, B. B., Lief, P. A. and Poet, R. (1948). The fate of procaine in man following its intravenous administration and methods for the estimation of procaine and diethylaminoethanol. *J. Pharmac. exp. Ther.* 94, 359–366

Bromage, P. R. (1965). A comparison of the hydrochloride and carbon dioxide salts of lidocaine and prilocaine in epidural analgesia. *Acta anaesth. scand.* Suppl. 16, 55–69

Catchlove, R. F. H. (1972). The influence of CO_2 and pH on local anaesthetic action. *J. Pharmac. exp. Ther.* 181, 298–309

Collinsworth, K. A., Strong, J. M., Atkinson, A. J., Winkle, R. A., Perlroth, F. and Harrison, D. C. (1975). Pharmacokinetics and metabolism of lidocaine in patients with renal failure. *Clin. Pharmac. Ther.* 18, 59–64

Covino, B. G. and Vassallo, H. G. (1976). *Local Anesthetics Mechanisms of Action and Clinical Use.* New York: Grune and Stratton

de Jong, R. H. and Heavner, J. E. (1971). Diazepam prevents local anesthetic seizures. *Anesthesiology* 34, 523–531

de Jong, R. H. and Heavner, J. E. (1973). Diazepam and lidocaine-induced cardio-vascular changes. *Anesthesiology* 39, 633–638

de Jong, R. H. and Heavner, J. E. (1974). Convulsions induced by local anesthetic – time course of diazepam prophylaxis. *Can. Anaesth. Soc. J.* 21, 153–158

de Jong, R. H. and Wagman, I. H. (1963). Physiological mechanisms of peripheral nerve block by local anesthetics. *Anesthesiology* 24, 684–727

de Jong, R. H., Robles, R. and Corbin, R. W. (1969). Central actions of lidocaine – synaptic transmission. *Anesthesiology* 30, 19–23

Einhorn, A. and Uhlfelder, E. (1909) Ueber den p-aminobenzöesäure diäthylester. *Liebigs Annln Chem.* 371, 131

Eidelberg, E., Lesse, H. and Gault, E. P. (1961). Convulsant effect of cocaine. *Fedn Proc.* 20, 322

Falk, E. (1890). Ueber nebenwirkungen und intoxication bei der anwendung neuerer arzneimittel. III Cocain. *Ther. Mh.* 4, 511–522

Fink, B. R. and Kish, S. J. (1976). Reversible inhibition of rapid axonal transport 'in vivo' by lidocaine hydrochloride. *Anesthesiology* 44, 139–146

Fink, B. R., Kennedy, R. D., Hendrickson, A. E. and Middaugh, M. E. (1972). Lidocaine inhibition of rapid axonal transport. *Anesthesiology* 36, 422–432

Finster, M., Morishima, H. O., Boyes, R. N. and Covino, B. G. (1972). The placental transfer of lidocaine and its uptake by fetal tissue. *Anesthesiology* 36, 159–163

Foldes, F. F., Molloy, R., McNall, P. G. and Koukal, L. R. (1960). Comparison of toxicity of intravenously given local anaesthetic agents in man. *J. Am. med. Ass.* 172, 1493–1498

Foldes, F. F., Foldes, V. M., Smith, J. C. and Zsigmund, E. K. (1963). The relation between plasma cholinesterase and prolonged apnoea caused by succinylcholine. *Anesthesiology* 24, 208–216

Franz, D. N. and Perry, R. S. (1974). Mechanisms for differential block among single myelinated and non myelinated axons by procaine. *J. Physiol., Lond.* 236, 193–210

Gaul, L. E. (1955). Cross sensitization from para-aminobenzoate in sunburn preventatives. *Anesthesiology* 16, 606–614

Geddes, I. C. (1965). Studies of the metabolism of Citanest ^{14}C. *Acta anaesth. scand.* Suppl. 16, 37–44

Goehl, T. J., Davenport, J. B. and Stanley, M. J. (1973). Distribution of biotransformation and excretion of bupivacaine in the rat and the monkey. *Xenobiotica* 3, 761–772

Halkin, H, Meffin, P., Melmon, K. L. and Rowland, M. (1975). Influence of congestive heart failure on blood levels of lidocaine and its active monodiethylated metabolite. *Clin. Pharmac. Ther.* 17, 669–676

Halsey, M. J. and Wardley-Smith, B. (1975). Pressure reversal of narcoses produced by anaesthetics, narcotics and tranquillisers. *Nature, Lond.* 257, 811–813

Halstead, W. S. (1885). Practical comments on the use and abuse of cocaine; suggested by its invariably successful employment in more than a thousand minor surgical operations. *N.Y. med. J.* 42, 294–295

Hansson, E., Hoffman, N. P. and Kristerson, L. (1965). Fate of mepivacaine in the body. II. Excretion and biotransformation. *Acta pharmac. tox.* 22, 213–223

Haschke, R. H. and Fink, B. R. (1975). Lidocaine effects on brain mitochondrial metabolism 'in vitro'. *Anesthesiology* 42, 737–740

Hollunger, G (1960). On the metabolism of lidocaine. II. The biotransformation of lidocaine. *Acta pharmac. tox.* 17, 365–373

Iversen, L. L. (1965). Inhibition of noradrenaline uptake by drugs. *J. Pharm. Pharmac.* 17, 62–64

Jack, J. J. B. (1975). Physiology of peripheral nerve fibres in relation to their size. *Br. J. Anaesth.* 47, 173–182

Johnson, S. M. and Miller, K. W. (1970). Antagonism of pressure and anaesthesia. *Nature, Lond.* 228, 75–76

Jörfeldt, L., Löfstrom, B., Pernow, B. and Wahren, J. (1970). The effect of mepivacaine and lidocaine on forearm resistance and capacitance vessels in man. *Acta anaesth. scand.* 14, 183–201

Kabela, E. (1973). The effects of lidocaine on potassium efflux from various tissues of dog heart. *J. Pharmac. exp. Ther.* 184, 611–618

Keenaghan, J. B. and Boyes, R. N. (1972). The tissue distribution metabolism and excretion of lidocaine in rats, guineapigs, dogs and man. *J. Pharmac. exp. Ther.* 180, 454–463

Kendig, J. J. and Cohen, E. N. (1977). Pressure antagonism to nerve conduction block by anesthetic agents. *Anesthesiology* 47, 6–10

Kennedy, W. F., Sawyer, T. K., Gerbershagen, H. V., Cutter, R. E., Allen, G. D. and Bonica, J. J. (1969). Systemic cardiovascular and renal hemodynamic alterations during peridural anesthesia in normal man. *Anesthesiology* 31, 414–421

Kennedy, W. F., Everett, G. B., Cobb, L. A. and Allen, G. D. (1971). Simultaneous systemic and hepatic hemodynamic measurements during high peridural anesthesia in normal man. *Anesth. Analg., Cleve.* 50, 1069–1077

Kerkut, G A., Shapira, A. and Walker, R. J. (1967). The transport of ^{14}C-labelled material from CNS to and from muscle along a nerve trunk. *Comp. Biochem. Physiol.* 23, 729–748

Klein, S. W., Sutherland, R. I. L. and Morch, J. E. (1968). Haemodynamic effects of intravenous lidocaine in man. *Can. med. Ass. J.* 99, 472–475

Koller, C. (1884). On the use of cocaine for production of anaesthesia on the eye. *Lancet* ii, 990–992

Lofgren, N. (1948). *Studies on Local Anaesthetics: Xylocaine.* Stockholm: Haeggstroms

Malagodi, M. H., Munson, E. S. and Embro, W. J. (1977). Relation of etidocaine and bupivacaine toxicity to rate of infusion in rhesus monkeys. *Br. J. Anaesth.* 49, 121–125

Maykut, M. O. and Kalow, W. (1955). Experiments with animals on the combined action of procaine and barbiturates. *Can. Anaesth. Soc. J.* 2, 109–115

Meffin, P. and Thomas, J. (1973). The relative rates of formation of the phenolic metabolites of mepivacaine in man. *Xenobiotica* 3, 625–632

Meffin, P., Robertson, A. V., Thomas, J. and Winkler, J. (1973). Neutral metabolites of mepivacaine in humans. *Xenobiotica* 3, 191–196

Meymaris, E. (1975). Chemical anatomy of the nerve membrane. *Br. J. Anaesth.* 47, 164–172

Miska, A. L., Patel, M. N., Alluri, V. R., Mulé, S. J. and Nyak, P. K. (1976). Disposition and metabolism of (^{3}H) cocaine in acutely and chronically treated dogs. *Xenobiotica* 6, 537–552

Moore, D. C., Bridenbaugh, L. D., Bagdi, P. A., Bridenhaugh, P. O. and Stander, H. (1968). The present status of spinal (subarachnoid) and epidural (peridural) block. *Anesth. Analg., Cleve.* 47, 40–49

Munson, E. S., Tucker, W. K., Ausinsch, B. and Malagodi, M. H. (1975). Etidocaine, bupivacaine and lidocaine seizure thresholds in monkeys. *Anesthesiology* 42, 471–478

Nayak, P. K., Miska, A. L. and Mulé, S. J. (1976). Physiological disposition and biotransformation of (^{3}H) cocaine in acutely and chronically treated rats. *J. Pharmac. exp. Ther.* 196, 556–569

Ochs, S. and Hollingsworth, D. (1971). Dependence of fast axoplasmic transport in nerve on oxidative metabolism. *J. Neurochem.* 18, 107–114

Olch, P. D. (1975). William S. Halsted and local anesthetics: contributions and complications. *Anesthesiology* 42, 479–486

Papahadjopoulous, D. (1972). Studies on the mechanism of action of local anaesthetics with phospholipid model membranes. *Biochim. biophys. Acta* 265, 169–186

Poppers, P. J. (1975). Evaluation of local anaesthetic agents for required anaesthesia in obstetrics. *Br. J. Anaesth.* 47, 322–327

Reidenberg, M. M., James, M. and Dring, L. G. (1972). The rate of procaine hydrolysis in serum of normal subjects and diseased patients. *Clin. Pharmac. Ther.* 13, 279–284

Reynolds, F. (1971). A comparison of the potential toxicity of bupivacaine, lignocaine and mepivacaine during epidural blockade. *Br. J. Anaesth.* 43, 567–572

Ritchie, J. M., Ritchie, B. and Greengard, P. (1965a). The active structure of local anesthetics. *J. Pharmac. exp. Ther.* 150, 152–159

Ritchie, J. M., Ritchie, B. and Greengard, P. (1965b). The effects of nerve sheath on the action of local anesthetics. *J. Pharmac. exp. Ther.* 150, 160–164

Robinson, W. M. and Jenkins, L. C. (1975). Central nervous system effects of bupivacaine. *Can. Anaesth. Soc. J.* 22, 358–369

Sakabe, T., Maekawa, T., Ishikawa, T. and Takeshita, H. (1974). The effects of lidocaine on canine cerebral metabolism and circulation related to the electroencephalogram. *Anesthesiology* 40, 433–441

Seeman, P. (1972). The membrane actions of anesthetics and tranquillizers. *Pharmac. Rev.* 24, 583–655

Skou, J. C. (1954a). Local anaesthetics. I. The blocking potencies of some local anaesthetics and of butyl alcohol determined on peripheral nerves. *Acta pharmac. tox.* 10, 281—291

Skou, J. C. (1954b). Local anaesthetics. V. The action of local anaesthetics on monomolecular layers of stearic acid. *Acta pharmac. tox.* 10, 317—324

Skou, J. C. (1954c). Local anaesthetics. VI. Relation between blocking potency and penetration of a monomolecular layer of lipoids from nerves. *Acta pharmac. tox.* 10, 325—337

Skou, J. C. (1958). Relation between the ability of various compounds to block nervous conduction and their penetration into a monomolecular layer of nerve tissue lipids. *Biochim. biophys. Acta* 30, 625—629

Smith, E. R. and Duce, B. R. (1971). Acute antiarrhythmic and toxic effects in mice and dogs of 2-ethylamino-2',6'-acetoxylidine (L-86), a metabolite of lidocaine. *Fedn Proc.* 30, 227

Stritchartz, G. R. (1973). The inhibition of sodium currents in myelinated nerve by quaternary derivatives of lidocaine. *J. gen. Physiol.* 62, 37—57

Strong, J. M., Parker, M. and Atkinson, A. J. (1973). Identification of glycinexylidide in patients treated with intravenous lidocaine. *Clin. Pharmac. Ther.* 14, 67—72

Strong, J. M., Mayfield, D. E., Atkinson, A. J., Burris, B. C., Raymon, F. and Webster, L. T. (1975). Pharmacological activity, metabolism and pharmacokinetics of glycinexylidide. *Clin. Pharmac. Ther.* 17, 184—194

Sugimoto, T., Schaal, S. F., Dunn, N. M. and Wallace, A. G. (1969). Electrophysiologic effects of lidocaine in awake dogs. *J. Pharmac. exp. Ther.* 166, 146—150

Takman, B. (1975). The chemistry of local anaesthetic agents. Classification of blocking agents. *Br. J. Anaesth.* 47, 183—190

Tasaki, I. (1953). *Nervous Transmission,* pp. 99—106. Springfield, Ill: Charles C Thomas

Tasaki, I., Watanabe, A. and Hallet, M. (1972). Fluorescence of squid axon membrane with hydrophobic probes. *J. membrane Biol.* 8, 109—132

Thomas, J., Morgan, D. and Vine, J. (1976). Metabolism of etidocaine in man. *Xenobiotica* 6, 39—48

Thomas, J., Long, G., Moore, G. and Morgan, D. (1976). Plasma protein binding and placental transfer of bupivacaine. *Clin. Pharmac. Ther.* 19, 426—434

Thomson, P. D., Rowland, M. and Melmon, K. L. (1971). The influence of heart failure, liver disease and renal failure on the disposition of lidocaine in man. *Am. Heart J.* 82, 417—421

Trevan, J. W. and Booch, E. (1927). The relation of hydrogen ion concentration to the action of the local anaesthetics. *Br. J. exp. Path.* 8, 307—315

Usubiaga, J. E., Wikinski, J., Ferrero, R., Usubiaga, L. E. and Wikinski, R. (1966). Local anesthetic-induced convulsions in man . . . an electroencephalographic study. *Anesth. Analg. curr. Res.* 45, 611—620

Van der Kleijn, E. and Wijffels, C. C. G. (1971). Whole body and regional brain distribution of diazepam in newborn rhesus monkeys. *Archs int. Pharmacodyn. Thér.* 192, 255—264

Waggoner, A. (1976). Optical probes of membrane potential. *J. membrane Biol.* 27, 317—334

Wagman, I. H., de Jong, R. H. and Prince, D. A. (1968). Effects of lidocaine on spontaneous cortical and subcortical electrical activity. *Archs Neurol.* 18, 277—290

Wagner, H. H. and Ulbricht, W. (1976). Saxitoxin and procaine act independently on separate sites of the sodium channel. *Pflügers Arch. ges. Physiol.* 364, 65—70

Weiss, P. and Hiscoe, H. B. (1948). Experiments on the mechanism of nerve growth. *J. exp. Zool.* 107, 315—395

White, C. W., Dearborn, E. H. and Swiss, E. D. (1955). The role of the liver in the disposition of procaine in the dog. *J. Pharm. exp. Ther.* 113, 470—474

18 Spinal and extradural analgesia
R. Bryce-Smith

OPERATIVE INDICATIONS

Spinal and extradural analgesia may be used interchangeably for many surgical operations and, within this field, it is almost impossible to present clear indications for one or the other method. There is well agreed support for both techniques for pelvic, perineal and lower limb surgery — in fact, for most operations below the umbilicus. But even enthusiasts for local analgesia will question the advantages in upper abdominal or thoracic surgery, although the literature will show no lack of such employment. Much of this support depends on the non-involvement of the respiratory tract, particularly in the presence of lung disease, when compared with general anaesthesia. This assumption disregards the reduced ventilatory efficiency and paralysis of the muscles of respiration which follows a high block and which may be further aggravated by the position of the patient. Hypoxia is thus caused which, with an accompanying fall in blood pressure, may be disastrous to some patients. Further, any limitation of active coughing in the presence of increased secretions will only aggravate the situation and suggest most strongly that a general anaesthetic, with adequate oxygenation, ventilatory assistance and ability to aspirate secretions, would be preferable. Obviously the employment of local analgesia does not preclude the concurrent use of general anaesthesia, and in the majority of instances a combined approach will be preferable to all concerned. Indeed, there are few occasions when retention of consciousness is essential for life. Sedation at least is advisable in all but those exceptional circumstances and, whenever possible, the wishes of the patient for unconsciousness should be met. Before pursuing any course of action, it is often salutory to place oneself in the patient's position and consider whether you would appreciate what is intended.

As in so many positions, common sense can provide a better answer than hard and fast rules. Where, however, an advantage may be gained by prolongation of the block, say, to control postoperative pain, the insertion of a catheter will permit repeated injections — and the extradural route is to be preferred in these cases.

OBSTETRICS

This aspect of pain relief offers perhaps the most extensive use of both spinal and extradural analgesia. A full and detailed account of this application will be found in Chapter 72.

THERAPEUTIC INDICATIONS

It is perhaps in the realm of therapeutic applications that specific choices between extradural and spinal analgesia can be made with some confidence.

Postoperative pain

The introduction of bupivacaine and its prolonged effects have encouraged the use of extradural analgesia in the control of postoperative pain. Ideally, this should be conducted by means of serial injections through an indwelling catheter and continued for as long as necessary, but the practical difficulties of arranging 'top-up' injections are not easily overcome. Even a single dose may serve the purpose of starting the patient off free of pain for the first few postoperative hours and is well worthwhile. Either procedure may be used regardless of the method of anaesthesia chosen for the surgery itself.

The value of a continuous thoracic block has been well demonstrated (Simpson *et al.*, 1961) even with the relatively short-acting lignocaine. It is excellent in the presence of severe pain which would otherwise be controlled only by heavy doses of centrally acting analgesics which would be sufficient to cause respiratory depression. Since this type of block can be segmental, minimal falls of blood pressure occur and intercostal paralysis is limited. It is therefore ideal after thoracotomy, high abdominal incisions and in the presence of fractured ribs (Lloyd and Rucklidge, 1969).

At the other end of the extradural space, a continuous sacral block may usefully be employed in the relief of posthaemorrhoidectomy pain and after open prostatectomy and a variety of orthopaedic procedures on the lower limbs.

Chronic pain

The precision with which an intradural injection of small volumes of solution may be made is a clear advantage in the deposition of neurolytic solutions. These include phenol, alcohol, silver nitrate and *m*-chlorocresol. Each has its place in the control of chronic pain, as does the use of barbotage (Lloyd, Hughes and Davies-Jones, 1972), or the injection of ice-cold or other hypertonic solutions (Hitchcock, 1967).

As a preliminary to a more permanent interruption of nerve fibres, the injection of a conventional spinal solution may be a valuable diagnostic

guide (Lloyd, 1976). It might be noted here that occasionally an intra-
thecal block may aggravate phantom limb pains (Leatherdale, 1956); and
the use of neurolytic solutions, even after causing an apparently complete
sensory loss, may have little if any effect on this distressing condition.

Extradural blockade has a limited use in the management of chronic
pain, save in one or two isolated circumstances. The employment of
neurolytic solutions has been universally disappointing and is not recommended. Nevertheless, Lipton (1976) has suggested that it is not unreasonable to institute serial injections of local analgesics through an
indwelling catheter, conducted by a patient's relatives, during the final
stages of a terminal illness with the patient at home.

Perhaps the main use of an extradural blockade in the treatment of the
more chronic types of pain is in types of 'sciatica'. Here the introduction
of 80 mg of methylprednisolone, with or without large volumes of local
analgesic solution or saline, has been advocated. It is probable that the
steroid is the most useful component of any mixture, although it is
claimed that larger volumes of solution may be helpful in breaking down
adhesions. The treatment may be repeated if necessary and the results are
often encouraging (Swerdlow and Sayle-Creer, 1970).

Renal colic

Renal colic can cause violent pain as a stone, often small, is passed down
the ureter. Pain becomes worse if the stone impacts, and is usually associated with ureteric spasm. The institution of a continuous extradural
block will immediately relieve the pain and the accompanying spasm.
This allows spontaneous passage of a stone which, it is claimed, may
occur in 55% of patients (Lloyd and Carrie, 1965).

Prolonged dilatation of the bladder

Encouraging results have been obtained by providing prolonged (two or
more hours) dilatation of the bladder where the bladder is unstable and
and where frequency may be the result of some types of carcinoma
(Ramsden *et al.*, 1976). The stimulation from this distension is considerable and is best managed by a continuous lumbar extradural block
which can be maintained for as long as the distension is planned. It has
been suggested that concurrent use of a caudal as well as lumbar extradural block may have certain advantages (Brown, Arthurs and Glashan,
1974), since the blockade may have to be extensive. To give complete
pain relief, it may be necessary not only to block the sacral nerves, but to
go as high as T8. During the course of distension, the patient must be
carefully observed, with regular monitoring of the blood pressure. This is
not only in the general interests of the patient, but also in an attempt to
match the distending pressure against the systolic blood pressure. Ideally,
a degree of hypotension of the order of 80 mmHg is desirable.

TECHNIQUE

Lumbar approach

The technique of lumbar puncture should be sufficiently well known and has been described in great detail by a number of authors, one of the best known being Macintosh and Lee (1973). It is perhaps the attention to small details and an understanding of the anatomy which spell success with the avoidance of unnecessary difficulties. The position of the patient, with maximum flexion of the spine, is the first requirement, followed by careful identification of an interspinous space. The needle should always be inserted slightly cephalad, with accurate direction determined once it has passed through the skin. This can be facilitated by ensuring that the operator's eye is at the same level as the needle.

Although the L2—3 or L3—4 interspaces are usually chosen, and these are recognized by counting from the intercristal line, the actual level is of less importance than choosing a well defined space, bearing in mind that the cord ends at the second lumbar vertebra. At first sight, it is easier to introduce the needle in the midline when, as it is advanced, it passes through the supraspinous ligaments before reaching the ligamentum flavum. However, a lateral approach, starting 1 cm lateral to the spine, with a medial direction so that it reaches the midline only at the ligamentum flavum, avoids the tough and sometimes calcified ligaments and has much to recommend it. With this method, the needle is not gripped so firmly and the sensation of resistance offered by the ligamentum flavum is more easily recognized.

To this point, approach to the lumbar extradural space is identical to that of lumbar puncture, but the needle must be arrested before the dura is penetrated. This requires accurate tactile appreciation of the ligamentum flavum, a feat clearly favouring the lateral approach, especially when a large-bore Tuohy needle is used. Recognition of the extradural space may be facilitated by the sudden loss of resistance to the injection of air (Flowers, Hellman and Hingson, 1949) or saline (Dogliotti, 1933) or by the presence of a negative pressure (Heldt and Moloney, 1928). Doubts have been expressed about the very existence of the negative pressure (Dawkins and Steel, 1971) and it is suggested that it may be found in only about 70% of patients. Thus, more and more, reliance is placed on the 'loss of resistance' test, using finger pressure on the barrel of a well fitting syringe, rather than such devices as a spring-loaded syringe (Brunner and Iklé, 1949), a balloon (Macintosh, 1950) or a spring-loaded stylet (Macintosh, 1953) which, while excellent, have practical failings and may not always be available.

The loss of resistance, confirmed by the free passage of a catheter, may be applied to extradural injections performed at other levels, although the introduction of a needle will require a different technique.

Thoracic approach

The obliquity of the spinous processes prevents a midline approach to the extradural space and a lateral approach is obligatory. It is achieved by identifying the appropriate level and inserting the needle vertically, 1 cm lateral to the chosen spine. It will then strike the lamina of the vertebra below. By directing the needle medially and cephalad, it may be 'walked' across the surface of the bone until it ultimately reaches the ligamentum flavum, which is pierced in the midline. Using a Tuohy needle, the rounded side of the bevel (opposite to the side opening) must be presented to the dura over which it will glide, making puncture almost impossible.

Caudal approach

With the patient in the prone or left lateral position, the sacral cornua are identified with the first and third fingers of the left hand. The middle finger palpates the smooth, posterior aspect of the coccyx and slides upward until the ridge outlining the rim of the sacral hiatus is reached. In a child, on whom a single-dose technique is intended, as for post-circumcision pain (Davenport, 1973; Kay, 1974), a 21 gauge needle is inserted vertically, just caudad to the middle finger, where it will pierce the sacrococcygeal membrane and the injection is made immediately.

When it is intended to insert a catheter in an adult, demanding the use of a large-bore needle, the above technique must be modified. Once more the needle is inserted at right angles to the skin, but about 1 cm more caudad. The hub is now depressed in a series of steps toward the buttocks. Pressure is maintained until the needle assumes the general direction of the caudal canal and the point finally slips through the sacrococcygeal membrane. The space may be recognized by the free injection of air or saline and a catheter should run easily beyond the tip of the needle. It should not, however, be advanced more than about 5 cm for fear of impinging on an obstruction which might deflect it through one of the intervertebral foramina.

By recognizing the posterior, inferior iliac crests, the lumbosacral angle may be determined. A catheter inserted to this level overcomes the posterior angulation of the sacrum and the consequent leak of local analgesic solution through the anterior sacral foramina (Bryce-Smith, 1954). This allows injections to be made which will achieve any height of block required without the use of large volumes of solution. In effect, the injection is made only one or two vertebral spaces inferior to a standard lumbar extradural approach. The same results may therefore be expected by adding an additional 3—5 ml of solution to that considered to be the correct volume for a block at L3—4 interspace. Such an approach may be invaluable in patients who are grossly arthritic or whose spines are fused, making a lumbar extradural injection impossible.

Rarely, a dural tap may be performed inadvertently. This occurs, not as a rule in consequence of advancing the needle too far, but to a developmental abnormality in which the cord and dura remain tethered to the coccyx. In such instances, cerebrospinal fluid will flow the moment the needle passes through the sacral coccygeal membrane (Dawkins, 1969).

LOCAL ANALGESIC SOLUTIONS

Use of local analgesic solution, or indeed any drug, requires in the UK the approval of the Committee of Safety of Medicines, and the corresponding body in other countries. This limitation is appreciated by an author and the examination candidate, if not the enthusiastic investigator. The list of drugs may be further shortened by availability and, perhaps even more important, general acceptance by anaesthetists on the merits of convenience, reliability and good results. Thus, for extradural analgesia, little else is used (in the UK) but lignocaine and bupivacaine, while for spinal analgesia, cinchocaine, prilocaine or mepivacaine are the only choices. All are well established drugs whose properties require no reiteration.

Solutions for spinal analgesia

In the UK, only hyperbaric solutions are used or, indeed, are obtainable for spinal analgesia. Most so-called light preparations are now believed to approximate isobaric solutions and thus achieve distribution within the cerebrospinal fluid by volumetric displacement rather than by gravity control (Macintosh and Lee, 1973). It is thus comparatively simple to learn a standard technique which requires but minor modifications to suit the particular analgesic agent chosen and achieve a predictable result. Such generalizations will apply to the majority of patients. There is little doubt that the relative specific gravity of the injected solution to that of the cerebrospinal fluid (sp. gr. 1.004), permitting gravity control of the agent by the patient's posture, is the major factor in determining spinal spread. However, experiments suggest that differences between cinchocaine (sp. gr. 1.025), prilocaine (sp. gr. 1.024) and mepivacaine (sp. gr. 1.035) play little part in the speed with which such solutions reach their destinations, particularly when the distance to be travelled by the solution is short.

Only where it is intended to achieve higher blocks and the distance which the solution must travel exceeds 10 cm, does the relative baricity have any significance. Thus, most preparations will take about 20 ± 5 s to travel 10 cm, say, the distance from the site of lumbar puncture to the bottom of the dural sac. But in achieving a high spinal, with a run of perhaps 20 cm, the heavier solution will require only 60 s compared with the lighter solutions which take 90 s to travel the same distance. However, the specific gravity of cerebrospinal fluid can vary appreciably, as can the viscosity. Both of these factors are further influenced by the temperature of the cerebrospinal fluid and that of the injected solution — the latter being usually administered at room temperature but quickly reaching that of body temperature. This effect, together with the dilution of the local anaesthetic by cerebrospinal fluid, also accounts for the slower onset of analgesia in high blocks. Possibly, too, the rate of circulation of cerebrospinal fluid, normally slow but greatly increased by a raised cerebrospinal fluid pressure, the result of a subarachnoid injection or increased peridural venous pressure, may exert some influence (Lofgren, 1975). The significance of these factors is not fully understood, but they could be responsible for the occasional unexpected behaviour of spinal analgesia, for example, in the pregnant woman at term or the seriously dehydrated patient. At the other end of the scale, fluid retention would also cause gross alterations in the mechanics, composition, viscosity and specific gravity of their respective cerebrospinal fluid (Bryce-Smith, 1976).

TABLE 18.1. Comparison of commonly used spinal analgesic drugs

	Concentration	Glucose	Sp. gr. at 37°C	Onset of full analgesia (min)	Complete recovery (min)
Amethocaine	0.2%	6.0%	1.060	7.0	120
Lignocaine	5.0%	7.5%	1.035	4.5	95
Cinchocaine	0.5%	6.0%	1.025	5.0	130
Prilocaine	5.0%	5.0%	1.022	3.0	110
Mepivacaine	4.0%	9.5%	1.035	3.0	100

* The specific gravity of cerebrospinal fluid is 1.004

The details of lignocaine are included because it is such a widely used preparation in other parts of the world, as is amethocaine, although sometimes only in a limited form in prepacked, sterile, spinal analgesia kits.

Bupivacaine, while used extensively for epidural analgesia, has not been popular for spinal analgesia, although reports imply that it can be used safely for this purpose (Ekblom and Widman, 1966). It is suggested that extensive protein binding may be the cause of its prolonged effect. Since an accidental spinal may occur during the performance of an extradural block, it is well to realize that full recovery may take as long as nine hours (Gillies and Morgan, 1973).

Extradural analgesic solutions

The rather complicated physicochemical properties which apply in spinal analgesia are not seen in extradural analgesia where one is concerned solely with the volume injected and the concentration of the drug which determine the quality of the analgesia. Distribution of solution depends almost exclusively on the volume although it may be difficult to determine precisely what this should be in a given patient. Numerous formulae have been suggested, although these are open to question because the total capacity of the extradural space cannot be accurately determined. The extradural space extends from the base of the skull to the sacral hiatus. It is of course only a potential space, being filled with fat, areolar tissue, blood vessels (from which blood may be displaced) and the spinal nerves.

Although classically it may be described as that part of the vertebral canal not occupied by the dural sac and its contents, this definition does not allow for the extravertebral extensions through the intervertebral foramina at all levels. Thus the extradural space has no precise limits and hence estimates of its volume must be treated with caution. By the same token, formulae to determine the volume of local analgesic solution to achieve a given level can only provide guidelines.

Attempts to determine the capacity of the extradural space have been made. Originally, iodized oil (Lipiodol) was injected and the volume related to the radiological appearances (Sicard and Forestier, 1921). Later, sodium iodide, more accurately representing a local analgesic solution, was used in fresh cadavers and gave a figure of 118 ml for the complete extradural space (Farr, 1926). From this one might attempt to estimate the required dose of a solution required to produce a given effect. However, neither this nor the formula suggested by Bromage (1954) has stood the test of time. Most workers now try to place the site of injection as near as possible to the midpoint of the segments to be blocked (Bonica *et al.*, 1957) and then think in terms of 1–1.5 ml of solution per segment with a total of 12–15 ml of solution. In a caudal extradural this figure will be raised to about 20 ml. Volumes much in excess of these figures will in any case approximate to toxic doses. No method exists of predetermining the size of the intervertebral foramina and, consequently, the amount of solution which will 'leak' alongside the nerves. The bony foramina as shown radiologically are no indication of their effective size which will be determined by the extent of ligamentous encroachment, the superior costotransverse and radiate ligaments in the thoracic region being the most important. At other anatomical levels some limitation is effected by the apposition of the anterior and medial scalene muscles in the cervical region and the relation of the psoas muscle to the lumbar foramina.

At the sacral level, the multifidus and sacrospinalis muscles complete the closure of the posterior sacral foramina, permitting only the passage of the posterior primary rami of the spinal nerves. But anteriorly, the pyriformis muscle interdigitates with the anterior sacral foramina (the equivalent to the lateral intervertebral foramina at other levels) but leaves them unobstructed. However, it is only in the sacral region that the foramina are totally patent and this explains why large quantities of solution may be required to produce anything other than involvement of the sacral nerves when caudal analgesia is employed. The situation is aggravated by the posterior curve of the sacrum relative to the lumbar portion of the vertebral canal so that with a patient lying supine it becomes necessary to fill the sacral canal before solution can overflow past the lumbosacral angle, an almost impossible task because of the constant leakage around the sacral roots. The analogy of trying to fill a bath with the plug out is most apt. The difficulty can readily be overcome by the use of a catheter inserted to the region of the lumbosacral angle, shown by the position of the posteroinferior iliac spines which are usually apparent as two dimples on either side of the midline.

Whatever level of extradural analgesia is established, the choice of lignocaine or bupivacaine will usually be determined by the duration of analgesia required. In many instances, bupivacaine will obviate the necessity of establishing a continuous block. Since, however, the effects of bupivacaine are long lasting, it may be advisable to establish the level of analgesia in the first instance by the use of a shorter-acting drug and so establish the volume required for subsequent use.

SITE OF ACTION

When a local analgesic solution is deposited in the subarachnoid space, there is no difficulty in appreciating that the cerebrospinal fluid acts as a vehicle carrying the drug to the spinal nerves as they leave the substance of the cord. The dorsal root ganglia may be affected directly, but it is of greater importance that the dorsal and ventral roots are bathed in the solution much as in any other form of peripheral nerve block.

In the extradural space, solutions may act theoretically in three different ways: by passing through the dura mater; by affecting the nerves after losing their dural cover (i.e. in the paravertebral spaces); or in the so-called 'ink-cuff' zones. The last refer to that area where the dura is thinning out to become perineurium, and which has been found to permit the passage of colloidal carbon particles and presumably, more easily, crystaloid molecules (Woollam and Millen, 1953). Experiments by Frumin *et al.* (1953) have shown that when an extradural injection is made, the local analgesic drug may be demonstrated in the cerebrospinal fluid at a different level. But whether the concentration is sufficient to achieve the degree of analgesia usually seen, is open to question (Sarnoff and Arrowood, 1946). It has also been shown that during the onset of extradural analgesia, zones of delayed effect, corresponding to the distribution of intercostal nerves, may be seen (Bryce-Smith, 1954). This suggests a restriction to flow in the region of the respective intervertebral foramina, presumably ligaments.

However, the 'ink zone' theory appears to satisfy both observations (1) that local analgesics can enter the cerebrospinal fluid at the periphery of the dural sleeve, and (2) that this sleeve may be compressed as it passes through the foramen. In most instances, the spinal nerves pass freely through the intervertebral foramina and dural extensions can be encountered during the performance of a paravertebral block. It is suggested that the drip of cerebrospinal fluid from a paravertebral needle does not necessarily indicate that the vertebral portion of the dura has been punctured as was once thought (Macintosh and Bryce-Smith, 1962), but rather that the dural sleeve has extended more laterally than usual. This opinion is supported by the confident prediction that if a dural tap is performed once during a series of paravertebral injections, it will probably occur at other levels in the same patient.

Obstruction at the intervertebral foramen could also explain the phenomenon of the unblocked segment, which is sometimes completely unaffected by further injection or by changing the position of the patient.

It has been estimated that an unblocked segment will be encountered in about 6.5% of all extradurals and most commonly at the T12—L1 levels (Ducrow, 1971). A different local analgesic drug may be tried, but as a rule effective analgesia can be achieved only by a paravertebral block of the appropriate nerve.

COMPLICATIONS

Apart from the technical difficulty of locating the subarachnoid space, there can be immediate consequences of establishing extradural or intra-dural analgesia. They are hypotension, respiratory failure and a total spinal blockade, all clearly dependent on the extent of the analgesia produced. Since a total or high spinal may well be intended as a means of deliberately lowering the blood pressure, it can only be considered a complication if it occurs unexpectedly. On the other hand, falls in blood pressure and, to a lesser extent, reduction in respiratory efficiency, can occur with almost any block in which the technique and management have been impeccable.

Hypotension

A fall in blood pressure will be dependent on the extent of the sym-pathetic paralysis and hence the size of the peripheral pool. At the same time, any block which rises above the L1 segment will effectively denervate the adrenal glands without causing peripheral vasodilation of more than the lower limbs. In all instances, the adoption of a head-down position, together with a rapid intravenous infusion of fluid, should quickly restore the situation. If necessary, a vasopressor, such as methoxamine (Vasoxine) or metaraminol (Aramine), may be administered intravenously.

Respiratory failure

Any form of local analgesic block which rises above the L1 segment will involve the trunk and will necessarily affect the intercostal nerves. The degree of intercostal paralysis may be further aggravated by the position of the patient. While the diaphragm should remain able to function until the blockade reaches the C3 level, it may not in practice be effective if abdominal distension, due to any cause, splints its movement. Clearly, too, the consequences will be more significant in any patient suffering from respiratory disease; thus local analgesia, while not directly influencing the respiratory tract, may not be preferable to general anaesthesia. Simi-larly, a thoracic block to relieve postoperative discomfort or the pain of fractured ribs must be limited in extent if serious respiratory paralysis (and hypotension) is to be avoided.

Oxygen given by a light-weight facemask in mild degrees of respiratory depression may be sufficient, but any other circumstances may well demand positive pressure ventilation after intubation which may require that the patient is rendered unconscious. In the case of a total spinal block, intubation and ventilation must be considered the first step and in most instances will not require the use of a general anaesthetic or muscle relaxant.

Neurological complications

It is perhaps in this field, more than any other, that the differences between intra- and extradural blockade become most significant. Clearly, the integrity of the dura mater is the important factor and since this necessarily influences the attitude, not only of anaesthetists, but also the general public, it is necessary to review the facts as far as they are understood.

FOLLOWING SPINAL ANALGESIA

Headache ranks high as a cause of distress to the patient. It is now generally accepted that the majority of postspinal headaches are due to the leakage of cerebrospinal fluid through the puncture hole in the dura mater. Thus, the water cushion supporting the brain becomes deficient, allowing the brain to pull on the tentorium cerebellum and surrounding blood vessels. Fortunately, the headache is rarely due to an underlying meningitis and is less often seen today following the adoption of a more careful technique and in the use of a fine gauge needle.

Transient paralysis of all the cranial nerves other than the first and tenth has been reported, but, with the exception of the sixth nerve, these are extremely rare. Abducent palsy should perhaps be regarded more correctly as a complication of extradural analgesia, as it is more likely to occur after an inadvertent dural tap with a large gauge needle (e.g. a Tuohy) prior to the insertion of an extradural catheter. It is suggested that the mechanism is due to a sudden loss of the CSF cushion of the brain, allowing the sixth nerve, in its long intracranial course, to become stretched across the petrous portion of the temporal bone (Bryce-Smith and Macintosh, 1951).

Although perhaps not a complication, for the effects are so transient and possibly not even noticed by the patient, is the development of a Horner's syndrome. It has been reported after lumbar extradural (Mohan, Lloyd and Potter, 1973) and caudal blocks (Mohan and Potter, 1975). It probably occurs more frequently than has been imagined, but hitherto the explanations for this phenomenon have not been altogether convincing.

However, it is the more serious permanent neurological damage which is of far greater significance and which is less well understood. These complications were reviewed fairly recently (Greene, 1961), and it was found that the frequency with which they occur has fallen appreciably during the last few decades. Pathologically, these complications are due to involvement of the meninges or the nerve tissue itself. Usually, however, both elements exist but with predominance of one type or the other. Thus arachnoiditis would seem to be more likely where the concentration of the local analgesic used was high, and the cauda equina is most frequently involved. The nerve lesion tends to be chronic in onset but may become progressively worse. Only when the meningeal reaction is inflammatory may one expect an acute reaction.

When nerve tissue is primarily involved, the usual picture is of destruction of the myelin nerve roots or cord with minimal meningeal reaction giving a picture of a non-progressive neurological deficit.

Radiculitis due to direct trauma with a needle is unlikely to occur in the corda equina region since the nerves are free-lying. At higher levels it is possibly due to the introduction of the needle too far laterally, although cord may be involved if the puncture is midline but made above the level of the second lumbar vertebra.

In examining the possible causative factors in these disasters, there would seem to be few which cannot be greatly minimized by scrupulous attention to asepsis, technique and employment of acceptable analgesic preparations. On comparing the supposed factors, a remarkable similarity is seen between these and the deliberate procedures now employed in the control of chronic pain. In a roundabout way it would seem that we are now making use of past misfortunes to interfere deliberately with nerve conduction and offer benefit to others. Conversely, if it is now recognized that certain procedures can cause nerve damage, then it should be possible to avoid such damage in normal spinal analgesia (Bryce-Smith, 1976).

FOLLOWING EXTRADURAL ANALGESIA

The complications described in the section above are almost exclusively the sequelae of spinal analgesia and have not been ascribed to extradural blockade. However, this latter technique carries with it the now well recognized anterior spinal artery syndrome, in which the posterior columns of the cord are spared (Annotation, 1958; Davis, Soloman and Levene, 1958). It seems likely that this condition may follow a period of hypotension in which the flow in the long anterior spinal artery becomes so reduced that intravascular clotting occurs. Thus, it is not surprising that occasionally the condition is progressive as the extent of the thrombus increases (Wells, 1966).

Haematoma

Haematomata may be caused by the introduction of any needle whether or not an analgesic drug has been injected. It has also been reported after general anaesthesia and in circumstances not even associated with surgical operations at all (Current Comment, 1948; Sinclair, 1954). Clearly, the concurrent use of anticoagulant therapy should preclude the use of spinal or extradural analgesia since the resultant pressure effect of the haematoma within the vertebral canal, particularly in the extradural space, may compress the cord, causing a paraplegia. Since an increasing number of patients are now receiving pre- and postoperative anticoagulant therapy to avoid the possibility of deep vein thrombosis or pulmonary embolus, one may be placed in something of a dilemma. Common sense suggests that if the therapy is to be effective in preventing thrombus formation, there must necessarily be an increased bleeding tendency and, further, there should be a realization that the response to any given dose of a drug varies from person to person. Thus a subcutaneous dose of heparin which may have no apparent effect in one person may cause complete lack of clotting in another. One must therefore advise that no needles should be introduced for spinal or extradural analgesia, nor indeed for any 'deep' local analgesic techniques, without first determining the clotting or bleeding state of the patient. In the absence of laboratory facilities, simple bleeding times (using a spring-loaded lance to give a standard puncture in the ear or finger) or the clotting time, may be used by anyone to give a rough guide.

Infection

Infection by either method is possible and of the gravest possible consequence. It is a serious complication, whatever the cause, and there is little to choose between the gravity of meningitis after a spinal tap and an extradural abscess following an extradural injection with a consequent pressure paraplegia. Unless the sterility of the equipment, drugs and technique can be completely guaranteed, neither method should even be contemplated.

Toxicity

The dose of analgesic solution injected is only likely to approach toxic levels during extradural analgesia. The amount used in spinal analgesia is insignificant.

In few other circumstances is it common practice to inject such a large volume of local analgesic solution of a relatively high concentration into a vascular area as in the extradural space, no matter which route is chosen. Thus, the possibility of a toxic reaction must always be borne in mind and the appropriate means of resuscitation must be immediately to hand.

Pre-existing central nervous system disease

While it may be considered unwise to risk the recrudescence of a pre-existing or dormant lesion, there is no properly documented instance in which this has occurred following spinal analgesia (Macintosh and Lee,

1973). For the peace of mind of the operator, and the patient, it is probably as well to choose extradural analgesia should some form of block be required in these patients.

Catheter breakage

Although comparatively rare with modern catheters, breakage still occurs in a limited number of circumstances. In the case of extradural analgesia it would seem that no action should be taken other than to inform the patient's general practitioner and make a careful record of the accident on the patient's notes (Atkinson, 1976). Attempts at finding the broken end are likely to result in a profitless laminectomy since fragments of catheter are notoriously difficult to locate in the tissues and migrate by virtue of muscle action to unexpected places. Only if the break has occurred at the skin margin may it be permitted to seek the fragment just below the skin with the use of a simple infiltration of local solution. Should a fracture occur during the conduct of a continuous spinal, a very different situation arises as there is a risk of a CSF fistula with consequent infection. Thus no choice remains but to carry out a full-scale exploration.

References

Annotation (1958). Occlusion of anterior spinal artery. *Lancet* ii, 515

Atkinson, R. S. (1976). Extradural block. In *Practical Regional Analgesia,* p. 136. J. A. Lee and R. Bryce-Smith (ed.). Amsterdam: Elsevier

Bonica, J. J., Backup, P. H., Anderson, C. E., Hadfield, D., Crepps, W. F. and Monk, B. F. (1957). Peridural block: analysis of 3637 cases and a review. *Anesthesiology* 18, 747–784

Bromage, P. R. (1954). *Spinal Epidural Analgesia,* p. 81. Edinburgh: Livingstone

Brown, P. R., Arthurs, G. J. and Glashan, R. W. (1974). Epidural analgesia in the treatment of bladder carcinoma. *Anaesthesia* 29, 422–428

Brunner, C. and Iklé, A. (1949). Beitrag zur peridural-anästhesie. *Schweiz. med. Wschr.* 79, 799–801

Bryce-Smith, R. (1954). The spread of solutions in the extradural space. *Anaesthesia* 9, 201–205

Bryce-Smith, R. (1976). The enigmas of spinal analgesia. *Proc. R. Soc. Med.* 69, 75–82

Bryce-Smith, R. and Macintosh, R. R. (1951). Sixth nerve palsy after lumbar puncture and spinal analgesia. *Br. med. J.* 1, 275–276

Current Comment (1948). Paraplegia following inhalation anesthesia. *Anesthesiology* 9, 439–440

Davenport, H. T. (1973). *Paediatric Anaesthesia,* 2nd edn, p. 143. London: Heinemann

Davies, A., Soloman, B. and Levene, A. (1958). Paraplegia following epidural anaesthesia. *Br. med. J.* 2, 654–657

Dawkins, C. J. M. (1969). An analysis of the complications of extradural and caudal block. *Anaesthesia* 24, 554–563

Dawkins, C. J. M. and Steel, G. C. (1971). Thoracic extradural block for upper abdominal surgery. *Anaesthesia* 26, 41–48

Dogliotti, A. M. (1933). Segmental peridural anesthesia. *Am. J. Surg.* 20, 107–118

Ducrow, M. (1971). The occurrence of unblocked segments during continuous lumbar epidural analgesia. *Br. J. Anaesth.* 43, 1172–1173

Ekblom, L. and Widman, B. (1966). LAC-43 and tetracaine in spinal anaesthesia. *Acta anaesth. scand.* Suppl. 23, 419–425

Farr, R. E. (1926). Sacral anesthesia. *Archs Surg., Chicago* 12, 715–726

Flowers, C. E., Hellman, L. M. and Hingson, R. A. (1949). Continuous peridural anesthesia and analgesia for labour, delivery and caesarean section. *Anesth. Analg. curr. Res.* 28, 181–189

Frumin, M. J., Schwartz, H., Burns, J. J., Brodie, B. B. and Papper, E. M. (1953). The appearance of procaine in the spinal fluid during peridural block in man. *J. Pharmac. exp. Ther.* 109, 102–105

Gillies, I. D. S. and Morgan, M. (1973). Accidental total spinal analgesia with bupivacaine. *Anaesthesia* 28, 441–445

Greene, N. M. (1961). Neurological sequelae of spinal anesthesia. *Anesthesiology* 22, 682–698

Heldt, T. J. and Moloney, J. C. (1928). Negative pressure in epidural space. *Am. J. med. Sci.* 175, 371–376

Hitchcock, E. (1967). Hypothermic subarachnoid injection for intractable pain. *Lancet* i, 1133–1135

Kay, B. (1974). Caudal block for postoperative pain relief in children. *Anaesthesia* 29, 610–611

Leatherdale, R. A. L. (1956). Phantom limb pain. *Anaesthesia* 11, 249–251

Lipton, S. (1976). Pain relief. In *Recent Advances in Anaesthesia and Analgesia,* p. 240. C. L. Hewer and R. S. Atkinson (ed.). Edinburgh: Churchill Livingstone

Lloyd, J. W. (1976). Management of intractable pain. In *Practical Regional Analgesia,* pp. 216–217. J. A. Lee and R. Bryce-Smith (ed.). Amsterdam: Elsevier

Lloyd, J. W. and Carrie, L. E. S. (1965). A method of treating renal colic. *Proc. R. Soc. Med.* 58, 634

Lloyd, J. W., Hughes, J. T. and Davies-Jones, G. A. B. (1972). The relief of severe intractable pain by barbotage of the of the cerebro-spinal fluid. *Lancet* i, 354–355

Lloyd, J. W. and Rucklidge, M. A. (1969). Management of closed chest injuries. *Br. J. Surg.* 56, 721–722

Lofgren, J. (1975). *Intracranial Pressure,* 2nd edn, p. 75. N. Lundberg (ed.). Berlin: Springer

Macintosh, R. R. (1950). Extradural space indicator. *Anaesthesia* 6, 98–99

Macintosh, R. R. (1953). Extradural space indicator. *Br. med. J.* 1, 398

Macintosh, R. R. and Bryce-Smith, R. (1962). *Local Analgesia: Abdominal Surgery,* 2nd edn, p. 53. Edinburgh: Livingstone

Macintosh, R. R. and Lee, J. A. (1973). *Lumbar Puncture and Spinal Analgesia,* 3rd edn, pp. 133, 167. Edinburgh: Churchill Livingstone

Mohan, J. and Potter, J. M. (1975). Pupillary constriction and ptosis following caudal epidural analgesia. *Anaesthesia* 30, 769–773

Mohan, J., Lloyd, J. W. and Potter, J. M. (1973). Pupillary constriction following extradural analgesia. *Injury* 5, 151–152

Ramsden, P. D., Smith, J. C., Dunn, M. and Ardran, G. M. (1976). Distension therapy for the unstable bladder. *Br. J. Urol.* 48, 623–629

Sarnoff, S. J. and Arrowood, J. (1946). Differential spinal block. *Surgery* 20, 150–159

Sicard, A. and Forestier, J. (1921). Radiographic method for exploration of the epidural space using lipiodol. *Revue neurol.* 37, 1264–1266

Simpson, B. R., Parkhouse, J., Marshall, R. and Lambrechts, W. (1961). Extradural analgesia and the prevention of postoperative respiratory complications. *Br. J. Anaesth.* 33, 628–641

Sinclair, B. J. (1954). Ascending spinal paralysis following hysterectomy under general anaesthesia. *Anaesthesia* 9, 286–287

Swerdlow, M. and Sayle-Creer, W. (1970). A study of extradural medication in the relief of the lumbosciatic syndrome. *Anaesthesia* 25, 341–345

Wells, C. E. C. (1966). Clinical aspects of spinovascular disease. *Proc. R. Soc. Med.* 59, 790–795

Woollam, D. H. M. and Millen, J. W. (1953). An anatomical approach to poliomyelitis. *Lancet* i, 364–367

19 Clinical use of nerve blocks in relation to surgery
Clive Jolly

The use of nerve blocks to relieve pain before and after surgery is becoming more widely recognized and, although general anaesthesia is often a first choice for pain relief during surgery, local analgesia still has a role because of its simplicity and safety. An increasing use of nerve blocks may be due to the popularity of epidural analgesia in obstetrics and the formation of pain relief clinics where much of the work has been centred around nerve blocking techniques.

This chapter discusses the role of nerve blocks with an emphasis on the practical aspects of this branch of anaesthesia. Indications and selected individual techniques are described.

ADVANTAGES AND DISADVANTAGES

In situations where long operating lists are necessary to cope with a heavy surgical workload some anaesthetists have simplified their techniques and quote the time needed to induce local analgesia as a disadvantage. There is no doubt that nerve blocks cannot be hurried but careful organization can eliminate this disadvantage. A patient scheduled for regional analgesia can be brought to the theatre about half an hour before the estimated finishing time of the previous operation. The block can be carried out in the induction or anaesthetic room without pressure of time and the patient can then be sedated and left in the charge of a nurse while the local analgesia takes effect.

In the accident and emergency department the use of local analgesia confers more flexibility upon the work of the department. The hazard of inducing general anaesthesia in the presence of a full stomach can mean long delays between a patient arriving in the department and being considered to be in a safe state for induction of general anaesthesia. A four-hour wait is the conventional time allowed but this is very unreliable. The hazard of regurgitation and inhalation of stomach contents can be eliminated by the use of local analgesia, and the timing of the operation can be at the convenience of patient, surgeon and anaesthetist. Although it is preferable for the anaesthetist to be present during the operation, this is not essential provided he is sure that the block has taken effect and the patient has not suffered any side-effects of the injection.

The skill required to use local analgesic techniques is not difficult to acquire but it does need practice. The law of diminishing returns applies in that the fewer blocks an individual anaesthetist uses, the less reliable is the result. The anaesthetist must have some motivation to use local techniques and to keep using them despite disappointing results with the first few cases. (Intravenous regional analgesia is the only 'block' requiring no special skill and should be used more frequently.) This, however, applies to all new techniques, and anaesthetists must make a decision whether to use local analgesia more frequently or not, after considering the possible indications for these techniques. Certainly if a busy hospital has no anaesthetist using local analgesia, then possible indications for their use will be passed by. The discussion of indications later in this chapter will show that these are more frequent than is sometimes realized.

If they are given a choice, patients in the UK will usually opt for general anaesthesia rather than local analgesia. This is partly because of a fear of being awake and aware of the frightening aspect of operating theatres. This dramatic side of medicine is popular viewing on television but definitely unpopular when the centre of attraction is oneself. In practice, however, few patients have an absolute dread of local analgesia. Some patients, on the other hand, have a fear of general anaesthesia and would prefer to be awake during the operation. This is why a preoperative visit is essential when the procedure should be explained, the patient reassured and a well timed premedication prescribed. Sedation is discussed more fully later in the chapter because it is so important to the success of a nerve block.

The surgeon's views on local analgesia are important. Some surgeons find it difficult to work with a conscious patient. They find that the necessity to watch their conversation is distracting, and there is no doubt that a quiet theatre is a factor helping with the success of a nerve block. Unless local analgesia is essential to the patient's life, then it is unwise to persist with this choice of pain relief in these circumstances. The opposite may be the case, however. Some surgeons prefer local analgesia for certain operations, and combinations such as retrobulbar block with neuroleptanalgesia for lens extraction, epidural block for lower abdominal surgery and brachial plexus block for tendon repairs are examples of situations in which surgeons often urge the anaesthetist to use local techniques. In many cases, surgeons who are not accustomed to operating upon patients who have had a regional nerve block are surprised at the intensity of the analgesia and the efficiency of the covering sedation.

Another quoted disadvantage of local analgesia is the rare complication of a nerve palsy. This is a matter of some concern to a few anaesthetists but it has to be remembered that a rare complication of general anaesthesia is cardiac arrest and death, or severe brain damage. Generally, the complications of local analgesia are few and it is a remarkably safe procedure.

The advantages and disadvantages are seldom clear-cut but correct management of the local analgesic technique will obviate some of the disadvantages. This aspect will now be considered.

TECHNIQUE

A meticulous technique is of the greatest importance to the success of a local nerve block. This fact is too often forgotten but may explain why one anaesthetist will succeed with local analgesia while his colleagues can never seem to make these techniques work.

Preparation and sedation

The patient should always be visited before operation, to explain the procedure and to tell him what to expect. It should especially be mentioned that the patient may feel touch but that this is normal and does not mean that the block is not working well. If the patient is told he will feel nothing and some sensation of touch is still present then he may well assume that pain will follow.

Sedation should be prescribed. Diazepam has proved an excellent drug for this purpose and has the added advantage of providing marked amnesia. The degree of drowsiness is variable but if it is not marked there is still absence of anxiety and seemingly alert patients will have no memory of the preanaesthetic period. In a very few instances diazepam seems to stimulate patients; if this is so then further sedation must be added. The timing of the administration of the diazepam is critical and one hour before induction gives the best results (Assaf, Dundee and Gamble, 1975; Gamble, Dundee and Assaf, 1975). An oral dose of 20 mg is suitable for the average adult.

The opiates are still widely used for premedication but have the drawback of causing nausea in some people. However, the addition of the powerful antiemetic drug droperidol counteracts this side-effect and also induces a neuroleptic type of sedation. A reliable sedation routinely used by the author for ophthalmic surgery is as follows: 45 minutes before expected induction of local analgesia, an intramuscular injection of papaveretum 10—20 mg with droperidol 5—10 mg is given. On arrival in theatre the sedation is increased if necessary, using fentanyl and droperidol. For this purpose a mixture of fentanyl 0.1 mg and droperidol 10 mg is diluted with water to 5 ml. One ml increments are given intravenously until the sedation is considered to be satisfactory. Diazepam 2.5 mg is always given just before induction of local analgesia and provides a greatly increased incidence of amnesia.

The timing of the nerve block should be such that the anaesthetist can work without pressure. The local analgesic may take 20 minutes to achieve its optimum effect and this should be taken into account.

Equipment and drugs

These should be checked before the anaesthetic is started. The most difficult piece of equipment to find may be a suitable needle. The conventional 21 gauge 3.5 cm intravenous needle will usually be adequate for brachial plexus and stellate ganglion blocks. Smaller needles as employed for intravenous injection can be used for other nerve blocks. Longer needles may be needed in obese patients and for paravertebral blocks. Even if few nerve blocks are carried out, every hospital should have available a plentiful supply of disposable needles such as, for example: 20 gauge 6.5 cm and 20 gauge 9 cm. If a lumbar sympathetic block is to be carried out, then a 13 cm needle is necessary; these are not readily available as disposable needles but can be kept separately sterilized in long glass tubes sealed at the central sterile supply department.

Markers to indicate depth of insertion of the needle are essential for accuracy in some blocks. Small squares of thin rubber are very effective since they grip the needle firmly but can be moved easily along its length.

Ampoules of local analgesic solution should be provided in sterile packs. Standardization of local analgesic drugs within an anaesthetic department is a simple procedure and the few solutions needed can be sterilized in the central sterile supply department and distributed to theatres, accident and emergency and outpatient departments.

The question of sterility is important. The standard may fall when many nerve blocks are carried out, but the anaesthetist should aim to be just as meticulous with his technique as his surgical colleagues are with even the simplest operation.

Procedure

It is best to identify bony landmarks before preparing the operation site. In the obese patient this may be difficult, and essential bone markings such as the spinous processes of the vertebrae should be marked with a skin pencil. The skin can then be washed with the antiseptic fluid of choice which will dry and sterilize the skin while the anaesthetist scrubs up. If, during the course of the nerve block, the needle has to pass deeply into the tissues or if some probing has to be done to identify a deep bony landmark, then the needle should be inserted slowly while injecting a dilute local analgesic solution. Lignocaine 0.25%, or its equivalent, is adequate but the maximum dosage level should be kept in mind. The aim is to cause little or no pain to the patient. In a few blocks it is less painful to identify the position of the landmarks and then insert the needle smoothly and swiftly. A stellate ganglion block from the anterior approach is an example of this technique.

Before making the final injection, an aspiration test should be made to ensure that the needle point is not within a blood vessel. A test dose of about 2 ml is made, with the wait of a few minutes if there is any doubt as to the position of the needle. This is particularly necessary if there is a possibility that the injection may enter the subarachnoid space; for example, in stellate ganglion or cervical plexus blocks. During infiltration analgesia the correct technique is to keep the needle moving and inject local analgesic solution all the time.

After the block has been completed, testing for skin sensation to see if the block has worked should be unobtrusive. The patient needs to feel that the doctor is confident of his treatment. Similarly, surgeons should be discouraged from making such remarks as: 'I am cutting you now, tell me if it hurts'.

Quiet confidence is the keynote in management of local analgesia, remembering that, during the performance of the nerve block, the patient is awake and may be frightened despite premedication.

INDICATIONS

Outpatient surgery

With the increasing surgical workload there is a shortage in many hospitals of beds, nurses and anaesthetists. One of the solutions has been to have the patient come into hospital in the morning and return home after surgery (Dean and Wilkinson, 1969; Williams, 1969; Calnan and Martin, 1971). This has made the task of the anaesthetist more, and not less, difficult. To provide good operating conditions with the patient alert and ready to leave hospital a few hours later is not always easy. Here, the increasing use of local analgesia can be a great help and also results in more confidence and a high percentage of successful nerve blocks.

In 'Necessity into choice' Nicholls (1977) makes this point clear when discussing herniorraphy under local analgesia. The following are examples where the use of local analgesia is possible: all operations on the upper limb under brachial plexus block or intravenous regional analgesia; some trunk operations under intercostal block with reinforcing local infiltration; herniorraphy under local analgesia; and foot operations under ankle block. Intravenous diazepam in small doses can be used as sedation during the operation if required and will leave no appreciable hangover. Another advantage of local analgesia is the removal of the hazard of a full stomach. Not every patient is reliable and instructions concerning food and drink are sometimes disregarded.

Accident and emergency department

The hazard of the full stomach using general anaesthesia is ever present in this department and the conventional four-hour wait from meal to surgery is by no means an adequate safeguard. The choice of local analgesia means that the patient can be operated upon without having to wait for his stomach to empty and his treatment can be fitted into the routine of a busy department. It is sensible to choose the anaesthesia to suit the patient's convenience and the doctor's time.

Analgesia for serious injuries to extremities

Patients who have severe but localized injury to hand, arm, foot or leg may suffer severe pain. The movement involved in transferring these patients from accident departments to operating theatres can be distressing. Often there is a waiting period while the theatre is made available. Opiates can be given but these are not totally effective in preventing severe pain, and local analgesia is seldom used for pain relief. It may be that this indication for nerve block is unconventional, certainly there is no clinical contraindication. Brachial plexus block, sciatic nerve block (by the anterior approach), femoral and obturator nerve block can all be carried out in the accident department. The patient should then be pain-free until operation. In these circumstances, even if the nerve block is not completely effective, the pain relief will be impressive. Campbell (1977) mentions local analgesia in this context when discussing the immediate hospital care of the injured, and Berry (1977) describes the use of femoral nerve block to give analgesia to patients with fractures of the femur.

Disaster and emergency situations

There has been some discussion about the best method of anaesthesia in disaster situations where existing anaesthetic services are overwhelmed. Selective use of local analgesia will allow patients undergoing operation to be supervised by trained ancillary staff while anaesthetists can administer general anaesthesia to more ill patients.

Shortage of trained staff

The use of intercostal block was found to be valuable by Farman, Gool and Scott (1962). Working in West Africa they had difficulty in training technicians in the management of anaesthesia using muscle relaxants. An alternative and satisfactory technique was instituted. The technician, supervised by a doctor, induced anaesthesia and intubated using either suxamethonium or ether. The surgeon then administered a bilateral intercostal nerve block. This provided excellent muscle relaxation and the general anaesthesia with spontaneous respiration was easily managed by the technician. This historic technique of intercostal nerve block covered by light general anaesthesia can be used with good results even within present-day circumstances.

Embolectomy

Removal of an embolus from the femoral artery is a not uncommon operation. In many cases these patients are very ill and general anaesthesia is hazardous. Local infiltration is usually the choice in these circumstances but regional nerve block is more satisfactory, and a femoral nerve block combined with obturator nerve block provides good operating conditions without distress to the patient (Gjessing and Harley, 1969).

Ophthalmic surgery

Ophthalmic surgery is so often carried out under local analgesia that the fact is rarely commented upon. Here is a situation where the operation site is small in area, well circumscribed and has a nerve supply which can be easily blocked with a local analgesic technique. In lens extraction for cataract there is a particular need for anaesthesia which avoids post-operative coughing, straining or vomiting. Neuroleptanalgesia is frequently used and can give impressive results. What is so often forgotten is that an essential part of the technique is the local analgesia that is induced. The neuroleptanalgesia provides the sedation which should accompany even perfect local analgesia. The surgeon usually induces local analgesia but there is no reason why the anaesthetist should not carry out this technique. In a busy ophthalmic operating list this division of labour is often more sensible since time can be allowed for the nerve block to work without delaying the operating list.

Medical indications

Patients with serious medical illness as opposed to surgical disease often need operations or diagnostic investigations, and local analgesia has advantages because there is so little upset of the respiratory or cardio-vascular systems. The management of anaesthesia in a poor-risk patient using intercostal nerve block for muscle relaxation is described in Clinical Anesthesia Conference (1969). The advantage of this method of local analgesia is the absence of hypotension which may be caused when other nerve-blocking techniques such as epidural or subarachnoid block are used.

Examples of diagnostic investigations under local analgesia are brachial plexus block for the provision of shunts in uraemic patients undergoing dialysis (Bromage and Gertel, 1972) and axillary brachial plexus block for cardiac catheterization in young children (Ross and Williams, 1970).

Postoperative analgesia

Postoperative pain following abdominal and thoracic operations may not be totally relieved by intramuscular injections of analgesics, and there is no doubt that the most complete relief of pain is obtained by using epidural analgesia. Some anaesthetists are reluctant to use this technique since frequent top-up injections are needed and there is a hazard of hypotension due to block of the sympathetic nervous system. Skilled nursing care and careful observation are necessary for this technique and a shortage of nursing staff and a heavy workload on the surgical wards may make the valuable technique of epidural analgesia hazardous. Another approach has been to use intercostal nerve block with the long-acting drug bupivacaine, which gives analgesia for 8—12 hours (Moore, 1975; Cronin and Davies, 1976; Humphreys and Kay, 1976). The large number of injections is a disadvantage but, with care, this is not distressing to the patient. If repeated once or twice then the most uncomfortable postoperative period can be covered.

Pain following oral surgery has been treated with nerve block using lignocaine and dextran (Meyer and Chinn, 1968). The action of the dextran is not clearly understood but its addition to lignocaine appears to prolong the action of the local analgesic (Loder, 1962).

Pain relief after herniorraphy can be relieved by blocking the ilio-inguinal and iliohypogastric nerves immediately after induction of general anaesthesia. This is a very simple technique almost free from complications.

Fractured ribs

Intercostal nerve block is being used in the treatment of chest injury with multiple fractured ribs (Campbell, 1977). In selected cases this form of pain relief avoids the use of intermittent positive pressure respiration which carries its own morbidity and mortality (Trinkle *et al.*, 1975).

Tracheal intubation

Patients with intestinal obstruction and in danger of regurgitation and inhalation of stomach contents are usually managed by rapid induction of anaesthesia with cricoid pressure. An alternative technique is to intubate the patient under topical anaesthesia before induction, thus ensuring that the trachea is sealed before intravenous induction agents are administered. This technique is particularly applicable to the near-moribund patient where even the most careful induction may cause serious cardiovascular depression. Thomas (1969) has reviewed 25 patients intubated under local analgesia, and Wycoff (1959) has described the technique in detail.

Skin grafting

The anterior aspect of the thigh is a most convenient skin graft donor site and a wide area is available. This procedure can be carried out under local analgesia since the femoral nerve and lateral cutaneous nerve of thigh are easy to block. The drawback hitherto has been the difficulty in blocking the obturator nerve and overlap of distribution may cause discomfort. Winnie (1975) has described a technique whereby the lumbar plexus can be blocked with one injection. This obviously has implications for other operations in this area.

CONTRAINDICATIONS AND COMPLICATIONS

If an anaesthetist is to carry out any nerve block, it is essential that he should be aware of the contraindications and how to treat ensuing complications. It is of interest that while there are several contraindications to subarachnoid and epidural blocks (principally because of the effect on the sympathetic nervous system causing hypotension), there is no absolute contraindication to regional analgesia. This is some indication of the safety of local analgesia. Relative contraindications which must be mentioned are determined patient opposition, allergy to a particular agent which would contraindicate its use and anticoagulant therapy.

Preoperative use of subcutaneous heparin to protect against postoperative venous thrombosis (Nicolaides *et al.*, 1972) is sometimes considered to be a possible contraindication. However, the proponents of prophylactic heparin say that there is no increased oozing during operation, and this should apply to the site of local analgesia. Extra care, however, should be taken to avoid unnecessary movement of the needle within the tissues. The use of intravenous regional analgesia is, of course, in no way contraindicated by anticoagulant therapy.

Complications

General complications of regional analgesia include broken needles, sepsis and injection of the wrong solution, but the most dangerous complication is overdose of local analgesic. Doctors who prescribe drugs with care and knowledge often have an illogical blind spot when using local analgesics. This is particularly the case when drugs such as lignocaine are employed for topical anaesthesia in investigations such as bronchoscopy. Cocaine, for example, has an upper dose limit by weight, for a fit adult, of 200 mg (3 mg·kg^{-1}) and since it is often used in concentration of 10% for topical analgesia, then the dose by volume is as low as 2 ml. The fact that absorption through mucous membranes can be very rapid should be remembered, and safe upper limits of dosages apply in exactly the same quantity for topical anaesthesia as for parenteral administration.

Absolute overdose is inexcusable. The upper dosage of lignocaine is 200 mg (3 mg·kg^{-1}) if used alone and 500 mg (7 mg·kg^{-1}) if adrenaline is added. In the case of bupivacaine the upper dose limit is 140 mg (2 mg·kg^{-1}) with or without adrenaline. However, these dose limits apply to the average fit adult, and elderly, small, ill patients and children will tolerate correspondingly less. Berger, Tyler and Harrod (1974) quote two deaths where 400 mg of lignocaine was used without adrenaline, showing that these dose limits are not just theoretical supposition. The rule that 1 ml of 1% solution contains 10 mg simplifies calculation of weight of drug from concentration.

Relative overdose can also occur if a safe amount of drug is accidentally injected into a blood vessel.

Effects of overdose

The result of overdose is always stimulation followed by depression. This may affect the cardiovascular system resulting in hypotension and temporary loss of consciousness, or the central nervous system where the drama of a convulsive attack tends to overshadow the following depression.

Convulsions cause death by anoxia and therefore the first priority is to stop the fit. Thiopentone is readily available but adds cardiovascular depression to the cerebral depression which follows the stimulation. Suxamethonium is safer but best of all is diazepam which reduces the increased activity in the central nervous system.

In each case apnoea will follow cessation of convulsions and intermittent positive pressure ventilation must be carried out. It is an inviolable rule that local analgesia should not be carried out without resuscitation equipment available. This means relevant drugs and apparatus to carry out intermittent positive pressure ventilation. If treatment is rapidly instituted then the patient is not seriously affected by this complication.

Cardiovascular depression is treated with intravenous infusion and oxygen, while vasopressors are used only if necessary and in very small doses to avoid a hypertensive reaction.

It can be seen from the foregoing that it is wise to insert an indwelling needle into a vein before carrying out any block, with the exception of techniques, such as those used for conservative dentistry, where a very small dose of local analgesic is injected.

SPECIFIC TECHNIQUES

Space precludes the detailed description of regional analgesic techniques but there are many books published on this subject, some of which are mentioned in the Further reading list at the end of this chapter. A few techniques are described briefly, with an emphasis on a practical approach to the problems involved.

Supraclavicular brachial plexus block

The possibility of pneumothorax deters some anaesthetists from carrying out this valuable and simple block but the incidence is low, below 1%, in most published reports. The technique described by Ball (1962) reduces the incidence of this complication and is a more logical approach to the plexus.

The anaesthetist stands at the head of the table rather than at the side. Point of injection is 1 cm above the midpoint of the clavicle. The needle is inserted downwards and caudally but not backwards or medially. The aim is to touch the first rib close behind the subclavian artery where injection of local analgesic is made. If paraesthesiae are obtained then the point of the needle is moved a very small distance and the whole amount of 20—30 ml of local analgesic is injected. Injection is thereby made into the fascial envelope covering the plexus. If no paraesthesiae are felt then the needle is stepped back on the rib, injecting 8 ml of local analgesic at a time, completing the injection as above if paraesthesiae are elicited. Up to 20 minutes should be allowed for the block to take effect.

Axillary brachial plexus block

This approach is safer than the supraclavicular and more acceptable to the patient since paraesthesiae are less necessary for the block's success. Anaesthetists often find it less easy than the supraclavicular approach and with a lower incidence of success. The following comments should be helpful.

With the arm abducted at right angles and the elbow flexed, the axillary artery is palpated and traced as high in the axilla as possible. The forefinger of the anaesthetist's left hand is placed on the artery in this position and the needle is inserted, without the syringe attached, at an acute angle to the skin (i.e. nearly parallel to the finger). A slight 'give' is felt when the sheath is pierced. The needle should then oscillate in time with the arterial pulse and this is the most valuable sign that the needle is placed correctly. The needle can then be held with the fingers of the left hand while a syringe is attached and injection is made. An alternative is to use a Labat syringe with rings on the barrel when the syringe is kept attached to the needle while the needle is placed in position. Aspiration before injection can be made with less risk of displacing the needle. The Labat syringe tends to be overlooked in favour of disposable syringes but it is a most useful instrument and deserves wider use. A tourniquet tied distal to the injection site encourages spread of local analgesic upwards where the musculocutaneous nerve leaves the fascial sheath. Winnie (1975) estimates the amount of local analgesic required (in millilitres) to be half the patients height in inches.*

Intravenous regional analgesia

This technique, for analgesia of the upper limb, deserves much wider use since it is reliable and needs minimal skill (Kennedy, Duthie and Parbrook, 1965; Thorne-Alquist, 1971). It is more successful if a rubber tourniquet is used to empty the venous blood from the limb as opposed to simple elevation of the arm. A helpful modification when the lesion is painful is to use an inflatable splint to compress the arm (Finlay, 1977). Two cuffs are needed, otherwise the presence of a tight cuff over a sensitive area will distress the patient. An indwelling needle is inserted into a vein before the tourniquet is applied, and when the veins are empty the upper cuff is inflated to a pressure above the systolic blood pressure. Injection of 0.5% lignocaine or prilocaine, at a dosage of approximately 40 ml, is then made.

* 1 inch = 2.54 cm.

After five minutes the lower cuff is inflated above the systolic blood pressure and the upper cuff is deflated. This means that the tight cuff, which has to be kept inflated for the duration of the operation, is around an analgesic area of the arm. At least 15 minutes should elapse after completion of the injection before the lower cuff is deflated. The incidence of reaction to possible spread of local analgesic into the general circulation is very low.

This technique can be used for analgesia of the lower limb but it is less satisfactory. Dosage of local analgesic for the lower limb is 60—80 ml.

Intercostal nerve block

If this technique is to be carried out for laparotomy then the patient has a general anaesthetic induced first and a cuffed endotracheal tube inserted. Spontaneous respiration is allowed during the operation since abdominal muscular relaxation follows block of the intercostal nerves. The patient remains supine and his arms are abducted with the elbows flexed. The arms are supported in this position by an assistant. This position must not be extreme and the test is to put oneself in this situation to see how far the arms will abduct and flex without discomfort. This manoeuvre exposes the lateral aspects of the chest, and intercostal nerve block can then be carried out in the midaxillary line without the patient having to be moved. It must be remembered that the lateral cutaneous branches may not be affected by block at this level but, since a general anaesthetic is induced, this is of no importance.

The needles used are 21 gauge 3.5 cm. Up to six needles are used; after each nerve is blocked the needle is withdrawn to skin level and left hanging in position until the end of the procedure. This acts as a marker to indicate which ribs have been blocked.

About 3 ml of 0.25% bupivacaine is adequate for each nerve block. If 0.5% is considered necessary for a large man it must be remembered that the dose injected will be above the 140 mg dose quoted as a maximum. In this case the amount injected at each site should be reduced to 2.5 ml. Lignocaine 0.5% can be used with adrenaline.

Femoral and obturator nerve block

Femoral nerve block is very simple to carry out. The nerve lies lateral to the artery (NAVY: i.e. nerve, artery, vein and 'Y' where the legs join the body), and 10 ml of local analgesic injected 1—2 cm lateral to the palpated artery pulsation will give an effective block.

Obturator nerve block is less easy. Textbooks on local analgesia should be studied carefully and the anatomical drawings visualized in the anaesthetist's mind. Point of injection is 1 cm below and lateral to the pubic tubercle. A 21 gauge 3.5 cm needle is inserted at right angles to the skin and injection of dilute local analgesic is made until the advancing needle touches bone. The needle is then replaced by an 8 cm needle which is inserted with the hub depressed toward the thigh and moved medially.

Bone is not touched and, at about twice the depth of the previous needle insertion, 10 ml of 0.5% bupivacaine or 1% lignocaine with adrenaline is made. As the needle is withdrawn, a further 10 ml of local analgesic is injected. Reduction of the power of abduction of the leg indicates a successful nerve block.

Winnie (1975) describes a technique whereby both blocks can be carried out through one approach by injecting a local analgesic solution into the fascial sleeve surrounding the femoral and obturator nerves.

References

Assaf, C. A. E., Dundee, J. W. and Gamble, J. A. S. (1975). The influence of the route of administration on the clinical action of diazepam. *Anaesthesia* 30, 152–158

Ball, H. J. C. (1962). Brachial plexus block. A modified supra-clavicular approach. *Anaesthesia* 17, 269–273

Berger, G. S., Tyler, C. W. and Harrod, E. K. (1974). Maternal deaths associated with paracervical block anesthesia. *Am. J. Obstet. Gynec.* 118, 1142

Berry, F. R. (1977). Analgesia in patients with fractured shaft of femur. *Anaesthesia* 32, 576–577

Bromage, P. R. and Gertel, M. (1972). Brachial plexus anesthesia in chronic renal failure. *Anesthesiology* 36, 488–493

Calnan, J. and Martin, P. (1971). Development and practice of an autonomous minor surgery unit in a general hospital. *Br. med. J.* 1, 92–96

Campbell, D. (1977). Immediate hospital care of the injured. *Br. J. Anaesth.* 49, 673–679

Clinical Anesthesia Conference (1969). Regional anesthesia in a poor risk patient. *N.Y. St. J. Med.* 69, 2678–2679

Cronin, K. D. and Davies, M. J. (1976). Intercostal block for postoperative pain relief. *Anaesth. Intens. Care* 4, 259–261

Dean, D. and Wilkinson, B. R. (1969). Outpatient operations. As the GP sees it. *Br. med. J.* 1, 176–177

Farman, J. V., Gool, R. Y. and Scott, D. B. (1962). Intercostal block in abdominal surgery – a method for the single handed surgeon. *Lancet* i, 879–881

Finlay, H. (1977). A modification of Bier's intravenous analgesia. *Anaesthesia* 32, 357–358

Gamble, J. A. S., Dundee, J. W. and Assaf, C. A. E. (1975). Plasma diazepam levels after single dose, oral and intramuscular administration. *Anaesthesia* 30, 164–169

Gjessing, J. and Harley, N. (1969). Sciatic and femoral nerve block with mepivacaine for surgery on the lower limb. *Anaesthesia* 24, 213–218

Humphreys, C. S. and Kay, H. (1976). The control of postoperative wound pain with the use of bupivacaine injections. *J. Urol.* 116, 618–619

Kennedy, B. R., Duthie, A. M. and Parbrook, C. D. (1965). Intravenous regional analgesia – an appraisal. *Br. med. J.* 1, 954–957

Loder, R. E. (1962). A long acting local anaesthetic solution for the relief of pain after thoracotomy. *Thorax* 17, 375–376

Meyer, R. A. and Chinn, M. A. (1968). Prolonged postoperative analgesia with regional nerve blocks. *J. Oral Surg.* 26, 182–184

Moore, D. C. (1975). Intercostal nerve block for postoperative somatic pain following surgery of the thorax and upper abdomen. *Br. J. Anaesth.* 47, 284–286

Nicholls, J. C. (1977). Necessity into choice. An appraisal of inguinal herniorrhaphy under local anaesthesia. *Ann. R. Coll. Surg.* 59, 124–127

Nicolaides, A. N., Desai, S., Douglas, J. N., Fourides, G., Dupont, P. A., Lewis, J. D., Dodsworth, H., Luck, R. J. and Jamieson, C. W. (1972). Small doses of subcutaneous sodium heparin in preventing deep venous thrombosis after major surgery. *Lancet* ii, 890–893

Ross, D. M. and Williams, D. O. (1970). Combined axillary plexus block and basal sedation for cardiac catheterisation in young children. *Br. Heart J.* 32, 195–197

Thomas, J. L. (1969). Awake intubation (indications, techniques and a review of 25 patients). *Anaesthesia* 24, 28–35

Thorne-Alquist, A. M. (1971). Intravenous regional anaesthesia. *Acta anaesth. scand.* Suppl. 40

Trinkle, J. K., Richardson, J. D., Franz, J. L., Grover, F. L., Arom, K. V. and Holstrom, F. M. G. (1975). Management of flail chest without mechanical ventilation. *Ann. thorac. Surg.* 19, 355–363

Williams, J. A. (1969). Out-patients operations. 1. The surgeon's view. *Br. med. J.* 1, 174–175

Winnie, A. P. (1975). Regional anesthesia. *Surg. Clins N. Am.* 55, 861–892

Wycoff, C. C. (1959). Aspiration during anesthesia, its prevention. *Curr. Res. Anesth. Analg.* 38, 5–13

Further reading

Bonica, J. J. (1969). *Clinical Anesthesia,* Vol. 1. *Regional Anesthesia: Recent Advances and Current Status.* Oxford: Blackwell

de Jong, R. H. (1970). *Physiology and Pharmacology of Local Anesthesia.* Springfield, Ill: Charles C Thomas

Eriksson, E. (1969). *Illustrated Handbook of Local Anaesthesia.* London: Lloyd-Luke

Jolly, C. (1962). *Local Analgesia.* London: H. K. Lewis

Lee, J. A. and Bruce-Smith, R. (1976). *Practical Regional Analgesia.* Monographs in Anesthesiology, Vol. 5. Amsterdam and Oxford: Excerpta Medica

Macintosh, R. and Bryce-Smith, R. (1962). *Local Analgesia: Abdominal Surgery,* 2nd edn. Edinburgh: Livingstone

Macintosh, R. and Mushin, W. W. (1967). *Local Analgesia: Brachial Plexus,* 4th edn. Edinburgh: Livingstone

Macintosh, R. and Ostlere, M. (1955). *Local Analgesia: Head and Neck.* Edinburgh: Livingstone

Moore, D. C. (1967). *Regional Block,* 4th edn. Springfield, Ill: Charles C Thomas

III The respiratory system

20 **Structural basis of lung function**
Norman C. Staub

GENERAL RELATIONSHIPS

The classic textbooks of lung structure and pathology describe the gross anatomy of the lung reasonably well. Other books, such as those by Weibel and by Cumming and Hunt, are concerned with quantitative histology and special anatomy. While these are valuable, the view of the whole lung tends to get lost in the details. The *American Review of Respiratory Diseases*, since 1974, has published a remarkable series of monthly reviews entitled, 'State of the Art', on a wide variety of pulmonary subjects. None, however, has dealt with over-all lung structure.

The normal adult human lungs weigh about 1000 g, of which 500 g is blood, and 500 g is lung tissue. At functional residual capacity (FRC), normally 3 litres, the over-all density of the lung is 0.25 $g \cdot ml^{-1}$. Every radiologist knows, or should, that the chest x-ray shows predominantly the shadows of blood vessels and larger airways. Alveolar structures (the actual respiratory portion of the lung) cannot be resolved. *Figure 20.1* shows a normal upright chest x-ray.

In the upright position, the lung averages 27 cm high at TLC but in the range of normal breathing (FRC) the over-all height is approximately 24 cm. In the lying position, as shown in *Figure 20.2*, the maximum anterior—posterior lung dimension at FRC is 20 cm.

The position of the heart in relation to the lungs is important. For example, what does it mean to say that the mean pulmonary artery pressure in man is approximately 1.9 kPa (19 cmH_2O)? Clearly, with the lung 24 cm high at FRC, pulmonary artery pressure cannot be 1.9 kPa everywhere. The same must also be true of pulmonary venous pressure.

West (1970) has described lung zones based upon the relationships between pulmonary arterial (Ppa), left atrial (Pla), and alveolar (Palv) pressures. In zone I, Palv > Ppa > Pla. There is no blood flow. In zone II, Ppa > Palv > Pla. Alveolar pressure regulates flow (Starling resistor effect). In zone III, Ppa > Pla > Palv. Flow is independent of alveolar pressure.

There is no zone I in the normal adult human lung. For example, in

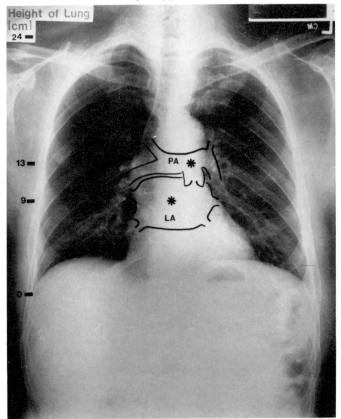

Figure 20.1
Chest x-ray taken in the standing position at FRC in a normal adult.
Total lung height is shown (cm) measured from costodiaphragmatic
angle to the tubercle of first rib. Main pulmonary artery (PA), its
branches and left atrium (LA) outlined. Asterisks (*) indicate
points where pressures are usually measured. PA pressure must
exceed 1.1 kPa (11 cmH$_2$O) in order to have lung apex perfused.
However, only 2% of total lung mass is in the top 10% of lung
height. The zone II/III boundary would be at 13 cm up the lung if
LA pressure is 0.4 kPa (4 cmH$_2$O). Thus, 70% of lung mass is below
this level. PA and LA pressures at the bottom of the lung are 1.3 and
0.9 kPa (13 and 9 cmH$_2$O) higher, respectively, than at the level of
measurement

Figure 20.1, the distance from the pulmonary artery bifurcation (where
pressure is usually measured) to the top of the lung is 12 cm. Thus, even
at the top of the lung, average pulmonary arterial pressure is about
0.7 kPa (7 cmH$_2$O) above alveolar pressure.

What is less obvious is that there is not much zone II in the normal
human lung either. In *Figure 20.1*, the height of the lung above the left
atrium is 15 cm and in the lying position (*Figure 20.2*), it is 10 cm. If *P*la
averages 1.1 kPa (11 cmH$_2$O) in the lying position and 0.3–0.4 kPA (3–4
cmH$_2$O) in the upright position, then the zone II/III boundary is only

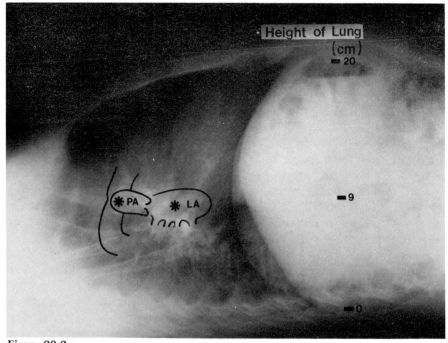

Figure 20.2
Chest x-ray taken in the lateral position lying down, at FRC. Same
subject as in Figure 20.1. Usual positions of PA and LA catheters for
pressure measurements are indicated by the asterisks (*). Because
pulmonary artery (PA) and left atrial (LA) pressures are higher,
essentially all of the lung is in zone III in the supine position

11—12 cm below the top of the lung in the upright position, and all of the
lung is in zone III in the lying position.

We must also consider the distribution of the lung mass within the
chest. Most of the lung is below the level of the zone II/III boundary in
the upright position. Based upon an old autopsy study of 50 adult humans,
I have computed that in the upright position about 60% of the lung mass
is below the left atrium. In the normal upright human, 70—75% of the
lung will be in zone III.

During positive pressure breathing, alveolar pressure rises relative to
left atrial pressure. The exact relationship depends on lung compliance
(effect on pleural pressure) and venous return (effect on cardiac output).
Nevertheless, as P_{alv} rises, more of the lung enters zone II. When attempting
to obtain a measure of left atrial pressure, via a pulmonary wedge catheter,
one must be certain that the catheter is in the zone III portion of the lung
in order to obtain a valid measure. This is not difficult to do in the normal
lung, especially in the usual lying position. But during positive pressure
breathing, there may be considerable uncertainty about the interpretation
of a wedge pressure.

AIRWAYS

There are three major groups of pulmonary airways: cartilagenous bronchi, membranous bronchioles and gas exchange ducts.

The summated volume of the bronchi below the trachea accounts for nearly half of the anatomical dead space as measured by single breath tests. Most of the remainder lies above the carina (trachea, glottis, pharynx, nose or mouth). The bronchioles, while exceedingly numerous, are very short and narrow. Although they are said to account for approximately 25% of the total anatomical dead space when measured histologically, in life they normally contribute far less, due to mechanical mixing of gas in the distal airways by the cardiac impulse. The gas exchange ducts, by definition, do not contribute to the anatomical dead space.

Of the air flow resistance distal to the carina, over 90% is localized within the cartilagenous bronchi in healthy normal adults. This is a complete reversal from the concepts of most respiratory physiologists 15 years ago. The change in view is due to quantitative measures of airway dimensions and to direct measurements of the pressure drop along the airways during air flow. The total cross-sectional area of the airway increases and gas flow velocity decreases rapidly in the bronchioles. The functional significance is that the alveoli of a lung segment are ventilated chiefly in proportion to their individual distensibilities (compliance) since airway resistance is common; that is, central.

Since the contribution of the bronchioles to air flow resistance is small, they would, as a group, have to be markedly constricted before over-all breathing resistance changed much. However, the distribution of ventilation among adjacent lung segments could be influenced by unequal alterations in bronchiolar diameter. Although there has been a great deal of investigation about regional differences in ventilation, not much is known about uneven ventilation among adjacent respiratory units.

The functional capabilities of the airways, not only in terms of smooth muscle tone, but also in terms of fluid and mucous secretion and propulsion of the mucociliary layer by the ciliated epithelium, are being examined vigorously. The distribution, function and regulation of the numerous individual cell types within the airway are shedding new light on specific functional details.

The smooth muscle and glands of the bronchi receive their motor innervation from the parasympathetic division of the autonomic nervous system over the vagus nerve. During normal breathing there is slight tonic airway constriction and little evidence for changes in large airway diameter. The main function of the external innervation to the smooth muscle may be to maintain a balance between anatomical dead space and air flow resistance. A small dead space improves the efficiency of alveolar ventilation but at the expense of increased work of breathing. An additional possibility is that reflex contraction of the large airways stiffens them against external collapse as may occur with forced expiration and coughing. The cough receptors are located in the trachea and main bronchi.

The bronchioles possess an abundant innervation although much of it is sympathetic vasomotor or from sensory receptors. It is uncertain how much parasympathetic motor innervation actually extends to the smooth muscle in the smallest airways. Experiments that demonstrate active, neurally mediated, constriction of bronchi do not show significant bronchiolar effects. Bronchiolar smooth muscle responds to local influences (H^+, CO_2, particulates, chemicals). For example, when the pulmonary circulation to a lung unit is occluded, ventilation to that unit decreases because of bronchiolar constriction. The fall of P_{CO_2} in the gas phase seems to be an important regulating factor.

The bronchioles in the normal lung are not constricted during breathing. Textbook pictures of collapsed, routinely prepared lungs give a false impression of airway shape and tone.

Because the bronchioles are directly attached to the connective tissue framework of the lung, they should passively dilate and constrict with increases and decreases in lung volume, respectively. At low lung volumes, they are narrower and their contribution to total air flow resistance is increased.

An important aspect of airway function is their nutritional blood supply. Both the cartilagenous and membranous airways in man receive a systemic (bronchial artery) blood supply in contrast to the gas exchange ducts which are fed by the pulmonary circulation. The venous effluent of the bronchial capillary network goes mainly into the pulmonary veins contributing to the physiological shunt-like effect.

Under some anaesthetic conditions, bronchial flow may increase but, in the absence of any increase in airway tissue oxygen consumption, calculated venous admixture from this cause is not affected.

The blood supply pattern is important because it provides an additional mechanism for discreet response among airways. Any substance related to or injected into the systemic veins would have its first and most concentrated action on the gas exchange ducts. In pulmonary embolism release of serotonin from the clot or release of endogenous lung histamine may cause selective alveolar duct and respiratory bronchiolar constriction. This has the effect of decreasing local compliance and ventilation without significantly affecting total airway resistance.

The transition from terminal bronchioles to respiratory bronchioles and alveolar ducts is sudden. *Figure 20.3* shows an example. We know little about the appearance and growth of alveoli except that during childhood, new alveoli and alveolar ducts are formed from bronchioles; that is, the lung grows centripetally and the number of bronchioles decreases from birth to adulthood.

Some investigators believe that the bronchiolar—alveolar junctions may represent areas of special function in terms of the clearance of cells, particulates and fluids.

ALVEOLI

The terminal respiratory unit (TRU) in the human lung consists of several alveolar ducts together with their accompanying alveoli. The unit, based

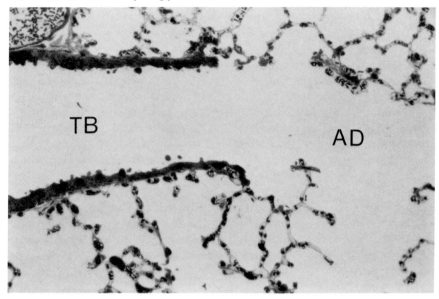

Figure 20.3
The transition from terminal bronchiolar (TB) epithelium to the
alveolar epithelium of the alveolar duct (AD) is abrupt. The bronchiole consists of a thin layer of connective tissue fibres continuous
with those of the adjacent alveolar walls, a discontinuous layer of
smooth muscle cells and secretory cells (Clara cells). The latter
account for the bumps seen along the TB lining. Normally, there
are no goblet cells at this level. (Mouse lung, 1 μm section, toluidine
blue, 150×)

upon combined anatomical and physiological grounds, was first described
by Hayek (1960) and contains 100 alveolar ducts and 2000 alveoli. At
FRC the unit is 3.5 mm in diameter with a volume of 0.02 ml. There are
150 000 such units in the normal adult human lung. The 'alveolus' of
which the physiologist speaks, is such a structure, not the anatomical
alveolus. The acinus, popular among pathologists, is somewhat larger.
Each acinus probably contains 10–12 ventilation units (TRUs).

In man there are about 300 million anatomical alveoli and 15 million
alveolar ducts. The alveolar gas volume is distributed between the alveoli
and ducts in the proportion of 2:1. *Figure 20.4* shows a section through
a ventilation unit.

The pattern of ventilation in the TRU is of interest. There is good
evidence, over the major range of lung volume, that fresh air ventilation is
confined to the alveolar ducts. The anatomical alveoli undergo gas exchange
by diffusion, which is a very rapid process over the short distances in the
TRU. The consequences of this pattern are that the anatomical alveoli
serve as a buffer volume to damp out large swings in end-capillary gas
tensions and that large particles, such as dust and medicinal aerosols, are
unlikely to reach or to deposit upon the main alveolar surfaces. Anaesthetic gases, of course, do reach the alveolar capillary membrane since

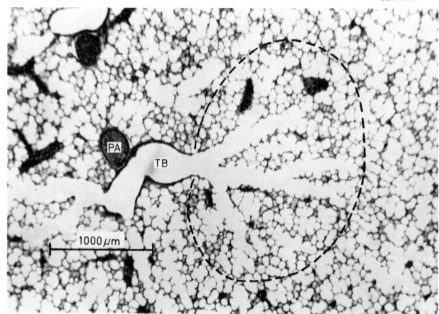

Figure 20.4
The terminal respiratory unit (the physiologist's 'alveolus') consisting
of the alveolar ducts and alveoli arising from a respiratory bronchiole.
The figure shows the unit in only one plane; the whole unit is
roughly spherical as the dotted outline suggests. Note the intimate
relation of the small vessels to the air spaces. TB, terminal bronchiole;
PA, pulmonary artery. (Guinea-pig, frozen, fixed, thin section)

their diffusion coefficients in air are similar to those of oxygen and
carbon dioxide.

Figure 20.5 is centred on an alveolar duct and its associated alveoli.
The diameter of the duct is about equal to the depth of the alveoli. There
has been much discussion about sequential ventilation in recent years. It
is clear that the pattern of mass ventilation into alveolar ducts followed
by diffusive exchange with adjacent alveoli is an example of sequential
ventilation. However, in the normal lung, the diffusion coefficients of
molecules in the gas phase is so rapid that there is no detectable difference
in partial pressures between alveolar duct and alveolar air within the
same TRU.

It is important to remember that the alveolar duct is functionally an
airway as well as a large fraction of the alveolar gas exchange volume.
The alveolar duct rings (see *Figure 20.5*) contain smooth muscle and have
the potential to regulate TRU volume and distensibility.

As the volume of gas in the lung changes, the TRU structures (anatomical
alveoli and alveolar ducts) change in volume and shape. Until recently the
consensus was that the ducts were the distensible structures. The alveoli
were thought to change shape but not volume as the alveolar ducts
expanded. The limited pleural surface view of the lung as it inflated and
deflated was compatible with such a scheme. The physiological argument

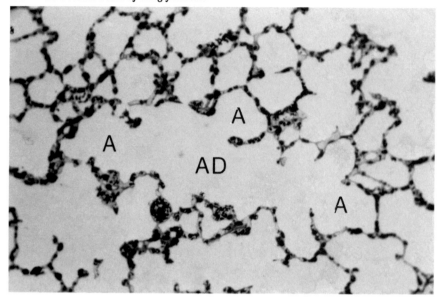

Figure 20.5
Alveolar duct (AD) and its associated alveoli (A). The duct is 100 μm
diameter as is the depth of the alveoli. Ducts are ventilated with
fresh air by convection (bulk flow). The alveoli are ventilated by
end-expiratory air from the AD. O_2 diffuses into and CO_2 diffuses
out of the alveoli so rapidly, over the short distances involved, that
no measurable oxygen or carbon dioxide tension gradients exist.
(Mouse, 1 μm section, toluidine blue, 150×)

in favour of that concept was that ventilation of only the duct prevented
sudden swings in blood gas tension but even more influential was the fact
that if the alveoli expanded, the alveolar walls must stretch, thereby
lengthening the capillaries and increasing pulmonary vascular resistance.

It is now clear that the old view is incorrect. Over the range of residual
volume (RV) to total lung capacity (TLC), the anatomical alveoli and
alveolar ducts show nearly proportional changes in volume. Their specific
compliances ($\Delta V/V\Delta P$), are the same. The inspired fresh air fills the ducts
while the alveoli fill with the end-expiratory alveolar duct gas.

Figure 20.5 shows that the anatomical alveolus is not spherical, as
depicted in models, but is a complex geometric structure with flat walls
and sharp curvature at the junctions between adjacent walls. This shape is
maintained until volumes below 25% of TLC are reached. *Figure 20.6*
shows pictures of the alveoli along the deflation pressure—volume curve of
the lung. The change in alveolar size is readily apparent. Shape changes are
obvious below 25% of TLC but quantitative analysis shows a change even
at 35% volume (FRC). The alveolar walls fold up at low lung volume.

Since linear dimensions change as the cube root of volume, increasing
alveolus volume from RV to TLC (a four-fold increase) only lengthens
the pulmonary capillaries by 0.6. Compared to other forces affecting
pulmonary vascular resistance, such a change is insignificant.

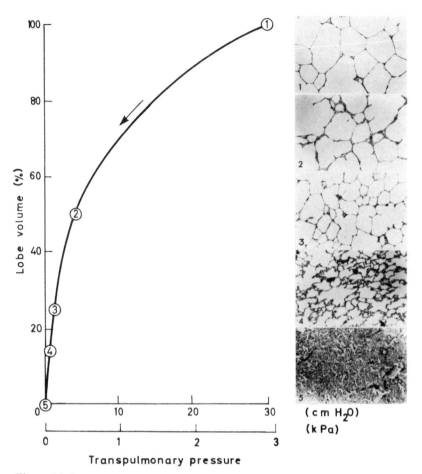

Figure 20.6
Alveolus and alveolar duct volume and shape changes at representative points along the air deflation, pressure—volume curve of lung.
The completely atelectatic lung is also shown. Volume changes
proportionally in alveolar ducts and alveoli between 100% *V* and
25% *V*. Alveolus shape begins to change at 35–40% *V* (near FRC).
(Cat, isolated lobes, frozen, fixed, thin sections, all at the same
magnification)

The isolated lung allowed to deflate passively does not become completely airless, but retains a minimal volume of 10–14% of TLC when
transpulmonary pressure is zero. Formerly, it was believed that airway
closure was responsible for the retained gas. From both anatomical and
physiological evidence, it is now apparent that the airways are not normally
closed at minimal volume. The reason for the volume retention is simply
that the elastic stresses (recoil) of the lung are zero. In *Figure 20.6*,
compare the completely airless lung with the one at minimal volume.
    The phenomenon of 'closing volume' has been explained as being due
to airway closure in lung units at low volume. If this is true, then either

the airways are under active smooth muscle constrictor tone, or the pleural pressure has gone positive relative to airway pressure, thereby compressing the lung.

The phenomenon of atelectasis does not usually involve individual alveoli. It is generally a phenomenon of a relatively large unit, possibly the TRU or even the acinus. Since even at zero transpulmonary pressure the gas volume of the units is not zero, additional causative factors must be involved in the development of 'spontaneous' atelectasis. A partial list of such factors includes the above mentioned airway closure by smooth muscle contraction, mucosal oedema or mucous plugs and prolongation of the low volume state (hypoventilation) which is conducive to a rise in the alveolar air—liquid interfacial tension, and fluid accumulation. These factors are accentuated by high alveolar Po_2 which favours rapid gas absorption by the blood distal to an obstruction.

The lung in the thorax is seldom at a uniform volume throughout. To say that the lung is at FRC does not mean that all TRUs are at FRC. As can be seen from a pressure—volume curve of the lung, units at low volume tend to be stiffer than units at intermediate volumes. This means that it is necessary to generate higher inflation pressures before these low volume units inflate. It is instructive to watch areas of compression atelectasis in the lung at thoracotomy as the anaesthetist inflates the lung. The well inflated lung does nearly all the 'breathing'. The compressed areas do not inflate.

On the other hand, over a period of time, atelectatic units within the lung spontaneously reinflate. This is partly explained by the forces generated through the structural interdependence between adjacent lung units.

PULMONARY CIRCULATION

In man, the pulmonary arteries travel adjacent to and branch with the airways down to the level of the TRU; that is, to the level of the respiratory bronchiole. In contrast, the pulmonary veins lie in the connective tissue septae at the periphery of the lung lobules as far from the artery and airway as is anatomically possible. At any level, the pulmonary artery and airway supply a limited zone of respiratory tissue, whereas the veins drain portions of several such zones and receive the bronchial venous drainage as well.

Because the pulmonary vascular bed is part of the low pressure circulation, its distensibility properties are more closely related to veins than to systemic arteries. The pulmonary vascular bed shares in increments of circulating blood volume and in redistribution of blood volume with hydrostatic or vasoactive changes. For example, it is relatively easy to increase or decrease the intrapulmonary blood volume by approximately 50% by changes in the relation between intrathoracic and extrathoracic pressure (for example, postural changes).

Part of the pulmonary vascular bed's distensibility is actually a phenomenon of recruitment of new vessels. This can be attributed to the hydrostatic pressure gradient over the full height of the lung. Every radiologist knows that in left atrial hypertension (pulmonary venous congestion) the upper lobe veins become more nearly equal in size to those of the lower lobes.

Postnatally, the normal pulmonary circulation is a low resistance circuit. Vascular resistance is distributed approximately equally upstream and downstream from the alveolar wall microvessels; a distribution that is different from that of the systemic circulation. The resistance distribution can be altered drastically. Notable examples are

(1) alveolar hypoxia, wherein pulmonary vasoconstriction is almost entirely localized to the precapillary segment;
(2) during infusion of the vasoactive peptide 5-hydroxytryptamine (serotonin) which is predominantly a pulmonary venoconstricting agent; and
(3) during positive pressure breathing wherein resistance is mainly at the alveolar wall microvessels because the increased alveolar pressure compresses them.

Pulmonary microvascular pressure at the level of the left atrium is not equal to left atrial pressure but is approximately half way between that and pulmonary artery pressure. Likewise, microvascular pressure varies with height in the lung; being highest at the bottom.

Because resistance is low, blood flow through the gas exchange vessels is pulsatile. This has been measured directly by the uptake of very soluble gases and, recently, in spontaneously breathing dogs with a thoracic window the pulsatile flow has been filmed and the velocity of flow measured in the pleural capillaries. The average linear velocity of flow is approximately $1000~\mu m \cdot s^{-1}$.

The arteries within the TRU branch frequently, giving rise abruptly along their course to the extensive capillary net within the alveolar walls. The capillaries are relatively long and cross several alveoli of a given TRU before joining to become venules. The vast extent of the whole capillary bed and the length of the individual paths means a relatively long transit time for red cells (0.5–1.0 s), and confirms indirect physiological evidence that the exchange of oxygen and carbon dioxide between alveolar gas and individual erythrocytes, as they flow along the pulmonary capillaries, reaches equilibrium before the cells leave the exchange bed. Arterial hypoxaemia due to too rapid transit of red cells through the lung's microcirculation is seldom a significant clinical problem.

The pulmonary vessels can be divided into two groups. The *extra-alveolar vessels* are imbedded in a loose connective tissue sheath that permits them considerable independent motion. The loose connective tissue sheath is a potential space just as the pleural space is. The pulmonary lymphatic vessels are located there. In pulmonary oedema or in interstitial emphysema, the sheath may be distended by fluid or air (*Figure 20.7*). There is indirect evidence for a negative hydrostatic pressure in these loose connective sheaths of the lung. The pressure is considered

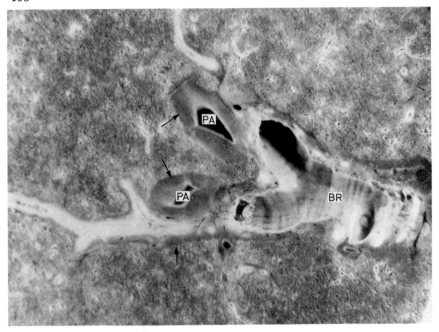

Figure 20.7
Interstitial pulmonary oedema to demonstrate the existence of the
perivascular and peribronchial loose connective tissue spaces. Small
bronchus (BR) and pulmonary arteries (PA). (Sheep, frozen,
unstained, 3.5×)

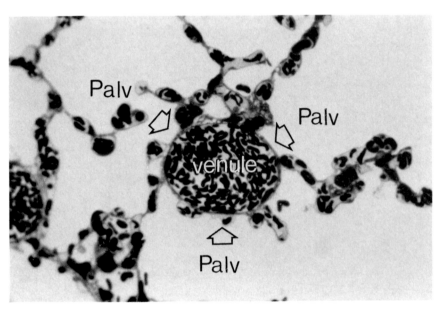

Figure 20.8
Intra-alveolar vessels include some arterioles and venules in addition
to capillaries. The venule shown here is approximately 50 μm
diameter. (Mouse, 1 μm section, toluidine blue, 450×)

to behave similar to pleural pressure, although not necessarily equal to it. The extra-alveolar vessels extend down to the beginning of the TRU.

The blood vessels of the TRU are included in the connective tissue framework of the unit and are subject to whatever forces operate at the alveolar level. They are referred to as *intra-alveolar vessels*. The effective hydrostatic pressure external to them is alveolar pressure. *Figure 20.8* shows that not all of the intra-alveolar vessels are capillaries.

Figure 20.9 is a model representing the two types of pulmonary vessels. The effects of positive pressure breathing on the two classes of vessels is

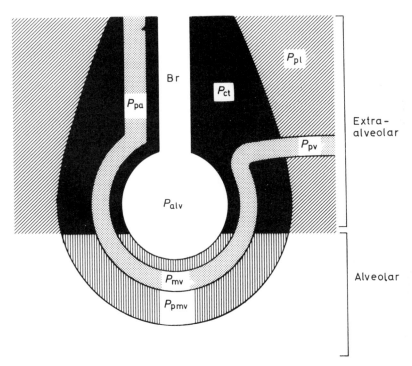

Figure 20.9
Lung pressures relevant to pulmonary circulation. When lung volume increases, the pleural (Ppl) and interstitial connective tissue (Pct) pressures around the extra-alveolar vessels decrease relative to pulmonary arterial (Ppa) and venous (Ppv). For alveolar vessels the pressures [alveolar, (Palv), microvascular (Pmv) and perimicrovascular (Ppmv)] all rise. Thus, the volume of extra-alveolar vessels tends to increase at the same time as the volume of alveolar vessels tends to decrease

different. When alveolar pressure is high relative to pulmonary artery pressure (zone I) the alveolar wall microvessels are directly compressed. On the other hand, the same high positive alveolar pressure tends to increase lung volume. Relative to alveolar pressure, the pressure around the extra-alveolar vessels decreases (behaving like pleural pressure) and they tend to enlarge.

Because of the importance of mechanical factors in the pulmonary circulation, there is a tendency to regard the pulmonary vascular bed as a completely passive system. However, active regulatory mechanisms do exist and, while not as striking as the passive events, are important. The key point seems to be that active regulation is predominantly a local mechanism to match perfusion to ventilation. Until recently, a stimulation of sympathetic vasomotor nerves to the lung was believed to have its major effect upon vascular distensibility. As a practical matter, since all of the cardiac output passes through the lung, over-all increases in pulmonary vascular resistance would seem to be counterproductive. Recent evidence indicates, however, that neurally mediated changes in resistance are probably more significant than had been thought.

Pulmonary vascular smooth muscle is sensitive to H^+ and low Po_2 but is relatively insensitive to noradrenaline. Pulmonary vascular smooth muscle is sensitive to circulating agents including prostaglandins and endotoxin.

Several years ago it was believed that the pulmonary venous smooth muscle was the most sensitive portion of the vascular bed. That belief was founded on a faulty appreciation of lung anatomy and depended upon models in which the pulmonary arteries were not related to the airways or alveolar gas. It is now clearly established that the pulmonary arteries are the usual site of vasomotor changes. This is particularly true of alveolar hypoxia where the site of vasoconstriction is entirely upstream from the alveolar wall microvessels. It is located in the small pulmonary arteries entering the TRU. One substance that has been shown to constrict pulmonary veins is 5-hydroxytryptamine.

An important question is whether the normal lung contains any anatomical connections between the pulmonary arteries and veins that permit some portion of blood flow to bypass the capillary network. Such vessels may occur as congenital or pathological developments. In the normal lung, such short circuits probably do not exist.

In addition to its gas exchange function, the lung is a blood filter. It must be frequently embolized by material from systemic vascular beds. For example, during intravascular coagulation or in processes involving platelet aggregation, the predominant site of removal of the microthrombi is the lung. The main reason for this is obvious, of course, in that 75% of the total circulating blood volume is in the venous circuit and the lung microvascular bed is the first set of small vessels through which the blood flows. Moderate numbers of microemboli generally produce no detectable dysfunction. At most they temporarily block flow to a TRU. The fate of such emboli is unclear. Some emboli are phagocytosed and removed into the lung tissue. Much of the stored foreign material (pigment) in lungs is believed to be of vascular origin. Some emboli can be degraded to small size, be passed through into the systemic circulation and be removed there. One example is the macroaggregated serum albumin used in lung scanning procedures. Larger accumulations of microemboli are believed to be important in the so-called adult respiratory distress syndrome. Following severe trauma, with or without a period of clinical shock, the lung may be extensively embolized by cellular fragments and pieces of clots washed out of the systemic microvascular bed. Pulmonary vascular resistance may be markedly increased and a common finding is interstitial and alveolar oedema. Although there has been much speculation and some evidence purporting to show that chemicals from the emboli themselves or generated by interactions between the emboli and pulmonary endothelium are responsible for the fluid leakage, it is possible, although unproven, that just the physical obstruction alone is sufficient to cause microvascular injury. Thoracic surgeons know that there are limits to the amount of lung tissue that can be resected without producing severe pulmonary hypertension and postoperative oedema. With sufficient embolization, the vascular bed is so restricted that the high pressure and velocity of blood flow through the open, perfused microcirculation harms the endothelial cells.

DIFFUSION

The high degree of alveolar partitioning of the lung has nothing whatsoever to do with ventilation. A simple sac replacing each TRU would work as well. The formation of alveoli can only be rationalized on the circulatory need to distribute a large quantity of blood into a very thin film as close to the gas phase as feasible so that the tissue resistance to gaseous diffusion is minimal.

How well this is accomplished is shown in *Figures 20.10* and *20.11*. The red blood cells in lung capillaries are, on the average, 1.6 μm from the

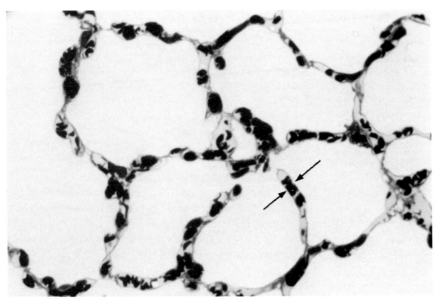

Figure 20.10
The air—blood interface for diffusion is revealed by this section
through several alveoli. More than 75% of the alveolar walls consist
of capillaries. The arrows indicate total alveolar wall thickness of
about 5 μm. Oxygen molecules diffuse into the blood from both
sides. Only those capillary segments containing moving red blood
cells participate in gas exchange. (Mouse, 1 μm section, toluidine blue, 500×)

gas phase. This dimension is critical because the diffusion of oxygen through lung tissue is many thousands of times slower than through the alveolar gas. The main criterion for the size of TRU is that oxygen diffusion in air is so fast relative to that in tissue that near equilibrium exists throughout the unit's gas phase.

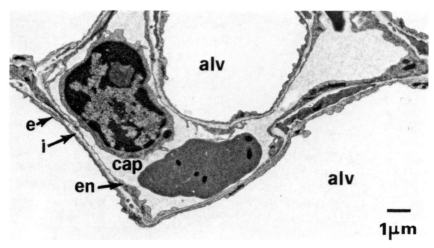

Figure 20.11
The alveolar wall showing the alveolar (alv) capillary (cap) path for
O_2 and CO_2 diffusion. In this low power electron micrograph the
the alveolar wall barrier consisting of alveolar epithelium (e),
interstitium (i) and endothelium (en) is less than 0.5 μm thick.
(Note 1 μm marker in lower right corner.) The main diffusion
barrier is in the plasma and red cell. The capillary segment shown
contains a red blood cell and a leucocyte. Only the membrane area
over red cells is relevant to gaseous diffusion. (Rat; preparation
courtesy Dr M. H. Williams, Cardiovascular Research Institute)

There has been much discussion about whether the blood within the alveolar walls is distributed in a sheet between the two opposing alveolar epithelial layers or in short, capillary segments. As a practical matter, a distinction between the two models is not critical. The important thing is that under zone III conditions (when the alveolar wall microvessels are all open and well filled with blood) more than 75% of the alveolar wall volume is blood. In *Figure 20.10* the alveolar wall cross-sections consist mainly of capillary segments containing red cells.

Only the portion of the alveolar wall containing red cells flowing in capillaries is useful in gas exchange. The human lung is said to possess a capillary capacity of 200 ml, but at rest only about one-third of it is used. This is especially true of the zone II portion of the human lung and explains the measured differences in diffusing capacity between the upper and lower halves of the lung. During exercise, more of the total capillary volume and diffusion surface are used. The active fraction of pulmonary capillaries is distributed both on a regional (hydrostatic) basis and randomly with a given TRU. Recruitment of more capillaries appears to be mainly a passive phenomenon in response to vascular and alveolar pressure changes.

The clinical measurement of carbon monoxide diffusing capacity is a useful addition to the pulmonary function armamentarium. But it is more helpful in studying the pulmonary microcirculation than it is in studying the physical process of diffusion. As noted before, the diffusion process is seldom the rate-limiting factor in gas exchange. The concept of 'alveolar capillary block' has little meaning in terms of diffusion.

LUNG CELLS

Because of the increasing interest in individual cell function in the lung it is worth briefly considering two cell types. These are the alveolar type II cell (granular pneumonocyte) and the alveolar macrophage.

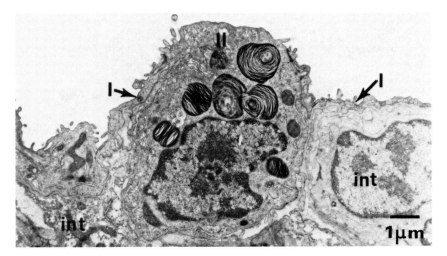

Figure 20.12
Alveolar type II cell (granular pneumonocyte). These cells are located in alveoli usually in the corners. They are a small but vital part of the alveolar epithelium. Note the junctions (I) between the cell and its neighbouring and alveolar pavement epithelial cells (type I cells). The laminated, osmiophilic inclusions of the type II cells are believed to be the source of the surface-active material. The cells are also the progenitors of the type I cell. Portions of two interstitial cells (int) are shown. The bar is 1 μm. (Rat; courtesy Dr M. H. Williams, Cardiovascular Research Institute)

The type II cell is characterized by the large, layered, osmiophilic inclusions (*Figure 20.12*). It is readily seen on routine lung sections, usually located in the alveolar corners. There is one type II cell per alveolus. Two major functional activities of these cells have been delineated. The osmiophilic inclusions appear to be the souce of the surface-active material lining the air–liquid interface of the alveoli. The cells are the stem cells from which the large alveolar epithelial cells (type I cells) originate. They respond to epithelial injury by multiplying rapidly and covering the air–blood barrier with a cuboidal layer.

The alveolar macrophages (*Figure 20.13*) are qualitatively similar to macrophages elsewhere although there are important quantitative differences. They are readily harvested from the alveoli in large numbers by lung lavage. They arise from undifferentiated cells in the lung, not from

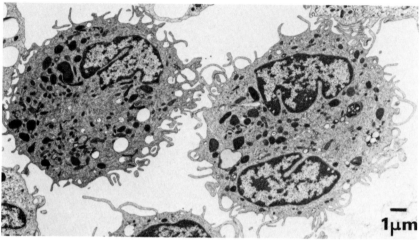

Figure 20.13
Alveolar macrophages obtained from alveolar lavage. There are no obvious ultrastructural differences between macrophages from various parts of the body. But functionally there are distinct differences. The bar is 1 μm. (Rat; courtesy Dr M. H. Williams, Cardiovascular Research Institute)

the alveolar epithelial type I or type II cells. They are important in removing (by phagocytosis) material from the alveoli. It used to be thought that most of these cells wandered out of the air spaces back into the lung interstitium, but it is more likely that most of them are cleared up in the airway.

LUNG MODEL

This brief presentation of the structural basis of lung function is concluded with a model of the lung (*Figure 20.14*), which meets the criterion of being faithful to structure while retaining sufficient simplicity to permit comprehension of function. The figure shows the classes of airways and blood vessels and their motor innervation. Two terminal respiratory units are shown in sufficient extent to indicate their complexity. The figure emphasizes the view that the matching of ventilation ($\dot{V}$) to perfusion ($\dot{Q}$) is the primary lesson to be learned about lung physiology.

The close identification of the terminal pulmonary arteries with a given TRU indicates why local adjustments of $\dot{V}/\dot{Q}$ within units can be made independently of over-all lung function. Changes in TRU ventilation will affect the chemical composition of the unit's vascular smooth muscle, leading to changes in perfusion that tend to restore $\dot{V}/\dot{Q}$. The corollary is

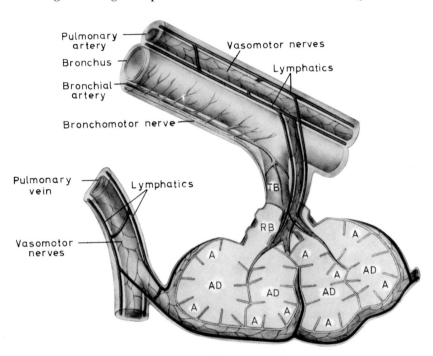

Figure 20.14
Lung model incorporating structure–function relationships. Three classes of airways and two classes of vessels are present. Note the relations of the bronchial blood supply, lymphatics and motor innervation, in so far as they are known. Possibilities for selective interactions that regulate local ventilation to perfusion become apparent in this model. The extent of the potential interstitial loose connective tissue spaces around the larger airways and vessels is shown by the exaggerated grey overlay. The space extends out to the beginning of the respiratory units along the airways, somewhat further into the units around the pulmonary arteries and around the entire circumference of the units along the pulmonary veins. The lymphatics are confined to this loose connective tissue space.
A, anatomical alveolus; AD, alveolar ducts; RB, respiratory bronchiole

also true; namely, that changes in unit perfusion will affect the forces governing ventilation. Some of the latter are rapid involving changes in bronchiolar tone; others are slow involving metabolic changes within alveolar type II cells that alter the turnover of surfactant.

The TRU regulates only the ratio of ventilation to perfusion. The total minute ventilation and cardiac output necessary for maintaining normal tissue gas tension are regulated centrally.

References and further reading

Breeze, R. G. and Wheeldon, E. B. (1977). The cells of the pulmonary airways. *Am. Rev. resp. Dis.* **116**, 705–777

Butler, J., Culver, B. H., Huseby, J. and Albert, R. (1977). The hemodynamics of pulmonary edema. *Am. Rev. resp. Dis.* **115** (part 2), 173–180

de Reuch, A. V. S. and O'Connor, M. (ed.) (1962). *CIBA Foundation Symposium on Structure and Function.* Boston: Little, Brown

Comroe, J. H., Jr. (1974). *Physiology of Respiration,* 2nd edn. Chicago: Yearbook Medical

Cumming, G. and Hunt, L. B. (ed.) (1968). *Form and Function in the Human Lung.* London: Livingstone

Hayek, H. V. (1960). *The Human Lung* (Trans. V. E. Krahl). New York: Hafner

Kato, M. and Staub, N. C. (1966). Response of small pulmonary arteries to unilobar hypoxia and hypercapnia. *Circulation Res.* **21**, 426–439

Krahl, V. E. (1964). Anatomy of the mammalian lung. In *Handbook of Physiology: Respiration I,* Chapter 6, pp. 213–284. W. O. Fenn and H. Rahn (ed.). Washington: Am. Physiol. Soc.

Macklin, C. C. (1954). Pulmonary sumps, dust accumulations, alveolar fluid and lymph vessels. *Acta anat.* **23**, 1–33

Miller, W. S. (1947). The lymphatics. In *The Lung,* 2nd edn, Chapter 6, pp. 89–118. Springfield: Thomas

Sobin, S. S., Tremer, H. M. and Fung, Y. C. (1970). Morphometric basis of the sheet flow concept of the pulmonary microvascular sheet in the cat. *Circulation Res.* **26**, 397–414

Spencer, H. (1968). *Pathology of the Lung; Excluding Pulmonary Tuberculosis,* 2nd edn. Oxford: Pergamon Press

Staub, N. C. (1963). The interdependence of pulmonary structure and function. *Anesthesiology* **24**, 831–854

Staub, N. C. (1969). Respiration. *A. Rev. Physiol.* **31**, 173–202

Staub, N. C. (1974). Pulmonary edema. *Physiol. Rev.* **54**, 678–811

Staub, N. C. (1975). Some aspects of airway structure and function. *Postgrad. med. J.* **51**, Suppl. 1, 21–30

Vaughan, T. R., Jr., DeMarino, E. M. and Staub, N. C. (1976). Indicator dilution lung water and capillary blood-volume in prolonged heavy exercise in normal men. *Am. Rev. resp. Dis.* **113**, 757–762

Weibel, E. R. (1963). *Morphometry of the Human Lung.* New York: Academic Press

West, J. B. (1970). *Ventilation/Blood Flow and Gas Exchange,* 2nd edn. Oxford: Blackwell

21 Hypoxia and oxygen transport
John F. Nunn

BIOLOGICAL ROLE OF OXYGEN

The development of aerobic metabolic pathways was a major landmark in evolution (Nunn, 1968). Nevertheless, primitive life forms depending on anaerobic metabolism appear to have existed for thousands of millions of years, and anaerobic metabolic pathways still function today alongside aerobic pathways in higher organisms.

The utilization of oxygen is ultimately dependent upon photosynthesis in plants, a process which releases oxygen as a byproduct. Although there is evidence that the present level of oxygen in the atmosphere inhibits the growth of plants, there is no doubt that it has conferred immense advantages on aerobic animal forms and permitted the development of all forms of animal life beyond the most primitive bacteria. Maintenance of life of all higher organisms depends upon the preservation of aerobic metabolism which thus becomes the most important responsibility of those caring for the unconscious patient.

Effect of oxygen on energy production

The use of aerobic as opposed to anaerobic metabolic pathways results in a very large increase in biological energy available from food fuels. The most familiar example is glucose metabolism, and the energy released may be considered in terms of the number of molecules of adenosine triphosphate (ATP) formed from adenosine diphosphate (ADP) by the addition of a high energy phosphate bond (see Chapter 2).

In the presence of oxygen and the necessary enzymes, contained in the mitochondria, glucose is converted entirely to carbon dioxide and water by means of the citric acid cycle and electron transport chain (the cytochrome system). In this process, one molecule of glucose results in the production of 38 molecules of ATP by the process known as oxidative phosphorylation. In the absence of oxygen, glucose is converted to lactic acid which is almost entirely ionized. Under these circumstances one molecule of glucose results in the net production of only two molecules of ATP. Anaerobic metabolism thus requires a 19-fold increase in the consumption of glucose for production of the same amount of biological energy.

Since there is a limit to the rate at which glucose can be transported into a cell, a severe reduction in the available biological energy is inevitable (see *Figure 2.4*) when aerobic metabolism is replaced by anaerobic metabolism in certain tissues. Cells with high energy utilization, such as neurons, liver cells and nephrons, cannot continue to function at the lower level of available energy and in due course will also suffer structural damage. In contrast, less vulnerable tissues such as skin, muscle and bone can survive long periods of oxygen deprivation resulting, for example, from the application of a tourniquet.

Effect of hypoxia on acid formation

In the absence of oxygen, glucose is metabolized to lactic acid which remains as an end-product until oxygenation is restored: two molecules of lactic acid are formed from one of glucose. At the pH of intracellular fluid, lactic acid is almost entirely ionized to hydrogen and lactate ions. The resulting intracellular acidosis may be sufficiently serious to interfere with the action of certain enzymes and may result in structural damage to cells quite apart from any effects of the accompanying reduction in ATP levels.

In tissues such as voluntary muscle, hydrogen and lactate ions are able to cross the cell membrane quite freely. Although this results in a generalized metabolic acidosis, the local intracellular acidosis is minimized. An entirely different situation applies in the brain where the blood—brain barrier hinders the free escape of hydrogen and lactate ions from the neurons into the jugular venous blood. The intracellular acidosis therefore persists and its extent is not fully revealed by studies of the jugular venous blood.

Greater structural damage follows acute hypoxia of neurons if the cells have previously been glucose depleted (Lindenberg, 1963; Geddes, 1967). This suggests that intracellular acidosis is more damaging than energy deprivation.

Mitochondrial P_{O_2} and the Pasteur point (see review by Cohen, 1972)

Oxygen is utilized almost entirely in the mitochondria where the P_{O_2} must be maintained above a critical level for aerobic metabolism to continue. This level, known as the Pasteur point, is of the order of 0.15—0.3 kPa (1—2 mmHg), or about 1% of the partial pressure of oxygen in the atmosphere (Chance, Schoener and Schindler, 1964). Probably, under normal circumstances, the mitochondrial P_{O_2} ranges from approximately 1 to 5 kPa (7.5—37.5 mmHg) depending on the activity of the cell and the proximity of individual mitochondria to the cell surface and the Po_2 of the blood in the nearest capillary. When the mitochondrial Po_2 is reduced, aerobic metabolism continues at the normal rate until the Pasteur point is reached, although this will occur at different times in the same cell depending upon the geometry of the relationship to its blood supply. Below the Pasteur point, there is usually an increase in anaerobic metabolism in an attempt to compensate for the reduction in ATP/ADP ratio which results from the reduction in aerobic metabolism.

The responsibility of the anaesthetist to maintain aerobic metabolism may thus be considered in terms of maintaining mitochondrial Po_2 above the Pasteur point in the most vulnerable organs, which include the brain, liver, kidney and heart. This depends on many factors which interact with one another in a complex fashion. A convenient starting point is to consider the steps of the oxygen tension gradient from the atmosphere to the mitochondrion.

THE OXYGEN CASCADE

The oxygen tension gradient from atmosphere to mitochondrion has been called the oxygen cascade and comprises alternating stages of *mass transport* (pulmonary ventilation and blood flow) and *diffusion* within the alveoli, across the alveolar/capillary membrane and between the systemic capillary and the site of utilization within the mitochondrion (*Figure 21.1*).

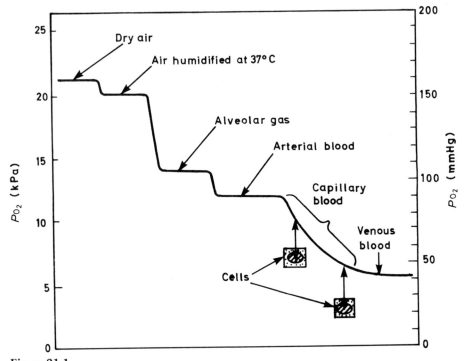

Figure 21.1
The oxygen cascade. The vertical arrows indicate a Po_2 gradient of 3 kPa (22.5 mmHg) between capillary and cells

Inspired gas to alveolar gas

Dry air, with an oxygen concentration of 20.93% at a barometric pressure of 101 kPa (760 mmHg) has a Po_2 of 21 kPa (158 mmHg). However, whether inspired dry or moist, air becomes saturated with water vapour at body temperature by the time it reaches the lower respiratory tract. By dilution the Po_2 is reduced to 20 kPa (150 mmHg) (*Figure 21.1*).

Alveolar gas always has a lower Po_2 than inspired gas, with the difference proportional to the ratio of the oxygen consumption ($\dot{V}o_2$) to the alveolar ventilation ($\dot{V}A$):

$$PAo_2 = PIo_2 - 95\, \frac{\dot{V}o_2}{\dot{V}A}\ \ \text{kPa}$$

PAo_2 is the alveolar gas Po_2.
PIo_2 is the inspired gas Po_2.
95 is the dry barometric pressure in kPa (713 in mmHg).
$\dot{V}o_2$ and $\dot{V}A$ must be expressed under the same conditions of temperature and pressure.

Under the conditions of anaesthesia, the major variable influencing the inspired/alveolar Po_2 difference is clearly the alveolar ventilation. Nevertheless, it is important to remember that an increased oxygen consumption in the presence of a fixed low alveolar ventilation will increase the difference and may lead to a catastrophic fall in alveolar Po_2.

Alveolar gas to arterial blood

The third step in the oxygen cascade (*Figure 21.1*) is between the alveolar gas (A) and the arterial blood (a). In the healthy conscious subject the (A–a) Po_2 difference is less than one kilopascal or only a few millimetres of mercury and of little practical importance. In pathological states, it may be increased by admixture of venous blood with arterial blood and by a mismatch of the relative distribution of inspired gas and pulmonary arterial blood. The (A–a) Po_2 difference is usually increased during routine anaesthesia, probably due to underventilation of dependent areas of the lung, caused by airway closure or narrowing. This results from the reduction in functional residual capacity which seems to be a consequence of routine anaesthesia. An increased alveolar–arterial Po_2 difference is a most important cause of arterial hypoxaemia in patients undergoing intensive therapy and in a wide range of complications of anaesthesia.

Arterial blood to cells

The first three steps of the oxygen cascade in *Figure 21.1* are common for the patient as a whole. The next step, from arterial blood to individual cells, is variable, not only between different organs but also between different cells within a particular organ. In effect this means that there is no one value for tissue P_{O_2} in an organ, and that there must be a very wide range of P_{O_2} values throughout the organ, with a mean value which cannot at present be measured.

This difficult concept is best considered in terms of the P_{O_2} gradient along a capillary. As oxygen is withdrawn by the surrounding cells, there is a progressive fall in oxygen *content* along the capillary, the magnitude of the fall depending upon the ratio of the tissue oxygen consumption to the blood flow. This results in a fall in *haemoglobin saturation* which depends upon the haemoglobin concentration in the blood. For example, if 5 ml of oxygen are withdrawn from 100 ml of blood, the saturation will fall by about 25% if the haemoglobin concentration is 14 $g \cdot dl^{-1}$ but by 50% if the haemoglobin concentration is only 7 $g \cdot dl^{-1}$. In turn, the fall of *saturation* governs the fall of *tension* in accord with the dissociation curve. As a result, the P_{O_2} falls more rapidly at the beginning of the capillary (*Figure 21.1*) where the saturation is on the flat part of the dissociation curve. Towards the venous end of the capillary the P_{O_2} fall is more gradual since the saturation is now approaching the venous point of the dissociation curve where the slope is steeper. There will be a spectrum of values for the venous P_{O_2} in different capillaries, different venules and different veins. An integrated mean venous P_{O_2} is attained in the mixed venous blood which may be sampled from right ventricle or pulmonary artery. Decline in P_{O_2} along a capillary is best shown in the liver sinusoids where danger of hypoxia increases towards the centrilobular vein.

Oxygen passes from capillaries to the mitochondria by diffusion and the geometry of the diffusion pathway can be considered reasonably constant over limited periods of time. Therefore, provided the oxygen consumption remains constant, the P_{O_2} gradient from capillary to mitochondrion will also be constant. The magnitude of this gradient must vary from one part of a cell to another, and the value of 3 kPa (22.5 mmHg) shown in *Figure 21.1* is intended as a working mean value. It may well be a reasonable value since a jugular venous P_{O_2} of 3 kPa (22.5 mmHg) is the minimum level for normal cerebral function.

CLASSIFICATION OF HYPOXIA

The account of the oxygen cascade indicates three major groups of causes of cellular hypoxia. Following the classification of Barcroft (1920), they are as follows:

'hypoxic' hypoxia, 'stagnant' hypoxia, and 'anaemic' hypoxia.*

Hypoxic hypoxia covers all conditions leading to a reduction of arterial P_{O_2}, including lowered barometric pressure, decreased concentration of oxygen in the inspired gas, hypoventilation and venous admixture.

* It is currently fashionable to describe a reduction of P_{O_2} as hypoxia rather than anoxia. To be consistent, a reduction in haemoglobin concentration should be described as hypaemia rather than anaemia but this term is not in general use.

Stagnant hypoxia means hypoperfusion, either regional or general.

Anaemic hypoxia includes any reduction of functioning haemoglobin concentration in the blood, such as anaemia, methaemoglobinaemia, and carbon monoxide poisoning.

Barcroft later introduced the term *histotoxic anoxia* to cover a failure of utilization of oxygen within the cell, such as might result from a poisoning of the cytochrome system with cyanide or carbon monoxide. Histotoxic anoxia will not be considered further in this chapter, although its relevance to anaesthesia is considered in Chapter 2.

It is important to realize that the types of hypoxia listed above are not mutually exclusive. For this reason they may be shown in a Venn diagram (*Figure 21.2*). Around the periphery are zones corresponding to a single

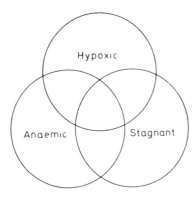

Figure 21.2
The classification of hypoxia arranged as a Venn diagram to show the combinations which are possible

type of hypoxia. Inside these zones are three triangular areas corresponding to combinations of two types of hypoxia: hypoxic plus stagnant; stagnant plus anaemic; and anaemic plus hypoxic. In the centre is a triangular space corresponding to a combination of all three types of hypoxia.

Clinical examples of these combinations are not hard to find. Haemorrhage results primarily in stagnant hypoxia due to failure of venous return, but this is later complicated by anaemic hypoxia when haemodilution occurs. In severe haemorrhage, hypoxic hypoxia is a terminal phenomenon when pulmonary perfusion fails (Freeman and Nunn, 1963), but may occur early in complicated trauma with, for example, crushed chest or airway obstruction.

Although types of hypoxia may coexist to the detriment of the patient, it is perhaps commoner to find one type of hypoxia partly compensated by an improvement in function under one of the other headings. For example, chronic hypoxia is normally accompanied by polycythaemia and anaemic hypoxia is generally associated with increased circulation. These changes tend to be general but local compensations also occur, particularly in the cerebral circulation which tends to maintain itself in the face of a wide range of physiological trespasses.

Consideration of the types of hypoxia in combination, as shown in *Figure 21.2*, offers a concrete example of the importance of considering the patient as a whole and not seeing a single malfunction in isolation.

This is particularly important when compensations are present and complications can be foreseen. It provides the basis for answering such questions as: 'Can I safely anaesthetize a patient with a haemoglobin of 8 g·dl^{-1}' or 'What is the lowest safe arterial P_{O_2}'.

Before proceeding to a quantitative consideration of combined forms of failure of oxygen transport, the different types of hypoxia will be considered in rather more detail.

HYPOXIC HYPOXIA

Definition

Hypoxic hypoxia is defined as a condition in which the arterial P_{O_2} is reduced. It therefore excludes uncomplicated anaemia in which the arterial oxygen content is reduced but the P_{O_2} is normal or even raised. It is difficult to define the normal arterial P_{O_2} since it declines with age, and there is also a fairly wide individual scatter of values about the mean for a particular age group. Furthermore, the P_{O_2} of an individual may vary markedly from time to time, depending on many factors including the activity of the subject. However, in general the arterial P_{O_2} should not be below 11 kPa (82.5 mmHg) in early adult life, with the lower limit of normal falling to 10 kPa (75 mmHg) at 60 years of age.

Causes

Causes of hypoxic hypoxia which affect primarily the alveolar P_{O_2} may be conveniently summarized in the following equation (Nunn, 1977):

$$P_{A_{O_2}} = (P_B - 6) \left(F_{I_{O_2}} - \frac{\dot{V}_{O_2}}{\dot{V}_A} \right) \text{ kPa}$$

BAROMETRIC PRESSURE

Barometric pressure (P_B) is a factor which can be ignored at sea level but is highly relevant to the care of patients at altitudes above about 2000 metres. Elevation of barometric pressure is practised in hyperbaric oxygen therapy. The constant 6 (kPa) represents water vapour pressure at body temperature. The corresponding value for mmHg is 47.

INSPIRED OXYGEN CONCENTRATION

Inspired oxygen concentration ($F_{I_{O_2}}$) (expressed as a fraction and not as a percentage) is a factor of the greatest importance, since it is the simplest and often most effective method of influencing a patient's oxygenation in therapy. Reductions in $F_{I_{O_2}}$ were once commonplace in 'gas–air' obstetric analgesia and in hypoxic dental anaesthesia, but should now occur only as a result of error or accident. If other factors remain constant, an elevation

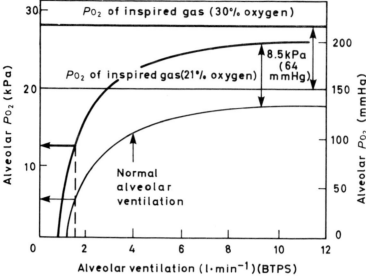

Figure 21.3
Alveolar P_{O_2} as a function of alveolar ventilation and inspired gas
P_{O_2}. The inspired P_{O_2} is shown as a horizontal line and the alveolar
P_{O_2} as a rectangular hyperbola which is asymptotic to the corresponding inspired gas P_{O_2}. The thin curve is for 21% oxygen in the
inspired gas and the thick curve for 30% oxygen. The two horizontal
arrows indicate the alveolar P_{O_2} at an alveolar ventilation of
1.5 l·min^{-1}. (Reproduced from Nunn, 1977, *Applied Respiratory
Physiology*)

of inspired oxygen concentration increases both inspired and alveolar P_{O_2}
by the same amount, approximately 1 kPa (7.5 mmHg) for 1% oxygen at
sea level (*Figure 21.3*). Thus 30% oxygen should result in an alveolar P_{O_2}
8.5 kPa (64 mmHg) higher than the value while breathing air, other
factors remaining unchanged. Clearly, under conditions of severe underventilation, this can represent the difference between a safe alveolar P_{O_2}
and one which is not compatible with life.

OXYGEN CONSUMPTION

Oxygen consumption ($\dot{V}_{O_2}$) receives too little consideration as a rule.
During uncomplicated anaesthesia, and in a patient at rest in bed, the
level is generally close to basal. However, highly significant increases occur
during pyrexia, shivering and convulsions, the rise due to a change in body
temperature being of the order of 7% per °C. Under these conditions it is
essential that the patient make the necessary increase in alveolar ventilation
(see below) or, failing that, the inspired oxygen concentration must be
increased as an emergency measure.

ALVEOLAR VENTILATION

Alveolar ventilation ($\dot{V}_A$) is well known to be a major factor influencing
alveolar P_{O_2}. However, it is not always appreciated that the relationship is

not linear but hyperbolic (*Figure 21.3*). As ventilation increases, the alveolar Po_2 approaches but never reaches the inspired Po_2. As ventilation decreases, the alveolar Po_2 falls along an ever-steepening curve with dramatic changes occurring in response to small changes in ventilation over the critical ranges of ventilation. Hyperventilation is not a very effective way of increasing alveolar Po_2, but hypoventilation is potentially a disastrous cause of hypoxia. Alveolar hypoventilation commonly results from a reduction of tidal volume or respiratory frequency but may also result from a severe increase in physiological dead space.

Alveolar Po_2 is also influenced by exchange of nitrogen and nitrous oxide (so-called diffusion hypoxia), but the changes are usually small and transient.

ALVEOLAR–ARTERIAL Po_2 DIFFERENCE

The alveolar–arterial Po_2 difference is the most important cause of hypoxic hypoxia under the conditions of anaesthesia and intensive therapy.

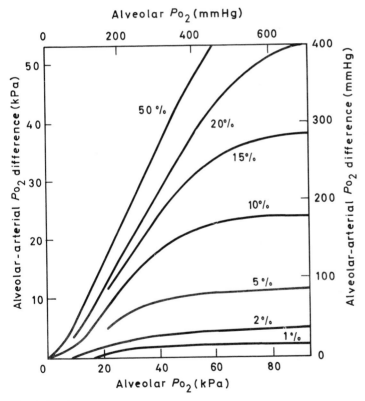

Figure 21.4
Influence of alveolar Po_2 and venous admixture (indicated as %) on alveolar–arterial Po_2 difference. Normal values are assumed for arterial–mixed venous oxygen content difference, haemoglobin concentration, etc. (Reproduced from Nunn, 1977, *Applied Respiratory Physiology*)

The main cause of an increased (A—a) Po_2 difference is admixture of venous blood with arterial blood such as may occur in congenital heart disease with right-to-left shunt, bronchial obstruction, pulmonary lobar collapse, increased bronchial circulation and so on. Another cause which does not usually result in such large Po_2 differences is a relative mismatch in distribution of inspired gas and pulmonary arterial blood. Inadequate diffusing capacity is no longer considered an important cause of increased (A—a) Po_2 difference in the resting patient at sea level (Staub, 1963).

The magnitude of the (A—a) Po_2 difference is influenced by many factors of which the most important are the venous admixture and the alveolar Po_2 (*Figure 21.4*). The subject is treated in greater depth by Nunn (1977).

STAGNANT HYPOXIA

Definition

The extreme form of stagnant hypoxia is circulatory arrest, with all intermediate grades up to normal perfusion. The adequacy of perfusion is conveniently considered as inversely proportional to the ratio of tissue oxygen consumption ($\dot{V}o_2$) to perfusion ($\dot{Q}$). This ratio equals the arterial/venous oxygen content difference:

$$\frac{\dot{V}o_2}{\dot{Q}} = Cao_2 - Cvo_2$$

where Cao_2 is the arterial oxygen content and Cvo_2 the venous oxygen content.

Applied to the body as a whole, this is the Fick equation and inadequate circulation in relation to the oxygen consumption may then be expressed in terms of the resultant desaturation of mixed venous blood.

Applied to regional blood flow, inadequate circulation is again related to desaturation of the venous blood and *Figure 21.1* shows how the tissue Po_2 is related to the venous Po_2. Some part of the tissue will have a Po_2 approximately 3 kPa (22.5 mmHg) below the venous Po_2 draining that area, provided there is no arterial/venous anastomosis in the organ which would result in a misleadingly high venous Po_2.

Cardiac output

Whole body hypoperfusion occurs classically in low output states such as hypovolaemia, constrictive pericarditis, mitral stenosis and myocardial ischaemia. Surprisingly, it has been found by several groups that aortic stenosis does not reduce the resting cardiac output below the normal range (Hancock and Fleming, 1960). *Increased* cardiac output is an essential compensation in anaemia and arterial hypoxaemia.

Regional blood flow

It is important to realize that individual organs cannot sense the cardiac output but only the arterial pressure. In fact, the brain retains reasonable perfusion under conditions in which there is a large reduction of cardiac output (Stone *et al.*, 1954) and this is probably also true of the heart.

Skin and muscle are usually sacrificed when cardiac output is reduced. Cutaneous hypoperfusion gives rise to the classic signs of 'shock' and is a good clinical indication of circulatory inadequacy. Hypoperfusion of voluntary muscle and other tissues gives rise to the lactacidosis which may be a grave complicating factor. It reduces myocardial contractility and incidentally makes a major contribution to the 'air hunger' of the shocked patient (Freeman and Nunn, 1963).

Liver and kidney have less effective circulatory homoeostatic mechanisms than brain and are frequently underperfused while cerebral blood flow is well maintained. Unfortunately, liver and kidney do not have the resistance to hypoxia of skin and muscle, and hypoxic damage to these organs may be critical for survival.

ANAEMIC HYPOXIA

Definition

Anaemic hypoxia refers to any condition in which there is a reduction in capacity of the haemoglobin to carry oxygen. There may be a reduction in the total quantity of haemoglobin or it may be partly converted to a form which cannot combine with oxygen. In addition, the dissociation curve may be so displaced that oxygen cannot be satisfactorily transported from lungs to tissues.

Significance

At normal arterial Po_2, haemoglobin (in normal concentration) carries about 20 ml of oxygen per dl of blood, while the corresponding level of dissolved oxygen is 0.3 ml. Thus the haemoglobin concentration is all-important for oxygen carriage by the blood, except during hyperbaric oxygenation when the dissolved oxygen may be raised to 6 ml·dl^{-1} when 100% oxygen is breathed at 3 atmospheres absolute pressure.

The effect of anaemia on tissue Po_2 may be explained as follows. If perfusion and tissue oxygen consumption remain normal, the *quantity* of oxygen removed from the blood remains the same but the *saturation* of the venous blood must be decreased below the normal value. Therefore, the capillary and venous Po_2 will be lower than normal and the pressure head for diffusion of oxygen into the tissues is reduced and so the tissue Po_2 is diminished. In many ways this situation is similar to hypoperfusion with normal haemoglobin (see above) which also results in increased oxygen extraction with diminished capillary and venous Po_2 and consequent reduction of tissue Po_2.

Anaemia

The most important cause of anaemic hypoxia is, of course, anaemia itself. The condition is so common and its recognition so simple that the haemoglobin concentration should always be measured before anaesthesia or surgery. Nevertheless, extensive experience in areas with endemic malnourishment and in the surgery of renal failure teaches that anaesthesia and major surgery may be carried out with chronic levels as low as 6 g·dl^{-1}. Even in the acute situation, isovolaemic anaemia appears less dangerous than other forms of hypoxia: Cullen and Eger (1970) found no biochemical evidence of tissue hypoxia following acute reduction of haematocrit to 10% in dogs. Survival at these levels is entirely dependent upon maintained hyperperfusion of all essential organs with a raised cardiac output. Therefore in accepting such patients, anaesthetist and surgeon must also accept responsibility for the maintenance of the high levels of tissue perfusion in the face of whatever may happen during the course of the surgical intervention. Preoperative transfusion with packed cells may be helpful but it is essential to avoid overloading the blood volume before surgery.

INACTIVE HAEMOGLOBIN

Haemoglobin may be effectively inactivated by carbon monoxide which combines with haemoglobin so strongly that it is only slowly displaced by oxygen.

Methaemoglobin is a form of haemoglobin in which the iron is in the trivalent ferric form instead of the divalent ferrous form: it is unable to combine with oxygen. Methaemoglobinaemia occurs in the idiopathic familial form but may also occur during anaesthesia as a result of the action of prilocaine (Scott, Owen and Richmond, 1964) or as a result of contamination of nitrous oxide with higher oxides of nitrogen (Greenbaum *et al.*, 1967). Reconversion to normal haemoglobin occurs rapidly with the injection of methylene blue or vitamin C. Sulphaemoglobin is also unable to combine with oxygen and cannot be readily reconverted to normal haemoglobin.

Shift of dissociation curve

The haemoglobin dissociation curve may be shifted to the left by alkalaemia (particularly low Pco_2), hypothermia and by decreased levels of 2,3-diphosphoglyceric acid. Amino-acid changes in the globin part of the molecule, and protein binding may also affect the curve.

When the arterial Po_2 is above about 8 kPa (60 mmHg), shifts in the

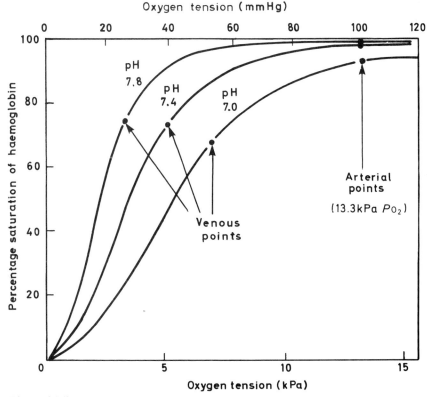

Figure 21.5
The oxyhaemoglobin dissociation curve at three values for pH
showing the effect on arterial and venous oxygen levels. In each
case it is assumed that the arterial Po_2 is 13.3 kPa (100 mmHg) and
the arteriovenous oxygen saturation difference is 25%. (Reproduced
from Nunn, 1977, *Applied Respiratory Physiology*)

dissociation curve cause only trivial changes in the oxygen content of the
arterial blood at a particular arterial Po_2. However, on the steep part of
the dissociation curve, the Po_2 at which oxygen is given up to the tissues
is markedly influenced, and shifts to the left can cause appreciable
reductions in venous and tissue Po_2 levels (*Figure 21.5*).

COMBINED STATES OF HYPOXIA

The concept of oxygen flux

It is helpful to consider the total quantity of oxygen delivered to the
body in each minute (Nunn, 1977). This equals the product of the cardiac
output and the arterial oxygen content. The latter approximates to the
product of the percentage saturation of the haemoglobin (divided by 100)
and the oxygen capacity of the haemoglobin (equal to the constant 1.31*

* The value 1.31 is based on the studies of Gregory (1974).

multiplied by the haemoglobin concentration). The dissolved oxygen is ignored in this simplified equation, which is acceptable provided the arterial Po_2 is less than 15 kPa (112.5 mmHg):

$$\frac{\text{oxygen}}{\text{flux}} = \frac{\text{cardiac}}{\text{output}} \times \frac{\text{haemoglobin saturation \%}}{100} \times 1.31 \times \frac{\text{haemoglobin}}{\text{concentration}}$$

Normal values at rest are as follows:

$$\underset{\text{ml·min}^{-1}}{1000} = \underset{\text{ml·min}^{-1}}{5500} \times \frac{95}{100} \times \underset{\text{ml·g}^{-1}}{1.31} \times \underset{\text{g·ml}^{-1}}{\frac{14.5}{100}}$$

In the resting state the oxygen consumption is of the order of 250 ml·min^{-1} or 25% of the oxygen flux. Therefore the mixed venous blood has a saturation level 25% below the arterial saturation, that is, 70% corresponding to a Po_2 of 5.3 kPa (40 mmHg). The large quantity of oxygen remaining in the venous blood provides a readily available store of oxygen which can be used without increasing cardiac output. However, any reduction in venous oxygen content must lower the venous Po_2 with consequent reduction in tissue Po_2. A certain reduction of venous Po_2 is acceptable without impairment of function, but reductions below 3 kPa (22.5 mmHg) may be associated with a partial change to anaerobic metabolism.

The oxygen flux equation is particularly useful for assessing the effects of combined forms of hypoxia as well as the effect of compensations such as polycythaemia. Since the oxygen flux is the product of three variables, it follows that a reduction of each to one-half of its normal value will lower the oxygen flux to one-eighth of its normal value. None of the three primary changes is in itself lethal but the combined effect results in an oxygen flux which is far below the minimum level for survival.

Reductions of oxygen saturation to 50% (Po_2 about 4 kPa or 30 mmHg) are unlikely to occur unnoticed, but corresponding reductions of cardiac output (to 2.75 l·min^{-1}) are apparently a normal feature of anaesthesia with artificial hyperventilation (Prys-Roberts *et al.*, 1967). Reductions of haemoglobin to 7 g·dl^{-1} are not unusual in hospital practice and are commonplace in the population at large in certain parts of the world.

The oxygen flux equation shows clearly that a reduction of both cardiac output and haemoglobin concentration is a particularly dangerous combination. For example, a cardiac output of 2.5 l·min^{-1} and a haemoglobin concentration of 10 g·dl^{-1} results in an oxygen flux which cannot rise above 330 ml·min^{-1} unless the patient breathes oxygen and even then can only reach 380 ml·min^{-1}; these low levels are likely to be lethal if maintained. Thus the answer to the question of anaesthetizing a patient with a low haemoglobin is that it depends upon the cardiac output and the saturation which can be maintained during the surgical intervention. If all goes well, an otherwise healthy patient with a haemoglobin of 7 g·dl^{-1} can survive major surgery but he cannot survive a sudden haemorrhage with reduction in cardiac output which would be withstood by a healthy patient. His life depends upon the maintenance of a raised cardiac output and this must be guaranteed during and after the period of surgical intervention. Similarly, patients with a critically low cardiac output are dependent upon maintaining a normal or raised haemoglobin level and high arterial Po_2.

Failure of oxygen transport is no less serious than an elevation of oxygen demand beyond the capacity of the oxygen transport of the patient. Consider, for example, a patient with mitral stenosis and a fixed low cardiac output of say 3 l·min^{-1}. Assuming he has a haemoglobin level of 14 g·dl^{-1} he has a maximum oxygen flux of 550 ml·min^{-1} while breathing air. This is sufficient for basal activity and short periods of mild exercise but would not sustain an oxygen consumption of more than about 400 ml. If, during an anaesthetic, such a patient were to convulse or if he were to shiver violently in the postoperative period, his oxygen demand might rise beyond his normal tolerance to a level which would result in severe venous desaturation with dangerous tissue hypoxia.

The oxygen flux equation is also valuable for consideration of oxygenation during cardiopulmonary bypass. Under these conditions the three variables are easily measured and the ratio of oxygen consumption to oxygen flux may be related to venous desaturation and lactic acid production.

In the paragraphs above, oxygen flux has been considered for the patient as a whole. In fact it is no less important to consider the regional oxygen flux, derived by the substitution of regional blood flow for cardiac output in the equation above. The most vulnerable organs must be considered and an adequate cardiac output avails nothing if these organs are underperfused.

INDICES OF HYPOXIA

It may be extremely difficult to obtain objective evidence of tissue hypoxia. It has been explained above why the mean tissue Po_2 is not amenable to direct measurement and the possibility of arteriovenous anastomoses limits the value of the measurement of the regional venous Po_2.

Evidence of anaerobic metabolism may be forthcoming from a change in the arteriovenous excess lactate difference (Huckabee, 1958), but the blood—brain barrier poses special difficulties in the case of the brain. Furthermore, increased lactate levels may result from causes other than hypoxia (Cohen, 1972).

Since anaerobic metabolism requires a 19-fold increase in glucose consumption for the same production of ATP, an increase in regional arteriovenous glucose difference may be the earliest sign of hypoxia. A more sophisticated measurement is the ratio of arteriovenous differences of oxygen and glucose. With full aerobic metabolism, the theoretical ratio is 6:1 (moles). A decrease indicates anaerobic metabolism. However, alternative metabolic pathways may be used in the brain and this will confuse the issue (Owen *et al.*, 1967).

Disappointment with biochemical evidence has led many to a study of function as an indication of tissue hypoxia. Fortunately this is easiest in the most vulnerable organ and in certain circumstances electroencephalography offers the possibility of early detection of cerebral hypoxia.

Few measurements of total oxygen flux have been made in man under conditions of extreme failure of oxygenation. However, it is likely that there is a critical oxygen flux, probably about 400 ml·min^{-1}, and measurement of this quantity might well prove helpful in estimating the degree of over-all hypoxia in a patient with more than one type of hypoxia.

MONITORING POLICY

Recognition of the problems of hypoxia is easier than the formulation of a method for assessment of the degree of over-all hypoxia in a patient whose oxygen flux is critically reduced. Such situations tend to arise quickly and the outcome may be fatal long before any measurements can be made. Full assessment requires a large number of measurements, some of which are difficult. The easy measurements include haemoglobin concentrations, arterial Po_2 (or saturation) and cardiac output. However, in many situations the key measurement may be cerebral, coronary or hepatic blood flow, none of which can be considered a bedside procedure.

The first measurement listed above, the haemoglobin concentration, should not present difficulty since the value changes relatively slowly and may be estimated before surgery. Arterial Po_2 is undoubtedly valuable in difficult situations and, in an emergency, it is always possible simply to inspect the colour of blood drawn from an artery. Minor degrees of hypoxia are readily detected by this method and serious arterial hypoxaemia should not be missed no matter what degree of cutaneous vasoconstriction exists.

Cardiac output cannot easily be measured in an emergency and reliance must therefore be placed on clinical observations which give indirect evidence of the cardiac output. Apart from the volume and force of the pulse, useful points are the pallor and temperature of the skin. In general it is unlikely that there is over-all hypoperfusion if the skin is pink and warm, although this will not exclude the possibility of regional circulatory failure. The finger plethysmograph in its various forms offers a semi-quantitative estimate of cutaneous blood flow but unfortunately most types which are currently popular cannot be calibrated.

Regrettably, regional blood flow through the vulnerable organs cannot be assessed by clinical means. Evidence of failure of oxygen flux to these regions is most commonly obtained by functional failure and, in the case of the brain, the level of consciousness and perhaps the electroencephalogram may be recorded.

Finally, a word of warning may be given against undue reliance on the blood pressure. A high pressure is no guarantee of adequacy of perfusion and neither is a low pressure necessarily associated with hypoperfusion, at least in the supine position. The vital factor is the vascular resistance. For example, release of noradrenaline may be associated with high blood pressure, high vascular resistance and hypoperfusion. In contrast, halothane and ganglionic blockade commonly result in hypotension with low vascular resistance and good tissue perfusion. The same degree of hypotension caused by haemorrhage is accompanied by intense vasoconstriction and failure of perfusion. Fortunately, these differences are usually evident in skin colour and temperature, and in skin capillary filling. These observations are, therefore, no less important than the blood pressure and must be taken into account in any scheme for monitoring the state of oxygenation of a patient. In fact, there are many situations where events move too quickly for measurement to play a part and the clinician must then rely on clinical bedside observations coupled with an understanding of the basic physiology.

References and further reading

Barcroft, J. (1920). Physiological effects of insufficient oxygen supply. *Nature, Lond.* 106, 125–129

Chance, B., Schoener, B. and Schindler, F. (1964). The intracellular oxidation–reduction state. In *Oxygen in the Animal Organism.* E. Neil (ed.). Oxford: Pergamon

Cohen, P. J. (1972). The metabolic function of oxygen and biochemical lesions of hypoxia. *Anesthesiology* 37, 148–177

Cullen, D. J. and Eger, E. I. (1970). The effects of hypoxia and isovolemic anemia on the halothane requirement (MAC) of dogs. III. The effects of acute isovolemic anemia. *Anesthesiology* 32, 46–50

Freeman, J. and Nunn, J. F. (1963). Ventilation-perfusion relationships after haemorrhage. *Clin. Sci.* 24, 135–147

Geddes, I. C. (1967). Recent studies in metabolic aspects of anaesthesia. In *Modern Trends in Anaesthesia* – 3. F. T. Evans and T. C. Gray (ed.). London: Butterworths

Greenbaum, R., Bay, J., Hargreaves, M. D., Kain, M. L., Kelman, G. R., Nunn, J. F., Prys-Roberts, C. and Siebold, K. (1967). Effects of higher oxides of nitrogen on the anaesthetised dog. *Br. J. Anaesth.* 39, 393–404

Gregory, I. C. (1974). The oxygen and carbon monoxide capacities of foetal and adult blood. *J. Physiol.* 236, 625–634

Hancock, E. W. and Fleming, P. R. (1960). Aortic stenosis. *Q. Jl Med.* 29, 209–234

Henderson, A. R. (1969). Biochemistry of hypoxia: current concepts. I: An introduction to biochemical pathways and their control. *Br. J. Anaesth.* 41, 245–250

Huckabee, W. W. (1958). Relationships of pyruvate and lactate during anaerobic metabolism. I: Effects of infusions of pyruvate or glucose and of hyperventilation. II: Exercise and formation of O_2-debt. III: Effect of breathing low-oxygen gases. *J. clin Invest.* 37, 244–254, 255–263, 264–271

Kelman, G. R. and Nunn, J. F. (1968). *Computer Produced Physiological Tables for calculations involving the relationships between blood oxygen tension and content.* London: Butterworths

Lindenberg, R. (1963). Patterns of CNS vulnerability in acute hypoxaemia. In *Selective Vulnerability of the Brain in Hypoxaemia.* J. P. Schade and W. H. McMenemy (ed.). Oxford: Blackwell

McDowall, D. G. (1969). Biochemistry of hypoxia: current concepts. II: Biochemical derangements associated with hypoxia and their measurement. *Br. J. Anaesth.* 41, 251–256

Nunn, J. F. (1968). The evolution of atmospheric oxygen. *Ann. R. Coll. Surg.* 43, 200–217

Nunn, J. F. (1977). *Applied Respiratory Physiology.* 2nd edn. London: Butterworths

Owen, O. E., Morgan, A. P., Kemp, H. G., Sullivan, J. M., Herrara, M. G. and Cahill, G. F. (1967). Brain metabolism during fasting. *J. clin. Invest.* 46, 1589–1595

Prys-Roberts, C., Kelman, G. R., Greenbaum, R. and Robinson, R. H. (1967). Circulatory influences of artificial ventilation during nitrous oxide anaesthesia in man. *Br. J. Anaesth.* 39, 533–548

Scott, D. B., Owen, J. A. and Richmond, J. (1964). Methaemoglobinaemia due to prilocaine. *Lancet* ii, 728–729

Staub, N. C. (1963). Alveolar-arterial oxygen tension gradient due to diffusion. *J. appl. Physiol.* 18, 673–680

Stone, H. H., MacKrell, T. N., Brandstater, B. J., Haidak, G. L. and Nemir, P. (1954). The effect of induced haemorrhage shock on the cerebral circulation and metabolism of man. *Surg. Forum* 5, 789–794

22 Hypercapnia
Cedric Prys-Roberts

The phylogenetic development of animal gas exchange organs has been largely influenced by two requirements: firstly, there is the need to keep arterial oxygen tension at a level which ensures adequate delivery of oxygen to the tissue cells, and secondly, there is the need to maintain an optimum ratio between the concentrations of hydroxyl $[OH^-]$ and hydrogen $[H^+]$ ions in the blood thus assuring appropriate neutrality of the tissue fluids (Rahn, 1967). Poikilothermic water breathers such as fish can only maintain adequate arterial Po_2 levels at the cost of 'ventilating' their gills with enormous volumes of water. As a result of this high ventilation and because of the relatively high solubility of carbon dioxide in cold water, their arterial CO_2 tensions are low and their bicarbonate concentrations are correspondingly reduced in order to maintain the optimum $[OH^-]/[H^+]$ at low but varying environmental temperatures. During the transition from water breathing to air breathing, the primitive amphibian lung, although adequate for oxygenation, had to be supplemented by skin respiration as an auxiliary gas exchange organ to cope with the rising CO_2 levels.

In an oxygen-rich atmosphere, man and other homoeotherms can satisfy their oxygen requirements at low levels of ventilation, and the fine adjustment of ventilation is thus pre-eminently geared to the maintenance of $[OH^-]/[H^+]$ ratio through carbon dioxide homoeostasis. The mechanisms for regulation of CO_2 elimination are complex, but ensure that in health the blood level of carbon dioxide is maintained within close limits. Hypercapnia is defined as an excess of carbon dioxide in the body, and implies a failure of these regulating mechanisms. The degree of hypercapnia which can be tolerated depends not only on the failure of such homoeostasis but also on the availability of oxygen. This consideration allows an arbitrary classification of hypercapnia into two grades:

moderate hypercapnia: Pco_2 range 5.3–13.3 kPa (40–100 mmHg)
severe hypercapnia: Pco_2 greater than 13.3 kPa (100 mmHg)

This classification emphasizes that a $Paco_2$ of more than 13.3 kPa is unlikely to occur *when a patient is breathing air*, since the dilution of oxygen in the alveolar gas by the raised carbon dioxide level causes severe hypoxia. It has also been observed that 13.3 kPa (100 mmHg) represents the upper limit of hypercapnia which is compatible with life in patients with severe lung disease (Refsum, 1963; McNicol and Campbell, 1965). Severe hypercapnia may therefore be regarded as an iatrogenic condition since a $PaCO_2$ of more than 13.3 kPa can only be prolonged in an oxygen-rich atmosphere, if a patient or animal either underventilates or breathes a high concentration of carbon dioxide. The upper limit of hypercapnia which has been described in man is about 33 kPa although there is little doubt that this level has been exceeded without recognition or documentation. The term 'supercarbia' was used by Graham, Hill and Nunn (1960) to describe a condition of spontaneous ventilation which supersedes ventilatory arrest in the dog at PCO_2 levels above 53 kPa (400 mmHg).

CAUSATION OF HYPERCAPNIA

Inadequate ventilation

The clearance of carbon dioxide from the blood passing through the lungs is determined by the alveolar ventilation ($\dot{V}A$) and its relation to carbon dioxide production ($\dot{V}CO_2$). The alveolar PCO_2 can be expressed:

$$PACO_2 = \frac{\dot{V}CO_2}{\dot{V}A} (PB - 6.27) \ (kPa) \tag{22.1}$$

Implicit in this equation is the fact that the partial pressure of CO_2 in both alveolar gas ($PACO_2$) and in arterial blood ($PaCO_2$) are reciprocally related to the alveolar ventilation. Reduction of ventilation leads to a hyperbolic rise in $PACO_2$, the final limit being determined by the actual level of alveolar ventilation. The rate of rise of $PACO_2$ is variable, usually between 0.1 and 0.2 kPa·min^{-1} (0.75–1.5 mmHg·min^{-1}) at normal levels of CO_2 production, regardless of whether the reduced alveolar ventilation is relative as a result of increased alveolar, anatomical or apparatus dead space, or absolute following a reduction of tidal ventilation.

In the presence of adequate oxygenation, there is no reason why the alveolar PCO_2 should not rise to over 70 kPa (525 mmHg), but there are few recorded instances of levels above 13.3 kPa (100 mmHg) during anaesthesia. Severe hypercapnia has been reported from hypoventilation during the early days of thoracic surgery, with maximum $PaCO_2$ levels as high as 31.5 kPa (236 mmHg). Moderate degrees of hypercapnia (PCO_2 6–10 kPa; 45–80 mmHg) are commonplace when patients are allowed to breathe spontaneously during anaesthesia, particularly when a face-mask contributes greatly to added dead space in the system. *Figure 22.1* shows a representative range of $PaCO_2$ values which have been observed in intubated man under a variety of anaesthetic agents.

Apnoea may be regarded as the extreme form of hypoventilation, and may be prolonged if mass-movement oxygenation (diffusion respiration) is employed. During this type of anaesthesia, $PaCO_2$ levels of more than

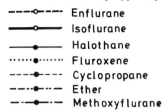

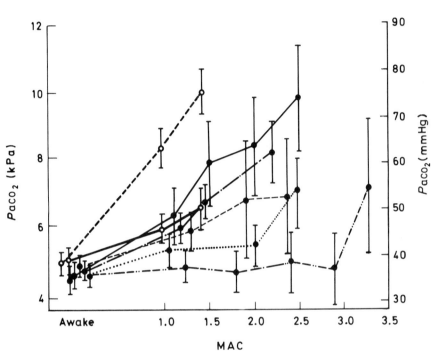

Figure 22.1
Comparison of mean $Pa{co}_2$ in spontaneously breathing patients
anaesthetized with various multiples of minimum alveolar concentrations (MAC) of diethyl ether (1 MAC = 1.9%), fluroxene (1 MAC
= 3.4%), cyclopropane (1 MAC = 9.0%), methoxyflurane (1 MAC =
0.2%), halothane (1 MAC = 0.7%), enflurane (1 MAC = 1.9%) and
isoflurane (1 MAC = 1.2%). Note the progressive increase of $PaCO_2$
with increasing multiples of MAC with each agent, but especially
with enflurane, halothane and isoflurane, compared with the lack of
ventilatory depression under 3 MAC of diethyl ether. (Modified
after Larson *et al.*, 1969, with the addition of data on enflurane and
isoflurane based on Calverley *et al.*, 1978, and Fourcade *et al.*,
1971)

26.6 kPa (200 mmHg) have been reported (Frumin, Epstein and Cohen,
1959), the rate of rise of $P{co}_2$ being between 0.4 and 0.7 kPa (3–5.3 mmHg)
per minute. Moderate degrees of hypercapnia (up to 10 kPa, 75 mmHg)
may occur as part of the compensation for the profound hypochloraemic
alkalosis resulting from uncorrected pyloric stenosis (Saunders *et al.*, 1974).

Rebreathing of exhaled carbon dioxide

Even when ventilation appears to be adequate, rebreathing may cause hypercapnia when the dead space of the apparatus is excessive, when very low gas flows (<3.0 l·min^{-1}) are used in Magill or Bain circuits, or as a result of defective carbon dioxide absorption in a circle system. During light anaesthesia, the challenge of rebreathing induced by added apparatus dead space is usually met by an increase in alveolar ventilation by the patient, so that PACO$_2$ does not necessarily increase significantly. It is important to realize, however, that such a ventilatory response may be suppressed at deep levels of anaesthesia, by the administration of opiate narcotics, and in patients with chronic obstructive airways disease in whom the hypercapnic drive to ventilation may be grossly diminished.

Severe hypercapnia (PACO$_2$ = 31.5 kPa, 236 mmHg) has been described when a patient rebreathed CO_2 as a result of defective apparatus, in which valves were missing from a circle absorber system and thus prevented the exhaled CO_2 being absorbed in a soda-lime canister. Excessive apparatus dead space may have contributed to other recorded cases of moderate and severe hypercapnia in patients whose high PACO$_2$ could otherwise only be explained by incredibly low alveolar ventilation. Under conditions of spontaneous ventilation through a facemask connected to a circle absorber system with a halothane vaporizer within the circle, PACO$_2$ levels between 8 and 21 kPa (60–157.5 mmHg) have been found despite higher than normal levels of minute ventilation, the latter resulting from tachypnoea with low tidal volumes. Hypercapnia was thus due to excessive apparatus dead space in the form of a facemask, and could probably have been reduced by endotracheal intubation. The rate at which PACO$_2$ will rise during total rebreathing is similar to that which occurs during apnoea, and is determined by the body storage capacity for CO_2 and the rate of its production by the tissues. Following a step decrease in ventilation, or addition of dead space, the build-up of CO_2 follows an exponential course which has at least two components and does not usually exceed 0.4 kPa (3 mmHg) in the first minute, and much less thereafter.

Inhalation of carbon dioxide

Inhalation of exogenous carbon dioxide differs from other causes of hypercapnia in that neither the extent nor the rate of rise of PACO$_2$ is limited by metabolic production of carbon dioxide. The maximum PACO$_2$ is thus limited only by atmospheric pressure and the oxygen requirement to maintain life, and a level of 80 kPa (600 mmHg) has been attained in the dog (Graham, Hill and Nunn, 1960) and could probably be achieved in man. Accidental severe hypercapnia from this cause may occur during anaesthesia, usually due to defective apparatus. Such an event was described by Prys-Roberts, Smith and Nunn (1967) in which a patient received a high concentration of CO_2 in the inspired gas due to the accidental opening of the control valve for carbon dioxide, which was not immediately recognized because the structure of the rotameter concealed the bobbin at the top of the tube. Despite a measured arterial P_{CO_2} of 33 kPa (248 mmHg), the patient did not appear to suffer any overt harm from the administration, nor from its rapid withdrawal. Similar levels of P_{CO_2} may have been attained for very short periods during psychiatric abreaction treatment by inhalation of 30% CO_2. There is always a danger that accidental severe hypercapnia may occur when carbon dioxide cylinders are routinely attached to anaesthetic machines. The use of 6% CO_2 in oxygen, or 12-litre Sparklet cylinders of CO_2, would prevent such accidents and would allow the anaesthetist the safe use of a valuable pharmacological tool for ventilatory stimulation.

Whatever the cause, moderate or severe hypercapnia presents a unique stress to the homoeostatic mechanisms of the intact animal, and it is surprising that survival is the rule rather than the exception, provided adequate oxygenation is possible. It would seem appropriate to quote a statement by Peters and Van Slyke (1931) that 'carbon dioxide excess is unlikely of itself to be of dangerous or even serious significance'. While this statement may well be true in many circumstances, the association of hypercapnia with other complications, particularly hypoxia, precludes the conclusion that hypercapnia of any degree is absolutely safe!

EFFECTS OF HYPERCAPNIA

The ubiquitous nature of carbon dioxide as the chief catabolite in the body accounts for its diverse effects and sites of action. Some of these actions are obviously of teleological importance in metabolic homoeostasis whereas others are clearly coincidental. From a physical standpoint, carbon dioxide might be expected to behave like inert gases and vapours in producing an inert gas narcotic effect according to its vapour pressure and fat solubility. Carbon dioxide is not an inert gas, however, and dissolves in the body fluids where it is stored in many forms. These depend on the nature of the fluid, but in all cases carbon dioxide is carried in simple solution according to Henry's law, and passes in and out of cells by diffusion along a partial pressure gradient. Carbonic acid is a weak acid, and its dissociation to H^+ and HCO_3^- ions only occurs to a significant degree if the H^+ ions are removed from the reaction by hydrogen ion acceptors such as haemoglobin and the other proteins. Where this occurs, particularly in the red cells of the blood, carbon dioxide is stored in the form of bicarbonate ions. Further storage of carbon dioxide occurs by its combination with haemoglobin and, to a lesser extent, with other proteins as carbamino compounds. Carbon dioxide is also stored in large quantities as calcium carbonate in bone.

In view of the dissociation of carbonic acid in blood and other body fluids, it is clear that carbon dioxide can exert physiological effects not only in its own right as a gaseous compound, but also through its more important role in the formation of hydrogen ions. Further difficulties arise in the interpretation of the effects of CO_2 excess, because it may have dual actions, firstly on control mechanisms which are teleologically linked to homoeostasis, and secondly direct effects upon target organs or tissues. In most cases, the net effect of hypercapnia is a balance between the one and the other, sometimes additive but at other times antagonistic.

The extrapolation of results obtained in one species to another is not always justified, since marked species differences exist. The value of observations in man of the effects of hypercapnia, often obtained under accidental and uncontrolled circumstances, is thus considerable, particularly in relation to anaesthesia where hypercapnia is common.

In many circumstances, there appears to be a continuous gradation of the effects of CO_2 from hypocapnia to hypercapnia; a discussion of the former will be found in Chapter 23. The rest of this chapter is specially concerned with those effects of hypercapnia which are related to anaesthesia and the care of paralysed, injured and unconscious patients in the intensive therapy unit.

Hypercapnia and the central nervous system

The effects of carbon dioxide on the central nervous system are complex, in that the total observed effect is a balance between at least five major actions: its effects on cerebral blood flow, and the secondary effects on cerebrospinal fluid pressure; its influence on intracellular pH in neurons, causing secondary effects within the cell, particularly those of the reticular activating system and hypothalamus; and finally it is presumed to exert an 'inert gas' narcotic effect.

CARBON DIOXIDE NARCOSIS

It is paradoxical that carbon dioxide was the first gas to be used in the search for surgical anaesthesia by Henry Hill Hickman in 1824. In this respect, carbon dioxide is unique in that it is the only known gas which produces reversible narcosis in higher animals by an effect other than the ordinary anaesthetic action which is common to other inert gases and vapours. Carbon dioxide exerts its narcotic effect through the formation of hydrogen ions and thus specifically reduces the pH of cerebrospinal fluid (Eisele, Eger and Muallem, 1967). Although narcosis can be better related to the CSF pH (*Figure 22.2*) than the blood P_{CO_2}, the effect of narcosis is directly related to the reduction of brain intracellular pH below a level of about 6.7 (Siesjö, Folbergrova and MacMillian, 1972), which is achieved at $P_{a_{CO_2}}$ values in excess of 27 kPa (202 mmHg). Because of the relative blood—brain barrier to ions the combination of either metabolic acidosis or alkalosis does not influence the onset of CO_2 narcosis (*Figure 22.2*) since the effect is dependent on the permeability of the blood—brain barrier to CO_2, and the ability of CO_2 to liberate hydrogen ions within the CSF. It is of considerable interest that progressive arterial hypercapnia up to $P_{a_{CO_2}}$ of 12.7 kPa (95 mmHg) does not reduce the

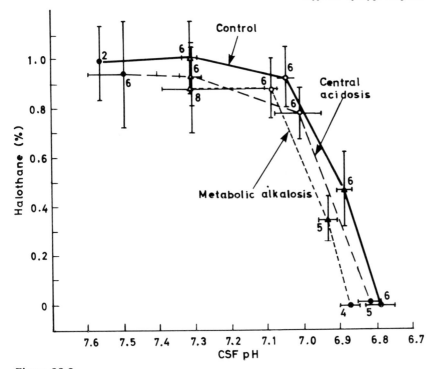

Figure 22.2
The requirement for halothane (minimum alveolar concentration,
MAC) in order to maintain anaesthesia in the dog at increasing levels
of arterial PCO_2, related to the pH of the cerebrospinal fluid. Range of
$Paco_2$ from 1.95 to 32.5 kPa (15–250 mmHg). Note that halothane
requirement does not alter significantly until CSF pH falls below
7.10, regardless of the pH of arterial blood which at this point was
7.05 in the control group, 6.85 in the central acidosis group and
7.25 in the metabolic alkalosis group. Halothane requirement was
zero when CSF pH fell below 6.90, thus signifying full CO_2 narcosis.
(Reproduced from Eisele, Eger and Muallem, 1967, by courtesy of
the Editor, *Anesthesiology*)

minimum alveolar concentration (MAC)* of halothane (*Figure 22.3*). This
conflicts with earlier qualitative studies which gave the impression that
moderate hypercapnia caused deepening of the anaesthetic level with
ether and with nitrous oxide. At higher levels of $Paco_2$, however, there is
progressive reduction of halothane MAC, and with carbon dioxide alone
in the dog, surgical anaesthesia equivalent to that obtained at MAC with
other agents is only achieved at a $Paco_2$ in excess of 26.6 kPa (200 mmHg).
This does not coincide with the considerably lower level of hypercapnia
at which consciousness is lost in man since, under the conditions of
ventilatory failure, a number of other factors tend to augment the narcotic
effects of CO_2. There is agreement, however, with the level of CSF pH in
monkeys which causes EEG changes characteristic of severe cortical
depression.

* The concept of MAC is defined in Chapter 3. *Ed.*

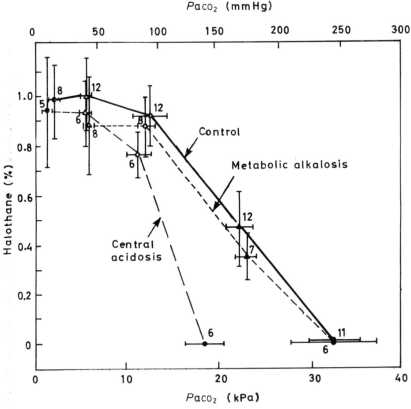

Figure 22.3
The requirement for halothane (minimum alveolar concentration,
MAC) related to increasing Pa_{CO_2} in the dog. No significant reduction
in halothane requirement occurred in any group until the arterial
P_{CO_2} exceeded 11.7 kPa (90 mmHg) regardless of the pH of the
arterial blood which was maintained between 7.1 and 7.3 in the
metabolic alkalosis group, and between 6.70 and 6.90 in the central
acidosis group. Note the wide difference of Pa_{CO_2} values at the point
of zero halothane requirement, that is, the point at which CO_2
narcosis is complete (18.5 kPa, 139 mmHg in the central acidosis
group and 32.7 kPa, 245 mmHg in the control group) (Reproduced
from Eisele, Eger and Muallem, 1967, by courtesy of the Editor,
Anesthesiology)

The state of narcosis achieved at Pa_{CO_2} levels below 26.6 kPa (200 mmHg)
differs from that produced by other gases and vapours. Hypercapnic
narcosis is associated with marked ventilatory and circulatory stimulation,
with increased muscle tone, and with cortical seizure activity. It was these
characteristics which finally deterred anaesthetists from their attempts to
use carbon dioxide as an anaesthetic, and thus ended a century of fruitless
attempts. This complex combination of depression and stimulation
emphasizes the multiplicity of neuronal effects produced by hypercapnia.

The depressant effects of carbon dioxide are probably due to at least
two effects: the first a direct inhibition of synaptic transmission in the
brain and spinal cord, and secondly the depressant effects of intracellular

function mediated by the reduction of intracellular pH (Siesjö, Folbergrova and MacMillan, 1972). Reduced intracellular pH is associated with disturbances of membrane electrolyte transport, interference with glucose utilization and substrate delivery, and intracellular amino-acid depletion. Although these changes have been investigated in detail for the brain, the mechanisms are almost certainly similar in other tissues. Acute hypercapnia (5% CO_2) causes a transient decrease in glycogen stores and an increase in glucose-6-phosphate and fructose-6-phosphate, but a marked decrease in the delivery of pyruvate and lactate (Folbergrova *et al.*, 1975). Similar substrate depletion is found in sustained moderate (5% CO_2) and severe (45% CO_2) hypercapnia, and also in hypoglycaemia (Folbergrova, MacMillan and Siesjö, 1972; Folbergrova, Pontén and Siesjö, 1974; Miller, Hawkins and Veech, 1975). In each of these circumstances these findings indicate inhibition of phosphofructokinase and a consequent marked impairment of the normal glycolytic pathway. In addition to the decrease in pyruvate, there is marked disturbance of the tricarboxylic acid cycle, with depletion of most intermediates, but an increase in succinate (Folbergrova *et al.*, 1975). A further consequence of the decreased delivery of pyruvate from the normal glycolytic pathway is the use of amino acids as an alternative source of pyruvate. Hypercapnia causes a marked decrease in

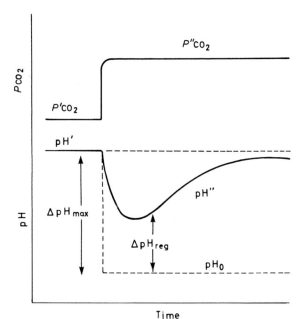

Figure 22.4
Diagram to illustrate the regulation of pH in a tissue compartment as a function of time during sustained hypercapnia. At any time, pH regulation (ΔpH_{reg}) is defined as the difference between the actual pH (pH$''$) and pH$_0$, the latter being the pH which would occur at the altered $P''CO_2$ if there was no tissue pH regulating mechanisms, that is, if the [HCO_3^-] remained constant. (From Siesjö, 1971, by courtesy of the Editor, *The Scandinavian Journal of Clinical and Laboratory Investigation*)

the amino-acid pool in brain cells and an increase in ammonia content due to the increased oxidative deamination. The latter is related to increased activity of aspartate amino transferase leading to glutamate depletion and an increase in aspartate formation (Folbergrova, Pontén and Siesjö, 1974; Folbergrova *et al.*, 1975).

The degrees of brain intracellular pH disturbance is dependent on the degree of intracellular buffering of the induced change of P_{CO_2} (Siesjö, 1971), but the changes of CSF pH induced by acute or sustained hypercapnia (Roncoroni, Roehr and Adaro, 1970; Messeter and Siesjö, 1971) lag behind those of the cells. The regulation of brain pH is time dependent (*Figure 22.4*) and for a given sustained level of pH, intracellular pH regulation reaches 90% of the theoretical possible value within three hours, and thereafter changes very little (*Figure 22.5*). By contrast the CSF pH follows the changes of intracellular pH with a considerable delay

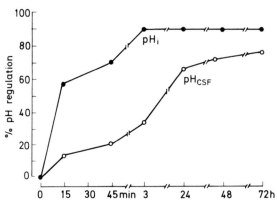

Figure 22.5
Patterns of the defence of intracellular pH (pH_i) and cerebrospinal fluid pH (pH_{CSF}) in response to sustained hypercapnia (Pa_{CO_2} about 11 kPa, 82.5 mmHg). The percentage pH regulation was defined as $100.\Delta pH_{reg}/\Delta pH$ max as shown in *Figure 22.4*. (From Siesjö, 1971, by courtesy of the Editor, *The Scandinavian Journal of Clinical and Laboratory Investigation*)

and does not appear to achieve better than 70–75% regulation. Three mechanisms contribute to the buffering of intracellular fluids in response to changes of P_{CO_2}: physicochemical buffering, consumption of organic acids, and transmembrane exchange of H^+ and HCO_3^- ions. The latter mechanism is only apparent in the slow correction of sustained perturbations of CO_2 (Siesjö, Folbergrova and MacMillan, 1972).

Stimulatory effects of hypercapnia on the central nervous system include excitation of the reticular activating system and its 'arousal' influence on the cortex, and enhanced activity of hypothalamic neurons. Woodbury *et al.* (1958) postulated three levels of brain excitability in response to hypercapnia: a stage of progressive depression up to a P_{CO_2} of 20 kPa (150 mmHg), a stage above this, of excitation during which convulsions may occur, and finally a stage of progressive depression of cerebral electrical activity supervenes at inhaled CO_2 concentrations of more than 40%. The elevated $Paco_2$ associated with spontaneous breathing during enflurane anaesthesia suppresses the electroencephalographic signs of cortical excitation typical of enflurane anaesthesia.

Autonomic effects of hypercapnia

Increased sympathetic adrenergic activity is responsible for many of the actions of carbon dioxide in the body (Skovsted, Price and Price, 1972), and this may be viewed as part of a generalized stress response to hypercapnia. Part of the response is mediated by neurogenic activity which liberates noradrenaline at adrenergic nerve endings, but there is also marked catecholamine secretion by the adrenal medulla, so that both adrenaline and noradrenaline are liberated into the circulating blood. During moderate hypercapnia, the plasma concentrations of both catecholamines increase proportionately, but at Pco_2 levels in excess of 26.6 kPa (200 mmHg) there is a relatively much greater liberation of adrenaline. These findings have been confirmed over a limited range of Pco_2 in humans. During anaesthesia the autonomic response is modified by the agent used; Price *et al.* (1960) found higher plasma catecholamine levels in response to hypercapnia in patients under cyclopropane anaesthesia compared with those under halothane. During moderate hypercapnia in the dog, reflexly induced pressor responses are enhanced compared with the eucapnic state, although the responses at all levels of Pco_2 are depressed by halothane anaesthesia (Prys-Roberts, unpublished observations). Plasma catecholamine levels remain elevated for some time after the termination of hypercapnia, although there are conflicting reports concerning the time course of their return to normal (Tenney and Lamb, 1965).

Hypercapnia also appears to modify the reactivity of the adrenergic neuroeffector junction. As with other effects, there is enhancement of many responses to infused catecholamines during moderate hypercapnia, but most authors are agreed that inhalation of more than 15% carbon dioxide depresses the chronotropic, inotropic and pressor responses to infused adrenaline. Conversely, it has been shown that inhibitory autonomic reflexes mediated through the parasympathetic pathway are enhanced by moderate hypercapnia (Ott and Shepherd, 1973). In conditions in which overactivity of the sympathetic nervous system occurs, such as in severe tetanus, the circulatory responses to moderate hypercapnia are greatly exaggerated, but show the characteristic parallel increase in heart rate, arterial pressure and central venous pressure (*Figure 22.6*).

Acid–base equilibrium during hypercapnia

Hypercapnia represents the greatest stress which is imposed on the homoeostatic mechanisms for maintenance of blood and tissue fluid neutrality. The lower limit of pH which can be tolerated with subsequent recovery is uncertain but is probably of the order of 6.50 in the arterial blood at a P_{CO_2} of 67 kPa (500 mmHg). An increase in alveolar P_{CO_2} from whatever cause results in a progressive build-up of the carbon dioxide stores, reflected in the increased P_{CO_2} of both arterial and mixed venous blood. In the intact animal, the dissociation of the carbonic acid formed within the red cells, and the buffering of the released H^+ ions by haemoglobin, result

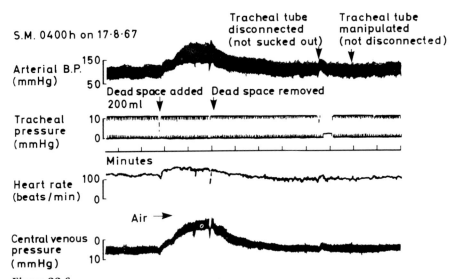

Figure 22.6
Exaggerated circulatory response to increased Pa_{CO_2} in a 10-year-old patient with severe tetanus treated by sedation, curarization and IPPV. The increase in Pa_{CO_2} occurred as the result of adding 200 ml of apparatus dead space to the inspiratory circuit of the ventilator. The immediate and parallel increase of heart rate, arterial pressure and central venous pressure is an exaggeration of the normal response to carbon dioxide observed in both conscious and anaesthetized humans during artificial ventilation. Cardiac output increased from 8.4 to 10.6 litres per minute. This response also illustrates the 'hypercapnic' effect of raising Pa_{CO_2} from 2.7 kPa (20 mmHg) to 5.4 kPa (41 mmHg) in a patient whose central and peripheral chemo-receptors had become reset to a low P_{CO_2} maintained for a number of days

in the formation of bicarbonate ions which leave the cell in exchange for chloride. As the plasma bicarbonate concentration $[HCO_3^-]$ exceeds that of the interstitial fluid (which has little independent buffering capacity), equilibration of bicarbonate concentration across the capillary membrane occurs. The resultant relationships between pH, P_{CO_2} and $[HCO_3^-]$ in the blood constitute the *in vivo* CO_2 dissociation curves (*Figure 22.7*). On theoretical grounds, the blood which most closely resembles the electro-lyte composition of the interstitial fluid is the mixed venous blood which represents the sum of all blood draining systemic capillaries which were in ionic equilibrium with the interstitial fluid (Michel, Lloyd and Cunningham, 1967; Prys-Roberts, 1968). The *in vivo* CO_2 dissociation curve of arterial blood differs in a predictable way from that of the mixed venous blood which is the true curve of the extracellular fluid (Roos and Thomas, 1967; Prys-Roberts, 1968).

When whole blood is exposed to changes of $P\text{CO}_2$ *in vitro*, the bicarbonate ions which are generated cannot be shared with an interstitial fluid pool, thus the CO_2 dissociation curves *in vitro* are quite different from, and do not accurately reflect the *in vivo* acid—base relations of the extracellular fluid (Böning, 1974; Böning *et al.*, 1974). Although this concept was introduced over 45 years ago (Shaw and Messer, 1932), it has only recently gained widespread acceptance, thus the widely held belief that hypercapnia caused metabolic acidosis can now be dispelled, since the indices used were not strictly independent of changes in $P\text{CO}_2$. There is no evidence that during uncomplicated nitrous oxide or halothane anaesthesia in man, nor during moderate hypothermia (28–30°C), hypercapnia causes any deviation from the normal *in vivo* dissociation curve (Prys-Roberts, Kelman and Nunn, 1966; Prys-Roberts, 1968).

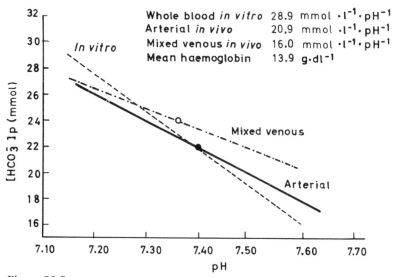

Figure 22.7
Human carbon dioxide dissociation curves of arterial and mixed venous blood *in vivo* during halothane anaesthesia, and the same blood exposed to similar changes of $P\text{CO}_2$ *in vitro*. The extremes of the *in vivo* lines represent changes of $P\text{CO}_2$ between 2 and 11.3 kPa (15 and 86 mmHg) in arterial blood. The slope of the mixed venous curve reflects the buffering of the extracellular fluid over the range of $P\text{CO}_2$ shown. (Data from Prys-Roberts, Kelman and Nunn, 1966; and Prys-Roberts, 1968)

Chronic hypercapnia, as found in patients with chronic ventilatory insufficiency, is associated with renal reabsorption of bicarbonate, thus maintaining a higher plasma $[HCO_3^-]$. The values of arterial blood pH are thus much higher for any given chronically sustained $P\text{CO}_2$ than they would be for the corresponding acute change of $P\text{CO}_2$ (Van Ypersele de Strihou, Brasseur and de Coninck, 1966). With increasing levels of chronic hypercapnia, there is an improvement in the ability to defend pH in response to an acute increase of P_{CO_2}, due to an improvement of the over-all buffering capacity of the body fluids (Goldstein, Gennari and Schwartz, 1971).

Hypercapnia and ventilation

From equation 22.1 it is clear that at a given CO_2 production, there is an 'ideal' value of alveolar ventilation which will maintain a 'normal' alveolar P_{CO_2}, but if the special case is considered where the inspired gas contains carbon dioxide:

$$F_{ACO_2} = F_{ICO_2} + \frac{\dot{V}_{CO_2}}{\dot{V}_A} \qquad (22.2)$$

As F_{ICO_2} approaches F_{ACO_2}, constancy of the latter is no longer maintained despite an increase in ventilation. The body tends to compromise by tolerating a slight increase in F_{ACO_2} rather than increasing alveolar ventilation to the point at which F_{ACO_2} is returned to normal. The response to increased metabolic CO_2 production apparently is more efficient, since ventilation is usually sufficient to maintain a normal F_{ACO_2} under conditions of raised $\dot{V}_{CO_2}$.

The relationship between the expired minute volume ($\dot{V}_E$) and the alveolar or arterial P_{CO_2} defines the carbon dioxide/ventilation dose/ response curve. The slope of this relation reflects the over-all sensitivity of the reflex ventilatory response to increased F_{ACO_2}, and its spatial position indicates the threshold of response to a given F_{ACO_2}. Even in normal man (*Figure 22.8a*) the slope of the CO_2 response is variable but tends to fall into one of four broad groups (Lambertsen, 1960). The slope and to some extent the position of the lines are also influenced by the level of alveolar oxygen, the position of the lines being moved to the left (*Figure 22.8b*) as the threshold response is reduced at low levels of alveolar oxygen. The stimulation of ventilation by increasing P_{CO_2} becomes maximal at inhaled CO_2 concentrations between 15 and 20% in the dog, and thereafter declines (*Figure 22.8d*). It is not known whether ventilatory arrest occurs in man in response to severe hypercapnia, and little guide can be obtained from the responses in other species. Ventilatory arrest occurs in the dog at a P_{ACO_2} between 26.6 and 53 kPa (200–400 mmHg) (Graham, Hill and Nunn, 1960), but the cat will continue to ventilate spontaneously even at a P_{CO_2} of 77 kPa (580 mmHg).

The normal ventilatory response to hypercapnia arises by two mechanisms: peripheral chemoreceptor response to increasing P_{CO_2} in arterial blood, and, more important, the response of neurons in the floor of the fourth ventricle of the brain to a reduction of the pH of cerebrospinal fluid (Mitchell *et al.*, 1963). Denervation of the peripheral chemoreceptors, the aortic and carotid bodies, only slightly depresses the hyperpnoea in response to CO_2 inhalation, and the main function of these receptors may be visualized as oxygen homoeostasis in arterial blood and compensation for metabolic acidosis by increased ventilation.

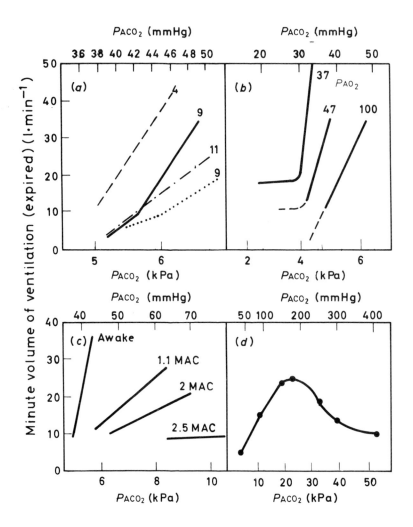

Figure 22.8
Carbon dioxide/ventilation dose/response curves under varying
circumstances. (*a*) Responses to inhaling carbon dioxide without
hypoxia in four groups of conscious human subjects (data derived
from Lambertsen, 1960). (*b*) Influence of hypoxia on the CO_2
response curves in conscious human subjects (P_{AO_2} values in mmHg)
(data from Nielsen and Smith, 1951). (*c*) Influence of increasing
depth of anaesthesia (as multiples of mean alveolar concentration,
MAC) on the CO_2 response curves in man (based on data from
Munson *et al.*, 1966). (*d*) CO_2 response curve between Pa_{CO_2} values of
5.3 kPa and 53 kPa (40 and 400 mmHg) in the dog, showing the
initial stimulatory response and subsequent return to normal
ventilation occurring at Pa_{CO_2} levels above 26.5 kPa (200 mmHg)
(based on data derived from Eisele, Eger and Muallem, 1967)

Anaesthesia is generally associated with suppression of the normal ventilatory responses to hypercapnia (*Figure 22.8c*), the CO_2 response curves being moved progressively to the right with increasing depth of anaesthesia, and the slope of the relation is also progressively depressed (Munson *et al.*, 1966; Larson *et al.*, 1969). Hypercapnia accentuates the ventilatory response to hypoxia and vice versa (Lloyd, Jukes and Cunningham, 1958), but halothane depresses this response markedly (Weiskopf, Raymond and Severinghaus, 1974). Patients with chronic hypercapnia ($P_{CO_2} > 7$ kPa (52 mmHg) have markedly flatter CO_2 response curves when compared with normal patients, or those with varying degrees of hypoxaemia but no hypercapnia (Kepron and Cherniack, 1973).

PULMONARY GAS EXCHANGE AND OXYGEN TRANSPORT

As a result of the hyperdynamic circulation during hypercapnia in anaesthetized man, the transport of oxygen between the lungs and the tissues is enhanced by the increased cardiac output, and is reflected in lower than normal arteriovenous oxygen content differences (Prys-Roberts *et al.*, 1968). As a consequence of the higher oxygen content of the mixed venous blood returning to the lungs, the contribution of shunted blood to venous admixture is reduced, thus the alveolar–arterial P_{O_2} difference is decreased. This effect is much less marked during hypercapnia than the opposite effect during hypocapnia. The slight increase in arterial P_{O_2} which occurs during hypercapnia is offset by the impaired uptake of oxygen by haemoglobin due to the Bohr effect on the oxygen dissociation curve. The gross displacement of the curve to the right during severe hypercapnia is sufficient to account for desaturation of arterial blood despite normal oxygen tensions (Prys-Roberts, Smith and Nunn, 1967).

Circulatory responses to hypercapnia

There now exists a voluminous literature on the effects of hypercapnia on the circulation in both conscious and anaesthetized man and in experimental animals. It is characteristic of the dual effects of carbon dioxide that the observed responses in any situation represent the balance between the depressant effects of the gas on target organs, and its excitatory effects mediated through the central excitation of the sympathetic nervous system. Thus, much of the conflict within this subject is apparent rather than real, and may be resolved if one considers the circumstances of each experiment in terms of species, age, type of anaesthesia, duration and severity of hypercapnia, mode of ventilation and so on.

It has long been recognized that increased P_{CO_2} and the associated acidosis causes a weakening of the force of myocardial contraction and a decrease in the beating frequency of the isolated heart. Hypercapnic acidosis decreases the contractility of isolated papillary muscles (Pannier and Brutsaert, 1968; Foëx and Fordham, 1972) but the effect is short-lived and there is a progressive recovery of function as the intracellular pH changes are buffered (*Figure 22.9*).

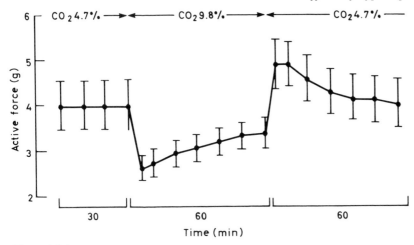

Figure 22.9
Response of isolated papillary muscle from a cat to a stepwise
increase of CO_2 in the perfusate (4.7–9.8%) and a stepwise return
to the original perfusate after 60 minutes. There is a progressive
recovery of active force with time, probably due to intracellular
buffering of the induced change of intracellular pH, reminiscent of
the response of brain cells shown in *Figure 22.4*. Following the step
return to a normal P_{CO_2} there is a marked overshoot of active force
followed again by a slow recovery to the baseline value. Mean values
± s.e.m. from 9 isometric cat papillary muscle preparations. (Based
on Foëx and Fordham, 1972, by courtesy of the authors)

Carbon dioxide excess has a depressant effect on peripheral vascular
smooth muscle, its effects being most marked on the precapillary resistance
section. The total peripheral vascular response during hypercapnia may be
modified by the simultaneous effects of adrenergic activity, on the same
vascular segments, and both may be further modified by the effects of
anaesthetics (Prys-Roberts, 1971).

HAEMODYNAMIC EFFECTS OF CARBON DIOXIDE IN THE CONSCIOUS STATE

An elevation of P_{aCO_2} from 5.2 to 6.7 kPa (39–50 mmHg) in conscious
man, during either spontaneous or controlled ventilation, causes marked
increase of heart rate and myocardial contractility, with consequent
increase of stroke volume and cardiac output, while systemic vascular
resistance is reduced (Cullen and Eger, 1974).

HAEMODYNAMIC EFFECTS OF CARBON DIOXIDE IN ANAESTHETIZED MAN

Volatile anaesthetics modify the haemodynamic effects of elevated P_{aCO_2}.
The direct effect of all anaesthetics is to impair myocardial contractility,
a property in common with high P_{CO_2}. Some anaesthetics enhance sympathetic activity (also a property in common with raised P_{CO_2}) and such
agents (cyclopropane, fluroxene, diethyl ether, isoflurane and enflurane)
enhance the sympathetic effects of raised P_{CO_2}, whereas nitrous oxide

and/or halothane do not (Prys-Roberts *et al.*, 1967; Prys-Roberts *et al.*, 1968; Cullen, Eger and Gregory, 1969; Cullen *et al.*, 1971; Fourcade *et al.*, 1971; Gregory *et al.*, 1974; Calverley *et al.*, 1978).

The effects of hypercapnia on cardiac performance are dependent on a further factor, the hydraulic impedance to left ventricular ejection (Gersh *et al.*, 1972). Systemic vascular resistance (SVR), the ratio of mean arterial pressure to cardiac output, is the main component of aortic input impedance. Hypercapnia is almost always associated with marked reduction of SVR and the non-pulsatile term of aortic input impedance, thus the depressant effects of anaesthetics and CO_2 on the ventricular muscle are to some extent offset.

The net effects in man are summarized in *Table 22.1* which emphasizes two constant features of the interaction of anaesthesia and hypercapnia and anaesthesia, increased cardiac output and reduced systemic vascular

TABLE 22.1. Cardiovascular responses to hypercapnia ($PaCO_2 = 8–11$ kPa, 60–83 mmHg) during various types of anaesthesia (1 MAC equivalent except for nitrous oxide). The increase of $PaCO_2$ in the conscious subjects was 1.5 kPa (11.5 mmHg) from a normal level of 5.2 kPa (38 mmHg).

	Heart rate	Contractility	Cardiac output	Systemic vascular resistance
Conscious	+ +	+ +	+ + +	−
Nitrous oxide	0	+	+ +	− −
Cyclopropane	+ + +	?	+ + +	− − −
Diethyl ether	+ +	+ +	+ + +	− −
Fluroxene	+	+ + +	+ + +	−
Halothane	0	+	+	−
Enflurane	+	+	+ +	− − −
Isoflurane	+ +	+ + +	+ + +	−

Key: +, <10% increase; + +, 10–25% increase; + + +, >25% increase; 0, no change; −, <10% decrease; − −, 10–25% decrease; − − −, >25% decrease.

resistance. Systemic vascular resistance decreases to a comparable degree with most anaesthetic agents but is most marked during enflurane anaesthesia and hypercapnia (Calverley *et al.*, 1978). The increase in cardiac output is most marked during anaesthesia with agents which enhance sympathetic activity and least marked with halothane or nitrous oxide. During halothane anaesthesia, the increase in cardiac output is mainly related to increased stroke volume secondary to the reduction in aortic input impedance (Foëx and Prys-Roberts, 1975a).

INTERACTION OF HYPERCAPNIA, ANAESTHESIA AND β-RECEPTOR BLOCKADE

Since the main sympathetic effects of hypercapnia are mediated through adrenergic β-receptors, the interaction of β-receptor antagonist drugs and hypercapnia is clinically important. It is also useful in the laboratory as a means of identifying the sympathetic component of the cardiovascular response to hypercapnia during anaesthesia. In the presence of β-receptor blockade, the effects of hypercapnia on sympathetic nervous activity are inhibited, leaving the direct myocardial depressant effects of carbon dioxide to produce additive effects with the anaesthetic agents (Foëx and Prys-Roberts, 1974).

During anaesthesia with halothane or nitrous oxide, the effects of a β-receptor antagonist (e.g. propranolol) are minimal if arterial $P\text{CO}_2$ is within the normal range. If a steady state of hypercapnia ($Pa\text{CO}_2$ = 10 kPa, 75 mmHg) is maintained during halothane or nitrous oxide anaesthesia, β-receptor blockade is associated with a marked decrease of myocardial contractility, stroke volume and cardiac output despite a modest increase in left ventricular pressure (Foëx and Prys-Roberts, 1974). Propranolol has a selectivity for peripheral vascular β-receptors rather than the heart, and since it does not block α-receptors, circulating catecholamines exert an unopposed vasoconstrictor effect on systemic blood vessels. Thus the combination of hypercapnia, anaesthesia and β-receptor blockade may be associated with an increase rather than a decrease of systemic vascular resistance.

It is customary to apply the term hypercapnia to elevated $P\text{CO}_2$ levels referred to the normal range of 4.8—5.6 kPa (36—42 mmHg). In patients under prolonged artificial ventilation, in whom the CO_2 stores have been chronically depleted by hyperventilation, there is progressive adaptation of chemoreceptor homoeostasis so that the circulation behaves in the same way as that of a normal man with a $Pa\text{CO}_2$ of 5.3 kPa (40 mmHg). However, if a dead space is added to the breathing circuit, thus raising the patient's $Pa\text{CO}_2$ acutely from 2.7 to 5.3 kPa (20—40 mmHg), the physiological responses observed are akin to those seen when normal man becomes moderately hypercapnic (Prys-Roberts, unpublished observations). The time course for the resetting of such adaptation is about two to four days, and rarely results in complete compensation of the acid—base disturbance in the blood (*Figure 22.6*).

ROLE OF HYPERCAPNIA IN THE INITIATION OF CARDIAC ARRHYTHMIA

It is widely recognized that hypercapnia is associated with alteration in cardiac rhythm and conduction in the presence of certain anaesthetic agents. In the conscious subject, cardiac arrhythmia is unusual at $Pa\text{CO}_2$ up to 11 kPa (80 mmHg), and above this the commonest change is to an A—V junctional rhythm with or without variable changes in T-wave deflection. It has been shown that the threshold of $Pa\text{CO}_2$ at which arrhythmia occurs may be modified by various anaesthetics. Thus Price *et al.* (1958) noted a mean threshold level at a $Pa\text{CO}_2$ of 7.7 kPa (58 mmHg, range 44—72) during cyclopropane anaesthesia, whereas the threshold range during halothane anaesthesia was considerably higher, and varied between 7.8 and 19 kPa (58 and 143 mmHg) with a mean level of 12.3 kPa (92 mmHg). The threshold may be further modified by the concentration of anaesthetic agent in use; episodes of arrhythmia during closed circuit halothane anaesthesia have been described as 'bizarre and alarming' even at moderate levels of hypercapnia.

Katz has recently implicated the increased sympathetic adrenergic activity as the main mechanism by which arrhythmia occurs, especially when an increase in heart rate cannot be mediated by the pacemaker, and nodal or ectopic foci predominate by default (Katz and Epstein, 1968). It has been reported that the sudden reduction of a high P_{CO_2} in dogs may initiate ventricular fibrillation, but these findings have not been universally confirmed, and there is much evidence to suggest that the response can be attributed to concomitant hypoxia occurring as a dilutional diffusion hypoxia when hypercapnia is terminated and followed by air breathing.

Hypercapnia and regional blood flow

CEREBRAL BLOOD FLOW

Following the classical work of Kety and Schmidt (1948), in which the vasodilator effects of hypercapnia on the cerebral circulation were defined, subsequent studies have both confirmed and modified the original general conclusion. Harper (1965) demonstrated that, in normotensive dogs, hypercapnia caused a marked increase in cerebral blood flow, but that this effect was absent in the hypotensive animal. Furthermore, he found that autoregulation of cerebral blood flow in response to changes in arterial pressure occurred in the eucapnic animal, but not in the hypercapnic animal. It was also evident that maximal cerebral vasodilatation occurred at fairly modest levels of P_{aCO_2} (10.7 kPa, 80 mmHg) in the dog. With acclimatization to prolonged hypercapnia the increased blood flow tends to return to the eucapnic level. The effect of carbon dioxide on the smooth muscle of the cerebral vessels is believed to be direct, since at constant P_{CO_2} variations in the pH of arterial blood do not significantly influence the cerebral blood flow.

In normal man, very high cerebral blood flows associated with marked cerebral vasodilatation have been reported when halothane anaesthesia is associated with hypercapnia (Christensen, Høedt-Rasmussen and Lassen, 1967). Their findings confirm the results of previous studies, but also draw attention to the potentiating effect of hypotension and hypercapnia in this respect, and the difference between the canine and human response.

SPLANCHNIC BLOOD FLOW

The influence of hypercapnia on pressure–flow relationships in the splanchnic and hepatic circulations varies considerably according to the anaesthetic agent used. During thiopentone and nitrous oxide anaesthesia, in which the sympathetic adrenergic mechanisms are not unduly suppressed, hypercapnia is associated with splanchnic vasoconstriction and reduced hepatic blood flow, whereas during halothane anaesthesia the balance is such that the direct vasodilator effect of carbon dioxide promotes splanchnic vasodilatation and a marked increase in hepatic blood flow (Epstein *et al.,* 1966).

LIMB BLOOD FLOW

The two major vascular circuits in the limbs are those to skin and skeletal muscle; in both circuits the response to hypercapnia is a balance between the direct vasodilator effects of CO_2 and the vasoconstrictor effects secondary to sympathetic adrenergic activity. During anaesthesia, the response is predominantly vasodilator in the skin circuit and vasoconstrictor in muscle.

PULMONARY CIRCULATION

Hypercapnia causes an increase in pulmonary artery pressure in most circumstances, and there is usually an associated increase in pulmonary blood flow (cardiac output). It has been customary to express pulmonary vascular resistance as the ratio of mean pulmonary artery pressure (pulmonary artery pressure–left atrial pressure) to pulmonary artery flow. Most investigators found that pulmonary vascular resistance, expressed in this way, was markedly increased during hypercapnia. It was further implied that such a change represented a pH-dependent pulmonary vasoconstriction (Barer, Howard and McCurrie, 1967). Although there is some evidence that CO_2 can exert a direct vasodilator effect on the pulmonary vasculature, it is generally believed that the effects of hypercapnia in the isolated lung are due to the vasoconstrictor effects of acids on the pre- and postcapillary vessels in the lung (Barer and Shaw, 1971).

The pulmonary circulation is characterized by the transmission of pulsatile flow through the capillary section into the pulmonary venous segment, to the extent that the pulsatile component of right ventricular power may comprise 20–50% of the total power output. For this reason, pulmonary vascular resistance calculated *in vivo* from measurements of pressure and flow may grossly underestimate the true impedance to the flow of blood through the lung (Milnor, Bergel and Bargainer, 1966). Analysis of the pulmonary vascular response to hypercapnia in terms of pulmonary input impedance (*Figure 22.10*) indicates that the changes in pulmonary arterial pressure do not result from vasoconstriction to the extent of a reduction of either pulmonary arteriolar calibre or distensibility (Foëx and Prys-Roberts, 1975b). It is clear that the effects of hypercapnia on the pulmonary circulation are considerably less marked than those of hypoxia or lung inflation.

CORONARY CIRCULATION

Although the coronary circulation is primarily organized to maintain coronary blood flow appropriate to myocardial O_2 consumption, a number of agents can cause dilatation or constriction of coronary arterioles.

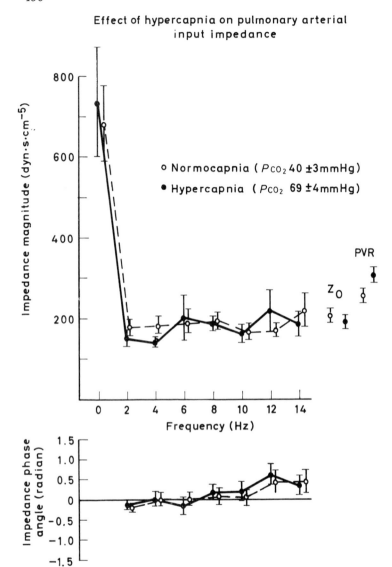

Figure 22.10

Pulmonary arterial input impedance spectra during normocapnia and hypercapnia (P_{CO_2} 5.3 and 9.2 kPa respectively) in the goat. Mean values ± s.e.m. from eight studies are shown in classes of 2 Hz band width. Note the small, insignificant difference between the values of impedance modulus at zero frequency. This modulus is the equivalent of pulmonary vascular resistance. Note also the lack of difference between the frequency dependent components of the spectra, and the lack of any phase difference. (From Foëx and Prys-Roberts, 1975b, by courtesy of the Editor, *Journal of Applied Physiology*)

Hypercapnia is associated with an increase in coronary blood flow which is disproportionate to the increase in left ventricular work and myocardial O_2 requirements (Foëx, unpublished observations). This effect is associated with a marked increase in coronary sinus Po_2 and a consequent decrease in the arteriovenous O_2 content difference across the coronary circulation.

Hypercapnia and body temperature

During the first 6–12 hours of sustained hypercapnia in response to breathing 15% carbon dioxide, body temperature falls by about 3°C but recovers to the original value over a period of three days (Schaefer *et al.*, 1975). The reduction of body temperature is due to:

(1) direct inhibition of cellular metabolism,
(2) increased heat loss due to the vasodilator effects of CO_2 on skin blood vessels, and
(3) a transient decrease, followed by a sustained increase in the nor-adrenaline content of cells in the hypothalamic region involved in thermoregulation.

Obstetric and neonatal implications of hypercapnia

The generalized circulatory effects of hypercapnia are reflected in changes in both maternal and fetal circulations with consequent effects on fetal oxygenation. Moderate hypercapnia in the human mother during caesarian section is associated with elevated umbilical vein Po_2 (Ivankovic, Elam and Huffman, 1970). In the sheep, maternal hypercapnia was shown to increase umbilical blood flow and to increase fetal umbilical vein Po_2 (Motoyama *et al.*, 1967). The neonatal lamb responds to hypercapnia in much the same way as the 1-year-old lamb and the adults of most species (Koivikko, 1969), producing a 30% increase of heart rate and cardiac output in response to an increase in $Paco_2$ from 5.4 to 10 kPa (41–75 mmHg)

RECOGNITION OF HYPERCAPNIA

Nunn (1961) has emphasized the difficulties involved in recognizing hypercapnia on the basis of clinical observation, and has stressed the need for direct measurement of CO_2 in arterial blood or alveolar gas as the only reliable and accurate method of estimating the degree of hypercapnia. Recent developments in methodology, and a widespread acceptance of blood gas analysis make the recognition of hypercapnia much easier than in the past. There are pitfalls for the unwary, however, in recognizing very high Pco_2 levels, particularly when the interpolation method of assessing

Pa_{CO_2} is used (Prys-Roberts, Smith and Nunn, 1967). The danger here is the linear extrapolation of the *in vitro* CO_2 dissociation curve beyond the limits of the calibrating gas mixtures, since the *in vitro* dissociation curve of whole blood is only approximately linear over a limited range. In general, the task is simply that of deciding whether the patient's Pa_{CO_2} is in excess of the normal range, and approximations to the nearest 1.3 kPa (10 mmHg) do not seriously affect the clinical outcome.

The reader may be inclined to believe that the physiological effects of moderate hypercapnia are if anything more beneficial than those of hyperventilation and the ensuing hypocapnia. However, the difficulty of ensuring that the degree of hypercapnia does not become excessive has influenced most anaesthetists to err on the side of safety and thus deliberately overventilate the patient rather than risk hypercapnia. In this matter it is convenience rather than physiological consideration which has determined the pattern of clinical practice.

References

Barer, G. R., Howard, P. and McCurrie, J. R. (1967). The effect of carbon dioxide and changes in blood pH on pulmonary vascular resistance in cats. *Clin. Sci.* 32, 361–376

Barer, G. R. and Shaw, J. W. (1971). Pulmonary vasodilator and vasoconstrictor actions of carbon dioxide. *J. Physiol.* 213, 633–645

Böning, D. (1974). The 'in vivo' and 'in vitro' CO_2 equilibration curves of blood during acute hypercapnia and hypocapnia. II Theoretical considerations. *Pflüg. Arch. ges. Physiol.* 350, 213–222

Böning, D., Schweigart, U., Nutz, V. and Stegemann, J. (1974). The 'in vivo' and 'in vitro' CO_2 equilibration curves of blood during acute hypercapnia and hypocapnia. I Experimental investigations. *Pflüg. Arch. ges. Physiol.* 350, 210–212

Calverley, R. K., Smith, N. T., Jones, C. W., Prys-Roberts, C. and Eger, E. I. (1978). Ventilatory and cardiovascular effects of enflurane anesthesia during spontaneous ventilation in man. *Anesth. Analg.* 57, 610–618

Christensen, M. S., Hóedt-Rasmussen, K. and Lassen, N. A. (1967). Cerebral vasodilatation by halothane anaesthesia in man and its potentiation by hypotension and hypercapnia. *Br. J. Anaesth.* 39, 927–934

Cullen, B. F., Eger, E. I., Smith, N. T., Sawyer, D. C. and Gregory, G. A. (1971). The circulatory response to hypercapnia during fluroxene anesthesia in man. *Anesthesiology* 34, 415–420

Cullen, D. J. and Eger, E. I. (1974). Cardiovascular effects of carbon dioxide in man. *Anesthesiology* 41, 345–349

Cullen, D. J., Eger, E. I. and Gregory, G. A. (1969). The cardiovascular effects of carbon dioxide in man, conscious and during cyclopropane anesthesia. *Anesthesiology* 31, 407–413

Eisele, J. H., Eger, E. I. and Muallem, M. (1967). Narcotic properties of carbon dioxide in the dog. *Anesthesiology* 28, 856–865

Epstein, R. M., Deutsch, S., Cooperman, L. H., Clement, A. J. and Price, H. L. (1966). Splanchnic circulation during halothane anesthesia and hypercapnia in normal man. *Anesthesiology* 27, 654–661

Foëx, P. and Fordham, R. M. M. (1972). Intrinsic myocardial recovery from the negative inotropic effects of acute hypercapnia. *Cardiovasc. Res.* 6, 257–262

Foëx, P. and Prys-Roberts, C. (1974). Interactions of beta-receptor blockade and P_{CO_2} levels in the anaesthetised dog. *Br. J. Anaesth.* 46, 397–404

Foëx, P. and Prys-Roberts, C. (1975a). Effect of CO_2 on myocardial contractility and aortic input impedance during anaesthesia. *Br. J. Anaesth.* 47, 669–678

Foëx, P. and Prys-Roberts, C. (1975b). Effects of changes in Pa_{CO_2} on pulmonary input impedance. *J. appl. Physiol.* 38, 52–57

Folbergrova, J., MacMillan, V. and Siesjö, B. K. (1972). The effect of hypercapnic acidosis upon some glycolytic and Krebs cycle intermediates in the rat brain. *J. Neurochem.* 19, 2507–2517

Folbergrova, J., Pontén, U. and Siesjö, B. K. (1974). Patterns of changes in brain carbohydrate metabolites, amino-acids and organic phosphates at increased carbon dioxide tensions. *J. Neurochem.* 22, 1115–1125

Folbergrova, J., Norberg, K., Quistorff, B. and Siesjö, B. K. (1975). Carbohydrate and amino-acid metabolism in rat cerebral cortex in moderate and extreme hypercapnia. *J. Neurochem.* 25, 457–462

Fourcade, H. E., Stevens, W. C., Larson, C. P., Cromwell, T. H., Bahlman, S. H., Hickey, R. F., Halsey, M. J. and Eger, E. I. (1971). The ventilatory effects of Forane, a new inhaled anesthetic. *Anesthesiology* 35, 26–31

Frumin, M. J., Epstein, R. M. and Cohen, G. (1959). Apnoeic oxygenation in man. *Anesthesiology* 20, 789–798

Gersh, B. J., Prys-Roberts, C., Reuben, S. R. and Schultz, D. L. (1972). The effects of halothane on the interactions between myocardial contractility, aortic impedance and left ventricular performance. II: Aortic input impedance, and the distribution of energy during ventricular ejection. *Br. J. Anaesth.* 44, 767–775

Goldstein, M. B., Gennari, F. J. and Schwartz, W. B. (1971). The influence of graded degrees of chronic hypercapnia on the acute carbon dioxide titration curve. *J. clin. Invest.* 50, 208–216

Graham, G. R., Hill, D. W. and Nunn, J. F. (1960). Die Wirkung hoher CO_2 – konzentrationen auf kreislauf und atmung. *Der Anaesthesist.* 9, 70–73

Gregory, G. A., Eger, E. I., Smith, N. T. and Cullen, B. F. (1974). The cardiovascular effects of carbon dioxide in man, awake and during diethyl ether anesthesia. *Anesthesiology* 40, 301–304

Harper, A. M. (1965). The interrelationship between $Paco_2$ and blood pressure in the regulation of blood flow through the cerebral cortex. In *Regional Blood Flow.* D. H. Ingvar and N. A. Lassen (ed.). Copenhagen: Munksgaard

Ivankovic, A. D., Elam, J. O. and Huffman, J. (1970). Effect of maternal hypercarbia on the newborn infant. *Am. J. Obstet. Gynec.* 107, 939–946

Katz, R. L. and Epstein, R. A. (1968). The interaction of anesthetic agents and adrenergic drugs to produce cardiac arrhythmias. *Anesthesiology* 29, 763–784

Kepron, W. and Cherniack, R. M. (1973). The ventilatory response to hypercapnia and to hypoxaemia in chronic obstructive lung disease. *Am. Rev. resp. Dis.* 108, 843–850

Kety, S. S. and Schmidt, C. F. (1948). The effect of altered tensions of carbon dioxide and oxygen on cerebral blood flow and cerebral oxygen consumption of normal young men. *J. clin. Invest.* 27, 484–492

Koivikko, A. (1969). Cardiovascular response of the neonatal lamb to hypoxia, hypercapnia and metabolic acidosis. *Acta paed. scand.* Suppl. 191

Lambertsen, C. J. (1960). Carbon dioxide and respiration in acid–base homeostasis. *Anesthesiology* 21, 642–651

Larson, C. P., Eger, E. I., Mullem, M., Buechel, D. R., Munson, E. S. and Eisele, J. H. (1969). The effects of diethyl ether and methoxyflurane on ventilation: II A comparative study in man. *Anesthesiology* 30, 174–184

Lloyd, B. B., Jukes, M. G. M. and Cunningham, D. J. C. (1958). Relation between alveolar oxygen pressure and the respiratory response to CO_2 in man. *Q. Jl exp. Physiol.* 43, 214–227

McNicol, M. W. and Campbell, E. J. M. (1965). Severity of respiratory failure: arterial blood gases in untreated patients. *Lancet* i, 336–338

Messeter, K. and Siesjö, B. K. (1971). Regulation of the csf pH in acute and sustained respiratory action. *Acta physiol. scand.* 83, 21–30

Michel, C. C., Lloyd, B. B. and Cunningham, D. J. C. (1966). The *in vivo* carbon dioxide dissociation curve of true plasma. *Resp. Physiol.* 1, 121–137

Miller, A. L., Hawkins, R. A. and Veech, R. L. (1975). Decreased rate of glucose utilization by rat brain *in vivo* after exposure to atmospheres containing high concentrations of CO_2. *J. Neurochem.* 25, 553–558

Milnor, W. B., Bergel, D. H. and Bargainer, J. D. (1966). Hydraulic power associated with pulmonary blood flow and its relation to heart rate. *Circulation Res.* 19, 467–480

Mitchell, R. A., Loeschke, H. H., Massion, W. H. and Severinghaus, J. W. (1963). Respiratory responses mediated through superficial chemosensitive areas on the medulla. *J. appl. Physiol.* 18, 523–533

Motoyama, E. K., Rivard, G., Acheson, F. and Cook, C. D. (1967). The effect of changes in maternal pH and Pco_2 on the Po_2 of fetal lambs. *Anesthesiology* 28, 891–903

Munson, E. S., Larson, C. P., Babad, A. A., Regan, M. J., Buechel, D. R. and Eger, E. I. (1966). The effects of halothane, fluroxene and cyclopropane on ventilation; A comparative study in man. *Anesthesiology* 27, 716–728

Nielsen, M. and Smith, H. (1951). Studies on the regulation of respiration in acute hypoxia. *Acta physiol. scand.* 24, 293–313

Nunn, J. F. (1961). The effects of hypercapnia. In *Modern Trends in Anaesthesia.* F. T. Evans and T. C. Gray (ed.). London: Butterworths

Ott, N. T. and Shepherd, J. T. (1973). Modifications of the aortic and vagal depressor reflexes by hypercapnia in the rabbit. *Circulation Res.* 33, 160–165

Pannier, J. L. and Brutsaert, D. L. (1968).
Contractility of isolated cat papillary muscle
and acid—base changes. *Archs int.
Pharmacodyn. Thér.* 172, 244—246

Peters, J. P. and Van Slyke, D. D. (1931).
Quantitative Clinical Chemistry, p. 950.
Baltimore: Williams and Wilkins

Price, H. L., Lurie, A. A., Jones, R. L., Price,
M. L. and Linde, H. W. (1958). Cyclopropane
anesthesia: epinephrine and norepinephrine
in initiation of ventricular arrhythmias by
CO_2 inhalation. *Anesthesiology* 19, 619—630

Price, H. L., Black, G. W., Sechzer, P. H. and
Linde, H. W. (1960). Modification by general
anesthetics (cyclopropane and halothane) of
circulatory and sympathoadrenal responses to
respiratory acidosis. *Ann. Surg.* 152,
1071—1077

Prys-Roberts, C. (1968). In-vivo CO_2 dissociation
curves of mixed venous and arterial blood in
anaesthetized man. *Br. J. Anaesth.* 40, 802

Prys-Roberts, C. (1971). Regulation of the
circulation. In *General Anaesthesia,* 3rd edn,
Vol. 1, Chapter 15, pp. 224—239. T. C. Gray
and J. F. Nunn (ed.). London: Butterworths

Prys-Roberts, C., Kelman, G. R. and Nunn, J. F.
(1966). Determination of the in-vivo carbon
dioxide titration curve of anaesthetized man.
Br. J. Anaesth. 38, 500—509

Prys-Roberts, C., Smith, W. D. A. and Nunn,
J. F. (1967). Accidental severe hypercapnia
during anaesthesia. *Br. J. Anaesth.* 39,
257—267

Prys-Roberts, C., Kelman, G. R., Greenbaum,
R. and Robinson, R. H. (1967). Circulatory
influences of artificial ventilation during
nitrous oxide anaesthesia in man. II Results:
The relative influence of mean intrathoracic
pressure and arterial carbon dioxide tension.
Br. J. Anaesth. 39, 533—548

Prys-Roberts, C., Kelman, G. R., Greenbaum, R.,
Kain, M. L. and Bay, J. (1968). Hemodynamics and alveolar—arterial Po_2 differences
at varying $Paco_2$ in anesthetized man. *J. appl.
Physiol.* 25, 80—87

Rahn, H. (1967). Gas transport from the external
environment to the cell. In *Development of
the Lung.* A. V. S. De Reuck and R. Porter
(ed.). London: Churchill

Refsum, H. E. (1963). Relationship between
state of consciousness and arterial hypoxaemia
and hypercapnia in patients with pulmonary
insufficiency, breathing air. *Clin. Sci.* 25,
361—367

Roncoroni, A., Roehr, E. F. and Adaro, F.
(1970). Acid—base equilibrium of cerebrospinal fluid in chronic respiratory acidosis
and provoked hypercapnia in relaxed patients.
Am. Rev. resp. Dis. 102, 790—800

Roos, A. and Thomas, L. J. (1967). The in-vitro
and in-vivo carbon dioxide dissociation curves
of true plasma. *Anesthesiology* 28,
1048—1063

Saunders, N. A., Carter, J., Scamps, P. and
Vandenberg, R. (1974). Severe hypercapnia
associated with metabolic alkalosis due to
pyloric stenosis. *Aust. N. Z. J. Med.* 4,
385—391

Schaefer, K. E., Messier, A. A., Morgan, C. and
Baker, G. T. (1975). Effect of chronic hyper-
capnia on body temperature regulation.
J. appl. Physiol. 38, 900—906

Shaw, L. A. and Messer, A. C. (1932). The
transfer of bicarbonate between the blood
and tissues caused by alteration of the carbon
dioxide concentration in the lungs. *Am. J.
Physiol.* 100, 122—136

Siesjö, B. K. (1971). Quantification of pH
regulation in hypercapnia and hypocapnia
(Editorial). *Scand. J. clin. Lab. Invest.* 28,
113—119

Siesjö, B. K., Folbergrova, J. and MacMillan, V.
(1972). The effect of hypercapnia upon
intracellular pH in the brain, evaluated by
the bicarbonate—carbonic acid method and
from the creatine phosphokinase equilibrium.
J. Neurochem. 19, 2483—2495

Skovsted, P., Price, M. L. and Price, H. L.
(1972). The effects of carbon dioxide on
preganglionic sympathetic activity during
halothane, methoxyflurane and cyclopropane
anesthesia. *Anesthesiology* 37, 70—75

Tenney, S. M. and Lamb, T. W. (1965). Physiological consequences of hypoventilation and
hyperventilation. In *Handbook of Physiology.
Respiration.* Section 1, Vol. 2, Chapter 37,
p. 998. Washington, DC: Am. Physiol. Soc.

Van Ypersele de Strihou, C., Brasseur, L. and
de Coninck, J. (1966). The carbon dioxide
response curve for chronic hypercapnia in
man. *New Engl. J. Med.* 275, 117—122

Weiskopf, R. B., Raymond, L. W. and
Severinghaus, J. W. (1974). Effects of
halothane on canine respiratory responses to
hypoxia with and without hypercarbia.
Anesthesiology 41, 350—360

Woodbury, D. M., Rollins, L. T., Gardner, M. D.,
Hirschi, W. L., Hogan, J. R., Rallison, M. L.,
Tanner, G. S. and Brodie, D. A. (1958).
Effects of carbon dioxide on brain excitability
and electrolytes. *Am. J. Physiol.* 192, 79—90

23 Hypocapnia
J. E. Utting

NORMAL VALUES AND DEFINITIONS

The normal range of arterial blood carbon dioxide tension (Pa_{CO_2}) is 4.8–5.9 kPa (36–44 mmHg); if the Pa_{CO_2} falls below 4.8 kPa (36 mmHg) a state of hypocapnia, hypocarbia or respiratory alkalosis is said to exist. In this chapter hypocapnia will be considered mainly in the context of anaesthesia accompanied by passive pulmonary hyperventilation. The term 'passive' indicates that hyperventilation is caused not by activity of the subject's respiratory muscles but by an external agency, for example by the anaesthetist squeezing the reservoir bag or by the action of a pulmonary ventilator. Passive pulmonary hyperventilation must be contrasted with 'active' pulmonary hyperventilation which is produced by the action of the subject's respiratory muscles. Not only are there mechanical differences between the two, but also it must be noted that active pulmonary hyperventilation involves muscular activity; caution is therefore required in taking data from one situation and applying it to the other. A degree of hypocapnia due to active pulmonary hyperventilation is common when patients are breathing spontaneously in light planes of anaesthesia, especially with diethyl ether. In less restricted terms, hypocapnia due to active pulmonary hyperventilation can be said to be a common biological phenomenon; it is seen, for example, in pregnancy, life at high altitudes and states of anxiety.

There is a tendency to use the term hyperventilation as a synonym for hypocapnia. Hyperventilation can be defined as a pulmonary ventilation in excess of that which would be required to keep the blood carbon dioxide tension within the normal limits under basal conditions. In the spontaneously breathing human volunteer, for example, inhalation of a mixture containing carbon dioxide will cause hyperventilation without hypocapnia, and passive pulmonary hyperventilation with a high carbon dioxide tension in the inspired gas will raise, not lower, the blood carbon dioxide tension.

HYPOCAPNIA IN ANAESTHESIA

Most patients anaesthetized by a technique involving artificial ventilation of the lungs are probably subjected to a degree of hypocapnia. It is often held that the hypocapnia contributes towards producing a fully anaesthetized patient, and is virtually harmless; indeed it has been described as a 'flexible adjunct to anaesthesia'.

The main argument against lowering the blood carbon dioxide tension rests on the possibility that this may cause cerebral hypoxia, since hypocapnia both decreases cerebral blood flow and shifts the oxygen dissociation curve to the left. There is also a reduction in cardiac output with a tendency to arterial hypoxaemia, intense vasoconstriction of some organs (for example, the skin) and an appreciable degree of biochemical disturbance. It has been suggested, too, that there may be difficulties in restarting spontaneous ventilation in patients whose blood carbon dioxide tension has been considerably lowered.

There is, however, no direct clinical evidence that hyperventilation as employed in anaesthetic practice is harmful to the patient. Any anaesthetic technique must be considered an assault on the patient's physiological and biological integrity, and hypocapnia may enable anaesthesia to be conducted with a lesser degree of drug-induced central nervous depression than would otherwise be the case. On the other hand, there is no reason to believe that the greater the degree of hypocapnia the greater will be the degree of central nervous depression produced. This, together with the fact that it is possible that mild degrees of hypocapnia may be innocuous and extreme degrees harmful, would argue against reducing the P_{CO_2} to the lowest level possible.

It must be noted that the state of quietude which is produced by passive pulmonary hyperventilation in patients undergoing surgical operations may not necessarily be due only to hypocapnia. There is evidence that rhythmic ventilation of the lungs may cause inhibition of spontaneous respiration even when the P_{aCO_2} is not allowed to fall (Katz and Wolf, 1964); this inhibition might well lead to a reduced tendency to arousal during surgical anaesthesia. Indeed it can be said that direct evidence suggests that hypocapnia does not increase the depth of anaesthesia, certainly with halothane (Bridges and Eger, 1966): the so-called minimum alveolar concentration (MAC) of that agent is not decreased in hypocapnia.

CENTRAL NERVOUS SYSTEM

In conscious human volunteers, hypocapnia produced either by active or by passive pulmonary hyperventilation is attended by signs of central nervous depression (Kety and Schmidt, 1946; Clutton-Brock, 1957; Robinson and Gray, 1961). Subjects show confusion and a stupid euphoria, which has been likened to mild alcoholic intoxication, and loss of consciousness occasionally occurs: pretibial analgesometry shows that a considerable degree of analgesia develops. Hypocapnia also causes reduction in the cerebral blood flow and a shift of the oxygen dissociation curve to the left. This has led to the view that the cerebral effects of hypocapnia are due to, or at least associated with, a state of cerebral hypoxia. This question will now be considered in some detail. In summary it can be said that profound hypocapnia is associated with a degree of cerebral hypoxaemia and there is little evidence that this occurs unless hypocapnia be extreme. There is little, if any, evidence that the cerebral effects of hypocapnia are *caused* by cerebral hypoxia: other mechanisms such as depression of the reticular system (Bonvallet and Dell, 1956) may be the cause.

Cerebral circulation

Carbon dioxide tension is the main determinant of cerebral vascular resistance and of cerebral blood flow (Chapter 33). An increase in Pa_{CO_2} causes a decrease in cerebral vascular resistance and an increase in blood flow; a decrease in Pa_{CO_2} an increase in cerebral vascular resistance and a decrease in cerebral blood flow. These changes tend to minimize changes in the carbon dioxide tension of the cerebral tissue.

This effect of hypocapnia is due to a direct action on the cerebral blood vessels. It is not caused by the sympathetic nerves, nor by the concomitant change in blood pH — indeed metabolic alkalosis causes slight cerebral vasodilatation not vasoconstriction. It is not caused by a fall in blood pressure for, though this may occur during hyperventilation, the degree is insufficient to account for the observed decreases in cerebral blood flow.

The reduction in cerebral blood flow produced by hypocapnia is considerable: thus a reduction of Pa_{CO_2} from normal to 2.7 kPa (20 mmHg) reduces cerebral blood flow in animals and man by the order of 40%. A reduction from 4 to 2.7 kPa causes a lesser percentage reduction in blood flow than does a reduction from 2.7 to 1.3 kPa, but there is no agreement in the literature as to whether there is a value for Pa_{CO_2} below which no further decrease in cerebral blood flow will take place (Wollman *et al.*, 1968). It has, however, been suggested that when cerebral vasoconstriction due to hypocapnia becomes more marked as the Pa_{CO_2} is progressively lowered, a point is reached at which cerebral hypoxaemia occurs and at this point hypoxaemia prevents any further vasoconstriction.

The Bohr effect

Hypocapnia increases blood pH and shifts the oxygen dissociation curve to the left — the Bohr effect. At normal levels of arterial blood oxygen tension (*c.* 13 kPa; 100 mmHg) there is little difference in the oxygen saturation of blood at different values of P_{CO_2}; the oxygen content of unit volume of blood is nearly the same whether the P_{CO_2} is 5.3 kPa (40 mmHg) or 2.7 kPa (20 mmHg). At a level of Pa_{O_2} corresponding roughly to the oxygen tension in mixed venous blood, however, oxygen saturation is substantially greater when the $P\text{co}_2$ is low. From this it follows that if a given amount of oxygen is extracted from a given volume of blood at $P\text{co}_2$ 2.7 kPa (20 mmHg) the final $P\text{o}_2$ will be less than if the same amount of oxygen is extracted from the same volume of blood at $P\text{co}_2$ 5.3 kPa (40 mmHg). In other words, in hypocapnia the jugular venous $P\text{o}_2$ would be less than it would be in normal conditions if the brain extracted the same amount of oxygen, even in the absence of cerebral vasoconstriction.

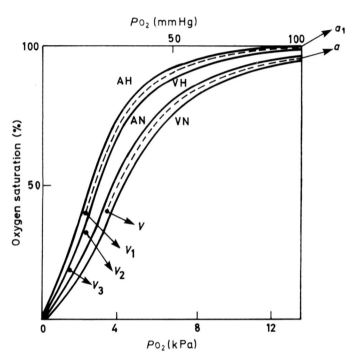

Figure 23.1
AN and VN are the arterial and venous dissociation curves in normo-carbia ($P\text{co}_2$ 5.3 and 6.1 kPa; 40 and 46 mmHg respectively); the functional curve is the dotted line a—v. The corresponding curves in hypocarbia are AH, VH and a_1—v_1, the last constructed on the assumption that about the same amount of O_2 is extracted in hypo-carbia as in normocarbia. If more CO_2 had been extracted from a given volume of blood (as in reduced blood flow), the venous point would move to v_2 or v_3. Note the $P\text{o}_2$ values corresponding to the various venous points (diagrammatic only)

In its passage through the capillary circulation, blood not only gives oxygen to the tissues but receives carbon dioxide from them; not only is the venous $P\text{o}_2$ less than the arterial, but the venous $P\text{co}_2$ is greater than the arterial. These ideas can easily be clarified by inspection of the oxygen dissociation curve in a standard textbook of physiology (or *Figure 23.1*).

Of much less importance to the anaesthetist is the fact that the decrease in hydrogen ion which is associated with hypocapnia results in an increase in the concentration of 2,3-diphosphoglycerate (2,3-DPG) in erythrocytes. This increase is gradual (it assumes importance, for example, on ascent to high altitude) and causes a shift of the oxygen dissociation curve to the right.

Jugular venous Po_2

Assuming that in hypocapnia cerebral oxygen consumption remains the same as in normal conditions, an assumption which, as will be seen later, is at least approximately true, it can be seen that there are two factors causing a reduction in jugular venous oxygen tension. First, cerebral vasoconstriction occurs; this diminishes the cerebral blood flow, and as the same volume of oxygen has to be extracted from a smaller volume of blood the Po_2 after extraction must be diminished. Second, hypocapnia shifts the oxygen dissociation curve to the left and this again would, even in the absence of cerebral vasoconstriction, cause a reduction in venous Po_2 from the level expected in the absence of hypocapnia.

It is possible to separate these two effects in terms of the reduction of jugular venous Po_2 which is found experimentally in hypocapnia. Thus Gotoh, Meyer and Takagi (1965) found that in subjects who reduced their arterial Pco_2 to about 2.7 kPa (20 mmHg) by active pulmonary hyperventilation, some 75% of the observed reduction of jugular venous Po_2 was due to the decreased cerebral blood flow and some 25% to the Bohr effect. Thus cerebral vasoconstriction is by far the more important of the two factors.

Little is known about the importance of the reduction in jugular venous Po_2 which occurs in hypocapnia, especially since cerebral oxygen consumption remains substantially unchanged. Nevertheless, it must mean that the oxygen tension in the environment of at least some of the cells in the brain is lower than it is in normal conditions.

Cerebral metabolism in hypocapnia

Early work (Kety and Schmidt, 1946) suggested that cerebral oxygen consumption remained the same during active pulmonary hyperventilation despite the reduction in cerebral blood flow and the Bohr effect. More recently, however, there has been some evidence of decreased cerebral oxygen consumption, but only in extreme degrees of hypocapnia. Thus Alexander, Smith and Strobel (1968) found a 10% decrease in cerebral oxygen consumption in extreme hypocapnia ($Paco_2$ c. 1.3 kPa; 10 mmHg) in volunteers subjected to passive pulmonary hyperventilation when anaesthetized with nitrous oxide and oxygen (70% and 30% respectively). These workers also found some increase in cerebral venous excess lactate. It was suggested that increased glucose uptake by the brain was due to anaerobic metabolism, and that despite this increase there was a net decrease in cerebral energy production of some 10%. More recently it has been found that the cerebral energy metabolism of rats is reduced substantially in extreme hypocapnia (Krgure *et al.*, 1975).

The EEG during hypocapnia

Hypocapnia causes the appearance of slow wave (delta rhythm) activity in the EEG (Gotoh, Meyer and Takagi, 1965; Stoddart, 1967). This change has been attributed both to cerebral hypocapnia *per se* and to cerebral hypoxaemia. In support of the latter hypothesis, it has been suggested that the appearance of slow wave activity during hypocapnia is correlated primarily with the reduction of jugular venous P_{O_2} and not with the reduction of P_{CO_2}. Interpretation of EEG changes, however, is notoriously difficult and much further work is needed before conclusive proof of either hypothesis can be established.

Tests of cerebral function after hypocapnia

If hypocapnia results in cerebral hypoxaemia, it might be expected that there would be some objective evidence of cerebral dysfunction after conditions have returned to normal. It is important to bear in mind that in anaesthetic practice passive pulmonary hyperventilation with a considerable degree of hypocapnia is a frequently used technique and is applied to patients of all ages. When light anaesthesia is used with hypocapnia, return of consciousness is prompt after the anaesthetic is discontinued, and this argues strongly against there having been any serious degree of cerebral hypoxaemia during the period of hypocapnia. Nevertheless, this argument is far from conclusive.

The critical flicker fusion test has been used in an attempt to obtain objective evidence of brain damage. The performance of this test is complicated, but the basic principle on which it depends is relatively simple. Flashes of light are perceived as discrete at slow frequencies. If the frequency of the flashes is increased, however, a stage is reached at which the light appears to the observer to be continuous, a phenomenon due to visual persistence. In some states of cerebral dysfunction (for example, in head injury) fusion is obtained at a decreased frequency compared with normal, and it is on this basis that critical flicker fusion has been used as a test of cerebral function. The method was improved and its sensitivity increased by using hexobarbitone. A small (subanaesthetic) dose of this does not decrease the critical value for flicker fusion in normal subjects, but in states of diffuse cerebral injury the critical flicker fusion rate may only be reduced after hexobarbitone has been administered.

Unfortunately, there is much about the critical flicker fusion test which is controversial and it is not universally accepted as a valid and accurate test for brain damage. An early report that there was a change in critical flicker fusion indicating slight brain damage in subjects after periods of hypocapnia (Allen and Morris, 1962) has been contradicted (Whitwam *et al.*, 1966).

CARDIOVASCULAR SYSTEM

The isolated heart

In the isolated heart, hypercapnia appears to diminish both the force and the rate of cardiac contraction. The effect of hypocapnia in these circumstances is less well documented but the evidence suggests that there is an increase in the force of cardiac contraction or no effect at all. In the isolated heart it seems probable that it is hydrogen ion concentration rather than carbon dioxide tension which is the important variable (Price, 1960).

Cardiac output in the intact subject

There is evidence that cardiac output increases during active hyperventilation in normal subjects, and this increase is associated with an increase in pulse rate. These changes are small or absent when hyperventilation is accompanied by the inhalation of 5% carbon dioxide (Burnum, Hickman and McIntosh, 1954).

Of more interest to the anaesthetist is the fact that hypocapnia induced by passive pulmonary hyperventilation in the anaesthetized patient causes a reduction in cardiac output (Theye, Milde and Michenfelder, 1966; Prys-Roberts *et al.*, 1967). This reduction is considerable, being in the order of 30% of the value obtained in normocarbia when the $P_{a_{CO_2}}$ is reduced to 2.7 kPa (20 mmHg). It is caused primarily by the reduction in the blood carbon dioxide tension itself, and not by an associated increase in intrathoracic pressure.

The mechanism of this reduction has not, as yet, been fully elucidated. There is no evidence that it is a response to decreased metabolic demand, for oxygen consumption in states of hypocapnia due to passive pulmonary hyperventilation does not decline. Hypocapnia, as has been indicated, does not reduce the force of contraction of the isolated heart, though it has been suggested that there may be myocardial depression in the intact subject. Prys-Roberts *et al.* (1967), however, found a decreased right atrial filling pressure during hypocapnia whereas it would be expected that, if decreased cardiac output were caused by myocardial depression, the right atrial filling pressure would be high.

Later work (Foëx and Prys-Roberts, 1975a,b) gave further evidence that myocardial contractility does not decrease in hypocapnia. The decrease in stroke volume may well be due to the increase in systemic vascular resistance which is associated with the decrease in carbon dioxide tension.

Cardiac rhythm and blood pressure

When hypocapnia is produced by passive pulmonary hyperventilation in lightly anaesthetized patients there is little tendency for cardiac arrhythmias to occur and the pulse rate remains much the same as in resting conditions. Mean arterial blood pressure declines somewhat, though this change is less remarkable than might be suggested by the decline in cardiac output because total peripheral resistance rises, as has been stated. It must, however, be emphasized that, under conditions in the operating theatre, surgical stimulation can cause reflex effects under light anaesthesia which may modify this pattern (by causing, for example, a rise in mean arterial pressure).

There is, however, evidence from the dog (Marshall *et al.*, 1976) which suggests that there is a decreased myocardial blood flow — a decrease associated with an increase in myocardial vascular resistance.

Peripheral circulation

Carbon dioxide has a dual effect on the peripheral circulation. Its direct action on vessels is usually to cause vasodilatation, but it also influences the calibre of the peripheral vessels by an action on the central nervous system. This central action is opposite in effect to the peripheral; carbon dioxide stimulates the vasomotor centre, causes an increased sympathetic discharge to the peripheral vessels, and thus tends to cause peripheral vasoconstriction. It is a useful, but not a completely valid, generalization to state that hypocapnia tends to cause peripheral vasoconstriction by a direct action on the vessels, and peripheral vasodilatation centrally by diminishing sympathetic activity. In these circumstances it is clearly even more dangerous than usual to transfer data obtained from the experimental subject to the human being; and as most of the peripheral circulation in the human is difficult to investigate, it is not surprising that knowledge of this subject is incomplete.

In the lightly anaesthetized human subject the total peripheral resistance increases during hypocapnia, in other words the sum effect on all the arterioles in the circulation is a decrease in calibre. Of the individual organs the brain has been considered already; that there is vasoconstriction in this organ might be expected since there is a relative paucity of sympathetic filaments supplying the cerebral vessels.

Blood flow through the forearm has been investigated in some detail, but the results are somewhat confusing. During hypocapnia there is an increase in blood flow through the limb; this increase is due to vasodilatation in the muscle, and is accompanied by cutaneous vasoconstriction. The vasodilatatioh of the muscle vessels is even greater when the nerves to the limb are blocked (a procedure which does not affect the cutaneous vasoconstriction) and is reduced but not abolished by the injection of a β-blocking agent (Brick, Hutchison and Roddie, 1966). This has led to the suggestion that vasodilatation in muscle vessels in the forearm may be due, in part at least, to a circulating adrenaline-like substance. This is a surprising finding since it is known that sympathetic activity and circulating plasma catecholamine concentrations are increased in conditions of carbon dioxide excess, and it would seem generally in accordance with the facts that the opposite is the case in hypocapnia and that in this state there is depression of the sympatheticoadrenal system.

Pulmonary circulation

The direct action of carbon dioxide on the vessels of the pulmonary circulation would seem to be the opposite to that which has been found in the systemic, and may be the basis of an important mechanism in the local regulation of pulmonary blood flow. Carbon dioxide excess in the fluid perfusing isolated lungs has been found usually to cause pulmonary vasoconstriction (Price, 1960). This would have the effect of diverting blood from poorly ventilated lung (where the local carbon dioxide tension will be high) to areas which are better ventilated (Chapter 24).

Alveolar–arterial oxygen tension differences

It is known that in normal physiological conditions there is a small difference between the oxygen tension in the alveoli and that in the arterial blood. This alveolar–arterial difference in oxygen tension, (A–a) Po_2 difference, is caused by the venous admixture effect: the mixture of arterial blood (which has fully exchanged in the lungs) with blood which has passed directly from the right to the left side of the circulation (for example, through a minute area of atelectatic lung), or which has been only partly arterialized because it has passed through an area of lung which is poorly perfused.

Alveolar–arterial oxygen tension differences are greater under anaesthesia than under ordinary physiological conditions, and they appear to increase when the blood carbon dioxide tension is reduced. It has been suggested that hypocapnia causes an increase in pulmonary shunting (Michenfelder, Fowler and Theye, 1966) and this may well be the case. Kelman *et al.* (1967), however, have emphasized the importance of the decrease in cardiac output which accompanies hypocapnia, and have suggested that there may be no need to invoke an increase in pulmonary shunting to explain the increase in alveolar–arterial oxygen tension differences. If the cardiac output goes down and oxygen consumption remains the same, mixed venous blood will have a lower oxygen content than before, since the same volume of oxygen has to be extracted by the tissues from a smaller volume of blood. Even in the presence of a shunt which forms a fixed proportion of the cardiac output, arterial oxygen tension will decline if the cardiac output declines because the shunted blood will be more desaturated. In fact in hypocapnia oxygen consumption increases.

Hyperventilation increases the alveolar oxygen tension since

$$Pa_{O_2} = Pi_{O_2} - \frac{Pa_{CO_2}}{R}$$

(where R is the respiratory exchange ratio). Thus a decrease in alveolar carbon dioxide tension will cause an increase in alveolar oxygen tension. It is not necessarily correct to assume, however, that this increase in the alveolar oxygen tension is associated with an increase in the arterial blood oxygen tension since hypocapnia is associated with an increased alveolar—arterial oxygen tension difference.

RESPIRATORY SYSTEM

Chemoreceptors

The carotid and aortic chemoreceptors react to changes both in PaO_2 and $PaCO_2$, but their response to the latter is much less than to the former. These peripheral chemoreceptors are responsible for the increased respiratory activity in response to hypoxaemia but are of quite secondary importance in respect of changes in the arterial blood carbon dioxide tension. There are, however, chemoreceptors in the central nervous system which are probably very closely associated with the respiratory neurons but separate from them, and situated on the ventral surface of the brain stem, and these are extremely sensitive to changes in $PaCO_2$; for example an increase of $PaCO_2$ of only 0.27—0.4 kPa (2—3 mmHg) will lead to a doubling of the alveolar ventilation through stimulation of these receptors. Hypocapnia, on the other hand, causes decreased activity of the respiratory neurons and respiratory depression.

The central chemoreceptors really monitor the hydrogen ion concentration of the cerebrospinal fluid (or possibly the interstitial fluid of the brain). Carbon dioxide readily passes through biological membranes (including those of the so-called blood—brain barrier), whereas hydrogen and bicarbonate ions do not. Thus an increase in $PaCO_2$ will be associated with an increased PCO_2 in the cerebrospinal fluid, and consequently an increase in H^+ there, whilst hypocapnia will cause the reverse. Changes in the concentration of bicarbonate ion in the cerebrospinal fluid are small in the short term (Paddle and Semple, 1969) but are important in such physiological conditions as acclimatization to high altitude.

Posthyperventilation apnoea

There is no doubt that animals subjected to hypocapnia may show periods of apnoea when hyperventilation ceases, and this apnoea may, indeed, be fatal. Opinions, however, differ whether or not there is normally a period of apnoea in the conscious subject following a period of active or passive pulmonary hyperventilation (Bainton and Mitchell, 1966). The results obtained depend largely on the experimental conditions employed; it is, for example, almost useless to employ an experimental subject who is aware of the purpose of the experiment.

Hypocapnia diminishes not only the blood carbon dioxide content but the carbon dioxide content of all the body tissues — the body's stores of carbon dioxide are depleted. After a period of hypocapnia, therefore, there must be a period of hypoventilation during which the carbon dioxide stores increase to their normal level. Hyperventilation does little to increase the body's stores of oxygen and, for this reason, during the period of hypoventilation there is a risk of arterial hypoxaemia if the subject is breathing air. This problem has been investigated by Sullivan, Patterson and Papper (1966): working with dogs they found that there was a period of hypoxaemia lasting for up to one hour after a period of passive pulmonary hyperventilation of an hour's duration. There is, however, little evidence that this occurs in the human after anaesthesia; probably here the blood carbon dioxide tension returns to near normal levels quite rapidly. Nevertheless, the possibility of hypoventilation after hypocapnia is of importance since it represents a further reason for considering the administration of oxygen in the immediate postoperative period if passive pulmonary hyperventilation has been employed.

Inflation and deflation receptors

It is important to distinguish the effects of hypocapnia from the effects of the mechanism by which the state of hypocapnia is produced. Thus it is necessary to consider the effects of rhythmic inflation of the lung on respiratory behaviour.

There are a number of receptors in the lung which feed back to the central nervous system information about the degree of inflation of the lung itself, and modify respiratory activity by so doing. Hering and Breuer showed over 100 years ago that inflation of the lungs inhibits inspiration and deflation inhibits expiration. It must, however, be noted that the Hering–Breuer reflex is relatively unimportant in man (Widdicombe, 1961).

The precise role of the pulmonary stretch and deflation receptors in intermittent positive pressure and intermittent positive–negative pressure respiration in the human subject has not been completely elucidated. Intermittent positive pressure respiration in the animal, however, has been found to lead to an inhibition of inspiratory activity which is not necessarily due to changes in blood pH and $P\text{CO}_2$. In the cat subjected to positive pressure ventilation, for example, the respiratory neuronal activity typically synchronized with the ventilator in two respiratory cycles; this, it was thought, was too rapid for there to have been any significant changes in the arterial blood gases (Robson, 1967). Inhibition of respiratory activity due to rhythmic inflation of the lungs has also been demonstrated in anaesthetized human patients (Katz and Wolf, 1964).

The initiation of spontaneous ventilation after hypocapnia

It has often been held that if hypocapnia is induced during anaesthesia, difficulty may be experienced in restarting spontaneous ventilation. It has been found, however, that if anaesthesia is maintained with nitrous oxide alone and no opiate premedication is given, spontaneous ventilation will recommence at a blood carbon dioxide tension considerably below normal when the neuromuscular block is reversed (Utting and Gray, 1962).

The problem is obviously a complex one. The volatile and gaseous anaesthetic agents (with the exception of nitrous oxide) all raise the apnoeic point, that is, they produce a situation in which spontaneous respiration will be resumed only at a higher Pa_{CO_2} than would be the case in their absence and the powerful narcotic drugs behave in a similar way (Ngai, 1967). On the other hand, a vast majority of afferent impulses tend to stimulate respiration even when the Pa_{CO_2} is low; surgical stimulation and the presence of an endotracheal tube are two examples familiar to the anaesthetist. In some circumstances, moreover, spontaneous ventilation will recommence at a lower level of blood carbon dioxide tension when the patient is awake than when he is asleep (Fink, 1961).

BIOCHEMICAL CHANGES

Oxygen uptake

Oxygen uptake (V_{O_2}) increases during hypocapnia, and this increase is not due only to an increase in the work due to the respiratory muscles (Karetzky and Cain, 1970). This increase might, it has been suggested, be of some importance in the presence of a shunt since the oxygen content of the shunted (mixed venous) blood would be decreased (Khambatta and Sullivan, 1973).

Plasma electrolytes

There is a decrease of both the plasma sodium and the plasma potassium during passive pulmonary hyperventilation. A decrease in plasma sodium of 5 mmol·l^{-1} would be not unusual, and a decrease of plasma potassium of the order of 0.5 mmol·l^{-1} for each 1.3 kPa (10 mmHg) decrease in Pa_{CO_2}.

It has been suggested that this decrease in plasma potassium may, in some circumstances, be of clinical importance in producing cardiac arrhythmias (Edwards, Winnie and Ramamurthy, 1977).

The cause of these changes is probably a movement of ions in and out of cells.

Changes in plasma chloride have been less well documented, though it seems probable that there is an increase in the plasma concentration of this ion during hypocapnia. This is what would be expected in terms of the chloride shift, since hypocapnia will decrease the 'actual bicarbonate' present in the plasma; this, in turn, will decrease the tendency for bicarbonate to enter cells and so exchange with chloride in so doing.

The effect of hypocapnia on serum calcium is dealt with below when tetany is considered.

Haematocrit and plasma water

Passive pulmonary hyperventilation leads to an increase in the haematocrit reading and to a decrease in plasma water (Robinson, 1961). The increased haematocrit cannot, however, be explained merely by a loss of water from the plasma; there must be an addition of red cells. The source of these added red cells and the mechanism of their addition to the circulating blood volume is not known.

TETANY

Passive pulmonary hyperventilation is not usually associated with signs of tetany: indeed tetany may be regarded as rare in anaesthetized patients and uncommon in conscious volunteers in whom hypocapnia is induced in this way. Nevertheless, in active pulmonary hyperventilation, both in volunteers and in patients, something resembling tetany occurs frequently.

It is not always true that the carpal spasm seen in active hyperventilation is due to tetany in the generally accepted sense, since it may occur in the absence of other signs of tetany (for example, Chvostek's sign may be negative).

True tetany is due to a decrease in the plasma-ionized calcium which causes an increase in neuromuscular excitability. Plasma calcium in actively hyperventilating volunteers has been investigated by Fanconi and Rose (1958). In hypocapnia induced in this way there is a slight rise in total plasma calcium, but a fall in plasma-ionized calcium.

It has been pointed out, however, that the concentration of ionized calcium in even severe hypocapnia is unlikely to be low enough to produce tetany (Tenney and Lamb, 1964). Probably true tetany is uncommon in hypocapnia.

METABOLIC ACIDOSIS

It has frequently been suggested that during hypocapnia there is a degree of tissue hypoxia. From this it is a reasonable step to suggest that any metabolic acidosis associated with hyperventilation might be due to anaerobic respiration of tissues which would result in an accumulation of lactic acid due to the incomplete combustion of carbohydrate material. A slight increase in blood lactic acid concentration in human volunteers who were actively hyperventilating was, indeed, demonstrated by Bock, Dill and Edwards (1932). Papadopoulos and Keats (1959) found some degree of metabolic acidosis in patients subjected to passive pulmonary hyperventilation but, though this was associated with an increase in blood lactic acid concentrations, the increase was insufficient to account for all of the metabolic acidosis.

Later work has tended to confirm that there is a small degree of metabolic acidosis during passive pulmonary hyperventilation and a slight increase in blood lactic acid concentration, an increase which is insufficient to account for the degree of metabolic acidosis which is found. On the other hand, Prys-Roberts, Kelman and Nunn (1966) did not find any evidence of metabolic acidosis or increase in blood lactate in lightly anaesthetized patients subjected to a short period of passive pulmonary hyperventilation with nitrous oxide anaesthesia (30% oxygen) and full muscle relaxation.

Any increase in blood lactic acid concentration, however, is not necessarily due to tissue hypoxia; an alternative source of lactic acid in a patient subjected to hypocapnia has been suggested by Danuta, Zborowska-Sluis and Dossetor (1967), who found that the increased blood lactic acid concentration associated with hyperventilation resulted, not from tissue hypoxia, but from stimulation of glycolysis in the red cells.

There is no evidence that fixed acids other than lactic acid (keto acids, phosphates, sulphates and so on) accumulate during hyperventilation. An increased renal excretion of bicarbonate is found as a compensatory response to long-term hypocapnia such as in life at high altitude, but in acute experiments there can hardly be sufficient time for a compensatory renal excretion of bicarbonate to take place to any great extent. Renal responses to hypocapnia, however, are quite complicated (Tenney and Lamb, 1964).

The concentration of blood lactic acid is not an accurate index of cellular hypoxia and it has been suggested (Huckabee, 1958) that 'excess lactate' is more reliable in this respect. Excess lactate has been studied in hypocapnia (Sykes and Cooke, 1965; Chamberlain and Lis, 1968) but, unfortunately, conflicting results have been obtained.

Cohen, Brackett and Schwartz (1964) detected small but appreciable differences in the behaviour of blood *in vitro* and *in vivo* during active hyperventilation. Prys-Roberts, Kelman and Nunn (1966), working with passively ventilated anaesthetized patients, are in agreement with the direction but not the magnitude of this change. Thus standard bicarbonate and base excess determined by interpolation *in vitro* may not give an absolutely accurate determination of conditions *in vivo* and the latter workers have, in fact, given a formula for correcting for this. It must, however, be emphasized most strongly that the difference between the behaviour of blood *in vivo* and *in vitro* is very small and in clinical circumstances it is safe to ignore it.

References

Alexander, S. C., Smith, T. C. and Strobel, G. (1968). Cerebral carbohydrate metabolism of man during respiratory and metabolic alkalosis. *J. appl. Physiol.* 24, 66–72

Allen, G. D. and Morris, L. E. (1962). Central nervous system effects of hyperventilation during anaesthesia. *Br. J. Anaesth.* 34, 296–304

Bainton, C. R. and Mitchell, R. A. (1966). Post-hyperventilation apnea in awake man. *J. appl. Physiol.* 21, 411–415

Bock, A. V., Dill, B. B. and Edwards, M. T. (1932). Lactid acid in the blood of resting man. *J. clin. Invest.* 11, 775–788

Bonvallet, T. M. and Dell, P. (1956). Proceedings of the Société d'electroencephlograph et des sciences connexes de langue Français. *Electroenceph. clin. Neurophysiol.* 8, 170–175

Brick, I., Hutchinson, K. J. and Roddie, I. C. (1966). The effect of beta adrenergic receptor blockade on the vasodilator response in the forearm of voluntary hyperventilation. *J. Physiol.* 187, 645–649

Bridges, B. E. and Eger, E. I. II (1966). The effect of hypocapnia on the level of halothane anesthesia in man. *Anesthesiology* 27(5), 634–637

Burnum, J. F., Hickman, J. B. and McIntosh, M. (1954). Effect of hypocapnia on arterial blood pressure. *Circulation* 9, 89–95

Chamberlain, J. H. and Lis, M. T. (1968). Observations of blood lactate and pyruvate levels and excess lactate production during and after anaesthesia with and without hyperventilation. *Br. J. Anaesth.* 40, 315–322

Clutton-Brock, J. (1957). The cerebral effects of over-ventilation. *Br. J. Anaesth.* 29, 111–115

Cohen, J. J., Brackett, N. C. and Schwartz, W. B. (1964). The nature of the carbon dioxide titration curve in the normal dog. *J. clin. Invest.* 43, 777–786

Danuta, T., Zborowska-Sluis, H. B. and Dossetor, J. B. (1967). Hyperlactatemia of hyperventilation. *J. appl. Physiol.* 22, 746–755

Edwards, R., Winnie, A. P. and Ramamurthy, S. (1977). Acute hypocapnic hypokalemia: An iatrogenic anesthetic complication. *Anesth. Analg., Cleve.* 56(6), 786–792

Fanconi, A. and Rose, G. A. (1958). The ionised, complexed and protein bound fractions of calcium in plasma. *Q. med. Rev.* 27, 463–494

Fink, B. R. (1961). The stimulant effect of wakefulness on respiration: Clinical aspects. *Br. J. Anaesth.* 33, 97–101

Foëx, P. and Prys-Roberts, C. (1975a). Effect of CO_2 myocardial centractility and aortic input impedance during anaesthesia. *Br. J. Anaesth.* 46(6), 669–678

Foëx, P. and Prys-Roberts, C. (1975b). Effects of changes in $Paco_2$ on pulmonary input impedance. *J. appl. Physiol.* 38(1), 156–162

Gotoh, F., Meyer, J. S. and Takagi, Y. (1965). Cerebral effects of hyperventilation in man. *Archs Neurol., Chicago* 12, 410–423

Huckabee, W. E. (1958). Relationship of pyruvate and lactate during anaerobic metabolism: Effects of infusion of pyruvate or glucose and of hyperventilation. *J. clin. Invest.* 37, 244–254

Karetzky, M. S. and Cain, S. M. (1970). Effect of carbon dioxide on oxygen uptake during hyperventilation in normal man. *J. appl. Physiol.* 28, 8–12

Katz, R. L. and Wolf, C. E. (1964). Neuromuscular and electromyographic studies in man: effects of hyperventilation, carbon dioxide inhalation and d-tubocurarine. *Anesthesiology* 25, 781–787

Kelman, G. R., Nunn, J. F., Prys-Roberts, C. and Greenbaum, R. (1967). The influence of cardiac output on arterial oxygenation: A theoretical study. *Br. J. Anaesth.* 39, 450–457

Kety, S. and Schmidt, C. F. (1946). The effects of active and passive hyperventilation on cerebral blood flow, cerebral oxygen consumption, cardiac output and blood pressure of normal man. *J. clin. Invest.* 25, 107–119

Khambatta, H. J. and Sullivan, S. F. (1973). Effects of respiratory alkalosis on oxygen consumption and oxygenation. *Anesthesiology* 38, 53–58

Krgure, K., Busto, R., Matsumoto, A., Scheinberg, P. and Reinmuth, O. M. (1975). Effect of hyperventilation on dynamics of cerebral energy metabolism. *Am. J. Physiol.* 228(6), 1862–1867

Marshall, M., Williams, W. G., Creighton, R. E., Volgyesi, G. A. and Steward, D. J. (1976). A technique for measuring regional myocardial blood flow and its application in determining the effects of hyperventilation and halothane. *Can. Anaesth. Soc. J.* 23(3), 244–251

Michenfelder, J. D., Fowler, W. S. and Theye, R. A. (1966). CO_2 levels and pulmonary shunting in anaesthetised man. *J. appl. Physiol.* 21, 1471–1476

Ngai, S. H. (1967). The pharmacological aspect of control of respiration. *Modern Trends in Anaesthesia – 3.* F. T. Evans and T. C. Gray (ed.). London: Butterworths

Paddle, J. S. and Semple, S. J. (1969). Changes in the bicarbonate concentration of lumbar and cisternal cerebrospinal fluid in man following acute hypocapnia and hypercapnia. *Br. J. Anaesth.* 41(10), 821–826

Papadopoulous, C. N. and Keats, A. S. (1959). The metabolic acidosis of hyperventilation produced by controlled respiration. *Anesthesiology* 20, 156–161

Price, H. L. (1960). Effects of carbon dioxide on the cardiovascular system. *Anesthesiology* 21, 652–663

Prys-Roberts, C., Kelman, G. R. and Nunn, J. F. (1966). Determination of the *in vivo* carbon dioxide titration curve of anaesthetised man. *Br. J. Anaesth.* 38, 500–509

Prys-Roberts, C., Kelman, G. R., Greenbaum, R. and Robinson, R. (1967). Circulatory influences of artificial ventilation during nitrous oxide anaesthesia in man. II: Results: the relative influence of mean intrathoracic pressure and arterial carbon dioxide tension. *Br. J. Anaesth.* 39, 533–547

Robinson, J. S. (1961). Some biochemical effects of passive hyperventilation. *Br. J. Anaesth.* 33, 69–76

Robinson, J. S. and Gray, T. C. (1961). Observations on the cerebral effects of passive hyperventilation. *Br. J. Anaesth.* 33, 62–68

Robson, J. G. (1967). The respiratory centres and their responses. In *Modern Trends in Anaesthesia* – 3. F. T. Evans and T. C. Gray (ed.). London: Butterworths

Stoddart, J. C. (1967). Electroencephalogram activity during voluntarily controlled alveolar hyperventilation. *Br. J. Anaesth.* 39, 2–10

Sullivan, S. F., Patterson, R. W. and Papper, E. M. (1966). Arterial CO_2 tension adjustment rates following hyperventilation. *J. appl. Physiol.* 21, 247–250

Sykes, M. K. and Cooke, P. M. (1965). The effects of hyperventilation on excess lactate production during anaesthesia. *Anesthesiology* 27, 778–782

Tenney, Y. S. M. and Lamb, T. W. (1964). Physiological consequences of hypoventilation and hyperventilation. *Handbook of Physiology*, Section 3: *Respiration*, Chapter 37, pp. 979–1010. Washington DC: Am. Physiol. Soc.

Theye, R. A., Milde, J. M. and Michenfelder, J. D. (1966). Effects of hypocapnia on cardiac output during anesthesia. *Anesthesiology* 27, 778–782

Utting, J. E. and Gray, T. C. (1962). The initiation of respiration after anaesthesia accompanied by passive pulmonary hyperventilation. *Br. J. Anaesth.* 34, 785–789

Whitwam, J. G., Boettner, R. B., Gilger, A. P. and Littel, A. S. (1966). Hyperventilation, brain damage and flicker. *Br. J. Anaesth.* 38, 846–852

Widdicombe, J. G. (1961). Respiratory reflexes in man and other mammalian species. *Clin. Sci.* 21, 163–170

Wollman, H., Smith, T. C., Stephen, G. W., Colton, E. T., Gleaton, H. E. and Alexander, S. G. (1968). Effects of extremes of respiratory and metabolic alkalosis on cerebral flow of man. *J. appl. Physiol.* 24, 60–65

24 Pulmonary circulation in relation to anaesthesia and pulmonary oedema
Norman A. Bergman

Pressure in the pulmonary artery is approximately one-sixth that in the aorta. Normal pulmonary artery pressures are about 2.6–4.0 kPa (20–30 mmHg) systolic and 0.9–1.6 kPa (7–12 mmHg) diastolic with a mean pressure of about 1.6–2.0 kPa (12–15 mmHg). Mean pressure in the left atrium is normally about 0.5–0.7 kPa (4–5 mmHg). In modern anaesthetic practice left atrial pressure is usually measured from a catheter 'wedged' in a pulmonary artery. Flow stops in that artery. The recorded pressure is that in the first distal communicating vessel and is considered to be a close estimate of mean left atrial pressure. Blood sampled through a wedge catheter cannot be regarded as representative of pulmonary venous blood because it has made two transits past alveoli. Mean pulmonary capillary pressure must be intermediate between that of pulmonary artery and left atrium, that is about 1.3 kPa (10 mmHg). Calculation of pulmonary vascular resistance requires simultaneous measurement of pulmonary blood flow (cardiac output) and pressure gradient across the pulmonary circuit (both pulmonary artery and left atrial pressures). Several peculiarities of the pulmonary circulation complicate interpretation of pulmonary haemodynamic measurements. Changes in pulmonary vascular resistance can be produced either actively, by vasomotion, or passively, by vascular distension. Thus caution must be exercised lest direct vasoactive properties be attributed to a drug which produced a pulmonary haemodynamic change by some indirect means. An example of this situation might be an agent which stimulates depth of respiration decreasing pleural pressure and passively distending the pulmonary circuit. Also, since the pressure gradient from pulmonary artery to left atrium is normally about 1.3 kPa (10 mmHg) significant changes in pulmonary vascular resistance can be associated with pressure changes of only 0.4–0.5 kPa (3–4 mmHg). Much information concerning the pulmonary circulation has become available in recent years.

VASOMOTION IN THE PULMONARY CIRCULATION

The pulmonary circulation is capable of changing its vasomotor tone in response to a variety of stimuli. Confusion regarding the response of the pulmonary circuit in many situations is being resolved by use of more sophisticated techniques in intact animals as well as studies using isolated perfused lungs, innervated perfused lungs, and muscle from pulmonary vessels (Bergofsky, 1974; Barer, 1976; Fishman, 1976a).

Under usual physiological conditions pulmonary vasculature probably has slight resting tone which may be maintained by locally elaborated neurohormones or other humoral agents. Administration of α-adrenergic blocking drugs in this circumstance causes a slight reduction in resting vascular tone and pulmonary vascular resistance. Adrenergic and cholinergic autonomic mechanisms are represented in the lung circulation. At present, the function of the cholinergic mechanism is not apparent. The adrenergic mechanism, however, is prominent in control of pulmonary vascular tone. Both α- and β-adrenergic receptors are present; α-receptors predominate both numerically and functionally.

Response to humoral agents and drugs

The complex systemic effects of many vasoactive substances sometimes obscure their action on the pulmonary circulation. Such direct pulmonary circulatory actions are frequently best observed in special isolated experimental preparations mentioned above. Adrenaline causes pulmonary vascular dilatation in small doses but vasoconstriction with larger doses. This dose-dependent phenomenon might be explained by a greater affinity of β-adrenergic receptors for adrenaline but with numerical and functional preponderance of α-receptors becoming evident at higher dosage levels. When adrenaline is given following prior administration of the α-adrenergic blocking drug phenoxybenzamine (Dibenzyline), vasodilatation occurs at dosages normally producing constriction in the unblocked preparation. Following β-adrenergic blockade with propranalol, the vasoconstrictor response to adrenaline is exaggerated. Noradrenaline causes pulmonary vasoconstruction. α-Adrenergic blockade reduces or abolishes this action but vasodilatation does not occur in the α-blocked preparation in response to noradrenaline. Isoprenaline (isoproterenol) causes a modest but significant pulmonary vasodilatation. Histamine is a potent pulmonary vasoconstrictor. Vascular effects of histamine in the lung can be modulated by autonomic blockade. α-Adrenergic blockade greatly attenuates histamine vasoconstriction while with β-adrenergic blockade the effect is markedly enhanced. It has been suggested that histamine might in some way utilize the α- and β-adrenergic mechanism for its vascular actions (Porcelli *et al.*, 1977). Serotonin (5-hydroxytryptamine) is another pulmonary vasoconstrictor. Constriction due to serotonin is enhanced by isoflurane, fluroxene, and nitrous oxide in isolated pulmonary artery strips (Benumof, Eurman and Wahrenbrock, 1977). Unlike histamine, the action of serotonin is uninfluenced by autonomic blockade. Angiotensin II, an octapeptide generated in the lung from angiotensin I, also acts as a vasoconstrictor in the pulmonary circuit. This action can be modulated by autonomic blockade in a manner qualitatively similar to but quantitatively less intense than that for histamine.

Prostaglandins E_1 and E_2 produce pulmonary vasodilatation. Other important pharmacological effects of these particular substances include peripheral circulatory dilatation and bronchodilatation. Prostaglandin $F_2\alpha$ is a pulmonary vasoconstrictor and also causes peripheral constriction and bronchoconstriction. Acetylcholine, when infused into the pulmonary artery, produces pulmonary vasodilatation. The effect is most pronounced in subjects with pulmonary hypertension such as may occur in mitral stenosis. Other drugs possessing pulmonary vasoconstrictor properties include phenylephrine and metaraminol. Aminophylline is a pulmonary vasodilator. As with acetylcholine, its vasodilating properties are most apparent when initial vascular tone is high.

HYPOXIC PULMONARY VASOCONSTRICTION AND RESPONSE TO HYPERCARBIA AND ACIDAEMIA

Hypoxia represents the most potent and, physiologically, probably the most important stimulus to pulmonary vasoconstriction described to date. This response of the pulmonary circulation to low oxygen tension is opposite to that of the systemic circulation where hypoxia causes vasodilatation. Acidaemia of both respiratory and metabolic origin also causes pulmonary vasoconstriction. The stimulus with acidaemia is probably hydrogen ion and not molecular carbon dioxide. Hypoxia and acidaemia act synergistically to influence the pulmonary circulation though the particular vascular segments upon which they act may differ. Alkalaemia causes pulmonary vasodilatation and blunts hypoxic pulmonary vasoconstriction (HPV).

The pressor response to hypoxia appears to involve two distinct mechanisms. The first of these is reflexly mediated by the autonomic nervous system with predominant site of action on large pulmonary arteries. The stimulus for the reflex is low arterial oxygen tension and receptors involved are the peripheral chemoreceptors (carotid bodies). Central connections occur in the hypothalamic area. Efferent stimuli travelling via sympathetic pathways act on large pulmonary arteries to alter physical properties of their walls, making them stiffer rather than to produce marked vasoconstriction. The second mechanism involved in hypoxic pulmonary vasoconstriction (HPV) operates locally so that the denervated lung still exhibits a marked pressor response to hypoxia. HPV occurs in small pulmonary vessels as a consequence of direct exposure to low oxygen tension. This occurs primarily in pulmonary arterioles of about 200 μm in size. These vessels are anatomically advantageously situated with relation to alveoli to permit detection of alveolar hypoxia. Low oxygen tension in alveoli is the usual stimulus to HPV but in extreme conditions very low mixed venous oxygen tension is an additional stimulus. Although some constriction of veins may occur with hypoxia, the predominant site of HPV appears to be on the arterial side of the pulmonary capillary.

The mechanism whereby small pulmonary vessels constrict in response to hypoxia remains obscure. It is postulated that a chemical mediator originating in the lung might be involved. There are a number of observations suggesting that release of histamine stored in mast cells in proximity to pulmonary arterioles might be the primary mechanism for HPV. There are, however, other observations which cannot be explained by invoking histamine as a mediator. Other arguments exist for assigning at least some role to other vasoactive substances present in the lung. Mediators transported to the lung from extrapulmonary sites might also be involved. Even if these do not directly trigger the pressor response to hypoxia, they may contribute to maintenance of basic vascular tone upon which HPV is superimposed. Innervated cellular structures have been identified in pulmonary epithelium of animals. These have been designated 'neuroepithelial bodies' and it has been postulated that they are neuro-receptor organs involved in detecting and responding to hypoxia (Lauweryns, Cokelaere and Theunynck, 1973). Events occurring in pulmonary arteriolar smooth muscle are also being examined for a possible role in triggering the pressor response to hypoxia. In pulmonary vasculature, hypoxia appears to stimulate metabolic activity and accelerate production of ATP. In other systemic vascular beds the action of hypoxia on metabolism is depressant. Low oxygen tension maintains the membrane of pulmonary vascular smooth muscle cells in a state of partial depolarization and also influences the role of calcium in excitation–contraction coupling (Bohr, 1977).

Physiological and pathophysiological aspects of HPV

Vasoconstriction in response to hypoxia in the pulmonary circuit subserves important homoeostatic mechanisms. With generalized hypoxia involving the entire lung, redistribution of blood flow occurs so that non-perfused areas in gravitationally disadvantaged lung regions begin to participate in gas exchange. Previously non-perfused blood vessels in other parts of the lung are recruited in addition. HPV also has a role in regional hypoxia. Localized increase in vascular resistance diverts blood from pulmonary units in which oxygen tension is low to those where ventilation might be better, thereby optimizing matching of ventilation and perfusion.

HPV is of interest and importance in several clinical situations. The response of the pulmonary circulation to hypoxia is an important component in the development of mountain sickness and cor pulmonale in many patients (Fishman, 1976b). Administration of bronchodilator aerosols containing β-adrenergic agonists, such as isoprenaline (isoproterenol), is frequently followed by decrease in systemic arterial oxygen tension. This is explained by action of the drug on pulmonary vasculature antagonizing HPV and thereby rendering matching of ventilation and blood flow less efficient. Patients with hepatic cirrhosis frequently have systemic arterial hypoxaemia. This has been explained by the action of vasodilator substances on the pulmonary circulation. These substances (possibly E-type prostaglandins) are produced in the splanchnic area and are normally inactivated by the liver. With liver disease, they reach the lung in concentrations sufficient to interfere with the homoeostatic functions subserved by HPV.

Patients with familial dysautonomia (Riley—Day syndrome) subjected to acute hypoxia are said to sustain systemic arterial hypoxaemia of a degree much more severe than in comparable individuals without this defect. It is speculated that the mechanism of HPV is lacking in patients with familial dysautonomia because of the widespread sensory receptor and autonomic deficiencies characterizing this condition. The exaggerated hypoxaemia occurs because the body fails to recognize and compensate for alveolar hypoxia. Patients with congenital heart disease in which ventricular septal defect is a feature may have increased right-to-left intracardiac shunt during hypoxia when pulmonary vascular resistance is further elevated by HPV. The shunt may be additionally exaggerated by a simultaneous decrease in peripheral resistance as might occur with administration of some anaesthetic agents. It is probable that HPV is the principal mechanism involved in reduction of blood flow through atelectatic lung (Benumof *et al.*, 1977).

Anaesthetic agents and hypoxic pulmonary vasoconstriction

Anaesthetic agents are capable of influencing hypoxic pulmonary vasoconstriction (HPV). Several groups of investigators have examined the effect of anaesthetic agents on HPV using preparations such as intact animals of various species, innervated lobes of lungs perfused *in situ* and isolated perfused lungs. Techniques used for assessing changes in pulmonary circulatory status in these studies include calculation of pulmonary vascular resistance from haemodynamic measurements, measurement of changes in pulmonary artery pressure at constant left atrial pressure and perfusion rate, use of electromagnetic flow meters applied to pulmonary vessels, and measurement of pulmonary excretion of intravenously administered radioactive gas from independently ventilated lungs. Results reported by different investigators and by the individual workers describing different studies are not always consistent. Discrepancies are most likely related to use of varying experimental preparations and techniques and species differences. Virtually all common anaesthetic agents have been investigated.

The most widely varying results have been reported for halothane. Some investigators report progressive, dose-dependent depression of HPV with this agent (Buckley *et al.*, 1964; Sykes *et al.*, 1973; Bredesen, Bjertnaes and Hauge, 1975). Other studies have found interference with HPV only at high concentrations of halothane, e.g. 3% (Loh, Sykes, and Chakrabarti,

1977). No effect upon, or enhancement of, HPV with halothane is reported by yet other workers (Benumof and Wahrenbrock, 1975; Mathers, Benumof and Wahrenbrock, 1977). Most investigators conclude that nitrous oxide inhibits HPV (Benumof and Wahrenbrock, 1975, Hurtig *et al.*, 1977; Mathers, Benumof and Wahrenbrock, 1977; Sykes *et al.*, 1977a, b). In a conflicting report, Buckley *et al.* (1964) describe enhancement of the pressor response to hypoxia during nitrous oxide administration. Lack of effect on HPV is also reported for enflurane at one and two MAC* (Mathers, Benumof and Wahrenbrock, 1977). Isoflurane and fluroxene exhibit dose-dependent inhibition of HPV (Benumof and Wahrenbrock, 1975; Mathers, Benumof and Wahrenbrock, 1977) as do methoxyflurane (Bredesen, Bjertnaes and Hauge, 1975, Sykes *et al.*, 1976), trichlorethylene (Sykes *et al.*, 1973; Sykes *et al.*, 1975) and diethyl ether (Sykes *et al.*, 1973; Sykes *et al.*, 1977; Loh, Sykes and Chakrabarti, 1977; Bredesen, Bjertnaes and Hauge, 1975). Various non-volatile anaesthetic drugs and adjuvants including thiopentone, ketamine, pethidine, lignocaine, chlorpromazine, fentanyl, droperidol, diazepam, pentazocine and pentobarbitone do not influence HPV (Benumof and Wahrenbrock, 1975; Bredesen, Bjertnaes and Hauge, 1975). However, the pulmonary pressor response to hypoxia was more consistently demonstrated after fentanyl–droperidol administration than after pentobarbitone (Susmano, Passovoy and Carleton, 1972).

Bjertnaes *et al.* (1976) have studied the influence of anaesthetic agents on HPV in man. They measured relative distribution of blood flow using lung scanning techniques following infusion of radioactive tagged albumin while the two lungs were ventilated with different gas mixtures via a Carlens' double lumen tube. When one lung was ventilated and nitrogen and the other with oxygen in the absence of volatile anaesthetic agents, percentage of cardiac output perfusing the hypoxic lung diminished markedly. When either diethyl ether or halothane was subsequently added to the nitrogen, percentage of cardiac output perfusing the hypoxic lung increased significantly. This was accompanied by a further fall in arterial oxygen tension. It was concluded that HPV is maintained in man but is highly impaired by the two inhalation agents studied.

In some circumstances, lungs in which the pressor response to hypoxia has been abolished by anaesthetic agents still exhibit vasoconstriction with acidaemia or noradrenaline administration (Sykes *et al.*, 1973). This is further evidence that varying sites and mechanisms might be involved in vasomotion in response to different stimuli. When studying isolated lobes, the effect of anaesthetic agents on HPV does not depend on whether the agent is confined to the lobe under investigation or administered to the entire lung (Mathers, Benumof and Wahrenbrock, 1977). Many studies on HPV and anaesthesia incorporate associated measurements of changes in arterial oxygen tension and shunt. Generally, these changes are predictable in a qualitative sense, but quantitatively frequently do not correlate very

---

*MAC — minimal alveolar concentration of an anaesthetic for suppressing response to a defined stimulus (see Chapter 3). *Ed.*

well with observed magnitudes of change in blood flow. This most probably relates to the complexity of physiological alterations which follow acute establishment of regional hypoxia.

Inhibition of HPV by anaesthetic agents may be of clinical significance. As discussed previously, HPV may be an important physiological mechanism involved in optimal matching of ventilation and blood flow in the lung. Interference with this mechanism by anaesthetic agents provides an attractive explanation, at least in part, for the increase in alveolar–arterial oxygen tension difference which frequently characterizes the anaesthetized state. Caution must be exercised, however, before accepting this explanation which implies that ventilation/perfusion relationships deteriorate during anaesthesia in man. To date, there is scant evidence that changes in ventilation/perfusion relationships are a significant cause of pulmonary dysfunction in anaesthetized patients. Also, impairment of oxygenation under clinical conditions in man occurs with intravenous anaesthesia in the absence of inhalational agents and also with inhalational agents which have not been shown to inhibit HPV. HPV and anaesthesia is a relatively new area of inquiry and further developments will be awaited with interest.

ANAESTHESIA AND PULMONARY HAEMODYNAMICS

Studies involving the pulmonary circulation during anaesthesia, although not nearly so numerous or comprehensive as those of the systemic circulation, are appearing with increasing frequency. Certain haemodynamic patterns associated with particular agents, techniques, and events occurring during anaesthesia are becoming evident.

Nitrous oxide does not appear to have any remarkable primary effect on the pulmonary circulation. Pulmonary haemodynamics were identical during air breathing and during inhalation of 50% N_2O, 30% N_2, 20% O_2 in dogs. A small decrease in pulmonary vascular resistance attributed to passive vascular dilatation secondary to increased left atrial pressure occurred in these dogs during inhalation of 80% N_2O, 20% O_2 (Dottori *et al.*, 1976a). No change in pulmonary haemodynamics was observed when nitrous oxide (60%) was added to 0.55% halothane in patients with valvular heart disease. When pulmonary pressures during anaesthesia in these patients were compared with values recorded at cardiac catheterization prior to surgery while breathing air, the only change reported was a decreased pulmonary vascular resistance during anaesthesia. This was interpreted as a passive change caused by increased left atrial pressure (Stoelting, Reis and Longnecker, 1972).

Pulmonary haemodynamics usually do not change appreciably during balanced anaesthetic techniques using nitrous oxide and various combinations of narcotics, barbiturates and muscle relaxants in patients whose left atrial pressure is normal preoperatively (Johnson, 1951; Wyant *et al.*, 1958; Dottori *et al.*, 1976b; Lappas *et al.*, 1976). Lappas *et al.* (1975) found small but significant increases in pulmonary artery pressure and pulmonary vascular resistance when nitrous oxide was inhaled by patients who had received large doses of morphine. These haemodynamic measurements, however, remained within the normal range. In patients with preanaesthetic left ventricular filling pressure greater than 1.6 kPa (12 mmHg), significant increases in pulmonary artery pressure and pulmonary vascular resistance were associated with balanced anaesthesia (Lappas *et al.*, 1976). In dogs, changes suggestive of pulmonary vasoconstriction followed administration of thialbarbitone (thiamylal) but not pentobarbitone (Goldberg *et al.*, 1968). Subarachnoid block is not associated with any characteristic changes in pulmonary haemodynamics in fit patients (Johnson, 1951).

Halothane, in the presence of adequate ventilation, has minimal effects on pulmonary haemodynamics. Small changes in pulmonary artery pressure and pulmonary vascular resistance observed during halothane anaesthesia could represent passive changes due to decreased cardiac output and elevated left atrial pressure or perhaps mild pulmonary constriction (Price *et al.*, 1969; Stoelting, Reis, and Longnecker, 1972; Fahmy *et al.*, 1976). Pulmonary artery pressures which were normal or only slightly elevated were observed in patients receiving methoxyflurane anaesthesia (mean value 2.4 kPa (18 mmHg); Flacke, Thompson and Read, 1976).

Active pulmonary vasoconstriction occurs during cyclopropane anaesthesia. Pulmonary artery pressure increases 0.5–1.3 kPa (4–10 mmHg) and pulmonary vascular resistance may double. Magnitude of these changes was greater at $F_{I}O_2$ = 0.25 than at $F_{I}O_2$ = 0.8. This suggests that variations in inspired oxygen tension over ranges entirely acceptable in clinical practice might still modulate pulmonary vascular tone. These changes in pulmonary haemodynamics during cyclopropane anaesthesia occur in addition to those caused by hypercarbia which can easily occur with unassisted respirations during use of this agent (Etsten *et al.*, 1953, Price *et al.*, 1969). Diethyl ether also causes active pulmonary vasoconstriction. Pulmonary vascular resistance increases markedly and pulmonary artery pressures greater than 4 kPa (30 mmHg) may be attained (Johnson, 1951; Wyant, Chang and Merriman, 1962).

Pulmonary hypertension with mean pulmonary artery pressure exceeding 4 kPa (30 mmHg) can accompany episodes of systemic hypertension during light general anaesthesia. This response is frequently associated with upper airway manipulation and endotracheal intubation or surgical stimulation. The mechanism is most likely reflex active pulmonary vasoconstriction and the pulmonary hypertension can be reversed with ganglionic blocking agents or vasodilators (Prys-Roberts *et al.*, 1971; Fahmy *et al.*, 1976; Lappas *et al.*, 1976). Smaller transient peaks in pulmonary artery pressure may occur with surgical incision and again at the termination of anaesthesia associated with endotracheal extubation (Sharefkin and MacArthur, 1972).

Hypercarbia during anaesthesia causes significant pulmonary hypertension. With either barbiturate-relaxant or halothane–nitrous oxide induction of anaesthesia, marked increases in pulmonary artery and left ventricular filling pressure occurred during respiratory acidaemia with pH_a less than 7.3. These changes are associated with comparable increases in right ventricular filling pressure (central venous pressure) (Sørensen and

Jacobsen, 1977). Flow patterns in pulmonary veins during the cardiac cycle in anaesthetized man resemble those in the caval system. On the left side of the circulation transient reversal of blood flow in pulmonary veins may occur in some patients during atrial systole. Peaks of blood flow from pulmonary veins into the left side of the heart occur during ventricular systole and again in midventricular diastole (Skagseth, 1976).

It is now possible to propose several tentative generalizations concerning behaviour of the pulmonary circulation during anaesthesia which are compatible with observations reported to date in man. Well managed, uncomplicated anaesthesia with agents and techniques currently in clinical use which are not characterized by stimulation of catecholamine release appear to lack or have very small direct effect on the pulmonary circulation. Changes in pulmonary artery pressure and pulmonary vascular resistance under these circumstances are frequently passive and measured values are not likely to be outside the normal range. A possible exception to this generalization may apply in patients with initially elevated pulmonary artery pressure (Lappas *et al.*, 1976). Significant increases in pulmonary artery pressure and pulmonary vascular resistance occur during anaesthesia associated with catecholamine release (diethyl ether and cyclopropane). These changes represent active vasoconstriction of pulmonary vessels and can be attributed primarily to α-adrenergic activity. Although some anaesthetics attenuate the response, hypoxia and respiratory acidaemia still cause pulmonary vasoconstriction in anaesthetized man and accentuate pulmonary hypertension due to other causes. High inspired oxygen concentrations might assist in reversal of pulmonary hypertension due to causes other than hypoxia. During anaesthesia, intense autonomic activity which produces systemic hypertension may also cause pulmonary hypertension which is responsive to treatment with ganglionic blocking drugs, vasodilators, and, presumably, increased anaesthetic depth.

Several consequences may ensue as a result of altered pulmonary haemodynamics during anaesthesia. When pulmonary artery pressure is increased, work and oxygen consumption of the right ventricle must increase to maintain its output against a higher afterload. If these additional demands cannot be met, right ventricular failure can occur. Also, increase in pulmonary artery pressure may alter the balance of forces favouring retention of fluid in the intravascular compartment to that favouring filtration of fluid into lung interstitial spaces. Mean pulmonary artery pressure which exceeded colloid osmotic pressure was observed in many patients during anaesthesia accompanied by hypercarbia (Sørensen and Jacobsen, 1977). Increases in both lung water and physiological shunt were observed under circumstances where pulmonary artery pressure remained elevated throughout an operative procedure (Byrick, Finlayson, and Noble, 1977). Thus, the potential for pulmonary oedema exists during sustained increases of pulmonary artery pressure during anaesthesia. Changes in pulmonary haemodynamics are associated with impaction of a femoral prosthesis during total hip replacement. Increase in mean pulmonary artery pressure and pulmonary vascular resistance occurred during peridural anaesthesia in both awake patients and in those receiving supplementary general anaesthesia with artificial ventilation (Modig and Malmberg, 1975).

PULMONARY OEDEMA

Factors influencing movement of fluid across pulmonary vascular walls are related in Starling's equation (Staub, 1974a, b):

$$Q_f = K [P_v - P_{pv}] - \sigma [\Pi_v - \Pi_{pv}]$$

where Q_f is net transmural fluid transfer, P_v and P_{pv} are respectively intravascular and perivascular (interstitial) hydrostatic pressures, Π_v and Π_{pv} are intravascular and perivascular colloid osmotic pressures and K and σ are constants relating to capillary membrane conductivity and reflectivity. P_v is normally about 1.3 kPa (10 mmHg). P_{pv} has been variously estimated as atmospheric or, alternatively, subatmospheric and considerably lower than pleural pressure. Π_v is normally about 3.0 kPa (22.5 mmHg). Π_{pv} depends on protein concentration in lung interstitial fluid and should usually be small. Thus, normal balance of forces favours retention of fluid in the intravascular compartment or only minimal filtration of fluid into the interstitial compartment. Staub (1974a, b) estimates that in man about 20 ml of fluid per hour might be transferred from intravascular to interstitial compartments. This fluid is collected and removed by pulmonary lymphatics and no water accumulates in the lung.

In some respects, pulmonary oedema may be regarded as an exaggeration of this dynamic fluid exchange which continuously operates under normal physiological conditions. Several stages in the pathogenesis of pulmonary oedema may be distinguished.

(1) Initially, accelerated transfer of fluid from intravascular to interstitial compartments occurs. Augmentation of lymph flow at this stage prevents accumulation of water in the lung. It is estimated (Staub, 1974a, b) that lymphatic flow from the lung might be capable of increasing to ten times its basal value.

(2) If the rate of filtration exceeds capacity of lymphatics, water accumulates in the interstitial compartment of the lung. At this stage, dilution of proteins in the extravascular compartment decreases interstitial osmotic pressure and tends in part to restore a balance of forces tending to favour intravascular retention of fluid.

(3) As pulmonary oedema progresses, fluid next appears in alveoli. Initially, quantity of fluid in individual affected alveoli is small and confined to the region of the angles between adjacent septa.

(4) Alveolar flooding is the next stage. When this occurs, it is an all-or-none phenomenon. One might observe alveoli completely filled with fluid while others have minimal fluid confined to septal angles or may be completely uninvolved. Half-filled alveoli do not occur.

(5) Finally, with florid pulmonary oedema, flooding is of sufficient magnitude so that foam appears in the tracheobronchial tree. This is frequently pink because of rupture of capillaries and increased diapadesis of erythrocytes.

Either increased intravascular pressure or increased permeability of blood vessel walls are primary mechanisms which can cause pulmonary oedema. When pressure in small pulmonary vessels is increased, as in left ventricular failure, balance of hydrostatic forces is altered to enhance filtration of fluid out of the vascular compartment. In the isolated, perfused dog lung, accumulation of lung water begins abruptly when pulmonary capillary pressure reaches 3.7 kPa (28 mmHg) and progressively increases as capillary pressure is further elevated (Gaar *et al.*, 1967). Increased vascular permeability in the lung occurs in situations such as chemical injury or bacterial endotoxaemia and may result in exudation of large volumes of oedema fluid of high protein content. Other secondary factors which influence transvascular movement of fluid may play a role in pulmonary oedema. Decreased colloid osmotic pressure associated with hypoproteinaemia lowers the intravascular pressure at which fluid transudation occurs in isolated dog lungs (Gaar *et al.*, 1967). It seems unlikely that diminished colloid osmotic pressure of itself can cause pulmonary oedema in clinical situations, but it may be expected to intensify the process initiated by one of the primary factors mentioned above. Similarly, pulmonary lymphatic obstruction, while unlikely to be a primary cause of oedema, might be an important contributing factor in some circumstances. The role of alteration in surface forces in the lung in relation to pulmonary oedema has not been established. So-called 'neurogenic pulmonary oedema' can occur in patients with head injury or other intracranial pathology. It is thought to be caused by intense, neurally mediated pulmonary vasoconstriction. Hypoxia does not increase permeability of pulmonary capillary membranes and there is no evidence that administration of oxygen helps restore permeability to an injured and 'leaky' capillary membrane. Recent and comprehensive reviews of pulmonary oedema and its pathogenesis contain further details (Staub, 1974a, b).

Pulmonary oedema and anaesthesia

The incidence of pulmonary oedema occurring during anaesthesia has been estimated at about 0.02–0.1%. Patients of all ages and of varying physical status may be affected and all commonly used anaesthetic agents have been involved. Only one-half of patients developing pulmonary oedema during anaesthesia have a history of heart disease (Cooperman and Price, 1970).

Several factors can precipitate pulmonary oedema during anaesthesia. Primary changes in cardiac performance can be associated with administration of drugs producing decreased cardiac contractility such as most potent volatile anaesthetic agents, barbiturates, etc. Cardiac efficiency can also be impaired by various arrhythmias, both spontaneous and drug induced, which impede cardiac filling. Tachycardia caused by atropine is particularly prone to initiate pulmonary oedema in patients whose cardiac output is limited by mitral stenosis and avoidance of atropine in these individuals has been advised. Another cause of pulmonary oedema during anaesthesia is overload of the pulmonary circulation caused by redistribution of blood from the peripheral systemic vascular beds to the pulmonary circuit. This redistribution can be initiated by administration of vasoconstrictor drugs or intense sympathetic activity. As mentioned previously, primary pulmonary vasoconstriction also occurs with intense sympathetic activity. Excessive subatmospheric intrathoracic pressure occurring during breathing against inspiratory obstruction may increase intrathoracic blood volume and induce pulmonary oedema.

Probably the most common cause of pulmonary oedema during anaesthesia is hypervolaemia due to excessive administration of parenteral fluids. Expansion of the intravascular compartment with large volumes of crystalloid solutions produces pulmonary oedema both by elevation of pulmonary vascular pressure and by dilution of plasma proteins. Intravascular absorption of large volumes of fluid may occur through open blood vessels during irrigation of hollow organs and is a particular hazard during transurethral prostatic resection.

Pulmonary oedema during anaesthesia may also result from altered permeability of vascular tissues in the lung. Factors which can alter vascular integrity include aspirated acid gastric juice and irritative and corrosive substances which may be inadvertently introduced into the lung during anaesthesia as impurities in anaesthetic gases. An example is nitrogen dioxide which on occasion has been a contaminant of nitrous oxide. The basis of pulmonary oedema associated with bacterial endotoxaemia is also altered vascular permeability. Pulmonary oedema can be a prominent feature of oxygen toxicity, lung trauma, blast injury, pulmonary burns, smoke inhalation, so-called adult respiratory distress syndrome and some types of pulmonary embolic phenomena such as amniotic fluid embolus. Pulmonary oedema has also been reported as a manifestation of an immune reaction during blood transfusion (Thompson *et al.*, 1971).

Clinical manifestations and treatment

Signs of pulmonary oedema during anaesthesia include increased respiratory frequency, decreased tidal volume, decreased respiratory compliance and increased respiratory resistance. During artificial ventilation, progressive impedance to ventilation can be noted. Evaluation of arterial blood gases confirms the deteriorating state of pulmonary gas exchange characteristic of pulmonary oedema. Râles may be absent during early interstitial phases but should become evident as fluid begins to occupy airways. In severe cases pink, frothy fluid appears at the mouth or endotracheal tube. As in the conscious patient, it is frequently difficult to distinguish between early pulmonary oedema and bronchoconstriction during anaesthesia. Additional diagnostic measures which might be used in this situation include roentgenographic examination and measurement of pulmonary capillary wedge or pulmonary artery end-diastolic pressures (Sharefkin and MacArthur, 1972). Central venous pressure measurement and inspection for distended neck veins frequently cannot be relied upon since right heart filling pressure may be normal in some cases of pulmonary oedema.

Management of pulmonary oedema associated with anaesthesia is generally directed toward attainment of four objectives. These are correction of the underlying cause, decrease of total and central blood volume, improving cardiac performance and improving pulmonary function. Initially, precipitating and aggravating causes of the pulmonary oedema should be identified if possible and corrected. This might include cessation of fluid administration, lowering of blood pressure, withdrawal or reversal of myocardial depressant drugs, etc. Measures useful for reducing central and total blood volume, and hence load imposed on the myocardium, include head-up posture, rotating venous occlusion tourniquets, phlebotomy, diuretics and vasodilators such as sodium nitroprusside, ganglionic blocking drugs, etc. Myocardial performance can be improved by administration of cardiac glycosides or dopamine when appropriate and correction of arrhythmias if present. Derangements of pulmonary function characteristic of pulmonary oedema can be treated with oxygen administration, mechanical removal of airway fluid and administration of positive pressure breathing with positive end-expiratory pressure as indicated. Obviously, specific treatment of pulmonary oedema will vary among patients depending upon their initial status and the aetiology of the condition. Where oedema has occurred as a result of injury to the pulmonary capillary membrane in a previously fit patient, as in aspiration of acid gastric contents, measures designed to decrease blood volume and improve myocardial performance are not likely to be particularly effective. Capability for measurement of left heart filling pressure (pulmonary capillary wedge pressure) is often useful in management of pulmonary oedema. Use of colloid solutions, such as albumin, and steroids in pulmonary oedema caused by 'leaky' membranes, while intuitively attractive, remains controversial.

Cooperman and Price (1970) found that most cases of pulmonary oedema associated with anaesthesia occur within the first hour following termination of anaesthesia. It is easy to imagine how several factors, such as hypertension due to returning pain sensibility, cessation of positive pressure breathing, excessive parenteral fluid administration, etc., can cumulate during this period of rapid physiological readjustment to produce pulmonary oedema. At this time, the rapid, shallow breathing of pulmonary oedema might be mistaken for residual action of neuromuscular blocking drugs.

References

Barer, G. (1976). The physiology of the pulmonary circulation and methods of study. *Pharmac. Ther. B.* 2, 247—273

Benumof, J. L., Eurman, P. and Wahrenbrock, E. A. (1977). In vitro interaction of serotonin and anesthetic drugs on isolated pulmonary artery strips. *1977 Annual Meeting Abstracts of Scientific Papers*, pp. 171—172. American Society of Anesthesiologists, Park Ridge, Ill.

Benumof, J. L. and Wahrenbrock, E. (1975). Local effects of anesthetics on regional hypoxic pulmonary vasoconstriction. *Anesthesiology* 43, 525—532

Benumof, J. L., Scanlon, T. S., Moyce, P. R. and Wahrenbrock, E. A. (1977). Mechanism of blood flow reduction through atelectatic lung. *1977 Annual Meeting Abstracts of Scientific Papers*, pp. 235—236. American Society of Anesthesiologists, Park Ridge, Ill.

Bergofsky, E. H. (1974). Mechanisms underlying vasomotor regulation of regional pulmonary blood flow in normal and disease states. *Am. J. Med.* 57, 378—394

Bjertnaes, L. J., Hauge, A., Nakken, K. F. and Bredesen, J. E. (1976). Hypoxic pulmonary vasoconstriction: Inhibition due to anesthesia. *Acta physiol. scand.* 96, 283—285

Bohr, D. (1977). The pulmonary hypoxic response. *Chest* 71 (2 Feb. Suppl.), 244—246

Bredesen, J., Bjertnaes, L. and Hauge, A. (1975). Effects of anesthetics on the pulmonary vasoconstrictor response to acute alveolar hypoxia. *Microvasc. Res.* 10, 236

Buckley, M. J., McLaughlin, J. S., Fort III, L., Saigusa, M. and Morrow, D. H. (1964). Effects of anesthetic agents on pulmonary vascular resistance during hypoxia. *Surg. Forum* 15, 183—184

Byrick, R. J., Finlayson, D. C. and Noble, W. H. (1977). Pulmonary arterial pressure increases during cardiopulmonary bypass, a potential cause of pulmonary edema. *Anesthesiology* 46, 433—435

Cooperman, L. H. and Price, H. L. (1970). Pulmonary edema in the operative and postoperative period: A review of 40 cases. *Ann. Surg.* 172, 883—891

Dottori, O., Haggendal, E., Linder, E., Nordström, G. and Seeman, T. (1976a). The haemodynamic effects of nitrous oxide anaesthesia on systemic and pulmonary circulation in dogs. *Acta anaesth. scand.* 20, 429—436

Dottori, O., Korsgren, M., Löf, A. and Wilhelmsen, L. (1976b). The haemodynamic effects of unsupplemented nitrous oxide—oxygen-relaxant anaesthesia in cardiac patients. *Acta anaesth. scand.* 20, 195—200

Etsten, B. E., Rheinlander, H. F., Reynolds, R. N. and Li, T. H. (1953). Effect of cyclopropane anesthesia on pulmonary artery pressure in humans. *Surg. Forum* 4, 649—654

Fahmy, N. R., Selwyn, A. S., Patel, D. and Lappas, D. G. (1976). Pulmonary vasomotor tone during general anesthesia and deliberate hypotension in man. *Anesthesiology* 45: 1, 3—13

Fishman, A. P. (1976a). Hypoxia on the pulmonary circulation. How and where it acts. *Circulation Res.* 38: 4, 221—231

Fishman, A. P. (1976b). State of the art. Chronic cor pulmonale. *Am. Rev. resp. Dis.* 114, 775—794

Flacke, J. W., Thompson, D. S. and Read, R. C. (1976). Influence of tidal volume and pulmonary artery occlusion on arterial oxygenation during endobronchial anesthesia. *Sth. med. J., Nashville* 69: 5, 619—626

Gaar, K. A., Taylor, A. E., Owens, L. J. and Guyton, A. C. (1967). Effect of capillary pressure and plasma protein on development of pulmonary edema. *Am. J. Physiol.* 213, 79—82

Goldberg, S. J., Linde, L. M., Gaal, P. G., Momma, K., Takahashi, M. and Sarna, G. (1968). Effects of barbiturates on pulmonary and systemic haemodynamics. *Cardiovasc. Res.* 2, 136—142

Hurtig, J. B., Tait, A. R., Loh, L. and Sykes, M. K. (1977). Reduction of hypoxic pulmonary vasoconstriction by nitrous oxide administration in the isolated perfused cat lung. *Can. Anaesth. Soc. J.* 24: 5, 540—548

Johnson, S. R. (1951). The effect of some anaesthetic agents on the circulation in man. *Acta chir. scand. Suppl.* 158

Lappas, D. G., Buckley, M. J., Laver, M. B., Daggett, W. M. and Lowenstein, E. (1975). Left ventricular performance and pulmonary circulation following addition of nitrous oxide to morphine during coronary-artery surgery. *Anesthesiology* 43: 1, 61—69

Lappas, D. G., Lowenstein, E., Waller, J., Fahmy, N. R. and Daggett, W. M. (1976). Hemodynamic effects of nitroprusside infusion during coronary artery operation in man. *Circulation* 54, III, 4—10

Lauweryns, J. M., Cokelaere, M. and Theunynck, P. (1973). Serotonin producing neuroepithelial bodies in rabbit respiratory mucosa. *Science, N. Y.* 180, 410—413

Loh, L., Sykes, M. K. and Chakrabarti, M. K. (1977). The effects of halothane and ether on the pulmonary circulation in the innervated perfused cat lung. *Br. J. Anaesth.* 49, 309—314

Mathers, J., Benumof, J. L. and Wahrenbrock, E. A. (1977). General anesthetics and regional hypoxic pulmonary vasoconstriction. *Anesthesiology* 46, 111—114

Modig, J. and Malmberg, P. (1975). Pulmonary and circulatory reactions during total hip replacement surgery. *Acta anaesth. scand.* 19, 219—237

Porcelli, R. J., Viau, A., Demeny, M., Naftchi, N. E. and Bergofsky, E. H. (1977). Relation between hypoxic pulmonary vasoconstriction, its humoral mediators and alpha—beta adrenergic receptors. *Chest* 71 (2 Feb. Suppl.), 249—251

Price, H. L., Cooperman, L. H., Warden, J. C., Morris, J. J. and Smith, T. C. (1969). Pulmonary hemodynamics during general anesthesia in man. *Anesthesiology* 30, 629—636

Prys-Roberts, C., Greene, L. T., Meloche, R. and Foëx, P. (1971). Studies of anaesthesia in relation to hypertension II: Haemodynamic consequences of induction and endotracheal intubation. *Br. J. Anaesth.* 43, 531—546

Sharefkin, J. B. and MacArthur, J. D. (1972). Pulmonary arterial pressure as a guide to the hemodynamic status of surgical patients. *Archs Surg., Chicago* 105, 699—704

Skagseth, E. (1976). Pulmonary vein flow pattern in man during thoracotomy. *Scand. J. thorac. cardiovasc. Surg.* 10, 36—42

Sørensen, M. B. and Jacobsen, E. (1977). Pulmonary hemodynamics during induction of anesthesia. *Anesthesiology* 46, 246—251

Staub, N. C. (1974a). 'State of the art' review. Pathogenesis of pulmonary edema. *Am. Rev. resp. Dis.* 109, 358—372

Staub, N. C. (1974b). Pulmonary edema. *Physiol. Rev.* 54, 678—811

Stoelting, R. K., Reis, R. R. and Longnecker, D. E. (1972). Hemodynamic responses to nitrous oxide—halothane and halothane in patients with valvular heart disease. *Anesthesiology* 37:4, 430—435

Susmano, A., Passovoy, M. and Carleton, R. A. (1972). Comparison of the effects of two anesthetic agents on the production of hypoxic pulmonary hypertension in dogs. *Am. Heart J.* 84:2, 203—207

Sykes, M. K., Davies, D. M., Chakrabarti, M. K. and Loh, L. (1973). The effects of halothane, trichloroethylene and ether on the hypoxic pressor response and pulmonary vascular resistance in the isolated, perfused cat lung. *Br. J. Anaesth.* 45, 655—663

Sykes, M. K., Arnot, R. N., Jastrzebski, J., Gibbs, J. M., Obdrzalek, J. and Hurtig, J. B. (1975). Reduction of hypoxic pulmonary vasoconstriction during trichloroethylene anaesthesia. *J. appl. Physiol.* 39:1, 103—108

Sykes, M. K., Davies, D. M., Loh, L., Jastrzebski, J. and Chakrabarti, M. K. (1976). The effect of methoxyflurane on pulmonary vascular resistance and hypoxic pulmonary vasoconstriction in the isolated perfused cat lung. *Br. J. Anaesth.* 48, 191—194

Sykes, M. K., Hurtig, J. B., Tait, A. R. and Chakrabarti, M. K. (1977a). Reduction of hypoxic pulmonary vasoconstriction during diethyl ether anaesthesia in the dog. *Br. J. Anaesth.* 49, 293—299

Sykes, M. K., Hurtig, J. B., Tait, A. R. and Chakrabarti, M. K. (1977b). Reduction of hypoxic pulmonary vasoconstriction in the dog during administration of nitrous oxide. *Br. J. Anaesth.* 49, 301—307

Thompson, J. S., Severson, C. D., Parmely, M. J., Marmorstein, B. L. and Simmons, A. (1971). Pulmonary 'hypersensitivity' reactions induced by transfusion of non-hl-a leukoagglutinins. *New Engl. J. Med.* 284, 1120—1125

Wyant, G. M., Chang, C. and Merriman, J. E. (1962). The effect of anaesthesia upon pulmonary circulation. *Anesth. Analg.* 41, 338—347

Wyant, G. M., Merriman, J. E., Kilduff, C. J. and Thomas, E. T. (1958). The cardiovascular effects of halothane. *Can. Anaesth. Soc. J.* 5:4, 384—402

25 The effects of anaesthesia on respiration
John F. Nunn

It has long been recognized that the inhalation of anaesthetics might have an adverse effect on breathing. Dr Beddoes, cited by Davy in 1800, remarked upon the purple colour of the blood flowing from leech bites during the inhalation of nitrous oxide and that report may claim to be the first observation of the effect of anaesthesia on gas exchange.

There are, in fact, a great number of effects of anaesthesia upon various aspects of the respiratory system and these will now be considered *seriatim*. Different aspects of the individual inhalational anaesthetics are considered in Chapter 8.

OXYGEN CONSUMPTION

During uncomplicated anaesthesia in healthy patients, oxygen consumption is about 15% below basal (Nunn and Matthews, 1959), as defined by the usual standards, which are based on the work of Aub and DuBois (1917). These standards were based on outpatients who had just walked in from the streets, and values obtained during anaesthesia are, in fact, approximately the same as those in well rested or sedated subjects (Robertson and Reid, 1952). Changes in organ oxygen consumption during anaesthesia have been reported by Theye (1972). The respiratory quotient is probably unaltered by anaesthesia except for patients receiving dextrose infusion in which case the respiratory quotient is usually unity.

Secondary factors such as thyroid function may alter the oxygen consumption but a most important factor is temperature, with values about 50% below basal at 31°C. Conversely hyperthermia increases oxygen consumption and very high values are attained in malignant hyperpyrexia. Oxygen consumption is markedly increased in shivering (Bay, Nunn and Prys-Roberts, 1968), during convulsions and also in agitated, restless patients undergoing intensive therapy.

For the maintenance of gaseous homoeostasis, alveolar ventilation must accord with the metabolic rate. Thus, during hypothermia, artificial ventilation commonly results in hypocapnia unless the minute volume is reduced. Similarly, in hypermetabolic states, ventilation must be increased.

CONTROL OF BREATHING

Effects on the respiratory rhythm

High blood concentrations of barbiturates cause apnoea by blocking the reciprocal innervation between the inspiratory and expiratory neurons (Robson, Houseley and Solis-Quiroga, 1963). Even light anaesthesia removes the effect of wakefulness which can have major effects on breathing (Nunn, 1977a).

Central chemoreceptor sensitivity to P_{CO_2}

Increasing concentrations of inhalational anaesthetics decrease the slope of the P_{CO_2}/ventilation response curve but the effect is quantitatively different for the commonly used inhalational agents (*Figure 25.1*). Thus at 1 MAC*, methoxyflurane and halothane cause much greater depression than diethyl ether. The effect at 1 MAC is least of all with cyclopropane, the difference perhaps being, in part, attributable to the different rates of secretion of catecholamines with these agents.

Depression of slope of the P_{CO_2}/ventilation response curve and perhaps a rightward shift of intercept also occurs with the opiates. This effect can be reversed by naloxone although the duration of action of opiates (even those which are said to be short acting) may outlast that of naloxone (see Chapter 54). Barbiturates may have a synergistic effect with opiates.

Peripheral chemoreceptor sensitivity to P_{O_2}

It was originally believed that the hypoxic drive was a rugged reflex which was unaffected by anaesthetics. This comforting belief, based on the administration of barbiturates to cats, has been shown to be untrue for halothane in dogs (Weiskopf, Raymond and Severinghaus, 1974) and man (Knill and Gelb, 1978). In fact, it is now clear that the hypoxia reflex is even more sensitive to anaesthetics than is the hypercapnic response. It should be stressed that hypoxic drive only becomes clinically relevant when the arterial P_{O_2} is less than 8 kPa (60 mmHg) and this should not arise in a satisfactory anaesthetic.

Reflex control of breathing

Anaesthesia is well known to depress or abolish the cough reflex. There appears to be no solid foundation for the belief that trichloroethylene

* The concept of MAC is defined in Chapter 3. *Ed.*

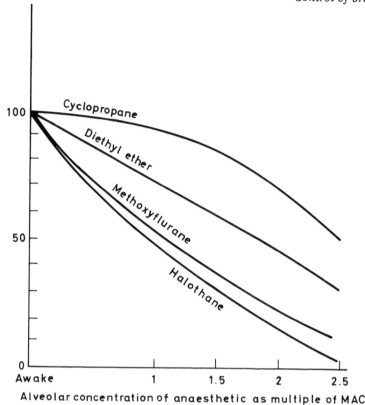

Figure 25.1
Depression of the slope of the awake P_{CO_2}/ventilation response
curve by increasing concentrations of various anaesthetics. The
concentrations of the anaesthetics are presented on an equinarcotic
scale. (Redrawn from Larson *et al.*, 1969)

causes tachypnoea as a result of sensitization of the pulmonary stretch
receptors (Ngai, Katz and Farhie, 1965). Expiratory resistance during
anaesthesia causes augmentation of the inspiratory effort of the consciously
breathing patient (Nunn and Ezi-Ashi, 1961). This is the exact opposite of
what would be expected if the Hering—Breuer reflex was active in man.

Breathing patterns

During anaesthesia with spontaneous respiration, the breathing pattern
differs from normal in several respects. Firstly, the expiratory muscles
usually become active although they are normally silent in the supine
conscious subject (Freund, Roos and Dodd, 1964). During anaesthesia,
inspiratory muscle tone ceases abruptly at the start of expiration so that
the expiratory waveform approximates to an exponential decay (Nunn,
1977b).

It has long been known that deepening anaesthesia is associated with
progressive loss of the intercostal component of breathing and this reduces

the relative contribution of the rib cage to the tidal volume (Jones *et al.*, 1979). It has now been shown that the normal ventilatory response to CO_2 is largely achieved by means of the intercostal muscles, and loss of their contribution accounts for much of the reduction of ventilatory response to rising P_{CO_2} observed during anaesthesia (Tusiewicz, Bryan and Froese, 1977).

Muscle spindles

It is commonly believed that the gamma motoneuron system is particularly sensitive to anaesthetic agents, and this accords with the loss of intercostal muscle activity during deepening anaesthesia, because the intercostals are rich in spindles while very few are found in the diaphragm. Nevertheless, the response of anaesthetized man to added resistance to breathing shows clear evidence of the type of adaptation to varying load which, in skeletal muscles, is typically mediated by spindles (Nunn and Ezi-Ashi, 1961). Subparalytic doses of neuromuscular blocking agents reduce the slope of the P_{CO_2}/ventilation response curve by interference with the motor system.

VENTILATION

Spontaneous respiration

Pulmonary ventilation can vary between very wide limits during anaesthesia. During spontaneous ventilation, the minute volume is governed primarily by the interplay between the respiratory depressant effect of the anaesthetic drugs and the driving effect of surgical stimulation, which is not totally suppressed even by deep anaesthesia (Eger *et al.*, 1972). Research studies of pulmonary ventilation during anaesthesia are often undertaken in the absence of surgical stimulation and therefore tend to emphasize the very low levels of ventilation which may occur. However, Nunn (1958) reported a mean minute volume of only 4.16 $l \cdot min^{-1}$ in a series of 26 intubated patients during surgery, with values of 2 $l \cdot min^{-1}$ being recorded on a number of occasions. Hypoventilation of this degree must inevitably result in hypercapnia, although the P_{CO_2} will rise comparatively slowly, with low values for the respiratory exchange ratio being recorded for at least the first hour of anaesthesia while carbon dioxide is being diverted to the rising body stores (Nunn, 1964).

Effect of endotracheal intubation

Endotracheal intubation not only bypasses about half of the patient's anatomical dead space but also results in the imposition of a smaller external apparatus dead space (see below). In a spontaneously breathing anaesthetized patient, removal of the endotracheal tube and substitution of a facemask without altering the depth of anaesthesia results in an increase of both ventilation and P_{CO_2}, the relative changes being governed by the P_{CO_2}/ventilation response curve thus:

$$\frac{\dot{V}\,(\text{mask}) \;-\; \dot{V}\,(\text{intubated})}{P_{CO_2}\,(\text{mask}) \;-\; P_{CO_2}\,(\text{intubated})} = \text{slope of } P_{CO_2}/\dot{V} \text{ response curve}$$

A mean change in minute volume from 4.9 to 5.9 l·min^{-1} was reported under these circumstances by Kain, Panday and Nunn (1969).

Artificial ventilation

During artificial ventilation of the anaesthetized patient, the selection of the minute volume is largely according to the whim of the anaesthetist. Approximately 6 l·min^{-1} minute volume will ensure a normal arterial P_{CO_2} in an average anaesthetized patient with an endotracheal tube and about 30 ml of apparatus dead space. However, anaesthetists tend to impose a wide range of minute volumes, commonly from 4 to 20 l·min^{-1} with corresponding variations in the P_{CO_2} (Nunn, 1958). Hypocapnia is often deliberately induced to enhance the depth of anaesthesia (see Chapter 23), or to reduce cerebral blood flow and intracranial pressure (see Chapter 33).

LUNG VOLUME AND FUNCTIONAL RESIDUAL CAPACITY

A consistent feature of all types of general anaesthesia is a reduction in functional residual capacity (FRC) by about 400 ml. The change from upright to supine position causes a reduction in FRC of about 800 ml so that the total reduction in FRC from upright (conscious) to supine (anaesthetized) is about 1.2 litres and sufficient to bring the lung volume close to residual volume. In many patients this will bring the end-expiratory level, if not the entire tidal range, below the closing capacity. This may be expected to result in areas of lung with greatly diminished or absent ventilation but with their circulation little changed. Following equilibration of trapped gas with pulmonary arterial blood, circulation through these areas will then constitute a shunt.

There can be little doubt that this phenomenon is a major factor in the increased alveolar–arterial P_{O_2} gradient observed during anaesthesia. Several workers have demonstrated a significant correlation between the decrease in FRC and the increase in alveolar–arterial (A–a) P_{O_2} gradient occurring after the induction of anaesthesia and also in the postoperative period.

Many features of the change in FRC have now been characterized and the reader is referred to Nunn (1977c). In summary, the FRC decreases very rapidly after induction and apparently remains constant until some time after recovery from anaesthesia. Oxygen absorption collapse does not seem to be a major aetiological factor and the decrease in FRC cannot be explained on the basis of trapped gas causing a measurement artifact. Changes are more marked in older patients but the decrease in FRC seems to be the same whether the anaesthetized patient is breathing spontaneously or paralysed and ventilated artificially (Hewlett *et al.*, 1974a). Expiratory muscle activity, although a common feature of anaesthesia with spontaneous breathing, does not appear to affect the magnitude of the change in FRC.

Cause of the change in FRC

Froese and Bryan (1974), using lateral chest radiography, have shown that, following the induction of anaesthesia with or without paralysis, the diaphragm rises into the chest by an amount roughly compatible with the decrease in lung volume (*Figure 25.2*). However, measurements of circumference of the chest have shown that the volume of the rib cage is only slightly decreased (Jones *et al.*, 1979).

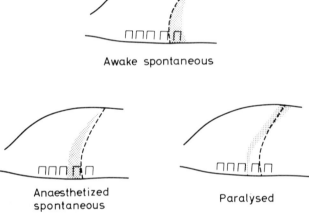

Awake spontaneous

Anaesthetized spontaneous

Paralysed

Figure 25.2
Position of the confines of the thoracic cavity shown by lateral chest radiography. The dashed line is the control position of the diaphragm at FRC in the supine position. Stippled area represents diaphragmatic excursion during tidal breathing. (Reproduced from Froese and Bryan, 1974, with permission of the authors and the Editor, *Anesthesiology*)

It is at present open to speculation why induction of anaesthesia should cause the end-expiratory position of the diaphragm to rise. One possibility is that the diaphragm is not fully relaxed at the end of expiration in the conscious supine subject. If this is the case, the changed pattern of breathing during anaesthesia with or without paralysis would accord with loss of any residual end-expiratory muscle tone. Unfortunately electro-myographic study of the diaphragm in man is difficult and studies in other species might not be relevant. A second possibility is increased pressure on the lower surface of the diaphragm due to altered distribution of blood volume away from the periphery towards the abdomen. This view is supported by the observations of Jones *et al.* (1979) that induction of anaesthesia resulted in only a small decrease in rib cage volume (−29 ml) and an increase in abdominal volume (+130 ml). The decrease in FRC occurs when thiopentone alone is used as the anaesthetic (Westbrook *et al.*, 1973), and therefore the explanation cannot be sought in terms of diffusion of nitrous oxide into closed gas compartments in the bowel.

There is ample evidence that the FRC can be restored to normal or above normal by the application of positive end-expiratory pressure (PEEP). Contrary to what might be expected, this does little to improve the arterial Po_2 during anaesthesia (Nunn, Bergman and Coleman, 1965; Whyche *et al.*, 1973). It seems probable that PEEP decreases the 'shunt' (usually about 10% during anaesthesia) but also decreases the cardiac output and therefore the mixed venous saturation. As a result there is a decreased shunt flow of more heavily desaturated blood so that the arterial Po_2 is unchanged.

Anaesthesia and the closing volume

Two studies have reported that the closing volume is unchanged following the induction of anaesthesia (Gilmour, Burnham and Craig, 1976; Hedenstierna, McCarthy and Bergström, 1976).

MECHANICAL PROPERTIES OF THE LUNGS

Airway resistance

Typical values for the total respiratory resistance during an uncomplicated anaesthetic are in the range $0.3–0.6$ $kPa \cdot l^{-1} \cdot s^{-1}$ ($3–6$ $cmH_2O \cdot l^{-1} \cdot s^{-1}$). Considerably higher values may be found in patients with obstructive airway disease or when bronchospasm complicates the anaesthetic. Minimal values are, however, about double the normal value in the conscious subject. The change is mainly due to the decrease in FRC referred to above. Airway resistance is a hyperbolic function of lung volume rising sharply as the lung volume decreases below the FRC (Nunn, 1977d).

In addition to this 'normal' increase in airway resistance following the induction of anaesthesia, there are many abnormal causes of increased airway resistance, some of which may be life threatening. These may be drug induced, caused by histamine release, foreign bodies, deformation of the respiratory tract, muscle spasm, secretions and so on. In addition, apparatus through which the patient breathes may become obstructed. Although limitations of space preclude a discussion of this important topic, it remains a major responsibility of the anaesthetist to ensure that airway resistance is minimal at all times. Major difficulties may arise in cases of severe bronchospasm arising from inhalation of gastric contents or as an abnormal response to a drug.

Compliance

It has been known for many years that the elastic recoil of the lungs (and therefore the whole respiratory system) is increased after the induction of anaesthesia. A typical value for static compliance of lungs + chest wall in the anaesthetized paralysed patient is 0.85 $l \cdot kPa^{-1}$ (85 $ml \cdot cmH_2O^{-1}$) compared with about 1.2 $l \cdot kPa^{-1}$ (120 $ml \cdot cmH_2O^{-1}$) in the supine conscious patient. The difference may be traced to the pulmonary compliance, the compliance of the relaxed chest wall being probably unchanged by the induction of anaesthesia.

The change in compliance is, like the change in airway resistance related to the change in lung volume, and it is helpful to consider the excellent study of Westbrook *et al.* (1973) who studied pressure/volume relationships in supine volunteers before and after the induction of anaesthesia and paralysis. They recorded pressure gradients across lungs and chest wall in relation to absolute lung volume. *Figure 25.3* shows their mean results at zero gas flow rates maintained for 3–7 seconds. The curves for

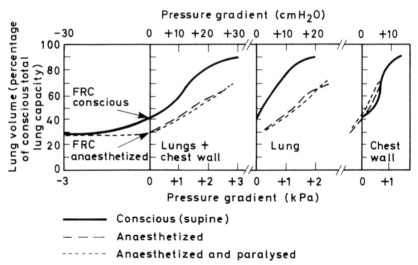

Figure 25.3
Pressure/volume relationships for supine volunteers before and after the induction of anaesthesia and paralysis. (Redrawn from the data of Westbrook *et al.*, 1973, except that the data for subatmospheric pressure have been derived from other sources)

lung + chest wall clearly show the reduction in FRC which follows the induction of anaesthesia and also the reduced slope of the pressure/volume curve (the compliance). It will also be seen that sustained inflation pressures of as much as 3 kPa (30 cmH_2O) will produce a lung volume of only 70% of total lung capacity as measured in the conscious subject. Inspection of the other two sets of curves will show that the major change is in the lungs rather than the chest wall. Institution of paralysis when the subjects were already anaesthetized did not cause major changes in any of the pressure/volume relationships, and the alterations were therefore primarily due to anaesthesia itself. It will also be seen from *Figure 25.3* that compliance, measured at lung volumes less than FRC, is extremely low during anaesthesia. Therefore the application of negative end-expiratory pressure (NEEP) will cause only small changes in lung volume. It was also noticed that the changes were not progressive during anaesthesia and could not be restored to control values by maximal inflation of the lungs.

DISTRIBUTION OF VENTILATION AND PERFUSION

Distribution of ventilation

During spontaneous respiration, the geometric pattern of the change in volume of the lung is influenced by the local action of the inspiratory muscles and the movements of the rib cage. During artificial ventilation the lungs and thoracic cage expand as a passive elastic body responding to the inflation pressure. It could only be coincidental if the geometric pattern of volume change was the same in each case.

Similar considerations apply to the differences between spontaneous breathing in conscious and anaesthetized patients. Differences in breathing patterns have been described above, and again it would not be surprising if these resulted in different regional patterns of inflation of the lung. It would, however, be an oversimplification to believe that regional lung ventilation simply followed changes in the outline of the confines of the thoracic cage since the lungs have considerable freedom to move within the thorax. It is, in fact, extremely difficult to define the pattern of distribution of gas within, for example, different lobes of the lungs.

In the lateral position, ventilation is preferentially distributed to the lower lung in the conscious subject breathing spontaneously. Rehder and Sessler (1973) have reported that this relationship is reversed in anaesthetized man, breathing spontaneously. In the paralysed artificially ventilated patient, the preferential ventilation of the lower lung is also lost (Rehder *et al.*, 1972; Rehder, Sessler and Rodarte, 1977). Gross changes may occur during thoracic surgery depending largely on the degree of retraction of the exposed lung (Nunn, 1961). Preferential ventilation of the upper lung is abolished by the application of positive end-expiratory pressure (PEEP) (Rehder, Wenthe and Sessler, 1973).

Regional ventilation (in terms of unit lung volume) has been studied *in horizontal slices of lung tissue* by the inhalation of ^{133}Xe. Hulands *et al.* (1970) found that anaesthesia and paralysis slightly increased the non-uniformity which is normally present (i.e. hyperventilation in the dependent and hypoventilation in the non-dependent parts of the lung of the supine subjects). However, the changes were minimal and of little functional relevance.

It is unlikely that these studies have covered every aspect of the effect of anaesthetics on distribution of ventilation. In particular, it is not possible at present to look at anything smaller than a horizontal slice of the lung a few centimetres thick and it is possible that maldistributions may be introduced within such a slice.

Distribution of pulmonary perfusion

In the conscious subject, perfusion is preferentially distributed to the dependent parts of the lung and this accords reasonably well with the distribution of ventilation. Hulands *et al.* (1970) reported no major changes when supine patients were anaesthetized and paralysed. There was no development of a zone I (absent perfusion) which might have provided an explanation of the increased alveolar dead space which is usually seen (see below).

The pulmonary hypoxic vasoconstrictor reflex may play a part in minimizing hypoxaemia due to maldistribution of pulmonary blood flow relative to ventilation. Certain anaesthetic agents may depress this reflex but reported results are highly variable and sometimes conflicting. They have been considered in detail in Chapter 24.

Distribution of ventilation/perfusion ratios ($\dot{V}/\dot{Q}$)

Maldistributions of either ventilation or perfusion are of little importance if both are equally affected so that ventilation/perfusion ratios remain normal in each functional unit of the lung. Considering whole lungs in the lateral position, $\dot{V}/\dot{Q}$ ratios are approximately equal in conscious man. Due to the change in distribution of ventilation described above, this ideal relationship is apparently lost during anaesthesia, with or without artificial ventilation and it may be grossly abnormal during thoracic surgery. In the supine position, Hulands *et al.* found slightly increased non-uniformity in $\dot{V}/\dot{Q}$ ratios in horizontal slices of the lung in three out of four patients. The changes were, however, insufficient to explain the full increase in alveolar–arterial $P\text{O}_2$ gradient which follows the induction of anaesthesia.

Understanding of the distribution of $\dot{V}/\dot{Q}$ ratios has been greatly enhanced by the technique developed by Dr West's group in San Diego. This method uses the retention and elimination of six inert tracer gases administered intravenously in solution and from this derives a distribution plot of blood flow and ventilation in relation to $\dot{V}/\dot{Q}$ ratios, examples of which are shown in *Figure 25.4*. The method can distinguish between true shunt and areas of very low $\dot{V}/\dot{Q}$ ratio (as shown for the lower graph in *Figure 25.4*).

The adaptation of this technique to the conditions of anaesthesia has presented a formidable technical challenge. In its original version (Wagner, Saltzman and West, 1974) halothane was one of the six tracer gases and it was necessary to replace this with enflurane so that the effect of halothane could be studied as an anaesthetic (Dueck, Rathbun and Wagner, 1978). Dueck *et al.* (1977) have studied a group of fairly elderly smokers before and then during halothane anaesthesia with artificial ventilation, paralysis being obtained with pancuronium. Following the induction of anaesthesia, the mean true shunt increased from 2.0% to 14% and the blood flow to areas of low (but not zero) $\dot{V}/\dot{Q}$ ratio increased from 2.5 to 16.0 units. No areas of high $\dot{V}/\dot{Q}$ ratio were created. In a personal communication

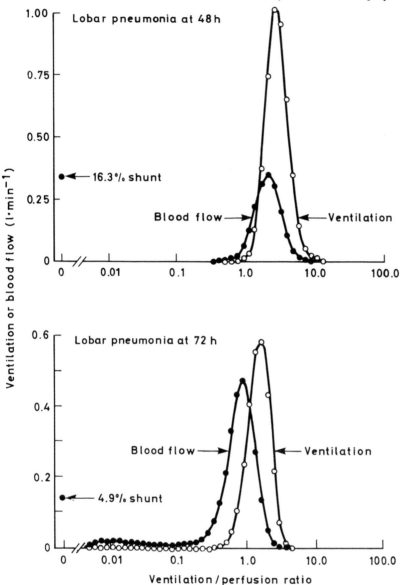

Figure 25.4
Distribution of ventilation and perfusion in relation to ventilation/
perfusion ratios in two subjects with lobar pneumonia. (From
Wagner *et al.*, 1975, by permission of the authors and the Editor,
the *Journal of Applied Physiology*)

Dueck reported that there was no consistent pattern of change: some
patients tended to develop a true shunt while other patients developed
areas of low $\dot{V}/\dot{Q}$ ratio. All changes were, however, roughly compatible
with the observed alveolar–arterial P_{O_2} gradient. During anaesthesia,
patients breathed 37% oxygen.

This most important study has clearly demonstrated that anaesthesia does in fact result in either increased shunts of areas of low $\dot{V}/\dot{Q}$ ratio, a change which had previously been inferred from the blood gas studies referred to below. It should also be noted that the changes reported by Dueck are consistent with those that would be expected in older patients from the decrease in FRC referred to above.

INDICES OF MALDISTRIBUTION

Dead space

During anaesthesia, the physiological dead space (V_D) *measured from the carina downwards* averages about 30% of the tidal volume (V_T) in patients without respiratory disease (Campbell, Nunn and Peckett, 1958).

This is about double the value in the normal conscious subject, in whom about 15% of the tidal volume is dead space below the carina and another 15% is dead space above the carina. Therefore it follows that, during anaesthesia, the intrapulmonary part of the physiological dead space is substantially increased. If the usual apparatus dead space is included, the V_D/V_T ratio of an anaesthetized patient with an endotracheal tube is about 50% and, if a facemask is used, the V_D/V_T ratio averages 67% (Kain, Panday and Nunn, 1969). This represents a substantial loss of efficiency of ventilation during anaesthesia and the effect is almost the same for anaesthetized patients breathing spontaneously as for those who are paralysed and ventilated artificially (Nunn and Hill, 1960).

The latter workers demonstrated that the increase in the physiological dead space during anaesthesia is in the alveolar rather than the anatomical compartment. Therefore, the explanation must lie in the ventilation of unperfused spaces at the alveolar level. Nevertheless, the mechanism of this has never been explained. There is no evidence for a reduction of pulmonary arterial pressure sufficient to deprive the uppermost parts of the lung of their perfusion and no areas of very high $\dot{V}/\dot{Q}$ ratio were found in the study of Dueck and his colleagues (see above).

Functionally, the effect of the increased V_D/V_T ratio is partly offset by the reduced metabolic rate which occurs during anaesthesia and partly by the use of an endotracheal tube which bypasses the dead space of the upper respiratory tract. During artificial ventilation it is almost always possible to increase the minute volume sufficiently to obtain carbon dioxide homoeostasis in spite of an increased V_D/V_T ratio. However, during anaesthesia with spontaneous respiration, the minute volume is often insufficient to keep the P_{CO_2} within normal limits and increases up to 10 kPa (75 mmHg) are a normal consequence of unassisted respiration in patients anaesthetized with halothane.

Pathological increases in V_D/V_T ratio may complicate anaesthesia and the most important causes are pulmonary embolism, pulmonary arterial hypotension and obstruction of a pulmonary artery with continuing ventilation.

Pulmonary shunting

Chapter 86 discusses the type of respiratory failure in which the increase in alveolar–arterial Po_2 gradient can be considered as being the result of a mixture of pulmonary arterial blood with pulmonary venous blood. This may be referred to simply as shunting. There can be little doubt that in many cases considered as 'shunting', there are areas of lung with $\dot{V}/\dot{Q}$ ratios which are very low but not zero. Indeed the study of Dueck *et al.* (1977) has shown that either or both types of dysfunction may follow the induction of anaesthesia.

The distinction between perfusion of areas with zero and very low $\dot{V}/\dot{Q}$ ratio is largely academic and compensation for the defect is normally by increasing the inspired oxygen concentration (FIo_2) in each case.

Soon after the development of the polarograph, it was shown that a moderate degree of 'shunting' was a normal feature of anaesthesia in patients without cardiorespiratory disease. This was manifest as an alveolar–arterial Po_2 gradient of about 20 kPa (150 mmHg) during the inhalation of high oxygen concentrations and it was shown that this was unlikely to be due to absorption collapse (Panday and Nunn, 1968). More sophisticated studies by other workers (cited in Nunn, 1977e) showed that there was a true shunt of the order of 10% of cardiac output in patients who had shunts within the normal range (2–6%) before the induction of anaesthesia. These measurements were based upon mixing equations using oxygen, and the indicated values for 'shunt' would include components due to perfusion of lung zones with very low $\dot{V}/\dot{Q}$ ratios.

For a given shunt, the alveolar–arterial Po_2 gradient is a function of the FIo_2. It is therefore convenient to plot arterial Po_2 values against FIo_2 during anaesthesia on an isoshunt diagram (*Figure 25.5*). Mean values for 15 studies fall along the 10% virtual shunt line and indicate that maintenance of an arterial Po_2 above the normal value requires, *inter alia*, a minimum FIo_2 of 30% during an uncomplicated anaesthetic. Considerably higher values are required during thoracic surgery or if there is any other cause of maldistribution of ventilation and perfusion. Pathological shunts may be present before anaesthesia or may arise as complications of anaesthesia from such causes as retained secretions, pulmonary collapse, pulmonary oedema, endobronchial intubation, etc.

HOMOEOSTASIS OF BLOOD GASES

Pco_2

Patients, left to breathe spontaneously during anaesthesia with nitrous oxide supplemented by either halothane or opiates, tend to develop hypercapnia. It is normal British practice to tolerate this hypercapnia, which does not usually exceed 10 kPa (75 mmHg) and does not appear to do the patient any detectable harm. In the United States, however, the hypoventilation is viewed with abhorrence and it is customary to assist

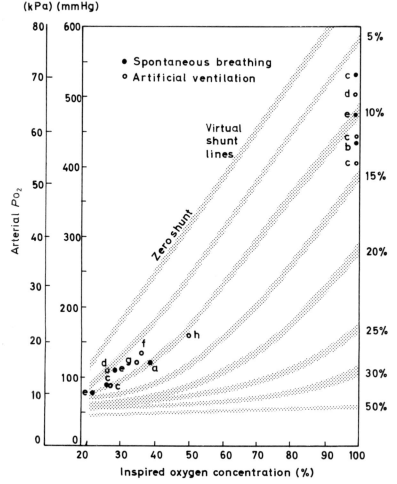

Figure 25.5
Mean values for arterial Po_2 plotted against inspired oxygen concentrations for 15 published studies of anaesthetized patients. (a) Michenfelder, Fowler and Theye, 1966; (b) Marshall *et al.*, 1969; (c) Price *et al.*, 1969; (d) Nunn, Bergman and Coleman, 1965; (e) Nunn, 1964; (f) Hewlett *et al.*, 1974b; (g) Theye and Tuohy, 1964; (h) Gold and Helrich, 1967

ventilation by manual compression of the reservoir bag. It must be reported that arterial Pco_2 levels as high as 21.3 kPa (160 mmHg) are apparently accepted by some anaesthetists in the course of routine closed circuit anaesthesia (Birt and Cole, 1965). The extreme level of 31.5 kPa (236 mmHg) was observed in the United States during thoracic surgery by Ellison, Ellison and Hamilton (1955).

During artificial ventilation, Pco_2 depends largely upon the ventilation which is selected by the anaesthetist. Monitoring of the arterial Pco_2 is unusual and is seldom necessary.

P_{O_2}

The normal approach to gaseous homoeostasis is to adjust the minute volume to obtain the required P_{CO_2} and then to adjust the F_{IO_2} to obtain the required P_{O_2}. Arterial P_{O_2} is not usually monitored during routine anaesthesia and is inferred from the minute volume and the F_{IO_2}, usually intuitively. It is therefore essential to err on the side of safety, to allow for those patients who show the largest alveolar—arterial P_{O_2} gradients. *Figure 25.5* shows that the *average* patient can be maintained with an arterial P_{O_2} of 13.3 kPa (100 mmHg) if the F_{IO_2} is 30%. Due to normal variability, however, this level of F_{IO_2} results in some patients having arterial P_{O_2} levels as low as 10 kPa (75 mmHg) during uncomplicated routine anaesthesia (Nunn, 1964; Nunn, Bergman and Coleman, 1965) and it may be felt preferable to maintain F_{IO_2} above 35%. It would appear to be unwise to reduce F_{IO_2} below 30%. A most dangerous situation develops when F_{IO_2} is unintentionally reduced due to malfunction of the anaesthetic circuit or oxygen supply.

Some anaesthetists prefer to use an F_{IO_2} in the range 90—100%. This ensures an alveolar P_{O_2} of about 85—90 kPa (640—675 mmHg) and an arterial P_{O_2} of at least 35 kPa (260 mmHg) in an uncomplicated anaesthetic. This virtually excludes the possibility of hypoxaemia, even in the presence of severe underventilation. Such an approach, however, also precludes the use of nitrous oxide and may result in absorption collapse of the lung under certain circumstances (Potgieter, 1959).

SUMMARY

Routine anaesthesia is associated with a variety of abnormalities of respiratory function. Many of these can be traced to a reduced intercostal muscle activity and to a decrease in the FRC although the cause of these changes is not fully understood. Gaseous homoeostasis is normally maintained by a combination of factors including the depression of the patient's metabolism, tracheal intubation, artificial ventilation and an increased F_{IO_2}. Monitoring of respiratory variables is unusual in routine anaesthetic practice and it is rare for mortality or morbidity to be due to the alterations in respiratory function in an uncomplicated anaesthetic.

In contrast, there are relatively uncommon situations during anaesthesia in which respiratory function may become a limiting factor for the patient's survival. Such situations include patients with gross pre-existing respiratory disease, certain types of surgery, malfunctions of anaesthetic equipment and some types of respiratory failure arising as complications during anaesthesia. These include bronchospasm, inhaled gastric contents and pulmonary oedema.

References

Aub, J. C. and DuBois, E. F. (1917). The basal metabolism of old men. *Archs intern. Med.* **19**, 823–831

Bay, J., Nunn, J. F. and Prys-Roberts, C. (1968). Factors influencing arterial P_{O_2} during recovery from anaesthesia. *Br. J. Anaesth.* **40**, 398–407

Birt, C. and Cole, P. V. (1965). Some physiological effects of closed circuit halothane anaesthesia. *Anaesthesia* **20**, 258–268

Campbell, E. J. M., Nunn, J. F. and Peckett, B. W. (1958). A comparison of artificial ventilation and spontaneous respiration with particular reference to ventilation–blood flow relationships. *Br. J. Anaesth.* **30**, 166–175

Davy, H. (1800). *Researches, Chemical and Philosophical; Chiefly concerning Nitrous Oxide, or Dephlogisticated Nitrous Air, and Its Respiration. A Facsimile Reproduction.* J. Johnson, London, reprinted by Butterworths, London 1972

Dueck, F., Rathbun, M. and Wagner, P. D. (1978). Chromatographic analysis of multiple tracer inert gases in the presence of anesthetic gases. *Anesthesiology* **49**, 31–36

Dueck, R., Rathbun, M., Clausen, J. and Wagner, P. D. (1977). *Altered Distribution of Pulmonary Ventilation and Blood Flow in Human Subjects following Induction of Inhalation Anesthesia.* Am. Soc. Anesthesiologists, Abstracts of Scientific papers, p. 223–224

Eger, E. L., Dolan, W. M., Stevens, W. C., Miller, R. D. and Way, W. L. (1972). Surgical stimulation antagonizes the respiratory depression produced by forane. *Anesthesiology* **36**, 544–549

Ellison, R. G., Ellison, L. T. and Hamilton, W. F. (1955). Analysis of respiratory acidosis during anaesthesia. *Ann. Surg.* **141**, 375–382

Freund, F., Roos, A. and Dodd, R. B. (1964). Expiratory activity of the abdominal muscles in man during general anesthesia. *J. appl. Physiol.* **19**, 693–697

Froese, A. B. and Bryan, A. C. (1974). Effects of anesthesia and paralysis on diaphragmatic mechanics in man. *Anesthesiology* **41**, 242–255

Gilmour, I., Burnham, M. and Craig, D. B. (1976). Closing capacity measurement during general anesthesia. *Anesthesiology* **45**, 477–482

Gold, M. I. and Helrich, M. (1967). Ventilation and blood gases in anaesthetized patients. *Can. Anaesth. Soc. J.* **14**, 424–434

Hedenstierna, G., McCarthy, G. and Bergström, M. (1976). Airway closure during mechanical ventilation. *Anesthesiology* **44**, 114–123

Hewlett, A. M., Hulands, G. H., Nunn, J. F. and Heath, J. R. (1974a). Functional residual capacity during anaesthesia. II. Spontaneous respiration. *Br. J. Anaesth.* **46**, 486–494

Hewlett, A. M., Hulands, G. H., Nunn, J. F. and Milledge, J. S. (1974b). Functional residual capacity during anaesthesia. III: Artificial ventilation. *Br. J. Anaesth.* **46**, 495–503

Hulands, G. H., Greene, R., Iliff, L. D. and Nunn, J. F. (1970). Influence of anaesthesia on the regional distribution of perfusion and ventilation in the lung. *Clin. Sci.* **38**, 451–460

Jones, J. G., Faithfull, D., Jordan, C. and Minty, B. (1979). Rib cage movement during halothane anaesthesia in man. *Br. J. Anaesth.* In Press

Kain, M. L., Panday, J. and Nunn, J. F. (1969). The effect of intubation on the deadspace during halothane anaesthesia. *Br. J. Anaesth.* **41**, 94–102

Knill, R. L. and Gelb, A. W. (1978). Ventilatory responses to hypoxia and hypercapnia during halothane sedation and anaesthesia in man. *Anesthesiology* **49**, 244–251

Larsen, C. P., Eger, E. I., Muallem, M., Buechel, D. R., Munson, E. S. and Eisele, J. H. (1969). The effects of diethyl ether and methoxyflurane on ventilation. *Anesthesiology* **30**, 174–184

Marshall, B. E., Cohen, P. J., Klingenmaier, C. H. and Aukberg, S. (1969). Pulmonary venous admixture before, during, and after halothane: oxygen anesthesia in man. *J. appl. Physiol.* **27**, 653–657

Michenfelder, J. D., Fowler, W. S. and Theye, R. A. (1966). CO_2 levels and pulmonary shunting in anesthetized man. *J. appl. Physiol.* **21**, 1471–1476

Ngai, S. H., Katz, R. L. and Farhie, S. E. (1965). Respiratory effects of trichlorethylene, halothane and methoxyflurane in the cat. *J. Pharmac. exp. Ther.* **148**, 123–130

Nunn, J. F. (1958). Ventilation and end-tidal carbon dioxide tension. *Anaesthesia* **13**, 124–137

Nunn, J. F. (1961). The distribution of inspired gas during thoracic surgery. *Ann. R. Coll. Surg.* **28**, 2–16

Nunn, J. F. (1964). Factors influencing the arterial oxygen tension during halothane anaesthesia with spontaneous respiration. *Br. J. Anaesth.* **36**, 327–341

Nunn, J. F. (1977). *Applied Respiratory Physiology*, 2nd edn. London: Butterworths. a – p. 30; b – p. 121; c – p. 67; d – p. 117; e – p. 301; f – p. 302

Nunn, J. F., Bergman, N. A. and Coleman, A. J. (1965). Factors influencing the arterial oxygen during anaesthesia with artificial ventilation. *Br. J. Anaesth.* **37**, 898–914

Nunn, J. F. and Ezi-Ashi, T. I. (1961). The respiratory effects of resistance to breathing in anesthetized man. *Anesthesiology* **22**, 174–185

Nunn, J. F. and Hill, D. W. (1960). Respiratory dead space and arterial to end-tidal CO_2 tension difference in anesthetized man. *J. appl. Physiol.* 15, 383–389

Nunn, J. F. and Matthews, R. L. (1959). Gaseous exchange during halothane anaesthesia: the steady respiratory state. *Br. J. Anaesth.* 31, 330–340

Panday, J. and Nunn, J. F. (1968). Failure to demonstrate progressive falls of arterial Po_2 during anaesthesia. *Anaesthesia* 23, 38–46

Potgieter, S. V. (1959). Atelectasis: its evolution during upper urinary tract surgery. *Br. J. Anaesth.* 31, 472–483

Price, H. L., Cooperman, L. H., Warden, J. C., Morris, J. J. and Smith, T. C. (1969). Pulmonary hemodynamics during general anesthesia in man. *Anesthesiology* 30, 629–636

Rehder, K. and Sessler, D. (1973). Function of each lung in spontaneously breathing man anesthetized with thiopental–meperidine. *Anesthesiology* 38, 320–327

Rehder, K., Sessler, D. and Rodarte, R. (1977). Regional intrapulmonary gas distribution in awake and anesthetized-paralyzed man. *J. appl. Physiol.* 42, 391–402

Rehder, K., Wenthe, F. M. and Sessler, A. D. (1973). Function of each lung during mechanical ventilation with ZEEP and with PEEP in man anesthetized with thiopental–meperidine. *Anesthesiology* 39, 597–606

Rehder, K., Hatch, D. J., Sessler, A. D. and Fowler, W. S. (1972). The function of each lung of anesthetized and paralyzed man during mechanical ventilation. *Anesthesiology* 37, 16–26

Robertson, J. D. and Reid, D. D. (1952). Standards for the basal metabolism of normal people in Britain. *Lancet* i, 940–943

Robson, J. G., Houseley, M. A. and Solis-Quiroga, O. H. (1963). The mechanism of respiratory arrest with sodium pentobarbital and sodium thiopental. *Ann. N.Y. Acad. Sci.* 109, 494–504

Theye, R. A. (1972). The contributions of individual organ systems to the decrease in whole-body $\dot{V}o_2$ with halothane. *Anesthesiology* 37, 367–372

Theye, R. A. and Tuohy, G. F. (1964). Oxygen uptake during light halothane anesthesia in man. *Anesthesiology* 25, 627–633

Tusiewicz, K., Bryan, A. C. and Froese, A. B. (1977). Contributions of changing rib cage – diaphragm interactions to the ventilatory depression of halothane anesthesia. *Anesthesiology* 47, 327–337

Wagner, P. D., Saltzman, H. A. and West, J. B. (1974). Measurement of continuous distribution of ventilation–perfusion ratios: theory. *J. appl. Physiol.* 36, 588–599

Wagner, P. D., Laravuso, R. B., Goldzimmer, E., Naumann, P. F. and West, J. B. (1975). Distributions of ventilation–perfusion ratios in dogs with normal and abnormal lungs. *J. appl. Physiol.* 38, 1099–1109

Weiskopf, R. B., Raymond, L. W. and Severinghaus, J. W. (1974). Effects of halothane on canine respiratory responses to hypoxia with and without hypercarbia. *Anesthesiology* 41, 350–360

Westbrook, P. R., Stubbs, S. E., Sessler, A. D., Rehder, K. and Hyatt, R. E. (1973). Effects of anesthesia and muscle paralysis on respiratory mechanics in normal man. *J. appl. Physiol.* 34, 81–86

Whyche, M. Q., Teichner, R. L., Kallos, T., Marshall, B. E. and Smith, T. C. (1973). Effects of continuous positive-pressure breathing on functional residual capacity and arterial oxygenation during intra-abdominal operations. *Anesthesiology* 38, 68–74

26 Anaesthesia and the patient with respiratory disease
James S. Milledge and John F. Nunn

One of the commonest problems encountered by anaesthetists on their preoperative rounds is the patient with chronic airways obstruction due to chronic bronchitis or emphysema. The advent of cleaner air in our cities and less tar in cigarettes may have reduced the severity of the problem in the community but in surgical wards the rising average age of patients has had the opposite effect. Adequate preoperative assessment of these and other patients with respiratory disease is important in order to identify those at risk so that they may be given adequate preoperative treatment, special care during anaesthesia and adequate treatment postoperatively, including artificial ventilation when indicated. Only very rarely will assessment mean a decision not to operate.

CLINICAL ASSESSMENT

From the point of view of anaesthesia, assessment is essentially in terms of function. Important points include the presence of actual or impending ventilatory failure, inability to clear secretions, loss of ventilatory response to CO_2, hypoxaemia and its causes.

History

It is unrealistic to expect the anaesthetist to take a long detailed history from patients, nor should this be necessary. The essential questions are:

Do you have a cough?
Do you bring up sputum (or phlegm)?
Do you get short of breath when walking uphill?
Do you smoke?

If any of the first three questions produces an affirmative answer, further questions should be put to find out how severe and of what duration is the cough, sputum and breathlessness. Patients with chronic bronchitis tend to minimize their symptoms and disability. They frequently deny any cough in answer to the first question, but they will often admit to being life-long smokers and then will allow that they do have a smoker's cough. They may deny breathlessness but later agree that they get puffed going upstairs and assume that this is natural for their age. During the brief history taking, note will be taken of any breathlessness at rest and of the ability to complete a sentence in one breath.

As in all cases, it is important to ascertain whether the patient is receiving any drugs which might influence the course of anaesthesia (see Chapter 48).

Examination

In most patients with chest disease the objective of the clinical examination will be (1) to assess the degree of airways obstruction, (2) to assess the degree of sputum retention. The clinical examination will also seek to exclude or confirm the presence of localized disease, e.g. an area of persistent coarse râles indicating an area of bronchiectasis, or an area of stony dullness and absent breath sounds indicating a pleural effusion.

SIGNS OF AIRWAYS OBSTRUCTION

In airways obstruction due to either bronchitis, emphysema or asthma, the chest is hyperinflated. The first group of signs of airways obstruction are, therefore, the signs of hyperinflation. On inspection the chest seems to be held in an inspiratory position with the ribs held up and out. This is best seen in the upper chest. There may be an increase in the normal dorsal kyphosis. These two effects cause an increase in the anteroposterior diameter of the chest. On percussion the note will be hyper-resonant and the diaphragmatic dullness will be lower than normal. However, both these are a matter of degree and, except in cases with gross changes, it is not possible to be certain of their significance. The best sign of hyper-inflation is the obliteration of the cardiac dullness. The hyperinflated lung intervenes sufficiently between the heart and chest wall to give a resonant note on percussion (and muffle the heart sounds). This is usually a quite definite sign, the cardiac dullness either is or is not obliterated and it correlates better than other signs with increase in functional residual capacity.

The most characteristic sign of airways obstruction is the production of high pitched rhonchi or wheezes. These are thought to be produced by the high velocity of air jetting through narrowed or collapsed airways. In many cases they can be heard from the foot of the bed and are usually easily audible with the stethoscope placed anywhere on the chest but they may not be heard in two circumstances where there is increased airways resistance. In some patients, well relaxed at rest, the tidal range may be just above the lung volume at which widespread airway closure occurs. If the patient breathes out a little further, expiratory wheezes are easily heard. The other situation is in very severe airways obstruction, usually due to asthma, when air flow through narrow bronchi may be too slow to produce audible wheeze. In a patient with obviously severe asthma a silent chest is a very sinister sign.

The third sign of airways obstruction is the prolongation of the expiratory phase of respiration. This is best elicited by asking the patient to take a deep breath and blow it all out quickly, i.e. a forced vital capacity manoeuvre. The examiner auscultates over the larynx using the bell of the stethoscope. Listening in this way to many patients one comes to appreciate the sound and duration of expiration from the normal bronchial tree. The sound lasts only one to two seconds and has no added high pitched wheezes. The increase in duration of expiration is very obvious, even with mild and moderate increases in airways resistance, and correlates well with FEV/VC ratios and with peak flow measurements (Lal, Ferguson and Campbell, 1964). In severe cases the patient is forced to take another breath before air flow stops so the actual duration no longer gives a true measure of his disability. During the same manoeuvre the wheezes can be easily heard and, in the two situations mentioned above, when they are absent in the ordinary chest examination this manoeuvre will bring them out.

SPUTUM RETENTION

The presence of sputum retained in the airways is revealed by the production of moist sounds, coarse râles. These tend to be heard best at the lung bases posteriorly, the most dependent part of the lung. If they clear on coughing it is likely that there is little bronchial pathology, whereas râles persisting after coughing may indicate bronchiectasis. Sputum retention may result in complete bronchial obstruction in part of the lung when, with no air entry, râles cannot be produced: therefore the absence of air entry with a diminished percussion note can be a sign of severe sputum retention. Any patient with a history of chronic sputum production should have physiotherapy as part of his preoperative preparation, and the physiotherapists will be able to give valuable help in assessing the patient's readiness for operation with respect to sputum retention. The sputum should be inspected and its colour and consistency noted. Patients with purulent sputum should have a short course of broad spectrum antibiotics before elective surgery. Fine crepitations in the lung bases suggest left ventricular failure requiring diuretic therapy before operation.

INVESTIGATIONS

Chest x-ray

The value of the preoperative chest x-ray lies mainly in the exclusion of unsuspected chest disease, such as pulmonary tuberculosis or carcinoma of the bronchus. In cases of chronic sputum production the x-ray may reveal opacities indicative of areas of bronchopneumonia which require preoperative treatment. Signs of hyperinflation will be seen in cases with increased airways obstruction and the heart size may be increased as part of the picture of cor pulmonale. The lung markings are usually rather prominent in bronchitis and there is often upper zone blood diversion, i.e. the vessels are more obvious in the upper than in the lower zones, a reversal of the usual pattern. In emphysema, areas of diminished lung markings are seen, especially in the bases, and in severe cases actual bullae may be seen.

Blood count

A high white count with increase in the polymorph neutrophils is suggestive of lung infection in these patients, and a haemoglobin above 16 g·dl^{-1} or haematocrit above 50% is suggestive of chronic hypoxia indicating the need for blood gas measurements.

Arterial blood gases

The primary function of the lung is to exchange oxygen and carbon dioxide between blood and air so as to supply the body with oxygen and excrete unwanted carbon dioxide. The partial pressure of O_2 and CO_2 in the arterial blood provide a good index of over-all lung function in relation to metabolic requirements. In simple terms there are three main patterns of derangement of blood gases, viz:

	P_{O_2}	P_{CO_2}
Hyperventilation	↑	↓
Hypoventilation	↓	↑
Shunting of transfer defect	↓	− or ↓

Hyperventilation is most commonly due to anxiety, which may well be due to fear or pain of the arterial puncture and is of no clinical importance.

Hypoventilation may be due either to a central depression, e.g. by drugs or chronically raised P_{CO_2}, or to pulmonary mechanical dysfunction. The commonest lung function disturbance leading to hypoventilation is chronic airways obstruction, as in chronic bronchitis. These patients are known as 'blue bloaters'. They are cyanosed, hypercapnic and over-weight. However, the relationship between airways obstruction and ventilation is complex, and patients at the other end of the spectrum — the 'pink puffers' with just as severe airways obstruction have more normal P_{O_2} and normal or low P_{CO_2}. They are very dyspnoeic, tend to be underweight and probably have more emphysema.

By transfer defect is meant those situations in which, although the bellows function of the lung is more or less normal, there is loss of efficiency in the transfer of gas from air to blood. These include the diffuse parenchymatous lung conditions such as sarcoidosis, fibrosing alveolitis, pneumoconiosis and shock lung, and more localized conditions such as collapse, bronchopneumonias and pulmonary emboli. The transfer defect results mainly in a reduction in arterial Po_2 while the Pco_2 typically remains normal or may be reduced. This is because although the transfer of CO_2 is also affected, hyperventilation results in more CO_2 being excreted from the normal part of the lung which compensates for the poor CO_2 transfer in more affected parts whereas, for O_2, because of the slope and shape of its dissociation curve, such compensation is not possible. For a detailed account of this mechanism see Nunn (1977). For practical purposes the transfer defects can be considered as if the hypoxaemia were due to shunting of a proportion of the cardiac output from the right to left sides of the heart, bypassing the gas exchanging parts of the lungs. From knowledge of the arterial Po_2, inspired Po_2 and blood haemoglobin concentration together with a measured or assumed value for arterial–mixed venous O_2 content difference, it is possible to calculate the value of this shunt as a fraction of the cardiac output (Nunn, 1977). It has been found (Lawler and Hewlett, 1978) that in most patients who are hypoxaemic in the intensive therapy unit, the value for this shunt remains, for practical purposes, unchanged as inspired Po_2 is changed from 21% to 100%. The practical value of this finding is that by measuring the arterial Po_2 at any known inspired O_2 concentration, the necessary inspired O_2 concentration to achieve a desired arterial Po_2 can be calculated.

In preoperative assessment it is usual to measure blood gases while breathing air. The importance of measuring the blood gases in patients with obstructive lung disease lies not only in assessing the severity and effect of their airways obstruction but also because it provides the best index of their postoperative requirement for ventilatory support. Milledge and Nunn (1975) found that in a series of 12 patients with severe airways obstruction ($FEV_{1.0}$ = 1 litre or less) given good preoperative preparation there was no problem *during* anaesthesia in any case. Patients with low arterial Po_2 (less than 7 kPa or 52.5 mmHg) but with normal or near normal Pco_2 (less than 6.5 kPa or 49 mmHg) need careful monitoring postoperatively with some added inspired oxygen. Such patients do not usually require ventilatory support, whereas patients with both hypoxaemia and hypercapnia (Pco_2 greater than 6.5 kPa or 49 mmHg) are likely to need ventilatory support for a time postoperatively. These patients also have a high risk of postoperative pulmonary complications (Stein *et al.*, 1962).

Lung function tests

The value of lung function tests is to provide a physiological diagnosis of the disturbance in lung function and an objective measure of its severity in patients. The commonest type of disability is that of increased airways resistance and fortunately the simplest tests of ventilatory capacity lung function, although not measuring the actual airways resistance, do give a good index of it.

BEDSIDE TESTS

These simple tests which can be performed at the bedside are:

The measurement of vital capacity (VC)
Forced expiratory volume one second ($FEV_{1.0}$)
Peak flow rate (PFR)

The vital capacity is measured by asking the patient to exhale fully from a full inspiration into a spirometer. This is first done slowly then as quickly as possible. In healthy subjects the VC will be the same whether expiration is slow or fast, but in patients with airways obstruction the slow VC is found to be larger. This is usually taken as a true VC. $FEV_{1.0}$ is measured at the same time. It is the volume of air expired during the first one second of a forced vital capacity. Finally the peak flow is also measured on a forced expiration, using a Wright's peak flow meter or similar apparatus. All these tests are repeated three to five times and the best results recorded.

The VC is reduced in both airways obstruction and in restrictive defects of the lung. The degree of reduction compared with predicted values gives a measure of the severity of the defect. $FEV_{1.0}$ is also reduced by both obstructive and restrictive defects but the reduction is more marked in airways obstruction. Thus, in restrictive defects $FEV_{1.0}$ is reduced *pari passu* with VC so that the ratio $FEV_{1.0}/VC$ remains normal, whilst in airways obstruction this ratio is reduced below the predicted value. Diagnosis of obstructive defect is made by inspection of the ratio $FEV_{1.0}/VC$ but, since VC is also reduced, the severity of obstruction is assessed by the actual value of the $FEV_{1.0}$ compared with the predicted value for that patient. Patients with $FEV_{1.0}$ less than 50% predicted have severe airways obstruction and are liable to have raised Pa_{CO_2} values.

Peak flow rate is affected by the same factors as $FEV_{1.0}$ and there is normally a close correlation between them (Ritchie, 1962). Knowing the PFR alone gives less information than does knowing both the $FEV_{1.0}$ and the VC but the peak flow meter is so portable that, for quick bedside assessment in cases of obvious airways obstruction, it is very valuable. It is easier for the patient because only the initial fraction of the forced expiration is required whereas complete forced expiration often provokes coughing. However, there are two points that need watching in making the measurement:

(1) If a full inspiration is not made the reduction is greater for PFR than for $FEV_{1.0}$ and
(2) there are a few patients with severe airways obstruction revealed by $FEV_{1.0}$ who achieve a spuriously high PFR by a sort of trick cough manoeuvre.

The PFR is especially useful in following the progress of a patient with, for instance, asthma and with the advent of new, inexpensive 'mini' meters we can look forward to routine charting of the PFR as easily as for blood pressure. It must be remembered that these tests do require patient co-operation and whoever makes the measurement needs considerable patience, in some cases, to achieve meaningful results. These tests are usually repeated after a bronchodilator so as to indicate the reversibility of any airways obstruction.

Impairment of ventilatory capacity has two distinct implications for anaesthesia. Firstly there is the possibility of ventilatory failure in the postoperative period. Secondly, peak expiratory flow may be reduced below the level required for clearing secretions. Each of these two developments may require that the patient be subjected to prolonged endotracheal intubation and artificial ventilation. Postoperative pulmonary complications are more likely to occur in patients with reduced ventilatory capacity as shown by a number of studies (Stein *et al.,* 1962; Andersen and Ghia, 1970; Lockwood, 1973; Appleberg, Gordon and Fatti, 1974). However, adequate preoperative treatment can reduce the incidence of these complications very considerably (Stein and Cassara, 1970). Even very severe ventilatory impairment with $FEV_{1.0}$ less than one litre is quite compatible with an uncomplicated anaesthesia and postoperative course if the P_{CO_2} is not significantly raised and the patient well prepared for surgery (Milledge and Nunn, 1975).

LUNG VOLUMES

The total lung capacity (TLC) and its subdivisions, reserve volume (RV), functional residual capacity (FRC) etc. are measured together by helium dilution in a closed circuit spirometer system. The same volumes can also be measured using a body plethysmograph. In airways obstruction, hyperinflation is shown by an increase in TLC, but FRC and RV are increased even more, due to early closure of small airways resulting in air trapping. Thus, the RV/TLC ratio is increased. These changes are most marked in cases of emphysema. Conversely, patients with a restrictive defect, e.g. pulmonary fibrosis, show a reduction in all lung volumes.

TRANSFER TEST

The standard method of measuring the transfer of gases by the lung is the single breath carbon monoxide transfer test (previously called the diffusing capacity for CO). The test is rather complicated, both in concept and technique. The measurement has been greatly simplified by the use of electronically automated apparatus resulting in good reproducibility. It is clinically a very useful test in diagnosing and following up patients with dominant transfer defects, such as sarcoidosis and fibrosing alveolitis. The interpretation of this test has been well reviewed by McHardy (1972).

The patient takes a single vital capacity breath of a mixture of helium, carbon monoxide (trace concentrations) and air. He holds his breath for ten seconds then exhales through the apparatus which collects a sample of gas after a preset volume has washed out the dead space. From the analysis of inspired and expired He and CO, and the volume inhaled, it is possible to calculate the transfer factor (the amount of CO transferred by the lungs from air to blood per minute per unit of driving pressure Pco). The factors involved in the transfer of CO are similar to those for oxygen whose transfer we are interested in but cannot measure. Patients with an isolated transfer defect have no ventilatory problems (by definition) and although they are breathless on exertion and hypoxaemic, they present the anaesthetist with no problem since their hypoxaemia is commonly relieved by only a moderate increase in inspired oxygen concentration. They must, of course, be given oxygen postoperatively.

TESTS OF REGIONAL LUNG FUNCTION

These tests are only likely to be of interest in cases where pulmonary surgery is contemplated and lung function is borderline. Even in such cases the results must be interpreted cautiously since the removal of a lobe or a lung would not leave the remaining lung function unaltered. Bronchospirometry, in which the ventilation VC and oxygen uptake of each lung is measured separately using a double lumen tube, was the earliest test in this group. It is possible in certain cases to confirm a clinical impression that, for instance, a lung destroyed by tuberculosis is non-functioning and might be removed without further impairment of lung function, but most centres have abandoned bronchospirometry because it really gives no information that could not be inferred from the clinical examination and chest x-ray. Also, it can be quite distressing for the patient.

Perfusion scans using intravenously injected ^{99m} technetium-labelled macroaggregates and a γ-camera are less traumatic for the patient and more informative. They are very useful in the diagnosis of pulmonary embolus though they cannot distinguish between perfusion defects due to vascular occlusion and those due to emphysema. The recently introduced krypton ventilation scan (Fazio and Jones, 1975) overcomes this latter problem. ^{81m}Krypton is inhaled continuously via a simple mask and, because of its short radioactive half-life (13 seconds), the concentration of radioactivity in any part of the lung is determined predominantly by the local ventilation. Thus a true ventilation scan is produced. Perfusion scans can be carried out simultaneously since the two isotopes have energy levels that are easily separable for the γ-camera. An area which is ventilated but not perfused is almost certainly the site of a pulmonary embolus. Changing patterns of perfusion and ventilation can be demonstrated in asthma before and after bronchodilator etc. The resolution of these scans is still poor compared with x-rays and at present, apart from their use in diagnosing pulmonary embolus, they have been of only limited use in clinical medicine. A drawback of the krypton ventilation scan is that the ^{81m}rubidium source needed to generate ^{81m}krypton cannot be available on a 24-hour, 7-days-a-week basis.

FLOW/VOLUME CURVES

In this test, the data buried in a simple spirometer trace of a forced vital capacity are displayed in such a way as to yield more information. Either the volume signal from a spirometer can be differentiated to give flow, or the flow signal from a pneumotachograph or other flow transducer can be integrated to give volume. The two signals are then plotted against each other to produce the flow/volume curve (*Figure 26.1*). From the curve it

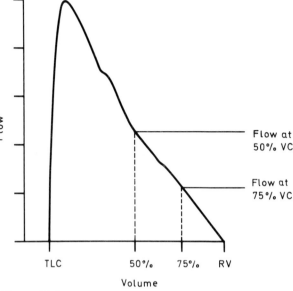

Figure 26.1
Flow/volume curve of a forced expiration in a normal subject. Note the almost straight descending limit. Indices derived from the curve are shown

is possible to read off the flow at any lung volume. It is thought that the flow is limited mainly by resistance in the large airways at large lung volumes and by resistance in small airways at small lung volumes. Thus, in early disease of the small airways, at a time when the peak flow and $FEV_{1.0}$ are not definitely abnormal, the tail of the flow/volume curve at small lung volumes may assume a concavity because flow in this region is disproportionately reduced. However, the between subject variation of these curves is very large and, at least in patients with quite severe airways obstruction, flow/volume curves have not yet been shown to add significantly to our assessment of their lung function.

CLOSING CAPACITY

If a vital capacity breath of oxygen is inhaled, it is distributed preferentially to the lung bases. This is because, since these basal areas carry the weight of the lung in expiration, they have the greater capacity to fill during inspiration, whereas the lung units in the apex being stretched partly open even in expiration cannot fill so much during inspiration. Thus, at full inspiration there is a gradient of oxygen concentration maximal at the base and minimal at the apex. The nitrogen concentration grades in the opposite way. Now if the subject exhales slowly past an N_2 meter into

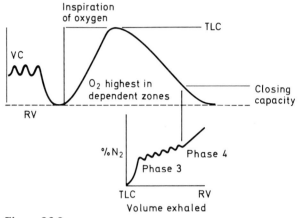

Figure 26.2
Measurement of closing balance by the resident gas technique (see text)

a spirometer, the nitrogen concentration is plotted against volume expired from TLC to RV. Four phases are seen in this trace (*Figure 26.2*):

(1) Zero nitrogen due to 100% oxygen in the dead space.
(2) Rapidly rising N_2 as the physiological dead space is washed out.
(3) The 'alveolar plateau' where N_2 rises slowly due to the fact that the lower part of the lung with low N_2 concentration tends to empty before the upper part of the lung. The slope of this line gives some index of the evenness of gas distribution in the lung, the steeper the slope the more uneven the distribution.
(4) An inflection in the line at the start of a steeper slope indicates the onset of airways closure in the dependent part of the lung, cutting off the contribution to the total expirate of those lung units with the lowest nitrogen concentration. Further expiration results in more airways closure and the line continues to rise.

The lung volume at which the inflection occurs between phases (3) and (4) is called the closing capacity. The volume from the inflection to RV as measured by this manoeuvre is known as the closing volume. RV measured separately is added to calculate closing capacity. Closing capacity is found to rise with age and to be larger in those who smoke. Thus, in the older subject, it may come to encroach on the tidal volume range. This may account for the reduction in Pao_2 with age, since blood which is perfusing areas of lung whose airways are closed during part of the respiratory cycle is, in effect, 'shunted' blood. This becomes more important as FRC is reduced on lying down and by anaesthesia.

The tests can also be carried out using a small bolus of a foreign gas (e.g. [133]Xe) inhaled at the start of inspiration and monitored during expiration with an appropriate detection device. The results are similar to the oxygen/nitrogen test described above. As a routine test, the closing volume suffers from poor reproducibility and a wide range of values in normal subjects.

VENTILATORY RESPONSE TO CO_2 – REBREATHING METHOD

The control of breathing is a complex interaction of neuronal and chemical factors. $P{CO_2}$ is an important factor, the effect of which can be easily measured. The method now most commonly used is the rebreathing method described and validated by Read (1967). The subject rebreathes for four minutes from a six-litre bag charged with 7% CO_2, 50% O_2, balance N_2. The rise in $P{CO_2}$ during rebreathing and the rising ventilation are recorded. The minute ventilation for each half minute is calculated and plotted against the $P{CO_2}$ for that half minute. After the first minute this plot is approximately linear and its slope gives a measure of the sensitivity of the subject's ventilatory response. The test can be made less tedious for the operator by using some form of direct ventilation measuring device and applying its output to the y-axis of an x–y recorder while the output of a CO_2 analyser is applied to the x-axis. The response line is then inscribed as the test is performed (Milledge, Minty and Duncalf, 1974).

There is a wide range of response in normal subjects, but reproducibility in a given individual is reasonably good (coefficient of variation about 20%) providing care is taken to have subjects truly at rest in quiet surroundings. Patients with obstructive airways disease have low CO_2 sensitivities, partly because of the increased work of breathing and partly because of central lack of sensitivity, especially in patients with chronic hypercapnia. This test has not yet found a place in routine lung function testing, but it is the test of choice in assessing the respiratory effects of drugs since it provides a far more sensitive test of respiratory depression than merely measuring the respiratory rate, minute volume or $Pa{CO_2}$ (Cormack, Milledge and Hanning, 1977).

OTHER TESTS

Other tests, such as the measurement of airways resistance and thoracic gas volumes in the body plethysmograph and tests of lung compliance, etc., still fall into the category of research procedures and are beyond the scope of this account.

EFFECTS OF PULMONARY SURGERY ON RESPIRATORY FUNCTION

An important aspect of preoperative assessment before pulmonary surgery is consideration of the likely effect of surgery on lung function. Prominent among the beneficial effects of pulmonary surgery are procedures to reduce secretions and purulent exudates. This the principal aim of lobectomy for bronchiectasis and drainage of a lung abscess. It may also be the cause of appreciable improvement of over-all lung function after resection for a bronchial carcinoma.

Removal of non-functional lung tissue may well cause an improvement or at least no deterioration of lung function. However, resection of functioning lung tissue may cause an appreciable and sometimes critical reduction in ventilatory capacity. The normal pair of lungs have a very large functional reserve. Nevertheless, sacrifice of functioning tissue must be avoided whenever possible, although the spread of neoplasm frequently makes wide excision essential.

Assessing the ability of a patient to withstand pneumonectomy can involve difficult decisions. If ventilatory function is reduced, much will depend on whether the lung to be resected makes an appreciable contribution to the total ventilatory capacity. If unilateral lung function studies in a patient with borderline respiratory function show that ventilation is equally divided between the two sides, then clearly pneumonectomy is likely to precipitate ventilatory failure. The difficult decisions arise when bronchial carcinoma coexists with chronic obstructive airway disease and also in advanced cases of pulmonary tuberculosis. One lung is normally able to take the entire pulmonary circulation, even during exercise, without causing pulmonary hypertension.

There are many forms of cardiac and pulmonary shunt in which venous blood reaches the left heart, causing arterial hypoxaemia. Resection of pulmonary shunts (such as neoplasms), like closure of intracardiac shunts, may be expected to improve the arterial oxygenation.

Modification of mechanical factors affecting ventilation

Improvement of ventilatory function can be expected to follow removal of large abdominal masses and correction of mechanical factors such as pulmonary decortication or fixation of a flail chest (Moore, 1975). However, certain procedures can cause a long-term impairment of ventilatory function and these include thoracoplasty and operations involving loss of diaphragm (such as palliative resections for extensive neoplasms).

Following lobectomy, the remaining lobes on that side rapidly expand to fill the vacant space. However, after pneumonectomy a space remains which is filled partly by mediastinal displacement and ascent of the diaphragm. Pleural fluid usually collects and there is a residual pneumothorax. In spite of this, ventilatory capacity after pneumonectomy is surprisingly good.

SHORT-TERM EFFECTS OF SURGERY

Whatever the long-term effects of surgery on lung function, it is important to remember that most operations are followed by a transient deterioration in pulmonary function (see Chapter 30). Apart from the effects of anaesthesia (considered below), ventilatory capacity and coughing may be markedly impaired by pain, dressings, drainage tubes, posture and so forth. Overtransfusion or postoperative fluid retention may precipitate pulmonary oedema, and tension pneumothorax may result from the formation of a valvular opening in either parietal or visceral pleura.

PREOPERATIVE PREPARATION

It is usually possible to do something to improve the condition of a patient's respiratory system before operation. When possible, in patients with chronic bronchitis, operation should be undertaken during periods of remission and it is best to avoid the winter months. It is useful to admit the patient several days before operation, particularly in the winter. The patient should be persuaded to stop smoking for as long as possible before operation.

Overt infection should be treated vigorously before operation, with a broad spectrum antibiotic such amoxycillin or co-trimoxazole (Septrin) or, preferably, with specific drugs following sensitivity tests (see Chapter 85). Regular preoperative bronchodilator therapy is valuable in patients with an appreciable element of spasm. Inhalation of an aerosol of a selective β_2 stimulator, such as salbutamol, is currently the most favoured technique.

PHYSIOTHERAPY

The value of breathing exercises is open to dispute but there is no doubt of the advantage of postural drainage before operation for patients with copious secretions. It is also important to establish rapport between patient and physiotherapist before surgery.

CORRECTION OF MECHANICAL FACTORS

Large pleural effusions should be drained before operation and a closed pneumothorax should be aspirated. It should be remembered that a closed pneumothorax will increase in volume when the patient inhales nitrous oxide (Hunter, 1955).

Premedication

Antisialogogues are helpful and almost essential for certain anaesthetic techniques in patients with chronic bronchitis. However, with large doses, secretions may be thickened and become difficult to clear either by coughing or by suction.

Opiates are contraindicated for patients with severe respiratory obstruction, and the longer acting drugs (such as morphine itself) impair the cough reflex in the postoperative period. Antihistamines with sedative side-effects are favoured, since they will prevent histamine-induced bronchospasm and also offer a satisfactory sedative and tranquillizing effect without respiratory depression. Promethazine, 20—50 mg (intramuscularly), is a suitable choice.

CHOICE OF ANAESTHESIA

No anaesthetic technique is unequivocally the best for all patients with the disabilities outlined above. All techniques have been used and all have their advocates. The choice may be considered as ranging between 'minimal interference' and 'maximal support' techniques (Holaday and Rattenborg, 1967).

Minimal interference techniques

The essence of minimal interference techniques is to keep the patient breathing spontaneously and to allow him to clear his own secretions. Techniques include regional analgesia and 'light' general anaesthesia, usually without endotracheal intubation. Sedation with diazepam is useful for reducing anxiety during surgery under regional anaesthesia. Minimal interference techniques are more likely to be selected for minor procedures and for operations on the lower abdomen and limbs which can be conveniently undertaken with regional anaesthesia.

ADVANTAGES

The advantages of this approach include the avoidance of any gross interference with the ciliary mechanism of the tracheobronchial tree, and also avoidance of the difficulties of re-establishing spontaneous respiration in a patient with abnormal control of breathing. There are also a few patients with air cysts or severe bullous emphysema who may show rapid enlargement of the cysts during artificial ventilation. These patients are more safely managed with spontaneous respiration except when the chest is open and the lungs exposed (Brown, 1966).

DISADVANTAGES

The disadvantages of this approach include the hazard of hypoventilation which may follow reduction of hypoxic drive or depression of respiratory neurons in a patient with critical reduction of ventilatory capacity. Without an endotracheal tube it is difficult or impossible to remove secretions by suction, and reliance must be placed on the patient's ability to clear his own airway. Control of arterial oxygenation may be difficult, since excess enrichment of the inspired gas with oxygen may cause apnoea. Ventilation may be more depressed than in normal patients during halothane anaesthesia (Pietak *et al.*, 1975).

Light general anaesthesia offers only limited surgical scope but regional anaesthetic techniques are widely applicable and may often be the technique of choice. It should, however, be remembered that patients with severe ventilatory failure may be unable to lie flat and refrain from coughing at intervals. In such patients laparotomy may not be feasible under epidural or spinal anaesthesia without general anaesthesia.

Maximal support techniques

In view of the important limitations of minimal interference techniques, there is an increasing tendency to manage patients with severe respiratory disease by anaesthesia, paralysis, endotracheal intubation, artificial ventilation and with reliance on suction for control of secretions. Under these conditions it is almost always possible to maintain an adequate alveolar ventilation with control of arterial $P\text{CO}_2$ at any required level. Only in exceptional cases is it impossible to maintain a satisfactory arterial $P\text{O}_2$ by increasing the concentration of oxygen in the inspired gas. Utting, Gray and Rees (1965) and Thornton (1969) recommend artificial ventilation during anaesthesia for all patients with chronic respiratory disease. In some patients, ventilation is improved by the use of positive end-expiratory pressure.

Maximal support techniques will usually be employed for major surgery, particularly of the abdomen. They will also be used for patients, already undergoing artificial ventilation, who require surgery. Such cases are not uncommon in intensive therapy units and include perforation of stress ulcers, drainage of subphrenic abscesses and institution of a feeding jejunostomy. Such interventions need have little adverse effect upon the state of the patient.

ADVANTAGES

Maximal support techniques should maintain satisfactory levels of all aspects of respiratory function throughout the operation. Exceptions include patients with extreme airway resistance and massive soiling of the tracheobronchial tree from a ruptured lung abscess but, in either event, the outlook is likely to be far better than with a minimal interference technique.

DISADVANTAGES

Many anaesthetists have experienced difficulty in re-establishing spontaneous respiration following paralysis of patients with severe respiratory disease. In such cases the first step is to ensure that neuromuscular conduction has been restored, and this should be tested by stimulation of a suitable motor nerve. Secondly, the drug history must be reviewed to exclude the possibility that apnoea is drug induced. The next stage is consideration of the $P\text{CO}_2$. Patients in respiratory failure have a high cerebrospinal fluid bicarbonate and are habituated to a high arterial

$P\text{co}_2$. It is very likely that $P\text{co}_2$ will be reduced to subnormal levels during artificial ventilation and some patients may not resume spontaneous breathing under these circumstances, particularly if they are still partially anaesthetized. The $P\text{co}_2$ should be restored to a level somewhat above the normal range and inhalation of 5% CO_2 is convenient for this purpose (Ivanov and Nunn, 1969).

The difficulty offered by a low $P\text{co}_2$ may be more theoretical than practical. Utting, Gray and Rees (1965) studied the resumption of breathing in a series of patients with preoperative hypercapnia. Following anaesthesia with hyperventilation and hypocapnia, their patients started to breathe at $P\text{co}_2$ values well below their preoperative level, and this was no doubt due to their anaesthetic technique, which avoided narcotics and the more potent inhalational agents. It is known that conscious patients will breathe spontaneously below their 'apnoeic' threshold $P\text{co}_2$ (Fink, 1961).

Some anaesthetists advocate a deliberate reduction of the inspired oxygen concentration to restart spontaneous breathing. This should be avoided if at all possible, but may have some theoretical basis in a 'blue bloater' who has lost his sensitivity to $P\text{co}_2$ and relies for his respiratory drive on an arterial $P\text{o}_2$ within the range 4–6 kPa (30–45 mmHg).

THE POSTOPERATIVE PERIOD

There are usually no insuperable difficulties in management of the problems which arise *during* anaesthesia in patients with even severe airways obstruction. Ventilation is under direct control and management of secretions is usually simple in an unconscious intubated patient. Inspired oxygen concentration is also under direct control and can be maintained close to 100% if required. This degree of control may be lost during the postoperative period when the patient is returned to the ward, although full control may be maintained by direct transfer to the intensive therapy unit with continued artificial ventilation during the early postoperative period. In cases of uncertainty it is usually safe to hold the patient in the recovery room long enough to make an assessment of the patient's ability to ventilate and control his secretions. However, in any case of doubt it is wise to transfer direct to the intensive therapy unit.

Assessment

PULMONARY VENTILATION

It is notoriously difficult to detect underventilation with the unaided senses and oxygen therapy may prevent the cyanosis which would otherwise indicate hypoventilation. Measurement· of minute volume with a Wright respirometer mounted on a facemask may be difficult in a semiconscious patient, and it is often simpler to measure the arterial $P\text{co}_2$. A postoperative elevation of $P\text{co}_2$ to 7 or 8 kPa (53 or 60 mmHg) can be regarded as within normal limits (Nunn and Payne, 1962) but it should also be remembered that, after a period of hyperventilation, P_{CO_2} rises very slowly when ventilation is reduced (Ivanov and Nunn, 1968). It is therefore unwise to assess the adequacy of ventilation on a single value for arterial P_{CO_2} measured soon after the return to spontaneous breathing.

HYPOXAEMIA

Except in gross hypoxia, cyanosis is an unreliable sign and, in any case of doubt, arterial P_{O_2} should be measured and the value related to the inspired oxygen concentration. It may be helpful to use a Ventimask so that the effective inspired oxygen concentration is known (Leigh, 1973). Quantification of shunting may be simplified by use of the isoshunt diagram (Benatar, Hewlett and Nunn, 1973).

SECRETIONS

Patients must be carefully watched for their ability to clear secretions. Severe expiratory airways obstruction may render the patient unable to cough effectively and his cilia may not have recovered from the effect of intubation and the inhalation of dry gas.

CHEST X-RAY

Chest x-ray is valuable for the exclusion of major defects of respiratory function such as tension pneumothorax, haemothorax, lobar collapse and so on. Unfortunately, the films must be taken under a difficult combination of circumstances with a supine patient and portable equipment. The patient's condition is likely to preclude his taking a maximal inspiration and holding his breath for the requisite time. The study of Prys-Roberts *et al.* (1967) showed some of the diagnostic limitations of radiography under these circumstances.

VENTILATORY CAPACITY

Peak expiratory flow rate and $FEV_{1.0}$ require careful interpretation when measured in the postoperative period. Low values may be due to residual narcosis, residual neuromuscular block, pain, increased airway resistance or mechanical factors (such as tension pneumothorax). Great caution is necessary when attempting to use measurements of ventilatory capacity to study any of these factors in isolation.

Management

HYPOVENTILATION

Hypoventilation requires a careful search for any cause which may be temporary, such as secretions, pneumothorax, residual neuromuscular blockage, excessive use of depressant drugs or pain. If it is clear that the patient cannot maintain an adequate ventilation in spite of the elimination of all such factors, it is usually necessary to maintain artificial ventilation. It is possible that clearance of secretions and reduction of dead space following intubation (Nunn, Campbell and Peckett, 1959) may be sufficient to restore a satisfactory alveolar ventilation without recourse to artificial ventilation.

PAIN

It is most important that ventilation and coughing should not be excessively impaired by pain. It is not unusual for ventilation and coughing to be improved by the administration of morphine after operation, but too large a dose may make matters worse. Very careful dosage is essential and, in difficult cases, the authors favour administration of the first injection of postoperative analgesic by the intravenous route, using a process of titration. The relief of pain is usually dramatic and one may observe directly the effect on ventilation and the patient's willingness to cough. Maximal respiratory depression occurs several minutes after an intravenous injection of morphine and the patient should not return to the ward for at least another 30 minutes.

Regional analgesia is an excellent method of postoperative pain relief for patients with respiratory disease. Spence, Smith and Harris (1968) found significantly better respiratory function in a group of patients with epidural analgesia than in a control group receiving opiates.

SECRETIONS

If a patient cannot control his secretions in the postoperative period it may become necessary to suck out the tracheobronchial tree at intervals. Unfortunately, this cannot be done without direct access to the trachea by bronchoscopy, intubation, tracheostomy or, less satisfactorily, by laryngoscopy. Fibreoptic bronchoscopy has greatly simplified treatment of collapse due to retained secretions (Milledge, 1976). In some cases it is preferable to perform a planned tracheostomy before the patient wakes from the anaesthetic. It is helpful to explain matters to the patient before operation and, under these conditions, tracheostomy is remarkably well tolerated and the wound heals easily.

PO_2

Control of the patient's PO_2 may be extremely difficult. There are patients with large shunts who require 100% oxygen in the inspired gas in order to maintain an acceptable arterial PO_2. However, when the main disability is alveolar hypoventilation, a very modest enrichment of the oxygen concentration of the inspired gas is usually sufficient to produce a satisfactory level of arterial PO_2 and administration of too high a concentration may cause apnoea. The essential features of the administration of oxygen to such a patient are easy access to a method of measurement of arterial Po_2, and means of controlling the inspired oxygen concentration within fairly close limits. By this means the inspired oxygen concentration may be titrated against the arterial Po_2 when hypoxaemia is due to shunting. In patients who have lost their respiratory sensitivity to carbon dioxide, skill is needed in steering the fine course between hypoxia and apnoea from loss of hypoxic respiratory drive.

CONCLUSION

This chapter has given no simple solution to the problem of how to anaesthetize patients with respiratory disease. Success lies rather in an understanding of the many difficulties which beset these unfortunate patients, and in the attention to detail by all members of the surgical and anaesthetic team throughout the period before, during and after surgery.

References

Anderson, N. B. and Ghia, J. (1970). Pulmonary function, cardiac status and postoperative course in relation to cardiopulmonary bypass. *J. thorac. cardiovasc. Surg.* 59, 474–483

Appleberg, M., Gordon, L. and Fatti, L. P. (1974). Preoperative pulmonary evaluation of surgical patients using the Vitalograph. *Br. J. Surg.* 16, 57–59

Benatar, S. R., Hewlett, A. M. and Nunn, J. F. (1973). The use of iso-shunt lines for control of oxygen therapy. *Br. J. Anaesth.* 45, 711–718

Brown, A. I. P. (1966). Anaesthesia for the respiratory cripple. *Proc. R. Soc. Med.* 59, 522–526

Cormack, R. S., Milledge, J. S. and Hanning, C. D. (1977). Respiratory effects and amnesia after premedication with morphine or lorazepam. *Br. J. Anaesth.* 49, 351–361

Fazio, F. and Jones, T. (1975). Assessment of regional ventilation by continuous inhalation of radioactive krypton – 81M. *Br. med. J.* 3, 673–676

Fink, B. R. (1961). Influence of cerebral activity in wakefulness on regulation of breathing. *J. appl. Physiol.* 16, 15–20

Holady, D. A. and Rattenborg, C. C. (1967). Selection of a method of anaesthesia for patients with pulmonary dysfunction. In *Lung Disease, Clinical Anaesthesia,* Vol. 1. D. A. Holaday (ed.). Oxford: Blackwell

Hunter, A. R. (1955). Problems of anaesthesia in artificial pneumothorax. *Proc. R. Soc. Med.* 48, 765–768

Ivanov, S. D. and Nunn, J. F. (1968). Influence of duration of hyperventilation on rise time of Pco_2 after step reduction of ventilation. *Resp. Physiol.* 4, 243–249

Ivanov, S. D. and Nunn, J. F. (1969). Methods of elevation of Pco_2 for restoration of spontaneous breathing after artificial ventilation of anaesthetised patients. *Br. J. Anaesth.* 41, 28–37

Lal, S., Ferguson, A. D. and Campbell, E. J. M. (1964). Forced expiratory time: A simple test for airways obstruction. *Br. med. J.* 1, 814–817

Lawler, P. J. and Hewlett, A. M. (1978). Clinical evaluation of the iso-shunt diagram. *Br. J. Anaesth.* 50, 77–78

Leigh, J. M. (1973). Variation in performance of oxygen therapy devices. *Ann. R. Coll. Surg.* 52, 234–253

Lockwood, P. (1973). The relationship between pre-operative lung function test results and post operative complications in carcinoma of the bronchus. *Respiration* 30, 105–116

McHardy, G. J. R. (1972). Diffusing capacity and pulmonary gas exchange. *Br. J. Dis. Chest* 66, 1–20

Milledge, J. S. (1976). Therapeutic fibreoptic bronchoscopy in intensive care. *Br. med. J.* 2, 1427–1429

Milledge, J. S., Minty, K. B. and Duncalf, D. (1974). On-line assessment of ventilatory response to carbon dioxide. *J. appl. Physiol.* 37, 596–599

Milledge, J. S. and Nunn, J. F. (1975). Criteria of fitness for anaesthesia in patients with chronic obstructive lung disease. *Br. med. J.* 3, 670–673

Moore, B. P. (1975). Operative stabilization of nonpenetrating chest injuries. *J. thorac. cardiovasc. Surg.* 70, 619–630

Nunn, J. F. (1977). *Applied Respiratory Physiology*, 2nd edn, pp. 277–291. London and Boston, Mass.: Butterworths

Nunn, J. F., Campbell, E. J. M. and Peckett, B. W. (1959). Anatomical subdivisions of the volume of respiratory dead space and effect of position of the jaw. *J. appl. Physiol.* 14, 174–176

Nunn, J. F. and Payne, J. P. (1962). Hypoxaemia after general anaesthesia. *Lancet* ii, 631–632

Pietak, S., Weenig, C. S., Hickey, R. F. and Fairley, H. B. (1975). Anesthetic effects on ventilation in patients with chronic obstructive pulmonary disease. *Anesthesiology* 42, 160–166

Prys-Roberts, C., Nunn, J. F., Dobson, R. H., Robinson, R. H., Greenbaum, R. and Harris, R. S. (1967). Radiologically undetectable pulmonary collapse in the supine position. *Lancet* ii, 399–401

Read, D. J. C. (1967). A clinical method for assessing the ventilatory response to carbon dioxide. *Australas. Ann. Med.* 16, 20–32

Ritchie, B. (1962). A comparison of forced expiratory volume and peak flow in clinical practice. *Lancet* ii, 271–273

Spence, A. A., Smith, G. and Harris, R. (1968). The influence of continuous extradural analgesia on lung function in the postoperative period. *Br. J. Anaesth.* 40, 801–802

Stein, M. and Cassara, E. L. (1970). Preoperative pulmonary evaluation and therapy for surgery patients. *J. Am. med. Ass.* 211, 787–790

Stein, M., Koota, G. M., Simon, M. and Frank, H. A. (1962). Pulmonary evaluation of surgical patients. *J. Am. med. Ass.* 181, 765–770

Thornton, J. A. (1969). The problem of general anaesthesia in patients with chronic respiratory disease. *Thorax* 24, 380

Utting, J. E., Gray, T. C. and Rees, G. J. (1965). Anaesthesia for the respiratory cripple. *Acta anaesth. scand.* 9, 29–38

27 Methods of oxygen therapy
Julian M. Leigh

The living body is no machine, but an organism constantly tending to maintain or revert to the normal, and the respite afforded by such measures as the temporary administration of oxygen is not wasted, but utilised for recuperation. (Haldane, 1917)

Those who prescribe oxygen must have a full understanding of the mechanisms of oxygen transport and of its disorders, and be aware of the complications which may accrue from injudicious therapy. These matters are dealt with in Chapters 21, 28 and 86. Currently, oxygen may be administered to *spontaneously breathing subjects* by various types of face-masks, catheters and cannulae, or by air—oxygen blow-over devices. Alternatively, the patient may be enclosed in an incubator, oxygen tent or hyperbaric chamber. Oxygen-enriched air may be supplied to a ventilator *during artificial ventilation*. Finally, when the lungs are very severely affected, oxygen may be delivered by *extracorporeal membrane oxygenation* if this is considered appropriate.

Adjuncts to oxygen therapy

A particular portion of the microcirculation which is affected by ischaemia may or may not be amenable to improvement by specific therapy. However, certain measures may be adopted to improve oxygen availability in addition to, and sometimes instead of, oxygen therapy.

(1) Cardiac output (tissue blood flow) may be increased by transfusions and infusions; digitalis, dopamine or other positive inotropic agents may be administered under appropriate circumstances.
(2) Arterial saturation may be improved by treating the lung pathology appropriately, i.e. reducing venous admixture by:
   (a) Physiotherapy.

    (b) Intubation (or bronchosopy) and suction, or tracheostomy and suction, and intermittent positive pressure ventilation (IPPV) with or without positive end-expiratory pressure (PEEP).

    (c) Antibiotics as necessary.

    (d) Sometimes steroids (humoral pneumonitis of various aetiologies).

    (e) Sometimes bronchodilators.

    (f) Treatment of congestive cardiac failure with digitalis and diuretics if appropriate.

    (g) The institution of continuous positive airway pressure (CPAP) when appropriate.

(3) Raise haemoglobin to normal or to the optimal value (see Chapter 53).

(4) Measures can also be taken to reduce tissue oxygen demands:

    (a) Paralysis and IPPV reduce the oxygen cost of breathing.

    (b) Digitalization reduces the oxygen uptake of heart muscle.

    (c) Prevention of hyperthermia avoids increasing oxygen requirements, e.g. by fanning or sponging, or both.

    (d) Induction of hypothermia, e.g. surface cooling to $30°C$ can reduce tissue oxygen requirements by up to 50%.

OXYGEN THERAPY FOR SPONTANEOUSLY BREATHING PATIENTS

The history of the administration of oxygen to patients has been beset with anomalies (Leigh, 1973a; 1974a) not the least of which have been uncertainties regarding dosage, of which the following extracts from the literature testify.

> The approach is one of advocacy based upon clinical experience allied to physiological considerations... I am only advocating care and precision in dosage and it is not usual to require controlled evidence that this is better than haphazard and imprecise dosage. (Campbell, 1963)

> If the concentration of oxygen which a patient is receiving is not known with a reasonable degree of accuracy, then the situation is analogous to the administration of an unknown quantity of a drug which may do harm if given in excess, or provide insufficient benefit if the dose is too small. (Scottish Home and Health Department, 1969)

> Oxygen has been taken for granted... on most occasions oxygen therapy can be instituted with ease and without too much thought... possibly administration of oxygen deserves much more thought than we now give it. (Ngai, 1972)

> HAFOE (high air flow with oxygen enrichment) provides a homogeneous inspired mixture, eliminates dead space, and obviates the need for a leak-free airway connection. It is the only practical method for obtaining controlled inspired O_2 in a mouth breathing patient. (Campbell and Minty, 1976)

Composition of inspired gas

An appreciation of the pattern of gas flow during spontaneous ventilation is fundamental to the consideration of the composition of inspired gas during oxygen therapy. A complete ventilatory cycle from the pneumotachogram of a resting subject is shown in *Figure 27.1*. There are

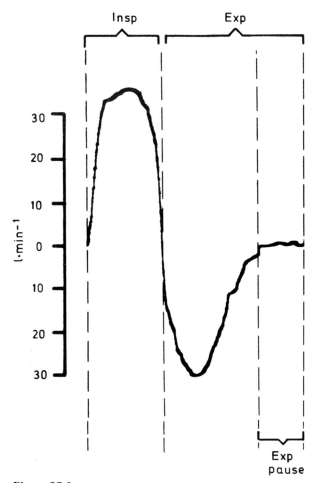

Figure 27.1
A single ventilatory flow waveform from the pneumotachogram of a resting subject

three obvious subdivisions: inspiratory flow, active expiratory flow, and the expiratory pause. The peak inspiratory flow rate is the key determinant of inspired concentration when the capacity of an oxygen therapy device is small compared to tidal volume. Total expiratory time attains more importance with increasing storage capacity of the various devices.

Figure 27.2 (a and b) shows inspiratory pneumotachograms from two healthy subjects of different bodily habitus. It is immediately obvious that there is between-subject variation in average peak inspiratory flow rate and within-subject variation in peak inspiratory flow rate, and that total expiratory time varies on a breath-to-breath basis due to variations in expiratory pause time.

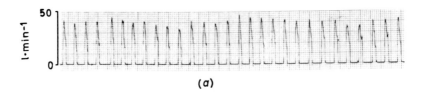

(*a*)

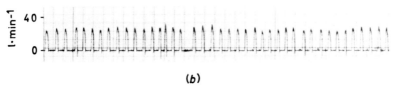

(*b*)

Figure 27.2
Inspiratory pneumotachograms in two subjects (*a*) male, 196 cm and 87.5 kg, FVC = 8.1 litres and FEV_1 = 5.25 litres; (*b*) female, 165 cm and 64.0 kg, FVC = 3.3 litres and FEV_1 = 2.87 litres. Recorded at a paper speed of $1\ mm \cdot s^{-1}$ (one minute = 12 large divisions). These traces clearly show both between- and within-subject variation in peak inspiratory flow rates, as well as variations in expiratory times

Oxygen therapy devices were classified (Leigh, 1970) depending on whether their performance was influenced by these variations, i.e. *variable performance devices,* or was independent of these variations, i.e. *fixed performance devices.*

Variable performance devices

These give uncontrolled (uncontrollable) oxygen therapy as they function only in relation to the wearer who *creates* the inspired mixture by the act of breathing. Various subject and device factors influence performance. The important *subject factors* are the inspiratory flow rate, which not only varies within each breath but attains a variable peak from breath to breath, and the duration of expiration and the expiratory pause. During the latter, oxygen concentration rises and carbon dioxide concentration falls within the storage capacity of the device. The *device factors* are oxygen flow rate, physical volume and vent resistance, where appropriate. The subtle interplay of these factors results in unpredictable oxygen dosage in a given patient at a given time. Thus, changes in arterial oxygen values within a subject may only reflect the influence of these variables rather than a true change in the state of the lungs under treatment. Furthermore, temporal variations in concentration also occur during any *single* inspiration (Leigh, 1973a, b; *Table 27.1*; Campbell and Minty, 1976). These temporal variations in turn must also affect regional alveolar concentration, because the regional distribution of inspired tidal volume tends to follow a fixed pattern (Grant, Jones and Hughes, 1974). This raises the possibility that there may be damage in some parts of the lung from too high a concentration and lack of benefit in others due to too low a concentration (Leigh, 1973a, b; Campbell and Minty, 1976).

TABLE 27.1. Values for within-breath and between-breath variation in oxygen concentration read from traces obtained with a rapid response oxygen analyser during spontaneous breathing using variable performance oxygen therapy devices

Type	Flow ($l \cdot min^{-1}$)	Within-breath variation Peak	Trough	Between-breath variation of end-tidal plateaux	No. of consecutive breaths
MC	5	60%	29%	37–42%	4
mask	10	95%	45%	54–64%	4
Poly-	5	65%	32%	51–54%	7
mask	10	82%	48%	61–66%	5

Variable performance devices may be subdivided functionally into three characteristic types:

(1) *no capacity systems* — nasal catheters and cannulae.
(2) *small capacity systems* — any device which consists of a mask shell only.
(3) *large capacity systems* — any device with a bag.

NO CAPACITY SYSTEM

When oxygen is delivered directly into the airway, with a nasal catheter or nasal cannulae, at a low flow rate of about 1 $l \cdot min^{-1}$ the ratio of oxygen flow to expiratory pause time does not permit sufficient storage of oxygen to affect the composition of the next inspiration. Under these circumstances, i.e. when peak inspiratory flow rate ($\dot{V}\hat{\imath}$) is larger than the oxygen flow rate ($\dot{V}FO_2$) and there is no storage capacity, the inspired oxygen concentration (FIO_2) achieved during a given inspiration is a pure function of $\dot{V}\hat{\imath}$ and $\dot{V}FO_2$, such that:

$$FIO_2 = 0.2093 + 1.242 \frac{\dot{V}FO_2}{\dot{V}\hat{\imath}}$$

Under these conditions, where $\dot{V}\hat{\imath} > \dot{V}FO_2$, breath-to-breath differences in FIO_2 are not marked. Therefore a given individual will achieve a reasonably constant though *unknown* FIO_2, but between-subject variation in FIO_2 will occur according to between-subject variation in average $\dot{V}\hat{\imath}$.

At *higher flow rates* (2–3 $l \cdot min^{-1}$) within-subject variation of FIO_2 occurs. Firstly, because the increasing ratio of $\dot{V}FO_2$ to $\dot{V}\hat{\imath}$ has a more significant affect, and secondly because significant storage of oxygen in the airway starts to occur during the expiratory pause. As the latter is variable in length, a variable amount of oxygen accumulates.

At flow rates higher than 3 l·min^{-1}, these devices are extremely uncomfortable for the user, especially when delivery is by nasopharyngeal catheter. In terms of patient acceptance, the binasal cannula at low flow rates was the most comfortable device tested in a survey by Kory *et al.* (1962).

SMALL CAPACITY SYSTEMS (e.g. Mary Catterall (MC), Edinburgh, Harris (OTU), Hudson)

Here apparatus dead space is added in the form of a mask shell. The air which is added to the oxygen during inspiration is drawn in through a vent which may be single or multiple. While some economy of expired oxygen is achieved (along with some retention of CO_2), some fresh oxygen is lost through the vent. These masks do not in fact provide a quantitative improvement in performance over catheters and cannulae, but they are more comfortable at higher gas flow rates.

Functional apparatus dead space is not synonymous with the physical volume of a given device. It is only equal to that part of the device from which alveolar gas is reinhaled. Its value depends upon factors similar to those affecting F_{IO_2} and it is therefore subject to a similar kind of variation.

Patients may respond to the imposition of apparatus dead space by an increase in alveolar ventilation and thus overcome its effect. On the other hand, it may be the cause of increasing asphyxia in patients with incipient or actual respiratory failure.

Rebreathing during clinical oxygen therapy is of a complex nature in which rebreathing of alveolar gas occurs mainly at the beginning of inspiration (Nunn and Newman, 1964). However, in general terms, functional apparatus dead space or rebreathing will be increased when the physical volume of the device is large, when the fresh oxygen flow is relatively low, when the expiratory pause is short, or when the respiratory resistance of the total effective vent is high — i.e. when the mask is close fitting.

The total vent resistance is a function, not only of the cross-sectional area of the vent which is a physical part of the mask design, but also of that leak area added by a poor fit to the face. Variations in the amount of this leak, from time to time during oxygen therapy, may be a considerable source of variation in performance of devices.

LARGE CAPACITY SYSTEMS (e.g. Boothby–Lovelace–Bulbulian (BLB), Oxyaire, Portogen, Pneumask, Polymask)

These devices are characterized by a rebreathing bag although the bag in the Portogen mask is a true reservoir bag, as there is a check valve between it and the mask shell. The Portogen is a modern lightweight version of the original Haldane mask. The Pneumask and Polymask are simply plastic rebreathing bags.

When considering the performance of the devices with bags, there are three sources of inspired oxygen — fresh oxygen flow which can accumulate throughout the respiratory cycle, expired gas retained in the dead space, and air coming through the vent. The concentration in the bag just before inspiration depends upon the expiratory time, the quality of the previous expirate, and loss of fresh gas from leaks. The ratio of gas taken from the bag to air taken through the vent depends on the relative resistance to flow and will also vary with the distending pressure in the bag throughout the respiratory cycle. Since the times, volumes, flows and resistances all vary, it is not surprising that the performance of devices in this group is exceedingly variable.

In practice the large capacity devices have largely been superseded by the small capacity devices (Leigh, 1973c).

Fixed performance devices

These devices allow controlled (known, fixed and selectable) oxygen dosage.

THEORY

To supply a subject with a constant inspired mixture, any device must either:

(1) be capable of exactly following the inspiratory flow waveform, or
(2) supply the gas mixture as a continuous flow in excess of peak inspiratory flow rate. This is referred to as 'high air flow with oxygen enrichment', or 'HAFOE'; it has the additional advantages of obviating the need for a leak-free airway connection and tending to eliminate dead space by venting the expirate (Campbell, 1960, Campbell and Gebbie, 1966).

Condition (1) may be met in three ways:

(a) By placing the individual in an environment of room proportions, containing the mixture.
(b) By using an anaesthetic-type circuit in which collapse of the reservoir bag during inspiration matches inspiratory flow.
(c) By using a device with a demand valve capable of delivering the gas mixture at inspiratory flow rate. A current example of such a device is the two-stage regulator for use with Entonox.

Condition (2) may be met in two ways:

(d) By the HAFOE system in which air is entrained by an oxygen venturi device.
(e) By the HAFOE system employing an air-blower humidifier to which oxygen can be added.
(f) By the HAFOE system employing a fan-driven air flow with a constant added oxygen stream (Flenley, Hutchison and Donald, 1963).

Oxygen rooms (a) were in vogue in the early 1920s (Leigh, 1974b) but are now generally ruled out on the grounds of practicality and expense. With air-blower humidifiers (e) it can be difficult to maintain a constant ratio of air to oxygen. The fan blower system (f) is somewhat impractical because of noise and bulk. Both (b) and (c) introduce apparatus dead space with the possibility of the rebreathing of alveolar gas. More importantly, these two systems require a leak-free airway connection, i.e., a close-fitting mask, which is a condition poorly tolerated by ill subjects. Thus (d) which does not require a tight-fitting mask remains the most acceptable and only practical method for delivering known concentrations to spontaneously breathing subjects.

REQUIREMENT FOR A HAFOE SYSTEM

The fraction of oxygen (F_{O_2}) given by a HAFOE device may be calculated from a simple mixing equation. This has been used to construct *Figure 27.3*

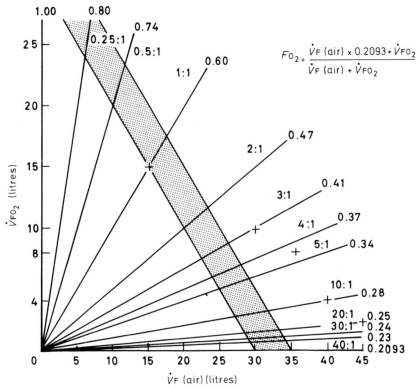

$$F_{O_2} = \frac{\dot{V}_F \text{ (air)} \times 0.2093 + \dot{V}_{F_{O_2}}}{\dot{V}_F \text{ (air)} + \dot{V}_{F_{O_2}}}$$

Figure 27.3
Mixing diagrams for different ratios of air/oxygen required for high air flow with oxygen enrichment (HAFOE). Mixing ratios are shown and the corresponding oxygen concentration (F_{O_2}) is shown to the right of each line. The shaded area approximates to *average* peak inspiratory flow rates found in healthy individuals. The sum of the co-ordinate values of any point on any isopleth represents the total flow. The crosses on the diagram represent the five definitive Mark 2 Ventimasks

which illustrates the implications when HAFOE is used to produce fixed performance (controlled) oxygen therapy. The mixing equation is given at the top right corner of the figure.

In this diagram the abscissa ($\dot{V}_{F(air)}$) represents flow of air only, for which F_{O_2} is 0.2093, and the ordinate ($\dot{V}_{FO_2}$) represents oxygen flow only, with an F_{O_2} of 1.0. The other isopleths in the diagram, radiating from the zero point, represent intermediate mixtures, for example, the 1:1 mixture giving an oxygen concentration of 60% ($F_{O_2} = 0.60$). The flows needed to produce any required mixture can be read from the axes from any point on the isopleth of the chosen percentage — the sum of the co-ordinate values of the point representing the total flow.

To give air–oxygen mixtures by the HAFOE principle, the total flow must always exceed average peak inspiratory flow rates. The shaded area on the graph is bounded by two lines, for each of which the total flow

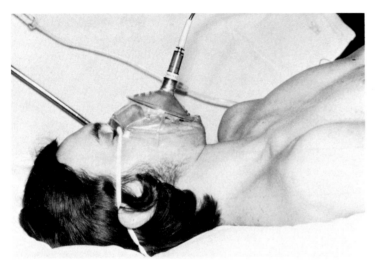

Figure 27.4
60% Ventimask: 15 l·min^{-1} of O_2 entrain an equal amount of air to produce a total flow of 30 l·min^{-1}

($\dot{V}_{F(air)}$ + $\dot{V}_{FO_2}$) is constant at 30 and 35 l·min^{-1} respectively. These values are convenient numbers in the neighbourhood of average peak inspiratory flow rates found in resting, *healthy* individuals (Leigh, 1973a, b). Thus, any device working on the HAFOE principle *must* have a total flow which is at least within but preferably to the right of the shaded area. (Pathological breathlessness is discussed later.)

The essential feature of a HAFOE oxygen therapy device is that it should blow oxygen mixtures at patients in excess of peak inspiratory flow rates, and its performance is thus independent of patient factors and of fit to the face. All operate on the venturi principle, in which a jet of pure oxygen entrains a *constant ratio* of room air to produce a fixed concentration mixture. Various devices of this type are obtainable (Ventimasks, *Figure 27.4* — Mixomasks, Multivents, Accurox and

Variomasks) and the range includes masks for 24, 26, 28, 30, 31, 35, 40, 50 and 60% oxygen. The characteristics of the British Ventimasks (Mark 2) are given in *Table 27.2*.

TABLE 27.2. Characteristics of the British Ventimasks (Mark 2)*

F_{IO_2} (%)	Entrainment ratio (air: O_2)	O_2 flow (l·min^{-1})	Air entrained (l·min^{-1})	Total flow (l·min^{-1})
24	23:1	2	46	48
28	10:1	4	40	44
35	4.6:1	8	36.8	44.8
40	3.1:1	10	30.1	40.1
60	1:1	15	15	30

* All these devices give a total flow $\geqslant 30$ l·min^{-1}. Note that different manufacturers recommend different O_2 flow rates for their individual venturi devices, and users must take care to observe the instructions that are clearly given with each type.

The upper limit of inspired oxygen concentration for spontaneously breathing patients is probably 60% (Campbell and Minty, 1976). Two reasons are adduced for this. Firstly, oxygen toxicity occurs more readily in *normal* lungs at levels above this (Chapter 28), and secondly, it is likely that the oxygenation of a patient who is hypoxaemic on such oxygen percentages would be better served by the institution of IPPV, irrespective of the fact that alveolar ventilation may be adequate or even increased.

HUMIDIFICATION OF VENTURI DEVICES

Humidification of the oxygen supply to a venturi device is not sensible. Not only may this give inadequate humidification of the *total* inspired gas but precipitation of water occurs within the venturi, thus interfering with the entrainment ratio and altering the concentration delivered. The manufacturers of the various types supply a 'humidity adaptor' which consists of a wide diameter cowling which can be fitted around the air entrainment ports. Humidified air can then be supplied to this cowling, e.g. from a blow-over humidifier for entrainment at the designated ratio.

The advantages of fixed performance or controlled oxygen therapy

Figure 27.5 shows arterial oxygen values measured in a patient breathing oxygen during the course of humoral pneumonitis associated with fat embolism syndrome. If these had been achieved using a variable perform-ance device, all that could be argued would be that arterial oxygenation was satisfactory. However, when they are considered in relation to the inspired oxygen which was being given in a controlled manner by HAFOE Ventimasks, it can be seen that the lungs were deteriorating from days 1–7. A further fall in Pa_{O_2} during days 6–8 would have necessitated IPPV and an improvement clearly commenced on day eight while the patient was using a newly available 60% Ventimask. Prior to that time, clinical practice would have been to commence IPPV rather than to use variable performance devices as one could not have been certain whether the patient was receiving 60% or 95% oxygen from the latter. Clearly the introduction of the 60% mask has allowed an improvement in the quality of management.

With the various venturi devices it is possible to give known oxygen

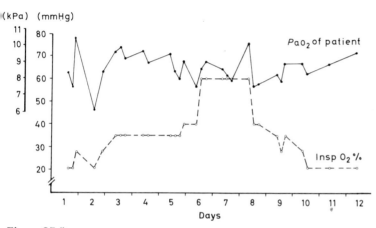

Figure 27.5
Pa_{O_2} and inspired O_2% in a case of fat embolism — spontaneously breathing with Ventimasks or air. The knowledge of oxygen concentrations during this illness permits the observer to conclude that, not only was arterial oxygenation reasonable during treatment but also, the lungs were deteriorating from days 1 to 7, and improvement clearly commenced on day 8

concentrations to all spontaneously breathing patients so that any measurements of oxygen in blood can be interpreted in the light of a true change within the patient who is being treated. Even so it has been argued (Bethune and Collis, 1977) that this is a defensible though extravagant ideal.

As the prescribed percentage of oxygen increases, the recommended oxygen flows of the commercially available devices tend to give less total flow (see *Table 27.2*). Although there is no reason why higher flows should not be used (other than in the interests of economy), it is well to consider peak inspiratory flow rates during dyspnoea.

Pathological and physiological dyspnoea

For more than 30 years, workers have examined pneumotachograms in an attempt to produce a 'form factor' which is defined as the ratio of peak inspiratory flow rate to minute volume. The advantage of this is that the 'form factor' can then be used to explore problems of respiratory mechanics under various circumstances. Some well known examples are given below (with the addition of the ellipse).

For the investigation of these matters it is necessary to assume that inspiration and expiration are equal in length and that there is no pause between each respiratory cycle:

Now the minute volume of ventilation $(\dot{V})$ = V_E/t, where V_E is the expired tidal volume and t is the duration of one respiratory cycle in minutes (i.e. seconds/60). If a peak inspiratory flow rate $(\dot{V}_I)$ is achieved when the tidal volume is inhaled in $t/2$ minutes and, if the inspiratory waveform is in the following forms, then the form factor $(\dot{V}_I/\dot{V}$ is as shown:

Waveform	Form factor
Any triangle	4
Sine wave	π
Ellipse	$8/\pi$
Square wave	2

The waveforms here refer to the shape of the pneumotachogram not the spirogram. They cover the waveforms described in the literature, i.e. triangles or peaks, domes and plateaux. These matters have been discussed in part by Cooper (1961) who employed the sine wave as the basis for a study of the effects on respiration of using breathing apparatus.

During normal breathing the duration of inspiration occupies less than half the respiratory cycle so that peak inspiratory flow rate in the normal subject at rest tends to be of the order of four times the minute volume (Cain and Otis, 1949).

Pathological respiratory insufficiency

Data on five patients who were in an intensive care unit with various lung affections were compared with five normal subjects (Leigh, 1973b).

The over-all average peak inspiratory flow rate for the group was 21.29 ± 2.14 $l \cdot min^{-1}$, which differed significantly $(p < 0.001)$ from normal subjects (31.44 ± 3.00 $l \cdot min^{-1}$).

These results suggest that in pathological dyspnoea the average peak inspiratory flow rates are reduced to obtain maximal mechanical efficiency, i.e., that the best compromise is reached between the demand for minute volume and the increased resistance to air flow occasioned by the underlying disease processes. The patients studied fall within the 'shallow breathing' type as described by Haldane. It may therefore be concluded that all patients of this type would be satisfied by the flow rates delivered by existing HAFOE devices. However, it is probable that in patients with 'air hunger' of pathological origin, such as that accompanying diabetic ketoacidosis, the peak inspiratory flows will be higher and resemble those seen during exercise.

The dyspnoea of exercise

Changes in average peak inspiratory flow rates during exercise have been well documented. For example, Silverman *et al.* (1951) found that in 18 healthy young men at extreme exertion, the average peak inspiratory

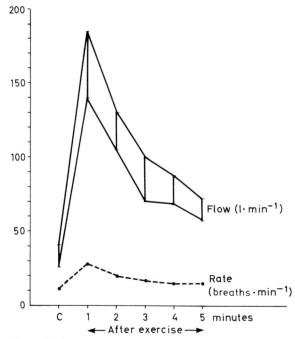

Figure 27.6
Range of peak inspiratory flow rates before strenuous exercise (C) and at one minute intervals thereafter — 29-year-old male subject

flow rate was 240 l·min^{-1}. *Figure 27.6* shows the range of peak inspiratory flow rates in a 29-year-old male at rest and then for a five-minute period after one minute of strenuous exercise. Peak inspiratory flow rates are given as the range within each minute of the recording. The broken line shows the respiration rate, C indicates control readings. The resting values show peak inspiratory flow rates ranging between 26 and 41 l·min^{-1} at a respiration rate of 11.5 per minute. In the first minute after the exercise period the peak inspiratory flow rates ranged from 140 to 185 l·min^{-1} at a respiration rate of 28 per minute. Clearly this kind of breathlessness is outside the scope of HAFOE devices, as currently available.

OXYGEN THERAPY DURING THE COURSE OF ARTIFICIAL VENTILATION

The need for careful control of the inspired oxygen concentration given to patients on ventilators in intensive therapy units has been recognized for over a decade (Pontoppidan and Berry, 1967).

When a patient is on a ventilator, oxygen from a flow meter usually passes to the machine which then delivers a mixture of room air and oxygen to him. Although the inspired oxygen concentration resulting from this type of delivery may be constant for long periods, it is not necessarily known. In addition, the assumption of a steady-state oxygen concentration may not always be valid with some pressure-cycled or patient-triggered machines, nor when compliance is fluctuating. Under these circumstances $\dot{V}$ will vary while oxygen flow ($\dot{V}FO_2$) will remain constant and FIO_2 at any time will be given by:

$$FIO_2 = \frac{0.2093\,(\dot{V} - \dot{V}FO_2) + \dot{V}FO_2}{\dot{V}}$$

With some modern ventilating systems the chosen oxygen concentration can be selected by premixing air and oxygen e.g. by using the Quantiflex air—oxygen mixer (Richardson, Chinn and Nunn, 1976). A constant

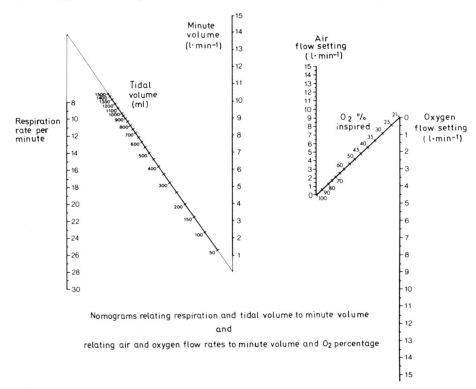

Nomograms relating respiration and tidal volume to minute volume

and

relating air and oxygen flow rates to minute volume and O_2 percentage

Figure 27.7
Nomogram designed for use with a minute volume divider run from separate air and oxygen supplies

mixture, given by the equation in *Figure 27.3*, is thus always available to the ventilator, irrespective of any change in the effective minute volume, so that this problem does not arise.

It is an essential part of good intensive therapy unit practice that inspired oxygen percentage is charted routinely with other parameters of ventilation, and certainly that 'blood gases' are always recorded together with the oxygen concentration at the time of blood sampling.

Where F_{IO_2} is not preselectable, it is desirable that the inspired oxygen concentration should be measured but, when this is not possible, a simple nomogram can be used. The nomogram in *Figure 27.7* has been designed for use with a minute volume divider run from separate air and oxygen supplies. A desired oxygen concentration can be achieved after selecting a chosen minute volume at the initiation of treatment or when oxygen concentration requires alteration during treatment. Alternatively, when looking after patients on ventilators which deliver room air with added oxygen from a flow meter, the nurse can determine the inspired oxygen percentage from values of oxygen flow rate and measured minute volume (or tidal volume × respiration rate).

OXYGEN THERAPY BY INCUBATOR

For small infants not on ventilators, an incubator is the only feasible method for giving continuous controlled oxygen therapy, although the concentration can fall rapidly to that of air when the access ports are opened. The oxygen concentration is obtained by means of an oxygen venturi entraining air to give usually 38% (although other venturis can be obtained for higher concentration). The flow rates are such that a complete air change occurs at least ten times per hour.

In addition, an incubator provides a completely controlled environment in respect of humidity and temperature. Infants, particularly premature ones, have poor temperature control mechanisms and a large surface area to body weight ratio — e.g. a 2 kg infant has a ratio of approximately 61 cm² of body surface for each 100 g of body weight, compared with a 76 kg adult, with a corresponding ratio of approximately 22 cm² per 100 g body weight. In a modern sophisticated servo incubator such as the Servo Incubator 79 (Vickers), a temperature-sensing baby probe feeds back to the air-heating system so that the baby's temperature can be adjusted to, or maintained at, a preset value within ± 0.25°C. The air temperature is regulated to no higher than 38°C and moreover is not permitted to rise more than 2°C above the baby's temperature. The relative humidity is maintained at 70%. Some users of incubators monitor the oxygen level with a polarographic or similar probe which is kept close to the baby's airway.

OXYGEN TENTS

The oxygen tent has apparently disappeared from use in adult oxygen therapy practice in Great Britain (Leigh, 1973c). Although, on occasions, small children will use a Ventimask, they are not usually sufficiently co-operative, and an oxygen tent may be the only practical method of raising the inspired oxygen concentration. Even so, a child in a tent may still be unco-operative, although clinical experience indicates that children who *really* require oxygen therapy tend to accept treatment readily. When a subject is in an oxygen tent access is restricted, so that nursing care and oxygen therapy may conflict.

Build-up of heat was a problem in early tents and the inflowing oxygen is now not only humidified but cooled to avoid this complication. In modern tents, especially those designed for children, complete air changes can be achieved 20 times per hour in theory, and concentrations in the region of 75% can be achieved if the tent is perfectly sealed. These tents usually incorporate a high output venturi-type nebulizer which circulates a 'cooling mist'. Cooling systems can be extremely efficient and temperatures within tents as much as $7°C$ below ambient can be obtained if so wished.

HYPERBARIC OXYGEN THERAPY (HOT)

Oxygenation of blood which has been shunted in the lungs occurs by way of the ideal pulmonary capillary blood flow ($\dot{Q}c$) which is optimally saturated. When the shunt ratio ($\dot{Q}s/\dot{Q}t$) is more than 40%, an FIO_2 of one is no longer capable of fulfilling this function. Logically, if PIO_2 is raised by raising atmospheric pressure, then arterial saturation may be considerably improved even with $\dot{Q}s/\dot{Q}t$ ratios as high as 50% (Nunn, 1977). As the haemoglobin capacity of the blood perfusing ventilated alveoli is used up, dissolved gas acts as the oxygenator but, as the quantity in solution is so low (0.3 $ml·dl^{-1}$ per 13.3 kPa (100 mmHg)) the pressure has to be raised considerably to achieve this. Pressures of $2.5-3.0$ ATA are thus required, at which the dissolved oxygen content is 5.6 $ml·dl^{-1}$. In theory, the oxygen consumption of the body (which amounts at rest to an extraction of 5 ml for every dl of blood circulated) could then be met by dissolved oxygen alone, independent of the presence of haemoglobin.

Oxygen under pressure may be given to a patient:

(1) in a large hyperbaric chamber sufficient to contain a number of personnel who breathe air while the patient is given 100% oxygen, or
(2) in an individual 'tank', pressurized with 100% oxygen.

The most common example of the latter consists of a double acrylic cylinder with internal dimensions of 214 cm in length and 59 cm diameter. The large oxygen chambers are less common than the individual 'tanks', for economic reasons, but therapy for the severely ill patient, who may be undergoing various forms of life-support treatment, may be logistically impossible in the latter.

Hyperoxia tends to lower cardiac output and produces vasoconstriction. Neither of these is desirable, although the latter can be overcome by vaso-dilator therapy. Additionally, the high values of capillary Po_2 which can be achieved are not necessarily sufficient to oxygenate ischaemic areas, although there is evidence (e.g. from the successful treatment of arrhythmias during HOT) to suggest that this may be important. Although trials are continuing in various centres throughout the world, the application of HOT where there is tissue ischaemia has, in general terms, proved to be disappointing.

Apart from the absolute value of HOT in industry, in the treatment of decompression sickness in its various forms, or during radiotherapy, where hyperoxia increases the radiosensitivity of some tumours, there are few, if any, established *mandatory* indications in medical practice. Its uses in medicine have included treatment of anaerobic infections, carbon monoxide poisoning or sulph- and methaemoglobinaemia, regional ischaemia from primary vascular causes or from crushing injuries, and cardiogenic shock especially with arrhythmias.

Central nervous system toxicity of oxygen, in the form of epileptiform fits (Paul Bert effect) is markedly increased at 3 ATA and fits can occur within 2–30 minutes in non-anaesthetized patients. HOT is thus usually given to conscious patients at 2–2.5 ATA for treatments of two hours interspersed with rest periods of one hour.

Hyperbaric conditions introduce the risk of decompression sickness and other hazards not only to patients but also to any personnel who may accompany them within the larger installations.

EXTRACORPOREAL MEMBRANE OXYGENATION (ECMO)

The use of ECMO in the treatment of acute respiratory failure has been reviewed by Newland (1977) and by Bregman (1977). Certain conditions which are potentially reversible, such as shock lung, fat embolism of the lung, pancreatitis, pneumonitis and infective pneumonia, still occasionally produce deaths even in young people. The techniques and expertise learned in 25 years of cardiopulmonary bypass have been utilized in the development of ECMO for such cases. As bubble and disc oxygenators are unsuitable, small low prime, high efficiency membrane oxygenators have been developed, although platelet consumption and thrombogenesis are still problems. As might be expected '. . . casual implementation of prolonged ECMO, using techniques and concepts taken unmodified from the cardiac theatres, is very likely to be unsuccessful for (technical) reasons unrelated to the patient's clinical condition' (Newland, 1977).

The results for the first decade or so (Gille, 1974; Gille and Bagniewski, 1976) seemed to be encouraging with a survival rate of 29 patients out of 232 (12.5%). However, a controlled multicentre study at present in progress in the USA, and promoted by the National Heart and Lung Institute (NHLI), shows a survival rate of 3 out of 36 patients (8%) with no significant difference from the mortality in the control group (Peirce, 1977).

The objective of ECMO is that hypoxia can be reduced, complications such as pneumothorax may be more manageable, potentially damaging ventilation pressures and oxygen concentrations may be reduced, and any accompanying circulatory failure or rise in pulmonary artery pressure can be mitigated and controlled in a more satisfactory fashion, all of which will prolong life and so permit the reversal of the underlying lung pathology when this is possible.

Management of the perfusion includes the following.

(1) Proximal and distal cannulation of both the femoral artery and femoral vein.
(2) High flow perfusion with a minimum of 50% of the patient's actual cardiac output, using a high capacity membrane lung together with an automated venoarterial perfusion circuit, with blood returning to the aortic arch or root of aorta.
(3) Control of coagulation by continuous infusion of heparin.
(4) Fail-safe perfusion controls with continuous 24-hour monitoring.
(5) Monitoring of the pulmonary artery and pulmonary wedge pressures, cardiac output, oxygen transport and utilization, in addition to more conventional blood gas measurements.
(6) Ability and readiness to employ adjunctive techniques such as hypothermia, hyperalimentation and haemodialysis.

This is all additional to the normal care provided in an intensive therapy unit.

SUMMARY

The object of oxygen therapy, whatever the method chosen, is to increase tissue oxygen availability. This may be difficult when the primary problem is tissue ischaemia. Logically, the concentration of oxygen should be selectable and unvarying in any situation of patient care since too much may be dangerous, too little may be inadequate, and both diagnostic and prognostic information is contained in the patients' response to its administration. Even assessment of the patient from the end of the bed is easier if his inspired oxygen concentration is known. Similarly, only when inspired oxygen is known and constant can serial measurements of oxygen in blood be interpreted in terms of improvement or otherwise in lung function (in the case of arterial measurements), or in terms of improvement or otherwise in the relationship between tissue blood flow and oxygen consumption (in the case of mixed venous measurements).

It would seem rational therefore that clinicians should always wish to use a fixed performance device for spontaneously breathing patients unless there are compelling reasons for not so doing — as for example in the treatment of children and infants.

For some time control over oxygen concentration has been an accepted practice during the management of patients on ventilators (Pontoppidan and Berry, 1967). The application of these ideas to spontaneously ventilating patients has only become possible more recently with the development of a realistic series of fixed performance venturi devices covering the clinical range.

Hyperbaric oxygen treatment is still not firmly established nor widely applied in medicine. Extracorporeal membrane oxygenation may have something to offer when tissue hypoxia is due to severe though theoretically reversible lung affections, but its value is still unproven.

References

Bethune, D. W. and Collis, J. M. (1977). Using oxygen masks. *Br. J. clin. Equip.* 2, 305–306

Bregman, D. (ed.) (1977). *Mechanical Support of the Failing Heart and Lungs.* New York: Appleton – Century – Crofts

Cain, S. M. and Otis, A. B. (1949). Some physiological effects resulting from added resistance to respiration. *J. aviat. Med.* 20, 149–160

Campbell, E. J. M. (1960). A method of controlled oxygen administration which reduces the risk of carbon dioxide retention. *Lancet* ii, 12–14

Campbell, E. J. M. (1963). Oxygen administration. *Anaesthesia* 18, 503–506

Campbell, E. J. M. and Gebbie, T. (1966). Masks and tent for providing controlled oxygen concentrations. *Lancet* i, 468–469

Campbell, E. J. M. and Minty, K. B. (1976). Controlled oxygen therapy at 60% concentration. Why and how. *Lancet* ii, 1199–1203

Cooper, E. A. (1961). *Behaviour of Respiratory Apparatus.* London: National Coal Board Medical Services

Flenley, D. C., Hutchison, D. C. S. and Donald, K. W. (1963). Behaviour of apparatus for oxygen administration. *Br. med. J.* 2, 1081–1088

Gille, J. P. (1974). L'assistance respiratoire par circulation extra-corporelle avec poumon artifical a membrane. *Bull. Physiopath. Resp.* 10, 373–410

Gille, J. P. and Bagniewski, A. (1976). Ten years of use of extracoporeal membrane oxygenation (ECMO) in treatment of acute respiratory insufficiency (ARI). *Trans Am. Soc. artif. internal Organs* 22, 102–109

Grant, R. J. B., Jones, M. A. and Hughes, J. M. B. (1974). Sequence of regional filling during a tidal breath in man. *J. appl. Physiol.* 37, 158–165

Haldane, J. S. (1917). The therapeutic administration of oxygen. *Br. med. J.* 1, 181–183

Kory, R. C., Bergmann, J. C., Sweet, R. D. and Smith, J. R. (1962). Comparative evaluation of oxygen therapy techniques. *J. Am. med. Ass.* 179, 767–772

Leigh, J. M. (1970). Variation in performance of oxygen therapy devices. *Anaesthesia* 25, 210–222

Leigh, J. M. (1973a). Towards the rational employment of 'the dephlogisticated air described by Priestley'. A study of variation in performance of oxygen therapy devices. *Ann. R. Coll. Surg.* 52, 234–253

Leigh, J. M. (1973b). *On the Performance of Oxygen Therapy Devices.* MD thesis. University of London

Leigh, J. M. (1973c). Present practice and current trends in oxygen therapy. *Anaesthesia* 28, 164–169

Leigh, J. M. (1974a). Ideas and anomalies in the evolution of modern oxygen therapy. *Anaesthesia* 29, 335–348

Leigh, J. M. (1974b). The evolution of oxygen therapy apparatus. *Anaesthesia* 29, 462–485

Newland, P. E. (1977). Extracorporeal membrane oxygenation in the treatment of respiratory failure – a review. *Anaesth. Intens. Care* 5, 99–112

Ngai, S. H. (1972). Editorial – Symposium on Oxygen. *Anesthesiology* 37, 99

Nunn, J. F. (1977). *Applied Respiratory Physiology,* 2nd edn. London: Butterworths

Nunn, J. F. and Newman, H. C. (1964). Inspired gas, rebreathing and apparatus dead space. *Br. J. Anaesth.* 36, 5–10

Peirce, E. C. II (1977). Extracorporeal membrane oxygenation for acute respiratory insufficiency: current status. In *Mechanical Support of the Failing Heart and Lungs,* p. 143. D. Bregman (ed.) New York: Appleton-Century-Crofts

Pontopiddan, H. and Berry, P. R. (1967). Regulation of the inspired oxygen concentration during artificial ventilation. *J. Am. med. Ass.* 201, 89–90

Richardson, F. J., Chinn, S. and Nunn, J. F. (1976). Performance and application of the Quantiflex air/oxygen mixer. *Br. J. Anaesth.* 48, 1057–1064

Scottish Home and Health Department (1969). *Uses and Dangers of Oxygen Therapy.* Edinburgh: HMSO

Silverman, L., Lee, G., Plotkin, T., Sawyers, L. A. and Yancey, A. R. (1951). Airflow measurements on human subjects with and without respiratory resistance at several work rates. *Archs ind. Hyg.* 3, 461–476

28 Oxygen toxicity
Graham Smith

Although oxygen is an essential element in the biological process of respiration, it produces several adverse effects which limit the safe exposure of an organism to hyperoxia. These effects are related predominantly to the partial pressure of oxygen and the duration of exposure, factors which were recognized almost one century ago by Paul Bert (1878). The relationship between pressure, duration of exposure and the development of toxicity is hyperbolic, probably for all types of oxygen toxicity, but it is particularly well recognized for the pulmonary and CNS manifestations (*Figure 28.1*).

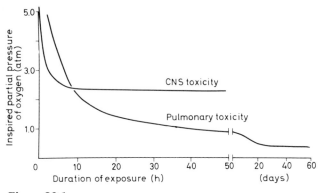

Figure 28.1
Approximate rate of development of pulmonary and CNS oxygen
toxicity as a function of the inspired partial pressure of oxygen

This hyperbolic relationship is specific to individual tissues and species and is responsible for many of the difficulties encountered in the conduct of research and in the appraisal of literature relating to oxygen toxicity. Very high hyperbaric pressures of oxygen cause damage rapidly, which is convenient for the research worker, but data obtained under these conditions are not necessarily applicable to the normobaric situation. Furthermore, investigations of the effect of long-term inhalation of oxygen at pressures of 0.5–0.8 atm demand control of environmental temperature, pressure, humidity and carbon dioxide and inert gas concentrations over a period of days or weeks. This requires considerable technical expertise which has been possible only in the last two decades.

Oxygen toxicity is a subject of such importance and widespread interest that many disciplines have contributed to the existing pool of knowledge. For those seeking detailed information, the most comprehensive reviews available are those on pulmonary oxygen toxicity by Clark and Lambertsen (1971a) and on the biochemical aspects of oxygen toxicity by Haugaard (1968). The clinician, however, should be referred to shorter reviews by Winter and Smith (1972), Clark (1974) and Smith and Shields (1975).

Raised partial pressures of oxygen produce adverse effects in many physiological functions (*Table 28.1*). Rapidly occurring changes which are

TABLE 28.1. Sites of adverse effects of hyperoxia

	Normobaric pressure of oxygen	*Hyperbaric pressure of oxygen*
'Physiological effects'	Ventilation. 'CO$_2$ narcosis' $\dot{V}/\dot{Q}$ changes Vasoconstriction Reduced buffering capacity of blood	
Lungs	Acute and chronic toxicity. Death	
Eye	Retrolental fibroplasia Retinal vasoconstriction	
CNS		Convulsions, coma, death
Endocrine		Adrenals ⎱ damage Thyroid ⎰
Blood	Depressed haemopoiesis	Haemolytic anaemia
Liver and kidney		Damage
Myocardium	Depressed contractility	Myocardial failure
Other		Toxic effects on all tissues, organs and enzyme systems

completely reversible may be produced in ventilation, the distribution of pulmonary ventilation and perfusion, and the cardiovascular system. Changes associated with structural damage (e.g. pulmonary oxygen toxicity or retrolental fibroplasia) are associated with a longer latency and recovery may be associated with residual damage. Although oxygen toxicity affects many organs and tissues (*Table 28.1*), it is the purpose of this chapter to review only those areas of clinical importance.

VENTILATION

The peripheral chemoreceptors contribute relatively little drive to ventilation under normal circumstances, although an increase in the inspired partial pressure of oxygen ($P\text{IO}_2$) has been shown to produce a small though sudden decrease in ventilation (DeJours *et al.*, 1959). However, patients dependent to a large extent on the hypoxic ventilatory drive, principally following long-standing chronic obstructive lung disease, may suffer severe hypoventilation as a result of a raised $P\text{IO}_2$ leading to hypercapnia and coma (Donald and Paton, 1955). This is termed 'carbon dioxide narcosis'.

In the normal individual a gradual increase in $P\text{IO}_2$ produces a progressive saturation of mixed venous blood which is not complete until the $P\text{IO}_2$ reaches 3 atm of oxygen. Conventionally, oxygen at a partial pressure of 303.9 kPa is said to have a pressure of 3 ATA or 3 atm. As oxyhaemoglobin is a poorer buffer than reduced haemoglobin, the carriage of CO_2 is reduced and the tissue $P\text{CO}_2$ increases. The increase in cerebral tissue $P\text{CO}_2$ causes increased central chemoreceptor stimulation and so leads to increased ventilation and systemic hypocapnia and arterial alkalosis (together with a CNS acidosis).

PULMONARY VENTILATION/PERFUSION ($\dot{V}/\dot{Q}$) CHANGES

Absorption collapse of alveoli is known to occur in human volunteers breathing 100% oxygen at 1 atm in situations where a considerable degree of airway closure has been induced deliberately (Nunn *et al.*, 1965; Greene, 1967; Nunn *et al.*, 1978). In addition, DuBois *et al.* (1966) have demonstrated in volunteers that the development of lung collapse is reduced by as little as 5% N_2 in the inspired gas.

Anaesthesia produces a reduction in functional residual capacity (FRC) and an increase in the extent of airway closure and therefore it might be expected that absorption collapse would occur more readily when 100% oxygen is used as the carrier gas. In patients *without cardiorespiratory disease*, experimental data suggest that the extent of any collapse would appear to be minimal. Although Dery *et al.* (1965) demonstrated an immediate decrease in the FRC of anaesthetized patients when 100% oxygen was introduced into the inspired gas, several more recent studies have not revealed any major differences in the FRC of anaesthetized patients breathing either 100% oxygen or 30–35% oxygen in nitrogen (Don *et al.*, 1970; Hewlett *et al.*, 1974).

Thus it would seem that in healthy patients in the supine position and in elderly patients undergoing surgery for fracture of the femoral neck (Wishart, Williams and Smith, 1977), the duration of oxygen breathing, or the extent of airway closure, are not sufficient to lead to detectable absorption collapse. However, thoracotomy and the lateral nephrectomy position (Potgieter, 1959) are associated with a considerable reduction in lung volume of the dependent lung and it is likely that collapse would occur in these situations.

In patients *with abnormal lungs*, alveolar collapse is more likely to occur as a result of pathologically induced airway closure. Thus, a small reduction in FRC was found with both 100% O_2 and 75% O_2 in patients in acute respiratory failure, but a similar effect was detectable only with 100% oxygen in normal subjects (Ramachandran and Fairley, 1970).

Recently, it has been shown that the most sensitive index of lung collapse in volunteers is the Pao_2 value during oxygen breathing (in comparison with radiography of the lungs or measurement of FRC) (Nunn *et al.*, 1978). Measurement of Pao_2 with an Fio_2 of 0.21 will be of value only when blood gas measurements prior to the period of oxygen breathing are available. Of some importance was the finding that collapsed alveoli were reinflated by several maximal inspirations (Nunn *et al.*, 1978).

In the last few years, it has been appreciated that oxygen produces alterations in $\dot{V}/\dot{Q}$ relationships in the lungs of patients in respiratory failure by mechanisms which do not involve lung collapse alone. Thus a progressive increase in Pio_2 has been shown to be accompanied by a progressive increase in venous admixture $(\dot{Q}_s/\dot{Q}_t)$ (Kerr, 1975). Although absorption collapse undoubtedly occurs, the use of positive end-expiratory

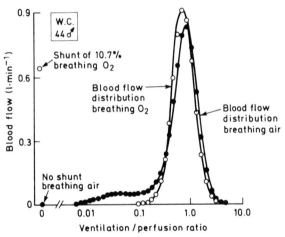

Figure 28.2
Distribution of pulmonary blood flow in a 44-year-old subject breathing air (closed circle) or 100% oxygen (open circle). (Reproduced by permission of the authors and publishers from Wagner *et al.* (1974). *J. clin. Invest.* 54, 54)

pressure (PEEP) was employed in several studies to exclude this as the sole mechanism of 'hyperoxic shunting' (Suter, Fairley and Schlobohm, 1975; Douglas *et al.*, 1976). Therefore, it seems likely that hyperoxia produces a redistribution of blood flow to non-ventilated areas. Alteration in the degree of hypoxic pulmonary vasoconstriction produced by an increase in mixed venous Po_2 (following an increase in Pao_2) is a possible mechanism (Smith, Cheney and Winter, 1974), but it should be stressed that the cause of 'hyperoxic shunting' is highly complex.

Recently, a technique has been developed for quantifying almost continuously the distributions of $\dot{V}/\dot{Q}$ ratios in the lungs of subjects by the steady state elimination of six 'inert' gases dissolved in dextrose and infused i.v. continuously (Wagner, Saltzman and West, 1974). Using this technique, the effect of inspiring 100% oxygen has been investigated (Wagner *et al.*, 1974). In the 44-year-old subject, depicted in *Figure 28.2*, while breathing air, there is a broad pattern of distribution of pulmonary blood flow including perfusion of lung units with $\dot{V}/\dot{Q}$ ratios of less than 0.1. The substitution of 100% oxygen for air caused an increase in shunt ratio to 10.7% within 30 minutes as a result of recruitment of the units with low $\dot{V}/\dot{Q}$ ratios. In the younger subjects, there are few units with such low $\dot{V}/\dot{Q}$ ratios and the increase in shunt was less marked. These changes developed during oxygen breathing with a normal respiratory pattern and they reversed rapidly on resumption of breathing air. Wagner *et al.* (1974) suggested that these changes resulted partly from the development of absorption collapse and partly from a release of hypoxic pulmonary vasoconstriction, a change which would enhance the development of atelectasis. Rapid reversibility of these changes is consistent with the demonstration that a few maximum inspirations were sufficient to re-expand lung units which had collapsed during oxygen breathing (Nunn *et al.*, 1978).

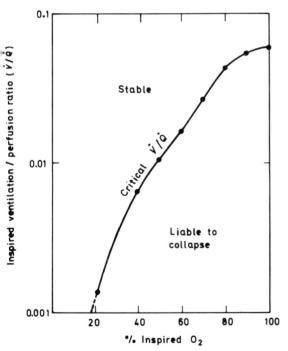

Figure 28.3
The relationship between the inspired oxygen concentration and the 'critical' $\dot{V}/\dot{Q}$ ratio. Note that as the F_{IO_2} increases, so does the $\dot{V}/\dot{Q}$ ratio which is unstable and therefore there are increasing numbers of lung units which have the potential to collapse as the F_{IO_2} increases. (Reproduced by permission of the authors and publisher from Dantzker, Wagner and West (1975). *J. appl. Physiol.* **38**, 886)

An extensive theoretical study has been made by complex computer techniques of absorption collapse occurring during oxygen breathing (Dantzker, Wagner and West, 1975). One can appreciate intuitively that as the ventilation of a lung unit gradually diminishes, a stage is reached where there is no gas flow from the unit during the expiratory phase as a result of absorption by blood perfusing that unit. At this stage, the unit is described as having a 'critical' $\dot{V}/\dot{Q}$ ratio. A further decrease in ventilation results in gas entering the unit during both inspiration and expiration and the unit is then described as 'unstable' since obstruction of the terminal airways will lead to collapse. The relationship of the critical $\dot{V}/\dot{Q}$ ratio to the inspired oxygen concentration is shown in *Figure 28.3*. As the F_{IO_2} increases, so does the $\dot{V}/\dot{Q}$ ratio which is critical. For young subjects, the lower limit of normal $\dot{V}/\dot{Q}$ is about 0.3 but, in the older subject, ratios in the range 0.1 to 0.01 may exist and so there is a potential for collapse when the inspired oxygen concentration exceeds 50%. The rate at which collapse occurs in lung units with unstable $\dot{V}/\dot{Q}$ ratios is shown in *Figure 28.4*. With 100% oxygen, collapse may occur in six

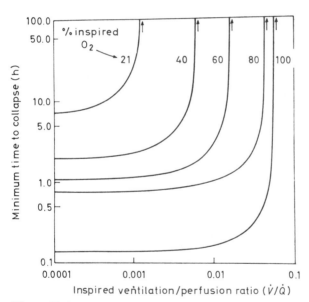

Figure 28.4
Calculations of the rate of collapse of unstable lung units ventilated with varying inspired oxygen concentrations. (Reproduced by permission of the authors and publisher from Dantzker, Wagner and West (1975). *J. appl. Physiol.* **38**, 886)

minutes whilst with 80% oxygen, collapse may occur in less than one hour. Similar considerations apply also to other gases which have a greater blood solubility than nitrogen, such as nitrous oxide, though the critical $\dot{V}/\dot{Q}$ will be much smaller and the rate of alveolar collapse much slower for this gas than for oxygen.

It should be stressed that this analysis of absorption collapse is a theoretical one. It does not take into account, for example, deformation of lung morphology during ventilation, a process which may alter the rate of development of alveolar collapse. Nonetheless, it provides valuable insight into an expanding body of data describing a progressive increase in $\dot{Q}_s/\dot{Q}_t$ with increasing F_{IO_2}.

The important clinical applications which emerge from this section on $\dot{V}/\dot{Q}$ effects may be summarized as follows.

(1) For patients with normal respiratory function, the use of 100% O_2 during anaesthesia does not appear to produce significant collapse in comparison with O_2/N_2 mixtures except in the dependent lung of patients in the lateral nephrectomy position or during thoracotomy.
(2) Although O_2/N_2O mixtures may induce theoretically greater lung collapse than O_2/N_2 mixtures, collapse does not occur during anaesthesia of patients for non-thoracic surgery. During thoracotomy, however, O_2/N_2 mixtures do produce less collapse of the dependent lung (Browne *et al.*, 1970).
(3) For patients with respiratory dysfunction:
    (a) An increase in P_{IO_2} produces an increase in venous admixture caused partly by absorption collapse.
    (b) Therefore, it is an undesirable practice to measure pulmonary shunt with a patient breathing 100% oxygen, and shunt fractions should be calculated using lower concentrations of oxygen.
    (c) The higher the inspired concentration of nitrogen, the less will be the extent of alveolar collapse. Although the pulmonary oxygen toxicity is related to the P_{AO_2} and not to the F_{IO_2}, the F_{IN_2} should be maintained as high as is compatible with a safe P_{aO_2}.

CARDIOVASCULAR EFFECTS

The effects of oxygen breathing on the cardiovascular system are related directly to the level of arterial P_{O_2} attained. Although oxygen at 1 atm has been reported to have little effect on cardiac output in spontaneously breathing patients (Barrett-Boyes and Wood, 1958), the bulk of data would suggest that cardiac output is diminished by 10–15% (Eggers *et al.*, 1962; Murray, 1964; Holt and Branscomb, 1965). With oxygen at 2 atm, cardiac output is depressed by 17% and at 3 atm by 20–25% (Cameron *et al.*, 1966). The depression in cardiac output is caused by a reduction in both stroke volume and heart rate. Mean arterial pressure is usually unchanged.

In animal preparations, oxygen has been demonstrated to diminish myocardial contractility at both normobaric and hyperbaric pressures (Daniell and Bagwell, 1968; Kioschos *et al.*, 1969). However, there is no evidence from studies of animals exposed to oxygen at 1 atm that myocardial failure develops (Smith, Lehan and Monks, 1963). With hyperbaric oxygen, however, it is possible that left ventricular failure may occur in some species, e.g. the rat, induced partly by the development of systemic hypertension (Wood *et al.*, 1972).

Oxygen at both normobaric and hyperbaric pressures produces vaso-constriction in all vascular beds. In the canine coronary circulation, oxygen produces severe vasoconstriction, even during haemorrhagic shock (Ledingham *et al.*, 1971).

Cerebral blood flow diminishes by 10% and 20% with 100% oxygen at 1 atm and 2 atm respectively. In spontaneously breathing man, the vaso-constrictive effect of oxygen is enhanced by the accompanying systemic hypocapnia, which has been described above (Ledingham, 1969).

Existing data suggest that in the human pulmonary circulation, oxygen produces vasodilatation in the presence of hypoxic pulmonary vasocon-striction, but little response in normal lungs (Smith and Shields, 1975). Studies of the long-term inhalation of oxygen by dogs at either 1 atm or 2 atm indicate that in the late stages of pulmonary oxygen toxicity, the pulmonary artery pressure may increase by a small amount (of the order of 0.5—0.7 kPa; 4—5 mmHg).

Other vascular beds, in which hyperoxia has been documented in producing vasoconstriction include the kidney, liver and limbs (Smith and Shields, 1975), although these effects are not clinically important. The vasoconstrictor action of oxygen is responsible for the disappointing results of clinical trials in which hyperbaric oxygen has been used as a means of improving tissue oxygenation.

The myocardial depressant action of oxygen may assume theoretical significance in the treatment of patients with myocardial infarction, but normobaric oxygen therapy is always indicated for these patients where hypoxaemia is present as the negative inotropic effect is related to a high arterial Po_2 (a Pao_2 in excess, say, of 40 kPa; 300 mmHg). The use of hyperbaric oxygen as a means of improving oxygenation around an area of infarction has been utilized in several clinical trials, but it would be fair to state that the results are equivocal (Ledingham, 1969). This conclusion is supported by the recent demonstration that oxygen at 2 atm did not alter significantly the size of acute infarcts in anaesthetized greyhounds (Marshall, Parratt and Ledingham, 1977).

ACUTE AND CHRONIC PULMONARY OXYGEN TOXICITY

Human volunteer studies

Oxygen breathing at 1 atm produces symptoms referable to the respiratory tract at times varying from a few hours to 20—30 hours of continuous exposure (*Figure 28.5*). The symptoms are those of mild, carinal irritation progressing to coughing, pain on deep inspiration and finally, dyspnoea so severe as to lead to the termination of oxygen exposure. However, the rate of development of symptoms is so variable as to be a poor index of oxygen tolerance. Extensive studies by Clark and Lambertsen (1971a,b) have suggested that reduction in vital capacity is the most useful and consistent physiological test of oxygen tolerance in human volunteers, but this test is obviously of little clinical use. Vital capacity decreases fairly quickly on exposure to oxygen (by 10% or so after 25 hours' exposure to 100% oxygen at 1 atm in 50% of subjects) and this may occur before the development of symptoms or of any other physiological changes. In addition, restoration of the vital capacity to normal may take several days after the period of oxygen exposure, during which time the subject may be otherwise normal.

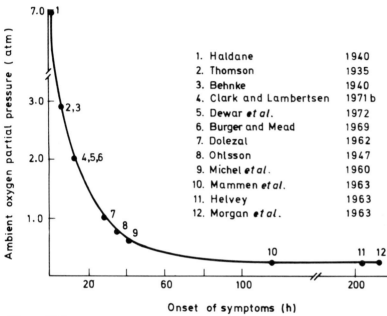

Figure 28.5
Rate of development of early oxygen toxicity in human volunteer studies. (Reproduced by permission of the authors and publishers from Smith and Shields (1975). *Pharmac. Ther. B* 1, 731—756, from which the references may be obtained)

Pulmonary function studies have failed to define clearly the mechanisms of reduction in vital capacity (which occurs mainly at the expense of the inspiratory reserve capacity), although a comprehensive physiological study has probably not been carried out in any single individual investigation. From various centres, studies with varying inspired partial pressures of oxygen have reported decreases in pulmonary compliance, carbon monoxide diffusing capacity and pulmonary capillary blood volume, and an increase in airways resistance. The interpretation of these findings and their relationship to vital capacity alteration are discussed in greater detail by Smith and Shields (1975).

Clinical studies

Pathological studies of oxygen toxicity in patients are confounded by major problems. Firstly, all such studies suffer from the disadvantage of being retrospective; secondly, the morphological changes produced by oxygen are non-specific and are similar to the changes produced by a variety of other injuries to the lungs; thirdly, there are no specific radiological or clinical features *ante mortem*.

Several studies have attempted to correlate the degree of *post mortem* histological abnormality with the inspired partial pressure of oxygen utilized for ventilating patients before death (Nash, Blennerhassett and Pontoppidan, 1967; Gould *et al.*, 1972). Of course, one assumes that patients treated with higher concentrations of oxygen had initially greater lung damage. Therefore, a relationship in such studies between histological changes and doses of oxygen may not be causal. Nevertheless, there is a striking similarity between the lesions seen in human lungs *post mortem* and those in animals exposed to high oxygen concentrations. In addition, some authors have attempted also to define in clinical studies the presence of an early exudative phase with damage to alveolar lining cells and endothelium with the development of interstitial oedema and hyaline membranes, followed by a later fibroproliferative phase. This later phase appears to be a non-specific reparative process in which there is septal thickening as a result of hyperplasia of the septal cells, increased collagen fibres and hyperplasia of the type 2 cells (Gould *et al.*, 1972; Anderson *et al.*, 1973).

These pathological features are characteristic also of the 'adult respiratory distress syndrome' or 'shock lung syndrome' which commonly may be produced by massive trauma, fat embolus, burns, shock, infection, direct lung injury and after surgery. It has been suggested that the lung has only a limited response to injury and this accounts for the similarity of *post mortem* features following a variety of different illnesses (Bachofen and Weibel, 1974).

The inherent deficiencies in all clinical studies have prevented the clear definition of the lower limit of safety of oxygen therapy. However, histological features compatible with oxygen toxicity have been noted in patients treated with 40% oxygen at 1 atm (Pratt, 1974; Sevitt, 1974). In an uncontrolled study of 12 patients who died at 7–61 months after treatment with self-administered low flow oxygen therapy at home, lesions compatible with oxygen toxicity were found in 50% of the patients, although these were not thought to contribute in any way to mortality (Petty, Stanford and Nott, 1971).

Animal studies

There is enormous species variation in susceptibility to oxygen toxicity and also wide intraspecies variation. In general, small animals are more susceptible than large ones: with 100% oxygen at 1 atm, rats and mice expire from pulmonary oxygen toxicity in one to two days, dogs in two to three days and monkeys in approximately two weeks.

Mammals exposed to 100% oxygen at 1 atm exhibit early respiratory distress followed by severe dyspnoea, coughing and cyanosis, gasping respiration in the terminal stages and finally death in apnoea. The pathological features in the lungs of such animals are shown in *Table 28.2*. This response, termed acute pulmonary oxygen toxicity, is produced by continuous exposure to relatively high doses of oxygen (of the order of 0.8–1.5 atm). Low doses of oxygen (exposure to 0.5–0.8 atm or even intermittent exposure to higher pressures) are associated with the development of chronic pulmonary oxygen toxicity, in which the characteristic

TABLE 28.2. Pathological features of acute pulmonary oxygen toxicity

Exudative phase (early)	Type 1 cell necrosis
	Endothelial cell damage
	Interstitial and perivascular oedema
	Hyaline membranes
	Intra-alveolar oedema
	Alveolar collapse
	Capillary congestion
Proliferative phase (late)	Hyperplasia of septal cells
	Fibrosis and fibroplastic proliferation
	Hyperplasia of type 2 cells

pathological features are those of septal thickening with capillary and type 2 alveolar epithelial cell hyperplasia.* It should be emphasized that the acute and chronic changes merely represent a spectrum of response and the two types of lesions may coexist in one animal.

The first change seen in both the rat and primate lung is endothelial damage followed by damage to the type 1 alveolar epithelial cell (Kistler, Caldwell and Weibel, 1967; Kapanci *et al.*, 1969; Kaplan *et al.*, 1969). This is accompanied by the development of interstitial and intra-alveolar oedema. The type 2 alveolar epithelial cells, thought to be responsible for the production of pulmonary surfactant, are relatively resistant to oxygen and at a later stage proliferate to reline the walls of the alveoli. These changes are responsible for the gross reduction in lung compliance and impairment of oxygen transfer seen during the later stages of oxygen toxicity.

Almost complete resolution of these changes may occur. In two monkeys exposed for 8 and 13 days to 100% oxygen at 1 atm and then gradually weaned back to ambient air, there was, after 56 and 84 days' recovery respectively, complete restoration of lung architecture apart from some focal scarring (Kapanci *et al.*, 1969).

Mechanisms of oxygen-induced lung damage

All the known mechanisms whereby damage may be produced in the lung are detailed in *Figure 28.6*.

Mucociliary transport in the trachea and bronchioles may be depressed

* See Chapter 20. *Ed.*

by oxygen (Laurenzi, Yin and Guarneri, 1968). In dogs, 100% oxygen at 1 atm was found to depress transport by 84% after six hours (Sackner *et al.*, 1976). A similar effect has been demonstrated also in man (Sackner *et al.*, 1975).

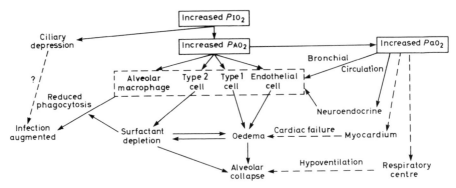

Figure 28.6
Mechanisms whereby oxygen may produce lung damage. ----- indicates routes for which evidence exists only with hyperbaric pressures of oxygen. (Considerably modified from Smith and Shields (1975). *Pharmac. Ther. B* 1, 731–756, by permission)

There is considerable interest currently in the effect of oxygen on pulmonary defence mechanisms. It has been shown that oxygen at 1 atm reduces the survival time of mice infected with either influenzal viral pneumonia (Ayers, Tierney and Imagawa, 1973) or diplococcal pneumonia (Angrick, Somerson and Weiss, 1974).

The alveolar macrophage exercises a scavenging function in the lung and helps to combat infection by ingesting bacteria which are then subjected to lytic enzymes. The alveolar macrophage of the mouse exhibits depressed phagocytic activity in response to 90% oxygen (Huber and La Force, 1970), but studies by Murphey *et al.* (1975) suggest that, *in vitro*, the alveolar macrophage is relatively resistant to oxygen. Further data is required to determine if the depression of phagocytic activity by macrophages *in vivo* is related to other changes produced during early oxygen toxicity; alteration in surfactant activity has been suggested as a possible mechanism (Huber, Goodenough and O'Connell, 1974).

There is little doubt that a raised alveolar Po_2 *per se* has a direct toxic effect on the cellular constituents of the lung architecture. However, a raised alveolar Po_2 may also produce lung damage indirectly by virtue of the concomitant elevation in arterial Po_2. An elevated Pao_2 may induce lung damage partly by virtue of a toxic level of oxygen in the bronchial circulation and partly by acting at sites outside the lungs. Central respiratory failure and direct myocardial depression produced by elevation of arterial Po_2 are of importance only with hyperbaric pressures of oxygen and will not be discussed further (see Winter and Smith, 1972).

There is considerable evidence that the general level of metabolic activity and the sympathoadrenal system are involved in the production of lung damage. Much of the evidence for this is derived from studies of exposure to hyperbaric oxygen in which hypophysectomy, adrenalectomy and sympatholytic drugs delay the development of pulmonary damage whilst ACTH, cortisone and sympathomimetic drugs increase the rate of development of lung damage. The mechanisms of these effects may be related to alteration in pulmonary arterial pressure and pulmonary trans-capillary pressures and capillary permeability with consequent alteration in the rate of development of interstitial and intra-alveolar oedema and also alteration in pulmonary repair processes. The data related to oxygen toxicity at normobaric pressures are less convincing.

Surfactant activity is depressed in oxygen toxicity. Research on the primary effects of oxygen on surfactant production as opposed to depression in activity secondary to changes such as exudative oedema, represents an area of considerable interest at the present time. Biochemical measurements on lipid components (Gilder and McSherry, 1974) and protein constituents (Gacad and Massaro, 1973) of surfactant reveal conflicting conclusions with regard to a primary effect of oxygen on the type 2 alveolar epithelial cells. However, strong circumstantial evidence from the ultrastructural abnormalities induced by oxygen in the type 2 cells (Massaro and Massaro, 1973; 1974) would suggest that it is reasonable to suppose at the present time that surfactant production is depressed directly by oxygen toxicity. In addition, surfactant activity is decreased secondary to exudative oedema accompanying the late stages of pulmonary oxygen toxicity.

Modification of pulmonary oxygen toxicity

If indirect mechanisms are important in the production of lung damage by oxygen, one would expect that intrapulmonary shunting (with a large $(A-a)$ Po_2 difference) would delay the development of oxygen toxicity. This question was first considered in 1967 by Winter *et al.* who produced a large $(A-a)$ Po_2 difference in dogs by the surgical creation of a right-to-left shunt. Operated dogs were found to be more tolerant to oxygen at 2.0–2.5 atm than non-operated control dogs. However, these findings were not confirmed with oxygen at 1 atm in similar experiments carried out by Ashbaugh (1971). This suggests that *in the absence of lung damage*, the indirect mechanisms are important only with hyperbaric pressure of oxygen.

Where *lung damage has been produced* in association with a measured or presumed increase in pulmonary shunting and reduction in arterial Po_2, tolerance was increased on exposure to oxygen at 1 atm (Smith, Winter and Wheelis, 1973). In addition, parenchymal lung damage produced in rats by prior exposure to hyperoxia (Wright *et al.*, 1966) or hypoxia (Brauer *et al.*, 1970) was also associated with increased oxygen tolerance at 1 atm. More recently, Brashear, Sharma and Deatley (1973) exposed rats to a period of hypoxia and found that these animals on subsequent exposure to oxygen at 1 atm exhibited greater oxygen tolerance than untreated control rats. Arterial blood sampling revealed that both the treated and untreated rats had the same arterial oxygen tensions confirming that in this particular study the mechanism of increased tolerance was not via the creation of an increased $(A-a)$ Po_2 difference.

These data suggest that in the rat, lung damage does not modify normobaric oxygen tolerance by reduction of the Pao_2 but that damaged lung tissue is more resistant to oxygen than normal lung. It is known that following damage to the lung, non-specific reparative processes include hyperplasia of the type 2 alveolar epithelial cells and these are more resistant to oxygen than the type 1 alveolar epithelial cells.

TABLE 28.3. Factors which modify pulmonary oxygen toxicity in animals*

Augmented damage or increased rate of development	*Decreased damage or decreased rate of development*
ACTH	γ-Aminobutyric acid (GABA)
CO_2 inhalation	Tris buffer
Convulsions	Antioxidants (vitamin E, vitamin C, methylene blue, etc.)
Cortisone and derivatives	Anaesthetic agents
Adrenaline and sympathomimetic drugs	Adrenergic blocking drugs
Thyroid hormones	Chlorpromazine and reserpine
Hyperthermia	Adrenalectomy
Paraquat	Hypophysectomy
X-irradiation	Altitude acclimatization
	Prior exposure to hyperoxia
	Phosgene
	Oleic acid

* For a more complete list and references, see Clark and Lambertsen (1971a)

There are a very large number of chemicals which alter pulmonary oxygen tolerance in experimental animals (Clark and Lambertsen, 1971a). Although most of these have no effect on lung structure, in general where lung structure is altered, oxygen tolerance is increased. The exception to this general statement is the substance paraquat. This herbicide potentiates the rate of development of fatal pulmonary oxygen toxicity (Fisher, Clements and Wright, 1973). In *Table 28.3* are listed some of the factors which have been shown to modify oxygen tolerance in experimental animals.

In the clinical context, there is no known substance which protects against pulmonary oxygen toxicity. The only known manoeuvre which increases tolerance in human volunteers to a given dose of oxygen is the use of intermittent as opposed to continuous exposure to that dose. However, extrapolation from animal data and knowledge that some patients have survived remarkably long periods of ventilation with 100% oxygen suggests that lung damage with associated arterial hypoxaemia *may* reduce the rate of development of oxygen toxicity in humans. However, in the absence of clinical data, it would seem prudent to treat patients with lung damage on the basis that their oxygen tolerance is the same as that of human volunteers and non-human primates.

It should be stressed also that, in the clinical context, toxicity is related to the partial pressure of inspired oxygen and not the concentration. Inert gases play an important role at normobaric pressures only by reducing the extent of absorption collapse (see above). However, in hyperbaric chambers, inert gases may increase oxygen tolerance by inducing inert gas narcosis, or decrease tolerance by causing increased gas density leading to an increase in Pa_{CO_2}.

Biochemical mechanisms of oxygen toxicity

In tissues, oxygen is reduced predominantly by the cytochrome and redox systems. However, a small amount is reduced to highly reactive free radicals including $O_2^{-\bullet}$ (superoxide radical) and $OH^\bullet$ which may be reduced to the much less reactive but still destructive substance H_2O_2. During the process of evolution, antioxidant defence mechanisms have developed including superoxide dismutase, catalases, peroxidases and α-tocopherol (vitamin E) which function in the following way:

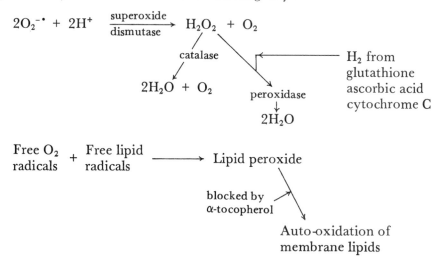

The production of free radicals is stimulated by oxygen, light and other forms of radiation including x-rays. It has been known for some time that antioxidants (glutathione, vitamin E, etc.) tend to delay the onset of oxygen toxicity (*Table 28.3*). Recently, it has been demonstrated that increased collagen content of lungs of rats exposed to 80%

oxygen for 41 and 84 days is produced by increased peroxidation of lipids in the lungs (Chvapil and Peng, 1975).

Of more interest, however, is the relationship which has been demonstrated between oxygen toxicity and superoxide dismutase (SD). Cells which contain a high concentration of SD are more resistant to oxygen than comparable cells containing a lower concentration of this enzyme (Gregory and Fridovich, 1973). Confirmation has been obtained in rats that the superoxide radical may be one of the primary agents in the biochemical basis of toxicity. Rats pretreated with 85% oxygen at 1 atm for seven days became resistant to 100% oxygen and had increased SD activity in their lungs. A progressive loss of tolerance was accompanied by a progressive reduction in the amount of pulmonary SD (Crapo and Tierney, 1974). In addition to increased SD levels, oxygen exposure has been shown to produce in the rat lung an increase in other antioxidant systems including glutathione peroxidase (Kimball *et al.,* 1976).

It should be stressed that oxygen poisoning at a biochemical level is a process of great complexity. Oxygen is a universal cellular poison which is as yet incompletely understood. The literature on the cellular mechanisms and biochemical aspects of oxygen toxicity is extensive and is reviewed by Haugaard (1968) and Davies and Davies (1965). Oxygen is known to inactivate many enzyme systems *in vitro*, but those which are thought to be important *in vivo* include oxidation of SH groups on essential enzymes, such as coenzyme A, peroxidation of lipids and inhibition of iron and SH containing flavoproteins. Thus, oxygen interferes with the tricarboxylic acid cycle, the electron transport system and oxidative phosphorylation in the mitochondria.

Clinical management of pulmonary oxygen toxicity

The clinician may suspect oxygen toxicity as a possible cause of lung damage *only* by knowing that the patient has been exposed to a toxic dose. Although it is not possible to state precisely the limits of toxicity for patients, an important prospective clinical study (Barber, Lee and Hamilton, 1970) suggested that in patients with head injury, impairment of arterial oxygenation with 100% oxygen did not occur before 40 hours. Therefore, one would suggest tentatively that a toxic dose (to produce structural damage) would be 100% oxygen for more than two days or 80% oxygen for several days. For practical purposes, the lower safe limit may be taken as 50% of 1 atm, and above this oxygen should be regarded as a cumulative toxic drug. As there is no treatment of oxygen toxicity, the only manoeuvre which the clinician may employ is to maintain the P_{IO_2} at the minimum compatible with adequate tissue oxygenation. This demands therapy aimed at producing a normal haemoglobin concentration and maintaining an adequate cardiac output by attention to fluid and electrolyte balance and inotropic support of the myocardium when necessary. In addition, the $(A-a)$ P_{O_2} difference may be reduced by the use of large tidal volumes, chest physiotherapy, bronchial toilet and perhaps the use of positive end-expiratory pressure on occasion. These measures also serve to reduce the extent of absorption collapse induced by oxygen breathing (see above). Detailed consideration of therapy falls outside the scope of this chapter.

CENTRAL NERVOUS SYSTEM TOXICITY

CNS oxygen toxicity, in the form of convulsions, occurs only at pressures in excess of 2.5 atm (*Figure 28.1*). It is a function of the arterial Po_2 and not the arterial oxygen content. The convulsions take the form of seizures very similar to those of grand mal epilepsy and furthermore they are also frequently but not invariably accompanied by premonitory signs. These include abnormalities of mood and behaviour, localized twitching especially around the face and head, and hallucinations (Donald, 1947; Lambertsen, 1965). The threshold for symptoms and convulsions varies enormously both between individuals and also in the same individual from day to day (Donald, 1947), but it would seem that the risk of convulsions is very slight for man for periods of two hours and one hour at pressures of less than 2.8 and 3.0 atm respectively. Pressures of oxygen in excess of 3.0 atm reduce the safe exposure limits dramatically (*Figure 28.1*). Apparently, the practical safety limits are shorter for subjects exposed to hyperbaric pressures under water in diving suits compared with exposure in dry hyperbaric chambers (Wood, 1969).

A wide variety of substances has been shown to exert a partially protective effect against the convulsive effects of hyperbaric oxygen in experimental animals (*Table 28.4*). Inhibition of many enzyme systems in the brain has been suggested as being solely or partially responsible for the convulsive effects of oxygen. Effects on the electron transfer system

TABLE 28.4. Substances which delay the onset of CNS oxygen toxicity in animals

Tris buffer

α-Tocopherol (vitamin E)

γ-Aminobutyric acid (GABA) and related compounds (glycine, alanine)

Arginine

Vitamin K

Anaesthetic agents

Antioxidants

Lithium

and on oxidative phosphorylation and alteration of the brain glutamate system represent the most fruitful sources of investigation. Recently, lithium has been shown to protect against oxygen convulsions by preventing depletion of brain glutamate and γ-aminobutyric acid (Bannister, Bhakthan and Singh, 1976).

RETROLENTAL FIBROPLASIA

Before four months of gestation, the human fetal retina does not possess blood vessels. Vascularization in the nasal region of the retina precedes the process in the temporal region, where it is not complete until one month after birth of the full term infant. During this period of immaturity, oxygen produces retinal vasoconstriction with obliteration of the most immature vessels. Subsequent exposure to air allows new vessel formation at the site of damage in the form of a proliferative retinopathy. Leakage of intravascular fluid leads to vitreoretinal adhesions, and even retinal detachment (Patz, 1976).

This condition (retrolental fibroplasia — RLF) was described first in 1942 but its association with oxygen therapy was not observed until 1951 (Campbell, 1951). Later, it became obvious that the dominant factor was not an F_{IO_2} in excess of 0.4, but an elevated retinal artery P_{O_2}. It is not known what the threshold of P_{aO_2} is for the development of retinal damage but an umbilical arterial P_{O_2} of 8–12 kPa (60–90 mmHg) has been said to be associated with only a very low incidence of RLF and no systemic hypoxia (Tasman, 1971).

Because frequent arterial sampling is difficult in babies, it has been suggested that ophthalmoscopic monitoring of vessel calibre may be a test of hyperoxia. It is suggested that if retinal vasoconstriction induced by oxygen gradually disappears 10–15 minutes after removal of the baby from the incubator, lowering of the F_{IO_2} will prevent retinal damage from occurring, but if constriction persists for longer than this period of time, retinal damage will occur. It seems clear that this is an adequate test of hyperoxia.

Careful assessment of the retinae of every infant exposed to hyperoxia in the paediatric intensive therapy unit should be undertaken by the ophthalmologist. Recently, of 384 infants exposed to hyperoxia under carefully controlled conditions, 68 were found subsequently to have some degree of RLF. Most resolved spontaneously to normal or near normal over a period of 38 months (Kingham, 1977).

It should be stressed that there are many factors involved in the development of RLF. Nonetheless, arterial hyperoxia is an important contributory factor. In a recent case report, the development of RLF was attributed to the short duration of hyperoxia encountered during general anaesthesia of a premature infant. However, as the authors acknowledged, it is difficult to substantiate a definite aetiological role for oxygen in this instance (Betts *et al.*, 1977).

References

Anderson, W. R., Strickland, M. B., Tsai, S. H. and Haglin, J. T. (1973). Light microscopic and ultrastructural study of the adverse effects of oxygen therapy on the neonate lung. *Am. J. Path.* **73**, 327–339

Angrick, E. J., Somerson, N. L. and Weiss, H. S. (1974). Oxygen effects on mortality of mice infected with diplococcus pneumoniae. *Aerospace Med.* **45**, 730–734

Ashbaugh, D. G. (1971). Oxygen toxicity in normal and hypoxemic dogs. *J. appl. Physiol.* **31**, 664–668

Ayers, L. N., Tierney, D. F. and Imagawa, D. (1973). Shortened survival of mice with influenza when given oxygen at one atmosphere. *Am. Rev. resp. Dis.* **107**, 955–961

Bachofen, M. and Weibel, E. R. (1974). Basic pattern of tissue repair in human lungs following unspecific injury. *Chest* **65**, 14S–19S

Banister, E. W., Bhakthan, N. M. G. and Singh, A. K. (1976). Lithium protection against oxygen toxicity in rats: ammonia and amino acid metabolism. *J. Physiol.* **260**, 587–596

Barber, R. E., Lee, J. and Hamilton, W. K. (1970). Oxygen toxicity in man. A prospective study in patients with irreversible brain damage. *New Engl. J. Med.* **283**, 1478–1484

Barratt-Boyes, B. G. and Wood, E. H. (1958). Cardiac output and related measurements and pressure values in the right heart and associated vessels, together with analysis of the hemodynamic response to the inhalation of high oxygen mixtures in healthy subjects. *J. Lab. clin. Med.* **51**, 72–90

Bert, P. (1878). *Barometric Pressure: Researches in Experimental Physiology*, p. 5. M. Hitchcock and F. A. Hitchcock (trans.) (1943). Columbus, Ohio: Langs College Book Co.

Betts, E. K., Downes, J. J., Schaffer, D. B. and Johns, R. (1977). Retrolental fibroplasia and oxygen administration during general anaesthesia. *Anesthesiology* **47**, 518–520

Brashear, R. E., Sharma, H. M. and Deatley, R. E. (1973). Prolonged survival breathing oxygen at ambient pressure. *Am. Rev. resp. Dis.* **108**, 701–704

Brauer, R. W., Parrish, D. E., Way, R. D., Pratt, P. C. and Pesotti, R. L. (1970). Protection by altitude acclimatisation against lung damage from exposure to oxygen at 825 mmHg. *J. appl. Physiol.* **28**, 474–481

Browne, D. R. G., Rochford, J., O'Connell, U. and Jones, J. G. (1970). The incidence of postoperative atelectasis in the dependent lung following thoracotomy; the value of added nitrogen. *Br. J. Anaesth.* **42**, 340–346

Cameron, A. J. V., Hutton, I., Kenmure, A. C. F. and Murdoch, W. R. (1966). Haemodynamic and metabolic effects of hyperbaric oxygen in myocardial infarction. *Lancet* **ii**, 833–837

Campbell, K. (1951). Intensive oxygen therapy as a possible cause of retrolental fibroplasia: a clinical approach. *Med. J. Aust.* **2**, 48–50

Chvapil, M. and Peng, Y. M. (1975). Oxygen and lung fibrosis. *Archs envir. Hlth* **30**, 528–532

Clark, J. M. (1974). The toxicity of oxygen. *Am. Rev. resp. Dis.* **110**, 40–49

Clark, J. M. and Lambertsen, C. J. (1971a). Pulmonary oxygen toxicity — a review. *Pharmac. Rev.* **23**, 37–133

Clark, J. M. and Lambertsen, C. J. (1971b). Rate of development of pulmonary O_2 toxicity in man during O_2 breathing at 2.0 ATA. *J. appl. Physiol.* **30**, 739–752

Crapo, J. D. and Tierney, D. F. (1974). Superoxide dismutase and pulmonary oxygen toxicity. *Am. J. Physiol.* **226**, 1401–1407

Daniell, H. B. and Bagwell, E. E. (1968). Effects of high oxygen on coronary flow and heart force. *Am. J. Physiol.* **214**, 1454–1459

Dantzker, D. R., Wagner, P. D. and West, J. B. (1975). Instability of lung units with low $\dot{V}A/\dot{Q}$ ratios during O_2 breathing. *J. appl. Physiol.* **38**, 886–895

Davies, Helen C. and Davies, R. E. (1965). Biochemical aspects of oxygen poisoning. In *Handbook of Physiology*, sect. 3, vol. 2, pp. 1047–1058. Washington DC: Am. Physiol. Soc.

DeJours, P., Girard, F., Labrousse, Y. and Teillac, A. (1959). Étude de la regulation de la ventilation de repos chez l'homme en haute altitude. *Revue fr. Etud. clin. biol.* **4**, 115–127

Dery, R., Pelletier, J., Jacques, A., Clavet, M. and Houde, J. (1965). Alveolar collapse induced by denitrogenation. *Can. Anaesth. Soc. J.* **12**, 531–544

Don, H. F., Wahba, M., Cuadrado, L. and Kelkar, K. (1970). The effects of anesthesia and 100 per cent oxygen on the functional residual capacity of the lungs. *Anesthesiology* **32**, 521–529

Donald, K. W. (1947). Oxygen poisoning in man. *Br. med. J.* **1**, 667–672

Donald, K. W. and Paton, W. D. M. (1955). Gases administered in artificial respiration. *Br. med. J.* **1**, 313–318

Douglas, M. E., Downs, J. B., Dannemiller, F. J., Hodges, M. R. and Munson, E. S. (1976). Change in pulmonary venous admixture with varying inspired oxygen. *Anaesth. Analg.* **55**, 688–695

Dubois, A. B., Turaids, T., Mammen, R. E. and Nobrega, F. T. (1966). Pulmonary atelectasis in subjects breathing oxygen at sea level or at simulated altitude. *J. appl. Physiol.* **21**, 828–836

Eggers, G. W. N., Paley, H. W., Leonard, J. J. and Waren, S. V. (1962). Hemodynamic responses to oxygen breathing in man. *J. appl. Physiol.* **17**, 75–79

Fisher, H. K., Clements, J. A. and Wright, R. R. (1973). Enhancement of oxygen toxicity by the herbicide paraquat. *Am. Rev. resp. Dis.* **107**, 246–252

Gacad, G. and Massaro, D. (1973). Hyperoxia: Influence on lung mechanics and protein synthesis. *J. clin. Invest.* **52**, 559–565

Gilder, H. and McSherry, C. K. (1974). Mechanisms of oxygen inhibition of pulmonary surfactant synthesis. *Surgery* **76**, 72–79

Gould, V. E., Tosco, R., Wheelis, R. F., Gould, N. S. and Kapanci, Y. (1972). Oxygen pneumonitis in man. Ultrastructural observations on the development of alveolar lesions. *Lab. Invest.* **26**, 499–508

Green, L. D. (1967). *The pathogenesis and physiological effects of pulmonary collapse induced by breathing oxygen and increased gravitational force.* PhD Thesis, University of London

Gregory, E. M. and Fridovich, J. (1973). Oxygen toxicity and the superoxide dismutase. *J. Bact.* **114**, 1193–1197

Haugaard, N. (1968). Cellular mechanisms of oxygen toxicity. *Physiol. Rev.* **48**, 311–373

Hewlett, A. M., Hulands, G. H., Nunn, J. F. and Heath, J. R. (1974). Functional residual capacity during anaesthesia. II: spontaneous respiration. *Br. J. Anaesth.* **46**, 486–494

Holt, J. H. and Branscomb, B. V. (1965). Hemodynamic responses to controlled 100% oxygen breathing in emphysema. *J. appl. Physiol.* **20**, 215–220

Huber, G., Goodenough, S. and O'Connell, D. (1974). Oxygen toxicity and bacterial infection in the lung: impairment of alveolar lining material versus alveolar macrophage bactericidal activity. *Clin. Res.* **22**, 506A

Huber, J. and LaForce, F. M. (1970). Progressive impairment of pulmonary antibacterial defence mechanisms associated with prolonged oxygen administration. *Ann. intern. Med.* **72**, 808

Kapanci, Y., Weibel, E. R., Kaplan, H. P. and Robinson, F. R. (1969). Pathogenesis and reversibility of the pulmonary lesions of oxygen toxicity in monkeys. II. Ultrastructural and morphometric studies. *Lab. Invest.* **20**, 101–118

Kaplan, H. P., Robinson, F. R., Kapanci, Y. and Weibel, E. R. (1969). Pathogenesis and reversibility of the pulmonary lesions of oxygen toxicity in monkeys. I: Clinical and light microscopic studies. *Lab. Invest.* **20**, 94–100

Kerr, J. H. (1975). Pulmonary oxygen transfer during I.P.P.V. in man. *Br. J. Anaesth.* **47**, 695–705

Kimball, R. E., Reddy, K., Peirce, T. H., Schwartz, L. W., Mustafa, M. G. and Cross, C. E. (1976). Oxygen toxicity: augmentation of antioxidant defense mechanism in rat lung. *Am. J. Physiol.* **230**, 1425–1431

Kingham, J. D. (1977). Acute retrolental fibroplasia. *Archs Ophthal., N.Y.* **95**, 39–47

Kioschos, J. M., Behar, V. S., Saltzman, H. A., Thompson, H. K., Myres, N. E., Smith, W. W. and McIntosh, H. D. (1969). Effect of hyperbaric oxygenation on left ventricular function. *Am. J. Physiol.* **216**, 161–166.

Kistler, G. S., Caldwell, P. R. B. and Weibel, E. R. (1967). Development of fine-structural damage to alveolar and capillary lining cells in oxygen-poisoned rat lungs. *J. Cell Biol.* **32**, 605–628

Lambertsen, C. J. (1965). Effects of oxygen at high partial pressure. In *Handbook of Physiology*, sect. 3, vol. 2, pp. 1027–1046. W. O. Fenn and H. Rahn (ed.). Washington DC: Am. Physiol. Soc.

Laurenzi, G. A., Yin, S. and Guarneri, J. J. (1968). Adverse effect of oxygen on tracheal mucus flow. *New Engl. J. Med.* **279**, 333–339

Ledingham, I.McA. (1969). Hyperbaric oxygenation. In *Recent Advances in Surgery*, pp. 295–338. S. Taylor (ed.). London: Churchill

Ledingham, I.McA., Parratt, J. R., Smith, G. and Vance, J. P. (1971). Haemodynamic and myocardial effects of hyperbaric oxygen in dogs subjected to haemorrhage. *Cardiovasc. Res.* **5**, 277–285

Marshall, R. J., Parratt, J. R. and Ledingham, I.McA. (1977). The effect of hyperbaric oxygen (2 ATA) on the haemodynamic, metabolic and electrocardiographic consequences of acute myocardial ischaemia in anaesthetised greyhounds. *J. Physiol.* **268**, 16P

Massaro, G. D. and Massaro, D. (1973). Pulmonary granular pneumocytes. Loss of mitochondrial granules during hyperoxia. *J. Cell Biol.* **59**, 246–250

Massaro, G. D. and Massaro, D. (1974). Adaptation to hyperoxia. Influence on protein synthesis by lung and on granular pneumocyte ultrastructure. *J. clin. Invest.* **53**, 705–709

Murphey, S. A., Hyams, J. S., Fisher, A. B. and Root, R. K. (1975). Effects of oxygen exposure on in vitro function of pulmonary alveolar macrophages. *J. clin. Invest.* **56**, 503–511

Murray, J. F. (1964). Systemic oxygen transport as a regulator of hemodynamics. *Clin. Res.* **12**, 190

Nash, G., Blennerhassett, J. B. and Pontoppidan, H. (1967). Pulmonary lesions associated with oxygen therapy and artificial ventilation. *New Engl. J. Med.* **276**, 368–374

Nunn, J. F., Coleman, A. J., Sachithanandan, T., Bergman, N. A. and Laws, J. W. (1965). Hypoxaemia and atelectasis produced by forced expiration. *Br. J. Anaesth.* **37**, 3–12

Nunn, J. F., Williams, I. P., Jones, J. G., Hewlett, A. M., Hulands, G. H. and Minty, B. D. (1978). Detection and reversal of pulmonary absorption collapse. *Br. J. Anaesth.* 50, 91–100

Patz, A. (1976). Current status of role of oxygen in retrolental fibroplasia. *Invest. Ophthalmol.* 15, 337–339

Petty, T. L., Stanford, R. E. and Nott, T. A. (1971). Continuous oxygen therapy in chronic airway obstruction: observations on possible oxygen toxicity and survival. *Ann. intern. Med.* 75, 361–367

Potgieter, S. V. (1959). Atelectasis: its evolution during upper urinary tract surgery. *Br. J. Anaesth.* 31, 472–483

Pratt, P. C. (1974). Pathology of pulmonary oxygen toxicity. *Am. Rev. resp. Dis.* 110, 51–57

Ramachandran, P. R. and Fairley, H. B. (1970); Changes in functional residual capacity during respiratory failure. *Can. Anaesth. Soc. J.* 17, 359–369

Sackner, M. A., Landa, J., Hirsch, J. and Zapata, A. (1975). Pulmonary effects of oxygen breathing. A 6-hour study in normal men. *Ann. intern. Med.* 82, 40–43

Sackner, M. A., Hirsch, J., Epstein, S. and Rynolin, A. M. (1976). Effect of oxygen in graded concentrations upon tracheal mucus velocity. A study in anesthetised dogs. *Chest* 69, 164–167

Sevitt, S. (1974). Diffuse and focal oxygen pneumonitis. A preliminary report on the threshold of pulmonary oxygen toxicity in man. *J. clin. Path.* 27, 21–30

Smith, C. W., Lehan, P. H. and Monks, J. J. (1963). Cardiopulmonary manifestations with high O_2 tensions at atmospheric pressure. *J. appl. Physiol.* 18, 849–853

Smith, G. and Shields, T. G. (1975). Oxygen toxicity. *Pharmac. Ther. B* 1, 731–756

Smith, G., Cheney, F. W. and Winter, P. M. (1974). The effect of change in cardiac output on intrapulmonary shunting. *Br. J. Anaesth.* 46, 337–342

Smith, G., Winter, P. M. and Wheelis, R. F. (1973). Increased normobaric oxygen tolerance of rabbits following oleic acid-induced lung damage. *J. appl. Physiol.* 35, 395–400

Suter, P. M., Fairley, H. B. and Schlobohm, R. M. (1975). Shunt, lung volume and perfusion during short periods of ventilation with oxygen. *Anesthesiology* 43, 617–627

Tasman, W. (1971). Retrolental fibroplasia. In *Retinal Diseases in Children*, pp. 105–120. W. Tasman (ed.). New York: Harper and Row

Wagner, P. D., Saltzman, H. A. and West, J. B. (1974). Measurement of continuous distributions of ventilation-perfusion ratios: theory. *J. appl. Physiol.* 36, 588–599

Wagner, P. D., Laravuso, R. B., Uhl, R. R. and West, J. B. (1974). Continuous distributions of ventilation-perfusion ratios in normal subjects breathing air and 100% O_2. *J. clin. Invest.* 54, 54–68

Winter, P. M. and Smith, G. (1972). The toxicity of oxygen. *Anesthesiology* 37, 210–241

Winter, P. M., Gupta, R. K., Michalski, A. H. and Lanphier, E. H. (1967). Modification of hyperbaric oxygen toxicity by experimental venous admixture. *J. appl. Physiol.* 23, 954–963

Wishart, H. Y., Williams, T. I. R. and Smith, G. (1977). A comparison of the effect of three anaesthetic techniques on postoperative arterial oxygenation in the elderly. *Br. J. Anaesth.* 49, 1259–1263

Wood, C. D., Perkins, G. F., Smith, A. G. and Reaux, J. M. (1972). Response of the cardiovascular system in oxygen toxicity. *Aerospace Med.* 43, 162–167

Wood, J. D. (1969). Oxygen toxicity. In *Physiology and Medicine of Diving and Compressed Air Work*, pp. 111–143. P. B. Bennett and D. H. Elliot (ed.). London: Balliere Tindal & Cassell

Wright, R. A., Weiss, H. S., Hiatt, E. P. and Rustagi, J. S. (1966). Risk of mortality in interrupted exposure to 100% O_2: role of air vs. lowered Po_2. *Am. J. Physiol.* 210, 1015–1020

29 Artificial ventilation
A. M. Hewlett

The knowledge that air may be made to pass artificially to and from a patient's lungs without help from the patient, has been known to mankind for centuries. Descriptions of such techniques have usually been associated with the resuscitation of the apparently dead, chiefly from drowning. Although the earliest descriptions of artificial ventilation involved the use of intermittent positive pressure ventilation (IPPV), via mouth to mouth breathing (Herholdt and Rafn, 1796) progress towards rhythmic lung inflation was hampered by the lack of a suitable means of sealing the airway, once cannulation of the trachea had been achieved. This was particularly important in the efforts to solve the 'pneumothorax problem' associated with open chest surgery. It was really this that set the scene for the invention of the wide-bore cuffed endotracheal tube, along with techniques for direct laryngoscopy, which in today's setting seem so absurdly simple and obvious. An excellent history of the development of thoracic anaesthesia was published in 1953 by Mushin and Rendell-Baker who demonstrate clearly how seemingly obvious developments have sometimes to be discovered and rediscovered many times before being universally accepted into common usage.

The clear advantages of 'controlled respiration' once it became a simple routine technique, paved the way for the invention of devices that would automatically inflate the lungs in a rhythmic manner. There were a few such devices in use as far back as 1909 (e.g. Janeway's apparatus — see Mushin and Rendell-Baker, 1953); but as the authors point out 'This early advocacy of what is now called "controlled respiration" appears to have escaped the notice of later investigators of this subject and the method was to lie dormant for some twenty-five years.' Progress was slowly maintained in the 1940s with the production of a few devices, but it was not until the stimulus of the poliomyelitis epidemics of the mid 1950s that development of efficient ventilators began to increase rapidly. Since then, a bewildering array of machines have been produced, some of which seem to have pursued sophistication as an end in itself. We are thus at present in the situation of having to decide whether to sacrifice robustness and simplicity for the sometimes dubious advantages that a highly sophisticated piece of apparatus may provide.

It is not intended in this chapter to describe the function of any particular ventilator nor to attempt to classify ventilators according to their mode of cycling, waveforms, etc., as these topics are exhaustively covered by Mushin *et al.* (1979). Rather the chapter will cover the more general aspects of artificial ventilation, with emphasis on its effects on the patient. Particular attention is paid to the over-riding aim, which is to optimize oxygen transport to the tissues. Greater details on physiological aspects can be found in Nunn (1977) and Sykes, McNicol and Campbell (1976).

INDICATIONS FOR ARTIFICIAL VENTILATION

The commonest indication for artificial ventilation is respiratory failure, which is discussed elsewhere (Chapter 86). However, this is by no means an invariable rule and, in spite of the many scientific advances in recent years, it still remains true that the decision to ventilate a patient artificially is essentially a clinical one, involving many criteria which cannot all be quantified.

The decision to ventilate may be made in any one of the following categories, which are listed in ascending order of immediacy.

Prophylactic ventilation

There is now some evidence that in certain disease entities, notably Gram-negative septicaemia, acute pancreatitis, fat embolism, etc., which are associated with a high incidence of so called 'shock lung' or adult respiratory distress syndrome (ARDS), that early ventilator treatment may minimize or prevent the onset of pulmonary interstitial oedema (Ledingham, 1975; Walker and Eiseman, 1975). Once established, this condition can progress inexorably to pulmonary fibrosis and complete failure of gas exchange. Ventilator treatment for such patients may often be started in the early stages of pulmonary deterioration, before there is obvious radiographic change or clinical abnormality. Evidence of intrapulmonary shunting, from measurement of the arterial Po_2 (Pao_2) is usually the first, and may be the only evidence of pulmonary dysfunction. Initially this may not be severe, and may be combined with a low or normal arterial Pco_2 ($Paco_2$).

In cases of *severe head injury*, some workers advocate immediate artificial ventilation, in spite of apparently normal respiratory function. The purpose is to prevent the onset of acute pulmonary oedema, and to minimize the rise in intracranial pressure resulting from bleeding or cerebral oedema, by deliberate hyperventilation (Brown, 1971; Turner and McDowall, 1976). This subject is dealt with in Chapter 23.

Clinical evidence of fatigue

Artificial ventilation may be instituted purely on clinical evidence of tiring, in spite of lung function and blood gas levels which are not grossly abnormal. The clinical signs of rising pulse, blood pressure and respiratory rate, together with increasing use of the accessory muscles of respiration and inability to cough should alert the operator to consider artificial ventilation. Failure to heed these signs often leads to an unseemly debâcle in which the patient has to be hastily intubated due to sudden deterioration. This is especially prone to occur in neuromuscular disorders such as acute infective polyneuritis, where the patient may maintain normal blood gas levels for some time, before sudden deterioration requires emergency intubation and ventilation.

Obvious deterioration of lung function

Probably the commonest indication for artificial ventilation is deterioration of blood gas levels, coupled with progressive signs of tiring. This is usually associated with increasing inability to clear secretions and increasing alveolar collapse.

Blood gas levels immediately threatening life

In the emergency situation of impending death from acute hypoxia, there is little choice but to institute artificial ventilation. The clinician may have observed the patient's progress to this point from any one of the previous three stages or he may be faced with an entirely unknown patient in whom there has been a sudden cardiac episode causing acute pulmonary oedema or indeed complete cardiorespiratory arrest. Whether the decision to ventilate will prove, in retrospect, to have been correct, is one that should not deter the operator at the time of the emergency (see Chapter 86).

MECHANICS OF ARTIFICIAL VENTILATION

At functional residual capacity (FRC) when the pressure at the mouth and in the alveoli is atmospheric, there is no tendency for gas to pass either into or out of the lungs. In this position the tendency for the lung to collapse (due to lung elasticity and the surface tension of the fluid—air interface in the alveoli) is exactly counterbalanced by the outward pull of the chest wall on the surface of the lung. Gas may now be made to pass into the lungs by:

(1) reducing the pressure in the alveoli by primary expansion of the chest cavity (spontaneous breathing, cuirass, whole body tank or electrophrenic respiration); or
(2) increasing the pressure at the mouth (IPPV).

Each method causes a pressure gradient between mouth and alveolus, resulting in flow of gas into the lungs. At the end of inspiration, providing enough time has been allowed for distribution, gas flow stops and the pressure in all the alveoli is the same as that at the mouth. The forces acting to impede this flow of gas into and out of the lungs must now be discussed.

From the point of view of expansion and contraction to produce tidal air flow, the lungs are passive organs that rely solely on work done on them by external forces. In the case of spontaneous respiration the work is done mainly by the diaphragm and intercostal muscles and, under normal resting conditions, all work is done during inspiration, expiration being passive. During IPPV the work is done by the breathing machine and again this is usually done during inspiration while expiration is generally passive.

Frictional resistance to gas flow

It is convenient to consider the work as done against two forms of resistance. During both inspiration and expiration, there is frictional resistance to gas flow through the air passages, to which may be added a small component due to the viscous resistance of the tissues. Since the pattern of gas flow is partly laminar and partly turbulent, the resistance increases with instantaneous flow rate. At the normal peak flow rate during quiet breathing (about 30 $l \cdot min^{-1}$) the pressure drop between alveolus and mouth is about 0.1 kPa (1 cmH_2O) in healthy patients. Airway resistance may achieve very high values indeed in certain pathological conditions, particularly asthma.

Elastic resistance to gas flow

During inspiration, work is also done to expand lungs and thorax from their resting position at FRC. In the healthy supine paralysed patient a sustained inflation pressure of 1 kPa (10 cmH_2O) will increase the lung volume by about 0.85 litres (*static compliance* 0.85 $l \cdot kPa^{-1}$). However, during an inflation of finite duration (as during a normal inspiration) it is necessary to consider the *dynamic compliance* which is normally about 70% of *static compliance*. The elasticity of the respiratory system can be divided into two components — that of the lungs which are tending to collapse and that of the chest wall which is normally tending to expand to a volume about 400 ml above FRC. FRC is thus the lung volume at which the elastic forces of lung and chest wall are equal and opposite. Decreased lung compliance, whether generalized or confined to discrete areas within the lung, has the effect of decreasing the FRC, leading to increased risk of airway closure and resulting venous admixture. IPPV and associated manoeuvres (see below) can reverse this to some extent by increasing the FRC. This is appropriate in the intensive therapy unit, but not during routine anaesthesia, where decreased compliance is an almost universal side-effect (see Chapter 25).

Work of breathing

Work done against elastic resistance during inspiration is stored as potential energy which is used to expel gas from the lungs during expiration, although this may be assisted by the expiratory muscles during spontaneous breathing or by a subatmospheric expiratory phase during artificial ventilation. The work required for a single normal breath is of the order of 1 joule. Therefore, at 20 breaths per minute, the power of breathing is only one-third of a watt, which requires barely 2% of the total metabolic requirements of the body. The work of breathing may however be greatly increased in a number of pathological states and it may be very difficult to assess the likelihood of a particular patient's musculature to be able to cope with the necessary workload. Their inability to do so may be a reflection of factors such as prolonged starvation, prolonged inactivity due to neuromuscular blocking drugs, and probably most important of all, muscular dysco-ordination, whereby the muscles act against each other (Chiang *et al.*, 1973).

The time constant

It is sometimes useful to consider the time constant for inflation and deflation. This equals the product of compliance and resistance and is of the order of 0.5 second for healthy lungs although it may be greatly increased in the presence of airway obstruction. With sustained pressure gradients, 95% of the total gas volume will actually flow during three time constants.

VOLUME REQUIREMENTS

The aim of artificial ventilation with a few exceptions is to keep the arterial P_{CO_2} and P_{O_2} as near to normal as possible. For the alveoli with an intact capillary blood supply, the following relationship holds true:

$$P_{AX} = P_{IX} \pm \left(\frac{\text{output or uptake of x}}{\text{alveolar ventilation}} \right) P_B \text{ dry} \qquad (29.1)$$

where P_{AX} is the partial pressure of gas x in the alveolar gas;
  P_{IX} is the partial pressure of gas x in the inspired gas;
  P_B is the barometric pressure.

Carbon dioxide

For *carbon dioxide,* where the first term on the right of the equation is usually zero, the alveolar P_{CO_2} is directly proportional to the CO_2 production, and inversely proportional to the alveolar ventilation. For a normal adult, with a basal CO_2 output of 180 ml·min^{-1}, the required alveolar ventilation is thus 3.2 l·min^{-1}. However, to ensure a supply of this volume of *fresh* gas to all the alveoli that have a capillary supply, the required total pulmonary ventilation must be increased by an amount sufficient to allow for 'wasted' gas. Wastage of gas, in a ventilatory sense, takes place at two sites.

(1) *In the conducting airways* gas exchange cannot take place, so that at the end of inspiration, fresh gas is left filling the spaces. At the end of expiration, alveolar gas remains to be inhaled first at the next breath. The wasted volume is here termed the anatomical dead space and (in millilitres) has a volume approximately equal to the weight of the patient expressed in pounds (1 pound = 0.45 kg). An endotracheal tube or tracheostomy bypasses approximately half of this volume. Functionally, the effective anatomical dead space is reduced during hypoventilation due to diffusion and the mixing effect of the heart beat (Nunn and Hill, 1960).

(2) *Alveoli which have impaired blood supply* continue to be inflated, but act as dead space, since no gas exchange is taking place. The classical situation in which this occurs is in the early stages of pulmonary embolism. The resulting air hunger due to the necessity of increasing the minute volume, is well known. Other more subtle causes are in reduced cardiac output states (most commonly due to hypovolaemia) where blood may not reach all the pulmonary capillaries, or where the mean intrathoracic pressure is high enough to cause a reduction in effective pulmonary artery perfusing pressure. Both these factors frequently operate in patients during IPPV so that most of them will have a greater dead space than normal and therefore require a minute volume greater than would normally be the case. This does not mean, however, that extraordinary attempts should be made to preserve a normal Pa_{CO_2}, if there is a very large dead space. This may not be feasible if a very high minute volume is necessary because of the danger of pulmonary barotrauma.

Oxygen

For *oxygen* where the first term on the right-hand side of equation (29.1) is not zero, it can be easily seen that the upper limit of the Pa_{O_2} must be the Pi_{O_2} since, with infinite ventilation the second term becomes zero. Thus the Pa_{O_2} is largely dependent on Pi_{O_2} and only to a smaller extent on the ventilation. It is only in conditions where there is an *extremely* high Pa_{CO_2}, such as in status asthmaticus, where significant compromising of the Pa_{O_2} could occur. In practice, in the intensive therapy unit (ITU), the ventilation level is adjusted to fix the Pa_{CO_2} and the Fi_{O_2} is then manipulated to adjust the Pa_{O_2}.

RESPIRATORY PATTERNS AND LUNG FUNCTION

Cournand *et al.* in 1948 investigated the effect of different respiratory patterns during artificial ventilation and outlined the basic principles of minimizing mean intrathoracic pressure to reduce interference with venous return.

Since that time, clinicians in the ITU have found that impairment of the venous return to the heart, although important, is not the only consideration. As well as this, in many conditions of serious lung disease, cardiac output is not as seriously affected by high mean intrathoracic pressures as was at first feared. Furthermore, it became apparent that there were positive advantages to gas exchange when the mean intrathoracic pressure was raised by the application of positive end-expiratory pressure (PEEP). The best pattern of ventilation is a compromise resulting from consideration of the several affected variables and, often as not, from trial and error. The over-riding aim is to maximize delivery of oxygen to the tissues, using the lowest possible F_{IO_2}. The issue resolves basically into a conflict between improving the arterial P_{O_2} and reducing the cardiac output, both of which usually result from raising the mean intrathoracic pressure.

Interference with venous return

Venous return to the heart depends on a pressure gradient between the peripheral venous system and the great veins in the thorax. Thus a rise in mean intrathoracic pressure causes a reduction in the supply of venous blood to the right side of the heart, if other factors remain constant. Cournand's principles are aimed at minimizing the rise in mean pressure with IPPV and are therefore basic to the proper conduct of artificial ventilation. However, his study was done using normal volunteers, in whom the changes in intrathoracic pressures could be expected to be transmitted to a large extent to the great veins. Many of the patients requiring ventilation, however, have some measure of obstructive airways disease, which tends to dissipate much of this pressure in overcoming resistance (Ambiavagar, Jones and Roberts, 1967). Excess inflation pressure is also dissipated in patients having reduced compliance due to severe intra-alveolar disease. This causes a large pressure gradient between the inside and outside of the alveolus, which prevents the transmission of the excess pressure to the great veins. Thus it may be only a small fraction of the inflation pressure which influences the venous return.

In the case of severe asthma requiring artificial ventilation, it is not the high inspiratory pressures *per se* that cause embarrassment to venous return, since they are poorly transmitted. It appears rather to be the continuously high alveolar pressures caused by gross expiratory resistance which raises pressure on the great veins. 'Air trapping' produces a gradual rise in FRC, until the flat part of the compliance curve is reached. In this range, very large pressure changes are necessary to effect even a small tidal flow and there is inevitably considerable obstruction to venous return.

Interference with pulmonary circulation

Possibly of greater importance in severe asthma and in the use of high intrathoracic pressures, is the compromising of the pulmonary capillary circulation. This can be severe enough to cause acute right ventricular failure with secondary reduction in left ventricular output. Lesser degrees of this phenomenon may account for the observed increase in physiological dead space (V_D) that sometimes occurs when high mean intrathoracic pressures are used, especially when pulmonary artery perfusion pressure is already low. This effect is not usually of significance at the pressures normally employed. In fact the reverse commonly happens; namely that on institution of IPPV, there is an effective decrease in the alveolar dead space, which is probably accounted for by redistribution of blood to areas of relative overventilation.

The institution of negative end-expiratory pressure (NEEP) can produce a mean intrathoracic pressure that is normal or below normal. This has been shown to have a beneficial effect on cardiac output (Maloney *et al.*, 1953). However, due to its tendency to cause proximal airway collapse, this manoeuvre tends to increase air trapping and an increased venous admixture often ensues (Velasquez and Farhi, 1964). As well as this, NEEP increases the tendency towards alveolar pulmonary oedema, by a direct negative pressure effect. In the presence of significant lung disease, therefore, other methods of maintaining cardiac performance are to be preferred.

IMPROVEMENT OF GAS EXCHANGE

IPPV and associated manoeuvres are usually instituted to improve gas exchange and maintain optimal oxygenation. There is rarely difficulty with elimination of carbon dioxide except in the case of severe asthma, massive pulmonary embolism or extremely severe reductions in cardiac output; but even in these conditions oxygenation is still of prime importance. In most other cases, the immediate changes brought about in V_D by efforts at improving oxygenation are of relatively minor significance, and can be compensated for by small adjustments in over-all minute volume.

Intrapulmonary shunting may be so severe that even the administration of 100% oxygen does not achieve an acceptable Pao_2. Because of the possibility of oxygen toxicity (Chapter 28) all efforts should be directed towards safe reduction of the F_{IO_2}. Essential to this is meticulous attention to chest physiotherapy, tracheobronchial toilet, treatment of infection, and appropriate fluid therapy (Chapter 86). Adjustment of flows and pressures of gas supplied to the patient is often highly effective in reducing venous admixture and suitable techniques are listed below. However, almost all such manoeuvres involve raising the mean intrathoracic pressure. This, as we have seen, causes variable degrees of reduction in cardiac output. Additional beneficial effects on the other hand, include decrease of lung water, re-expansion of collapsed lung, and decrease of the over-all resistance of the conducting airways.

Positive end-expiratory pressure (PEEP)

PEEP should be considered when more than 50% oxygen is required to maintain a satisfactory Pao_2 (Ashbaugh and Petty, 1973). By not allowing the pressure in the airways to fall below a specified level (usually 0.5–1 kPa or 5–10 cmH$_2$O) airways (and therefore alveoli) having a tendency to close, will be held open. This will reduce the degree of venous admixture by increasing the number of alveoli available for gas exchange. Because of decreased compliance of the lungs in many of the patients in whom PEEP is applied, there is poor transmission of the increased mean alveolar pressure to the thorax and thus the decrement in cardiac output may be insignificant. Indeed a few workers have successfully used PEEP pressures greatly in excess of 1 kPa (Kirby, Downes and Civetta, 1975). However, there is a risk of physical damage in applying such high pressures to the lungs.

Expiratory retard

This may be combined with PEEP. The aim is to slow down exhalation so that the flow rate is kept more even than the usual steep exponential fall. This tends to hold collapsing alveoli and airways open for longer, although in theory it does not prevent alveolar collapse when the pressure has fallen below the critical closing pressure. 'Air trapping' is reduced by preventing early collapse of more proximal airways as demonstrated by patients who employ pursed lips expiration. It is of maximum value in patients with obstructive airways disease who exhibit wheezing on exhalation. It can be useful in asthma provided care is taken to ensure that exhalation is complete before the next breath is delivered.

Increasing tidal volume

This should be done if possible by increasing the time allowed for inspiration, rather than increasing the inspiratory flow rate, which may exacerbate maldistribution (Baker, Colliss and Cowie, 1977).

Inspiratory hold

Most modern ventilators have the facility of 'inspiratory hold', which allows redistribution within the lung at maximum inspiration. The pattern is similar to the 'reverse ramp' (see below). Redistribution of gas will take place, if sufficient time is allowed, according to the relative compliances of the alveoli. This may be more favourable than the relative distribution which occurs during high flow, when distribution depends more on airway calibre than on alveolar compliance.

Variations in inspiratory flow patterns

Some modern ventilators allow a choice of inspiratory flow patterns to be made. The choice is usually between: ramp — gradually increasing flow; reverse ramp — fast flow followed by gradually decreasing flow; top hat — constant flow; and on some models, a modified sine wave flow pattern.

So far, extensive studies of the effects of variation of inspiratory wave-form have failed to show significant change in pulmonary shunt effect that cannot be accounted for simply by the change in mean intrathoracic pressure. There is some evidence that the reverse ramp pattern, which is essentially similar to an inspiratory hold, seems to be marginally better than others, although it appears to cause maximum interference with the cardiac output (Baker, Collis and Cowie, 1977).

High frequency positive pressure ventilation (HFPPV)

There is some evidence (Heijman *et al.*, 1972) that ventilation at a frequency of 60–100 pulses per minute can sustain adequate ventilation using conventional minute volumes. Using an expiratory resistance to maintain mean intrapulmonary pressure of between 0.05 and 0.25 kPa·cm^{-2}, the reduction in cardiac output was minimal compared with similar end-expiratory pressures used during conventional IPPV. There is at the moment, however, insufficient evidence showing whether this method is of clinical value in serious lung disease.

Respiratory patterns and resolution of lung pathology

Most studies on this topic are necessarily of short-term effects and there is little information on the effect of different waveforms on longer term resolution of pulmonary oedema, collapse, consolidation, etc. Unfortunately this type of information tends to be anecdotal, due to the difficulties of setting up a controlled prospective trial which is to have any statistical weight; but it would seem reasonable to assume that patterns producing the higher mean intrathoracic pressures and which promote optimum alveolar distribution should be the more effective. In this respect the reverse ramp or inspiratory hold would again seem to be the best of the available inspiratory waveforms.

OTHER MEANS OF IMPROVING Pa_{O_2} AND/OR TISSUE OXYGENATION

It must be stressed that improvement of Pa_{O_2} and tissue oxygenation does not lie solely in adjustment of minute volume, inspired oxygen concentration and the pattern of artificial ventilation, use of PEEP, etc. Chapter 86 reviews other longer term methods of minimizing shunt but it remains to consider the special importance of cardiac output.

Optimizing cardiac output

If peripheral utilization of oxygen remains constant, an increase in cardiac output causes an increase in mixed venous P_{O_2} ($P\bar{v}_{O_2}$). Thus any decrement to the Pa_{O_2} caused by a given shunt fraction will be decreased. Attention must therefore be paid to optimizing the performance of the heart, so that (1) oxygen delivery will be maximal for a given Pao_2 and (2) the effect on Pao_2 of intrapulmonary shunting will be minimized. Among the more important considerations are the following.

ELECTROLYTE AND ACID–BASE BALANCE

Myocardial function is especially sensitive to serum K^+. If the level is too high, depression of contractility occurs, if too low, there is a tendency toward arrhythmia. Metabolic acidosis causes depression of contractility, although this is not severe above pH 7.2. Indeed mild metabolic acidosis may be helpful to the delivery of oxygen to the tissues by its effect on the oxyhaemoglobin dissociation curve. Conversely, metabolic alkalosis adversely affects tissue oxygenation.

Intracellular metabolism must also be considered and attention paid to nutrition in the form of dextrose/insulin/K^+ regimens with or without other means of supplying energy and protein.

BLOOD VOLUME

It is now becoming increasingly obvious that adequate management of the severely shocked patient entails separate consideration on both sides of the heart. In the short term, it is the left heart that is of more immediate concern. It is thus important to obtain information on the left atrial pressure by measurement of the pulmonary capillary wedge pressure (PCWP). This entails insertion of a Swan–Ganz catheter into the pulmonary artery. Although care must be exercised in the interpretation of the PCWP when high levels of PEEP are being used (Roy *et al.*, 1977), an estimation of left atrial pressure is the best way to guide the clinician on the adequacy of circulating blood volume. Measurement of the PCWP also enables more accurate differentiation between pulmonary oedema due to pulmonary capillary dysfunction and that due to hydrostatic derangement.

PERIPHERAL VASODILATION

Cardiac output may be increased substantially by afterload reduction. This may be done using α-blocking agents such as phenoxybenzamine or direct peripherally acting drugs such as sodium nitroprusside. Extra blood volume is usually necessary and again the monitoring of the left atrial pressure is highly desirable during vasodilator therapy.

INOTROPIC DRUGS

Such drugs include digoxin, glucagon and the catecholamine-like compounds. In the latter group care must be exercised because of their stimulant effect on cardiac and tissue oxygen consumption, which may sometimes make matters worse. This is particularly true in pump failure due to myocardial infarction where there is a special danger of increasing infarct size. Dobutamine seems, at the time of writing, to be marginally better in this respect than other commonly used inotropic agents such as dopamine, although there is now an intensive search being conducted for a selective β_1 stimulant which causes minimal increase in myocardial oxygen consumption. Such a drug would thus be required to cause an increase in efficiency of myocardial contraction. In this respect, minimal chronotropic activity appears to be an important requirement.

STEROIDS

Steroids in high doses (e.g. methylprednisolone 30 mg·kg^{-1}) cause an increase in the cardiac output, associated with a decrease in pulmonary vascular resistance. There are also beneficial effects on the integrity of the pulmonary capillaries. The immediate effect on gas exchange is to cause an increase in intrapulmonary shunting due to the opening up of capillaries in poorly ventilated areas (Lozman *et al.*, 1975).

RAISING PaCO$_2$

A further manoeuvre commonly found to improve PaO$_2$ is to raise the PaCO$_2$, either by the insertion of a mechanical dead space or a reduction in the total ventilation. This effect must presumably also be due to an increase of cardiac output, but is clearly limited by the simultaneous increase in PACO$_2$ which occurs and possibly by deleterious effects on myocardial function occasioned by too great a reduction in pH.

Posture

Douglas *et al.* (1977) have recently shown that in some patients in acute respiratory failure, improved oxygenation may result from placing the patient in the prone position. The mechanism for this phenomenon is not entirely clear, but the increase in FRC probably plays an important part. It is also likely that there is some redistribution of blood to relatively well ventilated areas, which however, gradually become less well ventilated with increasing time in the dependent positions. Regular change of posture would thus seem beneficial and is indeed regarded as desirable in many units.

Decreasing peripheral oxygen consumption

Methods designed to decrease oxygen consumption include the familiar but highly important measures of muscle paralysis and sedation. Hypothermia (32°C) is occasionally successful in 'buying time' when all other measures have failed to produce adequate oxygenation.

Hyperbaric oxygen

Although hyperbaric oxygen seems an attractive means of improving oxygenation, there seem in practice to be very few indications for its use in severe lung disease (see Chapter 27).

Extracorporeal membrane oxygenation (ECMO)

Although now technically feasible, long-term oxygenation using bypass has not been shown to improve the mortality in serious lung disease (see Chapter 27).

ASSESSMENT OF OPTIMUM TISSUE OXYGEN DELIVERY

Once IPPV has been instituted and optimum cardiac performance is achieved, the necessity to use more than about 50% oxygen to achieve adequate Pao_2 should lead the clinician to consider the further manoeuvres referred to above. As we have seen, many of these, particularly PEEP, may cause some embarrassment to the cardiac output. In such a case there is usually a level of PEEP where oxygen carriage to the tissues ($\dot{Q} \times Cao_2$) is maximal. This point has been termed 'Best PEEP' by Suter, Fairley and Isenberg (1975).

Arterial Po_2 is only one factor regulating oxygen content, which in turn is only one aspect of oxygen carriage (see above). It may thus be misleading if considered in isolation from other factors, particularly haemoglobin concentration and cardiac output. In practice PEEP and associated manoeuvres are usually instituted initially because of an unacceptably low Pao_2. It does not necessarily follow, however, that an improved Pao_2 means better tissue oxygenation. Clinical impression is at best unreliable in severely shocked patients and direct measurement must be resorted to. The main ones are listed below.

Mixed venous Po_2 ($P\bar{v}o_2$)

The most direct method of assessment of oxygen delivery is to measure the $P\bar{v}o_2$, which involves use of a pulmonary artery catheter. While some workers consider this essential for effective patient care, others feel that less invasive methods are satisfactory although necessarily indirect.

Static compliance

Suter, Fairley and Isenberg (1975) have shown that 'Best PEEP' coincides with the point of maximum lung compliance, and advocate this as the most convenient method of selecting the level of PEEP.

Right atrial Po_2

Although more useful than a peripheral venous sample, the right atrial blood is not completely mixed and measured levels may fluctuate considerably, as the catheter samples different streams. It can only be used as a rough guide to over-all tissue oxygenation.

Indirect measurement of cardiac output

Transcutaneous aortovelography (TAV) has been reported to be useful in detection of changes in cardiac output (Bilton and Hanson, 1978). Quantitative measurements may be made only if a baseline has been established beforehand by direct measurement. The apparatus is easy to use and non-invasive. It will certainly record the point at which significant reduction of cardiac output is beginning to occur with increasing PEEP, although the level of best PEEP may be somewhat above this.

Direct measurement of cardiac output

Commonly used methods are the indocyanine green and thermal dilution techniques, both of which are capable of giving accurate measurements of cardiac output. Thermal dilution is now a relatively easy and reliable technique, and enables multiple repeated estimations. It does, however, entail use of the special Swan—Ganz catheter with a side port into the right atrium.

SPONTANEOUS RESPIRATION WITH IPPV

In the early stages of ventilator therapy, many patients require ventilation to be completely controlled. This is because of the need to break the vicious cycle of hypoxia and restlessness with increased peripheral oxygen consumption that patients with severe lung disease exhibit. When conditions become more stable it is often possible to allow return of some spontaneous respiratory activity even though ventilator treatment is still required.

Although it would seem likely that partial retention of spontaneous respiratory effort *should* be beneficial to the patient, there appears to be no evidence showing whether or not the integrity and bulk of the respiratory musculature is adversely affected by long-term inactivity. There *is* some evidence however that respiratory muscle co-ordination is affected by prolonged paralysis (Chiang *et al.,* 1973) but so far, any advantages in retaining partial spontaneous efforts have not been quantified. Other possible beneficial effects are (1) that cardiac function may be improved through a decreased mean intrathoracic pressure, and (2) that gas distribution could be improved due to the preferential distribution to dependent areas during spontaneous breathing and to the non-dependent regions during IPPV. Apart from this, the most obvious effect is that maintenance of spontaneous efforts often dramatically cuts down the amount of sedation that is necessary. Patients are thus able to be more responsive to nursing staff and are also more likely to be able to regulate their own respiratory condition.

It will be exceedingly difficult to prove whether or not patients achieve complete spontaneous respiration any faster if allowed to make spontaneous efforts throughout most of their illness. However, this should not deter clinicians from taking advantage of the other more tangible benefits that these techniques often provide. Neither should it prevent further study on the physiological effects which are largely unknown at the present time. There are two techniques for combining spontaneous breathing with IPPV.

Intermittent mandatory ventilation (IMV)

First proposed by Downs *et al.* (1973), this technique provides a reservoir from which the patient may take any number of spontaneous breaths, while over the same period receiving a preset number of breaths from the ventilator. As the patient's ability to breathe improves, the number of 'mandatory' breaths is gradually cut down, until complete spontaneous respiration is achieved. If the inspiratory reservoir is pressurized and a PEEP valve placed on the expiratory line, continuous positive airway pressure (CPAP) is possible for the spontaneous breaths. If, however, a PEEP valve is used without also pressurizing the inspiratory line, the patient is obliged to reduce his airway pressure to below atmospheric, from the PEEP level, with every inspiration. This could be advantageous from the point of view of cardiac output, but clearly adds considerably to the work of breathing at what may be a critical time.

Mandatory minute volume (MMV)

Hewlett, Platt and Terry (1977) have proposed an arrangement whereby the over-all minute volume is kept constant, and the patient is able to choose how much is supplied by spontaneous respiration, the remainder (if any) being provided by IPPV. A preset minute volume of gas is supplied to a reservoir from which the patient breathes spontaneously as much as he is able. The surplus is then delivered to a minute volume dividing ventilator, which then intermittently ventilates the patient with a preset tidal volume. The frequency of artificial ventilation thus depends on the flow delivered to the ventilator (i.e. preset $\dot{V}-$ spontaneous $\dot{V}$). CPAP and PEEP pressures may be set by a single manoeuvre. Ravenscroft (1978) has suggested a simpler method of administering MMV, which alters the tidal volume of the artificial breaths, rather than the frequency. However, CPAP is not possible with this method.

MMV has so far been found to be a useful adjunct to IPPV in approximately 70% of patients requiring artificial ventilation, particularly those whose ability to breathe varies from hour to hour (Hewlett, 1978). It is not a satisfactory technique in patients with a high dead space component in their spontaneous breathing (i.e. those with shallow, fast respirations) where IMV has been found to provide a more stable respiratory pattern. Both IMV and MMV offer the possibility of the patient taking an unobstructed inspiration and greatly help in preventing 'fighting the ventilator'. It could be argued that all patients on ventilators should be protected from the possibility of trying to breathe against a closed valve system.

'WEANING' FROM IPPV

Measurements of the work necessary to move the lungs and chest wall can now be made (Wilson, 1976). Furthermore there is data based on this measurement to show that predictions can be made with a fair degree of accuracy as to whether a patient at the beginning of his illness will require artificial ventilation (Proctor and Woolson, 1973; Chiang *et al.*, 1977). What is more uncertain is the prediction of a patient's ability to breathe spontaneously *after* artificial ventilation. At this stage, factors such as possible muscle wasting, dysco-ordination, apathy and ability to cough and sigh come strongly to the fore, forcing the clinician into a purely clinical decision to 'try and see'. Nevertheless Chiang *et al.* (1977) do review evidence to show that a patient's ability to sustain spontaneous ventilation correlates most closely with vital capacity and inspiratory force. Degree of venous admixture appeared to have no correlation and, regardless of the starting level of Pa_{CO_2}, patients who were weaned successfully had rises of Pa_{CO_2} of no more than 1 kPa (7.5 mmHg). Some of the evidence from other works is conflicting, particularly concerning cardiac output and its changes, although there is fairly general agreement on the following criteria being necessary for successfully re-establishing adequate spontaneous ventilation ('weaning'):

(1) adequate oxygenation with F_{IO_2} less than 0.4 and general stable condition;
(2) spontaneous minute ventilation at rest *less* than $10 \ l \cdot min^{-1}$;
(3) ability to double resting minute ventilation;
(4) ability to achieve an inspiratory force of 3 kPa (30 cmH$_2$O).

These measurements are simple and at least give a general guide to be assessed along with the other less definable factors mentioned above.

Excluding the use of IMV/MMV techniques, which to some extent side-step the issue, weaning is usually accomplished by gradually increasing periods of total spontaneous breathing. The use of CPAP is advocated by several workers as being beneficial at this stage (Feely *et al.*, 1975).

While it would be exceedingly difficult to prove that this method is less successful than those employing partial spontaneous breathing techniques, it is nonetheless true that there is often considerable physiological and psychological trauma attendant upon intermittent abrupt withdrawal of artificial ventilation. If spontaneous ventilation is not sustained with the first attempt at withdrawal, there is a strong case for institution of the more gradual approach which IMV or MMV allows.

The use of triggered ventilators for weaning purposes is tending to decrease. They have proved less than satisfactory mainly because of time delays between patient effort and ventilator response, lack of correlation between patient effort and ventilator tidal volume and perhaps of most importance, the ease with which the patient is able to master 'trick' movements which will trigger the machine but which are functionally quite unlike normal effective respiratory movements.

FURTHER DEVELOPMENT OF ARTIFICIAL VENTILATORS

Except at a few centres, availability of funds has now been outstripped by technological advance. The common dilemma is whether it is better for a unit to have only one type of ventilator, that is familiar to all, or to diversify so that students gain experience with many types. The most usual compromise, characteristic of centres with limited funds, is to have many of one type of simple, robust, and comparatively cheap ventilator, and a few more sophisticated ones for patients with more difficult respiratory problems.

An important reason for the prevailing lack of consensus among doctors as to the required performance of the ideal ventilator is the lack of precise feedback on many models of what the machine is actually doing at the time. This deficiency could be resolved by having a visual display, attachable to any ventilator, which shows waveforms for both flow and pressure. It is not helpful to be told that the 'reverse ramp' is the best flow pattern if there is no way of knowing whether or not the machine is producing it. It will be quickly found even by the most inexperienced operator, what each machine is capable of, and which factors really matter. It may thus be possible to judge the worth of more sophisticated machines and indeed which facilities are worth building into them.

References

Ambiavagar, M., Jones, E. S. and Roberts, D. V. (1967). Intermittent positive pressure ventilation in severe asthma; mechanical effects on the circulation. *Anaesthesia* **22**, 134–139

Ashbaugh, D. G. and Petty, T. L. (1973). Positive end-expiratory pressure: physiology, indications and contraindications. *J. thorac. cardiovasc. Surg.* **65**, 165–170

Baker, A. B., Colliss, J. E. and Cowie, R. W. (1977). Effects of varying inspiratory flow waveform and time in intermittent positive pressure ventilation. II: Various physiological variables. *Br. J. Anaesth.* **49**, 1221–1234

Bilton, A. H. and Hanson, G. C. (1978). Aortic velocity measurement in the care of the critically ill. In *Doppler Ultrasound in the Study of the Central and Peripheral Circulation*, Chapter 4, pp. 39–43. J. P. Woodcock and R. F. Sequeira (ed.). Bristol: University of Bristol Printing Unit

Brown, A. S. (1971). Intermittent positive pressure ventilation in the management of severe head injuries. In *International Symposium on Head Injuries*, p. 266. F. J. Gillingham and S. Obrador (ed.). Edinburgh: Churchill-Livingstone

Chiang, H., Pontoppidan, H., Wilson, R. S., Browne, D. R. G. and Katz, A. (1973). Respiratory muscle discoordination following prolonged mechanical ventilation. *Abstracts of Scientific Papers*, Annual Meeting of Am. Soc. Anesth., pp. 211–212

Cournand, A., Motley, H. L., Werko, L. and Richards, D. W. Jr (1948). Physiological studies of the effects of intermittent positive pressure breathing on the cardiac output in man. *Am. J. Physiol.* **152**, 162–174

Douglas, W., Rehder, K., Froukje, M. B., Sessler, A. D. and Marsh, M. M. (1977). Improved oxygenation in patient with acute respiratory failure: the prone position. *Am. Rev. resp. Dis.* **115**, 559–566

Downs, J. B., Klein, E. F. Jr., Desautels, D., Modell, J. H. and Kirby, R. R. (1973). Intermittent mandatory ventilation: A new approach to weaning patients from mechanical ventilators. *Chest* **64**, 331–335

Feeley, T. W., Saumarez, R., Klick, J. M., McNabb, G. T. and Skillman, J. J. (1975). Positive end-expiratory pressure in weaning patients from controlled ventilation: A prospective randomised trial. *Lancet* ii, 725–729

Heijman, K., Heijman, L., Jonzon, A., Sedin, G., Sjöstrand, U. and Widman, B. (1972). High frequency positive pressure ventilation during anaesthesia and routine surgery in man. *Acta anaesth. scand.* **16**, 176–187

Herholdt, J. D. and Rafn, C. G. (1796). *Life-saving methods for drowning persons.* Copenhagen H: Tikiob. Reprinted in 1960 by Aarhuus, Denmark Stiftsbogrrykkerie

Hewlett, A. M. (1978). *Mandatory minute volume.* Paper delivered to Intensive Care Society, May 1978

Hewlett, A. M., Platt, A. S. and Terry, V. G. (1977). Mandatory minute volume: A new concept in weaning from mechanical ventilation. *Anaesthesia* 32, 163–169

Kirby, R. R., Downes, J. B. and Civetta, J. M. (1975). High level positive end expiratory pressure (PEEP) in acute respiratory insufficiency. *Chest* 67, 156–163

Ledingham, I. McA. (1975). Septic shock. *Br. J. Surg.* 62, 777–780

Lozman, J., Dutton, R. E., English, M. and Powers, S. R. (1975). Cardiopulmonary adjustments following single high dosage administration of methylprednisolone in traumatised man. *Ann. Surg.* 181, 317–324

Maloney, J. V., Elam, J. O., Handford, S. W., Balla, G. A., Eastwood, D. W., Brown, E. S. and Ten Pas, R. H. (1953). Importance of negative pressure phase in mechanical respirators. *J. Am. med. Ass.* 152, 212–216

Mushin, W. W. and Rendell-Baker, L. (1953). *The Principles of Thoracic Anaesthesia Past and Present.* Oxford: Blackwell Scientific Publications

Mushin, W. W., Rendell-Baker, L., Thompson, P. W. and Mapleson, W. W. (1979). *Automatic Ventilation of the Lungs,* 3rd edn. Oxford: Blackwell Scientific Publications

Nunn, J. F. (1977). *Applied Respiratory Physiology,* 2nd edn. London: Butterworths

Nunn, J. F. and Hill, D. W. (1960). Respiratory dead space and arterial to end-tidal CO_2 tension difference in anaesthetised man. *J. appl. Physiol.* 15, 383–389

Proctor, H. J. and Woolson, B. A. (1973). Prediction of respiratory muscle fatigue by measurements of the work of breathing. *Surg. Gynec. Obstet.* 136, 367–370

Ravenscroft, P. J. (1978). Simple mandatory minute volume. *Anaesthesia* 33, 246–249

Roy, R., Powers, S. R., Feustel, P. J. and Dutton, R. E. (1977). Pulmonary wedge catheterization during positive end-expiratory pressure ventilation in the dog. *Anesthesiology* 46, 385–390

Suter, P. M., Fairley, H. B. and Isenberg, M. D. (1975). Optimum end-expiratory airway pressure in patients with acute pulmonary failure. *New Engl. J. Med.* 292, 284–289

Sykes, M. K., McNicol, M. W. and Campbell, E. J. M. (1976). *Respiratory Failure,* 2nd edn. Oxford: Blackwell Scientific Publications

Turner, J. M. and McDowall, D. G. (1976). The measurement of intracranial pressure. *Br. J. Anaesth.* 48, 735–740

Velasquez, T. and Farhi, L. E. (1964). Effect of negative pressure breathing on lung mechanics and venous admixture. *J. appl. Physiol.* 19, 665–671

Walker, L. and Eisman, B. (1975). The changing pattern of post-traumatic respiratory distress syndrome. *Ann. Surg.* 181, 693–697

Wilson, R. S. (1976). Monitoring the lung: mechanics and volume. *Anesthesiology* 45, 135–145

30 **Postoperative pulmonary complications**
Alastair A. Spence

After the first hour of recovery from anaesthesia and operation, patients who have undergone surgery of the limbs or body surface normally do not exhibit a deterioration of lung function with respect to the preoperative state. The presence of lung disorder in these patients is a sign that an accident, such as aspiration of gastric contents or thromboembolism, has occurred. By contrast, disturbance of lung function, often continuing for three to four days, is an inevitable accompaniment to abdominal surgery. This chapter will describe both the pulmonary sequelae and the complications which follow surgery; failure to recognize and to minimize the sequelae of abdominal surgery may be an important cause of complications also. The special problems of lung function following cardiac and thoracic operations are considered in Chapters 69 and 91.

Often, in the past, there may have been confusion as to the frequency of respiratory 'complications' after surgery. Most of the early resports depended on clinical assessment of the patient in which there was considerable scope for observer bias. For example, pyrexia is almost an inevitable accompaniment to a surgical incision. Production of purulent sputum is to be expected in smokers even in the absence of anaesthesia and surgery, as are expiratory rhonchi after upper abdominal surgery, even if convalescence is proceeding normally. Thus traditional statements that respiratory complications occur more frequently in the elderly, cigarette smokers, patients with pre-existing lung disease and the obese should be interpreted with caution. It is true that patients in these categories are more at risk, but the recognition of this fact and the adoption of suitable precautions is the key to safety.

Problems of the early postoperative period are considered further in Chapter 54.

THE NORMAL RESPONSE TO ANAESTHESIA AND OPERATION

Disturbance of oxygenation

DIFFUSION 'ANOXIA' (FINK EFFECT)

This term is applied to a transient (0.6–1.3 kPa or 5–10 mmHg) decrease in arterial Po_2 associated with a return to breathing air following nitrous oxide in oxygen. The primary cause is a dilution of the alveolar oxygen content as the more soluble nitrous oxide, leaving the tissues as a relatively greater amount, mixes with the less soluble nitrogen entering the tissues as a lesser amount; each gas moves along a similar tension gradient, although the directions of the gradients are opposite (Fink, 1955). A secondary factor, which prolongs and aggravates the effect, is alveolar hypoventilation, consequent upon dilution of the alveolar $P\text{CO}_2$ (Rackow, Salanitre and Frumin, 1961).

However, at worst, the reduction in $P\text{O}_2$ attributable to this effect lasts for not more than 10 minutes. It may be prevented completely by replacing the nitrous oxide of the anaesthetic gas mixture with oxygen for 1–2 minutes at the end of the surgical procedure. Such practice is commonplace. Of all the causes of a reduced arterial $P\text{O}_2$, the Fink effect is probably the most trivial; paradoxically it receives perhaps the most vigorous attention.

THE FIRST TWO HOURS AFTER OPERATION

For a variable time during this period, the proportion of right-to-left shunt within the lung is increased abnormally. Typically, when the patient breathes air, the arterial $P\text{O}_2$ is reduced by up to 4 kPa (30 mmHg) from the preoperative value (Nunn and Payne, 1962; Marshall and Millar, 1965). An exception is seen in young patients who have been anaesthetized for only a few minutes (Taylor, Scott and Donald, 1964); also, the elderly may be less affected than the middle age group (Wishart, Williams and Smith, 1977).

The mechanism of the defect is not understood fully, but is assumed to be a continuation of the factors which cause an increase in shunt during anaesthesia itself (Nunn, 1977). Thus there is an increased spread of the ventilation/perfusion ($\dot{V}/\dot{Q}$) relationship with the lung. In most cases, the arterial $P\text{O}_2$ can be restored to the preoperative value, at least, by increasing the inspired oxygen concentration to 35–40% (Conway and Payne, 1963).

Abdominal surgery

When patients with previously healthy lungs undergo abdominal surgery, there is impairment of oxygenation of the arterial blood for at least 48 hours after operation (Palmer and Gardiner, 1964). The magnitude of the deficiency is related to the site of the abdominal incision being least marked following surgery on the lower abdomen. It is worst following upper abdominal midline and paramedian incisions when the average reduction in arterial $P\text{O}_2$ (breathing air) is 3 kPa (22.5 mmHg) on the first postoperative day; in such patients, although there is a gradual improvement, the arterial $P\text{O}_2$ may not have returned to the preoperative value even by the fifth postoperative day (Spence and Smith, 1971).

Anscombe (1957) showed that patients recovering from abdominal surgery had a reduction in functional residual capacity (FRC). Alexander *et al.* (1973) confirmed this and found that, in parallel with the change in arterial P_{O_2}, the magnitude of the reduction in FRC was related to the surgical incision; decreases of 30% and 15% are typical values following cholecystectomy and inguinal herniorrhaphy respectively. Alexander *et al.* (1972) had shown that there was a significant correlation between the impairment of arterial P_{O_2} and the change in the relationship of FRC to closing volume in the early postoperative period (day one). Thus the temporary effect of abdominal surgery on the lung is similar to that of ageing in that there is an increase in gas trapping in the dependent, and most richly perfused, regions of the lung. This explains the finding of Georg, Hornum and Mellemgaard (1967) that the principal cause of impaired gas exchange after abdominal surgery was an increase in the scatter of $\dot{V}/\dot{Q}$ relationships in the lung, but reconciles the apparently differing view of Diament and Palmer (1967) that there is substantial right-to-left shunting of blood past collapsed lung tissue. Alexander *et al.* (1971) found that the change in the relationship of FRC to closing volume was less predictable on the second, compared with the first, postoperative day. This may be because absorption of trapped gas with alveolar collapse in the dependent regions of the lung so alters the forces acting on the airways that the tracer gas tests for the detection of 'closing volume' become virtually invalid.

Thus we can consider these longer term changes in the lung after abdominal surgery as occurring in two phases.

Phase 1

The resting lung volume (FRC) is reduced, gas is trapped, with consequent reduction in $\dot{V}/\dot{Q}$ in the dependent regions of the lung. This disorder of oxygenation is easily corrected by increasing the inspired oxygen concentration to 35—40%.

Phase 2

In some patients in whom the phase 1 effects are marked, there may be collapse of lung tissue in the areas of trapping, although this is unlikely to be obvious clinically in the first 24 hours after surgery. This situation is likely to be aggravated by retention of the normal secretion production of the bronchial mucosa, because of inability to cough freely, and suppression of the normal occasional deep breath and of the respiratory ciliary activity by drugs (Egbert and Bendixen, 1964), or a lack of humidification during anaesthesia (Burton, 1962). Thus the stage is set for bacterial invasion, particularly if there has been an infective process in the respiratory tract before operation, and pneumonia, characterized by familiar clinical and radiological signs. This is a process which can bring misery, and in some cases danger, to the patient and which inevitably delays his recovery from surgery.

The important lesson is that these later events are the development of a process which is initiated at the start of the postoperative period. Thus careful attention to measures which modify the phase 1 changes may contribute to a reduction in clinically obvious pulmonary morbidity.

CAUSES OF THE REDUCTION IN FRC

Wound pain

The pain of an abdominal incision causes a reflex increase in muscle tone. The abdominal muscles assist expiration; therefore spasm has a cuirass or corset-like effect on the thoracic cage (Anscombe, 1957). In support of this view, Bromage (1967) has shown that the relief of abdominal pain by extradural nerve block is associated with a reduction in the mean oesophageal pressure, taken to be an index of intrapleural pressure.

Abdominal distension

The loss of tone and motility of the gut following abdominal surgery causes an increase in pressure within the abdomen and elevation of the diaphragm. It is likely that this effect can be reduced, but not abolished, by avoiding the narcotic analgesics (Hymes *et al.*, 1973; Nimmo *et al.*, 1978). As much as four litres of air may be trapped within the abdomen (pneumoperitoneum) when the wound is closed. It is not uncommon to find radiologically detectable gas under the diaphragm as late as the third to fifth day after surgery. The problem as regards lung function is aggravated if the abdomen has been closed without drainage, since the gas may be under considerable pressure. Bevan (1961) has demonstrated a convincing relationship between the estimated volume of gas in the peritoneum and radiological evidence of lung collapse.

Intrapulmonary water

Jones, Lemen and Graf (1978) have shown that pulmonary venous congestion increases the closing volume in relation to the end-tidal position (FRC) in dogs. It is not clear if such changes contribute to the lung disorder following surgery, although attempts are being made to evaluate this aspect.

Posture

The relationship of FRC to closing volume is most favourable in the prone position and least favourable in the supine position (Le Blanc, Ruff and Milic-Emili, 1970).

PATIENTS SPECIALLY AT RISK

Cigarette smoking is associated with an increased production of secretions by the bronchial mucosa. Smokers may be expected to suffer a greater reduction in arterial Po_2 following operation compared with non-smokers (Marshall and Millar, 1965), probably because of an airways closing volume greater than would be predicted on the basis of age (Buist, van Fleet and Ross, 1973).

The patient who is grossly obese has an abnormally small FRC and is presumed to have an unfavourable relationship of end-tidal position to closing volume (Holley *et al.*, 1967). Thus the arterial Po_2 is often much less than in normal subjects of a similar age. The addition of the effects of a surgical operation on the lungs may cause life-threatening hypoxaemia in the first two to three postoperative days (Vaughan, Engelhardt and Wise, 1975). The problem of obesity is considered further in Chapter 46.

Dalrymple, Parbrook and Steel (1973) have suggested that a high 'neuroticism' score may be an index of susceptibility to pulmonary dysfunction after abdominal surgery.

THERAPEUTIC IMPLICATIONS

Much can be done by both anaesthetist and surgeon to lessen the factors which reduce FRC following abdominal surgery.

Abdominal pressure

When possible, the amount of air enclosed in the abdominal cavity should be reduced to a minimum. An abdominal drain will help to ensure that peritoneal gas is not under great pressure. If the abdomen is to be closed completely, suction may be applied at the time of the last peritoneal (sealing) suture. It may be that mixtures of nitrous oxide in oxygen given to relieve pain will also promote a reduction in the volume of enclosed gas (Alexander and Spence, 1973). The penalty of enclosing distended loops of bowel in the abdomen at laparotomy is obvious and, where other considerations permit, decompression is desirable. Abdominal binders are less common in modern practice, but are clearly undesirable if lung function is to be spared.

Posture

The patient should be nursed semi-recumbent rather than supine and early sitting and standing is to be encouraged.

Analgesia

Careful administration of narcotic analgesics so that pain relief is optimal will diminish the effect of pain on the lung and permit coughing and deep breathing. Alexander, Parikh and Spence (1973) showed a small improvement in pulmonary gas exchange and FRC when the total doses of narcotic analgesics were increased three-fold in comparison with routine practice in suitably selected patients, while Muneyuki *et al.* (1968) found that small doses of narcotic analgesics suitably titrated against the patient's observed pain spared the lung as effectively as extradural nerve block.

Abolition of wound pain by nerve blockade has long been regarded as highly effective in minimizing pulmonary disturbance after abdominal surgery (Cleland, 1949; Simpson *et al.*, 1961). Extradural block has conferred a small sparing effect on FRC and arterial Po_2 when compared with untreated pain (Sjögren and Wright, 1972; Wahba *et al.*, 1972) or casual administration of narcotic analgesics (Spence and Smith, 1971; Spence and Logan, 1975), but its chief value probably results from facilitating coughing and deep breathing (the phase 2 effects).

Hymes *et al.* (1973) found that the frequency of postoperative lung collapse was reduced when narcotic analgesia was replaced by trans-cutaneous electrical stimulation as the method of pain relief.

The use of gaseous analgesics such as nitrous oxide in oxygen would appear to spare lung function in at least three ways: the continuous depressant effects of the narcotics can be minimized or avoided, the patient breathes deeply once analgesia has commenced and there is the prospect of hastening the dispersal of gas from the peritoneum. In the author's hands, the technique is very satisfactory after upper abdominal surgery but there has been no formal evaluation of its merits.

Breathing exercises and physiotherapy

Much has been written about the need for deep breathing, percussion of the chest and assistance in the disposal of secretions from the bronchial tree in the postoperative period. The rationale of this therapy seems obvious and it is hardly surprising that its effectiveness is demonstrated easily in patients with pre-existing lung disease (Palmer and Sellick, 1953; Latimer *et al.*, 1971). Its value in patients with normal lungs before operation is questionable (Laszlo *et al.*, 1973; Pflug *et al.*, 1974) although unpublished studies in the author's laboratory have shown a late (day 5) sparing effect on FRC suggesting an attenuation of the phase 2 changes. The 'incentive' spirometer encourages the patient to breathe deeply and lessens the need for the attendance of a physiotherapist (Bartlett, Gazzaniga and Geraghty, 1973). In the debilitated patient, overzealous breathing exercises may seriously impair the cardiac output (Laws and McIntyre, 1969).

Several studies have suggested the use of doxapram infusions (for example doxapram 250 mg in 500 ml of 5% dextrose in water given over the first two hours after operation) as a pharmacological stimulus to deep breathing (Lees *et al.*, 1976).

Intermittent positive pressure breathing with a facemask or mouth-piece has no clear beneficial effect on postoperative lung function (Baxter and Levine, 1969; Cottrel and Siker, 1973).

THE PATIENT WITH PRE-EXISTING LUNG DISEASE

There have been no reports of large series of such patients. It is sometimes surprising — and a relief — to find that a patient with restrictive lung disease undergoing abdominal surgery may not suffer the mechanical changes in the lungs which have been described above in patients with normal or near normal lung function before operation. Occasional studies of such patients in the author's laboratory have often revealed little change in FRC as a result of operation and a gratifying maintenance of the arterial Po_2 at or near the preoperative value. Part of the explanation for this may be that the less compliant lung and thoracic cage are able to withstand the mechanical consequences of wound pain and abdominal distension. Furthermore, in many hospitals the patient with lung disease is likely to have received careful attention to the management of pain and the avoidance of bowel distension and pneumoperitoneum.

It should not be assumed, however, that patients with lung disease can undergo surgery without risk to arterial oxygenation in the postoperative period, and the only safe policy is regular measurement of the arterial Po_2 in the first 48 hours after surgery. A useful, if arbitrary, rule is that a patient in whom the arterial Po_2 is 8 kPa (60 mmHg) or less before surgery should maintain the preoperative value throughout the postoperative period. In the course of achieving this, skill in the provision of analgesia and breathing exercises, and care in the administration of oxygen may be required. If the best endeavours fail, the lungs should be ventilated artificially. In the writer's view, the use of controlled ventilation in the management of these patients is excessive at present. It seems a pity to court the dangers and expense associated with tracheal intubation and artificial ventilation if all the possibilities for facilitating spontaneous ventilation have not been tried. In a few hospitals throughout the world, 24-hour-stay postoperative care units have been established. These are particularly valuable for monitoring and treating the patient who is likely to require the maximum support necessary for a 'trial' of spontaneous breathing. These problems have been considered further in Chapter 26.

Adequacy of alveolar ventilation

If a patient has sustained a substantial loss of lung tissue as a result of disease or surgery, the ventilatory reserve may be so impaired, as a result of abdominal surgery, as to threaten carbon dioxide homoeostasis in addition to problems of oxygenation. A useful index of the risk is the preoperative vital capacity if it is remembered that an upper abdominal wound may cause a 50% reduction in this measurement. For example, a patient with only one functioning lung in which there is evidence of fibrosis as a result of a healed tuberculosis was found to have a preoperative vital capacity of 800 ml (Pao_2 8.2 kPa or 61.5 mmHg, $Paco_2$ 5.4 kPa or 40.5 mmHg) before upper abdominal surgery. The vital capacity decreased to 450 ml for three days following operation but gaseous homoeostasis was maintained by the use of thoracic extradural nerve block for 48 hours after surgery.

Any further loss of functioning lung tissue as a consequence of retained bronchial secretions with absorption collapse is an obvious risk to life in such patients. Thus narcotic analgesics should be avoided or, at least, administered in small doses intravenously so that the patient's ability to co-operate in breathing exercises and coughing is optimal. Several authors have described a substantial improvement in the postoperative vital capacity associated with successful techniques of analgesia (Simpson *et al.,* 1961) and Bromage (1955) has described a 'respiratory restoration factor' based on measurements of the vital capacity. However, such an improvement may not always occur. Spence and Smith (1971) found little improvement in vital capacity associated with extradural nerve block, although the quality of pain relief could not have been bettered. They attribute this lack of change to the dominant influence of factors causing abdominal distension and to the loss of motor power in the abdominal and lower intercostal muscles.

Again, it is the writer's opinion that artificial ventilation is not an easy option in the case of patients with restricted ventilation, although it is inevitable on occasions.

Bronchiectasis

This condition is less common nowadays, but patients with bronchiectatic cavities in the lung and copious production of pus pose a difficult problem of postoperative management following abdominal surgery. There is an obvious case for intensive treatment with antibiotics and breathing exercises to aid the disposal of pus before operation but, in spite of such treatment, a few patients have cavities which remain highly productive. Careful attention to pain relief after surgery is essential so that coughing is impeded as little as possible, for there is a real danger that, literally, the patient will drown in his own pus. This condition is perhaps the most obvious indication for the use of nerve block analgesia in the postoperative period. Similar considerations apply to the patient with excessive purulent sputum production associated with chronic bronchitis.

PULMONARY ASPIRATION (see also Chapter 75)

Aspiration of gastric contents to the lungs accounts for at least 10% of deaths attributable to anaesthesia (Edwards *et al.,* 1956; Bannister and Sattilaro, 1962). However, not all who aspirate during or after anaesthesia suffer damage to the lungs while sometimes there may be a mild bronchopneumonia with only slight systemic upset. The entry of solid matter to the bronchial tree may obstruct one of the larger bronchi — classically the right upper lobe bronchus — if the patient is in the supine position at the time of the accident. However, the greatly feared aspiration pneumonitis threatens life more than any of these and will be considered in greater detail.

Much of our understanding of the consequences of pulmonary aspiration comes from studies of animals, but it is easy to appreciate that an animal model may not typify all aspects of the already ill, perhaps elderly, patient in whom such disasters are particularly likely.

Laryngeal competence

Although massive regurgitation may overwhelm the larynx which is fully competent, certain types of patient are known to have impaired competence and to be specially liable to aspirate. These include all patients recovering from general anaesthesia, and certain sedatives such as diazepam (Tomlin, Howarth and Robinson, 1968; Carson *et al.*, 1973), those with a tracheal tube in place even when the cuff is inflated (Cameron, Reynolds and Zuidema, 1973), those from whom a tracheal tube has been removed after prolonged intubation (Davis and Cullen, 1974) and the elderly (Pontoppidan and Beecher, 1960).

The aspirate

It is generally assumed that the pH of the aspirate determines the severity of damage to the lung (Mendelson, 1946; Awe, Fletcher and Jacob, 1966), pH 3 or less being associated with aspiration pneumonitis. However, the continued occurrence of aspiration pneumonitis in obstetric practice (in which attempts to neutralize gastric acidity are almost routine nowadays) suggests that other unknown factors may influence the risk also.

As a rule, the larger the volume of aspirate, the poorer the prognosis. Sometimes, however, a patient will inhale a copious amount and recover with little after-effects, while a fatal pneumonitis may develop without any certainty on the part of the attendants that aspiration had occurred, suggesting that the volume had been small.

Lung changes

The water content of the pulmonary interstitium increases markedly so that the lung weight is more than doubled. The alveoli are filled with a haemorrhagic exudate, rich in protein and white blood cells. Microscopy reveals patchy necrosis of the entire alveolar—capillary membrane. The bronchial mucosa is congested and oedematous. In an experimental study in which 0.1 mol/l (0.1M) hydrochloric acid was instilled into the bronchial tree, in dogs, the pH of the bronchial secretions was highly acid initially but had returned to the neutral range by 30 minutes (Awe, Fletcher and Jacob, 1966). Following aspiration, the intrapulmonary shunt may be as much as 50% of the cardiac output (Cameron *et al.*, 1972).

Clinical features

In its worst form, pulmonary aspiration causes rapid respiratory and circulatory failure. If the patient has been breathing spontaneously, there is an initial period of apnoea followed by rapid shallow breathing and obvious distress. The arterial Po_2 is reduced markedly, usually sufficient to cause cyanosis. The arterial P_{CO_2} may be unchanged or increased. Bronchospasm is severe.

Circulatory collapse may occur with such speed that it is probably neurogenic in origin, although loss of water and blood constituents to the lung is the major factor subsequently. The haematocrit is increased. Severe metabolic acidosis supervenes rapidly. Gas exchange in the lungs may deteriorate over several days and, later, if ventilation is controlled mechanically, a marked decrease in lung compliance may be noted.

Initially, x-ray of the lung reveals patchy opacities which may be unilateral or bilateral. If the lung condition deteriorates further, opacification will have increased, sometimes to the stage at which both lung fields are virtually opaque. Thus the clinical and radiological changes in the lung in advanced forms of aspiration pneumonitis are indistinguishable from the imprecise condition known as the adult respiratory distress syndrome (ARDS).

Treatment

As a first aid measure, oxygen should be given using a facemask, but tracheal intubation is desirable since it permits endobronchial suction and facilitates artificial ventilation. Aminophylline 250 mg injected slowly i.v. may help to ease bronchospasm and lessen the work of breathing. A reliable intravenous cannula is essential, and the means of measuring central venous pressure desirable, in the treatment of the circulatory collapse. Early correction of metabolic acidosis with regular monitoring of the acid–base state is desirable.

Bronchoscopy is indicated only if it is considered that particulate matter has been aspirated also, and that it can be retrieved. There is little benefit and a possible risk of further damage to the lung from bronchial lavage, although volumes of isotonic saline not greater than 10 ml have been advocated (Hedley-Whyte *et al.*, 1976). Steroid lavage is of no value (Downs *et al.*, 1974).

There is controversy about the value of systemic steroids in reducing bronchial oedema and the alveolar exudate. Although many clinicians adopt this form of treatment on the grounds that, at least, it will cause no harm, the evidence from animal studies suggests that it is useless.

Cameron *et al.* (1968) found that intermittent positive pressure ventilation improved the survival of dogs in whom aspiration pneumonitis had been induced experimentally. In a similar study, Chapman *et al.* (1974) demonstrated the superiority of positive end-expiratory pressure. The general aim should be to maintain the arterial P_{O_2} as near as possible to the known or likely preoperative value subject to the need to avoid additional injury to the lung as a consequence of oxygen toxicity (see Chapter 28).

Secondary bacterial invasion may be an additional threat to recovery and samples of bronchial aspirates should be cultured by the bacteriologist. The use of prophylactic antibiotics cannot be shown to improve the course of the disease or reduce mortality, nevertheless many clinicians choose to administer a drug of the penicillin group (Cameron, Mitchell and Zuidema, 1973).

PULMONARY THROMBOEMBOLISM

Obstruction of the pulmonary arterial outflow by a thrombus or thrombi arising from the pelvic veins or the deep veins of the legs is an important cause of morbidity in the postoperative period. Massive embolism, in which the total flow to one or other lung is occluded, is the commonest cause of sudden death in the first ten days after surgery.

The frequency of pulmonary embolism is not known accurately because the diagnosis is notoriously difficult. Even at autopsy, the presence of smaller emboli may be missed, or there may be uncertainty as to the role of an obvious embolus in the death of a patient. In the International Multicentre Trial (1975) (of the effectiveness of calcium heparin in prophylaxis), 16 of 2076 general surgical patients, aged 40 years or more, for whom no special prophylactic measures had been taken, died of pulmonary embolism (16% of all postoperative deaths).

It is usually assumed, although by no means proved, that there is a relationship between the frequency of deep vein thrombosis and that of thromboembolism. The techniques of, and limitations to, the diagnosis of deep vein thrombosis have been reviewed by Browse (1978). The methods include the following.

(1) *Clinical examination* of the legs for swelling, dilatation of superficial veins and an increase in skin temperature; if there is inflammation in the vein wall, there will be pain and tenderness. McLachlin, Richards and Paterson (1962) found that, at best, these signs enabled a correct diagnosis in only 80% of a group of seriously ill patients whose veins were examined subsequently at autopsy.

(2) *Phlebography*, for which a radio-opaque contrast medium is injected into a superficial vein of the foot below a tourniquet (Thomas, 1972). Although this technique is not completely reliable, it is the standard method of investigation.

(3) *Doppler flow detector* — this is of value in diagnosing thrombi in the large veins above the calf. Unfortunately, it is least successful in detecting fresh thrombus formation — the very situation in which pulmonary embolism is likely.

Other techniques, having an application restricted to research studies, include: the fibrinogen uptake test (Flanc, Kakkar and Clarke, 1968); impedance plethysmography (Wheeler *et al.*, 1971); thermography (Cooke and Pilcher, 1974); isotope venography, using labelled albumin aggregates, with a γ-camera provides an opportunity to screen both the limbs and the lungs in the course of the same examination (Webber *et al.*, 1974).

Risk factors in deep vein thrombosis and thromboembolism

Death from thromboembolism occurs most often in patients over the age of 40 years (Registrar General, 1975), and the risk increases with age (Sevitt and Gallagher, 1961). There is an association with surgery in the obese, with heart failure and with cancer (Morris and Mitchell, 1977a), with the duration of operation and with major abdominal surgery (Flanc, Kakkar and Clarke, 1968; 1969), notably retropubic prostatectomy (Field, Kakkar and Nicholaides, 1972), with hip operations (Morris and Mitchell, 1976), and in patients with a history of previous venous thrombosis (Turnbull, 1960). Gibbs (1957) drew attention to injury including burns and found an association with the duration of immobilization in bed.

Pulmonary embolism is one of the common causes of maternal mortality and there is a strong association with operative delivery, notably caesarean section (Morris and Mitchell, 1977a). The risk of deep vein thrombosis is increased seven-fold in women who take oral contraceptives (Vessey and Doll, 1969), particularly those with a high oestrogen content (Inman *et al.*, 1970).

The diagnosis of pulmonary embolism

A massive embolus may cause death immediately by impeding the outflow from the right ventricle. In those who survive the immediate effects of embolism, there is a marked reduction in cardiac output and signs of intense sympathetic activity — cutaneous vasoconstriction, tachycardia, eyelid retraction, and proptosis. There is arterial hypoxaemia as a result of mismatching of ventilation to perfusion in the 'unaffected' lung tissue, but this may be aggravated further by right-to-left shunting if the foramen ovale has remained patent (Oakley, 1977). The arterial P_{CO_2} may be unchanged or decreased in spite of the fact that the pulmonary arterial obstruction causes a large increase in physiological deadspace. The arterial pressure may be maintained or reduced and the neck veins are distended. On auscultation of the heart right-sided gallop rhythm may be heard. The ECG is usually described as showing T-wave inversion in the right precordial leads associated with right axis shift. Other ECG changes may suggest posterior myocardial infarction and there may be peaked T waves in leads II and III. These features may not develop for several hours.

The radiographic appearances of the lungs are often unremarkable, although a high quality radiograph may reveal the absence of vascular markings in the unperfused region. Later, opacities may occur as a result of collapse of lung tissue or infarction.

The patient with smaller emboli in the periphery of the lung may have no symptoms or signs. However, infarction is likely to be accompanied by haemoptysis, chest pain (as a consequence of pleural inflammation), and dyspnoea. Later, a haemorrhagic pleural effusion may result. The importance of these smaller emboli is that they may herald subsequent small emboli or even massive embolism.

Differential diagnosis

The features of massive pulmonary embolism must be distinguished from those of severe acute myocardial infarction (in which the heart rate may be slowed, the arterial pressure reduced, and respiratory distress unusual) and acute tension pneumothorax. Acute right ventricular failure, in patients with chronic lung disease or pre-existing disease of the left ventricle, and acute cardiac tamponade, following surgery or trauma to the heart, may be confused with pulmonary embolism in respect of the initial signs.

Specialized techniques in diagnosis

PULMONARY ANGIOGRAPHY

Catheterization of the pulmonary artery via an arm vein and the injection of radio-opaque dye allows the pulmonary vasculature to be visualized and the extent of the occlusion to be determined. The measurement of increased pressures in the right side of the heart, in the course of inserting the catheter, may be an additional aid in diagnosis.

LUNG SCANS

In suitably equipped hospitals, intravenous injection of technetium-labelled macroaggregates of human serum albumin followed by scanning of the chest with a γ-camera will reveal perfusion defects after major embolism. This technique is not easy in patients who are very ill (Oakley, 1977).

The management of acute pulmonary embolism

MINOR EMBOLISM

The implications of the condition are an indication for careful examination of the veins of the legs to determine, if possible, the site and extent of venous thrombosis. Heparin and oral anticoagulants are the principal agents used in the treatment of deep vein thrombosis. The former is given intravenously in an initial dose of 10 000 units to produce an immediate prolongation of whole blood clotting time and treatment may be continued for as much as four to six days (Morris and Mitchell, 1978) by six-hourly injection or by continuous infusion. Oral anticoagulation with warfarin or phenindione is usually maintained for six weeks to three months.

Surgical removal of thrombi or plication of the vein proximal to an area of thrombosis may be considered (Browse, 1977). Thrombolytic therapy (Kakkar and Scully, 1978) is controversial; plasminogen activators such as streptokinase and urokinase convert plasminogen to plasmin while proteolytic enzymes such as plasmin and brinase cause direct fibrinolysis.

MASSIVE EMBOLISM

External cardiac massage may force the embolus onwards in the pulmonary arterial tree, thus minimizing the extent of obstruction (Heimbecker, Keon and Richards, 1973). Heparin in large doses (15 000 units) is given, for its serotonin blocking effect, to reduce pulmonary vascular and bronchial constriction (Miller, 1977). Oxygen should be administered by mask or, if that appears to be inadequate in preventing gross cyanosis, by controlled ventilation of the lungs.

A modified Trendelenberg operation has been advocated for immediate removal of the embolus (Clarke and Abrams, 1972). Reul and Beall (1974) have described a technique of partial femorofemoral bypass using a portable pump oxygenator as a prelude to pulmonary angiography and embolectomy with cardiopulmonary bypass.

Throughout the period of initial assessment and preparations for embolectomy, the patient should be nursed flat so that the return of blood to the right ventricle is not impaired. Rapid digitalization has been advocated (Soloff and Rodman, 1967). Miller, Hall and Paneth (1977) have drawn attention to the risks of venodilatation and cardiac depression associated with anaesthesia during preparation for pulmonary embolectomy.

There is evidence that fibrinolytic therapy can hasten the resolution of an embolus (The Urokinase Pulmonary Embolism Trial, 1973; Tibbut *et al.*, 1974). Active bleeding is an important contraindication to its use, although it is generally assumed that no increased risk is present beyond 48 hours after surgery. Streptokinase 250 000 units is given i.v. in the first 30 minutes of therapy followed by 100 000 units per hour for 48–72 hours (Miller, 1977). The thrombin clotting time should be measured before and at 12 hours and every 24 hours after commencing treatment. The values should be within two to four times the initial measurement.

Prophylaxis of venous thromboembolism

Morris and Mitchell (1978) have classified, in terms of the current evidence, the various methods that have been evaluated.

(1) STRONG EVIDENCE OF PREVENTION OF THROMBOSIS AND EMBOLISM

Oral anticoagulation is alone in this category, but the method is unpopular in surgical practice because of the risk of bleeding in the postoperative period and the need for regular laboratory supervision of the coagulation status.

(2) PREVENTION OF THROMBOSIS, BUT UNCERTAINTY ABOUT EMBOLISM

'Low dose' heparin (Sharnoff and DeBlasio, 1970; International Multi-centre Trial, 1975) is popular in current practice: 5000 units is given subcutaneously before operation and repeated twice daily after operation for two to five days.

Mechanical and electrical devices for stimulation of the calf muscles (Browse and Negus, 1970; Cotton and Roberts, 1975) are employed in some centres.

(3) CONFLICTING EVIDENCE IN RESPECT OF THROMBOSIS AND EMBOLISM

There have been claims and counter claims for the effectiveness of infusions of dextran 70 given during and after operation. A detailed study by Kline *et al.* (1975) found no influence of this treatment on overall surgical mortality or the frequency of venous thrombosis. However, dextran 70 did appear to reduce the frequency of fatal pulmonary embolism.

Aspirin and dipyridamole have been studied for their antithrombotic effect (Saltzman, Harris and Sanctis, 1971 Morris and Mitchell, 1977b) but the present view is that they are of little value.

(4) THEORETICALLY USEFUL

It is almost traditional practice that the patient should have leg exercise, massage and early ambulation after surgery. Although the efficacy of this has never been tested in a controlled trial (and is unlikely to be), it is notable that Flanc, Kakkar and Clarke (1969) found that specially vigorous measures of this type were of no obvious benefit.

'The Pill'

There has been confusion about the value of withdrawing oral contraceptives for three to four weeks before surgery. This practice is no longer recommended because some of the changes in clotting factors associated with oestrogens persist for weeks or months after discontinuing therapy (Poller, Thomson and Thomas, 1971). The additional risk of thrombosis in such patients should be minimized with the low dose subcutaneous heparin regimen (Editorial, 1976).

References

Alexander, J. I. and Spence, A. A. (1973). Apparent improvement in postoperative lung volumes by using the Entonox apparatus. A preliminary report. *Br. J. Anaesth.* 45, 90–92

Alexander, J. I., Parikh, R. K. and Spence, A. A. (1973). Postoperative analgesia and lung function: a comparison of narcotic analgesic regimens. *Br. J. Anaesth.* 45, 346–352

Alexander, J. I., Horton, P. W., Millar, W. T. and Spence, A. A. (1971). Lung volume changes in relation to airway closure in the postoperative period: a possible mechanism of postoperative hypoxaemia. *Br. J. Anaesth.* 43, 1196–1197 (Abstract)

Alexander, J. I., Horton, P. W., Millar, W. T., Parikh, R. K. and Spence, A. A. (1972). The effect of upper abdominal surgery on the relationship of airway closing point to end-tidal position. *Clin. Sci.* 43, 137–141

Alexander, J. I., Spence, A. A., Parikh, R. K. and Stuart, B. (1973). The role of airway closure in postoperative hypoxaemia. *Br. J. Anaesth.* 45, 34–40

Anscombe, A. R. (1957). *Pulmonary Complications of Abdominal Surgery.* London: Lloyd-Luke Ltd

Awe, W. C., Fletcher, W. S. and Jacob, S. E. (1966). The pathophysiology of aspiration pneumonitis. *Surgery, St. Louis* **60**, 232–238

Bannister, W. K. and Sattilaro, A. J. (1962). Vomiting and aspiration during anesthesia. *Anesthesiology* **23**, 251–264

Bartlett, R. H., Gazzaniga, A. B. and Geraghty, T. R. (1973). Respiratory maneuvres to prevent postoperative pulmonary complications. A critical review. *J. Am. med. Ass.* **224**, 1017–1021

Baxter, W. D. and Levine, R. S. (1969). An evaluation of intermittent positive pressure breathing in the prevention of postoperative pulmonary complications. *Archs Surg., Chicago* **98**, 795–798

Bevan, P. G. (1961). Postoperative pneumoperitoneum and pulmonary collapse. *Br. med. J.* **2**, 609–613

Bromage, P. R. (1955). Spirometry in assessment of analgesia after abdominal surgery: a method of comparing analgesic drugs. *Br. med. J.* **2**, 589–591

Bromage, P. R. (1967). Extradural analgesia for pain relief. *Br. J. Anaesth.* **39**, 721–729

Browse, N. L. (1977). What should I do about deep vein thrombosis and pulmonary embolism? *Ann. R. Coll. Surg.* **59**, 138–142

Browse, N. (1978). Diagnosis of deep vein thrombosis. *Br. med. Bull.* **34**, 163–167

Browse, N. L. and Negus, D. (1970). Prevention of postoperative leg vein thrombosis by electrical muscle stimulation. An evaluation with ^{125}I-labelled fibrinogen. *Br. med. J.* **3**, 615–618

Buist, A. S., van Fleet, D. L. and Ross, B. B. (1973). A comparison of conventional spirometric tests and the test of closing volume in an emphysema screening center. *Am. Rev. resp. Dis.* **107**, 735–743

Burton, J. D. K. (1962). Effects of dry anaesthetic gases on the respiratory mucous membrane. *Lancet* i, 235–238

Cameron, J. L., Mitchell, W. H. and Zuidema, G. D. (1973). Aspiration pneumonia: clinical outcome following documented aspiration. *Archs Surg., Chicago* **106**, 49–52

Cameron, J. L., Reynolds, J. and Zuidema, G. D. (1973). Aspiration in patients with tracheostomies. *Surgery Gynec. Obstet.* **136**, 68–70

Cameron, J. L., Sebor, J., Anderson, R. P. and Zuidema, G. D. (1968). Aspiration pneumonia: results of treatment by positive pressure ventilation in dogs. *J. Surg. Res.* **8**, 447–457

Cameron, J. L., Caldini, P., Toung, J. K. and Zuidema, G. D. (1972). Aspiration pneumonia: physiologic data following experimental aspiration. *Surgery, St Louis* **72**, 238–245

Carson, I. W., Moore, J., Balmer, J. P., Dundee, J. W. and McNabb, T. G. (1973). Laryngeal competence with Ketamine and other drugs. *Anesthesiology* **38**, 128–133

Chapman, R. L., Modell, J. H., Ruiz, B. C., Calderwood, H. W., Hood, C. I. and Graves, S. A. (1974). Effect of continuous positive pressure ventilation and steroids in aspiration of hydrochloric acid (pH 1.8) in dogs. *Anesth. Analg., Cleve.* **53**, 556–562

Clarke, D. B. and Abrams, L. D. (1972). Pulmonary embolectomy with venous inflow-occlusion. *Lancet* i, 767–769

Cleland, J. G. P. (1949). Continuous peridural and caudal analgesia in surgery and early ambulation. *NW. Med., Seattle* **48**, 26

Conway, C. M. and Payne, J. P. (1963). Postoperative hypoxaemia and oxygen therapy. *Br. med. J.* **1**, 844–845

Cooke, E. D. and Pilcher, M. F. (1974). Deep vein thrombosis: preclinical diagnosis by thermography. *Br. J. Surg.* **61**, 971–978

Cotton, L. T. and Roberts, V. C. (1975). Prophylaxis against deep vein thrombosis. *Br. med. J.* **2**, 499

Cottrel, J. E. and Siker, E. S. (1973). Preoperative intermittent positive pressure breathing therapy in patients with chronic obstructive lung disease: effect on postoperative pulmonary complications. *Anesth. Analg., Cleve.* **52**, 258–262

Dalrymple, D. G., Parbrook, G. D. and Steel, D. F. (1973). Factors predisposing to postoperative pain and pulmonary complications. A study of female patients undergoing elective cholecystectomy. *Br. J. Anaesth.* **45**, 589–597

Davis, F. G. and Cullen, D. J. (1974). Postextubation aspiration following prolonged intubation. *Annual Meeting of American Society of Anesthesiologists, Washington DC*, Abstract, pp 181–182

Diament, M. L. and Palmer, K. N. V. (1967). Venous-arterial pulmonary shunting as the principal cause of postoperative hypoxaemia. *Lancet* i, 15–17

Downs, J. B., Chapman, R. L., Modell, J. H. and Hood, C. I. (1974). An evaluation of steroid therapy in aspiration pneumonitis. *Anesthesiology* **40**, 129–135

Editorial (1976). Elective surgery and the pill. *Br. med. J.* **2**, 546

Edwards, G., Morton, H. J. V., Pask, E. A. and Wylie, W. D. (1956). Deaths associated with anaesthesia. A report of 1000 cases. *Anaesthesia* **11**, 194–220

Egbert, L. D. and Bendixen, H. H. (1964). Effect of morphine on breathing patterns. A possible factor in atelectasis. *J. Am. med. Ass.* **188**, 485–488

Field, C., Kakkar, V. V. and Nicholaides, A. N. (1972). *Thromboembolism: Diagnosis and Treatment*, p. 124. V. V. Kakkar and A. J. Jouhar (ed.) London: Churchill Livingstone

Fink, B. R. (1955). Diffusion anoxia. *Anesthesiology* **16**, 511–519

Flanc, C., Kakkar, V. V. and Clarke, M. B. (1968). The detection of venous thrombosis of the leg using ^{125}I-labelled fibrinogen. *Br. J. Surg.* 55, 742–747

Flanc, C., Kakkar, V. V. and Clarke, M. B. (1969). Postoperative deep-vein thrombosis effect of intensive prophylaxis. *Lancet* i, 477–479

Georg, J., Hornum, I. and Mellemgaard, K. (1967). The mechanism of hypoxaemia after laparotomy. *Thorax* 22, 382–386

Gibbs, N. M. (1957). Venous thrombosis of the lower limbs with particular reference to bedrest. *Br. J. Surg.* 45, 209–236

Hedley-Whyte, J., Burgess, G. E., Feeley, T. W. and Miller, M. G. (1976). *Applied Physiology of Respiratory Care*, p. 348. Boston: Little Brown Company

Heimbecker, R. O., Keon, W. J. and Richards, K. U. (1973). Massive pulmonary embolism. *Archs Surg., Chicago* 107, 740–746

Holley, H. S., Milic-Emili, J., Becklake, M. R. and Bates, D. V. (1967). Regional distribution of pulmonary ventilation and perfusion in obesity. *J. clin. Invest.* 47, 81–92

Hymes, A. C., Raab, D. E., Yonehiro, E. G., Nelson, G. D. and Printy, A. L. (1973). Electrical surface stimulation for the control of acute postoperative pain and the prevention of ileus. *Surg. Forum* 24, 447–449

Inman, W. H. W., Vessey, M. P., Westerholm, B. and Engelund, A. (1970). Thromboembolic disease and the steroidal content of oral contraceptives: a report to the Committee on Safety of Drugs. *Br. med. J.* 2, 203–209

International Multicentre Trial (1975). *Lancet* ii, 45–51

Jones, J. G., Lemen, R. and Graf, P. D. (1978). Changes in airway calibre following pulmonary venous congestion. *Br. J. Anaesth.* 50, 743–752

Kakkar, V. V. and Scully, M. F. (1978). Thrombolytic therapy. *Br. med. Bull.* 34, 191–199

Kline, A., Hughes, L. E., Campbell, H., Williams, A., Zlosnick, J. and Leach, K. G. (1975). Dextran 70 in prophylaxis of thromboembolic disease after surgery: a clinically oriented randomized double-blind trial. *Br. med. J.* 2, 109–112

Laszlo, G., Archer, G. G., Darrell, J. H., Dawson, J. M. and Fletcher, C. M. (1973). The diagnosis and prophylaxis of pulmonary complications of surgical operation. *Br. J. Surg.* 60, 129–134

Latimer, R. G., Dickman, M., Day, W. C., Gunn, M. L. and Schmidt, C. du W. (1971). Ventilatory patterns and pulmonary complications after upper abdominal surgery determined by preoperative and postoperative computerized spirometry and blood gas analysis. *Am. J. Surg.* 122, 622–632

Laws, A. K. and McIntyre, R. W. (1969). Chest physiotherapy: a physiological assessment during intermittent positive pressure ventilation in respiratory failure. *Can. Anaesth. Soc. J.* 16, 487–493

Leblanc, P., Ruff, F. and Milic-Emili, J. (1970). Effect of age and body position on 'airway closure' in man. *J. appl. Physiol.* 28, 448–451

Lees, N. W., Howie, H. B., Mellon, A., McKee, A. H. and McDiarmid, I. A. (1976). The influence of doxapram on postoperative pulmonary function in patients undergoing upper abdominal surgery. *Br. J. Anaesth.* 48, 1197–1200

McLachlin, J., Richards, T. and Paterson, J. C. (1962). An evaluation of clinical signs in the diagnosis of deep vein thrombosis. *Archs Surg.* 85, 738–742

Marshall, B. E. and Millar, R. A. (1965). Some factors influencing postoperative hypoxaemia. *Anaesthesia* 20, 408–427

Mendelson, C. L. (1946). Aspiration of stomach contents into lungs during obstetric anesthesia. *Am. J. Obstet. Gynec.* 52, 191–199

Miller, G. A. H. (1977). The management of acute pulmonary embolism. *Br. J. hosp. Med.* 18, 26–31

Miller, G. A. H., Hall, R. J. C. and Paneth, M. (1977). Pulmonary embolectomy, heparin, and streptokinase: their place in the treatment of acute massive pulmonary embolism. *Am. Heart J.* 93, 568–574

Morris, G. K. and Mitchell, J. R. A. (1976). Warfarin sodium in prevention of deep venous thrombosis and pulmonary embolism in patients with fractured neck of femur. *Lancet* ii, 869–872

Morris, G. K. and Mitchell, J. R. A. (1977a). The aetiology of pulmonary embolism and the identification of high risk groups. *Br. J. hosp. Med.* 18, 6–12

Morris, G. K. and Mitchell, J. R. A. (1977b). Preventing venous thromboembolism in elderly patients with hip fractures: studies of low-dose heparin, dipyridamole, aspirin and flurbiprofen. *Br. med. J.* 1, 535–537

Morris, G. K. and Mitchell, J. R. A. (1978). Clinical management of venous thromboembolism. *Br. med. Bull.* 34, 169–175

Muneyuki, M., Meda, Y., Urabe, N., Takeshita, H. and Inamoto, A. (1968). Postoperative pain relief and respiratory function in man: comparison between intermittent intravenous injections of meperidine and continuous lumbar epidural analgesia. *Anesthesiology* 29, 304–313

Nimmo, W. S., Littlewood, D. G., Scott, D. B. and Prescott, L. F. (1978). Gastric emptying following hysterectomy with extradural analgesia. *Br. J. Anaesth.* 50, 559–561

Nunn, J. F. (1977). *Applied Respiratory Physiology*, 2nd edn, pp. 301–304. London: Butterworths

Nunn, J. F. and Payne, J. P. (1962). Hypoxaemia after general anaesthesia. *Lancet* ii, 631–632

Oakley, C. (1977). The diagnosis of acute pulmonary embolism. *Br. J. hosp. Med.* 18, 15–24

Palmer, K. N. V. and Gardiner, A. J. S. (1964). Effect of partial gastrectomy on pulmonary physiology. *Br. med. J.* 1, 347–349

Palmer, K. N. V. and Sellick, B. A. (1953). The prevention of postoperative pulmonary atelectasis. *Lancet* i, 164–168

Pflug, A. E., Murphy, T. M., Butler, S. H. and Tucker, G. T. (1974). The effects of post-operative peridural analgesia on pulmonary therapy and pulmonary complications. *Anesthesiology* 41, 8–17

Pontoppidan, H. and Beecher, H. K. (1960). Progressive loss of protective reflexes in the airway with the advance of age. *J. Am. med. Ass.* 174, 2209–2213

Poller, L., Thomson, J. M. and Thomas, W. (1971). Oestrogen–progestogen oral contraception and blood clotting. A long term follow-up. *Br. med. J.* 4, 648–650

Rackow, H., Salanitre, E. and Frumin, M. J. (1961). Dilution of alveolar gases during nitrous oxide excretion in man. *J. appl. Physiol.* 16, 723–728

Registrar General (1975). *Registrar General's Statistical Review of England and Wales for the Year 1973.* Pt 1(a): Tables, medical. London: HMSO

Reul, G. J. and Beall, A. C. (1974). Emergency pulmonary embolectomy for massive pulmonary embolism. *Circulation* 50, Suppl. 2

Saltzman, E. W., Harris, W. H. and De Sanctis, R. W. (1971). Reduction in venous thromboembolism by agents affecting platelet function. *New Engl. J. Med.* 284, 1287–1292

Sevitt, S. and Gallagher, N. G. (1961). Venous thrombosis and pulmonary embolism: a clinico-pathological study in injured and burned patients. *Br. J. Surg.* 48, 475–489

Sharnoff, J. G. and DeBlasio, G. (1970). Prevention of fatal postoperative thromboembolism by heparin prophylaxis. *Lancet* ii, 1006–1007

Simpson, B. R., Parkhouse, J., Marshall, R. and Lambrechts, W. (1961). Extradural analgesia and the prevention of postoperative respiratory complications. *Br. J. Anaesth.* 33, 628–641

Sjögren, S. and Wright, B. (1972). Respiratory changes during continuous epidural blockade. *Acta anaesth. scand.* 16, 27–31

Soloff, L. A. and Rodman, T. (1967). Acute pulmonary embolism II. *Am. Heart J.* 74, 829–847

Spence, A. A. and Logan, D. A. (1975). Respiratory effects of extradural nerve block in the postoperative period. *Br. J. Anaesth.* 47, 281–283

Spence, A. A. and Smith, G. (1971). Postoperative analgesia and lung function. A comparison of morphine with extradural block. *Br. J. Anaesth.* 43, 144–148

Taylor, S. H., Scott, D. B. and Donald, K. W. (1964). Respiratory effects of general anaesthesia. *Lancet* i, 841–843

The Urokinase Pulmonary Embolism Trial (1973). *Circulation* 47, (Suppl. 2), 11

Thomas, M. L. (1972). Phlebography. *Archs Surg.* 104, 145–151

Tibbutt, D. A., Davies, J. A., Anderson, J. A. and others (1974). Comparison by controlled clinical trial of streptokinase and heparin in treatment of life threatening pulmonary embolism. *Br. med. J.* 1, 343–347

Tomlin, P. J., Howarth, F. H. and Robinson, J. S. (1968). Postoperative atelectasis and laryngeal incompetence. *Lancet* i, 1402–1405

Turnbull, A. C. (1960). *Thrombosis and Anticoagulant Therapy*, p. 61. W. Walker (ed). London: Livingstone

Vaughan, R. W., Engelhardt, R. C. and Wise, L. (1975). Postoperative alveolar-arterial oxygen tension difference: its relation to the operative incision in obese patients. *Anesth. Analg., Cleve.* 54, 433–437

Vessey, M. P. and Doll, R. (1969). Investigation of relation between use of oral contraceptives and thromboembolic disease: a further report. *Br. med. J.* 2, 651–657

Wahba, W. M., Craig, D. B., Don, H. F. and Becklake, M. R. (1972). The cardiorespiratory effects of thoracic epidural anaesthesia. *Can. Anaesth. Soc. J.* 19, 8–19

Webber, M. M., Pollak, E. W., Victery, W., Cragin, M., Renick, L. H. and Grollman, J. H. Jr (1974). Thrombosis detection by radionuclide particle (MAA) entrapment: correlation with fibrinogen uptake and venography. *Radiology* 111, 645–650

Wheeler, H. B., Mullick, S. C., Anderson, J. N. and Pearson, D. (1971). Diagnosis of occult deep vein thrombosis by a non-invasive bedside technique. *Surgery, St Louis* 70, 20–28

Wishart, H. Y., Williams, T. I. R. and Smith, G. (1977). A comparison of the effect of three anaesthetic techniques on postoperative arterial oxygenation in the elderly. *Br. J. Anaesth.* 49, 1259–1263

IV The circulatory system

31 Cardiac physiology
R. J. Linden

The physiology of the heart demands a fundamental understanding of how such a pump works. Its task is to pump an adequate supply of blood around the circulation. In this respect, inadequacy, or failure, is an inability to deliver enough oxygen and nutrients *to* the metabolizing tissues and to remove the formed waste products *from* the tissues. Adequacy or inadequacy, competence or failure, are therefore related to the extent of the activity of the tissues — to the extent of the oxygen consumption. The full range of consumption of oxygen is accomplished over a whole range of human activities from sleep or sedation, through rest in various postures to severe exercise.

Thus a full appreciation of the task of the heart will not be obtained until adequate explanations exist for the increase in cardiac output in the normal man from less than 5 $l \cdot min^{-1}$ to more than 30 $l \cdot min^{-1}$. But before attempting such explanations it is important to consider some of the fundamental components of the function of the heart.

THE CARDIAC CYCLE

For the explanations of cardiac function in this chapter it is assumed that the mechanisms concerned with the basic contractile processes of skeletal and cardiac muscle and of the electrical activity of the heart, including mechanisms involved in pacemaker potentials and conduction throughout the specialized tissues, are known to the reader. It is essential to appreciate that the electrical disturbance at the cell membrane *precedes* the mechanical contraction of the muscle.

The cardiac cycle in each chamber, each atrium and each ventricle, consists of a period of relaxation called *diastole* followed by a period of contraction called *systole*. During diastole the heart chambers fill with blood and during systole the blood is pumped forward into the next chamber or into the arteries.

ECG and events of the cardiac cycle

Figure 31.1 illustrates the various events observed during the cardiac cycle related to an electrocardiogram, the ECG being the resultant electrical

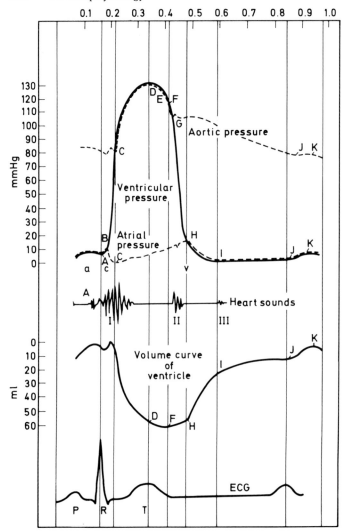

Figure 31.1
Events of the cardiac cycle. The phases are illustrated as follows:
A–C, isovolumetric contraction phase; C–D, maximum ejection;
D–F, reduced ejection. Diastole is divided into phases: F–G,
protodiastole; G–H, isovolumetric relaxation; H–I, rapid ventricular
filling; I–J, diastasis; J–K, filling by atrial contraction. a, c and r
refer to waves in atrial pressure pulse. (From Wiggers, 1952)

surface disturbance related to the electrical activity which flows over the
heart; this subdivision of the cardiac cycle was first suggested by Wiggers
(1921). It is important to study the diagram in detail and understand the
causes of all the events illustrated and to understand the relationships one
to the other, some of which are explained as follows. A rise in atrial pressure
begins a little after the origin of the P-wave which is caused by the spread

of depolarization across the atria and causes the atrial muscle to contract and raise the atrial pressure. Approximately 0.16 second after the P-wave, the QRS complex (depolarization of the ventricles) appears and initiates contraction of the ventricle, causing the ventricular pressure to begin to rise. It can be seen that the QRS complex begins slightly before the onset of ventricular contraction. Finally, one observes the ventricular T-wave in the ECG. This represents the stage of repolarization of the ventricles, at which time the ventricular muscle fibres begin to relax; thus the T-wave signals the end of the ventricular contraction approximately. A possible explanation for the T-wave and its changes has been postulated recently by Noble and Cohen (1978).

The atrium

Blood normally flows continually from the great veins into the atrium; guesses hazard that approximately 70% ot the flow occurs directly into the ventricles even before atrial contraction, and then atrial contraction causes an additional 30% of the filling of the ventricle. There are no reliable estimates of the contribution of atrial contraction to ventricular filling in conditions of rest to exercise but this must vary enormously, depending mainly on the degree of filling of the venous system, the heart rate and the extent of the activity in vagal and sympathetic nerves; thus the contribution of atrial contraction would be insignificant with the patient flat on his back, the heart rate slow and the venous system full, but might be an important force, in addition to ventricular suction, filling the ventricle at high heart rates, high sympathetic activity and low central venous pressures (Linden, 1963, 1965).

The atrial pressure curve consists of three major elevations labelled 'a', 'c' and 'v'; these can be seen in *Figure 31.1*. The a-wave is caused by the atrial contraction. The c-wave is caused mainly by two other factors: first, after the atrioventricular (AV) valves close they are caused to bulge further into the atrium because of the increase in pressure in the ventricles; second, the contraction of ventricular muscle pulls on the atrial muscle at the same time, creating increased tension in the atrial muscular structure which in turn results in an increase in pressure. The descending limb of the c-wave is caused by the continuing contraction of the ventricle pulling the valve ring down, creating a suction effect within the atrium. The v-wave results from a slow build up of blood in the atria during ventricular systole because the AV valves are closed. When the AV valves open, blood flows into the ventricles and the descending limb of the v-wave is observed.

The ventricles

During the descent of the a-wave of the atrial pressure pulse, the atrial muscle relaxes, causing a fall in pressure; pressure falls in the atrium below that in the ventricle and a momentary reverse flow causes the shutting of the AV valve (Little, 1951). Immediately following closure of the valve the ventricle contracts during the period of isovolumetric contraction, when both AV and aortic valves are closed, lasting about 0.03–0.05 second. Following this phase, pressure in the ventricle rises higher than that in the aorta and the aortic valve opens and ejection commences.

During the last quarter of ventricular systole almost no blood flows from the ventricles into the large arteries. The ventricular pressure falls to a value below that in the aorta during this protodiastolic period, causing the aortic valves to close; this is followed by a period of isovolumetric relaxation lasting about 0.04–0.08 second, during which both aortic valves and AV valves are closed. As soon as the pressure in the ventricle is below that in the atrium, the AV valves open and the ventricle fills rapidly, as shown by the ventricular volume curve in *Figure 31.1*. This is called the period of rapid filling of the ventricles. The period of rapid filling lasts approximately one-third of diastole at this heart rate; in the middle third only a small amount of blood normally flows into the ventricles and this period is called slow filling or diastasis; then atrial contraction adds a final thrust to the filling of the ventricle. It is obvious from the ventricular volume curve that filling is even more rapid than ejection and this is emphasized if we calculate the times of systole and diastole at fast heart rates and at high blood flows. For instance, at a heart rate of 180 beats per minute and an output of 25 l·min^{-1} during heavy exercise, the stroke volume is about 140 ml. With a cardiac cycle time of 0.33 s, of which systole lasts 0.2 s, it may be calculated that the 140 ml enters the ventricle in just over 0.1 s whereas ejection of that amount takes 0.2 s.

During diastole, filling of the ventricles normally increases the volume of each ventricle to about 140 ml. This volume is known as the end-diastolic volume. As the ventricle empties during systole the volume decreases by about 70 ml, which is called the stroke volume. The remaining volume in each ventricle (about 70–75 ml) is called the end-systolic volume or residual volume. When the heart contracts more strongly, the end-systolic (or residual) volume is encroached upon and may fall to as little as 10–30 ml. On the other hand, when large amounts of blood flow into the ventricle during diastole, the end-diastolic volume can become as great as 200 ml or more. Thus by increasing the end-diastolic volume and decreasing the end-systolic volume the stroke volume can be increased to more than double normal.

THE CORONARY CIRCULATION

Flow in any system, and no less in the coronary vessels, is based upon the perfusing pressure (driving pressure) and the resistance to flow. The perfusing pressure in the coronary system is the difference between pressure in the left main coronary artery (i.e. same as in the aorta) and the right atrial pressure. Coronary vascular resistance is determined not only by the vascular tone but also by the cyclic compression of the coronary vessels by the contracting muscle (Gregg and Fisher, 1963). Resistance caused by vascular tone varies indirectly with the fourth power of the mean calibre of the peripheral coronary vessels. The cyclic pattern of coronary flow is governed by (1) the aortic pulse pressure and (2) the restriction of flow resulting from physical compression of the coronary vessels by myocardial contraction. The instantaneous pattern at any time during systole is determined by the resultant of these two forces but it is the latter factor which ensures that the coronary blood flow pattern is different from anywhere else in the body. For further reading on this subject, consult Gregg (1950) and Rubio and Berne (1975).

Intramyocardial pressure

The intramyocardial pressure is determined by the magnitude of the intraventricular pressure development (Kirk and Honig, 1964; Buckberg and Kattus, 1973). Consequently, the fluctuations of coronary blood flow which occur during the cardiac cycle are more prominent in vessels supplying the left ventricle then in those supplying the right ventricle. At the onset of the isovolumetric contraction phase, the blood flow in the left coronary artery decreases abruptly and may actually flow backwards. With the onset of left ventricular ejection and the resulting rise of aortic pressure, coronary blood flow increases and reaches a systolic maximum shortly before the peak of the aortic pressure curve; flow then declines during the last part of systole. Approximately at the onset of the isovolumetric relaxation phase, coronary blood inflow rapidly increases to a peak value and then gradually decreases as it follows the pattern of the aortic pressure curve. Thus, in the normal left ventricle the largest fraction of the total coronary blood flow occurs during diastole (Gregg and Fisher, 1963). However, electromagnetic flowmeter studies have indicated that coronary flow in unanaesthetized dogs does continue during systole and contributes about 7–45% of the total flow (Gregg, Khouri and Kayford, 1965). This wide variation in flow reflects the changes which take place in the vigour of myocardial contraction in the same individual.

Compression of the coronary vessels by the contracting muscle can be demonstrated by comparing the coronary blood flow of the beating heart perfused at constant pressure with the flows achieved during ventricular asystole induced by vagal stimulation or ventricular fibrillation. At constant perfusion pressure the increase of coronary blood flow in the asystolic heart is about 50% above the control flow in the beating heart, and the extent of the rise of flow is taken to represent the magnitude of the mechanical or passive factors which restrict coronary flow (Berne, 1974).

Precise measurement of the pressure within the wall of the heart is difficult. However, some studies show that left ventricular intramyocardial pressure is greatest in the subendocardial muscle and falls off linearly to zero in the subepicardial levels of the heart (see, for example, Kirk and Honig, 1964). Systolic and diastolic subendocardial pressures may be equal to or greater than the intraventricular pressure, suggesting that the blood flow to the subendocardial layers occurs only during diastole, in contrast to the subepicardial muscle which is perfused during systole as well as during diastole. Despite these differences in epicardial and endocardial tissue pressures, both muscle layers normally receive equal flows (see, for example, Buckberg and Kattus, 1973). This is possible because the diastolic vascular resistance is lower in the endocardial layers; the same volume of blood per gram of tissue reaches the endocardium as reaches the epicardium since there is a greater diastolic than systolic flow to the endocardium. Several lines of evidence support the idea of graded subepicardial to subendocardial increase in systolic vascular resistance due to extravascular compression (for references, see Rubio and Berne, 1975). These include predominantly studies using radioactive microspheres. In addition, the right ventricular wall in contrast to the left ventricular wall is homogeneously perfused; aortic pressure and hence coronary perfusion pressure is at all times higher than right intraventricular pressure.

An important point of applied physiology is that the lower vascular tone of the subendocardial layers decreases the amount of additional vasodilatation that can be obtained when either myocardial oxygen requirement is increased or coronary blood flow is restricted. In either or both of these conditions a decrease in the ratio of subendocardial/ subepicardial flow may occur and is associated with (1) a reduction in contractility in the inner layers of the ventricular wall whereas the superficial muscles continue to develop normal or augmented contractile forces (Sonnenblick and Kirk, 1971), (2) an increased accumulation of lactate in subendocardial muscle layers (Griggs, Chen and Tchokoev, 1973) and (3) a further decrease in subendocardial muscle Po_2. Thus the deep layers are bound to show the effects of hypoxia earlier than the superficial layers.

EXTRAVASCULAR COMPRESSION AND INTRAVENTRICULAR PRESSURE

There is a relationship between intraventricular pressure and myocardial compression.

(1) Phasic changes in coronary blood flow associated with ventricular contraction are more prominent in left than in right ventricular flow curves.
(2) Asystole at constant coronary perfusion pressure results in increases in left and right coronary blood flow.
(3) In severe hypotension the systolic portion as well as the diastolic portion of the left coronary blood flow curve resembles the pattern of the aortic pressure curve.
(4) Left coronary blood flow ceases at a perfusion pressure of about 80 mmHg in systole and at 20 mmHg in diastole, whereas the cut-off pressure is less than 20 mmHg for right coronary flow in diastole and systole.
(5) Left intramyocardial pressure is greatest in the subendocardial layers and falls to zero at the epicardium.

(6) Strong stimulation of cardiac sympathetic nerves produces an increase in diastolic flow and a decrease in systolic flow (due to the tachycardia and the increase in intramyocardial pressure) often to a point where backflow is enhanced.

Coronary perfusion pressure

Coronary blood flow has been shown to correlate primarily with myocardial oxygen consumption and also with perfusion pressure. Studies in which coronary blood flow has been altered by changing coronary perfusion pressure have shown that a constant resistance to flow does not exist (see, for example, Berne, 1964). Under steady state conditions the coronary pressure–flow curve is convex, and nearly parallel, to the pressure axis over the physiological pressure range; that is, coronary blood flow tends to remain relatively constant despite the pressure change. However, at high pressures flow increases more rapidly, indicating a gradual reduction in resistance with elevation of perfusion pressure. This decrease in resistance to flow is due to distension of the vascular wall by increased transmural pressure. However, sudden and sustained changes in perfusion pressure give rise to abrupt changes in coronary blood flow in the same direction as the pressure. This transient increase in flow is not maintained and the flow returns to or toward the previous control level. It is this action which is termed autoregulation. The term autoregulation implies that steady state flow remains constant (perfect autoregulation) despite changes in perfusion pressure. However, in the heart only a moderate degree of autoregulation is typically observed in that the flow returns toward but not *to* the control level (Rubio and Berne, 1975).

Three mechanisms have been proposed to explain the phenomena of autoregulation of coronary blood flow: (1) the tissue pressure hypothesis proposes that autoregulation takes place through changes of the degree of compression of the thin-walled vessels due to increase (high perfusion pressure) or decrease (low perfusion pressure) in tissue pressure following changes in filtration; (2) the myogenic hypothesis proposes that an increase in the strain in the vascular smooth muscle produced by increase in perfused pressure stimulates the muscle to contract and the resultant increase in resistance returns blood flow to control levels; (3) the metabolic hypothesis proposes that coronary smooth muscle tone is controlled by vasodilator metabolite(s) released by parenchymal cells in response to their oxygen needs.

There is no direct evidence to support any of these hypotheses.

Myocardial oxygen consumption

There is a close relationship between the changes in coronary blood flow and the myocardial oxygen consumption (Eckenhoff *et al.*, 1947). The normal coronary sinus oxygen content is about 5 ml O_2 per 100 ml blood during enhanced myocardial metabolic activity and during reduced oxygen supply it can fall to levels as low as 1 ml O_2 per 100 ml blood (Scott, 1961). Among the determinants of myocardial oxygen consumption is the process of contraction itself; when cardiac work is increased by elevation of the aortic pressure, increasing the work done, myocardial oxygen consumption is increased more than when the work is increased due to an augmentation of cardiac output; that is, the development of pressure is more costly in terms of oxygen consumption than the increase in stroke volume. However, myocardial changes in oxygen consumption are not necessarily associated with changes in mechanical activity. Alterations in perfusion pressure in the arrested and beating dog or guinea-pig heart may elicit similar directional changes in coronary blood flow and oxygen usage without associated changes in contraction. The reason for this increase in myocardial oxygen consumption with increase in perfusion pressure has not been determined.

Hypoxia is a most powerful stimulus of coronary blood flow. However, the exact nature of the mechanism responsible for the reactive hyperaemia response is controversial and the vasodilatation is probably largely mediated by metabolic processes.

The nature of the process whereby the coronary blood flow is normally maintained at critical levels commensurate with the metabolic requirements of the myocardium is unknown. There is agreement that oxygen has an important effect on coronary resistance vessels as well as on other peripheral vessels. Two mechanisms have been proposed: (1) a direct effect of oxygen on the vascular smooth muscle cells of the arterial wall, and (2) an indirect effect through its action on parenchymal cells which produce vasodilator metabolites such as potassium, lactate, phosphate, adenosine; at the moment the mechanisms are unknown (Rubio and Berne, 1975).

Nervous regulation of coronary blood flow

Sympathetic and parasympathetic nerves innervate the coronary vessels. The direct effect of the stimulation of cardiac sympathetic nerves is coronary vasoconstriction and that of the parasympathetic, vasodilatation; these effects can be produced reflexly as well as by direct stimulation. This relatively simple relationship has not been easy to obtain and the literature is controversial. There has been difficulty in eliciting vasomotor responses of the coronary vessels to stimulation of autonomic nerves because the responses are usually masked by the effects of accompanying changes in metabolism, oxygen consumption, rate of pressure development during contraction (dP/dt), heart rate and systolic myocardial compression. However, the discovery of specific blockers of α and β receptors has been a major factor in resolving the problem of adrenergic humoral effect on coronary resistance vessels. Although sympathetic nervous activity results in constriction and vagal nerve activity in dilatation, both responses constitute only about 30—40% change in coronary resistance as compared with a five- to sixfold change in resistance caused by changes in metabolic activity (Rubio and Berne, 1975).

SYMPATHETIC EFFECTS

In paced and non-paced beating hearts and anaesthetized and unanaesthetized dogs or in fibrillating hearts, stimulation of stellate ganglia or intracoronary administration of noradrenaline produce an initial vasoconstriction followed by a vasodilatation. The delayed decrease in resistance is secondary to the concomitant increased myocardial activity associated with increases in metabolism, etc., enumerated above. Blocking the secondary myocardial response with β blockers reverses the dilator coronary responses to noradrenaline and a sustained nerve stimulation elicits only vasoconstriction; this vasoconstriction is blocked by a α-receptor antagonists (Feigl, 1967). A reflex decrease in spontaneous sympathetic firing by stimulation of carotid sinus nerves produces coronary dilatation, indicating that sympathetic nerves normally maintain a degree of coronary constriction which can be reflexly affected (Hackett *et al.*, 1972).

PARASYMPATHETIC EFFECTS

In non-paced, paced and fibrillating dog hearts stimulation of the peripheral cervical vagi produces a decrease in coronary resistance (Berne, DeGeest and Levy, 1965). These effects are blocked by atropine. In anaesthetized dogs, after cardiac β-receptor blockade and pacing, stimulation of aortic and carotid chemoreceptors with nicotine or cyanide produces a coronary vasodilatation that is abolished by bilateral vagotomy or atropine (Hackett *et al.*, 1972). Stimulation of the carotid sinus nerve after β-receptor blockade causes coronary vasodilatation which is reduced by vagotomy or administration of atropine (Hackett *et al.*, 1972). Thus the effect of activity in the vagal nerves on coronary vessels is vasodilatation and this can be evoked reflexly.

Isoprenaline, adrenaline and noradrenaline cause relaxation in isolated muscle strips of coronary vessels and the effects are blocked by β-receptor blockade which occasionally reveals a slight contraction (Zuberbuhler and Bohr, 1965). Noradrenaline is about ten times as potent as adrenaline in causing relaxation of muscle strips from the small coronary vessels. In isolated hearts perfused with blood but arrested with potassium, isoprenaline causes dilatation of the coronary vessels; the effect can be blocked by β-receptor blockade (Klock *et al.*, 1965). This evidence suggests the presence of β receptors in the coronary vessels. It is difficult to be precise about the role of the β receptors in the coronary arteries but at least they will respond to circulating catecholamines.

THE HEART AS A PUMP

The forces circulating the blood through the body emanate from three force pumps — the skeletal muscles together with the valved veins acting as one pump and the two pumps of the heart. It is important to realize that there are both central and peripheral factors (Guyton, 1963, 1968; Linden, 1963). Consideration of two extremes will illustrate the point.

Given an anaesthetized patient flat on his back, with chest and abdomen opened, when the other forces affecting venous return, gravity, muscle pumps, respiratory pumps have been removed, the sole remaining forces responsible for the circulation of the blood must reside in the heart — *vis a tergo* and *vis a fronte* — the forces from behind and in front. *Vis a tergo* is considered below and *vis a fronte*, the suction effect on venous return of the heart, has been discussed elsewhere (for references, see Linden, 1963). At the other end of the range where the cardiac output is 25 litres or more it is difficult not to attribute most of the force driving the blood round the circulation to the activity of the muscle pumps. It is of interest, therefore, to examine the mechanisms by which the main force pumps, the ventricles (regarding the atria as booster pumps), function. Bearing in mind that the main determinants of the changes in cardiac output are the changes in venous return, it is obvious that the main question really is how does the heart respond to the varying flows through it.

Heart rate and cardiac output

It is often stated that the cardiac output (CO) is related to the stroke volume (SV) and heart rate (HR), and an equation is usually given as

$$CO = SV \times HR$$

The heart rate and cardiac output are measured independently and the stroke volume is then calculated by dividing the cardiac output by the frequency of the beating of the heart. However, it does not necessarily follow that if the heart rate is increased the cardiac output will also increase; the heart rate and stroke volume are not independent variables; for instance, it is known that a simple increase in heart rate reduces stroke volume.

All the evidence suggests that a simple increase in heart rate does not result in an increase in cardiac output; it may be shown that an increase in HR from 40 beats per minute up to 70–90 beats per minute produces a small increase in output, but above this rate the cardiac output decreases a little until at 150 beats per minute it decreases even more (Linden, 1963; Linden and Snow, 1974).

An explanation of the above results resides in the relative changes of systole and diastole as the period of the cardiac cycle changes. When the heart rate is increased simply by electrical pacing, the period of systole remains constant and the period of diastole shortens. This shortening of diastole has little effect upon the filling of the ventricle, because only the period of diastasis (see *Figure 31.1*) is encroached upon, until the heart rate reaches about 70–90 beats per minute. Above this rate, further increases in heart rate encroach upon the period of rapid ventricular filling and results in a decrease in end-diastolic volume. Therefore the reduction in stroke volume always observed when the heart rate is increased by pacing may be accounted for in terms of Starling's law (see later).

STROKE VOLUME

Thus, looking at the equation again, if the heart rate is not responsible for the increased cardiac output of exercise then there must be changes in stroke volume. There are only two important mechanisms to be considered when examining the function of the ventricles: the mechanism involving Starling's law (Starling, 1918) and that resulting from the action of sympathetic nerves or catecholamines on the heart. No attempt will be made to describe the biochemical nature of the changes involved in these two mechanisms, only to describe the physical changes resulting from them so that their action may be recognized in the whole heart. These mechanisms can be recognized in isolated muscle.

Isolated cardiac muscle

The experimental work on isolated cardiac muscle has tended to follow in the steps of that on skeletal muscle with the consequence that experimental results obtained with cardiac muscle have been interpreted using models based upon characteristic skeletal muscle. There are, however, sufficient differences in the properties of cardiac and skeletal muscle to make such an interpretation along the lines of the classical theory based on skeletal muscle inadequate (see, for example, Brady, 1968; Ciba Symposium, 1974). However, it is not proposed in this chapter to give a

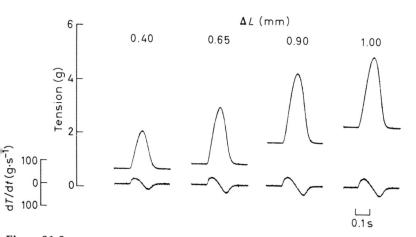

Figure 31.2
The effect of changes in initial length on the isometric twitch of an isolated papillary muscle from the right ventricle of a rabbit. The upper record is the tension (g) and the lower record the rate of change of tension (g·s^{-1}). The muscle was stimulated continuously at a rate of 30 per minute. The initial length of the muscle at zero resting tension was 5 mm. The initial length was then increased in a stepwise manner by the amounts shown above each record. The records are examples of single twitches when a steady state had been reached. (From Linden and Snow, 1974)

comprehensive review of cardiac muscle physiology or the possible intra-cellular explanations of the mechanisms of Starling's law. Suffice it to say that the acceptance in 1966 (Gordon, Huxley and Julian, 1966) of an explanation based on the number of cross-bridges pertinent to the Huxley sliding filament theory, has been challenged by assertions of an increase in the activation process, probably by calcium ions, and it is suggested that this activation process is related to the initial length of the muscle fibres. The interested reader is referred to Jewell (1977), Katz (1977) and Noble (1978). To understand Starling's law and how it is integrated into the heart acting as a pump, it is necessary first to consider the performance of isolated muscle in terms of changes in initial length.

Change in the initial length of cardiac muscle results in a change in the force of contraction. An example of this mechanism operating is given in *Figure 31.2*, where the effect of increasing initial length of a rabbit papillary muscle on tension developed during an isometric twitch is shown. As the resting length and therefore tension increase, the active tension is also increased. Relatively small changes in initial length result in large changes in active tension. The second mechanism available to cardiac muscle is that inotropic changes may be observed. For the purposes of

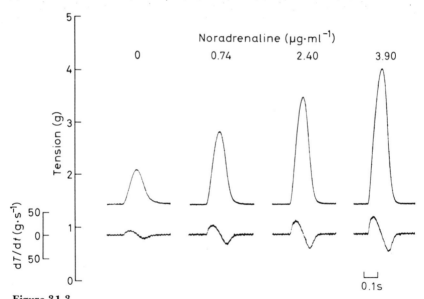

Figure 31.3
The effect of noradrenaline on the isometric twitch of an isolated papillary muscle from the right ventricle of a rabbit. The upper record is tension (g) and the lower record the rate of change of tension ($g \cdot s^{-1}$). The muscle was stimulated continuously at a rate of 30 per minute. The initial length of the muscle was constant at 5.5 mm. The concentration of noradrenaline in the fluid bathing the muscle was increased in a stepwise manner to the concentrations indicated above each record. The records are examples of single twitches when a steady state had been reached. (From Linden and Snow, 1974)

describing the physical changes in cardiac muscle on contraction a *reasonable definition* of an inotropic change is the change in the force of contraction of the cardiac muscle when it is altered other than by a change in initial length. An example of records illustrating an inotropic change are shown in *Figure 31.3*, where the effect of adding noradrenaline to the fluid bathing the muscle is to produce an increase in the force of contraction, as indicated by the active tension, from the same initial length. This operational definition of an inotropic change in isolated cardiac muscle is simply one of convenience; it enables the classification of agents which affect cardiac muscle and provides a basis for the measurement and interpretation of inotropic changes in the intact heart. Ideally it is desirable to define inotropic changes in terms of the underlying cellular and biochemical mechanisms. Such a definition is not possible at the present time; there is much speculation as to whether both the increased contraction caused by a change in initial length and the inotropic change have a common link in that activation is caused by calcium ions. For further reading the reader is recommended to consult Jewell (1977), Noble (1978) and the Ciba Symposium (1974).

The inotropic changes shown in *Figure 31.3* were produced by the addition of noradrenaline to the fluid bathing the muscle. Other agents of importance which produce inotropic changes are adrenaline, isoprenaline, calcium^{2+} and cardiac glycosides. Positive inotropic changes when demonstrated by an increase in either the peak isometric tension or dP/dt_{max} are usually accompanied by a small decrease in the duration of the twitch (*Figure 31.3*) but the degree to which the duration is altered in relation to the increase in peak tension is not the same for all inotropic agents. Typically, catecholamines tend to reduce the duration of the twitch whereas calcium ions and cardiac glycosides tend to increase the duration (Sonnenblick, 1962; Sonnenblick and Parmley, 1967). These differences in the action of agents capable of producing inotropic changes suggest that they do not all operate by the same final common path.

Inotropic changes may also be produced by changes in the frequency of contraction (Sonnenblick, 1962) and by altering the mechanical conditions under which the muscle is working (Parmley, Brutsaert and Sonnenblick, 1969). An example of this latter effect has been shown by Jewell and Rovell (1972), who found that if an isotonically contracting cardiac muscle is made to contract isometrically then the peak tension is increased for the first four to five isometric twitches. A reverse effect is seen when the muscle contracts isotonically again; thus a change in the mode of contraction — in this example, an increase in the tension in the muscle — has an inotropic effect. A possible explanation for the inotropic effects of increased frequency and of a change from isotonic to isometric contraction is that in both cases there is an increase in the uptake of calcium ions into the muscle cell (Langer, 1968; Kaufmann *et al.*, 1971).

Thus there are two mechanisms by which the ventricle may eject more blood: (1) Starling's law which relates the force of contraction to the initial length, and (2) a positive inotropic effect which occurs at a constant initial length.

Whole heart

Unfortunately, it is not possible to relate the quantitative changes observed in isolated muscle to measurements obtained in the whole heart; therefore, the following description of changes in the ventricle is dependent upon a qualitative approach. Thus the problem is largely one of attempting to assess the relative importance of the mechanisms demonstrated in isolated muscle in determining the function of the whole heart.

STARLING'S LAW

Starling (1918) originally stated his law in the following way: 'The Law of the Heart is thus the same as muscular tissue generally, that the energy of contraction, however measured is a function of the length of the muscle fibre'. Neither the energy of contraction nor the length of the muscle fibre can be measured in the whole heart, so the law cannot be verified. A reasonable approximation to the total energy of the contraction could be made if both the mechanical work done and the heat produced could be measured, as has been attempted in isolated cardiac muscle by Gibbs, Mommaerts and Ricchiuti (1967), who showed that the total energy released was related to the initial length of the muscle fibre. In the whole heart only the mechanical work done during the contraction (stroke work) is related to initial fibre length and the amount of energy produced as heat is usually ignored. The work done is usually estimated as the product of the stroke volume and the mean arterial pressure. However, stroke work estimated in this way is valid only if the kinetic energy of the blood leaving the heart is negligible and either the pressure or flow during the period of ejection is constant. Since neither pressure nor flow is constant during ejection, the calculation of stroke work as a simple product of stroke volume and mean pressure is only an approximation, and comparisons of stroke work, under different conditions of stroke volume and pressure, may lead to significant errors in quantitative interpretation of factors affecting stroke work. However, even though measurements of left ventricular function such as stroke work, stroke power and peak pressure do not actually measure the total energy of contraction, there are reasonable grounds based upon measurements in isolated muscle (see, for example, Gibbs, Mommaerts and Ricchiuti, 1967) to allow them to be used as indices of the energy of contraction.

Measurement of the initial length of the muscle fibres in the heart presents a problem as great as the measurement of the energy of contraction. In the left ventricle if the end-diastolic pressure is increased then so is the end-diastolic volume and therefore of necessity some, if not all, of the fibres will be stretched. In fact, measurement of dimensional changes, whether from the apex to the base or transversely, show an increase as the ventricle fills during diastole. However, it seems unlikely that, with the interdigitating layers of muscle in myocardium, muscle fibres regardless of their orientation will be stretched by the same amount; indeed, there is some evidence that they are not (Sonnenblick and Ross,

1967). Also, Fisher, Lee and Kavaler (1967) have shown that some fibres are further stretched during early systole and that the changes in end-diastolic volume play some part in determining whether a fibre is stretched or shortened during early systole.

The above considerations show that measurements of the size of the heart, whether of the volume or linear dimensions, only give a gross estimate of the initial fibre length and as such they may only be used as indices of fibre length. At the present time, then, Starling's law may only be demonstrated by showing the effects of changes in an index of fibre length upon an index of the energy of contraction; for example, the relationship between end-diastolic pressure in the left ventricle as an index of fibre length and stroke work as an index of the energy of contraction — thus as end-diastolic pressure is increased there is an increase in stroke work. However, the increments in stroke work are usually brought about by increments both in stroke volume and mean aortic pressure, and Sarnoff *et al.* (1960b) demonstrated that changes in mean aortic pressure produces an inotropic effect. In an isolated heart preparation in which heart rate and coronary blood flow were kept constant, they showed that an increase in aortic resistance resulted, after a few beats, in an increase in stroke work from the same end-diastolic pressure. *Figure 31.4* shows the

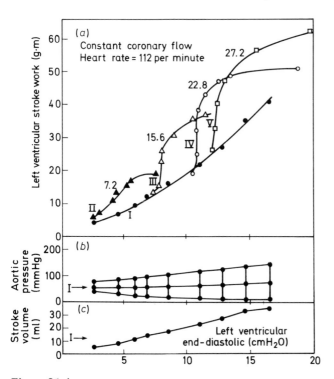

Figure 31.4
The inotropic effect of an increase in aortic pressure in the isolated dog's heart. Figures to the left of each curve in (*a*) indicate the stroke volumes in millilitres. For further explanation, see text. (From Sarnoff *et al.*, 1960b)

result of one experiment: the curve labelled I was obtained with the mean aortic pressure held approximately constant and the stroke work was increased by increasing the inflow to the heart. The constancy of the mean aortic pressure and the relationship of the stroke volume and the end-diastolic pressure in the ventricle are shown in (*b*) and (*c*). The relationship of the stroke volume to end-diastolic pressure in the ventricle is shown in (*c*) and the relationship between the left ventricular stroke work and the end-diastolic pressure is shown as curve I in (*a*); each of these relationships demonstrates the simple relationship of Starling's law: increasing end-diastolic pressure, and thus increasing end-diastolic length of the fibres, results in an increased force of contraction as indicated by increased stroke volume and the increased stroke work.

Figure 31.4 also illustrates the limitations of this particular set of indices. At each of the four different stroke volumes the aortic pressure was increased in a stepwise manner and at each stroke volume the relationship between stroke work and end-diastolic pressure is shown as curves II, III, IV, V in *Figure 31.4 (a)*. Each curve demonstrates a positive inotropic change with an increase in resistance to output from the left ventricle. It is apparent, then, that the demonstration of Starling's law by the relationship of stroke work to end-diastolic pressure also includes an extra amount of work that is not directly related to the initial length of the muscle fibre but to the afterload placed upon the heart (i.e. the mean aortic pressure). These relationships should not be used in any other way than to give a qualitative demonstration of Starling's law.

INOTROPIC CHANGES IN THE HEART

The quantitative measurement of inotropic changes in the whole heart is as difficult as measuring the changes in the initial length and force of contraction. There exists a variety of methods and no one particular method is ideal. A discussion of the various methods has recently been published (Linden and Snow, 1974). By definition, the index must not be influenced by changes in initial fibre length, which in the intact heart will be indicated either by end-diastolic pressure or some approximation to a measurement of end-diastolic volume. At the present time there seems little point in using complicated indices of inotropic changes until more is known about the mechanics of the intact ventricle. Under controlled conditions the maximum rate of change of ventricular pressure during isometric contraction phase (dP/dt_{max}) appears to be the most reliable provided it has been quantitatively validated in the preparation used.

As with the isolated cardiac muscle, inotropic effects in the intact heart may be produced in a variety of ways. The largest inotropic effects are produced either by stimulation of the cardiac sympathetic nerves or by the intravenous infusion of catecholamines. Relatively smaller inotropic changes may be produced by changes in either mean aortic pressure or heart rate.

INOTROPIC ACTIVITY IN AUTONOMIC NERVES TO THE HEART

In general, the effect of stimulating the sympathetic nerves to the heart is to cause an increase in the force of contraction of the muscle and an increase in heart rate; associated with these changes are an increase in cardiac output and in mean aortic pressure (for references, see Linden and Snow, 1974). Therefore, in order to quantify the direct inotropic effects of activity in the sympathetic nerves, it is necessary to keep both mean aortic pressure and heart rate constant. The relative chronotropic and inotropic effects of activity in the right and left cardiac sympathetic nerves in the dog are clearly illustrated by plotting the two responses (heart rate and dP/dt_{max}), obtained at each frequency of stimulation, against each other as shown in *Figure 31.5*. It may be seen that for a

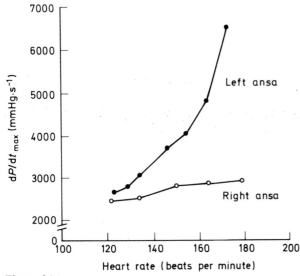

Figure 31.5
The relative chronotropic and inotropic effects of stimulating the right and left ansae subclaviae in the dog. Each point represents the values of the heart rate and dP/dt_{max} in response to a particular frequency of stimulation. (From Linden and Snow, 1974)

given increase in heart rate the inotropic effect produced by activity in the left ansa subclavia is about ten times that brought about by activity in the right ansa subclavia. Similar effects are obtained if inotropic changes are measured in the right ventricle.

The inotropic effect on ventricular muscle of activity in efferent vagal fibres to the heart is controversial. There is no doubt that in the dog vagal activity slows the heart and decreases the force of contraction of atrial muscle (see Linden, 1963, for discussion). It was also demonstrated that the relationship between end-diastolic pressure in the left ventricle and stroke work was not altered by activity in the vagus. This was confirmed by Furnival, Linden and Snow (1968), who compared the inotropic and chronotropic effects of stimulating the vagus nerves and found only small decreases in dP/dt_{max} of the order of 200–400 mmHg per second, which are not of great significance in a heart capable of functioning throughout the normal physiological range. However, such small changes may well be of significance in the failing heart or when the inotropic state is severely depressed as in the experiments of DeGeest *et al.* (1965). The effects in those small and absolute terms then become relatively important.

INOTROPIC EFFECT OF CATECHOLAMINES

Catecholamines are known to have both chronotropic and inotropic effects on the heart. If infused in the intact animal, the response of the heart may be modified by circulatory reflexes (baroreceptor reflexes) such that there may be a decrease in heart rate in response to an infusion of noradrenaline (Cobbold, Ginsburg and Paton, 1960). In order to assess the direct inotropic and chronotropic effects of circulatory catecholamines on the heart, the heart must be denervated and circulatory reflexes prevented from occurring. Also the inotropic effects in terms of dP/dt_{max} must be measured at a constant heart rate and mean arterial pressure. In experiments conforming to the above criteria it has been shown that the order of potency in producing both chronotropic and inotropic effects was isoprenaline greater than adrenaline, greater than noradrenaline (Furnival, Linden and Snow, 1971a). However, the relative chronotropic and inotropic effects of catecholamines were different; for any given increase in heart rate produced by the infusion of a catecholamine, noradrenaline produced a greater increase in dP/dt_{max} than either adrenaline or isoprenaline. Furnival, Linden and Snow (1971a) suggested that the different relative inotropic and chronotropic effects of circulating catecholamines occur because there is a greater density of adrenergic nerve endings in the sinoatrial node than in the muscle of the left ventricle associated with the different affinities of catecholamines for the uptake process into the sympathetic nerve fibres.

INOTROPIC EFFECTS ASSOCIATED WITH CIRCULATORY REFLEXES

A fall in pressure in the carotid sinus results in a reflex increase in heart rate and a positive inotropic response (Sarnoff *et al.*, 1960a; Levy *et al.*, 1966; Furnival, Linden and Snow, 1971b). Hainsworth and Karim (1972) have also demonstrated a similar positive inotropic effect on the ventricle in response to a fall in pressure in the arch of the aorta.

Stimulation of atrial receptors by distension of the vein–atrial junctions on both sides of the heart is known to result in a reflex increase in heart rate (Ledsome and Linden, 1964; Kappagoda, Linden and Snow, 1972). The efferent pathway of this reflex has been shown to be solely in the sympathetic nerves to the heart. It is therefore surprising that stimulation of atrial receptors at the pulmonary vein–atrial junctions does not result in any significant inotropic response (Furnival, Linden and Snow, 1971b).

REFLEXES FROM THE HEART

Many reflexes emanate from, and control, the cardiovascular system. They are usually grouped under one or other of two headings, depending on where the receptors or end-organs are sited: those reflexes from the vessels, such as the systemic arterial baroreceptor reflexes, and those from the heart. Those from the heart are considered here. This topic of reflexes from receptors in the heart has only recently come into prominence and short reviews have been published (Coleridge and Coleridge, 1972; Paintal, 1973; Shepherd, 1973; Linden, 1973, 1975); results of a symposium have been reported (Kidd, Hainsworth and Linden, 1979).

Over the years, various effects and functions have been attributed to receptors in the ventricles and atria. However, it seems now that some pattern of events has evolved. Broadly, two groups of effects are obtainable: stimulation of the ventricular receptors results in a decrease in heart rate and a fall in blood pressure; and stimulation of atrial receptors results in an increase in heart rate and in urine flow.

Throughout this section it must be remembered that before a stimulus/response sequence may be described as a reflex it must be demonstrated that there is an anatomical basis for such a reflex: it should be shown that there exists a nervous end-organ (a receptor), an afferent nerve, an efferent nerve and an effector organ. Not all the components of the reflexes have yet been established but there is sufficient evidence to warrant the acceptance of the reflexes and their qualitative effects.

Ventricular receptors

One approach to the problem of stimulation of cardiac receptors has been to use chemical substances by application and injection, in order to stimulate receptors in the ventricles of the heart. As long ago as 1867, Bezold and Hirt observed that the injection of veratrum produced apnoea, bradycardia and hypotension. Jarisch and his co-workers (e.g. Jarisch and Zotterman, 1948) confirmed these results and since that time these responses have been known as the Bezold–Jarisch reflex. Dawes (1947) localized some of the receptors responsible for the reflex bradycardia and hypotension to the left ventricle and later Dawes and Comroe (1954) suggested the reflex be called the 'coronary chemoreflex'.

Numerous investigations have described nerve endings in the ventricular epicardium and myocardium (e.g. King, 1939) but much of the published work represents drawings of slides and may contain much artefact. Miller and Kasahara (1964), in a careful study, concluded that there were no sensory endings in the myocardium; they assumed that the nerve fibres which they traced through the connective tissues of the septa between the muscles, extended ultimately into the endocardium. However, the very small nerve fibres have yet to be defined histologically.

Using physiological techniques to examine the discharge from fibres from the chambers of the heart, Coleridge, Coleridge and Kidd (1964) showed that there were two types of ventricular receptors — one with a pulsatile discharge in time with the heart beat and one with an irregular discharge. For various reasons little useful comment can be made about those with the cardiac rhythm: they are few in number and little else is known about them. As Paintal (1972) has suggested, the 'coronary artery' mechanoreceptors of Brown (1966) really belong to this group of receptors and are not true 'coronary' receptors. However, because Brown showed that stimulation of these receptors caused bradycardia and hypotension they can probably be included in the large group of systemic and pulmonary baroreceptors known to have this response.

The second type of ending described by Coleridge, Coleridge and Kidd (1964) was characterized by a sparse irregular discharge and is, at the moment, much more interesting. The discharge of these receptors is characterized by sparse irregular discharge into small nerve fibres which have a range of conduction velocities from $1-2$ m·s^{-1} and include a group of fibres known as C fibres.

It is now accepted that there are ventricular receptors which discharge irregularly into non-myelinated fibres (C fibres) in the vagi. They are distributed over the whole of the left ventricle in both epicardium and myocardium (Coleridge, Coleridge and Kidd, 1964; Sleight and Widdicombe, 1965; Muers and Sleight, 1972; Oberg and Thoren, 1972). They are activated by fairly gross changes. For instance, occlusion of the aorta (Muers and Sleight, 1972; Oberg and Thoren, 1972) resulting in high pressures, causes these endings to discharge. These investigators also referred to the eliciting of increased discharge in these small fibres in response to rapid infusions, electrical stimulation of cardiac nerves, intravenous or intracoronary injection of catecholamines, and the injection of drugs such as nicotine, veratridine and capsaicine. Strophanthin given intravenously was said to sensitize the receptors in a similar way to veratrum in that aortic occlusion led to a greater and more prolonged receptor activation after strophanthin administration than it did before. All these assaults on the myocardium are outside the physiological range and have provided little evidence so far of the natural physiological stimulus.

However, the investigators are usually convinced that a large distension of the ventricular myocardium or an intense contraction could provide an adequate stimulus; therefore it is not surprising that an increased receptor activity was observed in response to an ischaemic dilatation of the heart such as was observed when the coronary supply was occluded or during severe asphyxia (Thoren, 1972). Oberg and Thoren (1973) reported that stimulation of the ventricular receptors was followed by reflex effects on the heart rate and peripheral circulation such that bradycardia which occurs mainly as a result of increased vagal efferent discharge is considerably more evident than that effected by atrial baroreceptors for a given fall in blood pressure. The latter could be the underlying mechanism for the reflex vasodilatation associated with myocardial ischaemia (Constantin, 1963).

The generalized peripheral vasodilatation produced by the left ventricular receptors affects both the resistance and the capacitance vessels. The reflex adjustments in the renal vascular beds are relatively more pronounced when the ventricular receptors are activated than when arterial baroreceptors are stimulated. Thoren concluded that the over-all results implied that the afferent fibres from the left ventricular receptors seemed to be preferentially orientated toward central cardiovascular connections which affect heart rate and discharge in vasoconstrictor fibres to the kidney. A curious effect of intense activation of the left ventricular receptors is that it induced considerable relaxation of the stomach (Abrahamsson and Thoren, 1972).

It has also been reported that this reflex from the ventricular receptors is responsible for at least part of the bradycardia caused by digitalis glycosides (Sleight, Lall and Muers, 1969; Oberg and Thoren, 1972). The reflex bradycardia and hypotension caused by an injection of veratrum alkaloids (Bezold–Jarisch effect) are probably due to the chemical stimulation of the small nerve endings. Oberg and Thoren suggest that a rapid increase in ventricular volume might also activate these fibres by a distortion effect causing reflex bradycardia and that this is an explanation of the cause of vasovagal reactions. Furthermore, Koletat *et al.* (1967), from experiments in anaesthetized dogs, have suggested that the brady-cardia and hypotension observed at the time of myocardial infarction are brought about reflexly by an increase in discharge from the receptors in the infarcted area. In view of all this evidence, Sleight (1979) believes that 'the receptors are primarily excited by an increase in the force of contraction of the left ventricle or by intramyocardial tension'; thus they will be stimulated in a large heart, a vigorously contracting small heart or in certain pathological conditions.

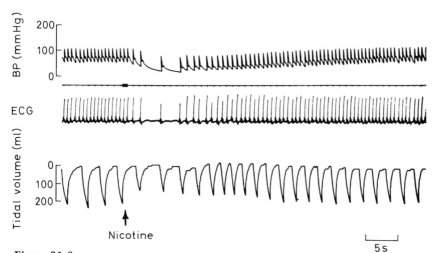

Figure 31.6
Conscious dog: indwelling pericardial and internal mammary arterial catheters. From above downwards: arterial BP (mmHg); electro-cardiogram and respiration (ml) measured with a spirometer (inspiration downwards); 25 μg of nicotine injected through the pericardial catheter. (From Sleight, 1964, by courtesy of the author)

Though the adequate stimulus to the ventricular receptors is in dispute, there is no doubt that stimulation of the receptors causes a reflex fall in blood pressure and heart rate. An example of such a response is shown in the beautiful demonstration of Sleight (1964). Knowing that nicotine and veratridine stimulated these receptors which discharge into small fibres, Sleight showed that in unanaesthetized dogs nicotine injected into the pericardium so as to stimulate the epicardial receptors did not cause 'pain' but resulted in a large fall in blood pressure and heart rate (*Figure 31.6*). Sleight (1979) has proposed possible physiological roles for these receptors.

Atrial receptors

Various reviews have commented on the function of atrial receptors (e.g. Coleridge and Coleridge, 1972; Paintal, 1973; Shepherd, 1973; Linden, 1975). Most of the histological attention has rightly been paid to the atrial endocardium which is the most profusely innervated area of the heart. The most characteristic features of this dense innervation are the wealth and variety of complex unencapsulated sensory endings found at the junctions of the superior and inferior vena cava and the right atrium and the pulmonary veins and the left atrium in both animals and man (Nonidez, 1937; Coleridge *et al.*, 1957; Holmes, 1957; Johnston, 1968). Paintal (1953, 1973), examining the physiological patterns of discharge of these atrial receptors, has described them as type A, mainly discharging in time with the a-wave of the atrial pressure pulse, type B, mainly in time with the v-wave, and an intermediate type. It is now considered that there are only two types — type B and intermediate — which have their receptors in the atrial endocardium (Kappagoda, Linden and Mary, 1977). Paintal considers the natural stimulus to these receptors to be a change in volume of the atrium.

Over the last 15 years it has become clear that stimulating atrial receptors in either the right or the left atrium results in an increase in heart rate. This increase in heart rate is reflex and it has been shown that the afferent nerves for this reflex are in the vagal nerves and the efferent nerves are solely in the sympathetic nerves to the sinoatrial node, there is no effect on the vagal efferent nerves nor it there a concomitant sympathetic discharge to ventricular muscle, and thus no positive inotropic effect. Stimulating the atrial receptors does not affect peripheral resistance and does not affect respiration (Linden, 1975).

Stimulation of right and left atrial receptors also results in an increase in urine flow. This again is a reflex response with afferent nerves in the vagal nerves and the efferent limb of this reflex is twofold. Stimulation of atrial receptors causes a decrease in the discharge in nerves to the kidney; the effect on the kidney of these changes in activity in these sympathetic nerves is unknown, but it is possible that they cause changes in blood flow (Mason and Ledsome, 1974) and therefore may be responsible for the changes in solute excretion observed during this diuresis but not wholly for the excretion of water (Lawrence, Ledsome and Mason, 1973). In addition, stimulation of atrial receptors causes a blood-borne agent to give rise to an increase in urine flow; the increase in urine flow was observed in animals in which the kidneys had been denervated and also in isolated perfused kidneys. It is thought that the blood-borne agent is not the anti-diuretic hormone because there is no consistent change in the level of antidiuretic hormone in the blood during stimulation of atrial receptors and also the increase in urine flow in response to stimulation of the receptors can be obtained in animals in which the postpituitary has been ablated (for references, see Linden, 1975). There is a possibility that this blood-borne agent is a diuretic substance.

There is no evidence yet on which to base a conclusion that these reflexes are involved in the regulation of blood volume.

References

Abrahamsson, H. and Thoren, P. (1972). Reflex relaxation of the stomach from receptors located in the heart. Analysis of receptors and afferents involved. *Acta physiol. scand.* 84, 197–207

Berne, R. M. (1964). Regulation of coronary blood flow. *Physiol. Rev.* 44, 1–29

Berne, R. M. (1974). In *Coronary Circulation in the Mammalian Myocardium*, pp. 251–281. G. A. Langer and A. Brady (ed.). New York: Wiley

Berne, R. M., DeGeest, H. and Levy, M. N. (1965). Influence of the cardiac nerves on coronary resistance. *Am. J. Physiol.* 208, 763–769

Bezold, A. von and Hirt, L. (1867). Ueber die physiologischen Wirkungen des essigsauren Veratrins. *Unters. physiol. Lab. Wurzburg.* 1, 75–156

Brady, A. J. (1968). Active state in cardiac muscle. *Physiol. Rev.* 48, 570–600

Brown, A. M. (1966). The depressor reflex arising from the left coronary artery of the cat. *J. Physiol. Lond.* 184, 825–836

Buckberg, G. D. and Kattus, A. A. (1973). Factors determining the distribution and adequacy of left ventricular myocardial blood flow. In *Current Topics in Coronary Research*, pp. 95–113. C. M. Bloor and A. A. Olsson (ed.). New York: Plenum Press

Ciba Symposium (1974). *The Physiological Basis of Starling's Law of the Heart*. London: North-Holland

Cobbold, A. F., Ginsburg, J. and Paton, A. (1960). Circulatory, respiratory and metabolic responses to isopropylnoradrenaline in man. *J. Physiol., Lond.* 151, 539–550

Coleridge, H. and Coleridge, J. C. G. (1972). Cardiovascular receptors. In *Modern Trends in Physiology – 1*, p. 245. C. B. B. Downman (ed.). London: Butterworths

Coleridge, H. M., Coleridge, J. C. G. and Kidd, C. (1964). Cardiac receptors in the dog with particular reference to two types of afferent endings in the ventricular wall. *J. Physiol., Lond.* 174, 323–339

Coleridge, J. C. G., Hemingway, A., Holmes, R. L. and Linden, R. J. (1957). The location of atrial receptors in the dog: a physiological and histological study. *J. Physiol., Lond.* 136, 174–197

Constantin, L. (1963). Extracardiac factors contributing to hypotension during coronary occlusion. *Am. J. Cardiol.* 11, 205–217

Dawes, G. S. (1947). Receptor areas in the coronary arteries and elsewhere as revealed by the use of veratridine. *J. Pharmac. exp. Ther.* 89, 325–342

Dawes, G. S. and Comroe, J. H. (1954). Chemo-reflexes from the heart and lungs. *Physiol. Rev.* 34, 167–201

DeGeest, H., Levy, M. N., Zieske, H. and Lipman, R. I. (1965). Depression of ventricular contractility by stimulation of the vagus nerves. *Circulation Res.* 17, 222–235

Eckenhoff, J. E., Hafkenschiel, J. H., Landmesser, C. M. and Harmel, N. (1947). Cardiac oxygen metabolism and control of the coronary circulation. *Am. J. Physiol.* 149, 634–649

Feigl, E. O. (1967). Sympathetic control of the coronary circulation. *Circulation Res.* 20, 262–271

Fisher, V. J., Lee, R. J. and Kavaler, F. (1967). The heterogenous contractile performance of the left ventricle. In *Factors Influencing Myocardial Contractility*, p. 133. R. D. Tanz, F. Kavaler and J. Roberts (ed.). New York: Academic.Press

Furnival, C. M., Linden, R. J. and Snow, H. M. (1968). The response of the left ventricle to stimulation of the vagus nerves. *J. Physiol., Lond.* 198, 100–101P

Furnival, C. M., Linden, R. J. and Snow, H. M. (1971a). The inotropic and chronotropic effects of catecholamines on the dog heart. *J. Physiol., Lond.* 214, 15–28

Furnival, C. M., Linden, R. J. and Snow, H. M. (1971b). Reflex effects on the heart of stimulating left atrial receptors. *J. Physiol., Lond.* 218, 447–463

Gibbs, C. L., Mommaerts, W. F. H. M. and Ricchiuti, N. V. (1967). Energetics of cardiac contractions. *J. Physiol., Lond.* 191, 25–46

Gordon, A. M., Huxley, A. F. and Julian, F. J. (1966). The variation in isometric tension with sarcomere length in vertebrate muscle fibres. *J. Physiol., Lond.* 184, 170–192

Gregg, D. E. (1950). *Coronary Circulation in Health and Disease.* Philadelphia: Lea & Febiger

Gregg, D. E. and Fisher, L. C. (1963). Blood supply to the heart. In *Handbook of Physiology, Circulation,* sect. 2, Vol. II, pp. 1517–1584. W. F. Hamilton and F. Dow (ed.). Washington, DC: American Physiol. Soc.

Gregg, D. E., Khouri, E. M. and Kayford, C. R. (1965). Systemic and coronary energetics in the resting unanesthetized dog. *Circulation Res.* 16, 102–113

Griggs, D. M. Jr., Chen, C. C. and Tchokoev, V. V. (1973). Subendocardial anerobic metabolism in experimental aortic stenosis. *Am. J. Physiol.* 224, 607–612

Guyton, A. C. (1963). *Circulatory Physiology: cardiac output and its regulation.* Philadelphia: W. B. Saunders

Guyton, A. C. (1968). Regulation of cardiac output. *Anesthesiology* 29, 314–326

Hackett, J. G., Abboud, F. M., Mark, A. L., Schmid, P. G. and Heistad, D. D. (1972). Coronary vascular responses to stimulation of chemoreceptors and baroreceptors. *Circulation Res.* 31, 8–17

Hainsworth, R. and Karim, F. (1972). Inotropic responses of the left ventricle to changes in aortic arch pressure in anaesthetized dogs. *J. Physiol., Lond.* 223, 213–228

Holmes, R. L. (1957). Structures in the atrial endocardium of the dog which stain with methylene blue, and the effects of unilateral vagotomy. *J. Anat.* 91, 259–266

Jarisch, A. and Zotterman, Y. (1948). Depressor reflexes from the heart. *Acta physiol. scand.* 16, 31–51

Jewell, B. R. (1977). A re-examination of the influence of muscle length on myocardial performance. *Circulation Res.* 40, 221–230

Jewell, B. R. and Rovell, J. M. (1972). Load-dependent changes in the contractility of isolated cardiac muscle. *J. Physiol., Lond.* 224, 50–51P

Johnston, B. D. (1968). Nerve endings in the human endocardium. *Am. J. Anat.* 122, 621–630

Kappagoda, C. T., Linden, R. J. and Mary, D. A. S. G. (1977). Atrial receptors in the dog and rabbit. *J. Physiol., Lond.* 272, 799–815

Kappagoda, C. T., Linden, R. J. and Snow, H. M. (1972). A reflex increase in heart rate from distension of the junction between the superior vena cava and the right atrium. *J. Physiol., Lond.* 220, 177–197

Katz, A. M. (1977). *Physiology of the Heart.* New York: Raven Press

Kaufmann, R. L., Antoni, H., Hennekes, R., Jacob, R., Kohlhardt, M. and Lab, M. J. (1971). Mechanical response of the mammalian myocardium to modifications of the action potential. *Cardiovascular Res.* 5, Suppl. 1, 64–70

Kidd, C., Hainsworth, R. and Linden, R. J. (1979). *Cardiac Receptors.* Cambridge: Cambridge University Press

King, A. B. (1939). Nerve-endings in the cardiac muscle of the rat. *Bull. Johns Hopkins Hosp.* 65, 489–499

Kirk, E. S. and Honig, C. R. (1964). An experimental and theoretical analysis of myocardial tissue pressure. *Am. J. Physiol.* 207, 361–367

Klock, F. J., Kaiser, G. A., Ross, J. and Braunwald, E. (1965). An intrinsic adrenergic vasodilator mechanism in the coronary vascular bed of the dog. *Circulation Res.* 16, 376–382

Koletat, T., Asianio, G., Tallarida, R. J. and Oppenheimer, M. J. (1967). Action potentials in the sensory vagus at the time of coronary infarction. *Am. J. Physiol.* 213, 71–78

Langer, G. A. (1968). Ion fluxes in cardiac excitation and contraction and their relation to myocardial contractility. *Physiol. Rev.* 48, 708–757

Lawrence, M., Ledsome, J. R. and Mason, J. M. (1973). The time course of the diuretic response to left atrial distension. *Quart. J. exp. Physiol.* 58, 219–227

Ledsome, J. R. and Linden, R. J. (1964). A reflex increase in heart rate from distension of the pulmonary vein–atrial junctions. *J. Physiol., Lond.* 170, 456–473

Levy, M. N., Ng, M., Lipman, K. I. and Zieske, H. (1966). Vagus nerves and baroreceptor control of ventricular performance. *Circulation Res.* 18, 101–106

Linden, R. J. (1963). The control of the output of the heart. In *Recent Advances in Physiology,* p. 330. R. Creese (ed.). London: Churchill

Linden, R. J. (1965). The regulation of the output of the mammalian heart. *Scient. Basis Med. A. Rev.* pp. 164–185

Linden, R. J. (1973). Function of cardiac receptors. *Circulation* 48, 463–480

Linden, R. J. (1975). Reflexes from the heart. *Progr. cardiovasc. Dis.* 18, 201–221

Linden, R. J. and Snow, H. M. (1974). The inotropic state of the heart. In *Recent Advances in Physiology*, p. 148. R. J. Linden (ed.) London: Churchill Livingstone

Little, R. C. (1951). Effect of atrial systole on ventricular pressure and closure of the A-V values. *Am. J. Physiol.* 166, 289–295

Mason, J. M. and Ledsome, J. R. (1974). Effects of obstruction of the mitral orifice on distension of the pulmonary vein–atrial junction on renal and hind-limb vascular resistance in the dog. *Circulation Res.* 35, 24–32

Miller, M. R. and Kasahara, M. (1964). Studies of nerve endings in the heart. *Am. J. Anat.* 115, 217–223

Muers, M. F. and Sleight, P. (1972). The reflex cardiovascular depression caused by occlusion of the coronary sinus in the dog. *J. Physiol., Lond.* 221, 259–282

Noble, D. and Cohen, I. (1978). The interpretation of the T wave of the electrocardiogram. *Cardiovasc. Res.* 12, 13–27

Noble, M. I. M. (1978). The Frank–Starling curve. *Clin. Sci. molec. Med.* 54, 1–7

Nonidez, J. F. (1937). Identification of the receptor areas in the venae cavae and pulmonary veins which initiate reflex cardiac acceleration (Bainbridge's reflex). *Am. J. Anat.* 61, 203–223

Oberg, B. and Thoren, P. (1972). Studies on left ventricular receptors, signalling in non-medullated vagal afferents. *Acta physiol. scand.* 85, 145–163

Oberg, B. and Thoren, P. (1973). Circulatory responses to stimulation of left ventricular receptors in the cat. *Acta physiol. scand.* 88, 8–22

Paintal, A. S. (1953). A study of right and left atrial receptors. *J. Physiol., Lond.* 120, 596–610

Paintal, A. S. (1972). Cardiovascular receptors. In *Enteroreceptors Handbook of Sensory Physiology*, pp. 1–45. E. Neil (ed.). Berlin: Springer-Verlag

Paintal, A. S. (1973). Vagal sensory receptors and their reflex effects. *Physiol. Rev.* 53, 159–227

Parmley, W. W., Brutsaert, D. L. and Sonnenblick, E. H. (1969). Effects of altered loading on contractile events in isolated cat papillary muscle. *Circulation Res.* 24, 521–532

Rubio, R. and Berne, R. M. (1975). Regulation of coronary blood flow. *Progr. Cardiovasc. Dis.* 18, 105–122

Sarnoff, S. J., Gilmore, J. P., Brockman, S. K., Linden, R. J. and Mitchell, J. H. (1960a). Regulation of ventricular contraction: influence of cardiac sympathetic and vagal nerve stimulation on atrial and ventricular dynamics. *Circulation Res.* 8, 1108–1122

Sarnoff, S. J., Mitchell, J. H., Gilmore, J. P. and Remensnyder, J. P. (1960b). Homeometric autoregulation in the heart. *Circulation Res.* 8, 1077–1091

Scott, J. C. (1961). Myocardial coefficient of oxygen utilization. *Circulation Res.* 9, 906–910

Shepherd, J. T. (1973). Intrathoracic reflexes. *Mayo Clin. Proc.* 48, 426–437

Sleight, P. (1964). A cardiovascular depressor reflex from the epicardium of the left ventricle in the dog. *J. Physiol., Lond.* 173, 321–343

Sleight, P. (1979). Possible physiological stimuli for ventricular receptors and their significance in man. In *Cardiac Receptors*, pp. 241–258. R. Hainsworth, C. Kidd and R. J. Linden (ed.). Cambridge: Cambridge University Press

Sleight, P. and Widdicombe, J. G. (1965). Action potentials in fibres from receptors in the epicardium and myocardium of the dog's left ventricle. *J. Physiol., Lond.* 181, 235–258

Sleight, P., Lall, A. and Muers, M. (1969). Reflex cardiovascular effects of epicardial stimulation by acetylstrophinthidin in dogs. *Circulation Res.* 25, 705–711

Sonnenblick, E. H. (1962). Force–velocity relations in mammalian heart muscle. *Am. J. Physiol.* 202, 931–939

Sonnenblick, E. H. and Kirk, E. S. (1971). Effects of hypoxia and ischaemia on myocardial contraction. *Cardiology* 56, 302–313

Sonnenblick, E. H. and Parmley, W. W. (1967). Active state in heart muscle: force–velocity–length relations, and the variable onset and duration of maximum active state. In *Factors Influencing Myocardial Contractility*, p. 65. R. D. Tanz, F. Kavaler and J. Roberts (ed.). New York: Academic Press

Sonnenblick, E. H. and Ross, J. (1967). Some ultra structural considerations in myocardial failure: sarcomere over extension and length dispersion. In *Factors Influencing Myocardial Contractility*, p. 43. R. D. Tanz, F. Kavaler and J. Roberts (ed.). New York: Academic Press

Starling, E. H. (1918). *The Linacre Lecture on the Law of the Heart.* London: Longmans, Green

Thoren, P. (1972). Left ventricular receptors activated by severe asphyxia and by coronary occlusion. *Acta physiol. scand.* 85, 455–463

Wiggers, C. J. (1921). Studies on the consecutive phases of the cardiac cycle. II. The laws governing the relative durations of ventricular systole and diastole. *Am. J. Physiol.* 56, 439–459

Wiggers, C. J. (1952). Circulatory dynamics. In *Physiologic Studies.* New York: Grune & Stratton

Zuberbuhler, R. C. and Bohr, D. F. (1965). Responses of coronary smooth muscle to catecholamines. *Circulation Res.* 16, 431–440

32 Cardiac arrhythmias
E. B. Raftery

THE CARDIAC MUSCLE ACTION POTENTIAL

As with all contractile tissues, contraction of the individual myocardial cell is accompanied by measurable electrical activity. Since the heart is continually active, this creates a field of electrical force at the surface of the chest which is constantly waxing and waning. Any two electrodes placed in this field will register a potential difference which also waxes and wanes. This potential difference, when amplified, is the electrocardiogram.

The electrical events which accompany contraction in the individual cell can be recorded by means of electrodes placed on the surface and inside the cell. At rest there is a potential difference across the cell membrane of -70 to -90 mV, which is the result of an active metabolic process which pumps sodium ions from the cell. Potassium ions move into the cell passively in order to balance this effect. When the cell becomes active, the permeability of the membrane to sodium ions suddenly increases, the sodium pump ceases to be active and sodium ions move along the concentration gradient into the cell, producing a rapid and complete depolarization. The resting potential rises to zero with a small overshoot. This is followed by a plateau which lasts about 150 ms during which complex ionic fluxes, chiefly involving calcium ions, take place. The resting potential is then restored as potassium ions move along their concentration gradient out of the cell. At the end of this process, the sodium pump reactivates and restores the resting ionic balance (*Figure 32.1*). This sequence is the pattern for nearly all the myocardial cells, but certain cells, particularly the specialized conducting tissue of the sinoatrial (SA) and atrioventricular (AV) nodes, and the His–Purkinje system, have the property of automaticity. The resting cell potential constantly drifts upwards until it reaches a threshold level (usually about -60 mV) when the 'sodium pump' is inhibited and the active electrical and mechanical events of contraction are triggered off (*Figure 32.2*). It is

638

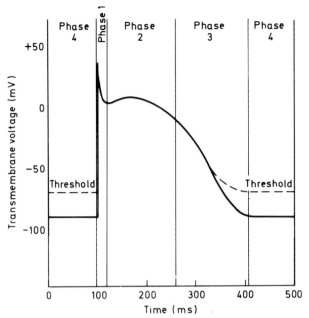

Figure 32.1
The electrical events of activation in a single cardiac muscle cell

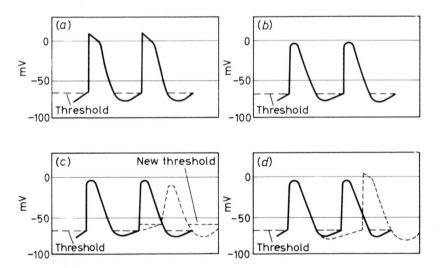

Figure 32.2
Action potentials from cardiac muscle cells with the property of
automaticity. (*a*) SA node cell. Note the continuous drift to threshold
which is the electrical basis for automaticity. (*b*) 'Working' myocardial
cell damaged by injury. Note the drifting resting potential which
represents a tendency to automaticity. (*c*) Group 1a drugs reduce
the rate of rise of the action potential and also raise the threshold
for inactivation of the sodium pump. The result is reduced automaticity. (*d*) Group 1b drugs produce the same effect by reducing
the rate at which drift takes place so that it takes longer to reach
threshold

important to realize that this threshold level can be raised or lowered by drugs or injury, and that automaticity in 'working' cells may be induced by these influences.

MECHANISMS OF ARRHYTHMIAS

Disorders of cardiac rhythm are seen in many different pathological disorders. However, the same arrhythmias are also often found in the absence of any detectable disease conditions, which suggests a single basic underlying mechanism which may be triggered by a wide variety of agents. It is still not possible to explain all arrhythmias by a single mechanism but the re-entry mechanism comes close to this idea.

The re-entry mechanism

This is best explained by consideration of the terminal Purkinje system. The terminal Purkinje cell divides into two radicals which communicate directly with a myocardial cell (*Figure 32.3*). Conduction down each radical takes place at the same speed; should something happen to slow or block conduction in one radical, the impulse reaches the myocardium by the remaining radical, and may spread from the myocardial cell to the damaged radical. It has been shown that in these circumstances retrograde conduction is common and the impulse may find the undamaged radical non-refractory and able to conduct the impulse back to the myocardial cell. In this way a self-perpetuating circus rhythm is set up. This mechanism is known to operate with macroscopic areas of damaged myocardium and parts of the His–Purkinje system, and re-entry has been clearly demonstrated to be the basic mechanism of supraventricular tachycardias, atrial flutter, ventricular tachycardia and types of ventricular ectopic beat.

Ectopic foci

Not all arrhythmias can be explained by re-entry. The mechanism of atrial fibrillation and random ventricular ectopic beats is almost certainly explained by areas of abnormal automaticity in damaged 'working' myocardial cells. In atrial fibrillation there are numerous such areas in the myocardium of the atria, bombarding the SA node with impulses. The traffic is such that many impulses die out in that complex structure, and penetration to the His bundle is irregular – hence the irregularity of the ventricular response. In random ectopic activity, areas of abnormal automaticity initiate conducted beats which interrupt the basic sinus rhythm in an irregular fashion.

Terminal Purkinje fibre system

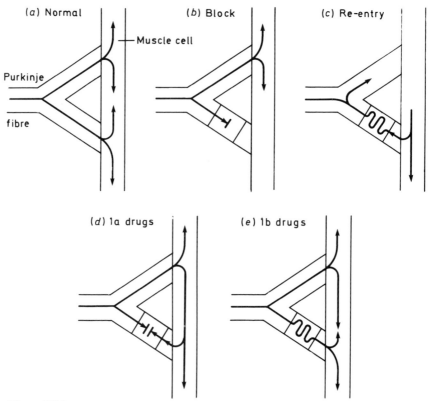

Figure 32.3
The mechanism of re-entry and the effects of drugs. (*a—c*) The way
in which a local circus rhythm can be established in single cells. The
same mechanism has been shown to be effective in large muscle
masses. (*d*) Group 1a drugs induce a bidirectional block and so
interrupt re-entry. (*e*) Group 1b drugs raise conductivity so that
antegrade conduction can take place and so interrupt re-entry

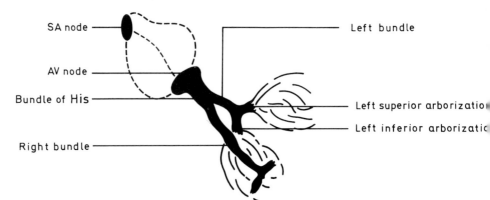

Figure 32.4
The specialized conducting tissue and the possible sites of heart
blocks

Heart block

The third major mechanism of arrhythmias is heart block. The normal sequence of myocardial contraction is depolarization spreading from the SA node across the atria to the AV node (*Figure 32.4*). Here there is a delay of a few milliseconds before the impulse spreads to the His bundle, and thence to the right and left bundles of specialized conduction tissue and to the Purkinje fibres, so reaching the myocardium. Interruption of this system at any point can give rise to one of the heart blocks considered below.

ANTIARRHYTHMIC DRUGS

The elucidation of the electrical events of the myocardial cell and the discovery of the re-entry mechanism have brought the classification of antiarrhythmic drugs within sight of a rational basis. They are now divided into four groups (Vaughan Williams, 1975): (1) membrane stabilizers; (2) β blockers; (3) drugs which increase the duration of the action potential; and (4) calcium antagonists.

1. Membrane stabilizers

These drugs reduce the rate of rise in phase I of the action potential, raise the threshold for activation and reduce the rate of resting potential drift (see *Figure 32.2*). There are two subgroups.

(a) Drugs in the first group convert unidirectional block in a damaged Purkinje cell into bidirectional block and so interrupt a re-entry mechanism. Examples: quinidine, procainamide (see *Figure 32.3*).
(b) Drugs in the second group reduce the level of block in a damaged Purkinje radical and thereby interrupt the re-entry mechanism. Examples: phenytoin, mexiletine, lignocaine (see *Figure 32.3*).

2. Beta blockers

Sympathetic activity increases cellular excitability by lowering the threshold, increasing the rate of resting potential drift and increasing automaticity. Beta-blocking drugs resist these effects by blocking the sympathetic transmitter (noradrenaline). Examples include propranolol, practolol and metoprolol.

3. Drugs which increase duration of the action potential

This effect prolongs the refractory period of the cell. Examples include disopyramide, amiodarone and bretylium.

4. Calcium antagonists

These drugs block the release of calcium from the sarcoplasmic reticulum and so make the cell less excitable. An example is verapamil.

This attempt to rationalize the classification and mode of action of these drugs has made it possible to select the appropriate agent in certain cases, but it must be admitted that, in practice, the selection of an anti-arrhythmic drug is still largely empirical.

SINUS RHYTHM

The normal configuration of the ECG complex with the normal limits of the time intervals is shown in *Figure 32.5*. The P-wave accompanies atrial systole and has two components due to right and left atrial depolarization. The P—R interval represents the conduction delay due to AV nodal delay and conduction down the His—Purkinje system to the myocardium. The QRS complex represents ventricular depolarization and contraction, while the ST segment and T-wave accompany repolarization. It should be noted that the QRS complex is metabolically passive and therefore closely reflects changes in electrical but not metabolic events. The ST segment and the T-wave involve expenditure of energy and are therefore more likely to reflect metabolic changes, whether local or systemic.

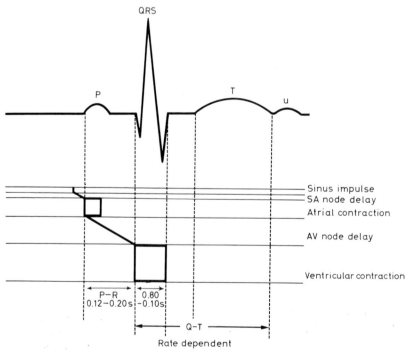

Figure 32.5
The normal configuration of the ECG complex

Sinus rhythm is under the control of the vagus (parasympathetic; inhibitory) and the sympathetic (stimulatory) nervous systems. Changes in the sinus rate are produced by changes in the balance of tone in the two systems. Slight variations in heart rate commonly occur in time with respiratory movements, and this normal variation in sinus rhythm is known as sinus arrhythmia (*Figure 32.6*).

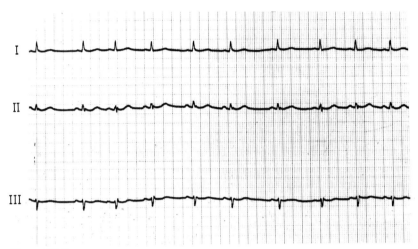

Figure 32.6
Sinus arrhythmia. Note the slowing of the sinus rate with inspiration

Sinus bradycardia is defined as sinus rhythm slower than 60 per minute. It commonly occurs in athletic individuals, and rarely has any pathological significance. However, slow heart rates are sometimes seen in conditions of low metabolic rate such as hypothyroidism and hypothermia. Under otherwise normal circumstances, rates of less than 40 per minute result in reduction of cardiac output.

Sinus tachycardia is defined as a resting sinus rhythm faster than 100 per minute. This is commonly due to sympathetic overactivity, and may be a sign of anxiety, thyrotoxicosis or incipient left ventricular failure. Rates in excess of 140 per minute will usually cause mechanical interference with maintenance of cardiac output.

Neither bradycardia nor tachycardia is necessarily disadvantageous to the individual, and treatment is not indicated unless there is a clear-cut underlying pathology or the heart rate is interfering with the maintenance of the cardiac output.

ECTOPIC RHYTHMS

There are three basic forms of ectopic activity.

(1) *Escape rhythms* — all cardiac cells have the potential for automaticity, but at a slower rate than the SA node. Should this normal pacemaker

default, a subsidiary pacemaker may make its appearance. An escape beat is always late and an escape rhythm is slower than the sinus rhythm.

(2) *Parasystolic rhythms* — if a subsidiary pacemaker develops the property of 'protection' (i.e. it is not discharged by the sinus beat) it may develop its own, slightly slower, rhythm in competition with the sinus pacemaker.

(3) *Extrasystolic rhythms* — intermittent activation of a re-entry pathway leads to premature beats with a close temporal link to the preceding sinus beat. Secondary foci or abnormal automaticity may also appear in the atria or ventricles, and may fire quite independently of the sinus node. This is the mechanism of ventricular ectopic beats.

Escape and parasystolic rhythms and supraventricular ectopics have little pathological significance and will not be considered further. Ventricular ectopic beats (*Figure 32.7*) may occur in normal individuals, as a result of excess tea, coffee or tobacco, certain drugs such as digitalis,

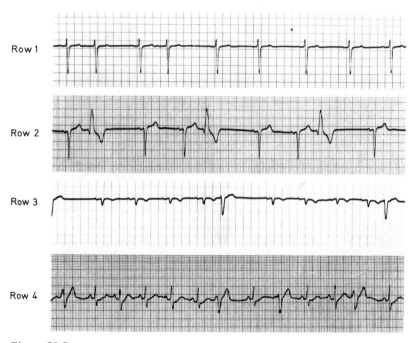

Figure 32.7
Row 1. Supraventricular ectopic beats. The QRS complex usually has the same shape as the sinus beat, but sometimes aberrant ventricular conduction alters the QRS shape. In these circumstances, the presence of an inverted P-wave strongly suggests that the beat is supraventricular. *Rows 2 and 3.* Ventricular ectopic beats originating in the right ventricle have the pattern of LBBB in lead V_1 (row 3); those originating in the left ventricle have the pattern of RBBB in lead V_1 (row 2). Re-entrant beats have a fixed temporal relationship with the preceding sinus beat. *Row 4.* Random ventricular ectopic beats have no fixed temporal relationship to the sinus beats and are thought to indicate a poor prognosis

myocarditis or ischaemic heart disease. In the last context, ectopic beats without a re-entry mechanism and arising from the left ventricle, are thought to be harbingers of more serious arrhythmias.

Treatment of these ectopic rhythms is the removal of the cause or, if this is not possible, then suppression with drugs. Ventricular ectopic beats may be very successfully suppressed with lignocaine (50 mg i.v.), as a bolus which may be followed by continuous intravenous administration of $1-3$ mg·min^{-1} of mexiletine (100 mg t.i.d. orally) or by disopyramide (100 mg t.i.d.). However, suppressive therapy is indicated only if there is clear evidence of serious underlying disease (e.g. ischaemic heart disease) which may predispose to more serious arrhythmias. Beta-blocking drugs have been shown to be very effective in suppressing ventricular ectopic beats arising during anaesthesia (Hellewell and Potts, 1965) but lignocaine is still the safest and most effective agent in this situation.

SUPRAVENTRICULAR TACHYARRHYTHMIAS (*Figure 32.8*)

1. Junctional tachycardias

This term is applied to extrasystolic tachycardias which may arise from single or multiple foci anywhere in the atrial or the AV node. These

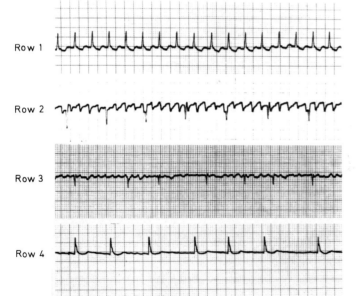

Figure 32.8
Row 1. Junctional tachycardias are characterized by abnormally shaped P-waves and complete regularity. *Row 2.* In atrial flutter the baseline is distorted by coarse 'sawtooth' waves, second degree heart block and a regular ventricular response. *Rows 3 and 4.* In atrial fibrillation the ventricular response is irregularly irregular and there is variation in QRS voltage. The baseline is distorted by chaotic f-waves which may be fine or coarse, but are best seen in leads V_1 and V_2

rhythms are essentially re-entrant in mechanism and can be found in healthy individuals, in association with established atrial fibrillation from any cause, after myocardial infarction and in digitalis toxicity, when there is commonly a degree of AV block. The heart rate is usually in excess of 160 beats per minute and these rhythms are generally very regular. This feature can be very important in making the distinction between ventricular tachycardia and junctional tachycardia with bundle branch block.

These rhythms are generally self-limiting, but prolonged attacks can usually be terminated by a variety of measures such as the Valsalva manoeuvre and eyeball compression, designed to increase vagal para-sympathetic tone. Digoxin 0.25 mg by mouth or intravenously will often terminate a resistant episode, but the β-blocking drugs (practolol 20 mg) intravenously are the treatment of choice for resistant tachycardias. Verapamil and phenytoin intravenously are often useful, but it is rarely necessary to employ them. Cholinergic drugs such as metacholine were once widely used but are now obsolete. It is sometimes necessary to use a direct current (d.c.) shock to restore sinus rhythm (see later).

2. Atrial flutter

In this rhythm the atria contract at about 300 beats per minute and the P-waves of the ECG are wide and bizarre, resulting in a 'sawtooth' appearance. There is usually an associated second degree AV block, with an even-numbered conduction ratio such as 2:1 or 4:1 and a regular ventricular rate. Odd-numbered conduction ratios are usually inconstant and result in an irregular ventricular response. This arrhythmia is commonly associated with atrial fibrillation and has the same causes.

The treatment of choice for a serious bout with rapid ventricular response is cardioversion with a d.c. shock, but otherwise digoxin is preferred. This drug increases the atrial rate until atrial fibrillation super-venes. When this happens and the drug is stopped, the heart commonly reverts to sinus rhythm for unknown reasons. Quinidine is sometimes used to slow the atrial rate, but when this is done it is essential to digitalize the patient beforehand in order to increase the degree of AV block and avoid the danger of an increased ventricular rate as the atrial rate slows.

3. Atrial fibrillation

Numerous ectopic foci throughout the atria bombard the AV node with impulses and produce varying second-degree block so that the ventricular rate is irregular. There is no organized atrial contraction, and the ECG baseline is distorted by bizarre and irregular waves (fibrillation or f-waves). This arrhythmia is quite common, and is found in association with rheumatic mitral valve disease, thyrotoxicosis, ischaemic heart disease, hypertension and cardiomyopathies. The arrhythmia is often paroxysmal, and there is frequently no apparent cause. The absence of co-ordinated atrial con-traction is important only when ventricular contractility is impaired, and the main haemodynamic disadvantage of this arrhythmia is seen when the ventricular rate is very rapid. The principal objective of treatment is not to restore sinus rhythm, which may be very difficult, but to control the ventricular response rate by depressing AV conduction and increasing the degree of block. In some patients, particularly those with thyrotoxicosis, digitalis alone may not be enough to control the ventricular response; in these cases the addition of a small dose of β blocker (e.g. propranolol 20 mg t.i.d.) is often effective. There is some danger of atrial thrombi and embolization with this arrhythmia, and some physicians use anticoagulants as prophylaxis against this. Attempts to restore sinus rhythm by d.c. conversion were very popular at one time, but are rarely successful for long periods of time.

VENTRICULAR TACHYARRHYTHMIAS (*Figure 32.9*)

1. Ventricular tachycardia

A series of three or more consecutive ventricular extrasystoles constitutes ventricular tachycardia. The rate is usually in excess of 160 per minute

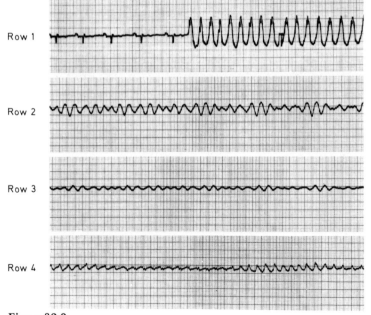

Figure 32.9
Row 1. Ventricular tachycardia is characterized by rapid wide beats which are usually slightly irregular. The artefact in the centre of this tracing is due to stopping of the ECG machine. *Rows 2 and 3.* Ventricular fibrillation is characterized by chaotic disorganized waves which may be coarse or fine. The finer the tracing, the more difficult it is to restore sinus rhythm. *Row 4.* Ventricular flutter: alternating bouts of coarse and fine, wide and disorganized beats

and the spacing of the beats is usually slightly irregular. The duration of each QRS complex is in excess of 0.12 second, with secondary ST and T changes of opposite polarity. Retrograde P-waves may sometimes be apparent.

Ventricular tachycardia is commonly associated with ischaemic heart disease, particularly acute infarction, and sometimes with hypertension and aortic valve disease. It is doubtful if it ever occurs in health. It is a dangerous arrhythmia because it is always accompanied by a profound fall in blood pressure and cardiac output, and is a common harbinger of ventricular fibrillation.

Prolonged episodes must be terminated as rapidly as possible by means of d.c. conversion or intravenous lignocaine (slow infusion up to a maximum of 800 mg) if conversion is not available or is impracticable. Lignocaine is usually effective, and the arrhythmia may then be prevented by means of a slow infusion (1.5 mg·min^{-1}) or by oral mexiletine (100 mg q.d.). Intravenous procainamide (250 mg) may be necessary but must not be given without ECG control so that the signs of overdosage (widening of the QRS) may be readily detected and the infusion stopped. Beta-blocking drugs are seldom effective (except in the instance of digitalis-induced ventricular tachycardia) and other drugs such as phenytoin and bretylium are sometimes used in very resistant cases.

2. Ventricular flutter

This is a rapid ventricular arrhythmia with very wide QRS complexes blending with wide T-waves to produce an effect like a sine wave. A variant with a continually recurring change of axis through 180° is referred to as 'torsades de point'. This is a terminal arrhythmia which can also be induced by a variety of drugs such as quinidine and chloroform.

3. Ventricular fibrillation

Multiple ventricular foci of pacemaker activity lead to a chaotic inco-ordinated activity which is inconsistent with life. The treatment is d.c. conversion and stabilization of the heart with intravenous lignocaine.

D.C. conversion

This method of dealing with tachyarrhythmias is commonly employed and many different types of defibrillator are available. For emergency situations such as ventricular fibrillation, the full power of the machine (usually 400 J) should be delivered with the first shock. For elective conversion, light anaesthesia with methohexitone or intravenous diazepam should be used and the smallest shock available (10 J) should be administered with a synchronizer to ensure that it is not placed any later than

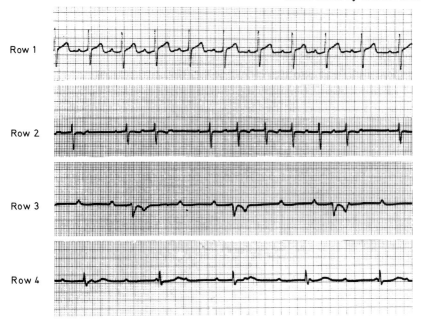

Figure 32.10
The heart blocks. *Row 1.* First degree (PR greater than 0.20 s).
Row 2. Mobitz type I (Wenckebach phenomenon); the P—R interval
increases in length with each beat until a beat is dropped. *Row 3.*
Mobitz type II (3:1 heart block). *Row 4.* Third degree (complete)
heart block calls for pacemaker insertion. Mobitz type II and third
degree block call for pacemaker insertion.

40 ms from the R-wave to avoid the danger of precipitating ventricular
fibrillation. Successive shocks up to 300 J may be necessary to effect
reversion to sinus rhythm. Elective reversion is best avoided if the patient
has had digitalis preparations, since this may precipitate ventricular
tachycardia and fibrillation.

DISTURBANCES OF CONDUCTION (see *Figure 32.4*)

1. Atrioventricular block

When a defect occurs in the specialized conduction tissue between the
atria and ventricles, AV block results (*Figure 32.10*). There are three types.

FIRST DEGREE

Here there is prolongation of the P—R interval beyond 0.20 second.

SECOND DEGREE

In this type there is intermittent interruption of conduction through the
AV node with dropped beats when P-waves are not followed by QRS
complexes. There are two types:

(1) *Mobitz I:* there is a progressive increase in the P–R interval with each beat until conduction fails and a beat is dropped (Wenckebach phenomenon). The sequence is then repeated.
(2) *Mobitz II:* there is a constant P–R interval in the beats before and after each dropped beat. This type has more serious implications than Mobitz type I.

THIRD DEGREE

Here none of the atrial beats is conducted, and the ventricles are paced by an ectopic pacemaker, usually in the bundle of His. The result is a slow heart rate which may place the patient in danger of standstill (Stokes–Adams attacks).

The commonest causes of AV block are idiopathic degeneration of the conducting system (Lanegre's disease) and ischaemic heart disease. Sclerotic processes from neighbouring structures (Levi's disease) and trauma are rarer causes.

2. Sinoatrial block

Disturbances of conduction from the sinoatrial pacemaker to the atrium can only be inferred from subsequent disturbance of P-waves. First, second and third degree block are recognizable but have little clinical significance. An important variety of this arrhythmia is sinoatrial disease, a condition commonly seen in elderly persons who exhibit sinoatrial block and suffer bouts of fast and slow arrhythmias of many types. These patients may be very symptomatic and often require pacemaker insertion.

3. Bundle branch block and the hemiblocks

Although not strictly arrhythmias, these conduction disturbances are so closely related that they are commonly included. The bundle of His divides into radicles on either side of interventricular septum — the right and left bundles. The right bundle is very long and does not divide until it reaches the apex of the right ventricle (see *Figure 32.4*). Here it rapidly disperses into a terminal Purkinje arborization. The left bundle is very short and rapidly breaks up into two wide bands — the superior and inferior arborizations — which sweep across the upper and lower surfaces of the left ventricle. Right bundle branch block produces a characteristic prolongation of the QRS beyond 0.12 s and a large secondary R-wave in V_1 due to late depolarization of the right ventricle (*Figure 32.11*). Left bundle branch block produces similar prolongation of the QRS interval with a characteristic, but less striking, secondary R-wave in lead V_6. A block placed in the superior left radicle shifts the electrical axis of the ECG to the left ($-30°$ or more = left axis deviation) while a block in the inferior arborization produces a shift to the right ($+90°$ or more = right axis deviation). These are referred to as the hemiblocks.

It is evident that complete heart block can be produced by a lesion in the bundle of His (the common situation) or by a combination of right and left bundle branch block, or by right bundle branch block and superior and inferior arborization block. These possibilities have little practical significance, but some combinations of minor blocks have serious prognostic implications. The combination of first degree heart block and left bundle branch block (*Figure 32.11*) is known to progress suddenly and unpredictably to complete heart block; the same is true for right bundle branch block and left superior hemiblock (causing left axis deviation, see *Figure 32.11*) and bilateral bundle branch block (alternating right and left bundle branch block). The combination of right bundle branch block and left inferior hemiblock does not appear to have the same dangers, while an isolated bundle branch block or hemiblock does not indicate impending serious arrhythmias.

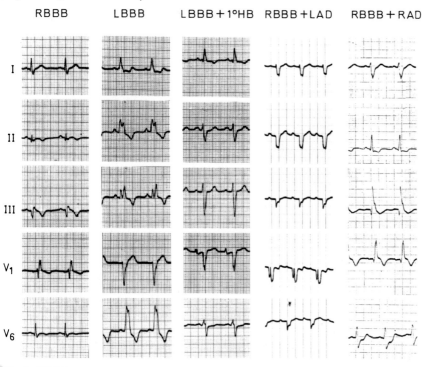

Figure 32.11
Conduction blocks and hemiblocks. The combinations of first degree heart block with bundle branch block and right bundle branch block with left axis deviation both suggest impending third degree heart block and call for pacemaker insertion

No specific treatment is indicated for the minor blocks. For complete heart block, if there are syncopal attacks or congestive heart failure, pacemaker insertion is the treatment of choice. Sympathomimetic drugs such as ephedrine or isoprenaline seldom do more than induce ventricular arrhythmias and are not to be recommended. Prophylaxis of the dangerous minor block combinations is widely practised in the USA, but not in

Britain. There is certainly a strong case for temporary pacemaker insertion in situations when complete heart block may be precipitated; for example, surgical procedures requiring general anaesthesia.

Modern pacemakers do not present undue difficulty for the anaesthetist. Some anaesthetic agents are reported to raise the threshold for cardiac stimulation, but the power output of modern units makes this a negligible problem. Interference from other electrical equipment is unlikely since pacemakers are well shielded, but diathermy, if used close to the unit, may be a problem. Interference produces a switch to a higher pacing mode rather than complete failure, so even diathermy is unlikely to produce unmanageable difficulties.

Pre-excitation (*Figure 32.12*)

There are two electrocardiographic syndromes which indicate the presence of an anatomical system which bypasses the AV node and allows the pacemaker impulse to reach the ventricles prematurely. These bypasses can conduct retrograde and antegrade, and the individual is subject to

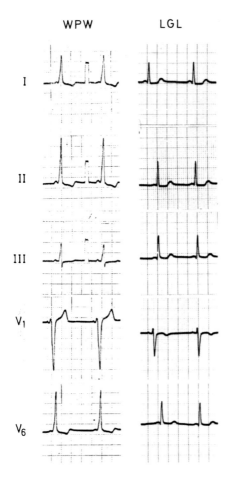

Figure 32.12
The Wolff–Parkinson–White (WPW) syndrome is characterized by a short P–R interval and a δ-wave between the P and the R. The Lown–Ganong–Levine (LGL) syndrome is characterized by a short P–R interval but no δ-wave

bouts of supraventricular tachycardia because of an inherent predisposition to re-entry. These are the Wolff—Parkinson—White syndrome, characterized by a δ-wave which interposes between the P-wave and the QRS, and the Lown—Ganong—Levine syndrome where the P—R interval is short, but there is no δ-wave. In these conditions, tachycardia can be readily controlled with disopyramide or verapamil, except in very rare cases where persistent tachycardias may require surgical division of the bypass band.

ARRHYTHMIAS AND THE ANAESTHETIST

There are three situations in which the anaesthetist may be concerned by disturbances of heart rhythm: preoperative, peroperative and postoperative.

Preoperative

A substantial proportion of patients have a rhythm disturbance which may or may not have been previously detected and treated. A preoperative ECG is essential if errors of judgement are to be avoided, and any patient with a suspicion of rhythm disturbance should be monitored throughout the operation and the postoperative period. If the arrhythmia is adequately controlled preoperatively, then no other special precautions are necessary; if not, then control must be established before the operation, provided always that there is time.

Peroperative (see review by Katz and Bigger, 1970)

AETIOLOGY

Arrhythmias commonly occur during anaesthesia, and are the result of interaction between many factors. These include certain types of mechanical stimulation, the pharmacological effects of anaesthetic agents, the use of agents such as suxamethonium, abnormal levels of electrolytes and a complex interaction of hypoxia, hypercapnia and circulating levels of catecholamines, the significance of which varies with different anaesthetic agents.

Certain operative procedures are more likely to provoke arrhythmias than others, and particular care is necessary during upper abdominal and thoracic surgery. Difficulties may also arise during ophthalmic surgery with pressure on the eyeball and traction on the extraocular muscles (see Chapter 63). Endotracheal intubation is perhaps the commonest cause of arrhythmias during anaesthesia and it is frequently associated with transient hypertension. Fortunately, the arrhythmias normally disappear rapidly when the tube is in place and, as a general rule, there is no need for treatment or prophylaxis with antiarrhythmic drugs.

Anaesthetics vary widely in their propensity to produce arrhythmias in the absence of other causes. Ethyl chloride and chloroform had a bad reputation while diethyl ether was considered safe in this respect. Halothane is intermediate. Suxamethonium and neostigmine can both produce severe bradycardia if the patient is not protected with atropine. In addition, suxamethonium may reduce the electrical threshold and sensitize the myocardium, producing ventricular arrhythmias during halothane anaesthesia. A contributory factor with suxamethonium may be the increase in plasma potassium concentration but both hyper- and hypokalaemia may cause a wide range of abnormalities of heart rhythm.

It is known that hypoxia, hypercapnia, increased catecholamine levels and certain anaesthetics can independently cause arrhythmias. However, hypoxia and hypercapnia as well as certain anaesthetics (particularly cyclopropane and diethyl ether) also raise the level of circulating catecholamines. The interactions are further complicated by the fact that a number of anaesthetics (particularly cyclopropane and the halogenated hydrocarbons) increase the sensitivity of the heart to circulating catecholamines. Hypercapnia in the presence of cyclopropane or halothane causes arrhythmias when the plasma catecholamine concentration is still below the level at which it will cause arrhythmias in the presence of a normal $P\text{CO}_2$ and there appear to be predictable $P\text{CO}_2$ thresholds at which arrhythmias first appear with these agents (see Chapter 22). A common problem is the use of exogenous catecholamines, such as adrenaline infiltration to reduce surgical bleeding. Doses of 100 μg (preferably in a dilution of at least 1:100 000) are considered safe during anaesthesia with halothane, trichloroethylene and methoxyflurane (references cited by Katz and Bigger, 1970). It should be remembered that tricyclic antidepressants greatly increase the circulating levels of endogenous catecholamines (Annotation, 1971).

TYPES OF ARRHYTHMIAS

Almost every type of arrhythmia has been reported during anaesthesia, in addition to sinus tachycardia and bradycardia. Common abnormalities include nodal rhythm, atrial and ventricular extrasystoles, and pulsus alternans. Less common are multifocal ventricular extrasystoles, pulsus bigeminus and atrial fibrillation. Heart block, ventricular tachycardia and fibrillation are fortunately rare.

INCIDENCE

In a large series of patients reported by Vanik and Davis (1968) new arrhythmias were observed during halothane anaesthesia in 16% of patients with no known preoperative heart disease, in 27% with known preoperative arrhythmias and in 34% with known preoperative heart disease but no arrhythmias. Most arrhythmias occurred during induction, and particularly during intubation, but the vast majority were benign and only 0.9% of arrhythmias detected by serial monitoring could be considered to be serious. Regional analgesia was found to be as likely as general anaesthesia to provoke arrhythmias.

TREATMENT

Most arrhythmias which are observed during anaesthesia do not require treatment. Supraventricular tachycardia may be controlled with β-receptor blockers and this may be necessary if the heart rate exceeds 140 per minute. Bradycardia below 40 per minute is best treated with atropine. Persistent and frequent ventricular extrasystoles (particularly multifocal) usually respond to β-receptor blocks but lignocaine (50 mg i.v. as a bolus) remains the safest and most effective drug for ventricular arrhythmias, while digoxin (to reduce the ventricular rate) is still the drug of choice for supraventricular arrhythmias. An intravenous pacemaker will be required in the event of complete heart block and a defibrillator must be kept available for emergency treatment of ventricular tachycardia or fibrillation. If there is a predisposing condition, such as known ischaemic heart disease, then operative ECG monitoring is mandatory. Insertion of a temporary pacemaker in the presence of a dangerous combination of minor blocks is wise.

Postoperative

Again, particular care must be taken in patients who have a predisposing condition, and careful monitoring in a suitable unit for 24 hours is essential.

It is said that patients rarely die because of arrhythmias induced during surgery, and this is undoubtedly true. However, arrhythmia control is so readily available that there is no reason why anyone should die from such a cause. Furthermore, there can be no reasonable doubt that maintenance of sinus rhythm and avoidance of arrhythmias make for less morbidity and more rapid recovery from a surgical procedure.

References

Annotation (1971). Cardiovascular complications from psychotropic drugs. *Br. med. J.* 1, 3

Hellewell, J. and Potts, M. W. (1965). Propranolol and ventricular arrhythmias with halothane. *Anaesthesia* 20, 269–274

Katz, R. L. and Bigger, J. T. (1970). Cardiac arrhythmias during anesthesia and operation. *Anesthesiology* 33, 193–213

Vanik, P. E. and Davis, H. S. (1968). Cardiac arrhythmias during halothane anesthesia. *Anesth. Analg. curr. Res.* 47, 299–307

Vaughan Williams, E. M. (1975). Classification of anti-dysrhythmic drugs. *Pharmac. Ther. B* 1, 115–138

Further reading

Bigger, J. T. Jr. (1973). Electrical properties of cardiac muscle and possible causes of cardiac arrhythmias. In *Cardiac Arrhythmias,* pp. 11–23. Hahnemann Symposia 25. L. S. Dreifus and W. Likoff (ed.). New York: Grune & Stratton

Stock, J. P. P. and Williams, D. O. (1974). *Diagnosis and Treatment of Cardiac Arrhythmias,* 3rd edn. London: Butterworths

Wit, A. L., Cranefield, P. F. and Hoffman, B. F. (1972). Slow conduction and re-entry in the ventricular conducting system. II. Single and sustained circus movement in networks of canine and bovine Purkinje fibers. *Circulation Res.* 30, 11–22

33 Cerebral blood flow

D. G. McDowall

APPLIED PHYSIOLOGY OF THE CEREBRAL CIRCULATION

This review of the applied physiology of the cerebral circulation begins with a description of the main factors which affect the cerebral blood flow (CBF) and then proceeds to consider the mechanisms by which CBF is controlled.

Effects of changes in blood pressure, cerebral venous pressure and cerebrospinal fluid pressure on cerebral blood flow

BLOOD PRESSURE

If the blood pressure is reduced rapidly, then CBF shows a proportionate acute fall. However, if the blood pressure is held at the new lowered value, CBF increases over the following 30–120 seconds. This phenomenon — the return of CBF to normal despite a lowering of blood pressure — is termed autoregulation. If blood pressure is only slowly reduced, then no change in CBF is seen until quite severe degrees of hypotension are reached. *Figure 33.1* is from the work of Fitch *et al.* (1976) and demonstrates the phenomenon of autoregulation in the baboon, an animal whose normal blood pressure is similar to that of man. It will be seen from this figure that mean blood pressure can be reduced to about 60% of its normal value (i.e. to a mean blood pressure of 7.3 kPa; 55 mmHg) before there is any appreciable fall in CBF. In man, the mean blood pressure below which CBF begins to fall has been put at 8 kPa (60 mmHg). Obviously, to achieve this CBF maintenance in the face of a falling blood pressure, the cerebral arterioles must relax and so lower the cerebrovascular resistance. When the lower limit of autoregulation is reached (i.e. at about 8 kPa (60 mmHg) mean blood pressure) it is envisaged that the cerebral arterioles are maximally dilated and can adjust no more.

The mechanism which produces the vascular dilatation in response to hypotension is not known but, from the facts given above, it is clear that it is one which takes between 30 and 120 seconds to act. There are two main hypotheses. The first states that the dilatation is due to the myogenic reflex; i.e. relaxation of muscular tone in an arteriole when the intravascular distending pressure is lowered. This is an intrinsic response of vascular smooth muscle to stretch and, since it is a response of *smooth muscle*, it is slow enough in action to fit into the observed time scale of

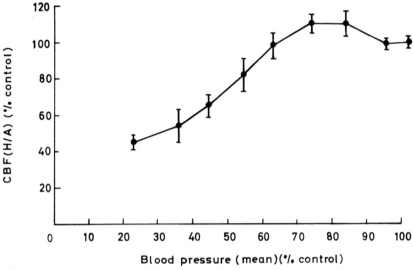

Figure 33.1
Autoregulation of cerebral blood flow in response to decreasing blood pressure by controlled haemorrhage in the baboon (mean ± standard error). (From Fitch *et al.*, 1976, by courtesy of the authors and the Editors of *Journal of Neurology, Neurosurgery and Psychiatry*)

autoregulation. The other hypothesis is the metabolic one which postulates that when CBF initially falls, due to blood pressure reduction, CO_2 accumulates in the cerebral tissue and this metabolically produced CO_2 dilates the cerebral arterioles, leading to a secondary adjustment of CBF to normal. This explanation would also fit into the observed time scale.

The response of the cerebral vasculature to reduction in blood pressure, however, varies with the method used to lower the pressure. If hypotension is produced by drugs such as trimetaphan, halothane or sodium nitroprusside, CBF is maintained at normal values to lower levels of blood pressure than is the case with haemorrhage (Fitch *et al.*, 1976). Indeed, amongst the hypotensive drugs themselves, there are differences in the effectiveness of autoregulation and, in particular, CBF is maintained to very low blood pressures during sodium nitroprusside hypotension; for example, at a mean pressure of 4.4–4.7 kPa (33–35 mmHg) in the cat, CBF did not differ significantly from the normotensive value (Maekawa, McDowall and Okuda, 1977; Michenfelder and Theye, 1977). These observations indicate that the mechanism of autoregulation cannot be as simple as the two classical theories would require. It has been suggested that the better maintained CBF during drug-induced as compared with haemorrhagic hypotension, is the result of increased sympathetic activity which accompanies bleeding, but which is not seen with hypotension due to ganglionic blockade (Fitch *et al.*, 1976). Sympathetic activity can produce some vasoconstriction (see below), particularly when the cerebro-vascular bed is widely dilated as it is during hypotension. This explanation would state that the sympathetic nervous system reduces the effectiveness of autoregulation in response to haemorrhage but does not affect the autoregulation to drug-induced hypotension.

Autoregulation includes not only the response to hypotension, but also the response to hypertension. Increases in blood pressure do not, except during the first 30–120 seconds, increase CBF, for the cerebral arterioles constrict to hold CBF constant. If the blood pressure is increased to very high levels, then eventually CBF increases. The blood pressure at which CBF breaks through the autoregulation mechanism in normal man is at a mean blood pressure of 130 mmHg. In patients with chronic hypertension, both the upper and the lower points on the autoregulation curve are elevated, due to hypertrophy of the smooth muscle of the arterioles, so that CBF begins to fall with hypotension and to rise with hypertension at higher levels of blood pressure than in normal man (Lassen and Christensen, 1976). In other words, the autoregulation sigmoid curve is shifted to the right in chronic hypertension.

Autoregulation is a feature of normal brain and it is a mechanism which is readily disturbed in abnormal situations. For example, loss of auto-regulation is seen during extreme hypercapnia or hypoxia, and also following extreme hypotension. The importance of a loss of autoregulation is, in part, that CBF falls with even a small reduction in blood pressure, but also that cerebral oedema may occur if the blood pressure increases, since the capillary bed is no longer protected by autoregulation against the transmission of high transmural pressure gradients.

VENOUS AND CEREBROSPINAL FLUID PRESSURES

The perfusion pressure of the brain, like that of any other organ, is not simply the mean arterial blood pressure, but is the arterial–venous pressure difference.

The venous pressure falls progressively as one passes downstream through the venous sinus system, until at the jugular bulb the pressure is only slightly above atmospheric pressure. This relationship to atmos-pheric pressure is established because in the supine, head-up or erect positions, the internal jugular veins are exposed to the atmospheric pressure in the neck. In the head-down position, however, the jugular veins become distended and the pressure on the jugular bulb is then related to the intrathoracic venous pressure and to the hydrostatic pressure of blood between the right atrium and the jugular bulb. In supine and head-up positions, transmission of intrathoracic pressure to the brain also occurs if blood is dammed back and distends the jugular veins, as in coughing, straining and in badly applied positive pressure ventilation.

If the cerebral venous pressure is elevated in any of these ways, the cerebral perfusion pressure is thereby reduced. The venous pressures achieved in coughing and straining can be very high and can lead to significant reductions in cerebral perfusion pressure which, fortunately, are usually short in duration. Elevations in cerebral venous pressure due, for example, to a tight expiratory valve during anaesthesia are more important because they are long-lasting and because the arterial blood pressure is also likely to be low.

Do increases in cerebral venous pressure reduce CBF? They must do so when the elevation in venous pressure is sufficient to reduce cerebral perfusion pressure below the lower autoregulatory limit. Lesser increases in cerebral venous pressure are compensated for by the mechanism of autoregulation in the same way as are falls in arterial blood pressure. Indeed, Jacobson, Harper and McDowall (1963) showed that moderate increases in cerebral venous pressure, up to 3 kPa (30 cmH$_2$O), are associated with increased CBF. Strange though this may at first seem, similar findings have been reported from physical studies of flow through collapsible tubing (Rodbard, 1955). This paradoxical increase in flow with increased outflow resistance is due to increased distension of the venous channels and to inhibition of the recurrent collapsibility of the thin-walled veins.

The effect of cerebrospinal fluid pressure on CBF is obviously an important one because of the increases in cerebrospinal fluid (CSF) pressure which occur with cerebral tumours and with subarachnoid haemorrhage and following cerebral trauma and ischaemia. Moderate elevations in CSF pressure (that is, those which leave cerebral perfusion pressure above the lower limit of autoregulation) are compensated for by relaxation of the cerebral arterioles, and therefore there is no change in CBF. Once CSF pressure increases sufficiently to lower cerebral perfusion pressure below the autoregulatory limits, then CBF falls progressively. In this regard, Kety, Shenkin and Schmidt (1948) showed that CBF was normal until CSF pressure exceeded 4.5 kPa (45 cmH$_2$O). When CSF pressure equals the arterial pressure, CBF must be zero and brain death becomes inevitable.

Effects of changes in blood gas tensions and blood pH on CBF

CARBON DIOXIDE

Elevating the arterial P_{CO_2} increases CBF, and lowering arterial P_{CO_2} reduces it. This relationship has been precisely delineated in the dog (Harper, 1965) and monkey (Reivich, 1964), and there is good evidence that the human circulation has a very similar flow—Pa_{CO_2} response to that of the monkey. The sensitivity of the cerebral vessels to Pa_{CO_2} is very great and equals about a 4% change in CBF for every 0.13 kPa (1 mmHg) change in Pa_{CO_2} in the range 4—8 kPa (30—60 mmHg) and the response is very rapid, being almost as quick as the initiating change in Pa_{CO_2} (Severinghaus and Lassen, 1967). At very high P_{CO_2} values flow sensitivity falls off, probably because the cerebral arterioles have reached a state of maximum dilatation. This occurs at values of Pa_{CO_2} in excess of 20 kPa (150 mmHg), when CBF is approximately two and one-half times normal.

At the other end of the scale, sensitivity to lowering of Pa_{CO_2} also falls off at very low levels of the latter. CBF reaches minimal values of about 45% of normal at Pa_{CO_2} of 2 kPa (15 mmHg) and further reductions have little effect. The basis of this limitation of hypocapnic vasoconstriction may be that the reduced CBF has produced a degree of tissue hypoxia which counteracts any further vasoconstriction. Supporting this view is the finding that the administration of hyperbaric oxygen allows CBF to fall even further with extreme hypocapnia (Reivich *et al.*, 1968). The question of the adequacy of cerebral perfusion during extreme hyperventilation is clearly a very important one to the anaesthetist, and this is discussed in detail in Chapter 23.

It is said that CO_2 responsiveness of the cerebral circulation is reduced during barbiturate anaesthesia, but equally important is the fact that under all forms of general anaesthesia, changes in Pa_{CO_2} continue to produce major alterations in CBF.

As a result of the marked CBF changes induced by Pa_{CO_2} alterations, the transit time of blood through the brain is affected, being increased by hypocapnia and decreased by hypercapnia. These changes in transit time can readily be seen during carotid angiography, and it is important to give the radiologist information about the arterial P_{CO_2} in any study done under general anaesthesia, so that the timing of the radiographs will be correct to allow visualization of the arterial, capillary and venous phases. The normal mode transit time of the cerebral circulation is in the range 6.5—10 seconds at normal P_{CO_2} but this is markedly affected by hypercapnia and hypocapnia.

The effects of blood CO_2 changes on cerebral vessels in spasm following, for example, subarachnoid haemorrhage are disputed. The vessels which are involved in spasm are medium and small arteries and not the arterioles. During vascular spasm the predominant site of flow control may therefore move to these larger vessels, which may differ from the arterioles in their response to CO_2. One factor which may be important here is that the segments of the arterial tree which go into spasm are richly supplied with adrenergic nerve fibres which do not penetrate in great numbers to the arteriolar segments (L. Symon, 1970, personal communication). This implies that if the larger arteries become the site of maximum cerebral vascular resistance, as a result of spasm, CBF control by P_{CO_2} and other factors may be markedly different fron normal.

This discussion has so far dealt only with acute changes in Pa_{CO_2}, but in clinical practice arterial P_{CO_2} may be either elevated (as in chronic respiratory failure) or reduced (as in ventilator therapy) for prolonged periods of time. Under these circumstances, CBF returns to its control values despite the maintained alteration in Pa_{CO_2}. Notwithstanding earlier experimental results, it now seems clear that the normalization of CBF during prolonged hypocapnia occurs at the same rate as the return to normal values of CSF pH. The adjustment of CSF pH in the presence of a maintained lowering of $Paco_2$ is produced by a fall in CSF bicarbonate. After 4 hours of hyperventilation in man, CBF has returned to 90% of its normocapnic value and complete normalization occurs by 6–12 hours (Severinghaus *et al.*, 1966; Raichle, Posner and Plum, 1970). From a clinical point of view these observations mean that during anaesthesia of short duration, CBF is still low at the end of 1–2 hours of hyperventilation, but this is not the case following very prolonged surgery. In the intensive therapy unit, patients treated by controlled hyperventilation have values of CBF after the first 12 hours which are determined by factors other than the lowered $Paco_2$.

As regards chronic hypercapnia, most patients in chronic respiratory failure have a normal CBF. The adaptation of CBF to prolonged hyper-capnia can be detected after 8–11 hours of elevated $Paco_2$ (Agnoli, 1968). The normalization of CBF during prolonged hypercapnia also closely follows the time course of the return to normal values of CSF pH produced by elevation of CSF bicarbonate.

HYPOXIA

The cerebral circulation does not respond to changes in Pao_2 close to the normal value, and this contrasts markedly with the sensitivity to changes in $Paco_2$. When the arterial Po_2 falls below 6.7 kPa (50 mmHg), cerebral vasodilatation occurs and increases rapidly with more severe hypoxia (*Figure 33.2*). At low values of Pao_2, CBF is more than twice normal. To

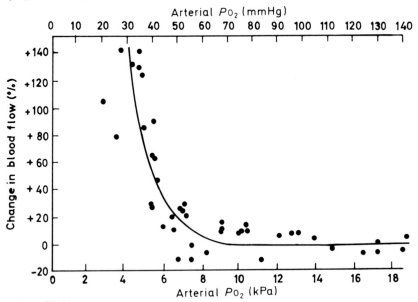

Figure 33.2
The effect of hypoxia on cerebral blood flow in the dog at constant $Paco_2$. (From McDowall, 1966b, by courtesy of the publishers)

appreciate the significance of these Po_2 values it is necessary to relate them to the known impairment of intellectual performance which occurs at arterial Po_2 values below 5.3 kPa (40 mmHg) (jugular venous $Po_2 \simeq$ 3.3 kPa or 25 mmHg) and the unconsciousness which occurs at 3.3 kPa (25 mmHg) (jugular venous $Po_2 \simeq$ 2.4 kPa or 18 mmHg). Of course during spontaneous ventilation, hypoxia causes overbreathing and the resultant hypocapnia shifts the CBF–Pao_2 relationship to the left. However, with extreme hypoxia, the effect of hypocapnia is negligible.

Hypoxic cerebral vasodilatation is a valuable protective mechanism for the brain since it reduces the resultant fall in cerebral available oxygen. It also means that the cerebral venous Po_2 associated with any given arterial Po_2 is higher than would otherwise be the case; in this way, cells in the 'lethal corners' have their oxygen supply maintained during moderate hypoxia.

The mechanism by which hypoxia produces cerebral vasodilatation has been assumed to be by means of tissue acidosis consequent upon the anaerobic production of lactic acid (see the section below on 'Mechanisms of cerebrovascular control'). Recently Borgstron, Johannsson and Siesjö (1975) have shown, however, that the CBF increase with hypoxia occurs before there is any detectable brain acidosis. It may be that, as in other situations, the factor which initiates the vascular resistance change is not the same one which maintains it. It remains likely that tissue acidosis fulfils the second of these roles.

Lactic acid escapes across the blood–brain barrier rather slowly, so the brain remains metabolically acid for some time after the correction of hypoxia. It has been shown that CBF remains elevated in the posthypoxic phase and returns to normal only when the metabolic acid–base state of the brain has been corrected (Betz and Heuser, 1967; Freeman and Ingvar, 1968). It is for this reason that a period of hypoxia is so much more serious than a period of hypoventilation during neurosurgery.

Hypoxia also directly dilates arterioles, as has been shown by studies on isolated vessels (Carrier, Walker and Guyton, 1964). However, a direct dilatory action would not account for the cerebral vasodilatation seen for some time after correction of arterial Po_2 to normal. This latter phenomenon is more easily explained in terms of the tissue pH hypothesis.

HYPEROXIA

Breathing 100% oxygen at normal barometric pressure reduces CBF by a little over 10%, while 100% oxygen at 2 atm absolute produces a 20% fall. The mechanism of this cerebral vasoconstriction with oxygen can partly be ascribed to the hyperventilation which accompanies hyperoxia. However, a reduction in CBF with hyperoxia has been shown to occur in animals during controlled ventilation and therefore at constant $Paco_2$. It thus appears that oxygen itself has a constrictive action on the cerebral vessels. It is possible that the effect is a direct and local one on the smooth muscle of the cerebral arteriole, since cerebral vessels *in vitro* constrict when the Po_2 of the perfusate is raised.

The significance of the vasoconstrictive action of oxygen should not be exaggerated, for there is no evidence that tissue oxygenation is ever impaired by oxygen therapy. The balance is always in favour of increased oxygen delivery to the brain, since CBF falls proportionately less than arterial oxygen content rises. Furthermore, there is evidence that in conditions of cerebral ischaemia, oxygen fails to exert its normal constrictive action. Cerebrovascular constriction does not increase proportionately with further elevation of Po_2, above 2 atm. Indeed, at 3 atm pressure, *under conditions of controlled ventilation*, there is a slight cerebral vasodilatation consequent upon the elevation in cerebral tissue Pco_2 which occurs as a result of the reduced CO_2-carrying capacity of highly oxygenated venous blood.

BLOOD pH

Metabolic changes in blood pH over the physiological range have very little, if any, effect on CBF. This is due to the slow transmission of hydrogen ions across the blood—brain barrier, which means that brain tissue pH is sheltered from the effects of acute changes in blood pH. There are limits to this brain protection, especially in the case of severe metabolic acidosis for, when blood pH falls below 7.30, brain tissue and CSF pH also fall (Mitchell *et al.*, 1964; Severinghaus, 1965). One would anticipate, therefore, that acute metabolic acidosis with pH below 7.30 would cause increased CBF due to brain tissue acidosis, but there is no evidence that this is so. Indeed, the evidence available demonstrates no CBF change even when blood pH is 'metabolically' lowered to 6.74 (Harper and Bell, 1963).

The brain is effectively protected against acute metabolic alkalosis in the blood, for very little change in brain pH occurs even when blood pH rises as high as 7.98 (Severinghaus, 1965). It is important to distinguish clearly between metabolic changes in blood pH and changes in cerebral tissue pH. These two do not immediately interact because of the blood—brain barrier which slows the exchange of hydrogen ions. Thus the blood can show a modest metabolic acidosis (arterial pH > 7.30) while cerebral tissue pH is within the normal range, and the converse can also occur, with CSF pH being more acid than arterial pH, as, for example, after a period of hypoxia or following a period of surgical interruption of cerebral perfusion. Blood pH does not influence arteriolar smooth muscle because of the interlocation of the blood—brain barrier. Brain tissue pH probably does affect arteriolar smooth muscle and may, in many instances, be involved in CBF control (see below).

Additional factors influencing CBF

CARDIAC OUTPUT

The volume of blood flowing through the brain is basically dependent on only two factors: (1) the cerebral perfusion pressure which, under normal conditions, is virtually the same as the mean arterial blood pressure; and (2) the cerebrovascular resistance. As cardiac output falls, blood pressure is at first maintained through sympathetic vasoconstriction in other vascular beds and CBF is thereby held at normal levels. With further reduction in cardiac output, blood pressure will begin to fall but CBF is still maintained via the local autoregulatory mechanism. Only when impairment of cardiac output is sufficient to lower the blood pressure below the autoregulatory limit does CBF become dependent upon cardiac output. Conversely, if cardiac output is increased (for example, by exercise), it has been repeatedly demonstrated that CBF is not altered.

In the case of the cerebral circulation, therefore, it is not very meaningful to suggest that cardiac output measurement is more important than blood pressure measurement.

BLOOD RHEOLOGY

If the red blood cell concentration of blood is reduced, cerebral vaso-dilatation occurs and CBF increases. This can be detected clinically in cases of severe anaemia. The question is to decide whether this increase in CBF results mechanically from the reduced blood viscosity or meta-bolically from the reduced arterial oxygen-carrying capacity. It seems that both mechanisms have a part to play in that, at haematocrit values below 30%, tissue hypoxia produces cerebral vasodilatation, while induced changes in blood viscosity also influence cerebral perfusion. For example, Thomas *et al.* (1977) showed that reduction of haematocrit (and therefore of blood viscosity) in polycythaemic patients increased CBF by 50%.

TEMPERATURE

Hypothermia reduces CBF at a rate of 6.7% in flow per degree Celsius reduction in temperature (Rosomoff, 1956), so that, in the clinical range of moderate hypothermia (28–30°C), CBF is approximately half normal. This reduction in flow with temperature may be due to changes in blood viscosity with cooling, to changes in arterial $P\text{CO}_2$ or to changes in cerebral metabolic rate. As regards arterial $P\text{CO}_2$, any patient cooled during controlled ventilation at constant minute volume will show a fall in $P\text{aCO}_2$ because total body CO_2 production falls. However, Forrester *et al.* (1964) have shown that even at constant arterial $P\text{CO}_2$, CBF at 30°C is reduced to 63% of that at 38°C. These workers further demonstrated that the responsive-ness of the cerebral vessels to alterations in $P\text{aCO}_2$ at 30°C was markedly reduced though not absent.

Cerebral metabolic rate also falls with cooling and does so in an expo-nential fashion, as would be predicted from *in vitro* studies (Michenfelder and Theye, 1968). At 28–30°C cerebral metabolism is approximately half the normal value. It is important to stress here the exponential nature of the relationship between temperature and cerebral metabolic activity, for it indicates that even quite modest reductions in temperature in clinical circumstances will have a major effect in reducing cerebral oxygen requirements.

Since, during hypothermia, CBF and cerebral metabolic activity fall together, arteriovenous oxygen differences across the brain remain relatively constant. Cerebral oxygenation, therefore, does not suffer during whole body moderate hypothermia. This conclusion is further supported by the absence of biochemical evidence of tissue hypoxia during hypothermia.

Hyperthermia, especially above $40°C$, leads to increased CBF and elevated cerebral metabolic activity.

Mechanisms of cerebrovascular control

It is a reasonable generalization to state that the cerebral circulation is more dependent on local intrinsic control and less influenced by extrinsic humoral and neurogenic factors than are other circulatory beds. This discussion will therefore deal first with intrinsic control and secondarily with recent discoveries of the influence of extrinsic factors.

CONTROL BY BRAIN EXTRACELLULAR FLUID pH

The pH of the extracellular fluid (ECF) of the brain has a major influence in controlling the vascular tone of the smooth muscle of small arteries and arterioles in the brain, as illustrated in *Figure 33.3*. Acidosis in the ECF produces dilatation and alkalosis constriction.

This relationship can be seen most readily in the response of CBF to changes in Pa_{CO_2}. Since CO_2 diffuses rapidly across the blood—brain barrier, hypercapnia causes a rapid extracellular pH shift in an acid direction, which results in vasodilatation and increased CBF, while hypocapnia induces the opposite sequence of changes.

The sequence of events with hypoxia has already been outlined, for hypoxia — at least in part — produces vasodilatation of the cerebral circulation through the anaerobic production of lactic acid with a consequent acidosis in ECF and CSF. Similarly, ischaemic hypoxia produces an acid shift in ECF pH which accounts for the cerebral hyperaemia which follows temporary surgical occlusion of intracranial arteries or of the internal carotid artery.

It is important to stress that the factor involved in cerebrovascular control is the pH of the ECF of the brain and not the pH of the arterial blood. Blood pH has little influence on CBF because of the slow movement of hydrogen ions or bicarbonate ions across the blood—brain barrier. It is thus possible to have an abnormal blood pH in the presence of a normal brain ECF pH, as in strenuous exercise. Alternatively, ECF pH of the brain can be acidotic following local cerebral circulatory arrest at a time when blood pH is normal.

The local concentrations of other ions additional to hydrogen ions can influence cerebrovascular tone. Particularly important is the local potassium ion concentration in the ECF, since ECF K^+ alters rapidly with neuronal activity. High tissue K^+ leads to vasodilatation and low K^+ constriction. In addition, Ca^{2+} ionic concentration has an effect on local CBF (Betz,

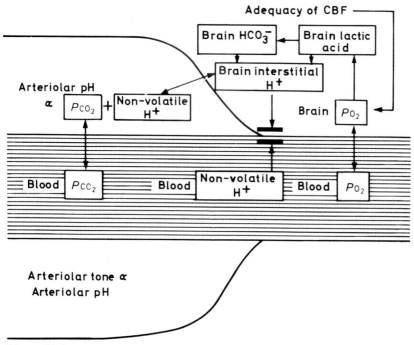

Figure 33.3
The brain tissue pH hypothesis of cerebral blood flow regulation.
On the left is represented an arteriole with its smooth muscle walls,
while on the right is a thin-walled capillary. The heavy bars on the
capillary represent the blood–brain barrier to free movement of
hydrogen ions. From this figure it can be seen that changes in blood
$P\text{co}_2$ influence the interstitial pH of the arteriolar smooth muscle by
diffusion through the vessel wall, while changes in blood H^+ ion
concentration do not directly affect interstitial pH. Diminution in
cerebral oxygen supply due to either hypoxic or ischaemic hypoxia
affects interstitial pH through the formation of lactic acid as a
consequence of increased anaerobic metabolism

1976), as does adenosine, which is formed from the breakdown of high
energy phosphates (Rubio, Berne and Winn, 1978).

INFLUENCE OF THE AUTONOMIC NERVOUS SYSTEM

There is now considerable evidence that the cervical sympathetic nervous
system has a vasoconstrictive action exerted mainly on the carotid and
vertebral arteries in the neck, on the branches of the circle of Willis, and
on the medium and small arteries on the brain surface. In addition, some
of the sympathetic fibres penetrate the brain with the arteries and terminate
near the arterioles. Harper *et al.* (1972) have postulated a scheme of dual
innervation of the cerebral vasculature, as illustrated in *Figure 33.4*, in
which the influence of the sympathetic nervous control is exercised on
the extraparenchymal (i.e. outside brain substance) arteries and veins,
while the metabolic control, which is illustrated in *Figure 33.3*, has its
main site of action at the arterioles and precapillary sphincters.

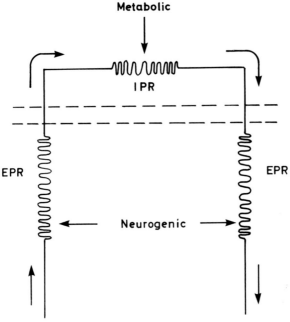

Figure 33.4
Dual control hypothesis of cerebral vascular resistance. In this schema
it is proposed that neurogenic influences are exerted on extraparenchymal arteries and veins, that is, the arteries and veins which lie on
the brain surface prior to penetration into brain tissue. Metabolic
control is considered to operate at the arteriolar level within brain
tissue. (From Harper *et al.*, 1972, by courtesy of the authors and
the Editors of *Archives of Neurology*)

This picture of sympathetic control of the cerebral circulation has been
complicated by the discovery of a separate component of the sympathetic
nervous system, which arises mainly in the locus coeruleus and is distributed
within the brain by adrenergic fibres which terminate close to the muscular
coat of small arteries and arterioles (Owman and Edvinsson, 1978). The
role of this system has not yet been elucidated.

It is important not to overemphasize the influence of sympathetic
nervous supply on CBF, for it is difficult to define any fall in CBF with
sympathetic stimulation, or any increase with sympathetic blockade
under normal resting conditions of CBF. The vasoconstrictive action,
which at most amounts to 20%, is seen most clearly when the circulation
is dilated by other factors, e.g. by hypercapnia (James, Millar and Purves,
1968). An important example of the sympathetic involvement in cerebrovascular control is the more efficient autoregulation found with drug-
induced hypotension, as compared with haemorrhagic hypotension,
which has been discussed above. It remains true, however, that by far the
most potent influence on the cerebral vasculature is the metabolic control
of the smooth muscle of the arterioles exercised by local tissue concentrations of hydrogen and other ions, particularly potassium.

Catecholamines circulating in the blood have little influence on CBF because they have difficulty in penetrating the blood—brain barrier. They may, however, influence CBF in areas of brain pathology where the blood—brain barrier has become incompetent, for then the catecholamines can cross into the brain tissue and affect the sympathetic transmitter receptors associated with the smooth muscle of the vessel walls (Mackenzie *et al.*, 1976).

Correlation between cerebral metabolic activity and cerebral blood flow

In the above discussion it has been implied on several occasions that a direct relationship exists between cerebral metabolic activity and CBF. There is evidence that this is in fact the case, for reductions in cerebral metabolic activity as measured by EEG frequency lead to similar reductions in CBF during barbiturate anaesthesia, while increased CBF has been demonstrated during the cerebral metabolic stimulation produced by convulsant and analeptic drugs. Under these conditions there appears to be a direct relationship between mean EEG frequency and CBF. Recently this has been shown to be true on a regional basis also, in that photic stimulation produces increased blood volume in the occipital lobe, and mental exercise results in localized changes in cerebral cortical blood volume — that is, volume changes indicative of cerebral vasodilatation at sites where increased metabolic activity is presumably induced (Risberg and Ingvar, 1968). Olesen (1971) has shown that voluntary muscular activity in one arm produces a focal increase in regional cerebral blood flow (rCBF) in the contralateral cortical motor area.

In sleep the changes are different, as between rapid eye movement (REM) sleep and slow wave sleep. In the former type of sleep, CBF is markedly increased while, in the latter, flow is increased slightly due to the mild hypercapnia which is present in this phase of sleep.

The connecting link between cerebral metabolic activity and CBF has long been ascribed to local tissue P_{CO_2}. Thus, increased regional cerebral activity, as is produced for example by photic stimulation, leads to a rise in local brain tissue P_{CO_2} and to local vasodilatation. The final signal is believed to be not P_{CO_2} itself, but an accompanying change in ECF pH of the smooth muscle of the arteriolar wall. There is much evidence in support of this concept of ECF pH acting as a link between metabolic activity and CBF, but there are some findings which indicate that it cannot be the complete mechanism. For example, the rapidity with which CBF increases at the start of an epileptiform convulsion seems to require a more rapidly changing signal than ECF pH (Astrup *et al.*, 1978). Similarly, when cerebral metabolism is reduced by Althesin injection, CBF begins to fall 2 seconds after the first EEG change, at a time when the maximum possible shift in tissue P_{CO_2} and pH is very small (Keaney *et al.*, 1978). For these reasons, some believe that there must be an additional initiating factor to trigger CBF change; one candidate for this role is the ECF K^+ concentration, since this alters rapidly with changes in neuronal activity.

This initial signal is probably backed up by a slower alteration of ECF pH which may provide the fine adjustment of the balance between flow and metabolism.

PATHOPHYSIOLOGY OF THE CEREBRAL CIRCULATION

So far we have considered the ways in which vascular tone is regulated in the normal cerebral circulation. This section will deal with the alterations in responsiveness shown by the abnormal cerebral circulation.

Circulation in and around intracranial tumours

Intracranial tumours can, of course, be very vascular or relatively avascular and so it is possible to detect many of them from regional changes in blood flow in the area of the tumour. One of the characteristics of tumour circulations is that, whether the flow is high or low, in certain parts of the tumour it is excessive for the local metabolic requirements. Since flow is in excess of oxygen uptake, local venous blood is highly oxygenated, giving the typical 'red veins' seen in and around intracranial tumours. This characteristic has been designated as 'luxury perfusion' or 'relative venous hyperoxia'. In addition to the level of resting flow in an intracranial tumour, the changes in flow produced by CO_2 and blood pressure alterations are also often abnormal. Thus, in tumour circulations, reduction of Pa_{CO_2} may lead to: (1) a smaller than the normal fall in regional blood flow; (2) no change in regional blood flow; or (3) actually an increase in regional blood flow. In addition, the tumour circulations may respond abnormally to variations in arterial blood pressure. The normal response is, as noted above, that CBF does not alter with either increase or moderate decrease in blood pressure due to intrinsic autoregulation of cerebral flow. This autoregulatory ability is often lost in tumour circulations, so an increase in blood pressure causes an increase in CBF and *vice versa*. In some tumours, both blood pressure and Pa_{CO_2} responsiveness are abnormal, but in others only one of the two responses is deranged. It is because of these abnormalities of response that, in using rCBF measurement in the detection of intracranial tumours, CBF is measured not only under resting conditions but also during acute alterations in Pa_{CO_2} and blood pressure.

It is believed that these alterations in rCBF in and around cerebral tumours can be explained by local tissue acidosis produced by the rapid growth and partially anaerobic metabolism of many intracranial tumours. Local tissue acidosis, as discussed above, produces local cerebral vasodilatation. In the presence of such local acidosis, lowering Pa_{CO_2} by hyperventilation may not elevate local tissue pH sufficiently to return it to within the regulatory range for cerebrovascular resistance. In this case, acute hypocapnia will then not reduce rCBF. It may even increase it if, by vasoconstricting the surrounding normal areas, the induced hypocapnia leads to a shift of perfusion toward the widely dilated and unresponsive arterioles of the tumour circulation. This mechanism has been termed 'inverse steal' or the 'Robin Hood effect', since blood is taken away from the well-to-do normal areas and given to the impoverished abnormal ones. It probably explains the improved angiographic visualization of tumour circulations observed by Samuel, Grange and Hawkins (1968) during hypocapnic anaesthesia. Hypercapnia sometimes produces the opposite effect — that is, a 'steal' of blood away from the tumour. This occurs if the degree of tissue acidosis in and around the tumour has already produced maximum arteriolar dilatation locally. Hypercapnia, then, by lowering the vascular resistance of the neighbouring normal vascular beds, leads to a diversion of flow away from the tumour circulation.

The failure of the tumour circulation to show normal autoregulation to blood pressure changes can be explained in a similar way. The local tissue acidosis in and around the tumour leads to maximal dilatation of the tumour vessels and so these vessels act as passive conduits through which the flow is controlled only by perfusion pressure.

There are still further special features of CBF in the presence of cerebral tumours which are even less well understood than those already discussed. One feature is that, in distant areas of normal brain on the same hemisphere as the tumour, cerebral perfusion is lowered.

Another feature is that marked alterations in flow occur which are related temporarily and perhaps causally with the appearance of 'plateau' waves. These plateau waves are waves of increased intracranial pressure (ICP) which occur intermittently in patients with intracranial tumours and which last for 5–20 minutes. At the peaks of these waves of elevated ICP, CBF is markedly reduced but cerebral blood volume is increased. Eventually, of course, with the inexorable expansion of an intracranial tumour, general ICP rises permanently and not just in the intermittent manner seen with plateau waves. The ICP may then reach a level at which general cerebral perfusion is reduced. In addition, however, the distortion of the brain produced by the tumour may lead to physical stretching and angulation of certain intracranial arteries sufficient to produce areas of ischaemia in the territories of the distorted vessels. The posterior cerebral artery seems to be frequently involved by such mechanical distortion.

Circulation in areas of partial vascular occlusion

If an intracranial vessel or an extracranial vessel in the neck carrying cerebral blood is partially obstructed, then the distal arterioles in the territory of supply dilate in an attempt to maintain flow. As the main vessel obstruction becomes more severe, the dilatory capacity of the intracranial vessels is eventually fully extended. In such circumstances the area supplied by the compromised vessel shows deranged responses to blood pressure and $PaCO_2$ changes, similar to those discussed in the section above, on tumour circulations. The circulation in such an area may be normal under resting conditions, but when blood pressure is acutely changed it may show loss of autoregulation and a passive pressure—flow relationship. Furthermore, hypocapnia may not reduce flow and may actually increase it because of the Robin Hood effect.

PHARMACOLOGY OF THE CEREBRAL CIRCULATION IN RELATION TO ANAESTHESIA

There is a large amount of information on the effects of anaesthetic drugs on CBF, $CMRo_2$ and ICP, and this is summarized in *Table 33.1.*

TABLE 33.1. Anaesthetic drug effects on CBF, ICP and $CMRo_2$

	CBF	ICP	$CMRo_2$	References
Induction drugs				
Thiopentone	↓	↓	↓	1–8
Althesin	↓	↓	↓	9–12
Ketamine	↑	↑	↑	13–22
Propanidid	↓	?	↓	23
Muscle relaxants				
Suxamethonium	?	↑	—	6, 24, 25
Tubocurarine	—	—	—	6, 33
Maintenance drugs: inhalational				
Nitrous oxide	↑	↑	— or ↓	6, 27–33, 38, 39, 40
Cyclopropane	— or ↑	↓ or ↑	↓	6, 7, 34
Halothane	↑	↑	↓	1, 6, 25, 26, 35–37, 41–45
Chloroform	↑	↑	↓	46–49
Trichloroethylene	↑	↑	↓	30, 44, 50–52
Diethyl ether	↑	↑	↓	6, 7, 46, 47, 53–61
Methoxyflurane	↑	↑	↓	62, 63
Fluroxene	?	↑	?	64
Isoflurane	↑	↑	↓	65, 66
Enflurane	↑	↑	↓	67, 68, 69
Maintenance drugs: intravenous				
Droperidol	↓	—	—	74, 75
Droperidol + phenoperidine (at constant $Paco_2$)	↓ or —	—	?	70–72
Fentanyl	↓	↓ or —	↓	74, 75, 76
Droperidol + fentanyl (at constant $Paco_2$)	↓ or —	↓ or —	↓	71, 73, 74, 77, 78
Morphine (at constant $Paco_2$)	↓ or —	↓ or —	↓ or —	79, 82, 83
Pentazocine (at constant $Paco_2$)	?	↓	?	84
Diazepam	↓	?	↓ or —	85, 86, 87

Opiate drugs

Opiate drugs have little effect on CBF or ICP at normal dose levels during controlled ventilation, but their potent respiratory depressant action causes increases in CBF and ICP when they are given to spontaneously breathing patients. At high dose levels during controlled ventilation, moderate cerebral metabolic depression occurs with an accompanying modest fall in CBF and ICP. It appears that droperidol, which is commonly used with an opiate during neuroleptanaesthesia, may have a specific cerebral vasoconstrictive action (Michenfelder and Theye, 1971).

Barbiturates

Changes in CBF have not been detected with sedative doses of barbiturates, provided alterations in $PaCO_2$ are taken into account. This failure may merely mean that the measurement techniques do not possess sufficient resolution to detect the small changes in flow which would seem to be likely with barbiturate sedation.

When barbiturates are given in doses sufficient to produce general anaesthesia, then CBF is certainly reduced. With a dose of thiopentone sufficient to produce light anaesthesia, CBF is reduced by about one-third of the normal conscious value. Deeper anaesthesia can reduce flow by as

Footnote to Table 33.1.

1. Gordon (1970); 2. Højgaard (1961); 3. Horsley (1937); 4. Landau *et al.* (1955); 5. Pierce *et al.* (1962); 6. Søndergard (1961); 7. Woringer, Brogly and Schneider (1951); 8. Shapiro *et al.* (1973); 9. Pickerodt *et al.* (1972); 10. Takahashi *et al.* (1973); 11. Turner *et al.* (1972); 12. Sari *et al.* (1976); 13. Dawson, Michenfelder and Theye (1971); 14. Evans *et al.* (1971); 15. Gardner, Dannemiller and Dean (1972); 16. Gibbs (1972); 17. List *et al.* (1972); 18. Sari, Okuda and Takeshita (1972a); 19. Shapiro, Wyte and Harris (1972); 20. Takeshita, Okuda and Sari (1972); 21. Wyte *et al.* (1972); 22. Hougaard, Hansen and Brodersen (1974); 23. Takeshita, Miyauchi and Ishikawa (1973); 24. Halldin and Wahlin (1959); 25. Marx, Andrews and Orkin (1962); 26. Wollman *et al.* (1964); 27. Henriksen and Jörgensen (1973); 28. Hulme and Cooper (1972); 29. Laitinen, Johansson and Tarkkanen (1967); 30. McDowall and Harper (1965); 31. Saidman and Eger (1965); 32. Theye and Michenfelder (1968); 33. Wollman *et al.* (1965); 34. Alexander *et al.* (1968); 35. Adams *et al.* (1972); 36. Christensen, Høedt-Rasmussen and Lassen (1967); 37. Galindo and Baldwin (1963); 38. Gordon and Greitz (1970); 39. Sakabe *et al.* (1978); 40. Sakabe *et al.* (1976); 41. Hunter (1964); 42. Jennett *et al.* (1969); 43. McDowall (1967a); 44. McDowall (1966a); 45. McHenry *et al.* (1966); 46. Finesinger and Cobb (1935); 47. Koopmans (1939); 48. McDowall (1965); 49. McDowall *et al.* (1966b); 50. McDowall and Harper (1969); 51. McDowall, Harper and Jacobson (1964); 52. Nowill, Stephen and Searles (1953); 53. Brennan (1938); 54. Finesinger (1932); 55. Lundberg, Kjallquist and Bien (1959); 56. McDowall (1967b); 57. Schmidt (1934); 58. Schmidt and Pierson (1934); 59. Sokoloff (1959); 60. White *et al.* (1942); 61. Woringer, Brogly and Dorgler (1954); 62. Fitch *et al.* (1969b); 63. Michenfelder and Theye (1973); 64. Jörgensen and Henriksen (1973); 65. Adams, Gronert and Michenfelder (1975); 66. Cucchiara, Theye and Michenfelder (1974); 67. Michenfelder and Cucchiara (1974); 68. Zattoni, Siani and Rivano (1973); 69. McKay *et al.* (1976); 70. Barker *et al.* (1968); 71. Fitch *et al.* (1969a); 72. Wilkinson and Browne (1970); 73. Kreuscher (1965); 74. Michenfelder and Theye (1971); 75. Misfeldt *et al.* (1976); 76. Moss *et al.* (1978); 77. Miller and Barker (1969); 78. Sari, Okuda and Takeshita (1972b); 79. Keats and Mithoefer (1955); 80. McCall and Taylor (1952); 81. Moyer *et al.* (1957); 82. Weitzner, McCoy and Binder (1963); 83. Takeshita, Michenfelder and Theye (1972); 84. Barker, Miller and Johnston (1972); 85. Cotev and Shalit (1975); 86. Carlsson *et al.* (1976); 87. Maekawa, Sakabe and Takeshita (1974)

much as 50%. Since equivalent reductions in cerebral metabolic rate occur at the same time, it is believed that CBF falls in the following way:

barbiturate anaesthesia
↓
reduced cerebral metabolic activity
↓
reduced cerebral CO_2 production
↓
tendency for cerebral tissue P_{CO_2} to fall
↓
resisted by cerebral vasoconstriction and reduced CBF

As a result of the reduced CBF and accompanying fall in cerebral blood volume, CSF pressure is reduced by barbiturate anaesthesia. It is for this reason that intermittent barbiturate administration has been recommended as a suitable technique for general anaesthesia in patients with intracranial tumours (see Chapter 64).

There is currently great interest in the possibility of protecting the brain against ischaemic damage by deep barbiturate anaesthesia. This putative protection would be afforded by the reduction in neuronal oxygen requirements, as a result of functional depression. As Michenfelder (1974) has shown, it follows from this concept that barbiturates can exert a protective effect only when neuronal activity is present. No protection can be expected when activity has been abolished by the severity of the ischaemia. At present a number of clinical trials of barbiturate protection of the brain are in progress in patients following severe head injury, cardiac arrest or cerebrovascular accident. An additional advantage of barbiturate treatment in these cases is the reduction in ICP produced. In using the treatment, care is necessary to avoid excessive falls in blood pressure, which would reduce the cerebral perfusion pressure and might make the brain ischaemia worse.

Althesin

The action of Althesin on CBF in normal brain is very similar to that of thiopentone and, like the latter drug, is probably secondary to cerebral metabolic depression. Rasmussen, Rosendal and Overgaard (1975) have demonstrated that, in *diseased* brain, Althesin may, in certain areas, actually increase rCBF. This unusual response may be a demonstration of a drug-induced inverse steal effect produced, as in the case of hypocapnic inverse steal, by a redistribution of rCBF from normal areas of brain to abnormal areas.

Ketamine

Ketamine increases CBF by a mechanism which is the mirror image of the picture seen with thiopentone and Althesin. The drug produces regional cerebral activation and, presumably, increased regional oxidative metabolism. The metabolic stimulation through the flow—metabolism linkage results in regional increases in CBF; ICP is also raised.

Inhalational general anaesthetics

The effect of nitrous oxide on CBF, though disputed, is probably one of vasodilatation with increased CBF and ICP (Henriksen and Jörgensen, 1973; Sakabe *et al.*, 1978). However, the effect seems to be prevented by the prior administration of barbiturates.

HALOTHANE

Halothane is a cerebral vasodilator at all clinical concentrations: 0.5% halothane increases flow by about 10%; 1% halothane by about 15%; and 2% halothane by about 25%. Higher concentrations of halothane usually depress blood pressure so greatly that CBF falls (*Figure 33.5*), and very low concentrations of halothane seem to have an opposite (i.e. a vasoconstrictor) effect (McDowall, Harper and Jacobson, 1963; Movita *et al.*, 1977).

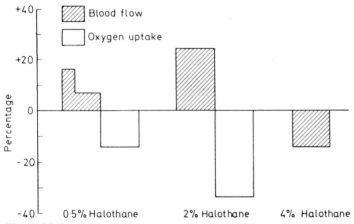

Figure 33.5
The effect of different concentrations of halothane on cerebral blood flow and cerebral oxygen uptake. (Values as percentage of control under unsupplemented nitrous oxide.) (From McDowall, 1967a, by courtesy of the Editor of *British Journal of Anaesthesia*)

There is a relationship between the concentration of halothane administered and the cerebral metabolic depression which occurs, in that 2% halothane depresses oxygen uptake (−30%) more than does 0.5% halothane (−15%). Recent evidence suggests that there is not a simple proportionate relationship between concentration and metabolic depression, since the depression reaches a maximum at 2% inspired halothane and further increases have little further effect.

TRICHLOROETHYLENE

Trichloroethylene is, like halothane, a cerebral vasodilator (*Figure 33.6*). The duration of the dilatory action requires further study, however, for in the dog it appears to be limited to about 30 minutes. Cerebral oxygen uptake is depressed by trichloroethylene. So, as with halothane, cerebral venous oxygen saturation rises.

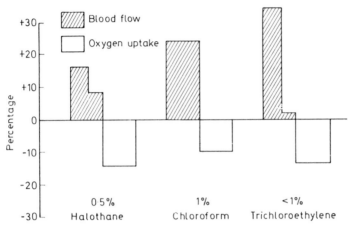

Figure 33.6
The effects of halothane, chloroform and trichloroethylene on cerebral blood flow and cerebral oxygen uptake. (Values as percentage of control under unsupplemented nitrous oxide.) (From McDowall, 1966a, by courtesy of the publishers)

ICP increases when trichloroethylene is administered and this effect is again accentuated in patients with intracranial space-occupying lesions. As regards the production of ICP changes, there is little to choose between halothane and trichloroethylene but, since the latter lowers the blood pressure less, cerebral perfusion pressure tends to be better maintained with it.

CHLOROFORM, ETHER AND METHOXYFLURANE

All these drugs are cerebral vasodilators and apparently also reduce cerebral metabolic rate. All produce increases in ICP which, in the case of methoxyflurane, have been shown to be substantially greater in patients with intracranial tumours (Fitch *et al.*, 1969b).

CYCLOPROPANE

According to the only report available on the influence of cyclopropane on the cerebral circulation (Alexander *et al.*, 1968), it behaves quite differently from volatile agents. Concentrations of 5 and 13% cyclopropane reduce both CBF and cerebral metabolic rate (similar to the effect of thiopentone), but 20% and 37% cyclopropane increase CBF, which is similar to the action of the volatile anaesthetics. The most surprising feature of this drug is that at the higher concentrations, the oxygen uptake of the brain is normal, despite the production of deep anaesthesia.

FLUROXENE, ISOFLURANE AND ENFLURANE

These newer volatile agents seem, like their predecessors, to be vasodilators, and for this reason they all increase ICP (Zattoni, Siani and Rivano, 1974). Enflurane has an additional action at concentrations greater than 2% when, especially in the presence of hypocapnia, it may produce convulsive-like activity on the EEG. When this occurs there is a further increase in CBF, due to the metabolic activation of the cerebral cortex (Michenfelder and Cuchiara, 1974).

OTHER FACTORS OPERATING DURING GENERAL ANAESTHESIA

The effects of the individual drugs used in anaesthesia on CBF have been discussed above, but it is important to remember that the influence of these drugs is small in comparison to the effects of alterations in $Pa\text{CO}_2$, blood pressure and temperature which often occur during general anaesthesia.

Changes in CSF pressure during anaesthesia

Any factor which dilates the cerebral vessels produces an elevation in CSF pressure because of the resultant increase in cerebral blood volume. Hypoxia and hypercapnia, therefore, cause large elevations of CSF pressure and it is for this reason that 'bad' anaesthesia produces 'tight' brains. Of the two, hypoxia is the worse, because its effect on cerebral vascular tone is not reversed immediately on correcting the Po_2 but is maintained for a considerable time by the persisting cerebral tissue acidosis. The causative hypoxia may not be hypoxic but ischaemic in origin, if a period of profound hypotension occurs during the induction of anaesthesia. The other ingredient of bad anaesthesia is increased expiratory resistance within the anaesthetic circuit. This has the effect of raising the mean intrathoracic pressure and, so, the cerebral venous pressure. The rise in the latter expands the cerebral veins, leading to increased cerebral blood volume and CSF pressure.

Even with perfect anaesthesia, however, there is still a proportion of cases in which the brain is congested and swollen when it is exposed. In some of these cases a vasodilatory volatile anaesthetic may be responsible but, in patients without intracranial space-occupying lesions, the changes in intracranial pressure produced by these drugs are small and are readily reversed by the concomitant use of hyperventilation. It must be admitted, therefore, that the causation of cerebral congestion and swelling in a proportion of cases is still not understood, for it can occur without any of the recognized factors being present.

The effect of volatile anaesthetic drugs in elevating ICP may be of clinical importance in patients with intracranial space-occupying lesions. It has been demonstrated that in these cases the administration of halothane, trichloroethylene or methoxyflurane produces large increases in ICP from starting levels (under unsupplemented nitrous oxide–oxygen) which are only slightly elevated above normal (Jennett *et al.,* 1969; Gordon, 1970). These changes are seen despite the maintenance of normocapnia by controlled ventilation. *Figure 33.7* shows the change in ICP

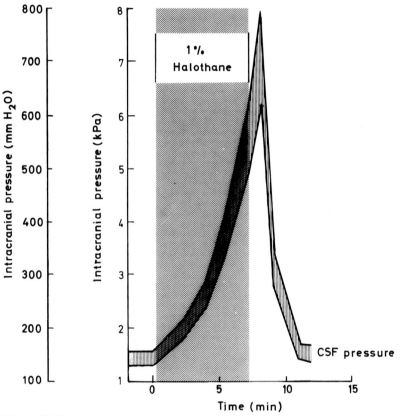

Figure 33.7
The increase in intracranial pressure produced in a patient with a cerebral tumour by 1% halothane during controlled normocapnic ventilation. (From Jennett, McDowall and Barker, 1967, by courtesy of the Editors of *Journal of Neurosurgery*)

produced by 1% halothane in a patient with an intracranial tumour. The features to note are the extent of the increase and the rapidity with which it occurred; equally important are the rapid fall on discontinuing halothane administration and the return to the starting level of pressure. Both of these latter points indicate that after short administrations of volatile anaesthetic drugs, there is no formation of cerebral oedema. All of the pressure change is due to rapid fluctuations in the intracranial blood volume. This may, however, not be the case after longer periods of volatile anaesthetic administration in patients with cerebral tumours.

These large intracranial pressure increases, which occur during the administration of volatile anaesthetics to patients with space-occupying lesions, may be of clinical importance through one of two mechanisms. First, the intracranial pressure rise may be greater in one intracranial compartment than another, so that brain shifts and perhaps brain herniation may be produced. Fitch and McDowall (1971) have demonstrated that, in dogs with artificial space-occupying lesions, the administration of halothane at constant $PaCO_2$ does produce increased gradients of intracranial pressure across the tentorium. Second, the cerebrovascular dilatation produced by the anaesthetic may not affect all the vessels around the tumour equally, because of loss of reactivity in certain areas. This loss of reactivity might arise from local cerebral tissue acidosis produced by tumour compression and oedema formation. The effect of unequal vasodilatation would be to steal blood from the acidotic compressed areas and give it to the adjacent healthy areas — the intracerebral steal effect again. As a consequence, further tissue acidosis and oedema may be produced. This effect would be further accentuated by the concomitant increase in ICP which must tend to compress the capillaries and veins in the area supplied by the non-reactive cerebral arterioles.

Many of these hazards can be reduced by hyperventilation prior to the administration of a volatile anaesthetic. Adams and colleagues (1972; Adams, Gronert and Michenfelder, 1975) believe that hyperventilation for 10 minutes before commencing halothane always prevents significant ICP increases, and that hyperventilation from the start of isoflurane administration will prevent ICP changes with this agent. However, with enflurane, Zattoni, Siani and Rivano (1974) observed increases in ICP despite hyperventilation. Other workers hold that any one of these volatile anaesthetics may produce a major increase in ICP, even during hyperventilation, if the intracranial compression produced by the brain pathology is severe enough (Jennett *et al.*, 1969; Gordon, 1970).

All are agreed that the presence of hypercapnia during the administration of a volatile anaesthetic, commonly the result of inadequate spontaneous ventilation, greatly accentuates the ICP changes and increases considerably the danger of brain shift and brain compression.

References

Adams, R. W., Gronert, G. A. and Michenfelder, J. D. (1975). Isoflurane and cerebrospinal fluid pressure. In *Intracranial Pressure — II*, pp. 334—336. N. Lundberg, U. Ponten and M. Brock (ed.). Berlin: Springer-Verlag

Adams, R. W., Gronert, G. A., Sundt, T. M. and Michenfelder, J. D. (1972). Halothane, hypocapnia and cerebrospinal fluid pressure in neurosurgery. *Anesthesiology* 37, 510—517

Agnoli, A. (1968). Adaptation of CBF during induced chronic normoxic respiratory acidosis. *Scand. J. clin. Lab. Invest.* Suppl. 102

Alexander, S. C., James, F. M., Colton, E. T., Gleaton, H. R. and Wollman, H. (1968). Effects of cyclopropane on cerebral blood flow and carbohydrate metabolism in man. *Anesthesiology* 29, 170 (Abstract)

Astrup, J., Heuser, D., Lassen, N. A., Nilsson, B., Norberg, K. and Siesjö, B. K. (1978). Evidence against H⁺ and K⁺ as main factors for the control of cerebral blood flow; a micro-electrode study. In *Cerebral Vascular Smooth Muscle and its Control*, pp. 313–332. Ciba Foundation Symposium No. 56. Katherine Elliott and Maeve O'Connor (ed.). Amsterdam: Elsevier/Excerpta Medica

Barker, J., Miller, J. D. and Johnston, I. H. (1972). The effect of pentazocine on pupillary size and intracranial pressure. *Br. J. Anaesth.* 44, 197–202

Barker, J., Harper, A. M., McDowall, D. G., Fitch, W. and Jennett, W. B. (1968). Cerebral blood flow, cerebrospinal fluid pressure and EEG activity during neuroleptanalgesia induced with dehydrobenzperidol and pheno-peridine. *Br. J. Anaesth.* 40, 143

Betz, E. (ed.). (1976). Ionic actions on vascular smooth muscle with special regard to brain vessels. Berlin: Springer-Verlag

Betz, E. and Heuser, D. (1967). Cerebral cortical blood flow during change of acid–base equilibrium of the brain. *J. appl. Physiol.* 23, 726–733

Borgstrom, L., Johansson, H. and Siesjö, B. K. (1975). Relationship between arterial Po_2 and cerebral blood flow in hypoxic hypoxia. *Acta physiol. scand.* 93, 423–432

Brennan, H. J. (1938). 'Gas oxygen' and cerebral congestion. *Lancet* i, 315–319

Carlsson, C., Hagerdal, M., Kaasik, A. E. and Siesjö, B. K. (1976). The effects of diazepam on cerebral blood flow and oxygen consumption in rats and its synergistic interaction with nitrous oxide. *Anesthesiology* 45, 319–325

Carrier, O., Walker, J. R. and Guyton, A. C. (1964). Role of oxygen in autoregulation of blood flow in isolated vessels. *Am. J. Physiol.* 206, 951–954

Christensen, M. S., Høedt-Rasmussen, K. and Lassen, N. A. (1967). Cerebral vasodilatation by halothane anaesthesia in man and its potentiation by hypotension and hypercapnia. *Br. J. Anaesth.* 39, 927–934

Cotev, S. and Shalit, M. N. (1975). Effects of diazepam on cerebral blood flow and oxygen uptake after head injury. *Anesthesiology* 43, 117–122

Cucchiara, R. F., Theye, R. A. and Michenfelder, J. D. (1974). The effects of isoflurane on canine cerebral metabolism and blood flow. *Anesthesiology* 40, 571–574

Dawson, B., Michenfelder, J. D. and Theye, R. A. (1971). Effects of ketamine on canine cerebral blood flow and metabolism: modification by prior administration of thiopental. *Anesth. Analg. curr. Res.* 50, 443–447

Evans, J., Rosen, M., Weeks, R. D. and Wise, C. (1971). Ketamine in neurosurgical procedures. *Lancet* i, 40–41

Finesinger, J. E. (1932). Cerebral circulation. XVIII. Effect of caffeine on the cerebral vessels. *Archs Neurol. Psychiat., Chicago* 28, 1290–1325

Finesinger, J. E. and Cobb, S. (1935). Cerebral circulation. XXXIV. The action of narcotic drugs on the pial vessels. *J. Pharmac. exp. Ther.* 53, 1–33

Fitch, W. and McDowall, D. G. (1971). Vaso-dilating anaesthetics and pressures in different compartments of the skull. In *Brain Hypoxia*, pp. 113–117. Clinics in Developmental Medicine, No. 39/40. J. B. Brierley and B. S. Meldrum (ed.). London: Heinemann Medical

Fitch, W., Barker, J., Jennett, W. B. and McDowall, D. G. (1969a). The influence of neuroleptanalgesic drugs on cerebrospinal fluid pressure. *Br. J. Anaesth.* 41, 800–806

Fitch, W., Barker, J., McDowall, D. G. and Jennett, W. B. (1969b). The effect of methoxyflurane on cerebrospinal fluid pressure in patients with and without intra-cranial space-occupying lesions. *Br. J. Anaesth.* 41, 564–572

Fitch, W., Ferguson, G. G., Sengupta, D., Garibi, J. and Harper, A. M. (1976). Auto-regulation of cerebral blood flow during controlled hypotension in baboons. *J. Neurol. Neurosurg. Psychiat.* 39, 1014–1022

Forrester, A. C., McDowall, D. G., Harper, A. M. and Nisbet, H. I. A. (1964). Cerebral blood flow during hypothermia with control of arterial carbon-dioxide tension. In *Proceedings, 3rd World Congress Anesthesiology* 3, 129–134

Freeman, J. and Ingvar, D. H. (1968). Elimi-nation by hypoxia of cerebral blood flow autoregulation and EEG relationship. *Expl Brain Res.* 5, 61–71

Galindo, A. and Baldwin, M. (1963). Intra-cranial pressure and internal carotid blood flow during halothane anesthesia in the dog. *Anesthesiology* 24, 318–326

Gardner, A. E., Dannemiller, F. J. and Dean, D. (1972). Intracranial cerebrospinal fluid pressure in man during ketamine anesthesia. *Anesth. Analg. curr. Res.* 51, 741–745

Gibbs, J. M. (1972). The effect of intravenous ketamine on cerebrospinal fluid pressure. *Br. J. Anaesth.* 44, 1298–1301

Gordon, E. (1970). The action of drugs on intracranial contents. In *Progress in Anaes-thesiology*, pp. 60–68. T. B. Boulton, R. Bryce-Smith, M. K. Sykes, G. B. Gillett and A. L. Revell (ed.). Amsterdam: Excerpta Medica

Gordon, E. and Greitz, T. (1970). The effect of nitrous oxide on the cerebrospinal fluid pressure during encephalography. *Br. J. Anaesth.* 42, 2–7

Halldin, M. and Wahlin, A. (1959). Effect of succinylcholine on the intraspinal fluid pressure. *Acta anaesth. scand.* 3, 155—161

Harper, A. M. (1965). Physiology of cerebral blood flow. *Br. J. Anaesth.* 37, 225—235

Harper, A. M. and Bell, R. A. (1963). The effect of metabolic acidosis and alkalosis on the blood flow through the cerebral cortex. *J. Neurol. Neurosurg. Psychiat.* 26, 341—344

Harper, A. M., Deshmukh, V. D., Rowan, J. D. and Jennett, W. B. (1972). The influence of sympathetic nervous activity on cerebral blood flow. *Archs Neurol., Chicago* 27, 1—6

Henriksen, H. T. and Jörgensen, P. B. (1973). The effects of nitrous oxide on intracranial pressure in patients with intracranial disorders. *Br. J. Anaesth.* 45, 486—492

Højgaard, K. (1961). Intracranial pressure during general anaesthesia. *Acta psychiat. neurol. scand.* 36, 582—600

Horsley, J. S. (1937). The intracranial pressure during barbital narcosis. *Lancet* i, 141—143

Hougaard, K., Hansen, A. and Brodersen, P. (1974). The effect of ketamine on regional cerebral blood flow in man. *Anesthesiology* 41, 562—567

Hulme, A. and Cooper, R. (1972). Changes in intracranial pressure and other variables during the induction of general anaesthesia. *Proc. R. Soc. Med.* 65, 883—890

Hunter, A. R. (1964). *Neurosurgical Anaesthesia*, p. 27. Oxford: Blackwell

Jacobson, I., Harper, A. M. and McDowall, D. G. (1963). Relationship between venous pressure and cortical blood flow. *Nature, Lond.* 200, 173—175

James, I. M., Millar, R. A. and Purves, M. J. (1968). Neural pathways involved in the control of cerebral blood flow in the baboon. *J. Physiol., Lond.* 196, 34P

Jennett, W. B., McDowall, D. G. and Barker, J. (1967). The effect of halothane on intracranial pressure in cerebral tumours. Report of two cases. *J. Neurosurg.* 26, 270—274

Jennett, W. B., Barker, J., Fitch, W. and McDowall, D. G. (1969). Effect of anaesthesia on intracranial pressure in patients with space-occupying lesions. *Lancet* i, 61—64

Jörgensen, P. B. and Henriksen, H. T. (1973). The effect of fluroxene on intracranial pressure in patients with intracranial space-occupying lesions. *Br. J. Anaesth.* 45, 599—602

Keaney, N. P., McDowall, D. G., Pickerodt, V. W. A., Turner, J. M., Lane, J. R., Okuda, Y., Deshmukh, V. D. and Coroneos, N. J. (1978). Time course of the cerebral circulatory response to metabolic depression. *Am. J. Physiol.* H74—H79

Keats, A. S. and Mithoefer, J. C. (1955). Mechanism of increased intracranial pressure induced by morphine. *New Engl. J. Med.* 252, 1110—1113

Kety, S. S., Shenkin, H. A. and Schmidt, C. F. (1948). The effects of increased intracranial pressure on cerebral circulatory functions in man. *J. clin. Invest.* 27, 493—499

Koopmans, S. (1939). Function of blood vessels in brain: effect of some narcotics, hormones and drugs. *Archs neerl. Physiol.* 24, 250—266

Kreuscher, H. (1965). *Hirndurchblutung unter Neuroleptanaesthesie*. Thesis, University of Mainz

Laitinen, L. V., Johansson, G. G. and Tarkkanen, L. (1967). The effect of nitrous oxide on pulsatile cerebral impedance and cerebral blood flow. *Br. J. Anaesth.* 39, 781—785

Landau, W. M., Freygang, W. H., Rowland, L. P., Sokoloff, L. and Kety, S. S. (1955). The local circulation of the living brain; values in the unanesthetized and anesthetized cat. *Trans. Am. neurol. Ass.* 80, 125—129

Lassen, N. A. and Christensen, M. S. (1976). Physiology of cerebral blood flow. *Br. J. Anaesth.* 48, 719—734

List, W. F., Crumrine, R. S., Cascorbi, H. F. and Weiss, W. H. (1972). Increased cerebrospinal fluid pressure after ketamine. *Anesthesiology* 36, 98—99 (Corresp.)

Lundberg, N., Kjallquist, A. and Bien, C. (1959). Reduction of increased intracranial pressure by hyperventilation. *Acta psychiat. neurol. scand.* Suppl. 139, 5—64

McCall, M. L. and Taylor, H. W. (1952). The effects of morphine sulphate on cerebral circulation and metabolism in normal and toxemic pregnant women. *Am. J. Obstet. Gynec.* 64, 1131—1136

McDowall, D. G. (1965). The effects of general anaesthetics on cerebral blood flow and cerebral metabolism. *Br. J. Anaesth.* 37, 236—245

McDowall, D. G. (1966a). Cerebral haemodynamics and metabolism during general anaesthesia. *Acta anaesth. scand.* Suppl. 25, 307—311

McDowall, D. G. (1966b). Inter-relationships between blood oxygen tension and cerebral blood flow. In *Oxygen Measurement in Blood and Tissues*, p. 205. J. P. Payne and D. W. Hill (ed.). London: Churchill

McDowall, D. G. (1967a). The effects of clinical concentrations of halothane on blood flow and oxygen uptake of the cerebral cortex. *Br. J. Anaesth.* 39, 186—196

McDowall, D. G. (1967b). *The influence of volatile anaesthetic drugs on the blood flow and oxygen uptake of the cerebral cortex and on cerebrospinal fluid pressure*. MD Thesis, University of Edinburgh

McDowall, D. G. and Harper, A. M. (1965). Blood flow and oxygen uptake of the cerebral cortex of the dog during anaesthesia with different volatile agents. *Acta neurol. scand.* Suppl. 14, 146—151

McDowall, D. G. and Harper, A. M. (1969). Cerebral oxygen uptake and cerebral blood flow during the action of certain anaesthetic agents. In *Pharmakologie der lokalen Gebirndurchblutung*, p. 108. E. Betz and R. Wüllenweber (ed.). München: Gräfeling

McDowall, D. G., Harper, A. M. and Jacobson, I. (1963). Cerebral blood flow during halothane anaesthesia. *Br. J. Anaesth.* 35, 394—402

McDowall, D. G., Harper, A. M. and Jacobson, I. (1964). Cerebral blood flow during trichloroethylene anaesthesia: a comparison with halothane. *Br. J. Anaesth.* 36, 11—18

McDowall, D. G., Harper, A. M., Bloor, K., Jennett, W. B., Ledingham, I. McA. and Jacobson, I. (1965). The influence of hyperbaric oxygen and chloroform anaesthesia on the oxygen tension of cerebral venous blood. In *Hyperbaric Oxygenation*, pp. 220—227. I. McA. Ledingham (ed.). Edinburgh: E. & S. Livingstone

McDowall, D. G., Okuda, Y., Heuser, D. and Keaney, N. P. (1978). Control of cerebral vascular smooth muscle during general anaesthesia. In *Cerebral Vascular Smooth Muscle and its Control*, pp. 257—273. Ciba Foundation Symposium No. 56. Katherine Elliott and Maeve O'Connor (ed.). Amsterdam: Elsevier/Excerpta Medica

McHenry, L. C., Slocum, H. C., Bivens, H. E., Mayes, H. A. and Hayes, G. (1965). Hyperventilation in awake and anesthetized man. *Archs Neurol., Chicago* 12, 270—277

McKay, R. D., Sundt, T. M., Michenfelder, J. D., Gronert, G. A., Messick, J. M., Sharbrough, F. W. and Piepgras, D. G. (1976). Internal carotid artery stump pressure and cerebral blood flow during carotid endarterectomy. *Anesthesiology* 45, 390—399

Mackenzie, E. T., McCulloch, J., O'Keane, M., Pickard, J. D. and Harper, A. M. (1976). Cerebral circulation and norepinephrine; relevance of the blood—brain barrier. *Am. J. Physiol.* 231, 483—488

Maekawa, T., McDowall, D. G. and Okuda, Y. (1977). Oxygen tension on the brain surface during hypotension induced by haemorrhage, trimetaphan or sodium nitroprusside. In *Cerebral Function, Metabolism and Circulation*, pp. 504—505. D. H. Ingvar and N. A. Lassen (ed.). Copenhagen: Munksgaard

Mackawa, T., Sakabe, T. and Takeshita, H. (1974). Diazepam blocks cerebral metabolic and circulatory responses to local anesthetic-induced seizures. *Anesthesiology* 41, 389—391

Marx, G. F., Andrews, C. and Orkin, L. R. (1962). Cerebrospinal fluid pressure during halothane anaesthesia. *Can. Anaesth. Soc. J.* 9, 239—245

Michenfelder, J. D. (1974). The interdependency of cerebral function and metabolic effects following maximum doses of thiopental in the dog. *Anesthesiology* 41, 231—236

Michenfelder, J. D. and Cucchiara, R. F. (1974). Canine cerebral oxygen consumption during enflurane anesthesia, and its modification during induced seizures. *Anesthesiology* 40, 575—580

Michenfelder, J. D. and Theye, R. A. (1968). Hypothermia: effect on canine brain and whole body metabolism. *Anesthesiology* 29, 1107—1112

Michenfelder, J. D. and Theye, R. A. (1971). Effects of fentanyl, droperidol and innovar on canine cerebral metabolism and blood flow. *Br. J. Anaesth.* 43, 630—635

Michenfelder, J. D. and Theye, R. A. (1973). Effects of methoxyflurane on canine cerebral metabolism and blood flow. *Anesthesiology* 38, 123—127

Michenfelder, J. D. and Theye, R. A. (1977). Canine systemic and cerebral effects of hypotension induced by haemorrhage, trimetaphan, halothane or nitroprusside. *Anesthesiology* 46, 188—195

Miller, J. D. and Barker, J. (1969). The effect of neuroleptanalgesic drugs on cerebral blood flow and metabolism. *Br. J. Anaesth.* 41, 554—555

Misfeldt, B. B., Jörgensen, P. B., Spotoft, H. and Rønde, F. (1976). The effects of droperidol and fentanyl on intracranial pressure and cerebral perfusion pressure in neurosurgical patients. *Br. J. Anaesth.* 48, 963—968

Mitchell, R. A., Bainton, C. R., Severinghaus, J. W. and Edelist, G. (1964). Respiratory response and CSF pH during disturbances in blood acid—base in awake dogs with denervated aortic and carotid bodies. *Physiologist, Wash.* 7, 208

Moss, E., Powell, D., Gibson, R. M. and McDowall, D. G. (1978). The effects of fentanyl on intracranial pressure and cerebral perfusion pressure during hypocapnia. *Br. J. Anaesth.* 50, 779—784

Movita, H., Nemoto, E. M., Bleyaert, A. L. and Stezoski, S. W. (1977). Brain blood flow autoregulation and metabolism during halothane anesthesia in monkeys. *Am. J. Physiol.* 233, H670—H676

Moyer, J. H., Pontius, R., Morris, G. and Hershberger, R. (1957). Effect of morphine and *N*-allylnormorphine on cerebral haemodynamics and oxygen consumption. *Circulation* 15, 379—384

Nowill, W. K., Stephen, C. R. and Searles, P. W. (1953). Evaluation of trichloroethylene as an anaesthetic aid and analgesic agent. *Archs Surg., Chicago* 66, 35—47

Olesen, J. (1971). Contralateral focal increase of cerebral blood flow in man during arm work. *Brain* 94, 635—646

Owman, C. and Edvinsson, L. (1978). Histochemical and pharmacological approach to the investigation of neurotransmitters with particular reference to the cerebrovascular bed. In *Cerebral Vascular Smooth Muscle and its Control*, pp. 275–304. Ciba Foundation Symposium No. 56. Katherine Elliott and Maeve O'Connor (ed.). Amsterdam: Elsevier/Excerpta Medica

Pickerodt, V. W. A., McDowall, D. G., Coroneos, N. J. and Keaney, N. P. (1972). Effect of Althesin on cerebral perfusion, cerebral metabolism and intracranial pressure in the anaesthetized baboon. *Br. J. Anaesth.* **44**, 751–757

Pierce, E. C., Lambertsen, C. J., Deutsch, S., Chase, P. E., Linde, H. W., Dripps, R. D. and Price, H. L. (1962). Cerebral circulation and metabolism during thiopental anesthesia and hyperventilation in man. *J. clin. Invest.* **41**, 1664–1671

Raichle, M. E., Posner, J. B. and Plum, F. (1970). Cerebral blood flow during and after hyperventilation. *Archs Neurol, Chicago* **23**, 394–403

Rasmussen, M. J., Rosendal, T. and Overgaard, J. (1975). Paradoxical responses of regional cerebral blood flow induced by the anaesthetic drug Althesin. In *Blood Flow and Metabolism in the Brain*, pp. 11.18–11.19. A. M. Harper, W. B. Jennett, J. D. Miller and J. O. Rowan (ed.). Edinburgh: Churchill Livingstone

Reivich, M. (1964). Arterial Pco_2 and cerebral hemodynamics. *Am. J. Physiol.* **206**, 25–35

Reivich, M., Dickson, J., Clark, J., Hedden, M. and Lambertsen, C. J. (1968). Role of hypoxia in cerebral circulatory and metabolic changes during hypocarbia in man; studies in hyperbaric milieu. *Scand. J. clin. Lab. Invest.* Suppl. 102

Risberg, J. and Ingvar, D. H. (1968). Regional changes in cerebral blood volume during mental activity. *Expl Brain Res.* **5**, 72–78

Rodbard, S. (1955). Flow through collapsible tubes; augmented flow produced by resistance at the outlet. *Circulation* **11**, 280–287

Rosomoff, H. L. (1956). Some effects of hypothermia on the normal and abnormal physiology of the nervous system. *Proc. R. Soc. Med.* **49**, 358–364

Rubio, R., Berne, R. M. and Winn, H. R. (1978). Production, metabolism and possible functions of adenosine in brain tissue *in situ*. In *Cerebral Vascular Smooth Muscle and its Control*, pp. 355–378. Ciba Foundation Symposium No. 56. Katherine Elliott and Maeve O'Connor (ed.). Amsterdam: Elsevier/Excerpta Medica

Saidman, L. J. and Eger, E. I. (1965). Change in cerebrospinal fluid pressure during pneumoencephalography under nitrous oxide anesthesia. *Anesthesiology* **26**, 67–72

Sakabe, T., Kuramoto, T., Kumagae, S. and Takeshita, H. (1976). Cerebral response to the addition of nitrous oxide to halothane in man. *Br. J. Anaesth.* **48**, 957–962

Sakabe, T., Kuramoto, T., Inoue, S. and Takeshita, H. (1978). Cerebral effects of nitrous oxide in the dog. *Anesthesiology* **48**, 195–200

Samuel, J. R., Grange, R. A. and Hawkins, J. D. (1968). Anaesthetic techniques for carotid angiography. *Anaesthesia* **23**, 543–551

Sari, A., Okuda, Y. and Takeshita, H. (1972a). The effect of ketamine on cerebrospinal fluid pressure. *Anesth. Analg. curr. Res.* **51**, 560–565

Sari, A., Okuda, Y. and Takeshita, H. (1972b). The effects of Thalamonal on cerebral circulation and oxygen consumption in man. *Br. J. Anaesth.* **44**, 330–334

Sari, A., Maekawa, T., Tahjo, M., Okuda, Y. and Takeshita, H. (1976). Effects of Althesin on cerebral blood flow and oxygen consumption in man. *Br. J. Anaesth.* **48**, 545–550

Schmidt, C. F. (1934). The intrinsic regulation of the circulation in the hypothalamus of the cat. *Am. J. Physiol.* **110**, 137–152

Schmidt, C. F. and Pierson, J. C. (1934). The intrinsic regulation of the blood vessels of the medulla oblongata. *Am. J. Physiol.* **108**, 241–263

Severinghaus, J. W. (1965). Regulation of pH on the cerebral cortex. *J. Physiol, Lond.* **181**, 35P

Severinghaus, J. W. and Lassen, N. (1967). Step hypocapnia to separate arterial from tissue Pco_2 in the regulation of cerebral blood flow. *Circulation Res.* **20**, 272–278

Severinghaus, J. W., Chiodi, H., Eger, E. I., Brandstater, B. and Hornbein, T. F. (1966). Cerebral blood flow in man at high altitude. *Circulation Res.* **19**, 274–282

Shapiro, H. M., Wyte, S. R. and Harris, A. B. (1972). Ketamine anaesthesia in patients with intracranial pathology. *Br. J. Anaesth.* **44**, 1200–1204

Shapiro, H. M., Galindo, A., Wyte, S. R. and Harris, A. B. (1973). Rapid intraoperative reduction of intracranial pressure with thiopentone. *Br. J. Anaesth.* **45**, 1057–1062

Sokoloff, L. (1959). The action of drugs on the cerebral circulation. *Pharmac. Rev.* **11**, 1–85

Søndergard, W. (1961). Intracranial pressure during general anaesthesia. *Dan. med. Bull.* **8**, 18–25

Takahashi, T., Takasaki, M., Namiki, A. and Dohi, S. (1973). Effects of Althesin on cerebrospinal fluid pressure. *Br. J. Anaesth.* **45**, 179–183

Takeshita, H., Michenfelder, J. D. and Theye, R. A. (1972). The effects of morphine and N-allylnormorphine on canine cerebral metabolism and circulation. *Anesthesiology* 37, 605—612

Takeshita, H., Miyauchi, F. and Ishikawa, T. (1973). Canine cerebral oxygen consumption studies related to electroencephalogram during propanid anesthesia. *Acta anaesth. scand.* 17, 227—237

Takeshita, H., Okuda, Y. and Sari, A. (1972). The effects of ketamine on cerebral circulation and metabolism in man. *Anesthesiology* 36, 69—75

Theye, R. A. and Michenfelder, H. D. (1968). The effect of nitrous oxide on canine cerebral metabolism. *Anesthesiology* 29, 1119—1124

Thomas, D. J., Marshall, J., Ross Russell, R. W., Wetherley-Mein, G., Du Boulay, G. H., Pearson, T. C., Symon, L. and Zilkha, E. (1977). Effect of haematocrit on cerebral blood flow in man. *Lancet* ii, 941—943

Turner, J. M., Coroneos, N. J., Gibson, R. M., Powell, D., Ness, M. A. and McDowall, D. G. (1972). The effect of Althesin on intracranial pressure in man. *Br. J. Anaesth.* 45, 168—171

Weitzner, S. W., McCoy, G. T. and Binder, L. S. (1963). Effects of morphine, levallorphan and respiratory gases on increased intracranial pressure. *Anesthesiology* 24, 291—298

White, J. C., Verlot, M., Selverstone, B. and Beecher, H. K. (1942). Changes in brain volume during anesthesia: the effects of anoxia and hypercapnia. *Archs Surg., Chicago* 44, 1—21

Wilkinson, I. M. S. and Browne, D. R. G. (1970). The influence of anaesthesia and arterial hypocapnia on regional blood flow in the normal human cerebral hemisphere. *Br. J. Anaesth.* 42, 472—482

Wollman, H., Alexander, S. C., Cohen, P. J., Chase, P. E., Melman, E. and Behar, M. G. (1964). Cerebral circulation of man during halothane anesthesia. *Anesthesiology* 25, 180—184

Wollman, H., Alexander, S. C., Cohen, P. J., Smith, T. C., Chase, P. E. and van der Molen, R. A. (1965). Cerebral circulation during general anesthesia and hyperventilation in man. *Anesthesiology* 26, 329—334

Woringer, E., Brogly, G. and Dorgler, R. (1954). New studies on the mechanisms of variation of venous and CSF pressures under the influence of certain general anaesthetics. *Anaesth. et Analg.* 11, 18—33

Woringer, E., Brogly, G. and Schneider, J. (1951). Study of the action of generally used anaesthetics on CSF pressure. *Anesth. et Analg.* 8, 649—662

Wyte, S. R., Shapiro, H. M., Turner, P. and Harris, A. B. (1972). Ketamine-induced intracranial hypertension. *Anesthesiology* 36, 174—176

Zattoni, J., Siani, C. and Rivano, C. (1973). The effects of Ethrane on intracranial pressure. In *Proceedings of the First European Symposium on Modern Anesthetic Agents,* pp. 272—279. P. Lawin and R. Beer (ed.). Berlin: Springer-Verlag

Zattoni, J., Siani, C. and Rivano, C. (1974). Effects of Ethrane on intracranial pressure. In *Ethrane,* pp. 272—279. P. Lawin and R. Beer (ed.). Berlin: Springer-Verlag

34 Preoperative assessment of the cardiovascular system
E. B. Raftery

The most important single factor in the reduction of surgical mortality and morbidity in the last 50 years has been the recognition that correct and careful preparation of the patient, whether in an emergency situation or for elective surgery, is essential. The ultimate responsibility for determining whether the patient is fit for anaesthesia, whether he will survive the postoperative period without significant deterioration and what form of treatment may be necessary to bring him to the appropriate state of readiness, rests squarely with the anaesthetist. It is estimated that 25–40% of all patients have medical diseases requiring treatment before operation (Kyei-Mensah and Thornton, 1974), a figure which clearly indicates the size of the problem.

As in all preoperative assessment, the most difficult part of the cardiovascular assessment is timing. There can be no doubt that the night before planned surgery is not the most appropriate time for the discovery of serious cardiac disease. Furthermore, it is not likely that the efforts of the surgical house officer, no matter how well intentioned, will be adequate in the detection of minor, but important, disease processes. It is sometimes argued that anaesthesia and surgery are very safe and the numbers of operative and perioperative deaths are so small that there is little point to preoperative assessment. This is fortunately true, but there is equally no doubt that postoperative morbidity is much improved if the patient has been properly prepared for the operation – a consideration of great importance in these days of elective and 'cosmetic' surgery.

Some anaesthetists (Burn, 1978) favour the concept of an outpatient clinic to which prospective surgical candidates are referred and where they can be assessed by the anaesthetist well ahead of time. This is hardly a practical proposition for all hospitals, but a reasonable compromise would be a cardiovascular questionnaire (Raftery, Cocker and Holland, 1971) to be completed by the surgical staff for all patients who are entered onto surgical waiting lists. These forms would be scanned by the anaesthetic staff and appropriate action taken if the answers were not satisfactory. In any case, no patient should go to surgery without an examination of the cardiovascular system, and for elective surgery, an ECG and chest x-ray should be available in every patient over the age of 45 years.

HISTORY

The three most important features of the cardiovascular history are the patient's smoking habits, a detailed statement of drugs being taken at the time of hospital admission and a specific question on the history of possible myocardial infarction in the previous year. Apart from the possibility of interaction between anaesthetic agents and drugs (particularly antihypertensive drugs), congestive heart failure and recent myocardial infarction carry a markedly increased risk of mortality and morbidity during and following anaesthesia (Tarhan *et al.*, 1972). Elective surgery in the first six months following myocardial infarction carries a 6% risk of perioperative reinfarction with an 80% mortality rate. The answers to these specific features are usually sufficient to clear the way for safe anaesthesia but specific inquiry into other cardiovascular symptoms may be necessary before a decision can be taken.

Dyspnoea

Patients will often reply positively to an enquiry for shortness of breath, and it is more informative to ask if there has been any change in their ability to perform everyday tasks such as housework or walking upstairs without undue dyspnoea over the previous year. Cardiac dyspnoea is closely associated with physical exertion and is seldom accompanied by wheezing. A history of deteriorating exercise tolerance should always be regarded with suspicion and lead to a search for abnormal cardiac physical signs. Attacks of episodic nocturnal dyspnoea may be suggestive of left ventricular failure but seldom occur without a background of deteriorating exercise tolerance.

A positive response to questioning for dyspnoea should lead to a search for a history of previous cardiac disease (such as rheumatic fever or myocardial infarction), and other cardiac symptoms such as ankle swelling. The causes of peripheral oedema are legion, and ankle swelling without exertional dyspnoea is seldom due to congestive heart failure.

Chest pain

Once again, this is a very common complaint but does not always indicate ischaemic heart disease. Anginal pain is characterized by its close relationship to exertion, substernal position radiating to the throat and jaw and the arms (particularly the left), and by its 'gripping' or 'crushing' nature.

However, anginal pain is notoriously variable and always requires confirmation by means of a 12-lead ECG. If this is normal despite a suspicious history, it is essential to have an exercise ECG before excluding the possibility of ischaemia.

The cardinal sign of myocardial ischaemia is flat depression of the ST segment which may be seen in any lead (*Figure 34.1*). There is complete

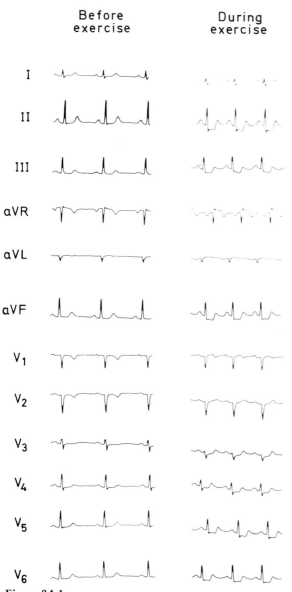

Figure 34.1

An ischaemic electrocardiogram. The left-hand column shows a normal ECG before exercise and the right-hand column shows very characteristic flat ST segment depression occurring in most leads during exercise. This appearance is characteristic of myocardial ischaemia agreement among cardiologists that depression of this kind greater than 1 mm below the isoelectric line is significant of obstructive coronary artery disease. There is less agreement about depression of less than 1 mm, particularly when the ST segment is not flat but slopes upward, and the opinion of an experienced cardiologist should always be sought if there is any doubt.

The importance of myocardial ischaemia to the anaesthetist lies in particular care to avoid abrupt falls in blood pressure and hypoxia under the anaesthetic, and the increased tendency for dangerous arrhythmias to be precipitated by the anaesthetic agent.

Minor symptoms

PALPITATIONS

A straightforward enquiry for this symptom will frequently elicit a positive response, particularly in the elderly, who suffer from paroxysmal arrhythmias much more frequently than is commonly realized. It is well known that anaesthetic agents provoke new arrhythmias more commonly in patients who have established arrhythmias (see Chapter 32), but it is not known if the same applies to paroxysmal sufferers. The resting ECG is commonly normal in patients with paroxysmal arrhythmias, but despite this it is mandatory that an ECG be available to the anaesthetist when the patient has a complaint of palpitations. If there is a suspicion of paroxysmal arrhythmias but no confirmatory evidence, then it is justifiable to proceed with the procedure, always bearing in mind the possibility of provoking arrhythmias with agents such as the halogenated hydrocarbons and local infiltration with catecholamines, and having lignocaine and a β blocker available for correction.

TIREDNESS AND FATIGUE

These symptoms are frequently associated with cardiac disease but are so common in other conditions, such as depression, that they are of no value in a cardiovascular assessment unless associated with major symptoms.

PHYSICAL EXAMINATION

The basic requirement of physical examination before anaesthesia is to uncover those conditions which are likely to increase an anaesthetic risk. These are hypertension, ischaemic heart disease, arrhythmias and heart failure from any cause.

Hypertension

Blood pressure measurement is one of the simplest and most informative procedures of any physical examination, and yet it is frequently carried out carelessly or even omitted by the surgical house-staff. No patient should go to surgery without a record of the blood pressure, even if only because of the comparative value if complications should arise. It is now established that blood pressure fluctuations during surgery are much greater in the uncontrolled than the controlled hypertensive (Prys-Roberts, Meloche and Foëx, 1971), no matter what agent has been used, and a diastolic pressure in excess of 15 kPa (110 mmHg) should always call for consideration of the urgency of the procedure and the possibility of preoperative cardiological referral.

The technique used for measuring blood pressure should always be the auscultatory method using a mercury-in-glass sphygmomanometer and recording the pressure at Korotkoff I (appearance of sound), IV (muffling) and V (disappearance). Korotkoff IV (muffling) is probably the best indicator of diastolic pressure, but it is often useful to have the Korotkoff V pressure as well, since a wide difference between the two will suggest vasodilated states with high cardiac output. A single high recording of blood pressure is of little value, particularly if the patient is nervous. The pulse rate is a useful clue to this state, and a good indicator for repeated readings.

It is now generally accepted that it is unwise to stop antihypertensive therapy before surgery, and even the disruption of reflexes produced by the β-blocking drugs is not a serious hazard during anaesthesia. However, the impact of surgery on the cardiovascular system is such that blood pressure often falls considerably during the postoperative period and may remain very low for a variable period up to six weeks. Thus it is wise to halve the dose of antihypertensive drugs postoperatively, and then adjust the dosage on a day-to-day basis, using a four-hourly pressure chart as a guide.

Myocardial ischaemia

The presence or absence of ischaemic heart disease cannot be detected by physical examination, although suspicion may be aroused by the presence of a fourth heart sound on auscultation of the heart. The diagnosis rests firmly upon the detection of characteristic changes in the ECG, either at rest or after exercise (see *Figure 34.1*), and the opinion of an experienced cardiologist should always be sought if there is any doubt.

Arrhythmias

The presence of cardiac arrhythmias can be deduced from irregularity of the pulse, and much can be inferred about the arrhythmias from the nature of the irregularity. However, once again the accurate diagnosis of the arrhythmia rests squarely with the electrocardiogram, and is of paramount importance (see Chapter 32). Right ventricular ectopic beats (Chapter 32) may be safely ignored, but left ventricular ectopic beats will call for active suppression with mexiletine (100 mg t.i.d.). Uncontrolled atrial fibrillation will require digoxin (0.25 mg twice daily orally for five days) to establish a controlled ventricular response before anaesthesia. Whenever a serious arrhythmia is discovered, the causes must be sought before anaesthesia is contemplated.

Heart failure

Heart failure is the one feature of the cardiovascular assessment which depends heavily on the results of physical examination. No patient should go to anaesthesia without a clear record of the presence or absence of pitting oedema of the ankles and sacrum, and the height of the jugular venous pressure must always be estimated. With the patient sitting at an angle of 45°, the right external jugular vein should be identified where it crosses the sternomastoid muscle. Light pressure with a finger just below the angle of the jaw stops the venous flow in the vessel, which then forms a conduit connecting indirectly with the right atrium. The upper level of the blood column can then be noted and referred by a horizontal line to the level of the sternal angle. A jugular venous pressure higher than 2 cm above the sternal angle is strongly suggestive of a raised central venous pressure. Estimations using the external jugular vein may be inaccurate because the vein traverses the fascia of the neck; therefore, a suspicion of raised venous pressure on the right side should be confirmed by a similar estimation on the left. Some authorities maintain that only the internal jugular vein should be used for venous pressure estimates because it is in direct communication with the right atrium with no possibility of fascial trapping, but the internal jugular cannot easily be occluded and it is seldom easily visible except in gross congestive heart failure.

A static column of blood connecting the jugular vein with the right atrium will show the pulsations which are present in that chamber and these can be detected by the naked eye. In sinus rhythm there is an a-wave which coincides with atrial systole and may be very large if there is pulmonary hypertension or pulmonary valve stenosis. The a-wave is closely followed by a second or v-wave which accompanies right atrial filling during systole. This wave may be markedly accentuated in tricuspid incompetence, whether organic or functional in origin.

A cardinal sign of congestive heart failure is an enlarged and tender liver which may be palpated below the right costal margin. Auscultation of the lung bases over the back may reveal the characteristic fine rales which are symptomatic of alveolar wall oedema resulting from the raised pulmonary venous pressure found in left ventricular failure. The characteristic auscultatory finding in the failing heart is a fourth heart sound, which may be obscured by murmurs and other sounds if there is an underlying organic valve lesion. (This is dealt with in more detail in the next section.) If there is any suspicion of heart failure, it is essential that a chest x-ray be examined for enlargement of the heart, hilar congestion, pleural effusion and the short straight-line opacities at the lung bases due to lymphatic congestion and known as Kerly B lines.

Examination of the venous system in the legs for evidence of varicose veins or chronic venous disease is always worth while in forecasting postoperative deep vein thrombosis and pulmonary embolization.

AUSCULTATION OF THE HEART

Skilled auscultation of the heart is not a basic requirement for the anaesthetist. Valve lesions do not predispose to anaesthetic or surgical complications, except in the case of cardiac surgery, and the fine points of precise diagnosis should be left to the cardiologist. However, it is important that the anaesthetist be able to time a murmur, since diastolic murmurs are always abnormal and demand a specialist referral at all times. Timing is readily made by simultaneous auscultation of the precordium and palpation of the carotid pulse.

Auscultation should be performed in all four classic areas — aortic, pulmonary, tricuspid and mitral (Oram, 1971) — with the object of identifying the first and second heart sounds, noting their intensity and observing the presence of additional sounds and murmurs.

Of particular importance to the anaesthetist is the detection of auscultatory signs of pulmonary hypertension and heart failure. In pulmonary hypertension the second heart sound in the pulmonary area is very loud and there may be additional signs of right ventricular hypertrophy such as a heaving precordial impulse to the left of the sternum. The most important auscultatory sign of heart failure is the fourth heart sound — a soft low-frequency noise which comes just before the first heart sound and is heard best in the mitral area. The importance of this sound can be appreciated by a brief explanation of its origin.

The atrium contracts at the end of the diastolic period of the cardiac cycle and abruptly increases the volume of the already full ventricle by about one-sixth. This sudden increase in stretch of the ventricular myocardium heralds the rapid shortening and ejection at the beginning of systole, and is accompanied by a sharp increase in ventricular pressure (the end-diastolic pressure). When the ventricular myocardium is normal, this atrial contribution to the events of systole is not critical and the absence of a co-ordinated atrial systole makes little difference to cardiac output or stroke output. However, when the myocardium is impaired, the atrial component of diastole and the increase in initial fibre length which it produces at the onset of systole play a vital role in the maintenance of an adequate stroke output. The vigour of atrial systole is increased and the force of ventricular filling produces vibrations which are interpreted by the ear as a sound (the fourth heart sound) which appears just before the first heart sound. Thus a fourth heart sound may be right or left ventricular in origin, and its appearance suggests myocardial failure. However, a fourth heart sound may be physiological, especially in thin-chested and young persons.

The third heart sound is a similar low-frequency noise which occurs much earlier in diastole, i.e. after the second heart sound. This sound is commonly physiological, especially in young persons, but is also associated with conditions in which there is dilatation of the ventricles (e.g. left-to-right shunts, mitral incompetence).

This is not the place for a dissertation on the types and significance of murmurs, but systolic murmurs are so common that the anaesthetist should be able to distinguish an innocent from an organic murmur. Innocent murmurs are soft, usually late systolic in timing and are most commonly located in the pulmonary area. They vary in intensity with position, often disappearing completely with exercise. Most importantly of all, they are not associated with any history of heart disease but are associated with a normal ECG and chest x-ray. Organic murmurs are loud, do not vary significantly with position and are almost always associated with a history of heart disease, an abnormal ECG and characteristic x-ray appearances. The problems presented by heart blocks and hemiblocks are dealt with in Chapter 32.

SUMMARY

The most important information required for a preoperative cardiovascular assessment is an accurate history — particularly of myocardial infarction — a knowledge of drugs being taken and their dosages, elimination of the signs of heart failure and an accurate measurement of the blood pressure. This information is best recorded at the time of entry on to the surgical waiting list, and passed to the anaesthetic staff for appropriate action. A chest x-ray and resting ECG are invaluable ancillary aids. Vigorous attention to blood pressure control, heart failure and control of serious arrhythmias are essential features of modern preoperative preparation.

References

Burn, J. M. B. (1978). Pre-operative care. *Br. J. hosp. Med.* **19**, 425—432

Kyei-Mensah, K. and Thornton, J. A. (1974). The incidence of medical disease in surgical patients. *Br. J. Anaesth.* **46**, 570—574

Oram, S. (1971). *Clinical Heart Disease*, pp. 65—105. London: Heinemann Medical

Prys-Roberts, C., Meloche, R. and Foëx, P. (1971). Studies of anaesthesia in relation to hypertension. I. Cardiovascular responses of treated and untreated patients. *Br. J. Anaesth.* **43**, 122—137

Raftery, E. B., Cocker, P. and Holland, W. W. (1971). Value of electrocardiogram in population studies. An attempt to improve interpretation. *Br. Heart J.* **33**, 837—840

Tarhan, S., Emerson, A. M., Taylor, W. F. and Gulliami, E. R. (1972). Myocardial infarction after general anesthesia. *J. Am. med. Ass.* **220**, 1451—1454

35 Anaesthesia for patients with cardiac disease and hypertension
G. W. Burton and H.G.R. Balmer

Cardiac disease and hypertension can markedly affect a patient's responses to anaesthesia and to surgery. The operative risk may be increased, depending upon the severity of the disease and the magnitude of the surgical procedure. Suitable preoperative treatment of the disease and appropriate management both during surgery and in the postoperative period can greatly reduce the risk, although it must be remembered that in some cases the therapy itself may modify the responses of the patient.

PREOPERATIVE PREPARATION OF THE PATIENT WITH HEART DISEASE

General management of cardiac failure

Cardiac failure is the state in which the heart is unable to maintain an adequate circulation despite there being a satisfactory filling pressure (see Chapter 31). The cardiac glycosides and diuretics remain the most important drugs used in its treatment, a full account of these drugs being given in Chapter 37.

Whenever possible, cardiac failure should be brought under control prior to surgery. Adequate rest can be a very useful adjunct to specific therapy; prolonged bed rest, however, predisposes to deep vein thrombosis and in most patients it may be preferable to restrict activity rather than to enforce complete bed rest. Patients in severe failure, especially those with pulmonary congestion and oedema, may benefit from a preoperative period of intermittent positive pressure ventilation (IPPV). The tendency towards pulmonary oedema will be reduced by the increased intra-alveolar pressure, and the work of breathing, which puts an extra load upon the heart, will be reduced. This is of particular value in infants, where the work of breathing can be considerable.

A large pericardial effusion can cause a high intrapericardial pressure, which limits the diastolic filling of the ventricles and thereby restricts the cardiac output. These patients have a high central venous pressure and may show a marked pulsus paradoxus. The very limited ability to compensate for the cardiovascular effects of anaesthetic agents makes it advisable to aspirate the fluid, and so relieve the raised intrapericardial pressure prior to attempting induction of anaesthesia. Pleural effusions or ascites may cause respiratory embarrassment and require preoperative drainage.

Preoperative therapy with the cardiac glycosides

An account of the cardiac glycosides and diuretics is given in Chapter 37. However, it should be mentioned here that anaesthesia and surgery, especially cardiac surgery, can affect a patient's tolerance to the cardiac glycosides. Their action may be greatly increased by a fall in plasma potassium, by a low P_{CO_2}, by drugs such as suxamethonium and the anticholinesterases, by catecholamines and by hypoxia (Selzer *et al.*, 1966). Because digoxin is excreted mainly by the kidneys, renal dysfunction can also lead to dangerous cumulative effects (see Chapter 37).

An arrhythmia which might have been caused by the toxic effects of a cardiac glycoside, or which may require an increased dosage for its control, can present diagnostic difficulties. Where such doubt exists, it may be useful to give potassium chloride (2 mmol) intravenously, which can be repeated after 4—6 minutes if the arrhythmia has not been controlled and there are no ECG signs of an elevated potassium. Should this not be successful, antidysrhythmic drugs may be used. At normal potassium levels the therapeutic range of digoxin is usually $1-2$ ng·ml^{-1} of blood.

Because of these dangers, the routine preoperative digitalization of all patients suspected of incipient heart failure is not to be recommended (Juler, Stemmer and Conolly, 1969). However, patients who are in heart failure and have a persistent tachycardia, especially if the heart is enlarged, may benefit greatly from preoperative digitalization. Normally the drug should be withdrawn 36 hours preoperatively, the reduced blood level at the time of surgery being offset by the increased sensitivity to the drug.

Cardiac glycoside therapy is contraindicated in conditions such as obstructive cardiomyopathy, constrictive pericarditis and incomplete heart block.

Myocardial ischaemia

Following myocardial infarction, the risk of anaesthesia decreases with the passage of time, but it is also related to the persistence of signs of myocardial injury. The risk is particularly high within the first 15 days (Fraser, Ramachandran and Davis, 1967). Goldman *et al.* (1977), reviewing the risks to cardiac patients undergoing non-cardiac operations, have demonstrated a higher than normal perioperative mortality in the period up to six months following a proven infarct. Sapala, Ponka and Duvernoy (1975) found an extremely high mortality in patients who still had an arrhythmia, heart block or congestive failure attributable to an infarct which had occurred during the three months prior to anaesthesia.

Re-infarction may not necessarily be associated with chest pain and carries a mortality rate of over 50% (Tarhan *et al.*, 1972). The risk appears to be independent of the type and duration of anaesthesia, but is greater in association with upper abdominal and thoracic operations.

Patients who have had a myocardial infarct more than six months previously, who are well compensated and free from cardiac failure and angina and who are in normal sinus rhythm, have only a slightly higher mortality risk than patients who are in a similar age group, are undergoing similar procedures and who have not had a myocardial infarct.

Should it be necessary to anaesthetize a patient shortly after myocardial infarction, or one who has severe myocardial ischaemia from any other cause, it is particularly important to take the utmost care to reduce to a minimum the inevitable depressant effects of anaesthesia upon the heart and circulation and to avoid causing hypoxia. It is possible that a certain degree of protection of the myocardium may be conferred by the slow intravenous administration of 200–300 ml of a glucose–insulin–potassium mixture (500 ml of 50% glucose, containing 80 units of insulin and 100 mmol of potassium chloride) (Opie and Owen, 1976). Further protection may be afforded by high dosage steroid administration, such as 30 mg·kg^{-1} of methylprednisolone (Lozman *et al.*, 1975).

THE CARDIAC GLYCOSIDES IN MYOCARDIAL ISCHAEMIA

The cardiac glycosides increase the myocardial oxygen consumption of the normal sized heart. However, the more important factor in oxygen requirement is the intramyocardial tension which is developed. Digitalization of the enlarged, failing heart increases its efficiency and so reduces the left ventricular end-diastolic volume. From Laplace's law, which relates wall tension to internal pressure, the smaller the size of the ventricular cavity, the lower will be the intramyocardial tension which is required to develop any particular systolic ejection pressure. The resultant fall in myocardial oxygen requirement is greater than any increase caused by the direct effect of the cardiac glycoside on the heart muscle.

Thus, when myocardial ischaemia is accompanied by heart failure and consequent increase in the left ventricular end-diastolic volume, digitalization may be beneficial, because of both its positive inotropic effect and the reduction in myocardial oxygen consumption; however, if the heart is not enlarged, the resultant increase in oxygen consumption can be harmful. A guide to the likelihood of benefit may be obtained from pulmonary wedge pressure measurements, using a flow-guided balloon-tipped catheter (see page 704). If the left ventricular filling pressure is over 2.4–2.7 kPa (18–20 mmHg) and fails to respond to the intravenous use of potent diuretics, digitalization should be undertaken.

Because of the increased sensitivity to the cardiac glycosides, only two-thirds of the standard dosage should be used (Mason, 1974).

Disorders of conduction

These are dealt with more fully in Chapter 32. Nevertheless, there are a few points of importance to the anaesthetist which should be mentioned here.

ATRIOVENTRICULAR BLOCK

First and second degree block, and less frequently third degree block, may result from the excessive electrophysiological effects of the cardiac glycosides, or it may be caused by excessive vagal tone. This type of block is frequently abolished by the use of large amounts of atropine (1.2 mg) given with the premedication; further amounts (0.3–0.6 mg) may be given intravenously if required. Ischaemic damage is the most common cause of third degree block and is sometimes the cause of second degree block. Right bundle block is not uncommon in otherwise healthy people, although it may be seen in some types of congenital heart disease or follow myocardial infarction. On the other hand, left bundle branch block is usually indicative of heart disease, most commonly of ischaemic origin.

Patients with the combination of heart block and cardiac failure can present a particularly difficult problem. The use of digitalis in patients with partial block can be dangerous, because it decreases the conduction velocity and prolongs the refractory period of nodal tissue. It is not contraindicated in complete heart block (third degree) or in bundle branch block, when its positive inotropic effects may be of value. Beta-adrenergic agonist drugs, such as isoprenaline, can be used to increase the idioventricular rate during anaesthesia induced with minimal amounts of an intravenous agent and maintained with nitrous oxide, oxygen and relaxant. However, β-stimulant drugs used in association with the halogenated hydrocarbons and cyclopropane can be dangerous, because of the possibility of producing ventricular fibrillation.

PACEMAKERS

If the patient has an unstable block, or is in failure, it is advisable to insert a pacemaker catheter into the heart under local anaesthesia preoperatively (Simon, 1977). The patient can then, if necessary, safely be digitalized and the heart rate controlled by the pacemaker. It may be safer to avoid the use of diathermy, because it can affect the performance of some pacemakers and cause ventricular fibrillation, although with modern pacemakers this is said to be unlikely.

ACCELERATED CONDUCTION

In the Wolff–Parkinson–White syndrome there is an accessory atrio-ventricular pathway and the rate of conduction from the atria to the ventricles is faster than normal, the P–R interval being less than 0.12 second. Patients with this syndrome are prone to recurrent attacks of supraventricular tachycardia, caused by re-entry (Wellens and Durber, 1975). Such attacks can be dangerous and difficult to treat, but usually they respond to lignocaine, disopyramide, amiodarone, verapamil or β-blocking agents. Atropine can restore a normal QRS complex by accelerating conduction through the AV node (Narula, 1973); however, it may precipitate a disproportionate tachycardia, making it preferable to use hyoscine for premedication (Hannington-Kiff, 1968).

Associated diseases

Heart failure may be secondary to, or aggravated by, other diseases which should be treated preoperatively. For example, it is common for respiratory disease to be associated with heart failure, and energetic treatment preoperatively will greatly reduce the risks of anaesthesia and surgery. Treatment of anaemia is important, but may be difficult because transfusion can easily overload the circulation; this problem can usually be avoided by giving frequent small quantities of packed cells and simultaneously administering potent diuretics. Thyrotoxicosis may be the cause of atrial fibrillation and heart failure and should be treated, as well as its cardiac effects. Hepatic and renal disease may be associated with large changes in plasma proteins and blood pH, and so alter the protein binding of drugs.

The effects of cardiac failure upon drug elimination

In heart failure the cardiac output is reduced, causing a corresponding fall in liver blood flow. Consequently there is a diminished ability to metabolize drugs, such as lignocaine and propranolol, which have a high hepatic clearance rate (Stenson, Constantino and Harrison, 1971). In addition to this, chronic hepatic congestion or hypoxia can impair the metabolic capacity of the liver (Nies, Shand and Wilkinson, 1976; Bond, 1978). Treatment of the heart failure may restore dosage requirements to more normal levels.

MANAGEMENT OF ANAESTHESIA

Patients with severe heart disease have a restricted ability to compensate for circulatory changes, and there may be narrow limits of tolerance to the effects of anaesthetic drugs, the stresses of surgery, blood loss and changes in posture. Preoperative preparation, with rest and drug therapy, may produce a dramatic improvement in the condition of the patient and so reduce the risk of operation. However, in some cases surgery may be urgent, not allowing sufficient time to achieve the full benefit of medical treatment, and in other patients the response to treatment may be limited.

It is important that anaesthesia is conducted well within the limits of tolerance set by the patient. Especially when there is a gross prolongation of the circulation time, it is essential to avoid sudden changes and to take extreme care in the use of drugs which could precipitate a fall in arterial pressure. Myocardial hypoxia is particularly dangerous and may be caused by a lowering of the arterial oxygen saturation, hypotension or an increase in the workload upon the heart. Should the oxygen supply to the heart become critical, a vicious circle can be set up, the falling cardiac output and blood pressure reducing the coronary blood flow and myocardial oxygen supply, leading to an accelerating circulatory collapse. Despite these problems, it is usually possible, with good premedication and appropriate choice and administration of drugs, to induce anaesthesia both pleasantly and safely.

Except for minor procedures, it is advisable to control pulmonary ventilation, using light anaesthesia and muscle relaxation. The induction of anaesthesia and endotracheal intubation must be smooth, taking care to avoid excessive sympathetic reflex activity, especially in patients who have a severe degree of heart failure or hypertension (see below).

In critically ill patients it is essential to avoid any undue fall in arterial blood pressure, and it is then safer to use a muscle relaxant, such as pancuronium, which does not cause systemic vasodilatation. Potent analgesics which have minimal cardiovascular effects, such as levorphanol and fentanyl, can be given intravenously in relatively large amounts, ensuring an adequate depth of anaesthesia in the presence of a high inspired oxygen concentration, and so avoiding the circulatory depressant effects which may be caused by inhalational agents.

In the poor-risk patient it is frequently advisable, postoperatively, to continue the control of ventilation until the cardiovascular system has become more stable. This also avoids any danger arising from respiratory inadequacy resulting from the persistent effects of either a muscle relaxant or a potent analgesic.

Premedication

It is important that patients with cardiac disease are adequately sedated before operation. This reduces the amount of anaesthetic agent required to induce anaesthesia, avoiding the sudden hypotensive effects which can be produced by larger amounts of intravenous agents and greatly facilitating induction of anaesthesia with a nitrous oxide—oxygen mixture. If the patient is inadequately sedated on arrival in the anaesthetic room, a gentle smooth induction can be achieved more easily by intravenous supplementation of the premedication.

Premedication in general is discussed in Chapter 47, although here it is necessary to mention some particular points in relation to the use of atropine. Both the antisialogogic and vagolytic effects can be beneficial.

However, in the Wolff–Parkinson–White syndrome (see page 697), and occasionally in severe mitral stenosis, a tachycardia can be dangerous and it may be advisable to avoid its use (see page 704).

Atropine is necessary in the premedication of patients receiving therapy with β-blocking drugs, to protect them from unopposed vagal activity. Similarly, it should be used in patients in whom vagal overactivity is causing adverse circulatory effects, such as some degree of heart block. In these patients the dosage of atropine should be high (at least 20 μg·kg^{-1}), in order to give the heart adequate protection. Atropine should also be included in the premedication of infants with cyanotic heart disease, bradycardia being relatively common especially during cardiac surgery and diagnostic catheterization. In these patients a fall in heart rate usually precedes any fall in arterial pressure; if the myocardium has become hypoxic, this bradycardia may not respond to atropine and relatively large amounts of isoprenaline or adrenaline may be required.

Problems associated with induction of anaesthesia

There are two types of patient who are particularly likely to present problems during induction: those in whom there is severe heart failure with a restricted cardiac output and slow circulation time, and patients with congenital heart disease where there is a right-to-left shunt together with a lesion restricting pulmonary perfusion.

PATIENTS WITH RESTRICTED CARDIAC OUTPUT

In patients with severe mitral or aortic valve disease or with constrictive pericarditis or a large pericardial effusion, the cardiac output is restricted and the circulation time prolonged. In such cases it is not uncommon to find an arm–brain circulation time of approximately one minute, and in very ill patients it can be as long as two to four minutes.

Patients with this severity of heart failure also show a greatly increased sensitivity to intravenous anaesthetic agents as regards their depressant effects both upon the level of consciousness and on the cardiovascular system. In order to avoid dangerous hypotension when anaesthesia is induced with an intravenous agent, the initial dosage must be kept very small and, before giving further increments, a note made both of its effects and of the time taken for its action to commence.

Suxamethonium is hydrolysed in the blood stream, and Harrison (1966) has shown that where there is a slow peripheral circulation, an initial dosage of 100 mg may be required to produce complete paralysis.

PATIENTS WITH RESTRICTED PULMONARY PERFUSION

Induction of anaesthesia can be particularly dangerous and difficult in patients who have a congenital cardiac defect with a large right-to-left shunt and restricted pulmonary perfusion as may be seen in Fallot's tetralogy, some cases of tricuspid atresia and patent ductus arteriosus with a reversed shunt. In these patients there is a free communication between the two ventricles (or pulmonary artery and aorta) and the amount of blood which flows to the lungs is dependent upon the relative outflow resistances of the systemic and pulmonary circulations. A reduction in pulmonary blood flow may be caused either by systemic hypotension, which lowers the resistance to outflow via the aorta, or by an increase in pulmonary vascular resistance, which may result from hypoxia or from the effects of a raised airway pressure (Strong, Keats and Cooley, 1966). An inadequate pulmonary blood flow produces hypoxia which, in turn, causes both a systemic hypotension and an increase in pulmonary vascular resistance, thereby increasing the right-to-left shunt and leading to a vicious circle.

An increase in right-to-left shunting is particularly likely to occur during the transition from spontaneous to controlled ventilation. This effect may be reduced by using pancuronium as the muscle relaxant, because of its lack of systemic vasodilator effects. It is also important to avoid an excessive airway pressure; it can be advantageous to ventilate the lungs at a slow rate, using a high inspired oxygen concentration and ensuring that the airway pressure is not raised during the expiratory pause. A stormy induction aggravates the situation and should be avoided by good preoperative sedation, although this must not cause undue respiratory depression.

If there is a potentially dangerous degree of hypotension, it must be treated immediately. For this, isoprenaline has the advantages both of increasing the cardiac output and of decreasing the pulmonary vascular resistance. The dosage depends upon the severity of the condition: although $0.5\ \mu g \cdot kg^{-1}$ would be considered to be large in normal patients, the severely hypoxic myocardium may require ten times this amount to produce an adequate effect; ventricular fibrillation appears to be less likely than in normal patients. If hypotension has been caused by peripheral vasodilatation, a direct-acting vasoconstrictor, such as metaraminol, can be used.

A reduction in pulmonary perfusion not only reduces the uptake of oxygen, but it also limits the uptake of anaesthetic agents from the lungs. If the shunt is large, an inhalational induction can be prolonged and very difficult unless the patient is very well sedated.

In these patients, therefore, premedication should be relatively heavy to facilitate induction, and should include sufficient atropine (at least $20\ \mu g \cdot kg^{-1}$) to reduce the risk of a bradycardia which could result in hypotension.

Techniques of induction of anaesthesia

NITROUS OXIDE

Gray and Riding (1957) showed that the dangers of circulatory depression caused by intravenous barbiturates can be avoided using a technique of preoxygenation followed by induction of anaesthesia with a non-hypoxic mixture of nitrous oxide and oxygen. When consciousness has been lost, a non-depolarizing relaxant is given and endotracheal intubation effected. Provided that the patient is well premedicated, this technique has much to commend it, although its use requires skill and experience. It is well tolerated by most patients and, because of the increased sensitivity to anaesthetic agents, a nitrous oxide induction is easier in the ill patient than it is in a fit person.

INTRAVENOUS BARBITURATE

An intravenous barbiturate has the advantage that most patients now expect to be anaesthetized in this way. In ill patients, it is vital to commence with a small amount of the drug and to allow for the slow circulation time (see page 699). The optimum dose is one which is sufficient to make the patient extremely drowsy and enable a facemask to be tolerated.

The choice of agent is much less important than the manner in which it is administered. Thus, though methohexitone may have a slightly more depressant effect upon the arterial pressure than thiopentone (Conway, Ellis and King, 1968), it may, on the other hand, be less likely to cause arrhythmias (Pitts *et al.*, 1965).

NARCOTIC ANALGESICS

High dosages of morphine (e.g. 1 mg·kg^{-1}) have been used, either alone or supplemented with diazepam, to induce anaesthesia in very ill patients (Lowenstein, 1971). Alternatively, levorphanol or fentanyl may be used, and cause less cardiovascular depression than does morphine. The respiratory depressant effects of these drugs are of little consequence when it is intended to continue pulmonary ventilation postoperatively.

DIAZEPAM

Fit patients may require large amounts of diazepam intravenously to render them unconscious, but in ill patients even a small dose may lower the blood pressure. The powerful sedative and anxiolytic properties make it an ideal component of premedication, but its role in the induction of anaesthesia in severely ill patients may be limited to the intravenous supplementation of the premedication, when patients are still very anxious.

ALTHESIN

Although causing few cardiovascular disturbances in healthy patients, Althesin causes as much hypotension as do the barbiturates when given to seriously ill cardiac patients (Harrison and Sellick, 1972).

KETAMINE

The direct effect of ketamine upon the myocardium is depressant (Chang, Chan and Ganendran, 1969; Chang, 1973) and its stimulant properties are dependent upon the sympathetic nervous system. The negative inotropic effects of ketamine are uncovered when the drug is given during the administration of sympatholytic agents such as halothane (Stanley, 1973). Thus, in patients in whom the sympathetic nervous system is actively compensating for cardiac disability, the direct myocardial depressant effects of ketamine can prove dangerous. However, its analgesic properties may prove to be useful when it is given as a slow intravenous infusion.

Muscle relaxants

Tubocurarine and, to a lesser extent, alcuronium lower the arterial blood pressure, principally by blocking transmission at autonomic ganglia (see Chapter 16).

Pancuronium has neither ganglion-blocking nor histamine-releasing effects. Its weak vagolytic action can increase the heart rate slightly and may raise the arterial pressure and cardiac output. It is particularly useful in the poor-risk patient, especially if a long period of relaxation is required.

Suxamethonium has a cholinergic effect and, in addition, potentiates the action of cardiac glycosides. In the patient who has not been completely digitalized, it may cause prolongation of the P—R interval, depression of the ST segment and T-wave flattening or inversion. Serious ventricular arrhythmias may be prevented by prior administration of a small amount (e.g. 2.5 mg) of tubocurarine (Dowdy and Fabian, 1963).

REVERSAL OF NEUROMUSCULAR BLOCKADE

In patients with severe cardiac decompensation it is often preferable not to attempt reversal of the muscle relaxant, but to continue IPPV post-operatively until cardiorespiratory function has become more stable. When reversal is attempted at the end of operation, it is frequently advisable to avoid causing a tachycardia from the unopposed effects of atropine. It is then preferable to give the atropine and neostigmine together, titrating their effects to maintain a steady heart rate. Should there be any doubt as to the adequacy of reversal, despite the use of a full dose of neostigmine (5 mg), it is advisable to reinstitute controlled ventilation until the effects of the drugs have worn off.

Pulmonary ventilation

Controlled ventilation, using light anaesthesia and muscle relaxation, avoids the cardiovascular depressant effects which can be caused by deep anaesthesia and it allows a better control of the arterial oxygen and carbon dioxide blood gas tensions. Controlled ventilation also reduces the work-load on the heart by removing the work of breathing, which can be considerable in patients with decreased pulmonary compliance, as may be found in advanced mitral disease or when there is a large left-to-right intracardiac shunt.

During anaesthesia there is increased mis-matching of ventilation and perfusion within the lungs and, therefore, the alveolar—arterial oxygen tension difference is increased. Sykes, Young and Robinson (1965) have shown that, during controlled ventilation, the effects of this venous admixture can be minimized by maintaining an inspired oxygen concentration of at least 30% and by using a high tidal volume. It must be kept in mind, however, that a high mean intrathoracic pressure, especially in a patient who is hypovolaemic, may reduce the venous return and thereby the cardiac output.

Prys-Roberts *et al.* (1967) have shown that if the P_{CO_2} is allowed to fall, there will be a fall in the cardiac output which is independent of the volume ventilation or the incorporation of a negative phase during expiration. A further disadvantage of a low P_{CO_2} is the shift to the left of the oxyhaemoglobin dissociation curve, which reduces the oxygen avail-ability to the tissues (see Chapter 23). A high P_{CO_2}, on the other hand, both stimulates the myocardium and may precipitate arrhythmias (see Chapter 22).

A minute volume of 5—7 litres usually produces an arterial P_{CO_2} within the desired range of 4.7—5.3 kPa (35—40 mmHg). In some patients the transfer of oxygen may be improved at higher minute volumes; this may be achieved, without lowering the P_{CO_2}, if the inspired gas contains a proportion of carbon dioxide. When a circle system is used, the soda-lime absorber may be turned off and the fresh gas inflow rate regulated accord-ing to the end-tidal P_{CO_2}.

Intravenous fluids and transfusion requirements

Many patients in heart failure have a low circulating blood volume, the arterial blood pressure and perfusion of the vital organs being maintained by vasoconstriction and a raised peripheral vascular resistance. The vaso-constriction may be reversed by anaesthetic agents, such patients being particularly susceptible to their effects. A dangerous fall in arterial pressure can usually be prevented, raising the blood volume by giving blood or other intravenous fluids; when effective, this is preferable to giving vaso-constrictor drugs, which increase the workload upon the myocardium. However, it is important to avoid a circulatory overload which could embarrass the heart, an unduly high filling pressure resulting in heart failure and a fall in cardiac output; if the left heart is failing, pulmonary oedema may be precipitated.

It is necessary, therefore, to monitor carefully the circulatory changes during major surgery in patients with heart failure. The optimum level of fluid replacement should be judged more from changes in the arterial and atrial or central venous pressures, rather than by relying solely upon estimates of blood loss. In left ventricular failure, a knowledge of the filling pressure of the left ventricle is of greater value than that of the right. It can be measured using a flow-directed balloon-tipped catheter, such as described by Swan, Ganz and others (Swan *et al.*, 1970), which is inserted via a peripheral vein and carried with the blood stream through the right side of the heart to the pulmonary artery. When the balloon is inflated to obstruct the flow of blood around it, the pulmonary 'wedge' pressure, measured from the tip of the catheter, reflects the pressure within the left atrium. From the catheter within the pulmonary artery, true mixed venous blood may be withdrawn, the arteriovenous oxygen content difference giving an indication of the cardiac output.

Sedation and analgesia

Adequate sedation is essential because it prevents restlessness, which would increase the workload on the heart. However, narcotic analgesics tend to produce peripheral vasodilatation and so to lower the arterial pressure, especially if the patient is hypovolaemic. This can cause a marked fall in cardiac output and blood pressure, particularly when the cardiac output is dependent upon a high left ventricular filling pressure. Great care should therefore be taken when giving narcotic analgesics to a patient who is in heart failure and who is also vasoconstricted.

Diamorphine (heroin) is a very good sedative and, because it produces less peripheral vasodilatation than does morphine, it has a less depressant effect upon the blood pressure (MacDonald *et al.*, 1967).

TREATMENT OF COMPLICATIONS

Changes in heart rate and rhythm

Disorders of rate and rhythm in general are discussed in Chapter 32. Here it remains to say that a tachycardia can lower the cardiac output by decreasing the diastolic filling time and thereby excessively reducing the stroke volume. Its treatment depends upon the cause; if it is due to excessive lightening of anaesthesia, it should respond to analgesic supplements.

A bradycardia can lower the cardiac output because the ventricular compliance decreases at high filling volumes, so that the increase in stroke volume does not compensate for the decrease in heart rate. If there is any element of vagal overactivity, the bradycardia should respond to atropine (0.3–0.6 mg i.v.); if it is due to hypoxia, it may respond to isoprenaline although, of course, attempts should also be made to eliminate the cause of the hypoxia.

Severe myocardial failure and hypotension

A low arterial pressure may be caused by a fall in cardiac output or by a reduction in the peripheral vascular resistance. Provided that perfusion of the myocardium and other vital organs is not impaired, it may be advantageous for there to be a low peripheral resistance, vasoconstrictor drugs being inappropriate because they would increase the workload upon the heart and raise the myocardial oxygen consumption. However, in some patients, the rise in arterial pressure produced by vasoconstriction may be beneficial, the resultant increase in coronary blood flow more than compensating for the greater workload on the heart.

Although it may be useful to have direct measurements of the cardiac output, an excessive fall in output and inadequate tissue perfusion may be inferred from a fall in the oxygen content of mixed venous blood (to less than 50–60% saturated), an increasing base deficit caused by the accumulation of lactic acid and other acid metabolites, or by a fall in urine output. A low cardiac output, causing an inadequate supply of oxygen to the tissues must be treated vigorously to avoid a progressive decline in the condition of the patient. The circulating blood volume should be brought to the optimum level (see above) and attempts made to raise the cardiac output and arterial pressure, using drugs such as the catecholamines and cardiac glycosides.

USE OF CATECHOLAMINES

The catecholamines should be given intravenously to avoid problems caused by the variability of absorption from the tissues. Initially, discrete bolus injections can be made into a running infusion, the amount being regulated according to the patient's response. For long-term circulatory support, the appropriate drug should be given as a continuous infusion via a central vein, to avoid tissue damage caused by drugs which have an intense local vasoconstrictor effect. Great care must be taken to avoid sudden high dosages, as may be caused by flushing a line containing a large amount of a potent drug.

Isoprenaline is a powerful β-adrenergic stimulant and is useful because it produces both an increase in cardiac output and a fall in total peripheral resistance. There is a wide variation in response to isoprenaline and initially only 5–10 μg should be given. Frequently a much higher dosage may be required, although in some patients even small amounts can cause an excessive tachycardia or an unstable rhythm.

Adrenaline has both α and β stimulant effects and is effective in many patients who do not respond well to isoprenaline, being of particular value in the acute situation intraoperatively. Initially, only 5–10 μg should be given but, as with isoprenaline, very much larger amounts may be required.

Noradrenaline is of particular value in patients who have a low arterial blood pressure caused by a low peripheral resistance, without severe depression of the cardiac output. The α-adrenergic stimulant effect raises the arterial pressure, increasing coronary perfusion and, thereby, the myocardial performance.

Dopamine and dobutamine are recently introduced synthetic catecholamine analogues, although dopamine occurs naturally in the body. They increase cardiac output with less tachycardia and peripheral vascular changes than those seen with isoprenaline and adrenaline infusions, and are to be preferred in the postoperative period. Dopamine is usually the drug of choice, although it may aggravate intrapulmonary venous admixture, increasing the alveolar—arterial oxygen tension difference. In the appropriate dose range the urine output is increased, but there is a loss of both sodium and potassium which probably involves a different mechanism of action from that which produces its cardiac effects (Goldberg, 1972; Robie and Goldberg, 1975).

USE OF THE CARDIAC GLYCOSIDES

The strength of myocardial contraction can also be increased by the positive inotropic action of a cardiac glycoside and, provided that the patient has not already been digitalized, it may be given intravenously. Ouabain can be a very useful drug in the failing heart but, although classed as rapidly acting, it takes some time before it becomes fully effective.

ACIDOSIS

The accumulation of acid metabolites lowers the pH and may thereby depress the myocardium, although a low pH does not prevent the heart from responding to catecholamines unless it is extreme. Experimentally, in the normal heart, it is unusual for the cardiac output to fall unless the blood pH is below 7.0 (Andersen, Border and Mouritzen, 1967). However, if the heart is already diseased, a fall in blood pH to below 7.2 should be corrected by sodium bicarbonate.

THE INTRA-AORTIC BALLOON PUMP

An inflatable balloon is placed within the aorta, usually via the femoral artery. By reference to an ECG monitor, inflation of the balloon is accurately timed to coincide with diastole and deflation with systole. The sudden deflation during systole greatly reduces the aortic impedance offered to left ventricular ejection and thereby reduces left ventricular work. Rapid inflation of the balloon at the beginning of diastole causes an abrupt pressure pulse to be transmitted up the aorta, increasing the coronary perfusion pressure during diastole.

The reduction in left ventricular work and increased coronary perfusion make it possible to sustain, for a limited period, patients who are in severe cardiogenic shock. It is therefore of value only when it can be anticipated that the impairment in cardiac function will be short-lived, being particularly useful in association with the operative correction of cardiac lesions and occasionally following myocardial infarction (Buckley *et al.*, 1973; Miller and Hall, 1975; Kaiser *et al.*, 1976).

Left ventricular failure and pulmonary oedema

In left ventricular failure, the ability of the left ventricle to empty during systole is impaired. The left ventricular end-diastolic volume increases, resulting in an elevated end-diastolic pressure and, therefore, a raised left atrial pressure. In addition to causing arteriolar constriction, an inadequate cardiac output produces a reflex constriction of the capacitance vessels, with consequent rise in the right atrial pressure and right ventricular output. Because of the left atrial back pressure this leads to pulmonary congestion and oedema. The resultant hypoxia may further restrict the myocardial oxygen supply, intensify the catecholamine release and so aggravate the left ventricular failure, creating a vicious circle, with falling cardiac output leading rapidly to death.

An excess of fluid leaves the pulmonary capillaries when the hydrostatic pressure of blood within them exceeds the sum of its colloid osmotic pressure and the intra-alveolar pressure. Emergency treatment must therefore be directed toward decreasing the intracapillary pressure and increasing the intra-alveolar pressure. Also, because pulmonary oedema impairs gas transfer, a high inspired oxygen concentration must be used.

The intra-alveolar pressure can be raised by increasing the airway pressure using IPPV and, if necessary, maintaining a positive phase during expiration (PEEP). The intracapillary pressure can be reduced by lowering the right atrial pressure; the left ventricular function curve (which clinically is taken to mean the relationship between ventricular output and atrial pressure – the so-called Starling relationship, discussed in Chapter 31) is flatter than that of the right ventricle so that a small fall in right atrial pressure, and hence right ventricular output, will cause a much greater fall in left atrial and pulmonary capillary pressures, thereby relieving the vicious circle which had caused the pulmonary oedema (Webb-Peploe and Shepherd, 1968).

The right atrial pressure can be lowered by giving vasodilator drugs, by venesection or by mechanically reducing venous return such as by trapping blood in the periphery with venous tourniquets, or by applying negative pressure to the lower half of the body (Potanin, 1967). Morphine and theophylline have traditionally been used in the treatment of acute left ventricular failure, their acute effect being mainly due to the production of a peripheral vasodilatation.

Fluid overload should be reduced by giving a potent diuretic. In addition, a cardiac glycoside may be of value, by increasing the efficiency of left ventricular function.

HYPERTENSION

The vast majority of patients with a pathologically raised blood pressure are suffering from essential hypertension. However, it should be verified that the raised arterial pressure is not the result of an associated condition – the most common being renal disease, while coarctation of the aorta, an endocrine dysfunction such as phaeochromocytoma or

Cushing's disease, a central nervous disorder such as the Guillain–Barré syndrome or a drug interaction (Foëx and Prys-Roberts, 1974) may occur.

A small group of patients suffer from malignant hypertension, where the small vessel disease has progressed to include necrotic areas in the arteriolar wall; this is associated with a very high arterial pressure, renal function is impaired and retinal changes may be seen. In these patients, life expectancy is short, and anaesthesia and surgery should be undertaken only when the patient's life is immediately at risk.

Marked haemodynamic responses to anaesthesia and surgery are relatively common in patients suffering from hypertension and ischaemic heart disease. These responses are particularly marked if the disease is untreated and they frequently occur during induction (Prys-Roberts, Meloche and Foëx, 1971; Prys-Roberts *et al.*, 1971). In severely hypertensive patients, even relatively minor surgery can be hazardous and it is advisable to monitor the arterial pressure directly, rather than to rely upon intermittent measurements obtained using indirect methods. Because major changes in pressure are likely to occur during induction of anaesthesia, it is also advisable to commence direct arterial pressure monitoring beforehand.

A severe, uncontrolled rise in blood pressure is particularly dangerous and may cause cerebrovascular injury or, by imposing a considerably increased workload on the heart, may lead to left ventricular failure with a rise in the left ventricular end-diastolic pressure and, perhaps, pulmonary oedema. If the intramural coronary arteries have been affected by the atheromatous process, the raised diastolic pressure may jeopardize the myocardial blood flow, especially in the subendocardial region, and produce ischaemic changes in the ECG. Decreasing the workload on the ventricle, by lowering the systemic vascular resistance, may relieve the failure and restore an adequate myocardial blood flow with reversal of the ECG changes (Prys-Roberts, 1977).

Myocardial ischaemia is usually evident from the conventional 12-lead ECG. In most instances, only one lead can be monitored during anaesthesia and intensive therapy; the CM_5 bipolar lead would appear to be the best single lead to show ischaemic changes in the ST segment and give a good demonstration of the P-wave and QRS complex (Blackburn *et al.*, 1967). The reference electrode (right arm lead) is placed over the manubrium sterni, the exploring electrode (left arm lead) in the V_5 position, over the fifth intercostal space in the anterior axillary line, and the earth (right lower limb lead) may conveniently be sited on the left shoulder; the ECG may then be displayed be selecting the lead I position.

The haemodynamic instability may also be shown by a marked fall in arterial pressure, it being important not to endanger perfusion of the cerebral or coronary vessels. Hypotension may result from an exaggerated response to anaesthetic agents or be caused by a low circulating blood volume. A marked fall in arterial pressure may be produced by only a modest blood loss, especially if the blood volume is restricted by pre-operative dehydration. The assessment of blood and other intravenous fluid requirements should be made from circulatory responses, rather than by relying solely upon estimates of the volume lost; measurement of the pulmonary wedge pressure (see page 704) is of particular value in assessing intravenous fluid requirements in patients with a diseased left ventricle (Gilbertson, 1974). A fall in arterial pressure may also result from a high mean intrathoracic pressure, by impeding the venous return to the heart, and it may be necessary to pay careful attention to the ventilation of the patient.

Every effort should be made to protect the hypertensive patient from this excessive haemodynamic instability and, where time permits, control of the hypertension should be achieved preoperatively. However, when emergency surgery is necessary in an untreated patient with advanced disease, some protection may be afforded by the intravenous administration of a β-blocking drug, such as propranolol (0.025—0.1 mg·kg^{-1}); this should be given slowly under ECG control and, unless there is a tachycardia, be preceded by atropine (1.2 mg). If there is evidence of heart failure or bronchospasm, it may be preferable to use a drug such as practolol, which has intrinsic stimulant activity and is cardioselective.

The drugs used in the treatment of hypertension are not found to cause undue problems of drug interaction with anaesthetic agents and, where care is taken, there is no evidence of their causing impaired cardiovascular performance during anaesthesia for general surgery (Prys-Roberts, 1976). However, care must be taken when vasopressor drugs are administered, because they can interact with some antihypertensive agents.

Even in the treated hypertensive patient, the blood pressure tends to be more labile than it is in the normal patient. During surgery, reflex autonomic activity, tending to raise the arterial pressure, can be reduced by increasing the depth of anaesthesia using intravenous analgesic drugs such as levorphanol and fentanyl, which have little effect upon the cardiovascular system, or by using low concentrations of volatile agents such as halothane, and by ensuring an adequate degree of muscle relaxation. Excessive autonomic activity may also be avoided when local anaesthetic techniques are employed as an adjunct to general anaesthesia.

If, despite these measures, there is a marked rise in arterial pressure, it is important to reduce the workload on the left ventricle by the careful administration of vasodilator agents. In a complex situation, a short-acting α-blocking drug, such as phentolamine or thymoxamine, or a slow infusion of sodium nitroprusside can be very useful (Tinker and Michenfelder, 1976). These drugs have the great advantage of possessing an action which is both rapid in onset and of short duration, so making it relatively safe to assess the over-all response of the cardiovascular system to vasodilatation. Having established the benefits produced by vasodilatation, it is then appropriate to give a longer acting drug, such as hydrallazine (20—40 mg slowly, given intravenously) or a ganglion-blocking drug, or to continue the infusion of sodium nitroprusside.

Left ventricular failure

Left ventricular failure occurs when there is a reduced ability of the left ventricle to empty against an unduly high resistance imposed by the systemic vasculature. The left ventricular end-diastolic pressure is raised and estimates of the pulmonary wedge pressure (see p. 704) give a far more reliable indication of the state of the left heart than may be obtained from the right side, by measuring the CVP. If left ventricular failure is causing pulmonary oedema and a fall in arterial oxygen tension, it should be treated as described on p. 707.

The systemic arterial pressure may be high, normal or low, because it is dependent not only upon the peripheral vascular resistance but also upon the cardiac output; this is likely to be reduced, particularly if pulmonary function has been affected and the arterial Po_2 is low.

Preoperative evidence of incipient left ventricular failure may not easily be elicited from a brief examination of the patient. However, in the hypertensive patient, some warning of the condition may be given by the history of a dry cough at night.

Left ventricular failure and pulmonary oedema may also be seen in the postoperative period. When the analgesia previously derived from the nitrous oxide and analgesic supplements wears off, the resultant increase in sympathetic activity can cause a marked rise in arterial pressure and, thereby, failure. In addition, the tendency toward pulmonary oedema may have been masked during IPPV, because of the raised intra-alveolar pressure. On return to spontaneous ventilation, the left ventricular failure may then become apparent and result in early postoperative collapse.

References

Andersen, M. N., Border, J. R. and Mouritzen, C. V. (1967). Acidosis, catecholamines and cardiovascular dynamics: when does acidosis require correction? *Ann. Surg.* 166, 344–354

Blackburn, H., Taylor, H. L., Okamoto, N., Rautaharju, P., Mitchell, P. L. and Kerkhof, A. C. (1967). Standardization of the exercise electrocardiogram. A systematic comparison of chest lead configurations employed for monitoring during exercise. In *Physical Activity and the Heart*, pp. 101–133. M. J. Karvonen and A. J. Barry (ed.). Springfield, Ill: Charles C Thomas

Bond, W. S. (1978). Clinical relevance of the effect of hepatic disease on drug disposition. *Am. J. hosp. Pharm.* 35, 406–414

Buckley, M. J., Craver, J. M., Gold, H. K., Mundth, E. D., Daggett, W. M. and Austen, W. G. (1973). Intra-aortic balloon pump assist for cardiogenic shock after cardio-pulmonary bypass. *Circulation* 48 Suppl. 3, 90–94

Chang, P. (1973). The effects of ketamine on the guineapig heart. *Br. J. Anaesth.* 45, 929–930

Chang, P., Chan, K. E. and Ganendran, A. (1969). Cardiovascular effects of 2-(o-chlorophenyl)-2-methylaminocyclohexane (C1–581) in rats. *Br. J. Anaesth.* 41, 391–395

Conway, C. M., Ellis, D. B. and King, N. W. (1968). A comparison of the acute haemodynamic effects of thiopentone, methohexitone and propanidid in the dog. *Br. J. Anaesth.* 40, 736–745

Dowdy, E. G. and Fabian, L. W. (1963). Ventricular arrhythmias induced by succinylcholine in digitalized patients. *Anesth. Analg. curr. Res.* 42, 501–513

Foëx, P. and Prys-Roberts, C. (1974). Anaesthesia and the hypertensive patient. *Br. J. Anaesth.* 46, 575–588

Fraser, J. G., Ramachandran, P. R. and Davis, H. S. (1967). Anesthesia and recent myocardial infarction. *J. Am. med. Ass.* 199, 318–320

Gilbertson, A. A. (1974). Pulmonary artery catheterization and wedge pressure measurement in the general intensive therapy unit. *Br. J. Anaesth.* 46, 97–104

Goldberg, L. I. (1972). Cardiovascular and renal actions of dopamine: potential clinical applications. *Pharmac. Rev.* 24, 1–29

Goldman, L., Caldera, D. L., Nussbaum, S. R., Southwick, F. S., Krogstad, D., Murray, B., Burke, D. S., O'Malley, T. A., Goroll, A. H., Caplan, C. H., Nolan, J., Carabello, B. and Slater, E. E. (1977). Multifactorial index of cardiac risk in non-cardiac surgical procedures. *New Engl. J. Med.* 297, 845–850

Gray, T. C. and Riding, J. E. (1957). Anaesthesia for mitral valvotomy. *Anaesthesia* 12, 129–147

Hannington-Kiff, J. G. (1968). The Wolff–Parkinson–White syndrome and general anaesthesia. *Br. J. Anaesth.* 40, 791–795

Harrison, G. G. (1966). The effect of cardiac lesions on the action of suxamethonium. *Anaesthesia* 21, 28–36

Harrison, S. G. C. and Sellick, B. A. (1972). Cardiovascular effects of Althesin in patients with cardiac pathology. *Br. J. Anaesth.* 44, 1205–1207

Juler, G. L., Stemmer, E. A. and Conolly, J. E. (1969). Complications of prophylactic digitalization in thoracic surgical patients. *J. thorac. cardiovasc. Surg.* 58, 352–358

Kaiser, G. C., Marco, J. D., Barner, H. B., Codd, J. E., Laks, H. and Willman, V. L. (1976). Intra-aortic balloon assistance. *Ann. thorac. Surg.* 21, 487–491

Lowenstein, E. (1971). Morphine 'anesthesia' – a perspective. *Anesthesiology* 35, 563–565

Lozman, J., Dutton, R. E., English, M. and Powers, S. R. Jr. (1975). Cardiopulmonary adjustment following single high dosage administration of methyl prednisolone in traumatized man. *Ann. Surg.* 181, 317–324

MacDonald, H. R., Rees, H. A., Muir, A. L., Lawrie, D. M., Burton, J. L. and Donald, K. W. (1967). Circulatory effects of heroin in patients with myocardial infarction. *Lancet* i, 1070–1074

Mason, D. T. (1974). Digitalis pharmacology and therapeutics: recent advances. *Ann. intern. Med.* 80, 520–530

Miller, M. G. and Hall, S. V. (1975). Intra-aortic balloon counterpulsation in a high-risk cardiac patient undergoing emergency gastrectomy. *Anesthesiology* 42, 103–105

Narula, O. S. (1973). Wolff--Parkinson–White syndrome: a review. *Circulation* 47, 872–887

Nies, A. S., Shand, D. G. and Wilkinson, G. R. (1976). Altered hepatic blood flow and drug disposition. *Clin. Pharmacokin.* 1, 135–155

Opie, L. H. and Owen, P. (1976). Effect of glucose–insulin–potassium infusions on arteriovenous differences of glucose and of free fatty acids and on tissue metabolic changes in dogs with developing myocardial infarction. *Am. J. Cardiol.* 38, 310–321

Pitts, F. N., Desmarais, G. M., Stewart, W. and Schaberg, K. (1965). Induction of anesthesia with methohexital and thiopental in electroconvulsive therapy. *New Engl. J. Med.* 273, 353–360

Potanin, C. (1967). Lower-body decompression in left heart failure. *Lancet* ii, 241–242

Prys-Roberts, C. (1976). Medical problems of surgical patients. Hypertension and ischaemic heart disease. *Ann. R. Coll. Surg. Engl.* 58, 465–472

Prys-Roberts, C. (1977). Vascular disease. Chapter 2 in *Medicine for Anaesthetists*. M. D. Vickers (ed.). Oxford: Blackwell

Prys-Roberts, C., Meloche, R. and Foëx, P. (1971). Studies of anaesthesia in relation to hypertension. I. Cardiovascular responses of treated and untreated patients. *Br. J. Anaesth.* 43, 122–137

Prys-Roberts, C., Kelman, G. R., Greenbaum, R. and Robinson, R. H. (1967). Circulatory influences of artificial ventilation during nitrous oxide anaesthesia in man. II. Results – the relative influence of mean intrathoracic pressure and arterial carbon dioxide tension. *Br. J. Anaesth.* 39, 533–548

Prys-Roberts, C., Greene, L. T., Meloche, R. and Foëx, P. (1971). Studies of anaesthesia in relation to hypertension. II. Haemodynamic consequences of induction and endotracheal intubation. *Br. J. Anaesth.* 43, 531–547

Robie, N. W. and Goldberg, L. I. (1975). Comparative systemic and regional hemodynamic effects of dopamine and dobutamine. *Am. Heart J.* 90, 340–345

Sapala, J. A., Ponka, J. L. and Duvernoy, W. F. C. (1975). Operative and non-operative risks in the cardiac patient. *J. Am. Geriat. Soc.* 23, 529–534

Selzer, A., Kelly, J. J., Gerbode, F., Kerth, W. J., Osborn, J. J. and Popper, R. W. (1966). Case against routine use of digitalis in patients undergoing cardiac surgery. *J. Am. med. Ass.* 195, 549–553

Simon, A. B. (1977). Perioperative management of the pacemaker patient. *Anesthesiology* 46, 127–131

Stanley, T. H. (1973). Blood pressure and pulse rate responses to ketamine during general anesthesia. *Anesthesiology* 39, 648–649

Stenson, R. E., Constantino, R. T. and Harrison, D. C. (1971). Interrelationships of hepatic blood flow, cardiac output, and blood levels of lidocaine in man. *Circulation* 43, 205–211

Strong, M. J., Keats, A. S. and Cooley, D. A. (1966). Anesthesia for cardiovascular surgery in infancy. *Anesthesiology* 27, 257–265

Swan, H. J. C., Ganz, W., Forrester, J., Marcus, H., Diamond, G. and Chonette, D. (1970). Catheterization of the heart in man with use of a flow-directed balloon-tipped catheter. *New Engl. J. Med.* 283, 447–451

Sykes, M. K., Young, W. E. and Robinson, B. E. (1965). Oxygenation during anaesthesia with controlled ventilation. *Br. J. Anaesth.* 37, 314–325

Tarhan, S., Moffitt, E. A., Taylor, W. F. and Giuliani, E. R. (1972). Myocardial infarction after general anesthesia. *J. Am. med. Ass.* 220, 1451–1454

Tinker, J. H. and Michenfelder, J. D. (1976). Sodium nitroprusside: pharmacology, toxicology and therapeutics. *Anesthesiology* 45, 340–354

Webb-Peploe, M. M. and Shepherd, J. T. (1968). Veins and their control. *New Engl. J. Med.* 278, 317–322

Wellens, H. J. J. and Durber, D. (1975). The role of an accessory atrioventricular pathway in reciprocal tachycardia. Observations in patients with and without the Wolff–Parkinson–White syndrome. *Circulation* 52, 58–72

36 Cardiopulmonary bypass
J. C. Richardson

Cardiopulmonary bypass is a technique which enables the heart and lungs to be excluded from the circulation whilst, at the same time, giving an adequate circulation to the rest of the body. This chapter gives a brief account of the use of cardiopulmonary bypass; further details on many of the subjects mentioned will be found in Chapters 32, 34, 35 and 37.

The clinical applications of the technique are, in the short term, open heart surgery, heart transplantation, myocardial revascularization (coronary artery surgery) and certain procedures which primarily involve the respiratory system (e.g. resection and replacement of the carinal area of the trachea). In the long term (and less commonly), bypass has been used in the support of the severely damaged myocardium (usually following open heart surgery or myocardial infarction) with the object of supporting it until it recovers its function, and in the maintenance of satisfactory levels of gaseous exchange following severe but temporary lung damage.

In order to exclude the heart and lungs from the circulation, the great veins in the chest (superior and inferior venae cavae) or the right atrium are cannulated and blood is allowed to flow through these cannulae to the pump—oxygenator ('heart—lung machine'). Here it is passed through an oxygenator and is then pumped back into the circulation via a cannula placed in the aorta or one of its major branches. In practice the usual site for this latter cannulation is the ascending thoracic aorta.

The heart—lung machine is provided with a means of maintaining the temperature of the patient at a predetermined level, and indeed of altering this temperature (upwards or downwards) as required. It is also provided with a number of sucker pumps which are used to aspirate blood from the heart cavities and pericardium during the surgical procedure and to discharge this blood into the oxygenator for return to the patient's circulation.

The materials from which those parts of the pump—oxygenator which are in contact with blood may be constructed are limited. For tubing and non-rigid oxygenators, silicone rubber, polyvinyl chloride and polytetrafluoroethylene are acceptable. For rigid components, stainless steel and polycarbonate are used. The components should have their internal surfaces finished to a high degree of polish, in order to minimize damage to the formed elements of the blood. If necessary, surfaces can be protected from contact with the blood by coating with a silicone (Antifoam A).

Pumps

The pumps used for short-term bypass are roller peristaltic (De Bakey) pumps which occlude and milk tubing containing blood against a track and thereby cause it to flow through the tubing. They have the advantages that the mechanical part of the pump does not come into contact with the blood and that the pump tube is disposable. The setting up of these pumps to achieve the correct degree of pressure on the tubing calls for some care, and 'overtightness' may lead to serious blood damage; this is particularly true of silicone rubber tubing in which the shear effect of the opposed surfaces of the tubes is particularly marked.

The design of pumps for long-term bypass and cardiac support is much more controversial and difficult, and many different devices have been suggested. Pneumatically driven 'artificial hearts' using a diaphragm as the pumping element and complete with valves which may be implanted within the chest have been used (Norman, 1976) but the most usual method of supporting a failing heart is with either a modified heart—lung machine and a De Bakey pump or an intra-aortic balloon pump (Webb, 1976). The use of an intra-aortic balloon pump (IABP) during and after operation has gained widespread acceptance in the management of high-risk operative patients with low output states due to reversible ventricular dysfunction (see Chapter 35). The technique involves the insertion into the aorta of a double balloon catheter, the balloons of which may be pneumatically inflated. The machine monitors the ECG and inflates the distal balloon as systole takes place, thus occluding the aorta. It then inflates the proximal balloon at the end of systole and, by occupying space within the occluded aorta, causes a rise in pressure, hence causing augmentation of the diastolic pressure; reports of survival rates vary from 13 to 70% (Norman, Cooley and Igo, 1977).

Oxygenators

All oxygenators are designed to expose a thin film of blood to a gas phase in order to allow oxygenation to take place and carbon dioxide to be eliminated. The early oxygenators employed multiple stainless steel rotating discs, the edge of which dipped into the blood and carried a thin film of the fluid through an atmosphere of oxygen. These disc oxygenators (such as the Kay Cross and the Gerbode) caused considerable blood damage and were extremely difficult to clean. They have been superseded by disposable oxygenators which use a different principle. Disposable oxygenators, which may be soft or rigid, are constructed of disposable plastic; they introduce a stream of small bubbles of gas into the blood flow. Gas exchange takes place between the blood and the bubble, and the resulting bubble–blood mixture is defoamed in a defoaming chamber which is coated with silicone antifoam. The blood is then allowed to collect in the distal part of the oxygenator before being returned to the patient.

A different concept, that of the membrane oxygenator, avoids the free gas/blood interface. In this device, which is disposable but extremely expensive, multiple thin films of blood are contained between very thin sheets of silicone rubber, separating the blood from the gas phase. The avoidance of free gas/blood interfaces minimizes blood damage, and avoids denaturing of protein and changes in the blood lipoproteins (Zapol *et al.*, 1972).

At the present time the main application of the membrane oxygenator is in the management of conditions in which serious but potentially reversible lung damage exists and (numerically, much more important) in the cardiac surgical treatment of small children (Hill *et al.*, 1972).

Whatever the type of oxygenator employed, gas input is adjusted to maintain satisfactory levels of gaseous exchange. Usually oxygen with added carbon dioxide is used, but in conditions of extreme hypothermia inert gas may be required to be added in order to remove sufficient carbon dioxide without producing extremely high oxygen levels. It is desirable that the gas flow through oxygenators be adjusted so that the blood gas levels in the patient approach normality. Poor oxygenation leads to acid–base disturbances and tissue damage, whilst high oxygen levels may be implicated in the production of gas microemboli, with subsequent neurological damage.

Heat exchangers

Because of the large surface area of heart–lung machines, considerable heat loss occurs. It may also be desirable to achieve levels of hypothermia during bypass procedures and therefore all equipment contains some kind of heat exchanger. This may be a separate device or may be incorporated in a disposable oxygenator. The blood is allowed to pass through multiple or concentric tubes which are surrounded by water maintained at a temperature appropriate to achieve the necessary levels of heat exchange. It is important to ensure that no leakage of water occurs into the blood through faults in heat exchangers.

Anticoagulation

In order that blood may be passed through the heart–lung machines without clotting, the patient must receive anticoagulants before being subjected to bypass. The anticoagulant used is heparin; this should be without preservative which may produce toxic effects. Various systems of heparinization are suggested. Satisfactory anticoagulation may be achieved with doses of 3 mg·kg^{-1} body weight or by the administration of 100 mg·m^{-2} of surface area. Heparin is destroyed quickly in the body — the half-life is in the order of one hour.

It is necessary to maintain adequate levels of heparinization throughout the bypass and this may be achieved by giving half the initial dose for each hour of bypass. The rate of heparin destruction *in vivo* is not constant and a fixed regimen, therefore, produces a somewhat unpredictable level of heparinization; the period of bypass may be prolonged. Recently more accurate means of assessing the level of heparinization have been developed. The most commonly used is to determine the coagulation time by a modified method (Hattersley, 1966; Jaberi, Bell and Benson, 1974). This 'activated' coagulation time should be maintained at a level of 480 seconds.

The reversal of heparinization at the end of bypass is achieved by the administration of protamine sulphate. If one of the arbitrary protocols of heparinization is employed, the protamine sulphate is administered at the rate of one-and-one-half to two times the initial dose of heparin. As protamine sulphate is in itself an anticoagulant, any inaccuracy in the estimation of residual heparin may lead to anticoagulation by excess protamine; therefore, it is desirable that an accurate assessment of residual heparin, using the activated coagulation time, be determined. Residual heparin may then be neutralized by administering protamine sulphate at the rate of 1.3 mg·ms^{-1} of residual heparin. Protamine sulphate should be administered intravenously and diluted with Ringer–lactate solution in order to avoid toxic effects such as fall in blood pressure and changes in the heart rate (Egerton and Robinson, 1961). It is usual to administer protamine sulphate in divided doses as its action is confined to the heparin in circulating blood. After the initial reversal, further heparin may be released from tissues and will be neutralized by the later dose of protamine.

Priming

Before the patient can be connected to the heart–lung machine, the apparatus must be filled with fluid and air must be excluded from the system. The early practitioners of bypass primed their apparatus with freshly drawn heparinized blood. This was demanding on donors and upon laboratory staff and was quickly replaced by various other methods. Initially, stored bank blood was used but, with the advent of disposable bubble oxygenators, primes using various mixtures of 5% dextrose and Ringer–lactate were adopted (Cooley, Beall and Grondin, 1962; Cooley, Beall and Hallman, 1965). A typical prime would allow the administration of 30–50 ml of 5% dextrose in Ringer–lactate solution per kilogram of body weight. In addition to the major priming solutions, sodium bicarbonate and heparin may be added.

The techniques of haemodilution enable bypass to be carried out with much less demand on the blood transfusion services. In addition, the viscosity of the blood is reduced, enabling better body perfusion to be achieved. Before bypass, the priming fluid should be warmed to approximately body temperature. When cannulation is completed and the air has been excluded from the apparatus and tubing, the patient is connected to the pump oxygenator and bypass is commenced. Flow rates of 2.4 l·m^{-2} body surface area are desirable, although this may be reduced under hypothermic conditions. In most currently used apparatus the flow from the machine is non-pulsatile. Certain authorities recommend that pulsatile flow offers advantages. Halley, Reemtsma and Creech (1958) demonstrated decreased oxygen consumption in the brain during non-pulsatile perfusion, and Clarke *et al.* (1968) demonstrated increased pulmonary vascular resistance and alveolar wall thickening after non-pulsatile bypass. Renal function and lymph flow is also improved by pulsatile flow.

Anaesthesia

Anaesthesia for open heart surgery must be administered in such a way as to cause as little disturbance to the circulation as possible. To this end, agents causing changes in blood pressure or heart rate or direct depressant action on the myocardium should be avoided. This subject is dealt with in Chapter 8.

Open heart surgery

Open heart surgery is carried out for the correction of congenital defects, repair or replacement of valves, repair of trauma, repair of damage due to myocardial infarction, revascularization of the myocardium and for cardiac transplant. Each of the procedures produces problems for the anaesthetist and for the person controlling the bypass.

Congenital defects tend to be treated in small children and babies. Critical congenital heart disease occurs in almost 11 000 babies in the USA each year and in more than two-thirds of these the anomalies are potentially correctable by open heart surgery. The technique of deep hypothermic circulatory arrest has greatly facilitated corrective cardiac surgery in these critically ill infants. Intracardiac repair of the most complicated cases known can now be performed accurately in a bloodless, motionless and relaxed heart. The technique of deep hypothermia with limited cardiopulmonary bypass and total circulatory arrest was originally described by Hikasa *et al.* (1967). The anaesthetized child is placed on bypass and cooled, using the pump oxygenator, to temperatures of 15–20°C, whereupon the heart is drained into the apparatus and total circulatory arrest is achieved. Surface cooling may also be used.

Valve surgery produces different problems. In particular, access to the aortic valve is through an incision in the aorta, and surgery at this site requires interruption of blood supply to the myocardium because of the necessity to place a cross-clamp across the aortic arch. The placing of this cross-clamp produces anoxic cardiac arrest; for single valve replacements lasting less than half an hour, this may be acceptable as a satisfactory technique although it may produce measurable and sometimes permanent myocardial damage (Reis *et al.*, 1969). The preservation of myocardial cellular viability during anoxia depends on the capacity of the heart to produce energy through anaerobic metabolism (Kubler and Spieckermann, 1970). For longer procedures there must be some protection of the myocardium. A degree of protection may be achieved if hypothermia is induced before the cross-clamp is placed on the aorta. Further protection may be achieved by applying mechanical coronary perfusion and hypothermia may be combined with coronary perfusion. More recently, anoxic cardiac arrest has been replaced by the instillation of cardioplegic solutions into the coronary arteries immediately after cross-clamping. This produces a flaccid heart, with good operating conditions, which subsequently shows little sign of damage after bypass. The solution used contains potassium, calcium, magnesium, heparin and bicarbonate as well as procaine, and is administered at 15°C (Tyers *et al.*, 1977).

In order to minimize movement of the heart, some surgeons use low voltage a.c. shocks to fibrillate the heart during surgery.

Surgery on the coronary arteries involves the replacement of the diseased artery by saphenous vein graft. During the procedure there is interruption of the blood supply to the myocardium. While grafting takes place, protection of the myocardium may be by hypothermia or cardioplegia. The repair of trauma of the heart produced either mechanically or following myocardial infarction presents no specific problem. Following surgery during which ventricular fibrillation is induced or the heart is arrested by anoxia, it is usually necessary to convert the ventricular fibrillation that ensues. This may be achieved by d.c. shock of approximately 45 J applied directly to the surface of the myocardium.

Management immediately after bypass

The low output syndrome develops after open heart surgery when the cardiac output is inadequate for the metabolic demands of the body. The causes are decreased myocardial contractility, hypovolaemia, acid—base imbalance, electrolyte disturbances, arrhythmias, inadequate ventilation, long-standing preoperative congestive heart failure, pulmonary hypertension and prolonged myocardial oxygen debt during a long perfusion.

The low cardiac output syndrome is manifested by hypotension, oliguria, peripheral vasoconstriction, cyanosis, raised CVP and metabolic acidosis. The main aim of treatment is to improve the cardiac output. This can be achieved by pharmacological stimulation of myocardial contractility by adjusting the fluid load in order to maintain the ventricular and diastolic fibre length, or by artificial pacing if rate is a limiting factor. Isoprenaline has been widely used and has proved effective in the management of the low cardiac output state. Adrenaline has received some attention, although it may introduce disproportionate peripheral and renal vasoconstriction.

Glucagon has been used, and recently dopamine (MacCannell *et al.*, 1966) and dobutamine, both synthetic catecholamines derived from isoprenaline, have become popular. These last two agents retain the positive inotropic effects of isoprenaline but lack strongly chronotropic and peripheral vasodilating effects.

Postoperative care

This subject is dealt with fully in Chapter 91. Here are appended a few notes related specifically to bypass procedures.

All patients subjected to open heart surgery should be cared for in an intensive therapy unit for at least the first 24 hours after bypass surgery. During this time, full monitoring should be maintained and system support as required should be available. In addition to arterial blood pressure, CVP, ECG, blood gas analysis, blood chemistry analysis, the monitoring of renal function and careful fluid balance, guidance to the state of the peripheral circulation may be obtained from the comparison of toe skin temperatures with body core temperatures. Any disparity suggests poor tissue perfusion and inadequate cardiac output, frequently associated with low circulating blood volume (Matthews, Meade and Evans, 1974).

Some authorities suggest that all patients should be subjected to IPPV for the first 24 hours after bypass but many units treat their patients as indicated by the results of their monitoring and use artificial pulmonary ventilation only in those patients who manifestly require it.

Complications of open heart surgery

Postoperative care of patients having had cardiac surgery is dealt with in Chapter 91. Here a few points of especial and more specific interest to cardiac bypass are outlined.

BLEEDING

Surgical bleeding is not uncommon and may be one of the factors leading to cardiac tamponade, which is an emergency requiring urgent treatment; it is manifested by a low output state with low arterial blood pressure and high CVP, poor or no urine output, accompanied in many cases by apparent cessation of drainage from the chest drainage tubes. All patients whose clotting studies are normal but who continue to bleed should be re-explored.

In addition to the above, haemorrhage may result from the changes which have been demonstrated in the normal blood clotting mechanism after open heart surgery in which extracorporeal circulation is used Gans and Krivit, 1962). The relevant importance attributed to thrombocytopenia, fibrinolysis and inadequate neutralization of heparin and to alteration of some blood clotting factors is varied. These problems may be related to damage, to blood constituents during cardiopulmonary bypass or to massive replacement transfusion. An early indication of damage to blood constituents may be haemolysis, leading to the appearance of free haemoglobin in the urine and quite rapidly to high levels of serum bilirubin in the postoperative period. Most clotting problems may be effectively treated by the administration of platelets, fresh-frozen concentrated human plasma, fresh blood or cryoprecipitated human antihaemophilic factor.

ACID–BASE DISTURBANCES

Poor perfusion, low output states and massive blood replacement together with pulmonary problems may all lead to changes in acid–base equilibrium in the postoperative period. Correction may be achieved by the administration of sodium bicarbonate (8.4%); the dose (in millilitres) is given approximately by the formula 0.3 × body weight in kilograms × the base deficit (in millimoles per litre).

RESPIRATORY

Many patients presenting for open heart surgery have a degree of lung damage which, in addition to alterations in haemodynamics, may produce postoperative respiratory difficulties. Inadequate physiotherapy before and after surgery may further complicate this problem, and postoperative respiratory problems are not unusual. The syndrome of 'pump lung' seems to be the result of a group of unrelated factors — including infection, massive blood transfusion and altered haemodynamic problems following bypass. This results in a diffuse pneumonitis or pulmonary oedema causing respiratory distress and poor oxygenation. Treatment may necessitate prolonged postoperative IPPV.

STRESS

Bleeding from the intestinal tract and, in particular, from acute peptic ulceration is reported after bypass and may be refractory to treatment.

EMBOLIC COMPLICATIONS

Emboli may be introduced into the circulation at any time during bypass and surgery. They may be due to several factors. For example, air may enter the heart during surgery; this requires determined efforts on the part of the surgeon to eliminate it before the beat is allowed to resume its function and discharge blood into the circulation. Oxygen, which is introduced from the heart–lung machine, may also cause gas embolism. Calcific and tissue emboli derived from debris produced during the removal of the diseased valve may get into the circulation and, finally, so may silicone antifoam particles from the surfaces of the heart–lung machine.

The most important results of the emboli are neurological and these are well described by Brierley (1963, 1967). The manifestations of these emboli vary from transient monoplegia to total brain death. Cases in which it is thought that brain damage has occurred or is likely to occur should be treated with an anticonvulsant such as phenobarbitone and large doses of steroids (dexamethasone). Brain damage has been reported following deep hypothermia (Bjork and Hultquist, 1960). It may also occur as a result of high SVC pressure and obstruction during bypass or as a result of failure to provide a satisfactory flow of oxygenated blood to the brain. The latter problem may arise from technical difficulties during perfusion.

PSYCHIATRIC

Many patients show some degree of disturbance following open heart surgery although in most cases this is minimal and transient, and perhaps may be attributed to the rather awesome experience to which they are subjected. The subject is well reviewed by Cohen (1967). There is evidence of a very few cases of permanent personality changes.

References

Bjork, V. O. and Hultquist, G. (1960). Brain damage in children after deep hypothermia for open heart surgery. *Thorax* 15, 284–291

Brierley, J. B. (1963). Neuropathological findings in patients dying after open heart surgery. *Thorax* 18, 291–304

Brierley, J. B. (1967). Brain damage complicating open heart surgery: a neuropathological study of 46 patients. *Proc. R. Soc. Med.* 60, 858–859

Clarke, C. P., Kahn, D. R., Dufek, J. et al. (1968). The effects of nonpulsatile blood flow on canine lungs. *Ann. thorac. Surg.* 6, 450–457

Cohen, S. I. (1967). Neurological complications of cardiac surgery and respiratory disorders: some psychiatric aspects. *Proc. R. Soc. Med.* 60, 859–860

Cooley, D. A., Beall, A. C. and Grondin, P. (1962). Open heart operations with disposable oxygenators, 5 per cent dextrose prime, and normothermia. *Surgery* 52, 713–719

Cooley, D. A., Beall, A. C. and Hallman, G. L. (1965). Open heart surgery using disposable plastic oxygenators, 5 per cent dextrose in water for priming, and maintenance of normothermia. *Ann. thorac. cardiovasc. Surg.* 4, 423–430

Egerton, W. S. and Robinson, C. L. N. (1961). The anti-heparin, anti-coagulant and hypotensive properties of hexadimethrine and protamine. *Lancet* ii, 635–637

Gans, H. and Krivit, W. (1962). Problems in haemostasis during open heart surgery. *Ann. Surg.* 155, 353–359

Halley, M. M., Reemstma, K. and Creech, O. (1958). Cerebral blood flow, metabolism, and brain volume in extracorporeal circulation. *J. thorac. Surg.* 36, 506–518

Hattersley, P. G. (1966). Activated coagulation time of whole blood. *J. Am. med. Ass.* 196, 436–440

Hikasa, Y. Shirotani, H., Mori, C. et al. (1967). Open heart surgery in infants with an aid of hypothermic anaesthesia. *Archs Jap. Chir.* 36, 495–508

Hill, J. D., O'Brien, T. G., Murray, J. J. et al. (1972). Prolonged extracorporeal oxygenation for acute post-traumatic respiratory failure. *New Engl. J. Med.* 286, 629–634

Jaberi, M., Bell, W. R. and Benson, D. W. (1974). Control of heparin therapy in open heart surgery. *J. thorac. cardiovasc. Surg.* 67, 133–141

Kubler, W. and Spieckermann, P. G. (1970). Regulation of glycolysis in the ischemic and the anoxic myocardium. *J. molec. cell. Cardiol.* 1, 351–377

MacCannell, K. L., McNay, J. L., Meyer, M. B. et al. (1966). Dopamine in the treatment of hypotension and shock. *New Engl. J. Med.* 275, 1389–1398

Matthews, H. R., Meade, J. B. and Evans, C. C. (1974). Peripheral vasoconstriction after open heart surgery. *Thorax* 29, 338–342

Norman, J. C. (1976). *The Clinical Application of Left Ventricular Assist Devices.* Report 1-HV-5-3006-1, pp. 1–239. (Available from the National Technical Information Service, 528 Port Royal Road, Springfield, Va 22151, USA)

Norman, J. C., Cooley, D. A. and Igo, S. R. (1977). Prognostic indices for survival during postcardiotomy intra-aortic balloon pumping. *J. thorac. cardiovasc. Surg.* **74**, 709–720

Reis, R. L., Staroscik, R. N., Rodger, B. M. *et al.* (1969). Left ventricular function after ischemic cardioplegia. *Archs Surg.* **99**, 815–820

Tyers, G. F. O., Manley, N. J., Williams, E. H. *et al.* (1977). Preliminary clinical experience with isotonic hypothermic potassium-induced arrest. *J. thorac. cardiovasc. Surg.* **74**, 674–681

Webb, W. R. (1976). Editorial: intra-aortic balloon pumping. *Ann. thorac. Surg.* **21**, 571–572

Zapol, W., Pontoppidan, H., McCullough, N. *et al.* (1972). Clinical membrane lung support for acute respiratory insufficiency. *Trans. Am. Soc. artif. intern. Organs* **18**, 553–560

Further reading

Ionescu, M. E. and Wooler, G. H. (1976). *Current Techniques in Extra-corporeal Circulation.* London: Butterworths

37 Cardiac drugs of importance in general anaesthesia
Clive P. Aber and B. C. Hovell

'To be forewarned is to be forearmed' — a most apt expression when considering the potential dangers of general anaesthesia in patients with established cardiovascular disease (Buckley and Jackson, 1961; Dack, 1963; Chamberlain and Edmonds-Seal, 1964; Skinner and Pearce, 1964; Marshall and Wyche, 1972; Tarhan *et al.*, 1972; Holdcroft and Hall, 1978). Although the majority of patients appear to tolerate the anaesthetic, the surgery and the postoperative period with little, if any, immediate deterioration of cardiac performance or the development of other cardiovascular complications, this is sometimes more an expression of human robustness than a measure of optimal medical care. Support for this harsh comment can be found in everyday clinical practice.

(1) *In the emergency situation,* often information is sparse with respect to the previous cardiovascular history and the current cardiac status or about long-term and immediate medications. The patient may then undergo an inadequate preoperative assessment by inexperienced junior medical staff who hand over to relatively untrained anaesthetists. As a consequence, a premature operation may be performed before an at-risk patient is in the best possible condition to withstand the further physiological trauma associated with general anaesthesia and surgery.

(2) *In elective procedures* potentially vulnerable groups of patients are: (a) those 'admitted overnight' or as 'day cases' for diagnostic procedures under general anaesthesia; (b) those offered general anaesthesia for dental treatment outside hospital where resuscitation facilities are often either absent or inadequate and, again, the anaesthetist may be relatively inexperienced; and (c) patients with untreated or inadequately controlled systemic hypertension or coronary artery disease who enter hospital for elective surgery.

Incomplete knowledge of the potential dangers of the wide range of cardiovascular drugs currently available (including interactions between anaesthetic and cardiovascular agents), fluctuating blood pressure levels and coronary blood flow, of the effects of acute withdrawal of drug therapy and of the depressive action of many anaesthetic agents on the myocardium are everyday areas of interest and concern even to the experienced physician and anaesthetist. The difference between the plasma and pharmacological half-life of any drug may also be misleading.

The agents most frequently encountered by anaesthetists are anti-hypertensives, β-receptor adrenergic blockers, digitalis preparations, diuretics and vasodilators. All of these are in common use in the treatment of patients with systemic hypertension, coronary artery disease, valvular and congenital heart disease, heart failure and recurrent arrhythmias (see Chapter 32). Occasionally, patients with permanent transvenous or epicardial pacing systems, who may also be receiving cardiovascular drugs, will require an anaesthetic. Alternatively, anaesthetists may have to use any of these preparations, either electively or in an emergency, to treat unexpected primary cardiovascular crises or to counteract complications attributable to previously administered cardiovascular drugs. In such circumstances the ability to answer such questions as 'what is the precise indication for drug intervention?', 'which agent is most appropriate?', 'what are the risks of using it?' is mandatory.

BETA-RECEPTOR ADRENERGIC BLOCKADE

All β-receptor adrenergic blocking agents produce a specific competitive reversible antagonism. Some of the more important physiological and pharmacological characteristics of this group of drugs are presented in *Tables 37.1 and 37.2.*

Cardioselective agents inhibit the cardiac β receptors ($β_1$) but exert little influence on the bronchial and vascular β receptors ($β_2$) when used in low

TABLE 37.1. Haemodynamic effects of chronic β blockade

(1)   Decreased heart rate
                       decreased pacemaker activity
                       reduced rate of conduction

(2)   Decreased contractility
                       decreased peak tension
                       decreased rate of tension development

(3)   Reduced blood pressure in resting subjects

(4)   Reduction in cardiac output as a result of (1) and (2)

(5)   Peripheral vascular resistance may be increased

As a result of these haemodynamic effects, a reduction in myocardial oxygen consumption is usually observed.

TABLE 37.2. Pharmacological properties of β blockade

	Cardioselectivity	Intrinsic sympathomimetic activity	Membrane-stabilizing action	Plasma half-life (h)	Usual oral dose range (mg)
Acebutolol (Sectral)	+	+	+	4–5	200–900
Metoprolol (Betaloc)	+	–	+	3–4	50–400
Practolol (Eraldin)	+	+	–	5–13	100–800
Atenolol (Tenormin)	+	–	–	6–9	50–300
Oxprenolol (Trasicor)	–	+	+	1–2	40–480
Alprenolol (Aptin)	–	+	+	2–3	40–320
Pindolol (Visken)	–	+	–	3–4	5–30
Propranolol (Inderal)	–	–	++	3–6	40–2000
Sotalol (Beta-Cardone)	–	–	–	5–6	80–480
Timolol (Blocadren)	–	–	–	4–5	5–45

dosage. However, in the higher doses frequently prescribed for the treatment of coronary heart disease, hypertension and some paroxysmal arrhythmias, comparatively little selectivity is witnessed.

Beta blockers which display *intrinsic sympathomimetic activity* (partial agonist effect) — that is, the capacity to stimulate β-adrenoreceptor sites in addition to occupying them — are theoretically less likely to promote cardiac insufficiency or severe bradycardia.

A further characteristic of some of these drugs is that they cause a decrease in the maximum rate of depolarization of the myocardial cells and also a lengthening of the effective refractory period. This is termed *the membrane stabilizing action* (quinidine-like activity or local anaesthetic effect). As a consequence, drugs in this subgroup are more likely to possess antiarrhythmic potential but to date this has been shown to have little clinical importance in the usual therapeutic doses.

It may be of future significance that β-blocking agents have been shown to possess other properties; for example, they may influence fibrolysis, platelet aggregation, carbohydrate metabolism, renin secretion, aldosterone activity and sodium retention. However, information is sparse with respect to these effects.

Cumulative clinical experience has shown that propranolol is most likely to promote heart failure and to cause bronchospasm, and therefore should be avoided where possible in patients with compromised myocardial function and known chronic obstructive lung disease. Propranolol and pindolol often cause central lethargy, and practolol, when used for any length of time, can induce a syndrome of systemic lupus erythematosus or fibrosing peritonitis, in addition to skin lesions. Oxprenolol and alprenolol are, on balance, most free of serious side-effects. The development of cold hands and feet and the exaggeration of peripheral vascular symptoms comprise another common side-effect of all β blockers.

Pharmacokinetics

The pharmacokinetic characteristics of the various β-blocking drugs are too complex to allow detailed description (Johnson and Regardh, 1976; Shand, 1976). However, some of the more important known features are presented. All are well absorbed after oral administration, and distribution is to the lungs and, to a lesser extent, to the liver, kidney and heart. Propranolol and oxprenolol penetrate the blood—brain barrier with ease but sotalol, practolol and atenolol do not. Propranolol and metoprolol are excreted in the urine after being almost completely metabolized, whereas alprenolol, practolol, atenolol, sotalol and timolol appear in the urine almost entirely in their non-metabolized forms. Only 45% of non-metabolized pindolol and a lesser proportion of tolamolol are excreted in this manner. Almost all of acebutolol and approximately 50% of atenolol are excreted via the gastrointestinal tract after both oral and intravenous administration. The half-life of the drugs is shown in *Table 37.2.*

Clinical use

The over-all effectiveness of any β blocker must be related to (1) the existing level of β-receptor stimulation at the time of administration, (2) the degree of dependence of the myocardium on β-adrenergic support at this time in order to maintain an adequate cardiac output (left ventricular function) and, of course (3) the dose, route of administration and particular agent employed.

Beta blockade alone or in combination with other drugs is now conventional therapy for coronary heart disease, systemic hypertension and certain arrhythmias. Less common therapeutic indications are hypertrophic obstructive cardiomyopathy, tetralogy of Fallot, phaeochromocytoma, hyperthyroidism, migraine, anxiety states and extra-pyramidal syndromes. The dose and frequency of administration vary considerably, according to the half-life of the drug favoured, from patient to patient and between different diseases (Waal-Manning, 1976).

Beta blockade and anaesthesia

Concern about the negative inotropic effect of propranolol (Tyers and Hughes, 1976) has caused anaesthetists to favour, when possible, the elective withdrawal of β blockade for at least 48 hours before the introduction of general anaesthesia, bearing in mind that all inhalational and intravenous anaesthetic agents are also myocardial depressants to a varying degree (Gersh *et al.*, 1970; Weaver, Bailey and Preston, 1970) (*Figure 37.1*) and that β blockade may prevent adequate compensatory

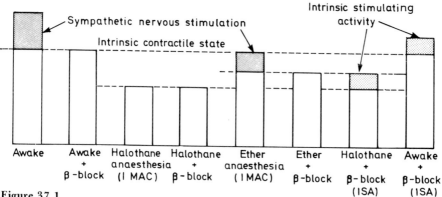

Figure 37.1
Schematic representation of the interaction between β-receptor blocking drugs and anaesthesia in animals and man. (The height of each column represents the contractile state of the myocardium.) MAC, the minimum alveolar concentration of an anaesthetic agent which just prevents a gross muscular response to a surgical incision in 50% of patients; ISA, intrinsic stimulating (sympathomimetic) activity of the β-receptor blocking drug. (Reproduced from Prys-Roberts *et al.*, 1973, by courtesy of Professor Prys-Roberts and the Editor of *British Journal of Anaesthesia*)

response to rapid changes in blood volume. This somewhat rigid attitude has to some extent also been conditioned by previous difficulty in continuing the administration of a β-blocking agent during anaesthesia and in the immediate postoperative period when many patients are often unable to accept oral treatment.

On the other hand, in practice it is now clear that abrupt withdrawal of β blockers, particularly in patients with coronary heart disease and hypertension, can prove disastrous. In the former group such action may invoke a very unstable coronary circulatory state, acute infarction or sudden death (Alderman *et al.*, 1974; Miller *et al.*, 1975; Mizgala and Counsell, 1976), patients with previously unstable angina being particularly at risk in this respect prior to revascularization surgery (Kaplan *et al.*, 1975). In hypertensive patients, marked blood pressure fluctuation has frequently been witnessed prior to and during induction of anaesthesia and at varying stages thereafter — for example, during extubation (Prys-Roberts *et al.*, 1973). This is more severe in the untreated and uncontrolled patients and therefore can be anticipated after withdrawal of β blockade.

In cardiac surgery propranolol can be administered until only a few hours before the operation without increasing the incidence of complications. Kaplan *et al.* (1975) reported 165 patients who underwent aortocoronary bypass grafting, two-thirds of whom had been receiving propranolol at an average dose of 120 mg (40—480 mg) daily until 24—48 hours before surgery, whereas in the remaining one-third propranolol had been discontinued for at least 48 hours. They observed no significant haemodynamic difference between the two groups during anaesthesia or during the postoperative phase. However, they comment that the most severely ill patients in their series, all of whom had preinfarction angina, required more inotropic support at the discontinuation of cardiopulmonary bypass; this, to some extent, may have reflected their preoperative level of β blockade rather than the duration of withdrawal of therapy. Similar observations in aortic coronary bypass surgery have been made by Moran *et al.* (1974) and Coltart *et al.* (1975). In general surgery, Kaplan and Dunbar (1976) likewise provide some evidence to suggest that continuation of β-blocking agents until certainly 12 hours before operation is safe. By contrast, Viljoen, Estafanous and Kellner (1972) firmly favoured the withdrawal of β blockers two weeks before surgery. However, this recommendation was made on a very small group of somewhat atypical patients.

Now that parenteral techniques for maintaining a satisfactory level of β blockade are being explored (McAllister, 1976) it should be possible to reduce the risk of ischaemic myocardial damage, hypertensive or hypotensive crises, and potentially lethal arrhythmias, both before and during surgery and in the immediate postoperative period.

Short-term prophylactic or therapeutic β blockade during general anaesthesia has attracted increasing interest in the past few years for several reasons. It has been used in attempts to stabilize the blood pressure during surgery in previously normotensive or hypertensive patients (Johnstone, 1966, 1971; Prys-Roberts *et al.*, 1973) and to prevent the development of major arrhythmias or excessive tachycardia in patients who are undergoing removal of a phaeochromocytoma (Robertson, 1965; Ross *et al.*, 1967; Bingham, Elliott and Lyons, 1972), thyroidectomy (Parsons and Jewitt, 1967; Shanks *et al.*, 1969; Michie, 1974), dental surgery (Rollason and Hall, 1973, Ryder, Charlton and Gorman, 1973), or cardiothoracic techniques (McClish *et al.*, 1968; Moran *et al.*, 1973). Use of β blockers during adrenaline infiltration has been described (Ikezono, Yasuda and Hattori, 1969) and these drugs have been used to protect the myocardium in patients with coronary heart disease. Finally, β blockade has been employed to abolish the reflex tachycardia that can occur during procedures involving the elective induction of hypotension with drugs such as hexamethonium, pentolinium, trimetaphan or sodium nitroprusside (Hale Enderby, 1974; Adams, 1975).

Contraindications to β blockage during general anaesthesia

The principal problems that result from the use of β-blocking agents are the direct consequence of the blockade *per se*. Contraindications to their use, therefore, include heart failure, cardiomegaly, chronic fixed or reversible obstructive lung disease, heart block (second and third degree), sinus bradycardia, in the acute stages of myocardial infarction, and metabolic acidosis (Petrie *et al.*, 1976).

Excessive β blockade during general anaesthesia

Precipitation of significant airways obstruction (bronchospasm) is unlikely if these drugs are withheld from known asthmatic and bronchitic patients. Should it develop, intravenous salbutamol or aminophylline usually promote rapid therapeutic benefit.

Excessive bradycardia or hypotension should be treated initially, and preferably early, by such simple measures as lightening the level of anaesthesia, appropriate repositioning of the patient (to aid venous return) and/or intravenous fluid administration. If these procedures fail to effect rapid haemodynamic improvement, more aggressive therapy is required: viz. (1) intravenous atropine (0.6—3.0 mg in divided doses); (2) intravenous isoprenaline by carefully controlled infusion (2—25 μg·min^{-1}); (3) intravenous salbutamol (2 mg immediately) or, rarely, (4) calcium chloride (250—1000 mg i.v. slowly) or aminophylline (250—500 mg i.v. immediately, then 1 mg·min^{-1} intravenous infusion, subject to the usual precautions with that drug).

The insertion of a transvenous pacing electrode may prove necessary — and occasionally the placing of such an electrode before surgery may be anticipated in the preoperative assessment.

Withdrawal of β blockade

If it is considered desirable to withdraw or reduce the level of β blockade prior to surgery, the dose should be lowered gradually over a period of 7–14 days under careful supervision, being prepared to re-establish previous dosage in the event of threatened 'rebound' (Shand, 1975). Simultaneous administration of isosorbide dinitrate (5–10 mg 6-hourly) during this withdrawal phase may afford additional protection.

ANTIHYPERTENSIVE AGENTS

The high incidence of systemic hypertension in Western populations means that many patients undergoing procedures under general anaesthesia will present with an elevated blood pressure, with or without evidence of target-organ (brain, heart, kidney) damage. What constitutes 'a raised blood pressure' for any given patient is not always easy to decide. Likewise, there remains a debate as to when to introduce therapy. A diastolic blood pressure of 110 mmHg or more and/or a systolic value of 160 mmHg or more in a patient under the age of 60 years merits consideration.

The anaesthetist may detect undiagnosed hypertension during the preoperative examination. Unless a life-threatening situation exists, this might dictate postponement of the procedure until the diagnosis is confirmed, appropriate investigations undertaken and satisfactory therapeutic control achieved. More usually, hypertension is known to be present but may not yet be under satisfactory control. Each of these hypertensive states has its own implications with respect to general anaesthesia.

For the past 25 years many anaesthetists have preferred hypertensive patients to arrive for anaesthesia in the untreated state, preoperative withdrawal of all antihypertensive agents with perhaps the exception of diuretics being favoured (Davison, 1951; Pickering, 1968; Grogono and Lee, 1970). The potential risks of 'an uncontrolled blood pressure' were held to be less than those of 'an uncontrolled anaesthetic'. However, more recent observations (Moyer, Brest and Nathanson, 1963; Hickler and Vandam, 2970; Prys-Roberts, Meloche and Foëx, 1971) have cast doubts about this attitude. The interaction between antihypertensive therapy and anaesthetic drugs has undoubtedly been exaggerated, is often predictable and therefore can usually be avoided; for example, extreme caution is required when administering pressor agents or using adrenaline infiltration in the hypertensive patient (Vlachakis, DeGuia and Mendlowitz, 1977). Furthermore, patients remaining on therapy show less extreme swings of blood pressure and heart rate during the anaesthetic and are less likely to exhibit arrhythmias.

Numerous antihypertensive drugs have emerged in recent years. Only those most commonly prescribed or of particular interest to anaesthetists are discussed.

Diuretics

These drugs promote both an initial and a sustained reduction of plasma and extracellular volumes by increasing renal loss of electrolytes and water (Leth, 1970; Dunstan, Tarazi and Bravo, 1974). They also may diminish the effect of sympathetic activity on the peripheral blood vessels (Hansen, 1968). In combination with other agents in the management of the more severe grades of hypertension, they exert a potentiating 'hypotensive' action.

The preparations most favoured in the long-term management of mild hypertension are the thiazide derivatives — chlorothiazide, hydrochlorothiazide, bendrofluazide and cyclopenthiazide — of moderate potency with a relatively slow onset of effect which may persist for up to 12 hours. The longer acting agents, methyclothiazide, polythiazide and chlorthalidone, are less often prescribed. They all promote diuresis by inhibiting sodium absorption in the cortical segment of the ascending loop of Henle. Because more sodium is then absorbed in the distal convoluted tubule in exchange for potassium and hydrogen ions, the development of hypokalaemia and alkalosis is common and may contribute to the anaesthetic risk.

The more rapidly acting and more potent diuretics with a shorter half-life, such as frusemide, ethacrynic acid and bumetanide, have little place in the treatment of hypertension. Similarly, the so-called 'potassium sparing' diuretics (spironolactone, triamterene and amiloride) have never commanded major acclaim as primary hypotensive agents but are sometimes offered along with other diuretics in an attempt to conserve potassium.

Symptomless hyperuricaemia is common as a consequence of diuretic therapy but rarely promotes gout unless there is a previous susceptibility or renal function is poor. Diuretics may cause hyperglycaemia and therefore may upset previously stable diabetic patients whether or not they were receiving oral hypoglycaemic agents or insulin.

Adrenergic neuron inhibitors

These antihypertensive agents inhibit the release of noradrenaline caused by action potentials in the terminals of the postganglionic sympathetic neurons. Guanethidine, bethanidine and debrisoquine all possess this property and are in relatively common use for moderate or severe hypertension.

Their antihypertensive effect is achieved by a fall in cardiac output and peripheral vascular resistance. This promotes characteristic postural (Chamberlain and Howard, 1964) and exercise hypotension (Khatri and Cohn, 1970) with, at times, deterioration in renal function. Bethanidine and debrisoquine produce their maximum effect within four hours of oral administration, have a relatively short half-life and therefore must be given in divided daily dosage. Guanethidine, on the other hand, with a longer half-life need only be given as a once daily regimen.

The side-effects of postural and exertional hypotension, diarrhoea and disturbance of renal and sexual function make these drugs less attractive for long-term use. It should also be noted that their hypotensive action is inhibited by tricyclic antidepressants. Conversely, the withdrawal of these psychotropic drugs may precipitate severe hypotension in patients who are also receiving bethanidine or debrisoquine.

Beta blockers (see also earlier section, 'Beta-receptor adrenergic blockade')

The mechanism whereby β-blocking drugs exert their antihypertensive effect is still unclear. Several possible, but as yet unproven, explanations have been forthcoming.

(1) Resetting of the baroreceptors (Prichard and Gillam, 1966, 1969).
(2) Chronic reduction of cardiac output (Hansson, 1973).
(3) A central effect (McMillin, 1973; Dollery and Lewis, 1976).
(4) An antirenin action (Bühler *et al.*, 1973, 1975).
(5) Reduction in plasma volume and the concentration of sodium in the arterial wall (Tarazi and Dunstan, 1972; Tarazi *et al.*, 1974).
(6) Adrenergic neuron blocking action (Barrett and Nunn, 1970).

Since, however, hypertension is a multifactoral disease and since some of the mechanisms may be dose dependent it would seem reasonable to suppose that one or more may apply in individual patients.

When combined with diuretics or vasodilators, an augmented hypotensive response is usual since the reflex tachycardia and increase in cardiac output frequently produced by these agents is either attenuated or blocked.

Propranolol and oxprenolol are examples of β blockers commonly employed in the treatment of hypertension (often in high doses).

Other antihypertensive agents

LABETALOL

This is a β blocker with some α-receptor blocking activity. Its value as an antihypertensive agent in chronic hypertension requires further evaluation (Prichard *et al.*, 1975).

ALPHA-METHYLDOPA

Whilst still a commonly employed antihypertensive agent in the UK, this drug is not prescribed so liberally elsewhere in Europe or in the USA.

Although it is moderately effective in the management of less severe grades of hypertension, its mode of action is as yet uncertain. Some central effect seems likely (Laverty, 1973).

After oral administration a reduction of peripheral vascular resistance has been described (Chamberlain and Howard, 1964), and a venopressor effect with venous pooling has also been reported (Mason and Braunwald, 1964). Only relatively minor and inconsistent changes of cardiac output have been observed.

Effective blood pressure control requires a daily dose of between 0.75 and 2.0 g. Nowadays few workers prescribe a higher dosage since the addition of a diuretic or some alternative antihypertensive agent is preferred.

Although postural and exertional falls in blood pressure occur, these are less evident than with the adrenergic neuron inhibitors.

Its clinical usefulness is limited by a fairly high therapeutic failure rate with moderate dosage, a substantial incidence of excessive fatiguability with, occasionally, the development of frank depression and the finding of a positive Coombs' test in 20% of patients receiving this drug — although overt autoimmune haemolytic anaemia is rare. Much less common side-effects include a 'hepatitis' syndrome, hyperpyrexia, a paradoxical pressor response and the appearance of a Parkinsonian syndrome.

Although opinions are commonly expressed that this antihypertensive agent promotes serious hypotension during anaesthesia, there is little in the literature to confirm this (Dodson, 1977).

Clonidine

Clonidine is a relatively mild antihypertensive drug which acts by stimulating α-adrenoreceptors in the hindbrain and thereby effecting a reduction in spontaneous sympathetic activity and increasing vagal tone (Henning, 1975). It rarely controls blood pressure on its own and it is usually necessary to add in a diuretic. Following oral administration (usual dose being 0.2–2.0 mg daily) its hypotensive effect can be seen in 30–60 minutes, reaching a peak in 2–4 hours, and it remains significantly effective for 6–12 hours. Renal function is preserved. Abrupt withdrawal can cause an exaggerated rise in blood pressure, sweating and an anxiety state within 8–24 hours (Honyor *et al.*, 1973). This situation is best treated by the administration of intravenous clonidine, phentolamine or propranolol.

VASODILATORS

Essentially, these agents cause peripheral vasodilatation by their direct actions with, as a consequence, a decrease in pre- and afterload on the heart. They are therefore used in acute/accelerated hypertension or in intractable heart failure (*Figure 37.2*).

Hydrallazine

This drug has a direct relaxation action on vascular smooth muscle (renal arterioles being particularly responsive) and thereby decreases peripheral vascular resistance. When used in high doses (600–800 mg daily), there is frequently a reflex increase in heart rate and cardiac output which may cause headache and palpitations, or angina in patients with coronary heart disease. Long-term administration in these higher doses may induce a subacute lupus-erythematosus-type syndrome but this is rarely observed with doses of 200 mg daily or less.

When given intravenously or intramuscularly (5—10 mg at a time), rapid falls in blood pressure can be obtained.

Hydrallazine combined with a β-blocking agent often proves very effective in the management of renal hypertension.

Prazosin

This is a moderately effective vasodilator but, unlike hydrallazine, does not cause a rise in cardiac output or tachycardia. Renal blood flow is maintained. However, severe postural hypotension and collapse have been witnessed shortly after starting therapy and as yet this preparation has not found widespread acclaim in the management of hypertension.

The initial dose must be small: 0.5—1.0 mg at bed time.

Diazoxide

Another agent which acts directly on vascular smooth muscle is diazoxide.

Bolus intravenous administration (300 mg) is recommended and can be repeated in about 20 minutes. This usually promotes a fall in blood pressure within 5 minutes which may persist for several hours (Finnerty, 1974). Reflex tachycardia and increase in cardiac output are frequently associated with this hypotensive response and may precipitate pulmonary oedema or myocardial ischaemia.

Since the maximum response is achieved within 20 minutes, blood pressure monitoring need only be continued for a relatively short period. Diazoxide causes hyperglycaemia.

Sodium nitroprusside, phentolamine and nitroglycerin

Successful and rapid haemodynamic manipulation with these other peripheral vasodilator agents has attracted considerable interest in recent years (Finnerty, 1974; Palmer and Lasseter, 1975; Helfant, 1976; Kaplan,

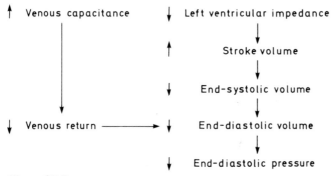

Figure 37.2
Haemodynamic changes with vasodilators

Dunbar and Jones, 1976). They have been used in the treatment of acute severe hypertension and in other situations where it would appear desirable to achieve rapid reduction in afterload (and to some extent preload); for example, when cardiac output has fallen as a consequence of acute myocardial infarction (provided the systemic blood pressure is not unduly low), or in acute left ventricular failure due to hypertension. The physiological mechanisms whereby these agents effect a reduction of cardiac work is shown in *Figure 37.2.*

Nitroprusside, phentolamine and nitroglycerin should be given by continuous dilute intravenous infusion using a constant infusion pump — the dose being titrated against the desired effect as reflected by the clinical progress and urinary output, preferably combined with meticulous haemodynamic monitoring to avoid extreme and rapid blood pressure fluctuations.

DOSES

Nitroprusside	$10-20$ μg·min^{-1} i.v.
Phentolamine	$0.1-2.0$ mg·min^{-1} i.v.
Nitroglycerin	$30-130$ μg·min^{-1} i.v.

Toxicity from sodium nitroprusside is uncommon unless a rapid infusion rate is employed, when severe acidosis and other metabolic changes thought to be due to cyanide intoxication and cellular hypoxia can occur (Greiss, Tremblay and Davies, 1976).

GANGLION-BLOCKING DRUGS

These drugs are now rarely, if ever, used for long-term management of established hypertension.

Pentolinium

When administered either subcutaneously or intramuscularly, pentolinium promotes a rapid fall in blood pressure. It is therefore still prescribed occasionally in the treatment of hypertensive crises, particularly when complicated by acute heart failure and pulmonary oedema. The dosage is 0.25 mg immediately, 0.5 mg half an hour later, followed by 1.0 mg every subsequent half hour until the desired effect is achieved.

Trimetaphan

Trimetaphan is an extremely short-acting ganglionic blocker often used to produce elective controlled hypotension during anaesthesia but, like pentolinium, can prove most effective in the management of hypertensive crises. Careful blood pressure monitoring is required after intravenous administration, the dose being $0.1-1.0$ mg·min^{-1}.

Since trimetaphan may cause histamine release, it should be avoided in patients who have a history of allergy.

Anaesthesia for patients on antihypertensive agents

If antihypertensive therapy is maintained throughout the period of general anaesthesia, special attention must be paid to the dose of the selected anaesthetic agent, which should be adequate but not excessive. An unduly rapid induction must be avoided, as must hypoxia, hypercarbia and excessive positive pressure ventilation. Other important points are that care must be taken in the positioning and handling of patients; also, blood pressure, heart rate and ECG must be sedulously monitored, as must blood and fluid balance. The use of appropriate vasopressor agents obviously requires great care.

DIGOXIN

Although the therapeutic value of digoxin in the treatment of congestive cardiac failure with atrial fibrillation and for some primary arrhythmic states is well established, the difference between the optimum therapeutic and toxic doses is small. Hospital and outpatient surveys have shown evidence of toxicity in up to 23% of patients (Carruthers, Kelly and McDevitt, 1974). However, improved knowledge of its pharmacokinetic characteristics (Shaw, 1977), the development of radioimmunoassay techniques (Koch-Weser, Duhme and Greenblatt, 1974) and the everyday use of electrocardiograms, have allowed more appropriate and safer prescribing habits.

Absorption, distribution and elimination

Since 1975, the pharmaceutical formulation of digoxin has been standardized to produce a reasonably constant bioavailability of at least 75% of the administered dose in one hour. Rapid absorption after ingestion is usual, with peak blood levels occurring at about 60 minutes. There is very little to be gained by intravenous administration. After intramuscular injections, which are often painful, there is often delay in absorption.

After intravenous injection, distribution mainly to the kidney, cardiac and skeletal muscle is complete in six hours. In the elderly with reduced renal function, plasma water and skeletal muscle mass, the plasma digoxin level may rise to toxic values if the usual adult dosage is prescribed.

Elimination is mainly via the kidney, approximately 37% of the drug being excreted daily. Only a very small percentage is metabolized. If renal function is poor, excretion is depressed proportional to the reduction in creatinine clearance and dosage must be reduced accordingly to prevent accumulation.

Plasma estimations

Plasma levels of between 0.8 and 2.6 ng·ml^{-1} are considered to be in the therapeutic range though evidence of toxicity can be observed with levels below this upper limit. In children a plasma level of up to 3.0 ng·ml^{-1} is still considered to be within the therapeutic range. Estimations should be made at least six hours after the last dose.

Dosage

A loading dose, if required for rapid digitalization, should be between two and three times the maintenance dose in the presence of normal renal function. Intravenous dosage should be 75% of the oral dose whether administered as a loading procedure or as maintenance therapy.

Adults
(1) Rapid oral digitalization: 0.75 mg loading dose, followed by 0.25 mg at 12-hourly intervals until either the ventricular rate has fallen to between 70 and 80 beats per minute or evidence of toxicity appears.
(2) Slow oral digitalization: 0.25 mg b.d. for 2–3 days, then 0.25 mg daily.
(3) Emergency intravenous digitalization: 0.5 mg as loading dose, followed by 0.125–0.250 mg daily.
(4) Usual maintenance dose: 0.125–0.500 mg daily.

Children
(1) Over 10 years of age, as for adults.
(2) Infants and children under 10 years of age: digitalization (all routes) 0.0125 mg·kg^{-1} body weight, repeated 6-hourly until therapeutic result obtained — 2 to 4 days usually being sufficient. Maintenance dose of up to 0.025 mg·kg^{-1} body weight daily.

Notes
(1) These recommendations are related to the digoxin preparations standardized after 1975.
(2) Ouabaine — previously used for rapid digitalization — is no longer available.
(3) Caution must be exercised when using the intravenous route if a patient has been receiving digoxin within the previous 10–14 days.

Toxicity

The more usual side-effects of digoxin are nausea, vomiting, anorexia, diarrhoea and a variety of arrhythmias, including ventricular ectopic activity (with bigeminus), sinus bradycardia, supraventricular tachycardias and AV conduction block of varying degrees. Occasionally, ventricular tachycardia and fibrillation or yellow vision (xanthopsia) occur. Increased sympathetic drive, hypokalaemia, hypercalcaemia, hypomagnesia, hypoxia, acid—base disturbance, hypothyroidism, insulin sensitivity and renal impairment predipose to drug intolerance, perhaps by effecting an increase in myocardial binding.

Although plasma digoxin levels may help confirm suspected toxicity, it should be appreciated that the relation between plasma levels, myocardial cell concentration and therapeutic effect is not always consistent. Furthermore, since equilibrium with the tissues is relatively slow, high (and therefore sometimes misleading) plasma levels may be found shortly after the onset of treatment before satisfactory digitalization has been achieved. However, in clinical practice, toxicity rarely develops so soon after the acute administration of this drug.

The commonest causes of intoxication are inadvertent and excessive dosage in the elderly or in hypokalaemia, a rapidly induced diuresis in heart failure and ill-conceived increments of digoxin for atrial fibrillation with an excessive ventricular rate or in the presence of supraventricular tachycardia.

Toxicity is relatively rare with plasma levels below 2 ng·ml^{-1} although there is an overlap between levels found in non-toxic and toxic patients. Therefore clinical awareness, combined with ECG monitoring, must be maintained before dosage adjustment, bearing in mind that similar symptoms, arrhythmias and S—T segment abnormalities in the electrocardiogram are common as part of the primary cardiac condition rather than necessarily being a manifestation of digoxin toxicity.

TREATMENT OF DIGOXIN TOXICITY

(1) Withdrawal of the drug is essential.
(2) Any predisposing factors such as electrolyte imbalance or hypoxia should be corrected.
(3) In the presence of ventricular arrhythmias (recurrent ventricular ectopic activity or ventricular tachycardia — fibrillation), one or more of the following antiarrythmic agents may be administered:
    (a) intravenous lignocaine 50—100 mg bolus;
    (b) intravenous phenytoin 50—250 mg over 5—10 minutes, or
    (c) cautious beta blockade.

D.C. countershock should be reserved for ventricular fibrillation or tachyarrhythmias with haemodynamic deterioration or those that have failed to respond to the other measures described.

Clinical use

Although the results of recent studies question the effectiveness of the positive inotropic action of digoxin when patients are in sinus rhythm (Knoebel, 1969; Davidson and Gibson, 1973), the benefit that can result from its chronotropic activity is beyond doubt.

Acute and chronic congestive cardiac failure, often with accompanying atrial fibrillation and rheumatic heart disease, are the commonest reasons for the administration of digoxin. This drug is also used solely or in combination with other antiarrhythmic agents to control paroxysmal tachycardia. In left heart failure following acute myocardial infarction with maintained sinus rhythm, the use of digoxin remains controversial and the evidence for and against is highly anecdotal. In hypertrophic obstructive cardiomyopathy digoxin should be avoided.

Prophylactic digoxin has also been advocated in certain classes of patients; for example, in the elderly or those who are undergoing thoracotomy, who may be considered to be at risk during or after surgery with respect to the development of heart failure, atrial fibrillation or paroxysmal supraventricular tachycardia (Deutsch and Dalen, 1969). However, there is little everyday support for the use of digoxin in this manner. Furthermore, diagnostic difficulties and subsequent problems in the management of perioperative arrhythmias would be anticipated under such circumstances. In contrast, withdrawal of digoxin in the preoperative phase in certain specialized fields (e.g. open heart surgery) to avoid the development of arrhythmias during cardiopulmonary bypass surgery is advised by Branthwaite (1977). Neither of these recommendations should be adopted routinely. A further account of digitalization in the preoperative period is given in Chapter 35.

GLYCERYL TRINITRATE AND ISOSORBIDE DINITRATE

These drugs are both commonly used, prophylactically and therapeutically, in the treatment of angina pectoris. They reduce cardiac work by lowering peripheral vascular resistance and, to some extent by improving coronary flow as a consequence of relaxation of responsive coronary vasculature and redistribution of coronary flow.

If administered in the immediate preoperative phase, the anaesthetist should be alert to the possible development of significant hypotension.

References

Adams, A. P. (1975). Techniques of vascular control for deliberate hypotension during anaesthesia. *Br. J. Anaesth.* 47, 777–792

Alderman, E. L., Coltart, D. J., Wettach, G. E. and Harrison, D. C. (1974). Coronary artery syndromes after sudden propranolol withdrawal. *Ann. intern. Med.* 81, 625–627

Barrett, A. M. and Nunn, B. (1970). Adrenergic neurone blocking properties of (±) − propranolol and (+) − propranolol. *J. Pharm. Pharmac.* 22, 806–810

Bingham, W., Elliott, J. and Lyons, S. M. (1972). Management of anaesthesia for phaeochromocytoma. *Anaesthesia* 27, 49–60

Branthwaite, M. A. (1977). *Anaesthesia for Cardiac Surgery and Allied Procedures*, p.33. Oxford: Blackwell Scientific

Buckley, J. J. and Jackson, J. A. (1961). Postoperative cardiac arrhythmias. *Anesthesiology* 22, 723–737

Bühler, F. R., Laragh, J. H., Vaughan, E. D., Brunwer, H. R., Gavros, H. and Baer, L. (1973). Antihypertensive action of propranolol: specific antirenin responses in high and normal renin forms of essential, renal, renovascular and malignant hypertension. *Am. J. Cardiol.* 32, 511–522

Bühler, F. R., Marbet, G., Patel, U. and Burkart, F. (1975). Renin-suppressing potency of various beta-adrenergic blocking agents at supine rest and during upright exercise. *Clin. Sci. molec. Med.* 48, 61S

Carruthers, S. G., Kelly, J. G. and McDevitt, D. G. (1974). Plasma digoxin concentrations in patients on admission to hospital. *Br. Heart J.* 36, 707–712

Chamberlain, D. A. and Edmonds-Seal, J. (1964). Effects of surgery under general anaesthesia on the electrocardiogram in ischaemic heart disease and hypertension. *Br. med. J.* 2, 784–787

Chamberlain, D. A. and Howard, J. (1964). Guanethidine and methyldopa: a haemodynamic study. *Br. Heart J.* 26, 528–536

Coltart, D. J., Cayen, M. N., Stinson, E. B., Goldman, R. H., Davies, R. O. and Harrison, D. C. (1975). Investigation of the safe withdrawal period for propranolol in patients scheduled for open heart surgery. *Br. Heart J.* 37, 1228–1234

Dack, S. (1963). Symposium on cardiovascular-pulmonary problems before and after surgery. II. Post-operative problems: Post-operative myocardial infarction. *Am. J. Cardiol.* 12, 423–430

Davidson, C. and Gibson, D. (1973). Clinical significance of positive inotropic action of digoxin in patients with left ventricular disease. *Br. Heart J.* 35, 970–976

Davison, M. H. A. (1951). Danger of methonium drugs. *Br. med. J.* 1, 584

Deutsch, S. and Dalen, J. E. (1969). Indications for prophylactic digitalization. *Anesthesiology* 30, 648–656

Dodson, M. E. (1977). Mechanisms of drug interactions. *Anaesthesia Rounds* No. 8, p. 15

Dollery, C. T. and Lewis, P. J. (1976). Central hypotensive effect of propranolol. *Postgrad. med. J.* 52, Suppl. 4, 116–120

Dunstan, H. P., Tarazi, R. C. and Bravo, E. L. (1974). Diuretic and diet treatment of hypertension. *Archs intern. Med.* 133, 1007–1013

Finnerty, F. A. Jr. (1974). Malignant hypertension. *Am. Heart J.* 88, 265–268

Gersh, B. J., Prys-Roberts, C., Reuben, S. R. and Baker, A. B. (1970). The relationship between depressed myocardial contractility and the stroke output of the canine heart during halothane anaesthesia. *Br. J. Anaesth.* 42, 560

Greiss, L., Tremblay, N. A. G. and Davies, D. W. (1976). The toxicity of sodium nitroprusside. *Can. Anaesth. Soc. J.* 23, 480–485

Grogono, A. W. and Lee, P. (1970). Danger lists for the anaesthetist: a revised version. *Anaesthesia* 25, 518–524

Hale Enderby, G. E. (1974). Pharmacological blockade. *Postgrad. med. J.* 50, 572–575

Hansen, J. (1968). Hydrochlorothiazide in the treatment of hypertension. The effects of blood volume, exchangeable sodium and blood pressure. *Acta med. scand.* 183, 317–321

Hansson, L. (1973). Beta-adrenergic blockade in essential hypertension. Effects of propranolol on haemodynamic parameters and plasma renin activity. *Acta med. scand.* Suppl. 55, 1–40

Helfant, R. H. (1976). Nitroglycerin: new concepts about an old drug. *Am. J. Med.* 60, 905–909

Henning, M. (1975). Central sympathetic transmitters and hypertension. *Clin. Sci. molec. Med.* 48, 195–203

Hickler, R. B. and Vandam, L. D. (1970). Hypertension. *Anesthesiology* 33, 214–228

Holdcroft, A. and Hall, G. M. (1978). Heat loss during anaesthesia. *Br. J. Anaesth.* 50, 157–164

Honyor, S. N., Hansson, L., Harrison, T. S. and Hoobler, S. W. (1973). Effects of clonidine withdrawal; possible mechanisms and suggestions for management. *Br. med. J.* 2, 209–211

Ikezono, E., Yasuda, K. and Hattori, Y. (1969). Effects of propranolol in epinephrine-induced arrhythmias during halothane anesthesia in man and cats. *Anesth. Analg. curr. Res.* 48, 598–604

Johnson, G. and Regardh, C. G. (1976). Clinical pharmacokinetics of beta-adrenoreceptor blocking drugs. *Clin. Pharmacokin.* 1, 233–236

Johnstone, M. (1966). Propranolol (Inderal) during halothane anaesthesia. *Br. J. Anaesth.* 38, 516–529

Johnstone, M. (1971). Oxprenolol (Trasicor) during halothane anaesthesia in surgical patients. *Br. J. Anaesth.* 43, 167–171

Kaplan, J. A. and Dunbar, R. W. (1976). Propranolol and surgical anesthesia. *Anesth. Analg. curr. Res.* 55, 1–5

Kaplan, J. A., Dunbar, R. W. and Jones, E. L. (1976). Nitroglycerin infusion during coronary artery surgery. *Anesthesiology* 45, 14–21

Kaplan, J. A., Dunbar, R. W., Bland, J. W., Sumpter, R. and Jones, E. L. (1975). Propranolol and cardiac surgery: a problem for the anesthesiologist. *Anesth. Analg. curr. Res.* 54, 571–578

Khatri, I. M. and Cohn, J. N. (1970). Mechanisms of exercise hypotension after sympathetic blockade. *Am. J. Cardiol.* 25, 329–338

Knoebel, S. B. (1969). In *Digitalis*. C. Fisch and B. Surawicz (ed.). New York: Grune & Stratton

Koch-Weser, J., Duhme, D. W. and Greenblatt, D. (1974). Influence of serum digoxin concentration measurements on frequency of digitoxicity. *Clin. Pharmac. Ther.* 16, 284–287

Laverty, R. (1973). The mechanism of action of some anti-hypertensive drugs. *Br. med. Bull.* 29, 152–157

Leth, A. (1970). Changes in pressure and extra-cellular volumes in patients with essential hypertension during long-term treatment with hydrochlorothiazide. *Circulation* 42, 479–485

McAllister, R. G. Jr. (1976). Intravenous propranolol administration: a method for rapidly achieving and sustaining desired plasma levels. *Clin. Pharmac. Ther.* 22, 517–523

McClish, A., Andrew, D., Moisan, A, and Morin, Y. (1968). Intravenous propranolol for cardiac disturbances in relation to halothane anaesthesia for cardiovascular surgery. *Can. med. Ass. J.* 99, 388

McMillin, W. P. (1973). Trasicor in the treatment of emotional stress. In *New Perspectives in Beta-blockade*, p. 313. D. M. Burley, J. H. Frier, R. K. Rondel and S. H. Taylor (ed.). Horsham: Ciba

Marshall, B. E. and Wyche, M. O. (1972). Hypoxemia during and after anesthesia. *Anesthesiology* 37, 178–209

Mason, D. T. and Braunwald, E. (1964). Effects of guanethidine, reserpine and methyldopa on reflex venous and arterial constriction in man. *J. clin. Invest.* 43, 1449–1463

Michie, W. (1974). The role of beta-adrenergic blockade in the management of thyrotoxicosis. *Ann. Acad. Med.* 3, 218–225

Miller, R. R., Olson, H. G., Amsterdam, E. A. and Mason, D. T. (1975). Propranolol with-drawal rebound phenomenon. *New Engl. J. Med.* 293, 416–418

Mizgala, H. F. and Counsell, J. (1976). Acute coronary syndromes following abrupt cessation of oral propranolol therapy. *Can. med. Ass. J.* 114, 1123–1126

Moran, J. M., Caralps, J. M., Mulet, J. and Pifarre, R. (1973). Propranolol and cardiac surgery. *New Engl. J. Med.* 289, 1254

Moran, J. M., Mulet, J., Caralps, J. M. and Pifarre, R. (1974). Coronary revascularization in patients receiving propranolol. *Circulation* 49–50, Suppl. 2, 116–120

Moyer, J. H., Brest, A. N. and Nathanson, D. (1963). Medical considerations in the hyper-tensive patient undergoing surgery. *Am. J. Cardiol.* 12, 286–292

Palmer, R. F. and Lasseter, K. C. (1975). Sodium nitroprusside. *New Engl. J. Med.* 292, 294–297

Parsons, V. and Jewitt, D. (1967). Beta-adrenergic blockade in the management of acute thyrotoxic crises, tachycardia and arrhythmias. *Postgrad. med. J.* 43, 756–762

Petrie, J. C., Galloway, D. B., Jeffers, T. A. and Webster, J. (1976). Adverse reactions to beta-blocking drugs: a review. *Postgrad. med. J.* 52, Suppl. 4, 63–69

Pickering, G. W. (1968). *High Blood Pressure,* 2nd edn. London: Churchill

Prichard, B. N. C. and Gillam, P. M. S. (1966). Propranolol in hypertension. *Am. J. Cardiol.* 18, 387

Prichard, B. N. C. and Gillam, P. M. S. (1969). Treatment of hypertension with propranolol. *Br. med. J.* 1, 7–16

Prichard, B. N. C., Thompson, F. O., Boakes, A. J. and Joekes, A. M. (1975). Some haemodynamic effects of compound AH5158 compared with propranolol, propranolol plus hydrallazine and diazoxide; the use of AH5158 in the treatment of hypertension. *Clin. Sci. molec. Med.* 48, 97–100

Prys-Roberts, C., Meloche, R. and Foëx, P. (1971). Studies of anaesthesia in relation to hypertension. I. Cardiovascular responses of treated and untreated patients. *Br. J. Anaesth.* 43, 122–137

Prys-Roberts, C., Foëx, P., Biro, G. P. and Roberts, J. G. (1973). Studies of anaesthesia in relation to hypertension. V. Adrenergic beta-receptor blockade. *Br. J. Anaesth.* 45, 671–680

Robertson, A. I. G. (1965). Pre- and post-operative care of patients with phaeochromocytomas. *Postgrad. med. J.* 41, 481–484

Rollason, W. N. and Hall, D. J. (1973). Dysrhythmias during inhalational anaesthesia for oral surgery. *Anaesthesia* 28, 139–145

Ross, E. J., Prichard, B. N. C., Kaufman, L., Robertson, A. I. G. and Harries, B. J. (1967). Pre-operative and operative management of patients with phaeochromocytomas. *Br. med. J.* 1, 191–198

Ryder, W., Charlton, J. E. and Gorman, P. B. W. (1973). Oral atropine and practolol pre-medication in dental anaesthesia. *Br. J. Anaesth.* 45, 745–749

Shand, D. (1975). Propranolol withdrawal. *New Engl. J. Med.* 293, 449–450

Shand, D. G. (1976). Pharmacokinetics of propranolol: a review. *Postgrad. med. J.* 52, Suppl. 4, 22–25

Shanks, R. G., Hadden, D. R., Lowe, D. C., McDevitt, D. G. and Montgomery, D. A. D. (1969). Controlled trial of propranolol in thyrotoxicosis. *Lancet* i, 993–994

Shaw, T. R. D. (1977). Clinical pharmaco-kinetics of digitalis. In *Recent Advances in Cardiology*, Vol. 7, pp. 425–445. J. Hamer (ed.). Edinburgh: Churchill Livingstone

Skinner, J. F. and Pearce, M. L. (1964). Surgical risk in the cardiac patient. *J. chronic Dis.* 17, 57–72

Tarazi, R. C. and Dunstan, H. P. (1972). Beta-adrenergic blockade in hypertension: practical and theoretical implications of long-term hemodynamic variations. *Am. J. Cardiol.* 29, 633–640

Tarazi, R. C., Ibrahim, M. M., Dunstan, H. P. and Ferraro, C. M. (1974). Cardiac factors in hypertension. *Circulation Res.* 34, Suppl. 1, 213–221

Tarhan, S., Moffit, E. A., Taylor, W. F. and Guiwani, E. R. (1972). Myocardial infarction after general anesthesia. *J. Am. med. Ass.* 220, 1451–1454

Tyers, G. F. O. and Hughes, H. C. (1976). Residual effects when chronic propranolol therapy is discontinued within 48 hours of cardiopulmonary by-pass. *Am. Heart J.* 91, 757–765

Viljoen, J. F., Estafanous, F. G. and Kellner, G. A. (1972). Propranolol and cardiac surgery. *J. thorac. cardiovasc. Surg.* 64, 826–830

Vlachakis, N. O., DeGuia, O. and Mendlowitz, M. (1977). Blood pressure responses to catecholamines during beta-adrenergic blockade with propranolol in hypertensive subjects. *Chest* 71, 38–43

Waal-Manning, H. J. (1976). Hypertension — which beta-blocker? *Drugs* 12, 412–441

Weaver, P. C., Bailey, J. S. and Preston, T. D. (1970). Coronary artery blood flow in the halothane depressed canine heart. *Br. J. Anaesth.* 42, 678–684

38 Autonomic drugs
Norton E. Williams

The autonomic nervous system is widely distributed throughout the body and controls the so-called automatic or vegetative functions such as circulation, respiration, digestion and the maintenance of body temperature. It can be conveniently divided on anatomical and physiological grounds into the following.

(1) *The parasympathetic system,* which leaves the CNS via cranial and sacral pathways, and is primarily concerned with conservation and restoration of energy. It slows the heart, lowers blood pressure and facilitates the digestion and absorption of nutrients, and the excretion of waste material.
(2) *The sympathetic system,* which emerges from the spinal cord in the thoracic and upper lumbar regions, and enables the body to be prepared for 'fight or flight'. Thus the heart rate is accelerated, blood pressure rises, there is shift of blood from skin and splanchnic vessels to skeletal muscle, and an increased availability in the plasma of 'energy providers', namely glucose and free fatty acids.

Central integration of these autonomic systems occurs in the medulla oblongata as far as respiration and blood pressure are concerned, and in the hypothalamus and related nuclei with regard to many of the other functions.

Drugs which influence autonomic activity do so for the most part by influencing neurohumoral transmission peripherally, either at ganglionic sites or at peripheral nerve endings and the effector organs which they supply. It is evident that many drugs have important effects (e.g. cardiac glycosides) or side-effects (e.g. neuromuscular blocking agents, tricyclic antidepressants) mediated at these sites. It is also clear that central regulation of autonomic activity will involve chemical transmission via acetylcholine, noradrenaline, dopamine and 5-hydroxytryptamine; this may be modified by drugs which may or may not have apparent peripheral autonomic activity. For example, the antihypertensive effects of methyl-dopa and clonidine almost certainly depend in part on an action within the hypothalamus. Nevertheless, it is convenient to discuss autonomic drugs as those whose primary action is to mimic or modify peripheral systems, and to classify them accordingly:

Parasympathomimetic drugs
Drugs which modify parasympathetic activity
Sympathomimetic drugs
Drugs which modify sympathetic activity

PARASYMPATHOMIMETIC DRUGS

Acetylcholine was synthesized by Baeyer in 1867. Dale (1914) observed that the effects of this substance mimicked closely the responses to stimulation of parasympathetic nerves, and introduced the term para sympathomimetic to characterize its effects. Loewi's cross-perfusion experiments (Loewi and Navratil, 1926) demonstrated the liberation into the circulating fluid of a substance which slowed the heart of the recipient frog. The substance was originally termed 'Vagustoff' and later identified as acetylcholine. The effect of acetylcholine thus liberated from post-ganglionic parasympathetic nerves bore a marked resemblance to that of the mushroom alkaloid, muscarine, and the term muscarinic became synonymous with parasympathomimetic. It subsequently became evident that acetylcholine was also the neurohumoral transmitter in all pre ganglionic fibres (sympathetic or parasympathetic), at the neuromuscular junction, in certain postganglionic sympathetic fibres such as vasodilator fibres and those to the sweat glands, as well as being involved in CNS transmission at some, but by no means all, synapses.

In spite of its extreme physiological importance, acetylcholine has little therapeutic application because of its diffuse effects and its evanescent action. It has been employed as a therapeutic convulsant in the manage-ment of schizophrenia (Cohen, Thale and Tissenbaum, 1944), and to provoke local axon responses when studying autonomic involvement in acute polyneuritis (Spalding and Crampton Smith, 1963). Other cholin-esters, such as propionylcholine and butyrylcholine, may be formed in the gut by bacterial action. They may inhibit acetylcholinesterase (AChE), and it has been suggested that the main physiological role of plasma cholinesterase may be the hydrolysis of these substances (Lehmann and Liddell, 1969).

Synthetic choline esters include acetyl-β-methylcholine (methacholine), carbachol and benzoylcholine. Methacholine is more slowly hydrolysed by AChE than its parent drug; it forms a useful substrate for direct estimation of red cell enzyme activity, and indirectly for the measurement of plasma edrophonium levels (Calvey *et al.*, 1976). It has also been used in the control of supraventricular arrhythmias. *Carbachol* is not destroyed by cholinesterases and is useful in the management of atony of bladder or bowel, especially in the postoperative period; its cardiac effects, after oral or subcutaneous administration, are less marked. *Benzoylcholine* is hydrolysed by plasma cholinesterase, and is commonly used for the estimation of levels of this enzyme.

Natural alkaloids which have parasympathomimetic activity include muscarine and arecoline which have no clinical uses, and pilocarpine, a useful miotic in the management of glaucoma.

Anticholinesterases will allow cumulation of acetylcholine at all its sites of action; increased parasympathomimetic activity will be one manifestation; however, a direct action of some of these drugs on the effector organ will also be a contributing factor (Riker and Wescoe, 1946). These compounds may combine with the AChE enzyme at two sites, anionic and esteratic, the latter having two components (*Figure 38.1*).

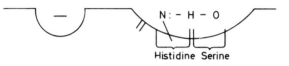

Histidine Serine

ANIONIC   ESTERATIC

Figure 38.1
Binding sites of acetylcholinesterase (AChE)

The anionic site attracts positively charged nitrogen atoms by electrostatic forces. The histidine component of the esteratic site allows for hydrogen bonding, whilst the serine grouping can produce covalent linkages with electrophilic carbon atoms.

Quaternary ammonium compounds block substrate attachment by reversible combination at the anionic site. In high dosage they may complicate the action of neuromuscular blocking agents.

Edrophonium combines at the anionic site, and by hydrogen bonding at the esteratic site; the compound formed is rapidly hydrolysable. The transient action of edrophonium makes it a useful diagnostic drug in the management of myasthenia gravis; it has occasionally been used in the treatment of paroxysmal atrial tachycardia.

Neostigmine and related carbamyl esters, like acetylcholine itself, combine at the anionic site and through the serine component of the esteratic site. An alcoholic moiety is initially split off, leaving a carbamylated enzyme which is then slowly hydrolysed (its half-life is roughly 40 000 000 times that of the acetylated enzyme (Wilson and Harrison, 1961)). The carbamates are known as 'competitive substrates' or 'acid-transferring inhibitors'.

Neostigmine, pyridostigmine and *ambenonium* can be used in the treatment of myasthenia gravis. Neostigmine is usually the drug of choice for reversal of neuromuscular blockade by non-depolarizing relaxants, although pyridostigmine may be a useful alternative (Katz, 1967; Lipmann and Rogoff, 1974).

The carbamates are also valuable for improving smooth muscle activity of bowel and bladder in the postoperative period. *Distigmine* is often used in this context and in the management of neurogenic bladders (Yeo, Southwell and Hindmarsh, 1973).

Physostigmine is the only non-ionized member of this group. It therefore readily crosses the blood—brain barrier, and has proved helpful in the treatment of poisoning by atropine compounds (Rumak, 1973) and by tricyclic antidepressants (Snyder, Blond and McWhirter, 1974).

Organophosphorous compounds usually combine with the enzyme at the esteratic site to form an extremely stable compound; virtually no hydrolysis occurs and return of enzyme activity depends upon the synthesis of new enzyme; they are thus potentially irreversible inhibitors. They have found widespread use as insecticides (along with newer carbamate compounds), and many of the more volatile agents in this group were synthesized during World War II with a view to development of chemical warfare. Poisoning by this group of substances will result in profound muscarinic effects as well as nicotinic manifestations, and treatment may include the use of atropine-like compounds, phenothiazines, anticonvulsants, cholinesterase reactivators such as pralidoxime and even carbamate compounds which will compete for the enzymatic site, and produce a more hydrolysable and therefore 'reversible' complex. One compound, *ecothiopate* (which combines at both sites) is a popular miotic. Its chronic usage has been associated with prolonged apnoea following suxamethonium (Pantuck, 1966).

DRUGS MODIFYING PARASYMPATHETIC ACTIVITY

Agents which modify parasympathetic activity are also known as parasympatholytic, anticholinergic or antimuscarinic drugs. Their main site of action is at effector organs innervated by postganglionic parasympathetic nerves, although some members of the group have important CNS effects; nicotinic effects are not significant, although experimentally atropine can modify depolarization at the motor end-plate (Katz and Miledi, 1973).

The naturally occurring alkaloids, atropine and hyoscine (scopolamine), are the most important members of this group. They are both organic esters of tropic acid and are chemically related to cocaine. They differ in their central effects and in the relative sensitivity of some effector organs (*Table 38.1*).

Atropine is also used to prevent muscarinic effects from administration of anticholinesterase drugs. It is often given with narcotic analgesics in the management of biliary and renal colic in the hope that it will relax smooth muscle, but it probably does not contribute greatly to the relief of pain. It is commonly employed as a mydriatic in the treatment of iridocyclitis or choroiditis; for diagnostic examination of the eye the shorter acting related compound, homatropine, is preferred. Its use is indicated in myocardial infarction where there is bradycardia associated with hypotension or premature ventricular beats (Adgey *et al.*, 1968).

Hyoscine (scopolamine) has central effects which have proved useful in the prophylaxis of motion sickness and other vestibular disorders; it produces 'twilight sleep' in association with narcotic analgesics, and its amnesic effect can be used to prevent awareness during obstetrical anaesthesia.

TABLE 38.1. Comparison of actions of atropine and hyoscine (scopolamine) in doses commonly used for premedication in adults

Site of action	Atropine 0.6 mg	Hyoscine (scopolamine) 0.4 mg
CNS	Cortical and medullary stimulation. Initial bradycardia due to vagal stimulation	Drowsiness; amnesia. Confusion in elderly patients
Eye	Less effect than hyoscine	Mydriasis and paralysis of accommodation
Respiratory	Bronchodilatation; increased V_D leads to raised rate and depth of respiration	Less marked bronchodilatation
Cardiovascular system	Some tachycardia after initial slowing; no slowing after i.v. injection; arrhythmias may occur	Less tachycardia and of shorter duration; arrhythmias unlikely
Antisialogogue effect	Less effective	More effective

Anticholinergic drugs have been widely used in the management of Parkinson's disease; they are still valuable in patients intolerant of levodopa and allied drugs, and especially in drug-induced Parkinsonism. *Benzhexol*, which appears to produce fewer peripheral side-effects than atropine, is a popular choice.

Semisynthetic and synthetic derivatives of the belladonna alkaloids include *atropine methonitrate, hyoscine butylbromide, propantheline,* and *dicyclomine.* These, being quaternary ammonium compounds, will not cross the blood—brain barrier; they also have significant ganglion-blocking effect. These properties have led to their development as antispasmodics in various gastrointestinal and genitourinary disorders; atropine methonitrate is a common constituent of various inhalant mixtures used in the treatment of bronchospasm. However, these drugs may produce significant side-effects due to their generalized antimuscarinic activity.

SYMPATHOMIMETIC DRUGS

In 1905, Langley, who a few years earlier had noted the similarity between effects of injection of adrenal gland extracts and sympathetic nerve stimulation, suggested that effector cells have excitatory or inhibitory 'receptor substances', and that the response to adrenaline depended upon which type of 'substance' was present. However, it was not until 1946 that von Euler showed that the substance in highly purified extracts of sympathetic nerves and effector organs bore a strong resemblance to noradrenaline. He proposed, and it was later confirmed, that noradrenaline is the predominant substance liberated at postganglionic sympathetic nerve endings, although small quantities of adrenaline may, on occasion, appear. By contrast, the adrenal medulla, supplied by preganglionic fibres liberating acetylcholine, has adrenaline as both its major catecholamine constituent and its secretion (approximately 80% in the adult), the remainder being noradrenaline.

In 1948, Ahlquist classified the receptor sites (or Langley's 'substances') as α and β on the basis of their response to six sympathomimetic amines. In general, α responses are excitatory (although there are α and β receptors for relaxation of intestinal smooth muscle)and β responses are inhibitory (with the notable exception of cardiac receptors). The differing sensitivities

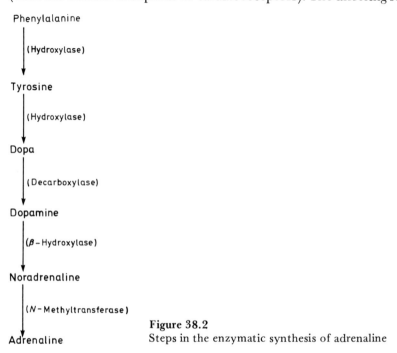

Figure 38.2
Steps in the enzymatic synthesis of adrenaline

of β receptors in various organs to stimulation and blockade led Lands and his coworkers (1967) to subdivide the β receptors into β_1 receptors in the heart and small intestine and β_2 receptors in bronchi and blood vessels.

The synthesis of adrenaline from phenylalanine was eventually demonstrated by Gurin and Delluva (1947); they gave radioactive-labelled precursor to rats and recovered radioactive adrenaline from the adrenal medulla. The synthesis takes place by the steps shown in *Figure 38.2*.

As the last three compounds are amines which can be represented by the general formula

$$ OH-\bigcirc\!\!\!-\overset{\beta}{CH}-\overset{\alpha}{CH}-NH $$
$$ \quad\quad OH \quad R \quad R \quad R $$

and as 3,4-dihydroxybenzene is also known as catechol, these substances along with isoprenaline constitute the important catecholamines.

It is now known that the key compound involved in the mediation of the metabolic effects of adrenaline and related compounds, and probably other pharmacodynamic actions, is cyclic adenosine 3′,5′-monophosphate (cyclic AMP). Catecholamines stimulate the enzyme adenylate cyclase to produce cyclic AMP from ATP (Sutherland and Rall, 1959). There is increasing evidence that the synthesis and release of many hormones is induced by intracellular accumulation of cyclic AMP and certain of the prostaglandins (PGE_2 and $PGF_{2\alpha}$).

Catecholamines

Adrenaline (epinephrine) induces the important physiological mechanisms of the 'fight or flight' response through α and β receptors. Usually, muscle blood flow is increased due to a β effect, but in high dosage, as after rapid intravenous infusion, there is a predominant effect on α receptors in muscle blood vessels and peripheral resistance is increased. This factor, coupled with its high arrhythmia potential, limits its employment in circulatory failure.

However, it has a wide variety of clinical uses. Alpha activity on skin and mucosal vessels makes it valuable as a nasal decongestant in allergic rhinitis, as a topical haemostat, and to reduce oedema and urticaria from drug hypersensitivity. It is the most commonly used vasoconstrictor added to local anaesthetic solutions. Powerful β activity leads to its use as a bronchodilator. It may be administered by subcutaneous injection (0.2–0.5 mg); intravenous injection is hazardous. It is found in various proprietary mixtures used as inhalants.

Rapid intravenous injection of adrenaline (0.5–1 mg) is used in the treatment of cardiac arrest. Theoretically, it should be most valuable in converting asystole (which has failed to respond to external cardiac massage) into fibrillation prior to the use of countershock; it may also help to render fine ventricular fibrillation more susceptible to defibrillation. Intracardiac adrenaline should be used only as a last resort (Chamberlain and Williams, 1976).

Noradrenaline (norepinephrine) exhibits almost exclusive α activity, and is also involved as a neurohumoral transmitter in certain tracts of the CNS. Intravenous infusion leads to an increased peripheral resistance, with elevated systolic and diastolic pressures, and usually a reflex slowing of the heart rate. The rationale for its use in the treatment of 'shock' associated with trauma, septicaemia and myocardial infarction is questionable, as compensatory vasoconstriction already occurs and elevated blood pressure results in further impairment of liver and renal blood flow. Noradrenaline can produce lethal shock in animals, and a similar effect is observed in man when this drug or other sympathomimetic amines are used injudiciously (Spoerel, Seleny and Williamson, 1964). Furthermore, extravasation may result in severe tissue necrosis.

Noradrenaline has also been used as a vasoconstrictor with local anaesthetics. It would appear to be theoretically superior to adrenaline, as arrhythmias are less likely. However, marked pressor responses have occurred after inadvertent intravenous injection, and death has been reported in a patient on concomitant tricyclic antidepressants (Boakes *et al.*, 1972).

Dopamine is the immediate precursor of noradrenaline, and is also an important transmitter in the CNS, especially the extrapyramidal system and the hypothalamus. Replenishment of dopamine stores is important in the treatment of Parkinsonism, but as dopamine does not readily cross the blood—brain barrier, its own precursor, L-dopa, is usually administered. Dopamine is the only catecholamine that specifically increases renal blood flow (Rosenblum, 1974); glomerular filtration rate, urinary output and sodium excretion are enhanced. This effect is abolished by haloperidol but not by propranolol, and it is suggested that the action is mediated through specific dopaminergic receptors; a similar mechanism may explain the increased splanchnic blood flow. It has positive β-receptor effects on the heart, but arrhythmias are less than with adrenaline or isoprenaline. It would appear to be a useful drug in the management of cardiogenic and toxaemic shock, in refractory congestive cardiac failure (Goldberg, 1974), and to improve circulation after cardiac surgery. It is administered by continuous infusion ($2–30$ mg·kg^{-1}. min^{-1}).

Dobutamine, a synthetic catecholamine, has been shown to have a marked positive inotropic action with little effect on rate (Jewitt *et al.*, 1974); it increases peripheral resistance.

Isoprenaline (isoproterenol) has a powerful action on β receptors, and almost no α effect. It therefore increases the rate and force of cardiac contraction whilst decreasing peripheral resistance. It is used in the management of low output states; however, arrhythmias are common, coronary blood flow will be reduced because of the fall in diastolic pressure, and renal blood flow may decrease due to diversion of blood to other vascular beds.

It is useful in the management of bronchial asthma; as well as the β effect, it may also directly inhibit antigen-induced release of histamine (Assem and Schild, 1969). It is usually administered by pressurized aerosol; oral or sublingual absorption is unreliable. Excessive usage of isoprenaline inhalers has been associated with an increased incidence of sudden death in asthmatic patients (Speizer, Doll and Strang, 1968), probably because of cardiac toxicity associated with severe hypoxia (Greenberg and Pines, 1967); a toxic effect of the fluorohydrocarbon propellants may be a contributing factor (Taylor and Harris, 1970). A theoretical disadvantage of isoprenaline is that vasodilatation of the bronchial mucosa may detract from the bronchodilator effect; a mixture containing a vasoconstrictor such as phenylephrine may be superior (Cushing and Miller, 1965).

Non-catecholamines

A large number of sympathomimetic amines have been synthesized for clinical use. They may be classified as follows.

DRUGS WITH MAINLY DIRECT ACTION

Via α receptors

Phenylephrine is used as a nasal decongestant, as a mydriatic and as a vasoconstrictor with local anaesthetic solutions.

Methoxamine is a powerful α-receptor stimulator which produces reflex slowing of the heart; it can thus be used to abolish attacks of paroxysmal atrial tachycardia. It is also of value in hypotensive states associated with sympathetic failure; for example, following spinal anaesthesia or ganglion-blockade hypotension.

Metaraminol is a similar drug, but sinus arrhythmia may occur during its use, and there may be a positive inotropic effect, presumably due to some β activity. Pulmonary blood pressure is elevated independently of cardiac output (Eckstein and Abboud, 1962).

Via β$_2$ receptors

These are drugs which have been developed primarily for the treatment of bronchial asthma, and include *salbutamol, orciprenaline, terbutaline* and *isoetharine* (actually a catecholamine). They are relatively specific for β$_2$ receptors, and have much less stimulant effect on the heart than does isoprenaline. They may be administered orally or via pressurized aerosols. Central side-effects including nervousness, tremor and drowsiness may occur; resistance to the effects of salbutamol after prolonged use has been demonstrated (Holgate and Tattersfield, 1977). The effect of these drugs on uterine smooth muscle has been utilized to delay delivery in premature labour (Liggins and Vaughan, 1973).

DRUGS WITH A MIXED (DIRECT AND INDIRECT) ACTION

This class of compounds is typified by ephedrine and by amphetamine and its substitutes. They possess α activity due to the release of noradrenaline stores in adrenergic nerve terminals, and β activity due to a direct effect on receptors (tachyphylaxis occurs presumably due to a depletion of these stores). They are well absorbed orally and cross the blood–brain barrier with ease; this accounts in part for their powerful CNS activity. They are resistant to the enzyme, monoamine oxidase, and in fact may inhibit its activity. Hypertensive crises leading to fatal intracranial haemorrhage have occurred when these drugs have been administered concurrently with the standard MAOIs (Goldberg, 1964).

Ephedrine occurs naturally in various plants, but can also be synthesized. Its peripheral actions make it useful in the prevention of syncope due to Stokes–Adams attacks and in the prophylaxis of hypotension following spinal anaesthesia. It is also available as a compound oral tablet or as a sustained release capsule for the management of asthma and related bronchospasm. It has been employed for its CNS effects in the management of narcolepsy and nocturnal enuresis.

Amphetamine's marked subjective CNS effects have led to widespread drug abuse, and it is now a controlled drug in the UK. It is a non-specific analeptic, and may be used to improve performance which has been reduced by fatigue; its use in the management of barbiturate poisoning is obsolete. It may also be employed in narcolepsy, Parkinsonism, certain psychogenic disorders and hyperkinetic states, and as an appetite suppressant in the management of obesity. A related drug, *fenfluramine*, which is used as an anorectic, causes drowsiness and therefore habituation does not occur; however, evidence suggests an interaction between fenfluramine and halothane in man (Bennett and Eltrincham, 1977). Fenfluramine is structurally related to both adrenaline and amphetamine, but appears to induce cardiac depression which may be associated with arrhythmias. Another related compound, *hydroxyamphetamine* does not readily enter the brain, and has been used in the management of hypotensive states. *Mephentermine* may be included in this group. It produces α and β effects and has been employed as a pressor agent, although tachyphylaxis will result after prolonged use, and convulsions may occur. Mucosal blanching and ulceration has been seen after local application.

DRUGS WHICH MODIFY SYMPATHETIC ACTIVITY

Ganglion-blocking drugs

These agents produce their effect by blocking postsynaptic receptor sites on autonomic ganglia. They include salts of *tetraethylammonium*, the *bis*-quaternary ammonium compounds *pentamethonium* and *hexamethonium*, the secondary and tertiary amines *pempidine* and *mecamylamine*, and the complex monosulphonium compound *trimetaphan*. At one time many of these drugs were extensively used in the treatment of hypertension, but presented the following disadvantages.

(1) The well ionized quaternary ammonium compounds are incompletely and unreliably absorbed from the gut.
(2) Preganglionic fibres to the adrenal medulla (mediated by ACh) are also blocked, and postural hypotension becomes a major problem.
(3) Autonomic ganglion blockade is non-selective (i.e. parasympathetic ganglia are blocked with equal ease). As many effector organs are predominantly under parasympathomimetic control, many undesirable side-effects such as tachycardia, paralytic ileus, urinary retention, xerostomia and visual disturbances will occur.

Trimetaphan (Arfonad) remains an important drug for use in controlled hypotension during surgery. It may also be valuable in the treatment of dissecting aneurysm or management of hypertensive crises, although drugs which act directly on vascular smooth muscle, such as sodium nitroprusside or diazoxide, may be preferable. Trimetaphan relies upon a direct action and the release of histamine, as well as its ganglion-blocking action, to produce the hypotensive effect.

The effects of ganglion-blocking agents at the neuromuscular junction are complex. In high dosage, neuromuscular blockade can be demonstrated in the cat (Bowman and Webb, 1972) and prolongation of neuromuscular blockade in man observed (Deacock and Hargrove, 1962); conversely, an anticurare effect on the rat diaphragm has been shown (Blackman, Gauldie and Milne, 1975); trimetaphan also depresses plasma cholinesterase and will prolong the effect of suxamethonium.

Drugs inhibiting adrenergic nerve endings

Noradrenaline is manufactured in the storage granules from its immediate precursor, dopamine, and is bound to an ATP—protein (chromogranin) complex in a 4:1 ratio. The arrival of an action potential at the nerve ending releases free noradrenaline which traverses the neuronal membrane to reach the postsynaptic (α or β) receptor sites. Excess noradrenaline is broken down to inactive metabolites by the enzyme catechol-O-methyltransferase (COMT). The remainder is returned by active transport to the axonal neuron, where there is some further destruction by monoamine oxidase, and re-enters the granular storage site (*Figure 38.3*).

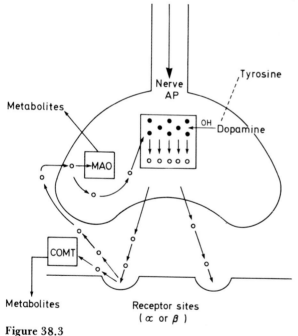

Figure 38.3
Synthesis, release and reuptake of noradrenaline at the adrenergic nerve terminal. AP, action potential; COMT, catechol-O-methyltransferase; MAO, monoamine oxidase. ●, bound noradrenaline; ○, unbound noradrenaline

The maintenance of a normal noradrenaline content therefore depends upon a balance between (1) its synthesis, storage and release from the granules, and (2) the reuptake of noradrenaline which has not been destroyed by enzymes. Increased plasma noradrenaline has been observed in some younger hypertensives, and may be a manifestation of an early phase in the development of hypertension (Sever *et al.*, 1977). Many drugs which are used extensively in the treatment of hypertension act by interfering with the noradrenaline balance, and eventually producing a depletion of noradrenaline storage at this site. They have proved superior to the ganglion-blocking drugs because parasympathetic nerves and preganglionic fibres to the medulla are unaffected, and side-effects are therefore fewer. The rauwolfia alkaloids (reserpine and its substituted derivatives) act mainly by blocking the uptake of dopamine, and the reuptake of noradrenaline into the storage granules. MAO destroys these

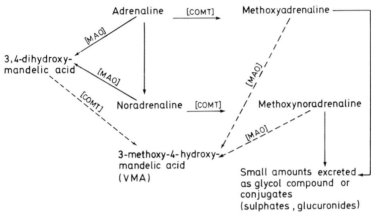

Figure 38.4
Metabolic pathways of adrenaline and noradrenaline. COMT, catechol-*O*-methyltransferase; MAO, monoamine oxidase

catecholamines, and there is eventual depletion of noradrenaline. A similar depletion occurs in the CNS, and this action is thought to be responsible for the major side-effect, depression, when relatively high doses are used. Rauwolfia alkaloids are therefore most effective when administered in relatively small doses for the treatment of mild to moderate hypertension (Goldberg, 1975).

α-Methyldopa was designed to compete in the normal synthetic pathways to noradrenaline, and result in the production of a 'false transmitter', α-methylnoradrenaline. It is now generally considered that the principal site of action of methyldopa is in the CNS; this also may be due to the formation of a false transmitter. Sedation is a relatively common side-effect and psychic depression has been described. Reactions of a drug-sensitivity type may also develop; 20% of patients show a positive Coombs' test, and haemolytic anaemia, drug fever and hepatitis can occur; retention of salt and water may result in oedema. However, it is a popular antihypertensive drug, and postural hypotension is infrequent. The monoamine oxidase inhibitor *pargyline* is used as an antihypertensive agent. Its mode of action is not clear, but one theory is that it allows accumulation of another 'false transmitter' octopamine at the nerve terminal. *α-Methyl-p-tyrosine*, which prevents noradrenaline synthesis by inhibiting the hydroxylation of tyrosine, appears to have little effect on the blood pressure of patients with essential hypertension (Engelman *et al.,* 1968). However, it has been used in the management of phaeochromocytoma with associated myocarditis (Bagnall, Salway and Jackson, 1976).

Guanethidine is thought to act within the storage granules. It is postulated that it displaces noradrenaline from the intragranular binding sites and prevents further uptake. Drugs which block active transport across the nerve membrane, such as cocaine, amphetamine and some tricyclic antidepressants, antagonize the effect of guanethidine. Following intravenous administration, there may initially be a pressor effect due to an increase in circulating noradrenaline. However, this will be followed by a fall in blood pressure which may last for several days. It does not cross the blood–brain barrier readily, and central effects are therefore rare. It is usually reserved for patients with more severe hypertension; postural hypotension, diarrhoea and failure of ejaculation are common side-effects. It has also been used to produce intravenous regional sympathetic block in the treatment of causalgic states (Hannington-Kiff, 1974).

An analogue, *bethanidine,* has a shorter duration of action and probably fewer side-effects. *Debrisoquine* is similar, but also possesses some MAOI activity. It was at one time proposed that the action potential in the adrenergic nerve led to the release of ACh, which itself stimulated the release of noradrenaline (Burn and Rand, 1959); *bretylium* was thought to block this mechanism. Present opinion suggests that the action of bretylium resembles that of guanethidine. Tolerance and the development of other side-effects preclude its use as an antihypertensive agent. Like guanethidine, it has significant local anaesthetic activity, and it has been employed in the treatment of cardiac arrhythmias.

Adrenergic blocking agents

These drugs block the postsynaptic receptor sites, and are classified as α or β blockers according to the type of receptor involved.

ALPHA-BLOCKING DRUGS

The earliest group of drugs found to possess α-blocking activity were the ergot alkaloids. However, they also produce marked stimulation of smooth muscle, which may be explained by a 'partial agonist' effect, and are of little value in this context. Haloalkylamines such as phenoxybenzamine and dibenamine, and the imidazolines phentolamine and tolazoline are used clinically for their α-blocking effect, although the imidazolines posses some stimulatory activity. As only α receptors are blocked, there will be an enhanced response to the circulating catecholamines via the unblocked β receptors, which usually manifests as tachycardia. This property limits their use as antihypertensive agents.

Alpha blockers have proved useful in the management of peripheral vascular disorders in which α-adrenergic vasoconstriction of skin vessels is predominant, such as Raynaud's phenomenon and acrocyanosis. They are of no value in the treatment of intermittent claudication; they merely divert muscle blood flow to skin, and exercise is a far more useful method of improving muscle blood flow.

Phenoxybenzamine has been used clinically in the management of 'shock'. Possible advantages are increased blood flow, with enhanced distribution and transfer of fluid from vascular to interstitial compartments, leading to an improved acid—base state. It has a prolonged duration of action, possibly due to chemical bonding at the receptor sites. It is preferably administered to slow infusion in a dose of 1 mg·kg^{-1}. *Thymoxamine* (1 mg·kg^{-1}) may be an alternative or the α-blocking properties of *chlorpromazine* (0.75 mg·kg^{-1}) may be utilized (Lees, 1976).

Phentolamine was once commonly employed in the diagnosis of phaeochromocytoma. False positive and false negative responses occur, and a more useful investigation is the estimation of urinary catecholamines and the major metabolite, 3-methoxy-4-hydroxymandelic acid (VMA) (*Figure 37.4*). Oral phenoxybenzamine is used in the preparation of such cases for surgery (or for long-term management of cases unsuitable for surgery), usually in combination with a β blocker. Phentolamine may be used intraoperatively to antagonize the hypertension occurring during manipulation of the tumour. However, severe hypotension may ensue following tumour removal, which may necessitate infusion of a vasopressor, and nitroprusside may be a rational alternative to phentolamine (Stamenković and Spierdijk, 1976). Haemorrhagic necrosis of phaeochromocytoma has been associated with phentolamine administration (Van Way *et al.*, 1976). *Labetalol*, which posses both α- and β-receptor blocking properties, may have some application in the management of phaeochromocytoma. Another α blocker, indoramin, has also been used in the prevention of migraine (Wainscott *et al.*, 1975) and exercise-induced asthma (Bianco *et al.*, 1974).

Clonidine is chemically related to tolazoline, and produces α-adrenergic blockade with partial agonist activity. However, its main hypotensive response associated with a bradycardia would appear to be mediated through the CNS. When used in the treatment of hypertension it may produce dry mouth, sedation and allergic manifestations. Postural hypotension is slight or absent. Sudden cessation of therapy often results in hyperirritability and a rebound hypertension (Hansson *et al.*, 1973); rapid reintroduction of the drug or treatment with α or β blockers may be necessary. In much smaller doses it is used in the treatment of migraine.

BETA-BLOCKING DRUGS

Powell and Slater (1958) showed that the dichloro analogue of isoprenaline produced some β-receptor blockade. This led to the development of many structurally related compounds which have had considerable vogue in the treatment of angina pectoris and hypertension. Pharmacological actions which varying members of the group exhibit include (1) a partial agonist effect (intrinsic sympathomimetic activity); (2) β_2-receptor blockade, which results in inhibition of the renin—angiotension system and in side-effects such as bronchospasm; and (3) a membrane-stabilizing or local anaesthetic effect (Prichard, 1978). These are summarized in *Table 38.2*.

Propranolol has proved valuable in the preoperative management of thyrotoxicosis and phaeochromocytoma, and in the prevention of arrhythmias during surgery (Johnstone, 1970). It is also used to prevent reflex

TABLE 38.2. Comparative pharmacological actions of the β-blocking drugs

	ISA	Specificity	MSA	Other
Dichloroisoprenaline	+			(1)
Pronethalol	+	−	+	(2)
Propranolol	−	−	+	
Practolol	+	+	−	(3)
Oxprenolol	+	−	+	
Timolol	−	−	−	
Sotalol	−	−	−	
Metoprolol	−	+	+	
Acebutolol	+	+	+	
Pindolol	+	−	−	
Atenolol	−	+	−	(4)
Labetalol	−	−	+	(5)
Alprenolol	+	−	+	

ISA, intrinsic sympathomimetic activity; MSA, membrane stabilizing activity.
(1) Not clinically used because of marked agonist properties.
(2) Withdrawn because of possible carcinogenic effects.
(3) Oral preparation withdrawn because of toxic effects (eye, peritoneal cavity).
(4) Prolonged half-life.
(5) Also has α-blocking properties.

tachycardia during induced ganglion blockade hypotension (Hellewell and Potts, 1966. Intravenous practolol is a useful alternative in these circumstances. Propranolol has also been employed in the management of pathological anxiety states (Granville-Grossman and Turner, 1966), to prevent the autonomic effects of anxiety which may mar public appearances, as an adjunct in the treatment of schizophrenia (Yorkston *et al.*, 1977) and in the treatment of atypical facial pain (Williams, 1977).

Antihypertensive drugs and anaesthesia

Many inhalational anaesthetic agents and neuromuscular blocking drugs exert important effects on the autonomic nervous system. It is not surprising that their administration to patients on pre-existing antihypertensive therapy initially gave cause for concern, and there were reports of hypotensive episodes, sometimes fatal, often vasopressor-resistant, and occurring typically during induction of anaesthesia. Withdrawal of therapy up to 14 days prior to surgery, with the attendant dangers of a rising blood pressure, or substitution with short-acting ganglion blocking agents, has been discussed (Dingle, 1966). Alternatively, tests to assess residual sympathetic activity, including the Valsalva manoeuvre, response to 'indirectly acting' sympathomimetic amines (Crandell, 1962) or tests for postural hypotension, can be used to detect patients at risk, although misleading results occur.

Further studies (Prys-Roberts, 1971) suggest that untreated or inadequately treated hypertensives are at special risk during anaesthesia, and recommend that control with antihypertensive therapy should be attained before elective surgery; pretreatment with β-blocking agents is advisable in more urgent circumstances.

References

Adgey, A. A. Jennifer, Geddes, J. S., Mulholland, H. C., Keegan, D. A. J. and Partridge, J. F. (1968). Incidence, significance, and management of early bradyarrhythmia complicating acute myocardial infarction. *Lancet* ii, 1097–1101

Ahlquist, R. P. (1948). A study of the adrenotropic receptors. *Am. J. Physiol.* 153, 586–600

Assem, E. S. K. and Schild, H. O. (1969). Inhibition by sympathomimetic amines of histamine release induced by antigen in passively sensitised human lung. *Nature, Lond.* 224, 1028–1029

Bagnall, W. E., Salway, J. G. and Jackson, E. W. (1976). Phaeochromocytoma with myocarditis managed with α-methyl-*p*-tyrosine. *Postgrad. med. J.* 52, 653

Bennett, J. A. and Eltrincham, R. J. (1977). Possible dangers of anaesthesia in patients receiving fenfluramine. Results of animal studies following a case of human cardiac arrest. *Anaesthesia* 32, 8–13

Bianco, S., Griffin, J. P., Kamburoff, P. L. and Prime, F. J. (1974). Prevention of exercise-induced asthma by indoramin. *Br. med. J.* 4, 18–20

Blackman, J. G., Gauldie, R. W. and Milne, R. J. (1975). Interaction of competitive antagonists: the anti-curare action of hexamethonium and other antagonists at the skeletal neuromuscular junction. *Br. J. Pharm.* 54, 91

Boakes, A. J., Laurence, D. R., Lovel, K. W., O'Neil, R. and Verrill, P. J. (1972). Adverse reactions to local anaesthetic/vasoconstrictor preparations. *Br. dent. J.* 133, 137–140

Bowman, W. C. and Webb, Sandra N. (1972). Neuromuscular blocking and ganglion blocking activities of some acetylcholine antagonists in the cat. *J. Pharm. Pharmac.* 24, 762–772

Burn, J. H. and Rand, M. J. (1959). Sympathetic postganglionic mechanism. *Nature, Lond.* 184, 163–165

Calvey, T. N., Williams, N. E., Muir, K. T. and Barber, H. E. (1976). Plasma concentration of edrophonium in man. *Clin. Pharmac. Ther.* 19, 813–820

Chamberlain, D. A. and Williams, J. H. (1976). Immediate care of cardiac emergencies. *Anaesthesia* 31, 758–763

Cohen, L. H., Thale, T. and Tissenbaum, M. J. (1944). Acetylcholine treatment of schizophrenia. *Archs Neurol. Psychiat.* 51, 171–175

Crandell, D. LeR. (1962). The anesthetic hazards in patients on antihypertensive therapy. *J. Am. med. Ass.* 179, 495–500

Cushing, I. E. and Miller, W. F. (1965). Nebulization therapy. In *Respiratory Therapy*, pp. 169–218. P. Safar (ed.). Clinical Anaesthesia series. Philadelphia: F. A. Davies

Dale, H. H. (1914). The action of certain esters and ethers of choline, and their relation to muscarine. *J. Pharmac. exp. Ther.* 6, 147–190

Deacock, A. R. de C. and Hargrove, R. L. (1962). The influence of certain ganglionic blocking agents on neuromuscular transmission. *Br. J. Anaesth.* 24, 357–362

Dingle, H. R. (1966). Antihypertensive drugs and anaesthesia. *Anaesthesia* 21, 151–172

Eckstein, J. W. and Abboud, F. M. (1962). Circulatory effects of the sympathomimetic amines. *Am. Heart J.* 63, 119–135

Engelman, K., Horwitz, D., Jécquier, E. and Sjoerdsma, A. (1968). Biochemical and pharmacological effects of α-methyltyrosine in man. *J. clin. Invest.* 47, 577–594

Goldberg, L. I. (1964). Monoamine oxidase inhibitors — adverse reactions and possible mechanisms. *J. Am. med. Ass.* 190, 456–462

Goldberg, L. I. (1974). Dopamine — clinical uses of an endogenous catecholamine. *New Engl. J. Med.* **291**, 707–710

Goldberg, L. I. (1975). Current therapy of hypertension — a pharmacologic approach. *Am. J. Med.* **58**, 489–494

Granville-Grossman, K. L. and Turner, P. (1966). The effect of propranolol or anxiety. *Lancet* i, 788

Greenberg, M. J. and Pines, A. (1967). Pressurised aerosols in asthma. *Br. med. J.* **1**, 563

Gurin, S. and Delluva, Adelaide (1947). The biological synthesis of radioactive adrenalin from phenylalanine. *J. Biol. Chem.* **170**, 545–550

Hannington-Kiff, J. G. (1974). Intravenous regional sympathetic block with guanethidine. *Lancet* i, 1019–1020

Hansson, L., Hunyor, S. N., Julius, S. and Hoobler, S. W. (1973). Blood pressure crisis following withdrawal of clonidine with special reference to arterial and urinary catecholamines, and suggestion for acute management. *Am. Heart J.* **85**, 605–610

Hellewell, J. and Potts, M. W. (1966). Propranolol during controlled hypotension. *Br. J. Anaesth.* **38**, 794–801

Holgate, S. T. and Tattersfield, A. E. (1977). Induction of bronchial beta-adrenergic resistance in normal man. *Br. J. clin. Pharm.* **4**, 385–386

Jewitt, J., Birkhead, J., Mitchell, A. and Dollery, C. (1974). Clinical cardiovascular pharmacology of dobutamine. *Lancet* ii, 363–367

Johnstone, M. (1970). Reflections on beta-adrenergic blockade in anaesthetics. *Br. J. Anaesth.* **42**, 262–269

Katz, Sir Bernard and Miledi, R. (1973). The effect of atropine on acetylcholine action at the neuromuscular junction. *Proc. R. Soc. Lond. B* **184**, 221–226

Katz, R. L. (1967). Pyridostigmin (Mestinon) as an antagonist of *d*-tubocurarine. *Anesthesiology* **28**, 528–534

Lands, A. M., Arnold, A., McCauliff, J. P., Ludvena, F. P. and Brown, R. G. Jr. (1967). Differentiation of receptor systems activated by sympathomimetic amines. *Nature, Lond.* **214**, 597–598

Langley, J. N. (1905). On the reaction of cells and of nerve-endings to certain poisons, chiefly as regards the reaction of striated muscles to nicotine and to curare. *J. Physiol., Lond.* **33**, 374–413

Lees, N. W. (1976). The diagnosis and treatment of endotoxic shock. *Anaesthesia* **31**, 941–945

Lehmann, H. and Liddell, J. (1969). Human cholinesterase (pseudocholinesterase): genetic variants and their recognition. *Br. J. Anaesth.* **41**, 235–244

Liggins, G. C. and Vaughan, G. S. (1973). Intravenous infusion of salbutamol in the management of premature labour. *J. Obstet. Gynaec. Br. Commonw.* **80**, 29–33

Lipmann, M. and Rogoff, R. C. (1974). A clinical evaluation of pyridostigmine bromide in the reversal of pancuronium. *Anaesth. Analg. curr. Res.* **53**, 20–23

Loewi, O. and Navratil, E. (1926). Über humorale Ubertragbarkeit der Herznervenwirkung. X. Mitteiling. Über das Schicksal des Vagusstoffs. *Pflügers Arch. ges. Physiol.* **214**, 678–688

Pantuck, E. J. (1966). Ecothiophate iodide eye drops and prolonged response to suxamethonium. *Br. J. Anaesth.* **38**, 406–407

Powell, C. E. and Slater, I. H. (1958). Blocking of inhibitory adrenergic receptors by a dichloro analogue of isoproterenol. *J. Pharmac. exp. Ther.* **122**, 480–488

Prichard, B. N. C. (1978). β-adrenergic receptor blockade in hypertension, past, present and future. *Br. J. clin. Pharmac.* **5**, 379–399

Prys-Roberts, C., Greene, L. T., Meloche, R. and Foëx, P. (1971). Studies of anaesthesia in relation to hypertension. II. Haemodynamic consequences of induction and endotracheal intubation. *Br. J. Anaesth.* **43**, 531–547

Riker, W. F. Jr. and Wescoe, W. C. (1946). The direct action of prostigmine on skeletal muscle: its relationship to the choline esters. *J. Pharmac. exp. Ther.* **88**, 58–66

Rosenblum, R. (1974). Physiological basis for the therapeutic use of catecholamines. *Am. Heart J.* **87**, 527–530

Rumack, B. H. (1973). Anticholinergic poisoning: treatment with physostigmine. *Pediatrics, Springfield* **52**, 449–451

Sever, P. S., Birch, M., Osikowska, B. and Tunbridge, R. D. G. (1977). Plasma noradrenaline in essential hypertension. *Lancet* i, 1078–1081

Snyder, B. D., Blond, L. and McWhirter, W. R. (1974). Reversal of amitriptyline intoxication by physostigmine. *J. Am. med. Ass.* **230**, 1433–1434

Spalding, J. M. K. and Crampton Smith, A. (1963). *Clinical Practice and Physiology of Artificial Respiration*, pp. 100–102. Oxford: Blackwell Scientific

Speizer, F. E., Doll, R. and Strang, L. G. (1968). Investigation into use of drugs preceding death from asthma. *Br. med. J.* **1**, 339–343

Spoerel, W. E., Seleny, F. L. and Williamson, R. D. (1964). Shock caused by continuous infusion of metaraminol bitartrate (Aramine). *Can. med. Ass. J.* **90**, 349–353

Stamenković, L. and Spierdijk, J. (1976). Anaesthesia in patients with phaeochromocytoma. *Anaesthesia* **31**, 941–945

Sutherland, E. W. and Rall, T. W. (1959). The relation of adenosine-3'5'phosphate and phosphorylase to the actions of catecholamines and other hormones. *Pharmac. Rev.* **12**, 265–269

Taylor, G. J. and Harris, W. S. (1970). Cardiac toxicity of aerosol propellants. *J. Am. med. Ass.* **214**, 81–85

Van Way, C. W. III, Faraci, R. P., Cleveland, H. C., Foster, J. F. and Scott, H. W. Jr. (1976). Haemorrhagic necrosis of phaeochromocytoma associated with phentolamine administration. *Ann. Surg.* **184**, 26–30

von Euler, U. S. (1946). A specific sympathomimetic ergone in adrenergic nerve fibres (sympathin) and its relations to adrenaline and nor-adrenaline. *Acta physiol. scand.* **12**, 73–97

Wainscott, Gillian, Volans, G. N., Wilkinson, Marcia and Faux, G. A. (1975). Indoramin in prevention of migraine. *Lancet* **ii**, 32–33

Williams, N. E. (1977). The role of drug therapy. In *Persistent Pain — Modern Methods of Treatment*, pp. 237–252. S. Lipton (ed.). London: Academic Press

Wilson, I. B. and Harrison, M. A. (1961). Turnover number of acetylcholinesterase. *J. Biol. Chem.* **236**, 2292–2295

Yeo, J., Southwell, P. and Hindmarsh, E. (1973). Preliminary report on the effect of distigmine bromide on the neurogenic bladder. *Med. J. Aust.* **1**, 116–120

Yorkston, N. J., Gruzelier, J. H., Zaki, S. A., Hollander, Doris, Pitcher, D. R. and Sergeant, H. G. S. (1977). Propranolol as an adjunct in the treatment of schizophrenia. *Lancet* **ii**, 575–577

V Renal, hepatic, endocrine and other systems

39 Anaesthesia and the kidney
J. E. Utting

Little is known about the effect of anaesthesia on the kidney and about anaesthesia for patients with renal dysfunction. Yet the subject is an important one, especially now when both renal dialysis and transplantation have, by keeping alive patients who would otherwise be dead, produced problems in anaesthesia which did not exist 20 years ago.

When discussing anaesthesia and the kidney it must be remembered that in the clinical situation anaesthesia is always accompanied by surgery. It is sometimes difficult to separate the effects of one from the other and sometimes there is confusion as a result. The clinical anaesthetist, however, is interested in the combined effects of both.

ANAESTHESIA, RENAL BLOOD FLOW, GLOMERULAR FILTRATION RATE

Measurements of renal blood flow during anaesthesia have usually been made using para-aminohippurate (PAH). The plasma clearance of PAH is assumed to be equal to the renal plasma flow; but this is only true if all the PAH is extracted from the blood by the kidney and there is none in renal venous blood. The extraction of PAH (E_{PAH}) is usually in the order of 90% — though in some circumstances, such, for example, as renal failure it may decline almost to nothing.

These facts must be kept in mind when dealing with accounts of renal blood flow during anaesthesia since these have usually been based on studies of PAH clearance, without E_{PAH} having been measured directly. Change of E_{PAH} during anaesthesia is a possibility which has not been adequately explored. A decreased removal of PAH from renal blood would make renal blood flow appear greater than it really was. In normal circumstances renal blood flow remains constant over a wide range of arterial blood pressure. This phenomenon is known as autoregulation and is probably a local phenomenon, occurring even in the isolated kidney.

The effect of anaesthetic agents on renal vascular resistance is of more interest than the effect on renal blood flow alone. Resistance is fundamentally pressure/flow and renal vascular resistance (RVR) is determined by dividing the pressure across the renal vessels by the renal blood flow (RBF); the pressure across the vessels is obtained by subtracting the mean pressure in the renal vein ($\overline{RV}$) from the mean pressure in the renal artery ($\overline{RAP}$).

$$\frac{\overline{RAP} - \overline{RV}}{RBF}$$

If an anaesthetic agent increases renal vascular resistance it may, of course, do so directly (by the action of the agent itself on the vessels) or indirectly (for example by stimulating secretion of catecholamines).

Glomerular filtration rate (GFR) is usually estimated using insulin clearance (or sometimes creatinine clearance); there is no reason to suppose that anaesthesia in any way invalidates the measurement of GFR. Both in normal circumstances and under anaesthesia GFR tends to be more nearly constant than does RBF.

The filtration fraction (FF) is the ratio of renal plasma flow to GFR. In normal physiological conditions the filtration fraction is about 0.2. If there is a change then it could be due to an alteration in the relative resistances offered by the afferent and efferent glomerular arterioles.

General anaesthesia

In general terms it can be said that general anaesthesia decreases both renal blood flow and glomerular filtration rate, the degree of decrease depending on depth of anaesthesia, though it must be emphasized at once that the effect is transitory (Miles *et al.*, 1952; Mazze *et al.*, 1963). It also decreases renal vascular resistance, and increases the filtration fraction. That this is due to the effects of anaesthesia itself and not of concomitant surgery has now been established in young, fit volunteers who were not subjected to surgery during the investigation (Deutsch *et al.*, 1966; Deutsch, Pierce and Vandam, 1967; Deutsch *et al.*, 1969). This recent work deserves further examination.

Not only was halothane and cyclopropane anaesthesia found to cause these changes but also techniques using non-depolarizing muscle relaxant drugs, when anaesthesia was maintained with nitrous oxide and oxygen (without supplementation) and pulmonary ventilation controlled. Furthermore, the changes found were considerable. Renal blood flow went down on average by about the same percentage in each of the studies: in the case of halothane (1.5%), for example, by 38%, cyclopropane (19%) by 42%, and nitrous oxide–relaxant by 36%. Glomerular filtration rate declined by 19% with halothane, by 39% with cyclopropane, and by 27% with the technique using nitrous oxide with a muscle relaxant. The filtration fraction, which in other studies has usually been shown to increase, was not statistically different, except in the case of halothane. Renal vascular resistance, however, was very markedly and significantly increased (with halothane by 69%, cyclopropane by 84% and N_2O—curare by 61%).

One other technique should be mentioned. A mixture of fentanyl and droperidol (with supplementary fentanyl) has been found to cause less disturbance of renal function (renal blood flow and glomerular filtration rate) than other techniques (Gorman and Craythorne, 1966). Further work is needed, however, to assess the clinical importance of this finding.

Finally, it should be mentioned that opinions differ as to whether autoregulation is abolished under general anaesthesia; it seems, however, that at least under some circumstances it is not. For example, autoregulation still occurs in the isolated, perfused kidney subjected to halothane (Bastron, Perkins and Pyne, 1977).

The cause of the decreased RBF and increased vascular resistance which occurs with anaesthesia is not known. It is possible, however, that the renin—angiotensin mechanism may be involved. It has been shown in the dog that a high intake of sodium in the diet, which inhibits the renin—angiotensin system, and some agents which block the mechanism may, in some circumstances, stop the fall in RBF and increased resistance associated with anaesthesia (Burger *et al.*, 1976).

Spinal and epidural analgesia

The effect of spinal and epidural analgesia (without adrenaline) has been studied in the rhesus monkey (Sivarajan *et al.*, 1975; Sivarajan, Amory and Lindbloom, 1976). Block only up to the level T10 caused significant hypotension but no significant decrease in renal blood flow in both cases: when the block extended up to T1, however, there was a significant decrease in renal blood flow.

Study of spinal analgesia in human volunteers (Kennedy, Sawyer and Gerbershagen, 1970) showed little change in renal blood flow and renal vascular resistance, though the latter did decline appreciably initially. The difference between various accounts in the literature is probably due, among other things, to differences in the height of the block. The effect of spinal and epidural analgesia in fit patients is probably benign provided the block is not too extensive.

Hypotensive anaesthesia

When hypotensive anaesthesia is induced with ganglion blocking agents renal blood flow initially declines but tends to return to near normal levels, presumably as further renal vasodilatation occurs. The glomerular filtration rate, on the other hand, remains depressed as long as the blood pressure is low (Miles *et al.*, 1952).

There is some sympathetic innervation to the renal vessels (though its physiological significance is debated); and it may be that the near constant blood flow is due to a decreased sympathetic tone secondary to autonomic blockade. It might be expected that glomerular filtration rate would decrease since filtration would go down if the pressure inside the glomerulus declines.

The effect of sodium nitroprusside has been compared with that of trimetaphan in the dog (Wang, Lui and Katz, 1977). It was found that a decrease in mean arterial pressure of between 30 and 40 mmHg was associated with an increased renal blood flow and decreased renal vascular resistance in the case of nitroprusside, but with a decreased flow and no change in renal vascular resistance when trimetaphan was used.

When hypotension is induced with halothane in dogs the decrease in arterial blood pressure is due mainly to a fall in cardiac output. During the period of hypotensive anaesthesia there is a slight renal vasodilatation, but during recovery renal vasoconstriction takes place (Engelman *et al.*, 1975).

Whatever the experimental results may be, however, they must not obscure the basic fact that in clinical practice hypotensive anaesthesia may be associated with renal failure if the hypotensive anaesthesia is not conducted competently. This is especially so when hypotension is induced in the elderly and those with poor renal function, and where hypotension is profound and long lasting (see Chapter 60).

NEPHROTOXICITY OF ANAESTHETIC AGENTS

Probably all general anaesthetic agents reduce renal function. Return to normal, however, is usually rapid after the anaesthetic has been discontinued, though some transitory decrease in renal function may be observed in the period after anaesthesia when ether is used (Jacobsen, Christiansen and Lunding, 1968) and this may be important in patients with poor renal function to start with.

In 1966 attention was drawn to a syndrome of renal failure which followed methoxyflurane anaesthesia, usually when high dosage had been used for long periods (Crandell, Pappas and Macdonald, 1966). A characteristic of this renal failure was a high urinary output (which did not respond to Pitressin) with volumes of 2.5–4 litres per day despite negative fluid balance (that is patients tended to become dehydrated and to lose weight). The urinary osmolarity was about equal to that of plasma, but in addition plasma sodium rose — perhaps because of losses of fluid other than urine (insensible perspiration, gastrointestinal secretion). In some, but not all of the patients, blood urea increased. Usually changes became apparent within 24 hours after anaesthesia and though the increased urinary output lasted but a few days in most patients in some it persisted for several weeks. Shortly after this report a number of reports of permanent renal dysfunction appeared (Panner, Freeman and Rath-Mayo, 1970; Hollenberg, McDonald and Cotran, 1972). Many of them were fatal.

Methoxyflurane anaesthesia is associated with an increased level of serum fluoride and of oxalic acid in plasma, both substances known to be nephrotoxic; it is widely accepted that this is due to metabolic degradation of the agents. It is now accepted, too, that these metabolic products of the degradation of methoxyflurane, and not the drug itself, are responsible for the renal toxicity of the agent. Metabolic pathways for the degradation of methoxyflurane products including fluoride and oxalic acid have been devised based on experimental findings and enzyme systems known to exist in man (Mazze, Trundell and Cousins, 1971).

The bulk of evidence now points to the probability that it is fluoride which is the more likely to be the primary cause of renal nephrotoxicity: indeed a similar picture of renal failure can be produced in rats poisoned with fluoride. There is evidence, however, that oxalic acid crystalluria occurs in renal biopsy specimens of patients with postoperative renal insufficiency following methoxyflurane (Frascino, Vanamee and Rosen, 1970). It may well be that the increased plasma level of oxalic acid produced by methoxyflurane may act as a secondary toxin.

The toxicity of methoxyflurane is increased by the aminoglycoside antibiotics gentamicin and kanamycin (Barr *et al.*, 1973; Mazze and Cousins, 1973) and tetracycline (Kuzucu, 1970). Agents which cause enzyme induction (such, for example, as phenobarbitone) may also increase toxicity of methoxyflurane by increasing its rate of metabolic degradation (Cousins and Mazze, 1973).

Methoxyflurane toxicity is, to some extent at least, dose dependent (Cousins, Nishimura and Mazze, 1972; Cousins and Mazze, 1973). It has been suggested (Mazze and Cousins, 1973) that the maximum exposure to the drug should be limited to '2.5 MAC hours' (that is end-expiratory methoxyflurane concentration in MAC units multiplied by the duration of the anaesthetic in hours) and that its use should be limited to special situations when low dosage can be attained, with two hours the maximum period of anaesthesia.

Nevertheless there must be room for doubt. It is a matter of weighing risks of using methoxyflurane with its known advantages. Many anaesthetists find no place for this agent in clinical practice.

SOME RENAL IMPLICATIONS OF SURGERY

A full treatment of fluid administration is beyond the scope of this chapter. However, one or two points of importance should be mentioned and more information sought in other chapters.

In the early 1960s it was suggested (Shires, Williams and Brown, 1961) that major surgery was associated with sequestration of extracellular fluid, giving rise to a reduction in the remainder. The fashion arose for infusing large volumes of fluid like Ringer-lactate during operation to replace this fluid loss. It is now realized that this concept needs modifying. True it is that major trauma can cause exudation, but this factor has, in many instances, been exaggerated. The danger from the overgenerous provision of crystalloid is, of course, pulmonary oedema. There is a tendency to retain water during and after surgery due to an increased secretion of antidiuretic hormone (ADH). If glomerular filtration rate is also decreased (as it is during anaesthesia) it is not surprising that urine production may be greatly decreased. Attempts to increase this to high levels may, in some circumstances, be ill-advised.

There is also a decrease in the excretion of sodium after anaesthesia and surgery, though this decrease is less than that of water. One cause, though not the only one, is the increased secretion of both glucocorticoids and aldosterone, the latter partly due to an increase in renin production. Other possible mechanisms for sodium retention are increased secretion of the so-called natriuretic hormone (the third factor) and the possible action of hormones locally on the kidney, such, for example, as the liberation of renin which might cause local liberation of angiotensin, which, by diverting blood from the superficial to the deep parts of the cortex might tend to increase sodium retention.

Jaundice

Renal failure can be precipitated by anaesthesia and surgery in patients with obstructive jaundice. This phenomenon is not to be confused with what was once called the hepatorenal syndrome; this latter term is best avoided as it appears to have been applied to a number of totally distinct conditions.

The cause of renal failure associated with jaundice is unknown. It does not seem to be due to bile thrombi blocking the tubules as was once thought. The use of mannitol, however, decreases the incidence and infusion of mannitol should probably be started before surgery. This subject is dealt with more fully in Chapter 40.

Mannitol

Mannitol is an osmotic diuretic. In animals it preserves glomerular filtration and urine flow when given before a period of hypotension which would otherwise have caused both to stop. It can also, in some circumstances, cause glomerular filtration to re-start during hypoperfusion of the kidney. Mannitol, therefore, is given prophylactically to patients who are at risk, such, for example, as those with obstructive jaundice, in aortic surgery and in patients who have suffered a period of haemorrhagic shock.

Caution is required with its use, however, because it causes a shift of water out of cells with an increase in extracellular fluid and circulating volume: this can give rise to pulmonary congestion or oedema, especially if there be anuria or oliguria which does not respond to the drug.

Shock

In hypovolaemia the blood pressure is initially well maintained because of compensatory vasoconstriction. The kidney shares in this vasoconstriction and (in the dog at least) blood flow through the kidney declines.

As blood loss continues and blood pressure begins to fall there is further reduction in renal blood flow (due to both decreased arterial blood pressure and increased renal vascular resistance). This decreased flow is especially marked in the renal cortex, in which there develops areas in which there is flow at all, thus probably explaining *post mortem* changes of patchy renal cortical necrosis (Carriere *et al.*, 1966).

Underfusion of the kidney is associated with a 'wash-out' of the high osmolarity of the renal medulla probably because of a relatively high flow through this part. This 'wash-out' results in a failure of the kidney to concentrate, and to a form of renal failure with a large volume of dilute urine; this may be long-lasting until recovery is complete.

The cause of decreased blood flow through the kidney in hypovolaemia is probably largely sympathetic stimulation (Bell and Harper, 1970) and catecholamine release (though there is some indication that the renin—angiotensin mechanism may also be involved). Stimulation of α receptors causes renal vasoconstriction, and of β receptors (more specifically β_2 receptors) vasodilation, though the latter effect is feeble. It is because the severe and persistent vasoconstriction associated with profound and prolonged shock is the product of both sympathetic activity and of catecholamine secretion that α-blocking drugs may sometimes be used.

Receptors which respond to dopamine have been discovered associated with the renal vasculature. These receptors mediate vasodilatation. Dopamine given at a low dosage rate causes both myocardial stimulation and renal vasodilatation. This renal vasodilatation may, of course, improve renal blood flow and urine output. Higher dose rates of dopamine, however, cause α-stimulation and, therefore, renal vasoconstriction.

THE ANAESTHETIST AND CHRONIC RENAL FAILURE

The prognosis of chronic renal failure has been greatly improved both by refinements of conservative treatment (attention to salt and water balance and to diet) and by dialysis and renal transplantation. For this reason increasing numbers of patients with this condition are being presented for surgery and the anaesthetist must know something of the problems involved. Fortunately he is now much more likely than formerly to be able to obtain the advice of a nephrologist and this advice should unhesitatingly be sought if practicable.

A wide variety of patients show, to a varying degree, some of the features outlined below. Some will be under treatment for chronic renal failure, some will be presented for investigations such as cystoscopy and ureteric catheterization, some will be on chronic dialysis, some will be presented for renal transplantation, some will have had renal transplants, and some may have rejected the transplant. Their condition will vary from very fit (as, for example, the successful transplant) to almost moribund (for example, patients anuric from bilateral renal calculi). The reader is referred to the articles of Goldsmith (1972) and Petrie (1972), on which a great deal of the following is based, for a fuller account of the importance of chronic renal failure and anaesthesia.

Salt and water balance

In chronic renal failure the ability of the kidney to maintain homoeostasis is reduced, and this fact is reflected in salt and water balance. Thus if too much sodium is taken it will be retained, together with water and this may cause, or contribute to, hypertension, oedema (systemic and pulmonary) and cardiac failure. Conversely if sodium loss is increased and/or intake diminished (for example, in gastrointestinal upset) sodium will not be adequately conserved and hyponatraemia will result. In some patients also sodium loss may be a conspicuous feature of the disease and an increased intake may be required.

As with sodium so, too, with water. Patients with chronic renal failure usually produce about two litres of urine a day. If they are given too much water, an especial danger with intravenous regimens, they excrete the load but slowly and water intoxication may result. If, on the other hand, their water intake is interrupted, as it will be before operation, they readily become dehydrated.

To maintain a patient with a chronic renal failure on an intravenous regimen is usually easy if he is in salt and water balance to begin with. The salt requirement is likely to be about the same as the daily intake had been in the days and weeks before he came to surgery — and this intake, the patient himself may well know if it has been worked out by a nephrologist. The water intake can be calculated on the basis of the urine output, together with an appropriate allowance for insensible perspiration — and this can be done on an hourly basis. For those awaiting surgery an infusion should be set up as soon as oral intake of water ceases, to minimize the danger of dehydration.

It is more difficult to manage the acutely ill patient who is not in water and salt balance. The history has to be considered, as well as the pathological findings. A low serum sodium usually indicates that the patient is overhydrated, the more likely diagnosis (treat by reducing fluid intake); but it may, less commonly, mean that there is sodium depletion (treat with hypertonic saline). Conversely a high serum sodium may indicate dehydration (treat with dextrose 5%) or, less likely, sodium excess (consider treatment with diuretics).

The central venous pressure (CVP) may be some value in assessing the patient's state and, especially, the response of the CVP to a small, rapid fluid load; for example, if this causes a rise in CVP it suggests that the patient is probably well hydrated. Sometimes a Swan–Ganz catheter may be used. The patient's weight, too, if known previously, may give an invaluable guide to the state of hydration.

Potassium

Hyperkalaemia usually occurs late in renal failure, but is probably the commonest immediate cause of death. It must be remembered that as the blood pH drops hydrogen ion enters cells and potassium is extruded from them. Hypercapnia must, therefore, be avoided, and moderate hypocapnia would appear to be desirable in an anaesthetic technique for states of hyperkalaemia.

In a grave emergency with a high serum K^+, spreading of the ECG complexes and, perhaps, ventricular extrasystoles, calcium gluconate i.v. affords the most rapid 'first aid' treatment, since the calcium ion is the physiological antagonist of the potassium ion. As a second line measure, when there is time to produce the mixture, the following may be given over a period of half an hour:

glucose 50%	100 ml
calcium gluconate 10%	100 ml
sodium bicarbonate 8.4%	100 ml
soluble insulin	24 units

Insulin causes potassium to enter cells (with glucose) and sodium bicarbonate is introduced into the mixture to decrease the extracellular hydrogen ion which has the same effect.

Cation exchange resins may be used later but it must be remembered that these cause hypernatraemia. Dialysis should be considered in every patient in whom the serum potassium has risen to 6 mmol·l^{-1}. Patients with a serum potassium of more than 7 mmol·l^{-1} and hypokalaemic changes in the ECG certainly require dialysis.

Metabolic acidosis

Retention of hydrogen ion occurs in renal failure because the acidic end-products of protein digestion cannot be eliminated by the kidney. A moderate degree of metabolic acidosis is usual in chronic renal failure (that is the actual bicarbonate is reduced to about 15 mmol·l^{-1}. Slow correction of this acidosis may be undertaken with bicarbonate solutions, but this also involves giving sodium and an appropriate allowance must be made when considering the sodium intake. If the plasma bicarbonate level has fallen below 15 mmol·l^{-1} dialysis will probably be required.

Anaemia and haemorrhage

Severe anaemia which is almost entirely refractory to medical treatment is invariable in advanced chronic renal failure and the haemoglobin level is usually some 7—9 g·dl^{-1}. It may improve considerably if adequate dialysis is established.

The tolerance of so low a haemoglobin level by patients with chronic renal failure is surprising, though less so when it is remembered that the viscosity of the blood is greatly decreased. Blood transfusion is hazardous; it may cause cardiac decompensation and it suppresses haemopoiesis. It should, therefore, be used only with great circumspection, for example, to replace blood lost at operation. Only blood which has been tested for

A-antigen ('safe blood') should be used: patients with chronic renal failure are very likely to harbour and transmit infectious hepatitis.

The tendency to haemorrhage in renal failure depends mainly on an increased capillary permeability, and on a functional platelet defect: this clears up with dialysis.

Pulmonary oedema – 'uraemic lung syndrome'

This can occur without there being a raised left atrial pressure and is probably due both to overhydration and increased pulmonary capillary permeability, not infrequently associated with hypoproteinaemia. Despite this it can usually be controlled by salt and water restriction.

Frank left ventricular failure can occur secondary to hypertension. In this case the usual treatment with diuretics may well not be successful or be inappropriate and dialysis may be the only practical alternative.

Hypertension

This is usually associated with retention of salt and water and responds to a reduction of body salt and water, either by restriction of intake or by dialysis. Sometimes it is necessary to give antihypertensive agents, of which methyldopa is probably the most widely used. Perhaps the best 'first aid' treatment of an acute and very high blood pressure is the intravenous administration of diazoxide 300 mg i.v. This, however, causes hyperglycaemia and is not useful as a long-term therapy.

Complications of hypertension of importance to the anaesthetist include left ventricular failure with pulmonary oedema and hypertensive encephalopathy (often with convulsions).

Cardiac failure

As with hypertension cardiac failure usually responds to restricting the intake of both water and salt. When using digitalis it must be remembered that though the initial dose may be the same as in normal patients the maintenance dose must be reduced to avoid toxicity (for example, to digoxin 0.25 mg every third day). This is because the alkaloid is excreted by the kidney.

Pericarditis

This used to be considered a terminal event in uraemia, but with modern methods of dialysis the outlook is good. Haemopericardium may occur from time to time and require paracentesis; this may be hazardous when there is a bleeding tendency.

Preoperative dialysis

The decision to subject a patient to haemodialysis has been mentioned several times but it must be emphasized that it is not merely based on biochemical findings. The signs associated with terminal uraemia also represent indications for dialysis. The appearance of Kussmaul's respiration is an example, and others are bleeding, muscular twitching and changes in consciousness (drowsiness and coma).

ANAESTHESIA FOR PATIENTS WITH RENAL DYSFUNCTION

Some of the main problems in anaesthetizing patients with renal dysfunction have been mentioned already; the patient may be anaemic, acidotic and overhydrated (occasionally dehydrated); he may have severe hypertension and the features that go with this, such, for example, as cardiac enlargement and pulmonary oedema. It remains to discuss what anaesthetic techniques should be employed in these patients.

Drugs

It is commonly thought that many of the drugs used in anaesthetic practice are excreted in significant amounts by the kidney. This is not so, though there is an important exception in the non-depolarizing muscle relaxants (and decamethonium) which are (see below). Even these drugs, however, can be used in patients with renal failure if they are used with care.

Most drugs are not eliminated by the kidney because they are weak electrolytes which are lipid-soluble in the un-ionized state. Though filtered to some extent through the glomerulus they will be largely reabsorbed by the other parts of the nephron. Many drugs are converted, usually in the liver, to more water-soluble derivatives which have little or no pharmacological activity and which are excreted by the kidney. Examples include the powerful narcotic analgesics, the barbiturates (except barbitone), benzodiazepines, phenothiazines, butyrophenone derivatives and ketamine: all of these are subjected to hepatic metabolism and the end-products excreted in the urine.

This leaves, in addition to the non-depolarizing muscle relaxants and decamethonium, only ganglion blocking drugs, aminoglycoside and other antibiotics, and digoxin as drugs which are important to the anaesthetist and which are eliminated by the kidney. There is a review of this subject by Prescot (1972).

Induction of anaesthesia

If a patient is very ill the anaesthetist may decide that an inhalational induction is safer than using an intravenous technique. In the majority of patients, however, an intravenous induction agent may be used safely though the dose must be small to avoid a fall in blood pressure which, in relevant cases, might prejudice renal blood supply. Thiopentone is commonly used, though Althesin has its adherents, as have other drugs. The so-called neuroleptic drugs may be used either to induce anaesthesia or as an aid to induction (see below).

Maintenance of anaesthesia

Nitrous oxide is the most useful inhalational agent for providing a basis for anaesthesia and reflex suppression, both in technique involving spontaneous and controlled pulmonary ventilation. Halothane, too, seems to be useful in renal failure. Its tendency to cause hypotension means that it must be used with discretion, but it is, with nitrous oxide, the agent most commonly used to maintain anaesthesia.

Trichloroethylene has been advocated because of its analgesic properties (Slawson, 1972); nevertheless many will find that this drug has disadvantages which militate against its use.

Spontaneous ventilation versus controlled ventilation

For many operations the use of thiopentone for induction, nitrous oxide and halothane for maintenance with the patient breathing spontaneously is adequate. Indeed renal transplantation can be undertaken in this way, though many would regard this as undesirable. In many circumstances this technique does not provide sufficient muscle relaxation for the surgeon to operate safely. Here the use of muscle relaxants becomes a necessity and, despite the difficulties with them, it is unwise to attempt to avoid their use in situations in which they are plainly indicated.

MUSCLE RELAXANTS

Of the muscle relaxants suxamethonium can cause a rise in serum potassium and this is a contraindication to its use when the serum potassium is elevated above normal. It is not, of course, contraindicated if the serum potassium is normal.

Non-depolarizing relaxants are difficult to assess (see Chapter 16). There is, at the moment, no reason to suppose that one is better than the other in renal failure except gallamine, which should be avoided. A theoretical study showed that prolonged curarization with tubocurarine is likely with large doses but not with small ones (Gibaldi, Levy and Hayton, 1972). This appears compatible with clinical evidence (Riordan and Gilbertson, 1971). It would seem, therefore, that when using non-depolarizing muscle relaxants in patients in renal failure, especially those for renal transplantation, it is advisable to use as small a dose as is compatible with the safe execution of the operation otherwise prolonged postoperative curarization may occur. This is best done by increasing the degree of central sedation and by using a correspondingly smaller dose of muscle relaxant drug.

Neostigmine with atropine should be given in the usual way to reverse neuromuscular block. Neostigmine, is, to some extent, excreted by the kidney, but its use in the doses associated with anaesthesia is not contra-indicated.

Neuroleptanalgesia

Such drugs as droperidol used with phenoperidine or fentanyl have great advantages in renal dysfunction. They provide a stable cardiovascular state, they act as powerful adjuvants to anaesthesia, they can reduce the amounts of muscle relaxant required and they are not excreted by the kidney. The use of fentanyl, with or without droperidol, is now widespread; the results obtained from it appear to be good provided the doses used are modest.

Problems

For renal transplantation it is commonly thought advisable to keep the central venous pressure at a higher level than other patients to attempt to stimulate urine function. Nonetheless the dangers of overhydration in a patient who is unable to compensate by renal excretion have got to be very carefully kept in mind. Similar considerations apply to attempts to stimulate the transplanted kidney to secrete urine with mannitol.

During renal transplantation it may be necessary to administer immuno-suppressive drugs such, for example, as hydrocortisone and sulphasalazine. The dosage of these will be decided by those who are responsible for the programme of immunosuppression, not by the anaesthetist.

Occasionally there is a catastrophic rise in arterial blood pressure during anaesthesia, though this is uncommon where adequate dialysis has been carried out before operation, as it is often associated with overhydration. Nevertheless even with adequate dialysis occasionally hypertension does become threatening. The drug of choice in reducing arterial blood pressure is probably diazoxide (see above). Nitroprusside is also used, but it is best left to those who have experience with it.

Blood loss, if it be anything other than trivial, must be replaced with a blood transfusion. It has already been pointed out that the use of 'safe' blood is mandatory.

Postoperative care

Because patients are anaemic the administration of oxygen in the immediate postoperative period would appear to be important, to minimize the danger of hypoxia (see Chapter 23).

Fluid balance postoperatively can be a difficult problem. As a rule the use of the regimen in which the urine volume is replaced and an allowance made for other losses (say 40 ml·h^{-1}) is that most frequently used.

Analgesic agents such as morphine may, of course, be given, but caution is obviously necessary in patients who are ill.

References

Barr, G. A., Mazze, R. I., Cousins, M. J. and Kose, K. J. (1973). An animal model for combined methoxyflurane and gentamicin nephrotoxicity. *Br. J. Anaesth.* 45, 306–312

Bastron, R. D., Perkins, R. M. and Pyne, J. L. (1977). Autoregulation of renal blood flow during halothane anaesthesia. *Anesthesiology* 46, 142–144

Bell, G. and Harper, A. M. (1970). Effect of haemorrhage on blood flow through renal cortex of the dog. *J. appl. Physiol.* 28, 583–587

Burger, B. M., Hopkins, T., Tulloch, A. and Hollenberg, N. K. (1976). The role of angiotensin in the canine renal vascular response to barbiturate anaesthesia. *Circulation Res.* 38, 196–202

Carriere, S., Thorburn, M. S., Morchoe, C. C. O. and Barger, A. C. (1966). Intrarenal distribution of blood flow in dogs during haemorrhagic hypotension. *Circulation Res.* 19, 167–179

Cousins, M. J. and Mazze, R. I. (1973). Anaesthesia, surgery and renal function, immediate and delayed effects. *Anaesth. Intens. Care* 1, No. 5, 355–373

Cousins, M. J., Nishimura, T. G. and Mazze, R. I. (1972). Renal effect of low-dose methoxyflurane with cardiopulmonary bypass. *Anesthesiology* 36, 286–292

Crandell, W. B., Pappas, S. G. and Macdonald, A. (1966). Nephrotoxicity associated with methoxyflurane anaesthesia. *Anesthesiology* 27, 591–607

Deutsch, S., Pierce, E. C. Jr. and Vandam, L. D. (1967). Cyclopropane effects on renal function in normal man. *Anesthesiology* 28, 547–558

Deutsch, S., Goldberg, M., Stephen, G. W. and Wu, W. H. (1966). Effects of halothane anaesthesia on renal function in normal man. *Anesthesiology* 27, 793–804

Deutsch, S., Bastron, R. D., Pierce, E. C. Jr. and Vandam, L. D. (1969). The effect of anaesthesia with thiopentone, nitrous oxide, narcotics and neuromuscular blocking drugs on renal function in normal man. *Br. J. Anaesth.* 41, 807–814

Engelman, R. M., Guy, H. H., Smith, S. J., Boyd, A. D., Narbay, R. D. and Turndorf, H. (1975). The effect of hypotensive anaesthesia on renal haemodynamics. *J. Surg. Res.* 18(3), 293–300

Frascino, J. A., Vanamee, P. and Rosen, P. P. (1970). Renal oxalosis and azotaemia after methoxyflurane anaesthesia. *New Engl. J. Med.* 283, 676–679

Gibaldi, M., Levy, G. and Hayton, W. (1972). Kinetics of the elimination and neuromuscular blinking effect of *d*- tubocurarine in man. *Anesthesiology* 36, 213–218

Goldsmith, H. J. (1972). The chemical pathology of renal failure. *Br. J. Anaesth.* 44, 259–265

Gorman, H. M. and Craythorne, N. W. B. (1966). The effects of a new neurolept-analgesic agent (Innovar) on renal function in man. *Acta anaesth. scand.* Suppl. 24, 111–117

Hollenberg, N. K., McDonald, F. D. and Cotran, R. (1972). Irreversible acute oliguric renal failure; a complication of methoxyflurane anaesthesia. *New Engl. J. Med.* 286, 877–879

Jacobsen, E., Christiansen, A. H. and Lunding, M. (1968). The role of the anaesthetist in the management of acute renal failure. *Br. J. Anaesth.* 40, 442–450

Kennedy, W. F. Jr., Sawyer, T. K. and Gerbershagen, H. U. (1970). Simultaneous systemic cardiovascular and renal haemodynamic measurements during high spinal anaesthesia in normal man. *Acta anaesth. scand.* Suppl. 37, 163–171

Kuzucu, E. Y. (1970). Methoxyflurane, tetracycline, and renal failure. *J. Am. med. Ass.* 211, 1162–1164

Mazze, R. I. and Cousins, M. J. (1973). Methoxyflurane nephrotoxicity – a study of dose-response in man. *J. Am. med. Ass.* 225, 1611–1616

Mazze, R. I., Trundell, J. R. and Cousins, M. J. (1971). Methoxyflurane metabolism and renal dysfunction: clinical correlation in man. *Anesthesiology* 35, 247–252

Mazze, R. I., Schwartz, F. D., Slocum, H. C. and Barry, M. G. (1963). Renal function during anesthesia and surgery; the effects of halothane anesthesia. *Anesthesiology* 24, 279–283

Miles, B. E., de Wardener, H. E., Churchill-Davidson, H. C. and Wylie, W. D. (1952). The effect of the renal circulation of pentamethonium bromide during anaesthesia. *Clin. Sci.* 11, 73–79

Panner, B. J., Freeman, R. B. and Rath-Mayo, L. A. (1970). Toxicity following methoxyflurane anesthesia. Clinical and pathological observations in two fatal cases. *J. Am med. Ass.* 214, 86–90

Petrie, J. J. B. (1972). The clinical features, complications and treatment of chronic renal failure. *Br. J. Anaesth.* 44, 266–276

Prescot, L. F. (1972). Mechanisms of renal excretion of drugs (with special reference to drugs used by anaesthetists). *Br. J. Anaesth.* 44, 246–251

Riordan, D. D. and Gilbertson, A. A. (1971). Prolonged curarisation in a patient with renal failure. *Br. J. Anaesth.* 43, 506–508

Shires, T., Williams, J. and Brown, F. (1961). Acute change in extracellular fluids associated with major surgical procedures. *Ann. Surg.* 154, 803–810

Sivarajan, M., Amory, D. W. and Lindbloom, L. E. (1976). Systemic and regional blood flow during epidural anesthesia without epinephrine in the rhesus monkey. *Anesthesiology* **45(3)**, 300–310

Sivarajan, M., Amory, D. W., Lindbloom, L. E. and Schwettmann, R. S. (1975). Systemic and regional blood flow changes during spinal anesthesia in the rhesus monkey. *Anesthesiology* **43(4)**, 78–88

Slawson, K. B. (1972). Anaesthesia for the patient in renal failure. *Br. J. Anaesth.* **44**, 277–282

Wang, H. H., Lui, L. M. P. and Katz, R. L. (1977). A comparison of the cardiovascular effects of sodium nitroprusside and trimethaphan. *Anesthesiology* **46**, 40–48

40 Anaesthesia for patients with diminished hepatic function
Leo Strunin

Adverse changes in liver function probably follow on most surgical procedures, whether carried out under a local or general anaesthetic. In the vast majority of cases these changes in function are of a minor nature, are rapidly reversed, and can be related to the extent of the surgical procedure (Clarke, Doggart and Lavery, 1976). Where there is pre-existing liver disease, anaesthesia and surgery may be followed by a severe deterioration in liver function and, on occasion, the development of acute liver failure. Preoperative assessment of liver function is not always straightforward and pre-existing liver disease may not be readily apparent. Nevertheless, a number of factors relevant to the anaesthetist when considering patients with potential liver dysfunction are important and consideration of these may reduce the risk of complications. Effects of anaesthetics on liver function are considered in Chapter 8.

DRUG METABOLISM

The central role of the liver in transforming lipid-soluble compounds into more water-soluble (polar) compounds is well recognized. This transformation is usually described as metabolism, or may be referred to as biological transformation or biotransformation. Although such metabolism is not usually concerned directly in producing anaesthesia, disturbance in liver function may lead to prolonged action of drugs. In addition, as the majority of drugs are protein bound at some stage during their passage in the body, any alteration in protein binding sites, such as may occur in certain forms of liver disease, may also adversely affect the action of drugs. Finally, drug metabolism usually gives rise to compounds with a higher molecular weight than the original substance. Biliary excretion of drug metabolites is an important route and may be interfered with in patients with biliary tract disease.

Premedication

It is often claimed that analgesic, sedative and narcotic drugs (in particular, morphine) should not be given to patients with liver disease. Such advice may be misleading. Patients with well compensated liver disease will tolerate such drugs well and it is only when decompression occurs that problems may arise. Of the liver function tests available, serum albumin may be a useful index (Branch *et al.*, 1976), low serum albumin levels being associated with prolonged action of drugs.

Pethidine, promethazine or diazepam may be used for premedication of patients with compensated liver disease. The response to pethidine may be helpful in determining what dose of this analgesic may be used in the postoperative period. Promethazine, a phenothiazine, can cause cholestatic jaundice (Hollister, 1957), however, the incidence of this complication is probably less than 0.5% of patients receiving the drug and is not related to the presence of pre-existing hepatic disease.

Intravenous induction agents

Agents such as thiopentone or Althesin, may be safely given to patients with compensated liver disease and prolonged action is unlikely (Ward, Adu-Gyamfi and Strunin, 1975). Indeed, increased doses may be required because of enhanced protein binding. However, as with all sedative drugs, there may be prolonged action and depression of conscious level when intravenous anaesthetic agents are administered to patients with decompensated liver disease. If there is any doubt concerning a patient's liver dysfunction, small doses only should be given.

Non-depolarizing neuromuscular blocking drugs

Patients with liver disease may be 'resistant' to non-depolarizing neuromuscular blocking drugs, such as *d*-tubocurarine (Dundee and Gray, 1953) and pancuronium (Nana, Cardan and Leitersdorfer, 1972; Ward, Adu-Gyamfi and Strunin, 1975).

The mechanism of 'curare resistance', necessitating increased doses, in patients with liver disease is not entirely clear. Explanations range from a low pseudocholinesterase concentration, to increased protein binding of drugs, to sequestration of drugs in the enlarged liver and spleen, often found in patients with chronic liver disease (Feldman, 1973). Both *d*-tubocurarine and pancuronium are mainly excreted in the urine (Agoston *et al.*, 1973; Kalow, 1953) and this may be relevant in patients with liver disease where there may be concomitant renal disturbance with altered volumes of distribution of drugs.

For the various reasons quoted above, large doses of non-depolarizing muscle relaxant drugs may be given to patients with liver damage and problems may be encountered in antagonizing their effects at the end of surgery. Facilities should therefore be available for ventilating such patients, if necessary, in the postoperative period.

Local anaesthetics

Amide-type drugs (for example lignocaine) are metabolized in the liver. Ester-type drugs (for example procaine) are primarily hydrolysed, either in the plasma or in the liver, by cholinesterase. In theory, therefore, patients with liver disease might have difficulty in metabolizing both types of local anaesthetic drugs. In practice, unwanted effects of local anaesthetics are almost entirely accounted for by overdosage, errors of techniques or the effects of vasoconstrictors, particularly adrenaline, and rarely by allergy to individual drugs (Strunin, 1975). Only when infusions of lignocaine are used in the treatment of cardiac arrhythmias does the presence of pre-existing liver disease decrease the dose requirement of lignocaine (Thomson, Rowlands and Melmon, 1971). Metabolism of local anaesthetics is further considered in Chapter 17.

Metabolism of inhalational anaesthetics is considered in Chapters 7 and 2.

EFFECTS OF ANAESTHESIA ON LIVER BLOOD FLOW

Since vasomotor control in the liver is minimal, a reduction in liver blood flow could be due to a decrease either in the portal vein or hepatic artery perfusion pressures. These in turn can be due to either increased splanchnic vascular resistance, reduced systemic arterial, or increased hepatic venous

TABLE 40.1. Factors influencing liver blood flow during anaesthesia and surgery

A General factors	B Sympathetic nervous system activity		
	Primary abnormality	Splanchnic vascular resistance	Liver blood flow
Fall in cardiac output	Hypoxia	Increased	Reduced
Ventilation	Hypercarbia	Increased	Reduced
Splanchnic reflexes	α-stimulation	Increased	Reduced
Anaesthetic agents	β-blockade	Increased	Reduced
Surgical manipulation	Ganglion blockade	No change	Reduced
	β-stimulation	Reduced	Increased

pressures, the latter arising, for example, due to right-sided heart failure. During anaesthesia and surgery a number of factors may affect the complex mechanisms involved in the control of liver blood flow (*Table 40.1*).

Ventilation

Libonati *et al.* (1973) have shown that one of the main factors controlling the ratio of change in blood flow of the liver during anaesthesia, to change in its oxygen consumption, is the level of arterial carbon dioxide tension. Both hyper- and hypoventilation lead to a fall in liver blood flow whereas the least effects are seen when normocarbia is maintained. The mechanical effects of intermittent positive pressure ventilation (IPPV) may in themselves obstruct blood flow through the liver.

Anaesthetic agents

In general, all anaesthetic agents, including spinal and extradural anaesthetic techniques, lead to a fall in liver blood flow accompanied by a fall in hepatic oxygen uptake. Despite quite marked falls in oxygen uptake, no evidence of hypoxia or anaerobic metabolism has been demonstrated in fit healthy volunteers (Price *et al.*, 1966; Libonati *et al.*, 1973). However, this may not be so for the patient with pre-existing liver disease or other illness.

There is very little information available on the effects of anaesthesia on liver blood flow in patients with hepatic disease. Patients with cirrhosis may have decreased liver blood flow and this may be further impaired by a portacaval shunt. Intestinal obstruction with distension also increases liver blood flow as does peritoneal infection (Gump, Price and Kinney, 1970).

For general anaesthesia in a patient with liver disease, oxygen–nitrous oxide plus relaxant with IPPV to normocapnia would seem to have the least effect on liver blood flow. Of the volatile anaesthetic agents so far studied, halothane would seem to be the least harmful. Nevertheless, the dose should be restricted, since liver blood flow will fall in proportion to the fall in arterial blood pressure produced by halothane. Both hypo- and hyperventilation seem undesirable, and methoxyflurane and cyclopropane are probably best avoided. Gelman (1976) has suggested that, although anaesthetic agents do have an effect on liver blood flow, the extent of the surgical manipulation is much more relevant in decreasing liver blood flow.

OBSTRUCTIVE JAUNDICE

In the patient who has an obstructive lesion of the biliary tree which is amenable to surgical treatment, general anaesthesia, particularly in children, may be required for certain diagnostic procedures such as needle biopsy of the liver, percutaneous cholangiography or laparoscopy. Eventually laparotomy for diagnostic and therapeutic purposes may be carried out and this presents certain anaesthetic problems.

Preoperative preparation

A prolonged prothrombin time is commonly found in the jaundiced patient and is usually due to non-absorption of vitamin K from the intestine due to a lack of bile salts. An additional factor may be hepato-cellular disease and this will be suggested by the finding of a low serum albumin concentration. Vitamin K_1, 10 mg intramuscularly, daily for three days preoperatively, should restore the prothrombin time to normal. If this does not occur and prothrombin time is persistently prolonged in excess of four seconds over the control value, it is likely that concomitant hepatocellular disease is present. In this case, fresh frozen plasma should be available and infused as necessary to reduce the risk of severe haemorrhage due to surgery or diagnostic procedures.

It is well recognized that there is an increased incidence of postoperative renal failure following anaesthesia and surgery in patients with preoperative jaundice (Dawson, 1965). Although the exact mechanism of such renal failure is not entirely clear it is likely that endotoxin produced from the patient's own bowel flora, caused by the reduction in bile salts resulting in biliary obstruction may be an important factor (Bailey, 1976). Dawson

TABLE 40.2. Use of mannitol to prevent postoperative renal failure in the jaundiced patient

Serum bilirubin (μmol.l^{-1})	Management
Over 20	Urinary catheter: monitor urine output (1) If urine output >50 ml·h^{-1}, no action (2) If urine output <50 ml·h^{-1} intravenous fluid load plus mannitol 5 or 10% i.v. until diuresis established
Over 140	Preoperative: antibiotics, restoration of fluid balance and urinary catheter Peroperative: CVP monitoring, fluid load, mannitol 5 or 10% i.v. to keep urine volume above 50 ml·h^{-1} Continue mannitol postoperatively (24—36 hours) to maintain diuresis

(1965) showed that postoperative renal failure could be prevented by inducing a diuresis preoperatively, and maintaining it peroperatively and in the immediate postoperative period with intravenous mannitol. By a suitable intravenous fluid regimen with administration of antibiotics and mannitol if necessary, it is possible to prevent postoperative renal failure in the jaundiced patient (*Table 40.2*). If the patient has been undergoing percutaneous cholangiography, the cardiovascular state should be carefully checked; infusion of plasma expanders may be necessary before induction of anaesthesia.

Pethidine and promethazine are suitable drugs to be given for pre-medication. If the patient has been on steroid therapy for the treatment of jaundice, then 100 mg of hydrocortisone hemisuccinate should be administered intramuscularly with premedication and continued thereafter six-hourly until steroid therapy is no longer required.

Anaesthesia

Table 40.3 shows an anaesthetic sequence which is suitable for patients with biliary obstruction undergoing laparotomy for therapeutic or diagnostic purposes (Ward, Adu-Gyamfi and Strunin, 1975). Anaesthesia may be induced by thiopentone or Althesin; increased doses may be required

TABLE 40.3. Anaesthetic sequence suitable for patients with biliary obstruction and/or chronic liver disease undergoing surgery

Preoperatively	Vitamin K$_1$ therapy
Premedication	Pethidine up to 100 mg, promethazine up to 25 mg (depending on weight and 'fitness' of patient) Hydrocortisone hemisuccinate 100 mg i.m. if patient on steroid therapy Antibiotics if patient is jaundiced
Induction	Thiopentone or Althesin
Muscle relaxant	Suxamethonium for emergency intubation Pancuronium or fazadinium for non-urgent case
Anaesthesia	Oxygen—nitrous oxide Spontaneous ventilation or IPPV to normocapnia Incremental pethidine or synthetic analogues
Monitoring	Urine via catheter and volumetric device Pulse, blood pressure and ECG Central venous pressure Temperature Fluid balance chart
Infusion	5% dextrose Blood, if necessary, via blood warmer
Immediate postoperative care	Oxygen therapy — IPPV if necessary Mannitol, antibiotics, physiotherapy

in the patient whose plasma proteins are abnormal. For all but the most minor procedures, central venous pressure should be monitored so that circulating blood volume may be maintained at the optimum but over-transfusion with mannitol avoided. A good anaesthetic record should be kept so that no confusion may arise in relation to the drugs administered during anaesthesia and changes in liver function postoperatively.

For rapid intubation, suxamethonium may be used and may be followed by pancuronium or fazadinium for more prolonged muscular relaxation.

These drugs are preferred to *d*-tubocurarine which may cause unacceptable hypotension, thus leading to a reduction in liver blood flow. Nitrous oxide—oxygen and halothane, with or without analgesic supplements, may be safely used in the jaundiced patient. Normocapnia should be maintained during IPPV and, since halothane reduces liver blood flow, the dose administered should be limited to avoid undue cardiovascular depression. When the cause of jaundice turns out to be viral in origin, anaesthesia is almost inevitably followed by a worsening of liver function, whatever anaesthetic agents are used.

Regional anaesthetic techniques should only be used after a careful check of the patient's prothrombin time and clotting factors, which may be abnormal. If a carcinoma of the head of the pancreas is found at laparotomy, splanchnic block under direct vision with 40—50 ml of 50% ethanol should be performed. This may be carried out easily by the surgeon and may prevent intractable pain in the postoperative period.

The postoperative period

A period of IPPV may be necessary until the effects of any neuromuscular blocking drugs have passed off. Oxygen should be administered to the spontaneously breathing patient for some hours postoperatively. If the response to the premedication drugs was uneventful, normal dosage of such drugs may be used for postoperative pain relief. If there is any doubt about the patient's conscious level small doses only should be given with careful monitoring. Urine output should be maintained if necessary by further mannitol infusion.

Cryptogenic infantile cholestasis

Type II cryptogenic infantile cholestasis is amenable to surgical correction by the Kasai operation (Kasai *et al.*, 1968). The operation is carried out within the first few months of life as soon as the diagnosis is established and consists of laparotomy with exposure of the major intrahepatic bile ducts by resection of a cone of liver tissue from the porta hepatitis, followed by direct anastomosis of the cuffed liver surface to a segment of the upper small intestine (Roux-en-Y operation) or to the gall bladder. The surgical procedure may be lengthy and blood loss may be marked. Anaesthesia should be carried out as detailed in *Table 40.3* with all precautions which are appropriate for anaesthetizing a neonate such as temperature control, an infant ventilator, microinfusion apparatus, careful estimation of blood loss and skilled postoperative nursing.

CHRONIC LIVER DISEASE

Chronic liver disease, hepatocellular disease or cirrhosis are often used interchangeably to describe the same thing. Cirrhosis is a pathological term and describes the changes which occur in the liver produced by a number of aetiological factors. Chronic liver disease may produce little alteration in liver function and only when some additional insult, often iatrogenic, produces further deterioration in liver function does the underlying disease state become clinically obvious. A constant feature of cirrhosis is increased resistance to flow of blood in the portal venous system resulting eventually in portal hypertension. In the later stages of chronic liver disease there may be progressive water retention, hyponatraemia, azotaemia and oliguria as a result of reduced renal plasma flow. Other signs which suggest that chronic liver disease has become decompensated include jaundice, oedema, ascites, a flapping tremor of the hands and changes in the neurological state progressing to coma (encephalopathy). A sudden change in size or shape of the liver may indicate that a hepatoma has developed. Three major problems may occur in the cirrhotic patient — encephalopathy, ascites and gastrointestinal haemorrhage. Other problems include infection, jaundice and vitamin deficiency. Drug metabolism is related to liver cell function. Forrest *et al.* (1977) have shown that the plasma half-lives of some drugs are correlated significantly with an increase of the vitamin K_1-corrected prothrombin time ratio and a reduction in serum albumin concentration in patients with chronic liver disease. There was no correlation with serum bilirubin concentration or serum aspartate aminotransferase activity. These findings suggest that impaired drug elimination is related to depressed hepatic protein synthesis.

TABLE 40.4. Grading of severity of liver disease (Pugh *et al.*, 1973)

Clinical and biochemical variables	Points scored for increasing abnormality		
	(1)	(2)	(3)
Encephalopathy (grade)	None	1 and 2	3 and 4
Bilirubin (μmol$\cdot$l^{-1})	<25	25–40	>40
Albumin (g$\cdot$l^{-1})	35	28–35	<28
Prothrombin time (seconds greater than control)	1–4	4–6	>6

Grade A	5–6 points
Grade B	7–9 points
Grade C	10–15 points

Patients with chronic liver disease may present for anaesthesia and surgery when their liver dysfunction is merely coincidental or as a direct result of some complication most commonly associated with portal hypertension. In the former situation, liver dysfunction may go unnoticed preoperatively and it may be perceived only when, in the postoperative period, detrimental changes in liver function occur. It is well recognized that anaesthesia and surgery may be precipitating factors in decompensating chronic liver disease. Routine liver function tests may be of little help in detecting compensated chronic liver disease preoperatively and a careful history and examination are often more revealing. Nevertheless, attempts have been made to estimate hepatic reserve and to determine the risk of surgery, particularly portosystemic shunting. *Table 40.4* illustrates a scheme whereby patients are graded as follows, 5–6 points are considered to be good operative risks (grade A); patients with 7, 8 or 9 points are moderate risks (grade B); and those with 10–15 points are poor operative risks (grade C). Where possible, only patients in the grade A category should be considered for anaesthesia and surgery. In certain circumstances, there may be some advantage in delaying surgery so the patient's condition may be improved. For example after a recent gastrointestinal haemorrhage, purgation and protein restriction with a restoration of blood volume may improve the patient's liver function.

Preoperative preparation

Although the grading system described above may be helpful, the appearance and general demeanour of the patient may be the best guide to his suitability for anaesthesia and surgery. Where the prothrombin time is prolonged, a course of vitamin K should be given before surgery and anaesthesia. If prothrombin activity is still abnormal, fresh frozen plasma should be administered just prior to induction of anaesthesia. Cross-matched blood as fresh as possible should be available in proportion to the surgical procedure planned. In patients who are HB$_s$Ag positive suitable precautions should be taken (see below).

In the well compensated patient the normal premedicant drugs, pethidine, promethazine or diazepam, are well tolerated, and, if endoscopy is contemplated, atropine may be given. Patients who have been on steroid therapy for autoimmune liver disease or for the treatment of jaundice, should be given additional hydrocortisone hemisuccinate at the time of premedication. In the jaundiced patient antibiotics and intravenous mannitol may be necessary.

Anaesthesia

Table 40.3 shows a suitable anaesthetic technique for minor and major surgical procedures in patients with chronic liver disease. In the ill patient, oxygen should be administered during induction of anaesthesia to allow for arteriovenous shunting, which is a feature of chronic liver disease. In patients with porphyria, thiopentone and Althesin should be avoided and ketamine is the intravenous induction agent of choice (Rizk, Jacobson and Silvay, 1977).

For minor surgical procedures, where intubation is not indicated, patients should be allowed to breathe spontaneously, using oxygen, nitrous oxide and halothane (see below).

For more prolonged procedures, or where muscle relaxation is indicated, neuromuscular blocking drugs may be used with IPPV and an attempt should be made to maintain normocapnia in order to minimize the effects on liver blood flow. Patients with liver disease do not tolerate blood loss well, and this may be severe during surgery particularly if portal hypertension is present. Central venous pressure should be monitored, blood pressure and pulse measured frequently, and adequate infusion lines established for blood transfusion. Blood should be administered early in the surgical procedure to give time for the citrate anticoagulant to be metabolized adequately by the liver and the blood should be passed through a warming coil before delivery to the patient. If blood transfusion is not required fluids containing sodium should be avoided and 5% dextrose in water is the intravenous fluid of choice.

HALOTHANE

Halothane is not contraindicated in patients with chronic liver disease. Indeed, in patients with biliary tract disease, fewer postoperative complications followed when halothane anaesthesia was used than when diethyl ether anaesthesia was used (Dawson *et al.*, 1963). However, since halothane may lower arterial blood pressure and thereby reduce liver blood flow, only low concentrations of the drug should be used. Once discontinued, the time interval for elimination of halothane is relatively short and this contrasts with the administration of intravenous drugs where difficulties may be encountered in relation to metabolism and excretion in patients with liver dysfunction.

When adrenaline is used for local infiltration the use of halothane is contraindicated. Local infiltration of the skin with a mixture of isotonic saline and adrenaline is commonly used in patients with portal hypertension to reduce bleeding from the skin and underlying structures during laparotomy.

Portal hypertension

Haemorrhage, usually from the upper gastrointestinal tract, is a common complication of portal hypertension. The general principles of management are directed towards resuscitation, control of haemorrhage, prevention of hepatic encephalopathy and, finally, assessment of the degree of portal hypertension with a view to elective surgery. Many patients are bleeding from oesophageal varices, but up to one-third are bleeding from lesions in other parts of the gastrointestinal tract. The precise diagnosis is made by fibreoptic endoscopy. Occasionally, a general anaesthetic may be indicated but diazepam intravenously is adequate although, in the severely ill patient, endoscopy may be performed without any sedation or anaesthesia.

Temporary control of haemorrhage from oesophageal varices is nearly always possible with a modified Sengstaken—Blakemore tube or the use of an infusion of vasopressin. In patients with jaundice, ascites and encephalopathy, gastrointestinal bleeding is usually an agonal symptom. The vital importance of good hepatic function is emphasized by the comparatively small risk to life in those patients with virtually normal livers who bleed from varices secondary to extrahepatic portal obstruction. Surgical treatment of oesophageal variceal haemorrhage may be by portosystemic shunting to reduce portal venous pressure or by obliterating the varices directly by suturing or with sclerosing material.

PORTOSYSTEMIC SHUNTS

Portosystemic shunts are generally only carried out in patients whose liver function is relatively good, i.e. grade A patients (see *Table 40.4*). The major anaesthetic problem during laparotomy is haemorrhage. This arises not only as a result of deficiency in clotting factors but also because of the high venous pressure, resulting from portal hypertension. The anaesthetic sequence described in *Table 40.3* is suitable for the surgical procedures associated with portosystemic shunting, e.g. portacaval or splenorenal or mesentericocaval anastomosis.

NON-SHUNT PROCEDURES

Non-shunt procedures involve, in the main, a direct approach to oeso-phageal varices and the procedure may well be carried out in patients who are considered unfit for major portosystemic shunting. Oesophageal transection involves opening the left chest and deflating the left lung to allow access to the oesophagus. Although a double lumen endotracheal tube may be an advantage, in those patients where there is any risk of bronchial haemorrhage a single lumen standard endotracheal tube should be used. The nasogastric tube should be passed only after the chest is opened and the surgeon has access to the oesophagus so that should haemorrhage occur it may be controlled.

Oesophageal injection of varices may be carried out via an oesophago-scope, either of the rigid or fibreoptic variety. Sclerosing material is injected, under direct vision, into the oesophageal tissue surrounding the varix. As an alternative, a catheter may be passed percutaneously into the liver and advanced via the portal vein into the major variceal supply vein. This latter procedure is usually carried out under radiological control (Scott *et al.*, 1976).

An anaesthetic technique suitable for injection of oesophageal varices via an oesophagoscope has been described by Ward, Davies and Strunin (1976). Since patients having injection of oesophageal varices may be grades B or C (*Table 40.4*) the minimum of drugs should be used. Diazepam and atropine are suitable for premedication and anaesthesia is induced with a small dose of either thiopentone or Althesin. Suxamethonium is used to facilitate endotracheal intubation. The endotracheal tube should be carefully positioned so that kinking does not occur during oesophago-scopy. An infusion should be set up through a large-bore cannula placed in a suitable peripheral vein and cross-matched blood as fresh as possible should always be available.

If the patient is being treated with a Sengstaken—Blakemore tube prior to injection of varices, this should be left in position until the trachea is intubated. In any event, a freshly tested Sengstaken–Blakemore tube should always be available for use in the postoperative period. At the end of the procedure, the endotracheal tube should be left in place until the patient is fully conscious and he should then be placed in the lateral position before extubation.

Postoperative period

Following anaesthesia and surgery, patients with chronic liver disease are particularly prone to develop a chest infection. The right lower lobe is a common site for problems following liver surgery. Nursing staff should be alerted to the presence of a chest drain which may be part of the surgical procedure since this might be unexpected in such patients. If analgesic or sedative drugs are necessary, their initial effect should be carefully assessed; it is preferable to commence with small doses.

MAJOR LIVER SURGERY

Anaesthesia may be required for patients with hepatic abscess, hepatic trauma, or liver resection for hepatic tumours and for orthoptic liver transplantation. In many instances liver function may be good but patients should be graded as previously described and a search made for the presence of HB_sAg (the surface antigen for hepatitis B — probably identical to Australia antigen). Since all the procedures will involve laparotomy, anaesthesia should follow the lines already described in *Table 40.3*. Haemorrhage may be a major problem. Adequate infusion lines should be established and central venous and arterial pressures should be monitored directly.

Hepatic tumours

During partial hepatectomy air embolus may occur as a result of damage to the hepatic veins; a CVP cannula should always be inserted so that any air may be aspirated. Venous obstruction by kinking of the inferior vena cava may cause hypotension, and activation of the fibrinolytic system may lead to fibrinogen depletion and increased bleeding.

In 25% of patients with carcinoid tumours, the carcinoid syndrome occurs with hepatic metastases. Mason and Steane (1976a, b) have reviewed the anaesthetic problems in anaesthetizing patients with the carcinoid syndrome during the removal of hepatic metastases. Delay in recovery from anaesthesia has been noticed in patients with carcinoid syndrome and may be related to the role of serotonin as a transmitter substance in the brain. The dose of anaesthetic drugs should be minimal and caution should be exercised with postoperative sedation. See also Chapter 43.

Orthoptic liver transplantation

Liver transplantation is a relatively rare event. To date (1978) some 75 operations have been carried out in the UK (Calne and Williams, 1977). The most common indications are hepatoma (hepatic carcinoma) and end-stage cirrhosis.

Organization is important; facilities have to be available, often at night, for acid–base, serum potassium, calcium and glucose estimations. Large quantities of blood are required (the initial order should be for at least 30 units), in addition to fresh frozen plasma to provide extra clotting factors. Fresh blood may also be necessary. If the recipient is HB_sAg positive, extra precautions (see below) will be necessary as well as a large dose of specific immunoglobulin for infusion during the anhepatic phase.

TABLE 40.5. Anaesthesia for orthoptic liver transplantation

Premedication	Pethidine, promethazine or diazepam, depending on fitness of patient

Vascular lines	(a) Radial artery cannula
	(b) Two central venous lines:
	    one for CVP monitoring
	    one for drug administration
	(c) Two intravenous infusion lines (at least 14 gauge)
	(d) An AV shunt if time permits

Monitoring	ECG: pulse rate and rhythm Temperature: nasal probe Arterial blood pressure Central venous pressure Regular arterial blood samples for: (a) acid–base assessment (b) serum potassium, calcium and glucose concentrations
Anaesthesia	(a) Preoxygenate if necessary (b) Vascular lines placed under local anaesthesia with 1% lignocaine (c) Induction with thiopentone: suxamethonium to facilitate intubation with cricoid pressure if necessary followed by pancuronium (d) Nasogastric tube (e) Oxygen–nitrous oxide IPPV to normocapnia (f) Increments of phenoperidine or fentanyl

Table 40.5 outlines the anaesthetic technique employed for liver transplantation at King's College Hospital, London. It is important to keep pace with blood loss, so that perfusion pressure of the transplanted liver is optimal. In this respect the Bently Autotransfuser is of great help. It need not be used in its autotransfusion capacity, but as a rapid infusion device. All blood should be warmed before administration and the patient should be on a warming blanket.

During surgery the inferior vena cava is clamped above the liver and the venous return to the heart drastically reduced; cardiac arrest may occur. On revascularization of the transplanted liver, air or cold infusion fluid with a high potassium content may be aspirated into the heart. Infusion of sodium bicarbonate, aspiration of air from the right atrium and administration of calcium as well as direct cardiac massage may be necessary to prevent cardiac arrhythmias.

Postoperatively, IPPV may be necessary and the patient should be nursed in isolation as immunosuppressant drugs are administered.

THE HB$_s$Ag POSITIVE PATIENT

Patients who have suffered an attack of virus B hepatitis may become carriers of the surface antigen for hepatitis B (HB$_s$Ag). There is a risk that such patients, particularly those with e antigen as well (that is antigen from the core of the hepatitis B virus), may infect theatre personnel. Precautions should begin as soon as the patient is sent for from the ward for transport to the operating theatre (Waterson, 1976). The patient should come straight into the operating theatre, not via the anaesthetic room. The number of personnel in the operating theatre should be kept to a minimum and all should wear disposable caps, masks, gowns, gloves and overshoes. Unnecessary injections or blood sampling should be avoided. Where possible disposable anaesthetic equipment should be used. Non-disposable items should be sterilized where appropriate by heating, ethylene oxide, or by the chemical disinfectant Diversol BX (Diversey Limited) which is a crystalline blend of chlorinated trisodium phosphate mixed with a bromine salt.

All patients with liver disease should be screened for HB$_s$Ag and the positive patients should be handled with the precautions outlined above. For further information on virus hepatitis see Strunin (1977).

Patients incubating viral hepatitis subjected to anaesthesia

Most studies of patients incubating viral hepatitis who are 'accidentally' subjected to anaesthesia and surgery suggest that liver function tends to deteriorate afterwards (Strunin, 1977). In general, it seems undesirable to anaesthetize such patients and the advent of immunological tests for both hepatitis A and B should reduce the incidence of these unnecessary events.

Experience of anaesthetizing patients with chronic liver disease, who happen to be carriers of HB$_s$Ag, does not suggest that any 'activation of virus' occurs following uneventful anaesthesia and surgery (Dykes, 1977).

ACUTE LIVER FAILURE

The role of the anaesthetist in the management of acute liver failure has been reviewed recently by Ward *et al.* (1977). On occasion general anaesthesia may be required for the insertion of vascular lines, placement of a subdural pressure transducer or rarely for tracheostomy. All analgesic and sedative drugs are avoided and, since the patients are always semi-comatose, an intravenous induction agent is unnecessary. Hyperventilation is a cardinal and probably protective feature of acute liver failure and should not be interfered with other than for the short apnoea period necessary for endotracheal intubation. The short-acting depolarizing neuromuscular blocking agent suxamethonium is used to facilitate passage of the endotracheal tube.

Spontaneous ventilation (increased minute volume supply of oxygen and nitrous oxide supply may be necessary) is desirable and minimal halothane may be added if nitrous oxide alone is not sufficient. Halothane should not be administered to any patient where there is the possibility that it may have been a precipitating factor in the acute liver failure. The anaesthesia time should be as short as possible and the endotracheal tube should be left *in situ* postoperatively as the patient's level of consciousness may decline temporarily and the risk of inhalation of stomach contents may therefore be increased.

PREVIOUS HISTORY OF JAUNDICE

If, at the preoperative visit, there is any suggestion from the history that liver dysfunction has occurred in the past, standard liver function tests should be carried out, including that for HB$_s$Ag. Most patients with a history of jaundice in the past will have suffered from viral hepatitis and provided they are HB$_s$Ag negative and their liver function tests are normal, are unlikely to present any major problem to the anaesthetist. A more difficult situation is where unexplained postoperative liver dysfunction has occurred recently and is linked to a specific anaesthetic drug, most commonly halothane. Under these circumstances, if a further anaesthetic is required, the patient's liver function should be carefully assessed and, if there is evidence that hepatitis is still present, surgery should be delayed if possible until the hepatitis has resolved. This will obviously depend on the circumstances, but the giving of any anaesthetic to a patient with acute hepatitis may be followed by further deterioration in liver function.

Repeated halothane anaesthesia

In a patient where liver function tests are normal and the history is one of unexplained jaundice or hepatitis following a previous halothane anaesthetic, present evidence suggests that halothane should be avoided subsequently. Nevertheless, the position is sufficiently confused to make the outcome, whatever anaesthetic is administered, by no means clear. For a detailed review of this topic, see Strunin (1977).

The best advice that can be given is that each case should be assessed as it arises and due attention given to the circumstances, medicolegal considerations, and the surgical procedure proposed. It should be noted that in the vast majority of patients who receive repeated halothane anaesthesia no untoward sequlae follow. Halothane is currently one of the safest and most acceptable anaesthetic agents available, and before it is discarded in favour of possibly less acceptable alternatives all the relative circumstances should be reviewed.

Halothane hepatotoxicity is considered in Chapter 8 and relevant aspects of biotransformation are discussed in Chapter 7.

References

Agoston, S., Vermeer, G. A., Kersten, V. W. and Meiger, D. K. F. (1973). The fate of pancuronium bromide in man. *Acta anaesth. scand.* 17, 267–275

Bailey, M. E. (1976). Endotoxin, bile salts and renal function in obstructive jaundice. *Br. J. Surg.* 63, 774–778

Branch, R. A., Morgan, M. H., James, J. and Read, A. E. (1976). Intravenous administration of diazepam in patients with chronic liver disease. *Gut* 17, 975–983

Calne, R. Y. and Williams, R. (1977). Orthoptic liver transplantation: the first 60 patients. *Br. med. J.* 1, 471–476

Clarke, R. S. J., Doggart, J. R. and Lavery, T. (1976). Changes in liver function after different types of surgery. *Br. J. Anaesth.* 48, 119–128

Dawson, J. L. (1965). Postoperative renal function in obstructive jaundice: effect of mannitol diuresis. *Br. med. J.* 1, 82–86

Dawson, B., Jones, R. R., Schnelle, N., Hartridge, V. B., Paulson, J. A., Adson, M. A. and Summerskill, W. H. J. (1963). Halothane and ether anesthesia in gall bladder and bile duct surgery. A retrospective study into mortality and hepatobiliary complications. *Anesth. Analg., Cleve.* 42, 759–770

Dundee, J. W. and Gray, T. C. (1953). Resistance to *d*-tubocurarine chloride in presence of liver disease. *Lancet* ii, 16–17

Dykes, M. H. M. (1977). Is halothane hepatitis chronic active hepatitis? *Anesthesiology* 46, 233–235

Feldman, S. A. (1973). Muscle relaxants. *Major Problems in Anaesthesia*, vol. 1. London: Saunders

Forrest, J. A., Finlayson, N. D. C., Adjepon-Yamoah, K. K. and Prescott, L. E. (1977). Antipyrine, paracetamol and lignocaine elimination in chronic liver disease. *Br. med. J.* 1, 1384–1387

Gelman, S. I. (1976). Disturbances in hepatic blood flow during anesthesia and surgery. *Archs Surg., Chicago* 111, 881–883

Gump, F. E., Price, J. B. and Kinney, J. M. (1970). Whole body and splanchnic blood flow and oxygen consumption in patients with intraperitoneal infection. *Ann Surg.* 171, 321–328

Hollister, L. E. (1957). Allergy to chlorpromazine manifested by jaundice. *Am. J. Med.* 28, 870–873

Kalow, W. (1953). Urinary excretion of *d*-tubocurarine in man. *J. Pharmac. exp. Ther.* 109, 74–82

Kasai, M., Kiman, S., Asakun, Y., Suzuki, H., Taira, Y. and Ohaski, E. (1968). Surgical treatment of biliary atresia. *J. pediat. Surg.* 3, 615–618

Libonati, M., Malsch, E., Price, H. L., Cooperman, L. H., Baum, S. and Harp, J. (1973). Splanchnic circulation during methoxyflurane anesthesia. *Anesthesiology* 38, 466–472

Mason, R. A. and Steane, P. A. (1976a). Carcinoid syndrome: its relevance for the anaesthetist. *Anaesthesia* 31, 228–242

Mason, R. A. and Steane, P. A. (1976b). Anaesthesia for a patient with carcinoid syndrome. *Anaesthesia* 31, 243–246

Nana, A., Cardan, E. and Leitersdorfer, T. T. (1972). Pancuronium bromide – its use in asthmatics and patients with liver disease. *Anaesthesia* 27, 154–158

Price, H. L., Deutsch, S., Davidson, I. A., Clement, A. H., Behar, M. G. and Epstein, R. M. (1966). Can general anesthetics produce splanchnic visceral hypoxia by reducing regional blood flow? *Anesthesiology* 27, 24–32

Pugh, R. N. H., Murray-Lyon, I. M., Dawson, J. L., Pietroni, M. C. and Williams, R. (1973). Transection of the oesophagus for bleeding varices. *Br. J. Surg.* 60, 646–649

Rizk, S. F., Jacobson, J. H. and Silvay, G. (1977). Ketamine as an induction agent for acute intermittent porphyria. *Anesthesiology* 46, 305–306

Scott, J., Long, R. G., Dick, R. and Sherlock, S. (1976). Percutaneous transhepatic obliteration of gastro-oesophageal varices. *Lancet* ii, 53–55

Strunin, L. (1975). Local anaesthetics. In *Meyler's Side Effects of Drugs 1972–1975*, vol. 8, Chapter 2. M. N. G. Dukes (ed.). Amsterdam, Oxford: Excerpta Medica

Strunin, L. (1977). The liver and anaesthesia. In *Major Problems in Anaesthesia*, vol. 3. London: Saunders

Thompson, D. D., Rowlands, M. and Melmon, K. L. (1971). The influence of heart failure, liver disease, and renal failure on the disposition of lidocaine in man. *Am. Heart J.* **22**, 417–421

Ward, M. E., Adu-Gyamfi, Y. and Strunin, L. (1975). Althesin and pancuronium in chronic liver disease. *Br. J. Anaesth.* **47**, 1199–1204

Ward, M. E., Davies, T. D. W. and Strunin, L. (1976). Anaesthesia for injection of oesophageal varices. *Ann. R. Coll. Surg.* **58**, 315–317

Ward, M. E., Trewby, P. N., Williams, R. and Strunin, L. (1977). Acute liver failure: experience in a special unit. *Anaesthesia* **32**, 228–239

Waterson, A. P. (1976). Hepatitis B as a hazard in anaesthetic practice. *Br. J. Anaesth.* **48**, 21–24

41 Diabetes in relation to anaesthesia

R.S. Ahearn and B.A. Walker

Diabetic patients can safely undergo surgical operations of all kinds. Certain diabetic complications, notably arterial degeneration, may increase the hazards of surgery but the metabolic disturbance itself adds scarcely anything to the risk, provided the diabetes is under good control before, during and after the operation. Preoperative preparation is required to ensure that the patient comes to operation free of ketosis and with the diabetes well controlled. On the day of operation the patient should reach the theatre with an empty stomach, a normal level of blood sugar and adequate glycogen reserves, the maintenance of these last two being ensured by the administration of soluble insulin and intravenous glucose if and when required. The diabetic state may be aggravated by any surgical operation to a degree depending on the duration of the operation, the patient's individual susceptibility to stress and the amount of associated shock and while the choice of anaesthetic agent will naturally depend on the type of operation contemplated, the propensity for certain drugs to raise the level of blood sugar, to cause postoperative vomiting or to damage the liver must be borne in mind.

Prevalance

Diabetes is sufficiently common to represent 2% or 3% of most population groups and, therefore, chance will ensure the presence of a few diabetics in any collection of patients coming for surgery. Indeed, there is evidence that this figure for prevalence is far too low. One survey in England found that 6% of the population studied had some minor deviation of the glucose tolerance test, sufficient to classify them as 'diabetic' by the accepted criteria of this test and this figure rose to 16% in those over 50 years of age (Working Party appointed by the College of General Practitioners, 1963).

Classification

It is now recognized that diabetes mellitus is a syndrome that comprises several disease entities. There are only two common phenotypic groups, however.

JUVENILE ONSET TYPE DIABETES

This usually develops during the first 40 years of life, but may occur at any age. The majority of these patients develop severe symptoms acutely, show a marked tendency to ketosis and a significantly diminished insulin output. Since administration of insulin is required for the survival of these patients, an alternative and preferable name for this group is insulin-dependent diabetes.

MATURITY ONSET TYPE DIABETES

This usually appears in middle-aged or elderly patients who are often obese. It can, however, appear at any age. Endogenous insulin is present to a lesser or greater extent, depending upon the degree of obesity, and for this reason ketosis rarely occurs. The primary treatment is dietary restriction, although this may need to be supplemented by oral hypoglycaemic compounds. An alternative name for this group is insulin-independent diabetes.

TABLE 41.1

Conventional insulin preparation	*Highly purified*	*Time course*		
		Onset	*Peak*	*Duration*
Neutral insulin B.P. Soluble	Leo Neutral Actrapid MC	½–1 h	3–6 h	6–8 h
Isophane insulin B.P.	Leo Retard	2 h	6–12 h	24 h
Biphasic insulin B.P.	Novo Rapitard	1 h	4–10 h	24 h
Insulin zinc suspension B.P. Semilente	Semitard MC	1 h	3–8 h	12–14 h
Insulin zinc suspension B.P. Lente	Monotard MC Lentard MC	2 h	6–12 h	24 h
Insulin zinc suspension B.P. Ultralente	Ultratard	5–7 h	10–20 h	36 h
Globin insulin	–		8–24 h	20–26 h
Protamine zinc insulin	–		18–24 h	36 h
Neutral 30%/Isophane 70%	Leo Mixtard RI	½–1 h	4–8 h	24 h

Commercial preparations of insulin

Apart from soluble insulin, there are many other preparations of insulin available, designed to have a more prolonged length of action, either by the addition of other proteins (such as globulin or protamine) or by using zinc suspensions. Further study has also shown that it is impurities in commercial insulin, rather than the insulin itself, that lead to antibody formation. Some of these impurities are precursors of insulin such as proinsulin and other intermediates like C-peptide, and are biologically inactive. Other impurities include glucagon, vasoactive intestinal poly-peptide (VIP) and pancreatic polypeptide (PP) (Bloom *et al.*, 1976). This knowledge has led to the development of purer forms of insulin which are much less liable to give rise to antibody formation. Products freed of proinsulin contain less than 20 parts per million of proinsulin. Mono-component insulin has been purified by chromatography and, when subjected to electrophoresis and chromatography, only the insulin band is seen. The proinsulin content is less than one part per million.

It is sometimes necessary to anaesthetize, as an emergency, a patient who has had his usual insulin preparation for that day and it is, therefore, essential to know the characteristics, and, in particular, the duration of action of the different insulin preparations. These are shown in *Table 41.1*.

THE DIABETIC AS A SURGICAL PATIENT

Although ketoacidotic coma may be precipitated by the trauma of surgery it is exceedingly rare for this to happen on a planned regimen to cover the operation. It must be remembered, however, that ketoacidotic coma carries a mortality of 5–10% even in special units and up to 30% elsewhere (Alberti and Hockaday, 1977). This complication must therefore be avoided at all costs, and it behoves all anaesthetists to be meticulous in the management of their diabetic patients before, during and after surgery. Minor operations call for just as much forethought as do those of a more serious nature. Indeed, unnecessary diabetic complications such as hypo-glycaemia, ketosis and postanaesthetic vomiting appear to occur more frequently following minor surgery, probably because less careful pre-cautions are taken. It cannot be too strongly emphasized that the real tragedies occur, not due to mismanagement of the diabetic regimen, but due to failure to provide such a regimen. Even in the best conditions, it is not unknown for a patient to reach theatre without having his urine tested, or for the anaesthetist to be unaware of the results of such a test.

Effects of anaesthetic drugs on diabetes

Anaesthetic drugs affect the blood sugar level, broadly speaking, in proportion to the degree of sympathetic stimulation they produce. Sympathetic stimulation results in release of catecholamines and an increased rate of glycogenolysis of both liver and skeletal muscle, causing a rise in blood sugar level.

The popular volatile agents of the past, chloroform and diethyl ether, cause a marked rise in blood sugar concentration (Adriani, 1946). Halothane, the most widely used volatile agent in practice today, causes only a slight increase. The same is true for trichloroethylene, methoxyflurane and enflurane.

Nitrous oxide has no effect on blood sugar concentration, provided hypoxia be avoided. Cyclopropane produces a measurable rise, though less marked and less prolonged than that seen with diethyl ether. The commonly used intravenous induction agents have virtually no affect on blood sugar (Murdoch, 1958). The same may be said of intravenous analgesics and neuromuscular blocking drugs.

The induction of anaesthesia may also influence blood sugar levels. A stormy induction due to an inhalational technique being used, or resulting from an inadequate dose of intravenous agent in a robust young patient, can cause a significant increase. On the other hand, a smooth induction followed by maintenance with drugs which have little metabolic effect will result in no change, or merely a slight rise.

The use of hypotensive anaesthesia with ganglion blockers or other drugs which suppress, partly or wholly, the sympathetic nervous system, may be hazardous as the autonomic response to hypoglycaemia will be prevented thereby, perhaps, delaying its recognition.

Aims in anaesthetizing diabetics

Just as the majority of diabetics lead relatively normal lives, if properly supervised, so they tolerate anaesthesia and surgery well, provided they receive care and attention. The aim must be to prepare the patient in such a way that he is non-ketotic, with a normal or only slightly raised blood sugar and, as far as possible, is calm and tranquil. This minimizes the increased release of catecholamines, which is a sequel of preoperative anxiety.

An anaesthetic technique should be chosen which will result in rapid return to consciousness and which will cause minimal sympathetic stimulation, while at the same time will not produce sympathetic blockade unless this is especially indicated. Techniques associated with severe respiratory depression produce a marked rise in the arterial carbon dioxide concentration. This causes increased release of catecholamines and sympathetic stimulation. Barbiturate induction, followed by nitrous oxide, oxygen and relaxant, where indicated, or nitrous oxide, oxygen and halothane is usually quite satisfactory. Either of these techniques has only a slight effect on blood sugar and recovery from anaesthetic is rapid. Hypotensive anaesthesia is permissible, if circumstances dictate, provided its hazards are recognized (see above).

Effect of surgery on diabetes

The effect of surgery, *per se,* on diabetes varies from patient to patient. Preoperative anxiety, accompanied by sympathetic stimulation, causes hyperglycaemia. Major abdominal surgery has a similar tendency, though peripheral or minor surgery has little or no effect.

The effects of the postoperative period are unpredictable. Insulin requirements may fall dramatically if a stressful factor has been removed by surgery. This may happen, for example, with the removal of an infected, gangrenous limb and a similar situation may arise after a caesarean section. In these circumstances hypoglycaemia may result within a few hours. Conversely, insulin requirements may increase due to postoperative infection and vomiting, if prolonged, may precipitate ketosis.

Rarely, mild diabetics treated with oral hypoglycaemic agents become hyperglycaemic and possibly ketotic after major surgery and may require insulin therapy for a short period. In the vast majority of cases, however, the postoperative period does not differ from that seen in non-diabetic patients.

MANAGEMENT OF DIABETICS UNDERGOING SURGERY UNDER GENERAL ANAESTHESIA

Insulin-independent diabetics are generally a relatively simple problem. Insulin-dependent diabetics, however, can present difficult problems. This group will be dealt with under three headings: the controlled diabetic undergoing elective surgery, the controlled diabetic undergoing emergency surgery and surgery in uncontrolled diabetes. This will be followed by a brief account of the treatment of ketoacidotic hyperglycaemic coma.

Insulin-independent diabetics

These are generally easy to manage. If patients are on oral hypoglycaemic drugs, these should be withheld on the day of operation. Postoperative urinalysis should be performed routinely, and, if indicated, a blood sugar level determined. Occasionally, a surgical operation in a patient with maturity onset diabetes may create a need for insulin, but this will be a temporary feature of the immediate postoperative period. Patients in this group undergoing emergency surgery who have already had their oral therapy for that day should have their blood sugar checked preoperatively; but usually no different regimen from that described above is necessary.

Although many of those normally maintained with oral agents (tolbutamide, chlorpropamide, diguanides, acetohexamide) can undergo most surgical procedures without any change in their routine, there are occasions when control with insulin is desirable. Again this is particularly so if postoperative infection is expected or if major surgery is contemplated, but also if surgery of any severity is planned and the diabetes is only barely controlled with the oral hypoglycaemic drugs. In such cases the latter should be replaced by soluble insulin and adequate time left for preoperative stabilization. One further point is related to the duration of action of the oral agents. This is in the region of 4—6 hours with diguanides, 6—12 hours with tolbutamide and 12—24 hours with acetohexamide. Chlorpropamide is bound to plasma protein and its action may persist for as long as 60 hours; a dose given on the day before operation may cause hypoglycaemia on the day of operation — or even on the following day — a possibility to be guarded against (Galloway and Shuman, 1963). Furthermore, patients controlled on chlorpropamide seldom need supplementary insulin on the day of operation whereas those on other oral agents may well do so.

The controlled insulin-dependent diabetic and elective surgery

MINOR OPERATIONS

The best time of day for surgery is either the first case in the morning or the first case in the afternoon. If the operation is a minor one, unlikely to interfere with eating and drinking and is being performed in the morning, food and insulin should be omitted until after surgery (Fletcher, Langman and Kellock, 1965). When the patient has recovered he may be given slightly less than his usual dose of insulin and some fluids, followed, if tolerated, by a light meal. Urinalysis should be performed as soon as possible, and a blood glucose estimation performed if this be indicated.

If the operation is in the afternoon, breakfast may be given, along with approximately a quarter of the patient's usual daily insulin dosage. A blood glucose estimation should be done in the late morning and, on this regimen, it should be moderately elevated. If not 50 ml of dextrose 50% should be given at the time of induction of anaesthesia.

Postoperatively the blood glucose level should always be checked. If satisfactory, the patient should be continued on his usual regimen. If the level exceeds 15 mmol·l^{-1} it will be necessary to institute the postoperative regimen described under major surgery (see below).

MAJOR OPERATIONS

Those diabetics who are on a long-acting insulin preparation (*Table 41.1*) are converted to soluble insulin given twice daily. This is most conveniently done in the 48 hours prior to surgery. Again, the operation should be first on the list, and it is prudent to check the fasting blood glucose level. The patient should be given approximately a quarter to a third of his total daily insulin requirement two hours prior to anaesthesia. This should be covered by glucose 25 g given as a 50% solution intravenously in order to prevent the onset of hypoglycaemia. A blood glucose level at the time of induction will guide the anaesthetist as to whether further glucose is necessary, the aim always being to prevent hypoglycaemia whilst the patient is unconscious.

In very long operations, such as reconstructive vascular surgery, blood glucose determination should be done during surgery. Insulin will need to be given if there is a serious rise in blood glucose (for example, by 10 mmol·l⁻¹ or more) but this rarely happens. A further blood glucose estimation is necessary in the immediate postoperative period and this may again indicate a need for insulin. The patient is then returned to the ward and the postoperative management will be determined by a number of factors. The first of these is whether he is able to tolerate his usual diet. Obviously, following major abdominal procedures, it is some time before oral feeding can be instituted. In the interim control must depend on frequent blood glucose estimations with insulin given accordingly.

The second factor is the change of insulin requirements due to the trauma of operation. This varies from patient to patient and therefore the dose of insulin cannot be determined in advance; one has to be guided by the patient's response to the first postoperative dose.

The third factor is the type of operation. In patients who have had urological surgery urine samples will not be available to act as a guideline and hence control must continue, based upon blood glucose estimations. Following other operations, such as orthopaedic procedures, urine samples will be available and may be used as the basis for a 'sliding scale' regimen in the interim until the patient is able to return to his usual regimen. A suitable sliding scale based on four-hourly urinalysis is:

2% glycosuria:	20 units of insulin
1½% glycosuria:	16 units of insulin
1% glycosuria:	12 units of insulin
under 1% glycosuria:	nil

If ketonuria is also present at any of the above levels of glycosuria, 10 units of insulin are added. It is wise to supplement the urinary findings by regular blood glucose assays and, in some diabetics who have very high insulin requirements, increased doses of insulin will need to be given. In those cases whose blood glucose remains over 25 mmol·l⁻¹, insulin dosage should be based solely on blood glucose levels. As soon as control is established, and the patient is eating normally, he should revert to twice daily soluble insulin and then back to his usual regimen.

The controlled insulin-dependent diabetic and emergency surgery

Emergency surgery may be necessary in the controlled diabetic. Such a patient may already have had his usual injection of a long acting insulin which is still exerting its effect. Under these circumstances, the need for further soluble insulin or intravenous glucose can only be determined with the aid of repeated blood glucose estimations. Postoperative management is similar to that of an elective operation (see above).

Surgery in uncontrolled diabetes

An elective operation must always be postponed if the diabetes is out of control and the patient must first be stabilized. It is fortunately rare for a patient in diabetic ketosis to require immediate surgery. There is, therefore, usually time to treat ketoacidosis before operation. It is, of course, common for a patient in severe diabetic ketosis to complain of severe abdominal pain (the 'diabetic abdomen'); but this pain subsides as the ketosis is treated and is not due to a surgical emergency. Fever and leucocytosis are common to both conditions. If doubt exists as to whether abdominal pain or ketosis is the primary event, it should be settled by commencing treatment of the ketosis immediately. As the ketosis lessens the abdominal pain will disappear, unless it is due to appendicitis or other surgical emergency which can then be dealt with.

Treatment of ketoacidotic hyperglycaemic coma

It must be remembered that only a proportion of patients with keto-acidosis actually present in coma and that more commonly the patient is merely drowsy. There is obvious hyperventilation and dehydration and the breath smells of acetone; the pulse is rapid, the blood pressure low and there is marked glycosuria and ketonuria. In addition the blood glucose is usually over 28 mmol·l^{-1}, the plasma bicarbonate is always below 12 mmol·l^{-1} and the arterial blood pH is decreased — it may be as low as 6.75.

Ketoacidotic coma results from a relative or absolute deficiency of insulin and insulin is the essential basis of therapy. The aim of treatment is to achieve effective serum concentrations of insulin of 20–200 mU·ml^{-1} as quickly as possible. The difficulty is that although the intravenous route is efficient insulin has a short half-life of four minutes and, therefore, continuous intravenous infusion is necessary (Sonksen *et al.*, 1972). Intermittent bolus injections do work, but cause wide swings of blood sugar. An alternative to continuous intravenous infusion is hourly intra-muscular injections (Alberti, Hockaday and Turner, 1973), for it has been shown that intramuscular insulin is slowly discharged into the blood stream and that hourly injections allow sufficient insulin to diffuse into the circulation to provide adequate blood levels. The absorption of insulin given by the usual subcutaneous route is far too variable under these conditions.

Thus the key major change that has occurred in the treatment of diabetic ketoacidosis in the last five years has been the demonstration of the effectiveness of low dose insulin regimens given either by continuous intravenous infusion or hourly intramuscular injections. This has led to the adoption of safe, simple and effective regimens in which the same dose of insulin is used for all patients regardless of previous treatment with insulin and regardless of initial blood sugar.

A suitable regimen for the treatment of severe ketoacidosis, modified from that suggested by Alberti and Hockaday (1977), is as follows:

INTRAVENOUS FLUIDS

Saline 1 litre in 30 minutes, followed by 1 litre in 1 hour, a further 1 litre in 2 hours, and, thereafter, 500 ml every 4 hours.

INSULIN

(1) *Intramuscular regimen:*
    give 20 units, then 5 units every hour. If no change in blood glucose occurs after 2 hours, change to intravenous regimen.
(2) *Intravenous regimen:*
    infuse soluble insulin 5 units per hour in saline 0.9% using a syringe pump. It is wise to add a small amount of albumin or a gelatine-based plasma expander in order to prevent losses by absorption on to infusion apparatus. If no response occurs within 2 hours, double the infusion rate.

POTASSIUM

Start administration of potassium 13 $mmol \cdot h^{-1}$ from the time of the first infusion. If plasma potassium falls below 4 $mmol \cdot l^{-1}$, change to potassium 26 $mmol \cdot h^{-1}$. If potassium rises above 6 $mmol \cdot l^{-1}$, stop infusion.

SODIUM BICARBONATE

If pH is below 7.1 give bicarbonate 50 mmol with potassium 13 mmol in 30 minutes (using Y connector to main saline infusion). If pH falls below 7.0 give sodium bicarbonate 100 mmol and potassium 26 mmol in 45 minutes. Determine arterial pH 30 minutes after bicarbonate administration and give further bicarbonate until pH is above 7.1.

ADDITIONAL POINTS

(1) Use ECG monitor throughout as a guide to potassium therapy.
(2) Ensure that an adequate circulating blood volume is maintained, if necessary by the use of central venous pressure monitoring and transfusion if required.
(3) Consider heparinization to prevent the onset of disseminated intravascular coagulation, which has an appreciable incidence in diabetic coma, particularly the hyperosmolar variety (Whelton, Walde and Harvard, 1971).
(4) When plasma glucose level falls below 14 $mmol \cdot l^{-1}$ change infusion fluid to glucose (5 $g \cdot dl^{-1}$). Change insulin to 5 units intramuscularly every 2 hours or 8 units intravenously every 4 hours. Use potassium 13 mmol per glucose 500 ml.
(5) Continue oral potassium replacement for 5—7 days.

RECENT DEVELOPMENTS

A recent development in the employment of continuous low dose infusion techniques is to use this method to maintain satisfactory blood glucose concentrations during a prolonged operation (or in the management of a difficult labour). The simultaneous infusion of dextrose and continuous low dose insulin facilitates the maintenance of blood glucose concentrations of between 5 and 10 mmol·l^{-1} as well as having the advantage of supplying adequate energy requirements.

Conclusions

It cannot be overemphasized that diabetic patients are put at grave risk when the state and progress of their diabetes has not been considered preoperatively by the anaesthetist. Serious anaesthetic problems seldom arise in the diabetic who has been adequately prepared. The regimens described are designed to ensure that the patient reaches theatre with a normal level of blood sugar and adequate glycogen reserves.

References

Adriani, J. (1946). *The Chemistry of Anaesthesia.* Oxford: Blackwell Scientific Publications

Alberti, K. G. M. M. and Hockaday, T. D. R. (1977). Diabetic coma: a reappraisal after five years. *Clin. Endocrinol. & Metab.* 6, 421–455

Alberti, K. G. M. M., Hockaday, T. D. R. and Turner, R. C. (1973). Small doses of intramuscular insulin in the treatment of diabetic 'coma'. *Lancet* ii, 515–522

Bloom, S. R., Adrian, T. E., Mitchell, S. J., Barnes, A. J. and Kohner, E. M. (1976). Dirty insulin, a stimulant to autoimmunity. *Diabetologia* 12, 381

Fletcher, J., Langman, M. J. S. and Kellock, T. D. (1965). Effect of surgery on blood sugar levels in diabetes mellitus. *Lancet* ii, 52–54

Galloway, J. A. and Shuman, C. R. (1963). Diabetes and surgery. A study of 667 cases. *Am. J. Med.* 34, 177–191

Murdoch, R. (1958). Anaesthesia and blood sugar in operations. *Scott. med. J.* 3, 205–211

Sonksen, P. H., Srivastava, M. C., Tompkins, C. V. and Nabarro, J. D. N. (1972). Growth hormone and cortisol responses to insulin infusion in patients with diabetes mellitus. *Lancet* ii, 155–160

Whelton, M. J., Walde, D. and Harvard, C. W. H. (1971). Hyperosmolar non-ketotic diabetic coma: with particular reference to vascular complications. *Br. med. J.* 1, 85–86

Working Party appointed by the College of General Practitioners (1963). Glucose tolerance and glycosuria in the general population. *Br. med. J.* 2, 655–659

42 Pituitary and adrenal glands in relation to anaesthesia
R. A. Millar

ENDOCRINE DISEASE AND ANAESTHESIA

Endocrinology is the science concerned with the secretion of intracellularly synthesized hormones into the circulation, where they are transported to nearby and distant sites of action. Recent and continuing advances in the technology of hormone measurement, adding radioimmunoassay and competitive protein binding to pre-existing fluorimetric methods, have improved the precision of diagnosis and treatment, and have increased understanding of the physiological background to clinical disease; they have also confirmed many endocrinological responses to surgical and anaesthetic 'stress' in normal patients. The purpose in this and the following chapter is to summarize the pathological basis and clinical features of endocrine disorders which may be presented to the anaesthetist, to consider their management throughout the perioperative period, and to mention briefly certain areas where new concepts and knowledge are developing. According to environment, an individual anaesthetist may be exposed to only a few of the many endocrine disorders in florid form, such as the commonest — diabetes and thyrotoxicosis. However, endocrinology permeates many other aspects of anaesthetic practice and clinical medicine, since disordered function can affect several organs in the body, and because corticosteroids are used widely for the control of inflammation and adverse immune reactions; in this context, their beneficial effects are often inseparable from the accompanying unwanted and perhaps dangerous hormonal activity.

The fact that, more and more frequently, endocrine manifestations of many disease processes are continuing to be recognized (for example, those involving autoimmune processes and aberrant hormone-secreting tumour cells), makes it impossible for the reviewer to cover all the clinical syndromes of possible importance in anaesthetic practice, nor can he provide reassurance that unexpected features may not occur, to which the anaesthetist should be alert.

PITUITARY GLAND AND HYPOTHALAMUS

The pituitary gland, composed of anterior and posterior lobes, of different embryological origin, lies within the sella turcica, bridged over by the layer of dura mater named the diaphragma sellae, with the optic chiasma above in the subarachnoid space, superior to which are the hypothalamus and third ventricle. Laterally, there are the optic tracts and cavernous sinuses, the internal carotid arteries, the first division of the trigeminal nerve, and the third, fourth, and sixth cranial nerves. Below lie the sphenoidal air sinuses. The hypothalamus connects vascularly, from its median eminence, by the portal vessels to the anterior lobe (adenohypophysis) which contains cells of three types — acidophil, basophil, and chromophobe; and structurally, by nerve fibres in the infundibular stalk, to the posterior lobe (neurohypophysis) which contains neuroglial fibres emanating from the supraoptic and paraventricular hypothalamic nuclei and with which are often included the median hypothalamic eminence and infundibular stalk.

Anterior lobe

The hormones secreted are each controlled by a hypothalamic releasing (R) and/or inhibiting (I) hormone (H, chemically identified) or factor (F, demonstrated biologically but not structurally):

(1) ACTH, adrenocorticotrophic hormone, from basophil cells (by CRF, corticotrophic releasing factor);

(2) TSH, thyroid-stimulating hormone, from basophil cells (by TRH);

(3) GH, growth hormone, somatotrophin, from acidophil cells (by GHRF and GHIH — somatostatin);

(4) MSH, melanocyte-stimulating hormone, from basophil cells (by MSHRF and MSHIF);

(5) LH, luteinizing, and FSH, follicle-stimulating hormone, from basophil cells (by LH/FSH–RH);

(6) prolactin, from acidophil cells (by PLRF and PLIF).

Recent progress in biochemical identification, including that by the 1978 Nobel laureates, is likely to identify as hormones several of these hypothalamic releasing factors.

The three main mechanisms controlling ACTH release from the basophil cells of the pituitary gland, under hypothalamic dominance, are: (a) 'stress', including pain and trauma, infection, anxiety, and hypoglycaemia; (b) negative feedback, by which plasma cortisol probably regulates the release of corticotrophin releasing factor (CRF) from the hypothalamus; (c) diurnal rhythm, a component of hypothalamic regulation which can be overcome by 'stress'.

Posterior lobe

Of the two hormones secreted after synthesis in the hypothalamus, ADH (antidiuretic hormone, inappropriately named 'vasopressin') maintains blood osmolality by increasing reabsorption of water by the distal renal tubules, while oxytocin contracts the parturient uterus. ADH secretion is regulated by hypothalamic osmoreceptors and by vascular receptors responsive to pressure or volume; hypotension does not result from destruction of the neurohypophysis. A third secretory product, the neurophysins, currently regarded as protein carriers and not known to have any intrinsic action, are packaged with the hormones in neuro-secretory granules.

Pituitary tumours

About 80% are chromophobe adenomas, usually non-secretory, and associated with hypopituitarism.

Eosinophil adenomas are associated with secretion of growth hormone (the most abundant of the anterior pituitary hormones) resulting in acromegaly (or giantism, if prior to epiphyseal union in children).

Basophil adenomas secrete ACTH and MSH, and may present as Cushing's disease. In patients treated by bilateral adrenalectomy and subsequently given steroid replacement, a pituitary adenoma may develop (Nelson's syndrome), causing large increases in ACTH and MSH, and local pressure effects which may necessitate surgical removal.

Craniopharyngiomas, usually occurring in children, are tumours or cysts, often calcified, which develop in cell rests in the sella turcica or suprasellar space, and commonly cause pressure effects on the pituitary lobes or stalk, the hypothalamus, or the visual tracts.

Other tumours, of the pineal gland, or ependymomas or meningiomas, may disturb pituitary function. Primary carcinoma of the pituitary gland is a rarity, but metastatic tumours may occur from sites such as breast, lung or kidney.

The clinical features of pituitary tumours vary according to the lesion and location within the gland, hypopituitarism being common as a result of partial destruction by enlarging tumours such as chromophobe adenomas. This may involve only some functions, although pituitary failure may be sequential, the first decline being in secretion of gonadotrophins, followed by growth hormone, ACTH, and then thyroid stimulating hormone.

Pituitary hyposecretion (hypopituitarism)

Apart from chromophobe adenoma, causes of hypopituitarism include simple cysts or other tumours, infection, granulomata (syphilis, sarcoidosis), and rarely Sheehan's syndrome (infarction occurring up to several years following postpartum uterine haemorrhage). Skull fractures are a not uncommon cause, as is surgical removal of a tumour of the gland, while hypophysectomy may be used to treat malignant disease.

The clinical features of hypopituitarism differ in several respects from those of Addison's disease; thus, although adrenal cortisol production is diminished through a lack of ACTH, changes in electrolyte balance are less notable because of the continued secretion of aldosterone. Pallor is usual in hypopituitarism, and is not explained by the normally mild normochromic anaemia which occurs. This sign is important in differentiating hypopituitarism from primary adrenal cortical failure (Addison's disease) wherein the negative feedback response to lowered levels of plasma cortisol causes oversecretion of MSH, resulting in pigmentation. In hypopituitarism some features of hypothyroidism may be present, while axillary, body and pubic hair is scanty.

The clinical features may also include hypoglycaemia, hypothermia, water intoxication and ventilatory failure. The danger of coma, often precipitated by infection or injury, should be emphasized to those working in intensive therapy units. If hypopituitarism is suspected, blood samples should be sent for assay of plasma cortisol (and ACTH, if feasible) as early as possible before treatment is started.

The treatment is the provision of substitution therapy in accord with the deficiencies which are observed clinically — hydrocortisone (cortisone, if urgency is less), followed by thyroxine.

Surgery of the anterior pituitary gland

The gland may be partially or completely destroyed or excised for the following conditions: acromegaly (eosinophil adenoma); Cushing's disease (basophil hyperplasia or tumour); chromophobe adenoma; Nelson's syndrome; craniopharyngioma; metastatic carcinoma of breast or prostate; and occasionally diabetic retinopathy.

In place of surgical hypophysectomy for relief of pain in invasive carcinoma, pituitary adenolysis has been produced by transnasal, trans-sphenoidal injection of 1–2 ml of absolute alcohol, under general anaesthesia (Corssen *et al.*, 1977).

Surgery may involve: (1) implantation of radioactive (β-emitting) yttrium ^{90}Y, or of more penetrating γ-emitting isotope seeds, or the use of cryosurgery, through a transnasal, anterior trans-sphenoidal approach, which can also be employed for standard surgical removal; (2) trans-frontal craniotomy and surgical removal.

Anaesthetic management of pituitary surgery

TRANS-SPHENOIDAL APPROACH TO THE PITUITARY
(Messick, Laws and Abboud, 1978)

The following aspects are relevant.

(1) Preoperative steroid administration.
(2) A risk of tracheal aspiration from nasal bleeding (and, possibly, CSF leakage) is minimized by the use of a moist posterior pharyngeal pack.

(3) Packing of the nasal cavities with local analgesic/adrenaline solutions may preclude the use of halothane or other interacting anaesthetic agents, or may necessitate the immediate availability of the β-adrenergic blocker, propranolol, which can be used to abolish cardiac arrhythmias induced by adrenaline absorption.

(4) The head-up position, often used, may induce postural hypotension. The dangers from venous air embolism should be reduced by means of a Doppler ultrasound monitor placed over the precordium, and its treatment by aspiration from the heart may be anticipated by insertion of a central venous catheter into the right atrium.

(5) ECG monitoring is required, and a direct display of intra-arterial pressure is desirable for full circulatory control.

TRANSFRONTAL CRANIOTOMY

This requires optimal exposure of the deep-lying structures within the anterior fossa, and therefore considerable retraction of the frontal lobes; thus the normal neuroanaesthetic technique will include:

(1) reduction of intracranial pressure (commenced preoperatively if required) by means of: mechanical ventilation to reduce Pa_{CO_2} to 3.3–4.0 kPa (25–30 mmHg); hypertonic mannitol or urea solutions; ventricular drainage, if indicated after removal of the frontal bone flap; lumbar spinal drainage by indwelling plastic catheter inserted before anaesthesia or surgery; and possibly general hypothermia, if favoured through circumstances or environment.

(2) full circulatory monitoring, including ECG, intra-arterial pressure, the application of a Doppler monitor to the precordium, and insertion of a central venous catheter.

(3) head-up position, to reduce venous bleeding.

(4) controlled hypotension, to approximately 8.0–10.7 kPa (60–80 mmHg) systolic, to assist in reducing bleeding and intracranial pressure. This is technically straightforward using halothane, specific vasodilators such as sodium nitroprusside may be chosen (by infusion of less than $8 \,\mu g \cdot kg^{-1} \cdot min^{-1}$) while glyceryl trinitrate ($100 \,\mu g \cdot ml^{-1}$) is gaining in popularity.

Certain features of acromegaly require full preanaesthetic assessment, consultation, and specific perioperative management:

(1) large body size, kyphosis, and muscular weakness; there is a greater risk of local pressure injury associated with movement of the patient, or with positioning on the operating table.

(2) enlarged mouth structures, involving distance from mouth to glottis, tongue size, and a reduced width or anteroposterior diameter of the cricoid cartilage (Hassan *et al.*, 1976). Airway difficulties in anaesthesia have been reviewed (Burn, 1972).

(3) impaired carbohydrate tolerance, or diabetes.

(4) arterial hypertension.

Diabetes insipidus

Presenting with features such as constant thirst (in conscious patients) and a large output of urine of low specific gravity, and attributable to damage to the neurohypophyseal mechanism for ADH production, this disease is associated with: (1) pituitary tumours (and may follow surgery for these); (2) craniopharyngioma; (3) basal skull fractures; (4) sequelae to encephalitis, meningitis, and syphilis; (5) undefined causes.

The polyuria (up to 20 litres in 24 hours) may result in marked dehydration and a raised plasma osmolarity, unless there is adequate water replacement.

A positive diagnosis can be made when the administration of vasopressin increases urinary osmolality or specific gravity (which will not occur, however, in the presence of renal tubular damage).

ADRENAL CORTEX

The three layers comprise, from without inwards:

(1) zona glomerulosa, which secretes aldosterone under the control primarily of the renin—angiotensin system. Aldosterone, the naturally occurring mineralocorticoid, causes sodium retention and potassium excretion, effects which are also shown by glucocorticoids in large doses (i.e. those used therapeutically for anti-inflammatory or immuno-suppressive actions);
(2) zona fasciculata; and
(3) zona reticularis, in both of which are synthesized the glucocorticoids, mainly hydrocortisone in man, under the control of ACTH.

Other hormones synthesized in the cortex include androgens, under pituitary control, whose anabolic (nitrogen-retaining) action is opposite to the catabolic action of glucocorticoids; and oestrogen and progesterone.

Adrenal hyperfunction

Cushing's syndrome, the name given to the symptoms and signs associated with prolonged exposure to elevated plasma corticosteroid levels, can result from changes within the adrenal cortex, either unilaterally as in the case of adenoma and carcinoma (about 20% of cases) or bilaterally as in ACTH-dependent hyperplasia (70% of cases, named Cushing's disease); or iatrogenically, from administration of excessive quantities of ACTH or of corticosteroids; or from the ectopic secretion of ACTH by tumours of non-endocrine tissue (10% of cases).

Whereas Cushing's disease (as classified above) is commoner in females, there is a predominance of males in the incidence of Cushing's syndrome secondary to ectopic ACTH production by tumours.

The clinical features of this condition are well known, especially the facial and bodily changes; those of main concern to the anaesthetist include the following manifestations of glucocorticoid excess:

(1) impaired glucose tolerance, manifest as hyperglycaemia, glycosuria, or diabetes mellitus;
(2) protein breakdown, leading to muscle weakness, easy bruising, osteoporosis and skeletal fragility;
(3) arterial hypertension;
(4) electrolyte changes – potassium loss, sodium gain.

In Cushing's disease involving an androgen-producing tumour, signs of glucocorticoid excess are replaced by virilization or feminization.

Production of ACTH ectopically by 'non-endocrine' tumour tissue causes a modified Cushing's syndrome, usually without the characteristic facial and bodily changes. High plasma levels of ACTH or MSH lead to brown pigmentation, and there may be potassium depletion and alkalosis.

Adrenal cortical insufficiency

Again, the cause may be within the adrenal glands, or due to disorders of the regulating mechanism in the anterior pituitary or hypothalamus.

Within the adrenal glands, congenital adrenal insufficiency presents at birth or in childhood; it results from a hydroxylase deficiency which leads (by negative feedback) to increased ACTH secretion and overproduction of compounds other than hydrocortisone and aldosterone, such as the androgenic steroids.

Acquired adrenal disease (Addison's) results mainly from autoimmune adrenalitis (about 80% of cases), less commonly now from tuberculous destruction, and from other causes including adrenal haemorrhage or infarction, metastatic carcinoma, amyloidosis, and haemochromatosis. The autoimmune form is associated with atrophy of all three zones of the adrenal cortex. Caseation and calcification are common in tuberculous destruction of the gland.

Autoimmune adrenalitis may be associated with other organ-specific autoimmune diseases, such as thyrotoxicosis, Hashimoto's thyroiditis, primary atrophic hypothyroidism, pernicious anaemia, premature ovarian failure, idiopathic hypoparathyroidism and diabetes mellitus. Bilateral adrenalectomy, undertaken previously as a therapeutic measure, is an obvious cause of adrenal insufficiency.

Adrenal hypofunction as a consequence of disordered pituitary and hypothalamic control may accompany trauma, infection, and space-occupying lesions close to these structures within the skull. Associated histopathological changes in the pituitary and hypothalamus, extending to complete necrosis, have been reported. In such secondary adrenal insufficiency, the secretion of ACTH and TSH is said to be more resistant to pituitary damage than is that of gonadotrophins or growth hormone.

Clinical features of adrenal insufficiency include hyperpigmentation (provided that adequate anterior pituitary function is maintained), weakness, weight loss, and gastrointestinal disturbances. Of especial relevance to anaesthetic practice are a systolic pressure usually below 110 mmHg, postural hypotension, impaired reflex circulatory control and possible sensitivity to narcotics.

TESTS OF ADRENAL SUFFICIENCY

These require measurement of plasma cortisol (which is now a semi-routine laboratory technique by fluorimetry), and if possible of ACTH. Factors to be considered are:

(1) low plasma cortisol (reflecting inadequate cortical output, or suppression by exogenous administration);
(2) presence of the normal diurnal rhythm (highest in the early morning, lowest in the late evening);
(3) response of cortisol to stimulation by ACTH or tetracosactrin (depot), this being a measure of adrenal cortical response only;
(4) response to insulin hypoglycaemia, to assess the entire afferent nervous, hypothalamic, pituitary, and adrenal cortical pathways;
(5) metyrapone test — a measure of the 'efferent' pathways: hypothalamus, pituitary, adrenal cortex, including feedback control.

High levels of plasma ACTH, with low cortisol, provide direct evidence of primary adrenocortical insufficiency.

TREATMENT OF ADRENOCORTICAL INSUFFICIENCY

Patients with Addison's disease, involving all three zones of the cortex, may require both glucocorticoid and mineralocorticoid replacement (therapy which is necessary to and causes regression of congenital hyperplasia). In secondary adrenocortical deficiency, glucocorticoid only is required.

For long continued glucocorticoid administration, the usual dosage is cortisol 20 mg at about 0800 and 10 mg at about 1800 hours, to mimic the normal diurnal variation. It is important to note that cortisone acetate, so widely used, must be metabolized by the liver to hydrocortisone, which requires several hours.

Mineralocorticoid replacement can be with fludrocortisone, 0.05–0.15 mg in one morning dose.

Patients on steroid treatment should carry a bracelet indicating the condition and dosage given. Infection requires an increased dose, as do even minor operations.

ACUTE ADRENAL CRISIS

Presenting as a medical emergency in intensive care units, or in relation to surgical procedures, this requires prompt treatment with hydrocortisone hemisuccinate given intravenously. Whenever possible (and to avoid misinterpretation of a sometimes nebulous clinical picture), a venous blood sample should be withdrawn before treatment for estimation of plasma cortisol and ACTH. According to the state of blood glucose and electrolytes, appropriate fluids should be given intravenously.

The widespread use of corticosteroids for their anti-inflammatory or immunosuppressive action in many diseases frequently brings them to the anaesthetist's attention. Certain points should be emphasized, in relation to normal clinical doses:

(1) that cortisone acetate is slower acting than hydrocortisone, the latter being the choice in emergency situations and in the perioperative period;
(2) that the anti-inflammatory (glucocorticoid) and mineralocorticoid effects of cortisone and hydrocortisone are about equal;
(3) that the glucocorticoid action of prednisone or prednisolone is about five times greater than that of hydrocortisone, but these drugs are much weaker mineralocorticoids (equivalent to about 16%);
(4) that betamethasone and dexamethasone are extremely potent gluco-corticoids (anti-inflammatory action 40 times that of hydrocortisone), and have very much less mineralocorticoid action;
(5) that fludrocortisone shows almost exclusive mineralocorticoid effects, and approximates to aldosterone (which is not in clinical use).

The complications and dangers of corticosteroid therapy, relative to anaesthetic practice, include:

(1) fluid retention;
(2) diabetes-like carbohydrate intolerance;
(3) osteoporosis;
(4) suppression of signs of major infection;
(5) impaired wound healing and easy bruising;
(6) peptic ulceration, of special importance in patients having gastric tube feeding in intensive care units;
(7) mental euphoria or depression;
(8) suppression, for example by the very commonly used anti-inflammatory glucocorticoid, betamethasone, of the release of corticosteroids from the adrenal gland.

CORTICOSTEROID THERAPY IN THE PERIOPERATIVE PERIOD

A regimen for administration of glucocorticoids is required for surgical patients in the following circumstances.

(1) When there is pre-existing deficiency or absence of secretion of endogenous hormones; examples of conditions causing primary and secondary adrenocortical insufficiency are Addison's disease and hypopituitarism respectively.
(2) If adrenocortical insufficiency will result from the operation performed, such as the removal of certain pituitary tumours, and adrenalectomy.
(3) As an addition to steroids already being administered for other conditions. A list of the latter is too extensive to enumerate, but includes diseases of collagen tissue (most commonly, rheumatoid

arthritis), leukaemias, ulcerative colitis, severe asthma and allergic conditions, and for immunosuppression in patients who have undergone organ transplantation.

In the first and second categories above, the treatment required perioperatively may include other hormone replacement, and will be influenced by participating medical and surgical opinion.

In the third category, the need for additional steroid administration is relative, and no doubt unnecessary at times. The requirement of 'steroid cover' is seldom supported by secure fact or measurement, even when hypotension of uncertain cause appears to be benefited by hydrocortisone administration. However, until more measurements are recorded in the literature, the recommendation must still be given to supply boosting doses throughout the perioperative period to patients who have been treated with steroids within the previous two months.

Many possible regimens for perioperative steroid administration have been suggested, often involving the use of cortisone acetate or prednisone, and a gradual reduction in dose in the postoperative period. Simpler schedules have been recommended by a few contributors to the anaesthetic literature, on the basis of measurements of plasma cortisol (Plumpton, Besser and Cole, 1969; Oyama, 1973). It is suggested that hydrocortisone hemisuccinate be used in basic doses of 100 mg intramuscularly, starting with the premedication, and continuing every six hours for three days after major surgery. The same drug should be available to the anaesthetist for intravenous use at any stage during surgery.

Whenever doubt exists about the use of pre- or intraoperative steroid administration, the anaesthetist may well be entitled to withhold the drug and maintain a state of alertness; such reliance on clinical judgement (medicolegal factors apart) can be compared with the ever present possibility that any anaesthetized patient will develop bradycardia or hypotension: this does not justify the routine preoperative 'covering' injection of atropine or of a vasopressor drug.

RENIN–ANGIOTENSIN–ALDOSTERONE SYSTEM

Renin, stored in the granules of the juxtaglomerular cells of the afferent arteriolar wall, is probably released on vasodilatation of the afferent arteriole, and conversely is inhibited by vasoconstriction (Peart, 1977). Major factors concerned with release are:

(1) vasodilators, including glucagon, bradykinin, prostaglandins, and frusemide;
(2) β-adrenergic stimulators, such as isoprenaline, adrenaline, and apparently noradrenaline in low dose;
(3) sympathetic stimulation, directly or reflexly (e.g. postural change);
(4) autoregulation – renal vasodilatation secondary to arterial hypotension;
(5) calcium efflux across the juxtaglomerular cell;
(6) block of mineralocorticoid activity, by spironolactone or sodium deprivation.

Inhibition of renin release results from:

(1) vasoconstrictors such as angiotensin and vasopressin;
(2) α-adrenergic stimulators including methoxamine, and noradrenaline in high dose;
(3) β-adrenergic blockade, by propranolol;
(4) 'autoregulation', i.e. renal vasoconstriction secondary to arterial hypertension;
(5) calcium influx across the juxtaglomerular cell;
(6) mineralocorticoid activity, by aldosterone, or a sodium load.

Renin interaction with substrate produces the decapeptide angiotensin 1, which is converted to the octapeptide angiotensin 2 mainly in the lung but also elsewhere, including the kidney. Angiotensin 3, now recognized, is known to be active and important in respect to aldosterone release, but has much less pressor action.

Angiotensin 2 stimulates all smooth muscle, including vascular, but probably has a minor role in normal circulatory homoeostasis. An important indirect action appears to be stimulation of the area postrema in the floor of the fourth ventricle, which raises arterial pressure through increases in cardiac output and peripheral resistance. Also, it causes thirst in animals.

Stimulation of aldosterone secretion by angiotensin represents a major controlling factor in sodium and water excretion.

In spite of several studies, the direct effect of anaesthetic agents on the renin—angiotensin system remains unclear, because of associated changes in arterial pressure; in rats, sodium nitroprusside was stated to stimulate renin release (Miller *et al.*, 1977).

Aldosteronism

The primary and secondary forms are distinct.

PRIMARY ALDOSTERONISM

Known as Conn's syndrome, and associated with an adrenocortical adenoma, this features arterial hypertension, hypokalaemia and muscle weakness, metabolic alkalosis, and low plasma renin activity. Surgical excision of the tumour is a definitive remedy for the patient as described by Conn, and can be associated with administration of the aldosterone antagonist, spironolactone.

Primary hyper-renism has also been described; as the term suggests, it is distinguished from Conn's syndrome by elevated plasma renin, released from one kidney. The condition, which can be caused by renal ischaemia from stenosis, or by a neoplasm, is stated to be treated successfully by nephrectomy; anaesthetic management has involved the use of sodium nitroprusside to control high arterial pressures (Christian and Naraghi, 1977).

SECONDARY ALDOSTERONISM

This occurs when renin secretion is increased (cf. the primary form), in disorders mainly associated with altered renal blood flow, or oedema. Such conditions include renovascular or malignant hypertension, the nephrotic syndrome, hepatic cirrhosis with ascites, and cardiac failure. Another distinction from primary aldosteronism is that arterial pressure may be normal. Spironolactone may be used, in addition to treatment of the causal disorder.

In a recent survey, Peart (1977) discusses briefly the role of the kidney in the metabolism of vitamin D (with its relationship to calcium and phosphorus), and refers to the likely existence of a renal erythropoietic hormone, the main releasing stimulus being hypoxia.

PHAEOCHROMOCYTOMA

This tumour of chromaffin tissue (derivation: 'dusky colour') secretes the catecholamines noradrenaline (mainly) and adrenaline; usually it is histologically benign but it is always potentially life threatening unless its presence is recognized, its site established, its effects controlled, and its surgical removal planned with care. The usual site is in the adrenal medulla, but about 10% may occur in aberrant tissue in relation to the abdominal sympathetic chain, the para-aortic areas, the carotid or aortic bodies, the glomus jugulare, not uncommonly in the urinary bladder, and very rarely within the cranial cavity; several case reports during pregnancy have been described. According to recent classifications (see below), adrenal phaeochromocytoma and similar tumours in other tissue can be classified as apudomas.

A review paper by ReMine *et al.* (1974), covers 138 cases over a 44-year period at the Mayo clinic. The tumours occurred at all ages, most commonly in the fifth decade, and slightly more frequently in females. Hypertension was present in 91% of cases, paroxysmally in 42%. Symptoms and signs did not correlate with the size, distribution, and location of the tumour. Associated conditions included gall-stones (23%) and neurofibromatosis (three cases); there were four patients with the 'Sipple syndrome' of bilateral phaeochromocytoma, medullary carcinoma of the thyroid, and hyperparathyroidism.

In view of the possible association, any case of neurofibromatosis should be screened for the presence of phaeochromocytoma (Krishna, 1975).

The diagnosis of phaeochromocytoma rests on the clinical signs, together with:

(1) radiographic demonstration of an adrenal tumour, by nephrotomography in particular, arteriography, or venography;
(2) measurement of high urinary concentrations of noradrenaline, adrenaline, and their metabolic end-products 2-methoxy-4-hydroxymandelic acid (VMA), metanephrine and normetanephrine;

(3) measurement of plasma catecholamines (recent radioenzymatic methods have greater sensitivity and specificity than previous fluorimetric techniques);

(4) selective withdrawal of blood samples from an inferior caval catheter may help to locate the tumour's position.

It is doubtful now if diagnostic pharmacological tests (involving histamine stimulation, phentolamine blockade, etc.), which were never fully satisfactory, have an important place in diagnosis.

Despite routine preoperative assessment, phaeochromocytoma may remain undetected and still produce an unexpected, life-threatening crisis (Rorie, 1975).

Preoperative preparation

(1) The anaesthetist should see the patient several days preoperatively, to assess all aspects of preparation, including any need for continuous moderate sedation.

(2) An α-adrenergic blocking agent is required. The most effective is phenoxybenzamine, which can be administered orally in doses of 40 mg, repeated as necessary to control arterial pressure over several days preceding operation. Phentolamine, a less potent drug, may be effective in the preoperative period in milder cases.

(3) As a result of the vasoconstrictor release induced by α-adrenergic blockade, intravenous fluids are likely to be required to maintain blood volume in optimum relation to circulatory capacity. Fluid administration should be adjusted according to electrolyte measurements, and a normal haemoglobin maintained.

(4) Many patients with phaeochromocytoma have been managed successfully without using β-adrenergic blocking drugs, and it is doubtful if they are essential in the preoperative period. If indicated, perhaps for the treatment of cardiac arrhythmias, they are unlikely to prove a hazard unless there is poorly controlled organic heart disease or incipient circulatory failure.

Anaesthetic management

Historically, most anaesthetic agents have been employed, and from the voluminous literature it is difficult to attribute special morbidity or mortality to any one. The mass of research findings which can be taken to contraindicate the use of certain anaesthetics must be balanced against the successful application of these same agents. It is easier for the investigator to criticize adversely the judgement of the clinical anaesthetist, or for the latter to denigrate certain research findings as of little practical importance, than it is to reconcile apparent controversy. Such reconciliation is possible, however, in arguing the case for using an agent such as halothane, even though it is a potential cause of both increased myocardial irritability and circulatory depression.

The following points are emphasized.

(1) Monitoring must include intra-arterial pressure recording and ECG, both begun before induction of anaesthesia; also central venous pressure.
(2) Blood loss must be fully replaced, and additional fluid administered according to central venous pressure and electrolyte measurements.
(3) Arterial pressure must be controllable by the anaesthetist, and experience has shown that this cannot be achieved by preoperative therapy alone; rather, the anaesthetic technique must include a reliable means of antagonizing the hypertensive action of catecholamines. This is not attainable by light anaesthesia using nitrous oxide, neuromuscular blockade, and narcotic or neuroleptic supplements, nor by epidural or spinal blockade. The intermittent injection of phentolamine has not proved consistently adequate during such techniques, while the continuous intravenous infusion of phenoxybenzamine is not well documented.*

Animal studies have suggested that hypotension induced by halothane results mainly from direct depression of cardiovascular end-organs. This agent, therefore, or another of similar potency such as enflurane, can be used deliberately to antagonize circulatory stimulation by noradrenaline and adrenaline. Halothane has been employed thus with success, by the author, and by many others contributing to the literature on phaeochromocytoma. Recovery from anaesthesia may be less rapid, but wild fluctuations in arterial pressure will have been avoided, provided that fluids and blood have been replaced.

The more valid argument against halothane rests on its sensitization of the myocardium to catecholamines, producing ventricular arrhythmias. Their occurrence, whenever a sufficiently large dose of adrenaline is injected by a surgeon into a vascular area such as the scalp, can easily be demonstrated; noradrenaline release by even mild carbon dioxide accumulation is probably also a firm reason for the common occurrence of ventricular ectopic beats in spontaneously breathing patients, and for their extreme rarity (in the absence of injected adrenaline or of ischaemic heart disease), in normal patients given halothane by mechanical ventilation.

Ventricular ectopic beats during mechanical ventilation with halothane, occurring in the minutes following adrenaline infiltration, can be abolished by intravenous injection of propranolol 1–2 mg. During surgery for phaeochromocytoma, β-receptor blockade can be induced similarly (although it may not be required) while administering halothane.

It is possible, in face of the published evidence of its higher threshold of interaction with injected catecholamines, and of its use in anaesthesia for phaeochromocytoma, that enflurane should be preferred to halothane (Kreul, Dauchot and Anton, 1976). The essential action, however, is the reversible antagonism of circulatory stimulation by catecholamines, and this is one outstanding *therapeutic* use of potent inhalation anaesthetic agents.

* Parenteral preparations of phenoxybenzamine are not available in some countries. *Ed.*

It is inappropriate to describe categorically a single technique of anaes-thetic induction and maintenance, but the following are recommendations based on the writer's personal experience of anaesthetizing patients with phaeochromocytoma, from direct observation of other methods of management, and from a perusal of publications too numerous to list here.

Following adequate preoperative sedation and α-adrenergic receptor blockade with phenoxybenzamine, a radial artery cannula is inserted using local anaesthesia, and arterial pressure is displayed on an oscilloscope. ECG electrodes are applied, and it is advisable to have a direct write-out of the electrocardiogram and arterial pressure for purposes of documen-tation. Thus, the preparation is similar to that for a cardiac or other major operation.

Induction of anaesthesia can be accomplished, probably equally satis-factorily in several ways, a primary purpose being to minimize or prevent the rises in arterial pressure, and tachycardia, evoked by endotracheal intubation.

(1) Using 1–4 ml of Innovar intravenously (100 μg fentanyl, 2.5 mg droperidol, per ml), 100% oxygen is inhaled, and ventilation is assisted. At this stage, it is possible to produce analgesia of the larynx and upper airway by transtracheal injection of 4 ml of 4% lignocaine, or less effectively by topical spray. Subsequently, additional 'Innovar' can be given to achieve full induction of anaesthesia and endotracheal intubation.

(2) As in the preceding account, but following an initial limited dose of neuroleptic drugs and transtracheal injection of lignocaine, thiopentone sodium is given for induction of anaesthesia, and for endotracheal intubation.

(3) Whether preceded by small doses of thiopentone or of neuroleptic drugs, full anaesthesia is induced with halothane or enflurane. Arterial pressure is monitored closely, and is lowered to approximately 10.7 kPa (80 mmHg) before endotracheal intubation is performed, to ensure deep anaesthesia and minimal circulatory stimulation by endotracheal intubation; this is helped by previous transtracheal injection or endo-tracheal instillation of lignocaine (the former manoeuvre is less consistently successful in the patient who is already anaesthetized with an inhalation agent).

Thereafter, after instituting mechanical ventilation, arterial pressure can be maintained at any desired level, preferably in the range 9–13 kPa (70–100 mmHg) systolic, by careful adjustment of the inspired halothane (or enflurane) concentration. Of the neuromuscular blocking agents available, *d*-tubocurarine chloride can be used safely, perhaps in smaller and more frequently repeated doses than usual.

A central venous catheter should be placed in the internal jugular or other vein, for pressure measurement.

Syringes to hand should contain propranolol 1–2 mg, and suitably diluted solutions of pressor drugs of choice (metaraminol, 1 mg·ml^{-1}, is convenient).

The need to use β-adrenergic blocking agents during operation should be prejudged from the incidence of ventricular arrhythmias, and from the anaesthetic concentration required to control arterial pressure, in the earlier stages of the surgical procedure. During tumour removal, an increase in inspired anaesthetic concentration, and intravenous propranolol, may be required to achieve full control.

Before and during surgical removal of an active phaeochromocytoma, blood and fluid replacement should be generous. Adequate surgical exposure may require nephrectomy, and the pleura may be opened.

Following tumour removal, the inspired anaesthetic concentration should be reduced to a minimum to limit the recovery period required. Depending on anaesthetic, surgical and environmental conditions, neuromuscular blockade may be reversed, or mechanical ventilation maintained into the postoperative period.

Close supervision of pulmonary ventilation, arterial pressure, fluid and electrolyte balance, and of body position, requires that these patients be observed in postoperative recovery or intensive care units.

The fascination and challenge to anaesthetists of phaeochromocytoma and other catecholamine-secreting tumours is well revealed in case reports which continue to appear with consistency in all the world's literature. Currently, the vogue for neuroleptanalgesia has led to use of this technique, in combination with antiadrenergic or hypotensive agents other than inhalation anaesthetics. Indeed, a few recent publications describe just such wide and irregular oscillations in arterial pressure as were reported in the anaesthetic literature of two decades ago; once observed, however, hypertensive episodes appear now to be better controlled, for example by sodium nitroprusside infusion. It is an interesting paradox that droperidol was associated with extreme hypertension in a patient with phaeochromocytoma, an effect which was antagonized by phenoxybenzamine (Sumikawa and Amakato, 1977).

Although only about 3% of chemodectomas (carotid body tumours) appear to be catecholamine secreting, the anaesthetic events during biopsy and subsequent removal of one such tumour have been described, arterial pressure showing the wide oscillations characteristic of so many operations for phaeochromocytoma (Clarke, Matheson, and Boddie, 1976). The anaesthetic management, based on fentanyl, droperidol, alcuronium, nitrous oxide, and phentolamine (preoperatively, α- and β-adrenergic blockers were used), did not inhibit acute hypertensive episodes, which were controlled with sodium nitroprusside. Similar techniques have been described in five other patients with phaeochromocytoma (Stamenkovic and Spierdijk, 1976), and extended in another to include insertion of a Swan–Ganz catheter for comprehensive cardiac monitoring (Darby and Prys-Roberts, 1976).

These recent publications present alternatives to the deep inhalation anaesthesia (with intrinsic control of arterial pressure) which the author has recommended for removal of phaeochromocytoma. Whether techniques employing neuroleptanalgesia, with sodium nitroprusside to control arterial pressure, can be considered as better regulated or safer, is conjectural.

ENDOCRINE SECRETION DURING ANAESTHESIA AND SURGERY

This subject has been reviewed elsewhere (Oyama, 1973; Millar, 1974; see also Chapter 52), and only a brief summary is appropriate here. Most surgical operations induce a pronounced rise in plasma cortisol, and several other hormones which are subject to regulation by the hypo-thalamic—anterior pituitary system. Plasma catecholamines are also increased, and a noteworthy feature (outside the scope of this section) is a state of relative glucose intolerance, in which several hormones may be implicated. It is clear, from many measurements of plasma cortisol, that abdominal surgery is associated with the most pronounced 'adreno-cortical stimulation'; also, that general anaesthetic agents, over a wide range of clinical doses, cannot modify radically these hormonal responses to surgery. However, spinal, epidural and probably other regional analgesic techniques appear to suppress rises in plasma cortisol, if only for the duration of the blockade. It is probable, therefore, that afferent stimu-lation, particularly strong during abdominal surgery and perhaps correlated roughly with the degree of postoperative pain which is expected, causes activation of the hypothalamus—anterior pituitary system with consequent release of several controlling hormones such as ACTH.

Inhalation anaesthetic agents, especially those which stimulate central sympathetic discharge (cyclopropane, diethyl ether), increase plasma cortisol in addition to catecholamines; since ACTH levels also rise, activation of the hypothalamus seems likely to be a basic mechanism in both responses. However, the rise in plasma cortisol evoked by general anaesthetics is less than that caused by major surgery.

As has been stated elsewhere, it is arguable whether such hormonal activation is beneficial to the patient, or merely represents responses which are pharmacological (in the case of the anaesthetic agents) or reactionary to physiologically abnormal surgical stimuli. Two comments are of possible relevance: first, that the perioperative use of dexamethasone suppresses cortisol secretion, without clear, unmanageable or persistent adverse effects, for example in neurosurgical patients; second, that the preoperative intramuscular injection of 100 mg hydrocortisone probably increases plasma cortisol to levels which are far in excess of those induced by surgery.

References

Burn, J. M. (1972). Airway difficulties asso-ciated with anaesthesia in acromegaly. *Br. J. Anaesth.* 44, 413–414

Christian, C. M. and Naraghi, M. (1977). Anes-thetic management of primary hyperrenism. *Anesthesiology* 46, 436–437

Clarke, A. D., Matheson, H. and Boddie, H. G. (1976). Removal of catecholamine-secreting chemodectoma. The use of neuroleptanaes-thesia, adrenergic blockade and sodium nitroprusside. *Anaesthesia* 31, 1225–1230

Corssen, G., Holcomb, M. C., Moustaffa, I., Langford, K., Vitek, T. J. and Ceballos, R. (1977). Alcohol-induced adenolysis of the pituitary gland: a new approach to control of intractable cancer pain. *Curr. Res. Anaesth. Analg.* 56, 414–421

Darby, S. and Prys-Roberts, C. (1976). Unusual presentation of phaeochromocytoma. Manage-ment of anaesthesia and cardiovascular monitoring. *Anaesthesia* 31, 913–916

Hassan, S. Z., Matz, G. A., Lawrence, A. M. and Collins, P. A. (1976). Laryngeal stenosis in acromegaly: a possible cause of airway difficulties associated with anesthesia. *Curr. Res. Anesth. Analg.* 55, 57–60

Kreul, J. F., Dauchot, P. J. and Anton, A. H. (1976). Hemodynamic and catecholamine studies during pheochromocytoma resection under enflurane anesthesia. *Anesthesiology* 44, 265–268

Krishna, G. (1975). Neurofibromatosis, renal hypertension, and cardiac dysrhythmias. Case History number 85. *Curr. Res. Anesth. Analg.* 54, 542–545

Messick, J. M., Laws, E. R. and Abboud, C. F. (1978). Anesthesia for transsphenoidal surgery of the hypophyseal region. *Curr. Res. Anesth. Analg.* 57, 206–215

Millar, R. A. (1974). Anaesthesia and endocrine secretion. In *Scientific Foundations of Anaesthesia*, 2nd edn. C. Scurr and S. Feldman (ed.). London: Heinemann Medical

Miller, E. D., Ackerly, J. A., Vaughan, E. D., Peach, M. J. and Epstein, R. M. (1977). The renin–angiotensin system during controlled hypotension with sodium nitroprusside. *Anesthesiology* 47, 257–262

Oyama, T. (1973). *Anesthetic Management of Endocrine Disease.* Berlin, Heidelberg, New York: Springer-Verlag

Peart, W. S. (1977). The kidney as an endocrine organ. *Lancet* ii, 543–547

Plumpton, F. S., Besser, G. M. and Cole, P. V. (1969). Corticosteroid treatment and surgery, 2. The management of steroid cover. *Anaesthesia* 24, 12–18

ReMine, W. H., Chong, G. C., Van Heerden, J. A., Sheps, S. C. and Harrison, E. G. (1974). Current management of pheochromocytoma. *Ann. Surg.* 179, 740–748

Rorie, D. K. (1975). Unsuspected phaeochromocytoma in a surgical patient. *Anesthesiology* 43, 363–365

Stamenkovic, L. and Spierdijk, J. (1976). Anaesthesia in patients with phaeochromocytoma. *Anaesthesia* 31, 941–945

Sumikawa, K. and Amakato, Y. (1977). The pressor effect of droperidol on a patient with pheochromocytoma. *Anesthesiology* 46, 359–361

43 Thyroid, parathyroid and other endocrine glands in relation to anaesthesia
R. A. Millar

THYROID GLAND

The two hormones secreted by the gland, thyroxine (T_4) and tri-iodothyronine (T_3), are bipeptides containing respectively four and three iodine atoms per molecule, and are stored in colloid vesicles as thyroglobulin. Thyroid stimulating hormone (TSH), released from the anterior pituitary under the control of thyrotrophin releasing factor (TRF) secreted by the hypothalamus, enhances the release of the thyroid hormones, and also their synthesis; weaker stimulation is produced by chorionic gonadotrophin. Through negative feedback, serum T_4 and T_3 exert some inhibitory influence on the pituitary and probably hypothalamus. Both hormones act widely to increase cellular metabolism, although T_3 is more potent and acts more rapidly because of weaker binding to serum proteins.

Hyperthyroidism (thyrotoxicosis)

This results from excessive production, probably at first of T_3 and later of both hormones. From the detection in serum of 'human specific thyroid stimulator', an IgG immunoglobin, thyrotoxicosis may now be considered to be an autoimmune disease. The thyroid vesicles are depleted of colloid, vascularity is increased, and there are epithelial changes. In most patients, there is diffuse hyperactivity, or multiple active nodules are interspersed with inactive areas. Occasionally, more commonly in older patients, there may be only one hyperactive nodule. As a result of negative feedback evoked by the high serum levels of T_3 and T_4, there is inhibition of the normal TSH secretion by the anterior pituitary.

The clinical features of hyperthyroidism of special concern to the anaesthetist include the following.

(1) Enlargement of the isthmus and two lateral lobes of the thyroid gland involves the upper trachea, cricoid and thyroid cartilages. There may be extension retrosternally, there is the possibility of tracheal compression or deviation before surgery, or collapse of tracheal rings at removal, and there may be trauma to one or both recurrent laryngeal nerves.

(2) Increased cardiac output, which will slow the rate of equilibration of inspired with alveolar, arterial and cerebral partial pressures of anaesthetic.

(3) Increased sensitivity to sympathetic stimulation, and to effects of catecholamines.

(4) Tachycardia, persisting during sleep.

(5) Cardiac arrhythmias, including atrial fibrillation especially in elderly patients (thyrotoxicosis is one of the three commonest causes).

(6) Abnormal glucose tolerance.

(7) Anxiety.

(8) Exophthalmos, the cause of which remains unknown.

(9) Thyrotoxic myopathy (weakness of proximal muscles of limbs).

(10) Thyrotoxic crisis (see below).

The diagnosis of hyperthyroidism, although outside the scope of this summary, can be based on various measurements as follows: T_4 (increased); T_3 (increased); effective thyroxine ratio (ETR), which integrates into one procedure the total serum thyroxine and the binding capacity of thyroid-binding proteins (increased); *in vivo* uptake of i.v. technetium (^{99m}Tc), or of radioactive iodine (^{131}I; ^{132}I) employing a scan technique; T_3 suppression test; serum TSH levels in response to TRH stimulation (suppression in thyrotoxicosis). Of less value now are measurements of protein-bound iodine (non-specific) and T_3 resin uptake (superseded by ETR).

NON-SURGICAL TREATMENT OF THYROTOXICOSIS

This includes the administration of antithyroid drugs, radioactive iodine, and β-adrenergic blocking agents.

Antithyroid drugs, which include carbimazole and methimazole (and the thiouracils as alternatives), act by blocking the binding of iodine to mono- and di-iodotyrosine (preceding the coupling of the latter to thyroglobulin). They are given initially in full suppressive doses for several weeks, and thereafter reduced, since overtreatment may increase the size of the gland through production of TSH by the anterior pituitary. It is believed, by restricting the use of these drugs as the sole definitive therapy to younger adults without marked thyroid enlargement, and by continuing for at least one year, that over 40% of thyrotoxic patients will show lasting remission. Toxicity of these antithyroid drugs extends from skin rashes to agranulocytosis and even red cell aplasia.

Radioactive iodine is often used for patients over 40 years; its single serious complication appears to be hypothyroidism, whose accumulative incidence increases linearly in subsequent years. It is avoided, empirically, in persons of reproductive age. Two or more months may be required for its effect to occur, and preferably its administration should not be preceded by that of carbimazole.

Beta-adrenergic blocking drugs cause symptomatic improvement by opposing sympathetic overactivity manifest as anxiety, tremor, palpitations, lid retraction, etc. Asthma is the main contraindication, while cardiac complications require special consideration. Propranolol, 40 mg three times a day, or higher, may be required.

PREPARATION AND ANAESTHETIC MANAGEMENT FOR SURGERY IN HYPERTHYROIDISM

(1) The aim, preoperatively, is that patients should be in a nearly normal (euthyroid) state; management depends upon the adequacy of this preparation, and may include immediate pretreatment with potassium iodide (60 mg orally, twice daily, for 14 days), to reduce thyroid function transiently and to diminish vascularity.

(2) The preoperative use of carbimazole or methimazole requires scrutiny of the haematological picture, and a search for any history of sore throat or other infection.

(3) Beta-adrenergic blocking agents, now used so commonly before cardiac surgery and manageable by the anaesthetist skilled in that field, need not prejudice safe anaesthesia, provided that cardiovascular function has been assessed adequately.

(4) Preoperative sedation should be sufficient to obtund anxiety.

(5) In addition to carrying out a normal preoperative visit and clinical examination, the anaesthetist must view the radiographs to detect tracheal compression or deviation. This, and retrosternal extension of the thyroid gland, may require special selection of a reinforced endotracheal tube.

(6) Since thiopentone may inhibit thyroxine production transiently (acting like the thiouracils), it can be considered as a suitable induction agent.

(7) Exophthalmos requires that the eyes be covered, by taping together the upper and lower lids, and applying a layer of petroleum jelly gauze.

(8) Heart rate, arterial pressure, ECG and body temperatures must be monitored.

(9) A head-up tilt (requested by some surgeons to minimize bleeding) increases the risk of venous air embolism, and may require that a suitable Doppler detector be applied to the precordium and that a central venous catheter be inserted for possible aspiration of air.

(10) Surgery may result in
   (a) damage to one or both recurrent laryngeal nerves. Inspection of the larynx, when there is unilateral palsy, shows the affected vocal cord in a central, immobile position. There will be post-operative hoarseness which shows slow recovery as the opposite

cord compensates. Bilateral involvement is a disaster, resulting in respiratory obstruction;

(b) haematoma, causing pressure on trachea or vascular structures in the neck;

(c) pneumothorax: when recognized, chest drainage may or may not be required; when suspected, an immediate chest film should be taken, if possible in the sitting position;

(d) trauma to, or removal of the parathyroid glands, which may be shown by mild hypocalcaemia in the postoperative period. Accidental removal is a leading cause of hypoparathyroidism.

About 80% of thyrotoxic patients treated by subtotal thyroidectomy should escape complications over a three to five year follow-up; in the remainder, depending on the amount of gland removed, there may be a recurrence of thyrotoxicosis or the development of hypothyroidism.

THYROTOXIC CRISIS

This 'storm' represents an acute manifestation of all the features of hyperthyroidism, and if untreated results in coma and death. It may occur soon after partial thyroidectomy in still hyperthyroid patients, after emergency operations (or infections) in any patient with untreated hyperthyroidism, and on withdrawing iodine therapy before achieving adequate control. The clinical features include:

(1) hyperpyrexia;
(2) confusion, restlessness, delirium; rarely, usually in older patients, apathy, and prostration;
(3) tachycardia; atrial fibrillation; cardiac failure;
(4) flushing and sweating;
(5) vomiting, diarrhoea, and abdominal pain;
(6) dehydration and ketosis.

Treatment is required urgently to reduce metabolic rate, lower temperature, restore or maintain acid—base balance, and correct fluid and electrolyte disturbances:

(1) Antithyroid drugs: carbimazole, 80—100 mg orally (gastric tube), followed by 20 mg six-hourly until control is achieved.

(2) Sodium iodide, 0.5 g in 2 ml distilled water, intravenously every 12 hours. On theoretical grounds, this should be preceded by antithyroid drugs in case iodides stimulate hormone synthesis.

(3) Beta-adrenergic blockade with propranolol 1—2 mg intravenously, increasing the dose as necessary, with caution in the presence of cardiac complications; 40 mg orally four times daily will establish continuing control of heart rate and reduce sympathetic overactivity.

(4) Surface cooling with ice packs, or more urgently by loose ice, fans, and gastric and bladder irrigation with cooled fluids.

(5) Sedation, for example with intravenous or intramuscular diazepam.

(6) Oxygenation by mask; depending on acid—base state, which requires assessment and control, mechanical ventilation may be advisable.

(7) Administration of fluids and appropriate amounts of glucose and electrolytes, according to requirements supported by measurements.

(8) In the presence of peripheral circulatory failure, hydrocortisone hemisuccinate 100 mg intravenously; higher doses, repeated as indicated, may be preferred.

The use of iodine as an urgent treatment in thyrotoxic crisis (and to reduce size and vascularity before surgery), contrasts with the development of non-toxic goitre in iodine-deficient areas of the world. Apparently, high plasma concentrations of inorganic iodides depress thyroid activity, with an action directly opposite to that of thyroid-stimulating hormone (TSH); it is not clear whether there is direct antagonism of TSH by high iodide concentrations, or if these inhibit thyroid-releasing factor (TRF) in the hypothalamus.

In a case report describing hyperthyroidism associated with a hydatidiform mole (Kim, Arakawa and McCann, 1976), a temperature rise following a 20 minute operation was attributed to a thyroid crisis, a normal state being restored after five days.

Goitre

Although there are many types of goitre (i.e. enlargement of the thyroid gland), those seen in anaesthetic practice comprise mainly the following: simple, cystic and adenomatous with or without calcification, thyrotoxic (see above) and carcinomatous; subacute and Hashimoto's thyroiditis also deserve mention.

Simple goitre may be associated with iodine deficiency, attributable to dietary lack (correctable by addition of table salt), to interference with absorption (calcium excess), or to a high intake of naturally occurring goitrogens (e.g. certain vegetables) which prevent iodine concentration in the thyroid. Antithyroid and other drugs, including PAS and sulphonamides, which interfere with the synthesis of thyroid hormones, and a prolonged intake of iodide-containing mixtures, may also cause goitre which is attributed to increased secretion of pituitary TSH.

Benign adenomas or cysts of the thyroid gland are usually removed surgically. Thyroid carcinoma presents early as a single nodule, whose histology cannot be identified without surgical removal, although it may show as a 'cold' area on thyroid scanning.

Medullary carcinoma of the thyroid is of special interest, being associated with increased circulating levels of plasma calcitonin, prostaglandins, or 5-hydroxytryptamine (5HT or serotonin), which cause flushing and abdominal symptoms. Although these tumours involve the parafollicular cells (C cells) of the thyroid, which secrete the polypeptide hormone calcitonin which lowers serum calcium concentration, hypocalcaemia is not a feature of medullary carcinoma of the thyroid.

Hypothyroidism

This may be primary, occurring mainly in middle-aged females, and due to Hashimoto's thyroiditis or atrophy (goitre may or may not be present); or secondary, due to failure of TSH production by the anterior pituitary or of TRH by the hypothalamus. In the primary forms, which may involve autoimmune mechanisms, myxoedema usually occurs (skin thickening from mucinous deposition), whereas it is less likely to be evident when the cause is pituitary hyposecretion.

Investigation of hypothyroidism shows that all patients have an elevated plasma TSH level; the ETR ratio is the single most suitable diagnostic procedure.

Treatment is with thyroxine 0.05 mg per day, increased gradually to 0.15–0.20 mg per day. Beta-adrenergic blocking drugs may be useful in the presence of ischaemic heart disease.

Clinical features of hypothyroidism of special note for the anaesthetist include:

(1) decreased metabolism, and reduced mental and physical activity;
(2) predisposition to pernicious anaemia;
(3) presence of a polyneuropathy;
(4) enlargement of the tongue;
(5) cardiovascular signs, usually including bradycardia unless there is circulatory failure, with which there may be tachycardia and cardiac enlargement;
(6) myocardial ischaemia;
(7) commonly, arterial hypertension because of arteriosclerosis;
(8) predisposition to hypothermia;
(9) mental signs;
(10) possibly, signs of pituitary or adrenal hypofunction.

MYXOEDEMATOUS COMA WITH HYPOTHERMIA

This is treated by

(1) slow warming to ensure a gradual rise in body temperature;
(2) T_3 given intravenously (as an infusion of 100 $\mu g \cdot l^{-1}$), associated with close cardiovascular monitoring;
(3) intravenous hydrocortisone, glucose and fluids.

PARATHYROID GLANDS

Hyperparathyroidism

The four parathyroid glands lie, elusively, on the posterior aspect of the thyroid, in its substance or within its sheath, related to the upper cornu of the thymus. Their blood supply is from the inferior thyroid arteries.

The integrated actions of parathyroid hormone, calcitonin (from the thyroid gland) and vitamin D are responsible for the control of the absorption, turnover in bone, and excretion, of calcium. Parathormone increases plasma calcium and lowers phosphate concentrations, respectively, by removal from bone and excretion by the kidney. Calcitonin's action on bone is opposite to that of parathyroid hormone.

Plasma calcium occurs in diffusible and non-diffusible forms, the former consisting mainly of ionized calcium, with a small amount in organic salts such as citrate and phosphate. Ionized calcium is the fraction involved in neuromuscular function. It should be noted that total plasma calcium can be low, yet the ionized fraction normal, when the protein bound component is reduced as a result of low plasma albumin. So also a raised total calcium concentration (above the normal 2.5 mmol·l^{-1} or 10 mg·dl^{-1}) does not necessarily indicate increased parathyroid activity. Adjustment for plasma albumin should be: subtract or add 0.0225 mmol·l^{-1} (0.09 mg·dl^{-1}) calcium for each 1 g·l^{-1} increase or decrease, respectively, from 46 g.l^{-1}.

Hyperparathyroidism may be primary, attributable to one or more adenomata, occasionally to hyperplasia or carcinoma. The secondary form is associated with renal failure. There is an increase in plasma calcium, up to 5 mmol·l^{-1} (20 mg·dl^{-1}), and a decline in inorganic phosphate toward 0.8 mmol·l^{-1} (2.5 mg·dl^{-1}). Urinary calcium is increased to above 5 mmol (200 mg) daily. Renal calculus is often a presenting feature in primary hyperparathyroidism, but this is a rare cause of a relatively common condition. Abdominal symptoms also occur, sometimes even with signs of peptic ulcer or acute pancreatitis. Bony cysts may be evident by radiography (osteitis fibrosa).

Diagnosis of hyperparathyroidism depends mainly on a raised plasma calcium concentration, repeated at intervals if necessary. If possible, radioimmune assay of parathormone should be carried out. In the differential diagnosis of hypercalcaemia, hyperparathyroidism must be distinguished from causes such as prolonged immobilization, bone metastases, Paget's disease, sarcoidosis, vitamin D excess and myelomatosis.

Removal of a parathyroid adenoma can be a surgical challenge, for reasons of anatomy and patience. Anaesthetic management is similar to that for thyroid surgery.

Hypoparathyroidism

This may occur transiently after partial thyroidectomy, or permanently after total resection of the thyroid. A decline in plasma calcium occurs within 24—48 hours of surgery. Rarely, it may represent an autoimmune condition, perhaps associated with other similarly induced endocrine disease.

Plasma calcium is reduced, and phosphate increased, and tetany occurs. Treatment with parathormone being unsatisfactory because of antibody formation, therapy involves vitamin D or substitutes. In an acute phase, calcium gluconate is given intravenously.

TETANY

This implies increased nervous excitability, due to a reduction in plasma ionized calcium (sometimes combined with magnesium depletion), which is aggravated by alkalaemia (which lowers the ionized calcium fraction) from respiratory or metabolic causes. Whereas children may show carpopedal and laryngeal spasm, and convulsions, only the first of these is usual in adults, together with cramp in the limbs and paraesthesiae. Treatment of tetany is initially by injection of 20 ml of 10% calcium gluconate intravenously (4.5 mmol), followed by correction of any existing alkalosis.

MYASTHENIA GRAVIS

This is a neuromuscular disorder characterized by fluctuating muscular fatigue, and an inability to sustain activity, which shows partial return of function with rest or the administration of cholinergic drugs.

Although the cause of the disease requires further clarification, studies in the past few years have confirmed that a basic defect is a reduction of the available acetylcholine receptors at neuromuscular junctions, resulting from autoimmune attack. Laboratory investigations have made use of α-bungarotoxin, which binds specifically and irreversibly to the active sites of acetylcholine receptors and can be labelled with radioactive iodine; and of the great numbers of acetylcholine receptors (which can be extracted and analysed biochemically), which are present in electric eels. Studies have been carried out on animal models and on muscle biopsied from myasthenics and controls. The conclusions suggest that a dominant defect in myasthenia gravis is at the postsynaptic area, where the geometric pattern of the receptor membrane is altered, with sparse folds and nerve terminals which are reduced in size. Although the acetylcholine vesicles have now been found to be of normal number and size, there is a reduced amplitude of the miniature end-plate potentials, supporting the hypothesis that a decrease of available acetylcholine receptors per se could account for the clinical and physiological features of myasthenia gravis. Since the number of acetylcholine—receptor interactions occurring in response to a nerve impulse normally exceeds the requirement to trigger an action potential, the condition can be seen to reduce the probability of such interaction; thus, the 'safety margin' of neuromuscular transmission is diminished in the myasthenic patient.

The initiation and mechanism of the autoimmune attack against acetylcholine receptors in human myasthenia gravis is not yet understood, although an animal model of 'experimental allergic myasthenia gravis' has been devised. A high proportion of patients have serum antibody directed against, and binding to skeletal muscle, and although this may also cross-react with cells of the thymus, there is no firm evidence that this antibody contributes directly to the pathogenesis. However, immunoglobulin fractions (IgG) from myasthenic patients, injected into mice, have been reported to reduce the amplitude of miniature end-plate potentials and the number of acetylcholine receptor sites. Evidence from tissue cultures suggests that both blockade and degradation of acetylcholine receptors occurs. Cell-mediated immune mechanisms, involving T and B lymphocytes, may be of importance, although present evidence favours the antibody-mediated process. Hypogammaglobulinaemia may be a feature.

While a role of the thymus in myasthenia gravis has been well considered, in view of pathological changes in the gland in about 75% of patients with the disease, and from favourable results of thymectomy, the processes involved are not understood. The changes are mainly 'hyperplasia' (increased germinal centre formation), a small number (up to 15%) showing gross or microscopic thymomas. Of interest is the presence in the thymus of skeletal muscle-like or 'myoid' cells, which may react with antimuscle antibody, and the finding that such cells, when grown in cultures, have surface acetylcholine receptors. Whether these cells could set off an autoimmune response, and the possibility of viral involvement, is speculative at present.

The reader is referred, for a full account of myasthenia gravis, to a recent comprehensive review (Drachman, 1978).

A small number of patients have thyrotoxicosis or Hashimoto's thyroiditis, and sometimes there is an association with rheumatoid arthritis, systemic lupus erythematosus, pernicious anaemia and diabetes mellitus.

The incidence of myasthenia gravis is as low as two to five cases per million of population per annum, females more often being affected, in an age range 15–50 years. Myasthenic patients may be classified as follows (Osserman, 1971):

(1) Neonatal, occurring transiently in about one of six infants of myasthenic mothers, and remitting spontaneously or with anticholinesterase treatment.
(2) Juvenile, from birth to puberty.
(3) Adult:
    (a) ocular only, limited to one eye, causing ptosis and diplopia;
    (b) mild generalized type, often mainly ocular and of slow onset;
    (c) moderate generalized, with progression from ocular to skeletal and respiratory muscles;
    (d) acute fulminating, with rapid onset of skeletal and respiratory muscle weakness.

Among the clinical features, muscle fatigue is dominant and an initially strong muscle movement tires quickly. This may occur at the end of a day or after exercise. The eye muscles, swallowing and speaking, and the proximal limb muscles are notably affected. Selective respiratory involvement is not characteristic, although asphyxia is obviously a potential cause of death. There is no sensory loss nor sign of an upper motoneuron lesion.

Pharmacological tests

(1) Edrophonium, 2—10 mg i.v., causes clinical improvement for periods up to about 5 min.
(2) Neostigmine 1—2 mg i.m., with 0.5—1.0 mg atropine. Improvement occurs in 10—15 min.
(3) In the 'regional curare test', a tourniquet is used to confine to one arm the effect of *d*-tubocurarine chloride, 0.2 mg/20 ml normal saline. Electromyography may be used; measurements of hand-grip strength show reductions of about 10% in normal subjects, and much greater effects (e.g. 60%) in myasthenics. Equipment for pulmonary ventilation should be to hand.

Treatment of myasthenia gravis

This is with neostigmine or pyridostigmine, the latter drug being slower in onset and more prolonged in action. Thymectomy is considered for any patients who do not respond to drug treatment. The use of steroids, which benefit the condition in many patients, requires individual management, and special indications which are more important than the attendant side-effects.

A retrospective review of 100 cases of transcervical thymectomy for myasthenia gravis (Girnar and Weinreich, 1976), showed that this operation had been used for patients without thymomas, the transthoracic approach being reserved for malignant or inaccessible tumours. However, a median sternotomy is probably now the recommended manoeuvre for all cases. Elective tracheostomy, formerly an invariable procedure, was not performed, and postoperative tracheostomy was required in less than 3% of patients. In an earlier series of 28 cases, routine preoperative tracheostomy had been commonly performed (Loach *et al.*, 1975), and it was concluded that mechanical ventilation was required in the post-operative period if the vital capacity was below 2 litres while on optimum anticholinesterase treatment preoperatively.

Anaesthetic management of thymectomy

(1) Preoperative respiratory function should be established by measurement, including blood gases and radiography.
(2) The patient's medication may be continued up to the immediate preoperative period.
(3) Premedication should be light, for example with diazepam 10 mg.
(4) The safest technique is to omit neuromuscular blocking drugs. This is facilitated, before endotracheal intubation, by injection of 4 ml of 4% lignocaine through the cricothyroid membrane, preferably in the conscious patient to ensure adequate coughing and spread, after full explanation and reassurance and the administration of small intravenous doses of narcotic or sedative drugs.

(5) For induction of anaesthesia, thiopentone sodium is convenient, or an inhalation technique can be used from the start, and continued until a deep plane of anaesthesia is reached. If lignocaine has not been injected transtracheally, it should now be sprayed on and through the vocal cords, after which endotracheal intubation should be as straight-forward as when neuromuscular blockers are used.

(6) Maintenance of anaesthesia with mechanical ventilation can be with halothane or enflurane with which adequate relaxation can be maintained and spontaneous respiration prevented.

(7) Resumption of spontaneous respiration at the end of surgery should permit extubation, provided that blood gases are monitored subsequently and that the equipment required for mechanical ventilation is kept at hand. Patients should be nursed postoperatively in an intensive therapy unit.

(8) Complications of thymectomy include haemorrhage and pneumothorax. Insertion of a chest drain is usually required before surgical closure, and a chest x-ray should always be taken immediately postoperatively.

(9) In theory, many drugs could adversely affect the myasthenic patient, such as antibiotics which reduce acetylcholine release, diuretics which cause potassium loss, and antiarrhythmic agents including quinidine and procainamide; electrolyte imbalance, especially of calcium, should also be considered.

CHOLINERGIC CRISIS

This is attributable to overdosage with neostigmine, and must be differentiated from a myasthenic crisis. A small dose of edrophonium makes the condition worse, but should improve myasthenic weakness. The features include the following.

(1) Generalized muscle weakness – similar to myasthenia.

(2) Parasympathetic overactivity of the gastrointestinal tract, shown by nausea, vomiting, and diarrhoea.

(3) Parasympathetic stimulation of secretions – sweating, salivation, and bronchorrhoea.

Treatment may include pulmonary ventilation and anticholinergic drugs.

Myasthenic syndrome

This is a condition of muscle weakness, occurring in association with several diseases, especially bronchial carcinoma, and probably with steroid administration. In contrast to the development of progressive fatigue on muscular activity, which is characteristic of myasthenia gravis, the weakness and neuromuscular changes show improvement with exercise and can be demonstrated electromyographically.

ENDOCRINE MANIFESTATIONS OF MALIGNANT DISEASE

There are several reasons for hormone secretion to be modified in malignant disease. Thus, in such a predicament there can be primary overactivity of a gland such as the anterior pituitary; there can be secondary deposits in the glands, leading to hyposecretion, causing such conditions as diabetes insipidus or adrenal insufficiency in association with the metastases of a bronchial carcinoma to posterior pituitary and adrenal glands respectively. There can also be endocrine manifestations, without direct involvement of the glands, as a result of hormone production by ectopic cells. From recent work on the APUD cell concept (see below), the production of amines and peptides by non-endocrine tissue is being recognized to a steadily increasing extent.

Whatever the origin, the clinical features of increased levels of plasma ACTH (and cortisol) may include muscle weakness, carbohydrate intolerance, hypertension, oedema and pigmentation. Such a picture may be seen in medullary carcinoma of the thyroid gland, whereas in oat cell bronchial neoplasms there is insufficient time for the florid manifestations to develop. Treatment, which may obviously include removal of the primary tumour (demanding adequate preoperative assessment by the anaesthetist), could also involve adrenalectomy; potassium-sparing diuretics, and metyrapone, may be indicated.

In cases of increased secretion of ADH, there will be dilutional hyponatraemia and an osmolarity which is low in plasma and high in urine. Puffy oedema may be present, and patients may have headache, nausea and vomiting, and be apathetic. The diagnosis can be confirmed by demonstrating a raised serum ADH level by radioimmune assay. Treatment, apart from possible removal of the primary tumour, may involve water restriction and the use of lithium to block renal tubular transport.

In patients with hypercalcaemia, plasma parathormone levels may be raised, and clinical features resemble those of hyperparathyroidism. In such cases, osteolytic bone metastases are common. Phosphate may be given orally to reduce calcium absorption. A calciferol-like steroid may be secreted by certain tumours.

A raised plasma level of thyroid-stimulating hormone (TSH) characterizes secondary thyrotoxicosis; this, and the absence of eye signs, distinguishes it from the primary condition wherein TSH is suppressed through the feedback mechanism. Involvement of erythropoietin may result in erythrocytosis.

The following summarizes the endocrine manifestations of malignant disease.

(1) It is an uncommon feature, occurring for example, in perhaps 2% of

bronchial carcinomata compared to a 3% incidence of CNS involvement in this condition.

(2) The endocrine picture is subtle, not florid.

(3) Several symptoms and signs mimic the primary disease.

(4) Many types of tumour are involved.

(5) Several hormones may be produced by one tumour.

(6) Some improvement in the patient's condition may be attainable, even when treatment of the primary disease is impossible.

There should be a thorough preoperative assessment by the anaesthetist.

At the present stage, the APUD cell concept appears complex, but should increase understanding of the mechanism of ectopic and aberrant hormone production. The writer must rely heavily on recently published work, including notable reviews by Tischler *et al.* (1977) and Whitwam (1977). The title APUD is an acronym derived from the three most important characteristics of these cells: amine content; amine precursor uptake; and amino-acid decarboxylation. Additional features include characteristic chemical and ultrastructures, and specific immunofluorescence. The APUD cells are proven or presumptive derivatives of neuroectoderm. They have similarities to nerve cells, and they can be grouped into central and peripheral divisions. The central division consists of neurosecretory cells found in hypothalamus, pituitary and pineal glands. The peripheral division includes cells of the sympathetic nervous system and adrenal medulla, and others found in gut, pancreas, thyroid (type C cells), probably parathyroid, carotid body, skin (melanocytes), lungs (type P) and urogenital tract. Many peptides produced in the gut are also found in the brain, and could be neurotransmitters; vasoactive intestinal peptide (VIP) may be one such. Similarly, somatostatin (the hypothalamic inhibitor of growth hormone release) has been identified in stomach and pancreas and can inhibit intestinal peptides such as insulin, glucagon and gastrin.

It is possible to regard peripherally situated cells of the APUD series as fulfilling a primitive neuroendocrine function in an earlier evolutionary period, and perhaps in present times as a potentially active component of the nervous system. If cells of neuroectodermal origin are initially programmed for neuroendocrine activity, it must be presumed that their actual function depends on their environment.

It has been reported recently that APUD cells are present in normal lung, the speculation being made that liberated peptides could have a role in ventilation/perfusion disturbances, pulmonary oedema and similar conditions.

Apudoma

This term was applied first to an ACTH-secreting medullary carcinoma of the thyroid, but has been extended to describe any neoplasm of APUD cells. Acceptance of the APUD concept suggests the term 'parahormone' for the deviant secretions by non-endocrine tissue.

According to published information (for references, see Whitwam, 1977) the apudomas include tumours of only a few of the orthodox endocrine glands: pituitary adenomas, producing only the normal homones of this gland; medullary carcinoma of thyroid, and adenoma of pancreatic islet cells, from which both normal and parahormones are secreted; and thymoma, secreting only parahormones. Other cell groups classifiable as apudomas, secreting normal and/or parahormones, include carcinoid tumours of intestine, oat cell and bronchial carcinoma, chemodectoma, paraganglioma, ganglioneuroblastoma and melanoma. In this classification, phaeochromocytoma is also included.

Hormone liberation by APUD cells results in syndromes such as Cushing's (most common); Schwartz—Bartter (ectopic ADH); WDHA (VIP secretion associated with watery diarrhoea, hypokalaemia and achlorhydria); and Zollinger—Ellison (gastrin is implicated).

Multiple endocrine adenopathy (MEA) is the term applied to the concurrence of two or more endocrine tumours. These are classifiable as MEA type I, involving parathyroid and pituitary glands, pancreas, and possibly others; and MEA type 2 (Sipple's syndrome) comprising medullary carcinoma of the thyroid, phaeochromocytoma and signs of hyperparathyroidism.

Carcinoid syndrome

This is seen in only about 25% of carcinoid tumours, some 40 cases having been described in the anaesthetic literature, wherein a comprehensive review and accompanying case report have recently been published (Mason and Steane, 1976). Carcinoid tumours may occur anywhere in the intestinal tract, but most commonly in appendix or ileum, and a majority which produce the syndrome have metastasized to the liver.

Features of the syndrome include flushing, bronchospasm, diarrhoea, hypertension or biphasic pressure changes, and cardiovascular collapse; valvular lesions of the heart may be present. Descriptions have included a pink flush, with hypertension and tachycardia; or a blue flush, with hypotension and bradycardia.

Causative substances in the carcinoid syndrome include serotonin (5-hydroxytryptamine, confirmed by increased urinary excretion of 5-hydroxyindole acetic acid), but more recently several others have been implicated: histamine (especially in gastric tumours), bradykinins (whose half-life is brief and formation is linked to the enzyme kallikrein), prostaglandin, calcitonin, probably the 'normal' gastrointestinal hormone gastrin, glucagon and enteroglucagon, the vascularly reacting substance VIP, and such 'parahormones' as ACTH, ADH, MSH and HCG (human chorionic gonadotrophin).

Treatment of the carcinoid syndrome may include drugs which are antagonistic to 5-hydroxytryptamine such as methotrimeprazine, chlorpromazine, and possibly droperidol; and to bradykinin, such as aprotinin 200 000 units intravenously.

Surgical treatment of carcinoid involves removal of the primary tumour, whenever possible, together with hepatic metastases (e.g. by lobectomy). Ligation of the hepatic artery has been performed (Patel, Millar and Warner, 1977).

In anaesthetic management, drugs which are capable of releasing histamine such as morphine, d-tubocurarine, and possibly Althesin, should probably be avoided. If liver involvement is extensive enough to reduce cholinesterase production, the use of suxamethonium is inadvisable. Drugs affecting arterial pressure, including catecholamines and other pressor agents, if used, may require careful titration to avoid interaction with the several substances liberated by carcinoid tumours.

In the space available, it has been impossible to cover all aspects of endocrine disease of relevance to anaesthetic practice. It will be obvious that many new facts are being acquired about the structure, function and localization of those hypothalamic releasing and inhibiting hormones on which pituitary function is largely dependent; also, that new classifications are being sought and developed for peripheral tissue cells which are capable, in certain disordered circumstances, of releasing those hormones normally secreted by the orthodox neuroendocrine system.

References

Drachman, D. B. (1978). Myasthenia gravis. *New Engl. J. Med.* **298**, 136−142; 186−193

Girnar, D. S. and Weinreich, A. I. (1976). Anesthesia for transcervical thymectomy in myasthenia gravis. *Curr. Res. Anesth. Analg.* **55**, 13−17

Kim, J. M., Arakawa, K. and McCann, V. (1976). Severe hyperthyroidism associated with hydatidiform mole. *Anesthesiology* **44**, 445−448

Loach, A. B., Young, A. C., Spalding, J. M. K. and Smith, A. C. (1975). Postoperative management after thymectomy. *Br. med. J.* **1**, 309−312

Mason, R. A. and Steane, P. A. (1976). Carcinoid syndrome: its relevance to the anaesthetist. *Anaesthesia* **31**, 228−242

Osserman, K. E. (1971). Studies in myasthenia gravis − review of a twenty-year experience in over 1,200 patients. *Mount Sinai J. Med.* **38**, 538−572

Patel, A. U., Miller, R. and Warner, R. R. P. (1977). Anesthesia for ligation of the hepatic artery in a patient with carcinoid symdrome. *Anesthesiology* **47**, 303−305

Tischler, A. S., Dichter, M. A., Biales, B. and Greene, L. A. (1977). Neuroendocrine neoplasms and their cells of origin. *New Engl. J. Med.* **296**, 919−925

Whitwam, J. G. (1977). APUD cells and the apudomas. A concept relevant to anaesthesia and endocrinology. *Anaesthesia* **32**, 879−888

44 Acid–base balance in relation to anaesthesia
D. R. Bevan

The proliferation of sophisticated electronic equipment has made the measurement of pH and gas tensions of any body fluid quick, accurate and reproducible. Unfortunately, such ease of measurement conceals the clinician's confusion and his difficulty in relating the simple measurement to the clinical state of the patient. The clinician's confusion arises from two causes. First, acid–base terminology is based upon complicated physicochemical concepts which are seldom understood. Second, the multiplicity of 'simple' diagrams and associated jargon has evolved attempting to separate the metabolic and respiratory components from any set of acid–base data. The confusion has been compounded by the erroneous assumption that the change in pH which occurs in blood tonometered with gases of differing CO_2 tensions is similar to the change in whole body pH which occurs when the $P{CO_2}$ of the patient is altered.

TERMINOLOGY

ACIDS AND BASES

In lay terms, the property of acidity is associated with the sour taste of a solution. Some solutions are more sour, and hence more acid, than others. Chemically, the acidity of a substance, e.g. HC1, $H_2PO_4^-$, is related to its ability to ionize in solution to give hydrogen ions (H^+) and residual anions (A^-):

$$HA \rightleftharpoons H^+ + A^-$$

Consequently, the more H^+ that can be produced the more acid the solution.

In 1964 the New York Academy of Sciences defined an acid as a proton donor and a base as a proton acceptor.

BUFFERS

Buffers are substances which, by their presence in solution, increase the amount of acid or base which must be added to that solution to cause a unit change in H^+ concentration. The important buffers in biological systems are haemoglobin, plasma proteins, phosphates and the carbonic acid—bicarbonate systems.

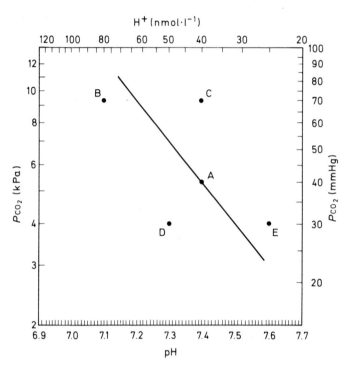

Figure 44.1
Sets of pH—$P\text{CO}_2$ acid—base data (see text)

TABLE 44.1. Sets of pH—$P\text{CO}_2$ acid—base data (see text)

	pH	*PCO₂*		*Respiratory status*	*Metabolic status*	*Over-all status*
		kPa	*mmHg*			
A	7.4	5.3	40	Normal	Normal	Normal
B	7.1	9.3	70	Acidosis	Acidosis	Acidaemia
C	7.4	9.3	70	Acidosis	Alkalosis	Normal
D	7.3	4	30	Alkalosis	Acidosis	Acidaemia
E	7.6	4	30	Alkalosis	Alkalosis	Alkalaemia

Acidosis, alkalosis and acidaemia, alkalaemia

The terms acidosis, acidaemia and alkalosis, alkalaemia are often used interchangeably, but this is not correct.

Acidaemia should be defined as existing if the arterial pH is less than 7.35. Similarly, an alkalaemia is present if the pH is above 7.45. If a primary non-respiratory (metabolic) tendency towards acidaemia is accompanied by a tendency towards respiratory alkalaemia so that the resulting pH still lies within the normal range, the acid–base state should be known as non-respiratory acidosis accompanied by a respiratory alkalosis. By definition, if the P_{CO_2} is above 6.0 kPa (45 mmHg) or less than 4.7 kPa (35 mmHg) a respiratory acidosis or alkalosis, respectively, is present. If the set of pH–P_{CO_2} values produces a point on the *in vivo* CO_2 titration curve to the left or right of the normal curve, then a metabolic acidosis or alkalosis, respectively, is present.

For example, consider the sets of values in *Table 44.1,* which accompanies *Figure 44.1.*

SI units

Using the Système Internationale (SI) nomenclature, acidity is expressed in nmol·l^{-1} instead of pH units. Nevertheless, Waddell and Bates (1969) have criticized such a change because: (1) the measurement is made according to a standard, operational pH scale; (2) biological activity is related to the chemical potential exerted by H$^+$ and, hence, is logarithmic in nature; (3) as blood pH values in the population are probably normally distributed, the distribution of H$^+$ concentration, nmol·l^{-1}, will be skewed. Thus, ideally, H$^+$ concentration should be converted to pH units before parametric statistical analysis (calculation of mean, s.d. and use of Student's 't' test) is performed.

ASSESSMENT OF ACIDITY

The range of hydrogen ion (H$^+$) concentrations found in aqueous bodily solutions is large, 10^{-1}–10^{-15} mol·l^{-1}. For convenience, these concentrations are expressed by exponential arithmetic (*Table 44.2*).

TABLE 44.2. Conversion of H$^+$ concentration (mol·l^{-1} and nmol·l^{-1}) to pH units

$[H^+]$ (mol·l^{-1})	pH	$[H^+]$ (nmol·l^{-1})
0.001 = 10^{-3}	3	1 000 000
0.000 01 = 10^{-5}	5	10 000
0.000 000 1 = 10^{-7}	7	100
0.000 000 001 = 10^{-9}	9	1

$$[H^+] = 10^{-p} = \frac{1}{10^p}$$

$$pH = -\log[H^+]$$

([H^+] is the concentration of H^+. The H^+ exponent, p, is the initial letter of the words potenz, puissance or power; Sorensen, 1909).

One basic difficulty is that it is not possible to measure either the actual H^+ concentration or its activity in biological systems. The pH numbers, produced by electrometric measurement, are defined by an operational scale based upon standard buffer solutions at fixed temperatures of measurement (Bates, 1964). They do not relate precisely to H^+ concentration or activity.

The normal value for arterial pH in man, at a Pa_{CO_2} of 5.3 kPa (40 mmHg) is 7.4 with a range of 7.35–7.45. For venous blood the range is 7.32–7.42.

DETERMINANTS OF pH

During cellular metabolism the acidic products from catabolism flow into the alkaline extracellular fluid. In the resting subject catabolism of carbohydrates and fats produces an acid load of approximately 15 000–20 000 mmol per day which is excreted by the lungs as carbon dioxide. Protein catabolism leads to the additional production of 50–80 mmol per day of non-volatile acids, mostly sulphuric and phosphoric acids, which are excreted by the kidney. Incomplete oxidation of carbohydrate and fats in disease states leads to the production of more non-volatile acid, such as lactic acid in anaerobic metabolism and keto acids in diabetes mellitus.

Buffering

As non-volatile acids are released, their effect is buffered by the action of bicarbonate in the extravascular extracellular fluid (ECF) and in the blood by bicarbonate (50%), haemoglobin (35%), plasma protein (6%) and phosphates. The net effect of the balance between acid production, excretion and buffering is reflected in the ECF pH.

BICARBONATE–CARBONIC ACID SYSTEM

The addition of H^+ or CO_2 to ECF leads to the production of carbonic acid:

$$H^+ + HCO_3^- \rightleftharpoons H_2CO_3 \rightleftharpoons H_2O + CO_2 \tag{44.1}$$

according to the law of mass action;

$$\frac{[H^+] \times [HCO_3^-]}{[H_2CO_3]} = \text{constant } K \tag{44.2}$$

or

$$pH = pK + \log \frac{[HCO_3^-]}{[H_2CO_3]} \tag{44.3}$$

(Henderson, 1908; Hasselbalch, 1917)

The buffering capability of such a system is optimal at a pH near its pK. The pK for the bicarbonate–carbonic acid system is 6.2. Consequently, it is a relatively weak buffer at physiological pH (7.4). Its importance lies in the ability of carbonic acid to produce CO_2 which is excreted via the lungs. The addition of H^+ and elimination of CO_2 drives equation 44.1 to the right.

The bicarbonate–carbonic acid system forms the cornerstone of acid–base control as carbonic acid can be formed by the addition of either CO_2 (respiratory acid load) or non-volatile acids (metabolic or non-respiratory load).

HAEMOGLOBIN

Haemoglobin acts as a buffer mainly due to the presence of histidine residues whose pK lie in the physiological range of pH. Its buffering capacity alters with the oxygenation of haemoglobin. Reduction of haemoglobin causes it to become more basic and, hence, allows it to buffer more H^+ than oxyhaemoglobin (Nunn, 1977).

CO_2 carriage (*Figure 44.2*)

As CO_2 is released, it is carried to the lungs, for excretion, by the blood in three forms.

(1) DISSOLVED CO_2

The solubility coefficient of CO_2 in plasma is 0.23 mmol·l^{-1}·kPa^{-1} (0.03 mmol·l^{-1}·mmHg^{-1}). Therefore, at a Pa_{CO_2} of 5.3 kPa (40 mmHg) at 37°C, 1.2 mmol·l^{-1} of carbon dioxide is carried by plasma. The concentration of H_2CO_3 in plasma is only 1/1000 that of the total concentration of CO_2 so that equation 44.3 may be rewritten:

$$pH = pK^1 + \log \frac{[HCO_3^-]}{\alpha P_{CO_2}} \quad (\alpha = \text{sol. coeff. for } CO_2) \tag{44.4}$$

(2) BICARBONATE

Addition of CO_2 to blood drives equation 44.1 to the left. The production of HCO_3^- is achieved mainly in the red cell where the reaction is catalysed by carbonic anhydrase. Bicarbonate diffuses from the red cell to be replaced by Cl^- ions. The H^+ produced by the formation of HCO_3^- is

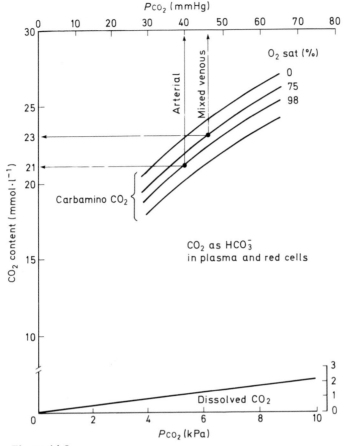

Figure 44.2
Carriage of CO_2 in blood

buffered by haemoglobin. Consequently, HCO_3^- production is increased in the presence of reduced haemoglobin.

(3) CARBAMINO COMPOUNDS

Carbon dioxide combines with the terminal amino groups of haemoglobin to form carbamino compounds. Although the total amount of CO_2 carried by carbamino compounds is small (1.7 $mmol·l^{-1}$ in venous blood) the AV CO_2 carbamino difference (0.6 $mmol·l^{-1}$) accounts for one-third of the total AV CO_2 content difference. Carbamino carriage is also augmented by reduced haemoglobin.

Renal acid excretion

The presence of carbonic anhydrase (CA) in renal tubular cells encourages the production of H^+:

$$CO_2 + H_2O \overset{CA}{\rightleftharpoons} H_2CO_3 \rightleftharpoons H^+ + HCO_3^-$$

Most of this H^+ passes into the proximal tubule where it neutralizes most of the 5000 mmol per day HCO_3^- of the glomerular filtrate. The CO_2 produced diffuses back into the tubular cell. Although no net H^+ excretion results, this action prevents loss of filtered base. Smaller amounts of H^+ are secreted into the distal tubule and collecting ducts to make the urine as acid as pH 4.6.

Approximately 30 mmol of H^+ are excreted each day as 'titratable acid', bound to urinary phosphate buffer. The phosphate of the glomerular filtrate, in the monohydrogen form (HPO_4^{2-}), buffers H^+:

$$HPO_4^{2-} + H^+ \rightleftharpoons H_2PO_4^-$$

Normally a further 50—60 mmol per day, which may be increased to 500 mmol per day, is excreted as urinary ammonium (NH_4^+) formed by the combination of H^+ and NH_3 in the tubular cell. The NH_3 is synthesized in the distal tubular cell from glutamine. Thus the maximum renal acid secretion, as seen in diabetic ketoacidosis, is approximately 700—750 mmol per day (Pitts, 1974) of which two-thirds is NH_4^+ and one-third titratable acid.

SAMPLING FOR ACID—BASE DETERMINATION

The acid—base status of most body tissue is reflected in that tissue's venous blood. (The brain is an important exception to this rule as lactate produced by anaerobic metabolism is confined by the blood—brain barrier to the brain cells and cerebrospinal fluid.) Thus the assessment of whole-body acid—base status may be determined by analysis of mixed venous blood. As this can only be achieved by pulmonary artery or, at least, right ventricular sampling, most investigators use arterial blood as 'oxygenated mixed venous blood'. This has the additional advantage that the arterial Po_2 may be determined from the same sample.

An alternative, which is particularly useful in small chilren, is to use a sample of capillary blood. If this is taken from a warm, vasodilated part of the periphery, usually the hand or heel, it has been shown that the Pco_2 is within 0.07 kPa (0.5 mmHg) and the pH within 0.005 units of simultaneously obtained arterial samples. Capillary sampling is unsuitable for Po_2 determination.

The estimation of intracellular and CSF acid—base status will be considered separately.

ASSESSMENT OF ACID—BASE STATE

In vivo CO_2 titration

Consideration of the Henderson—Hasselbalch equation 44.4 is the core to the understanding of acid—base balance. Both metabolic and respiratory factors are represented. Unfortunately, some established methods of assessing acid–base balance have linked pH to the molar concentrations of bicarbonate and carbonic acid in plasma or blood *in vitro* and assumed that similar changes would be found *in vivo*. In addition, it is now appreciated that the constants in the equation cannot be predicted accurately.

Nevertheless, the equation allows us to expect that an *in vivo* alteration of P_{CO_2} will be associated with a predictable change in pH. Such an association has been confirmed in animals and in man (Prys-Roberts, Kelman and Nunn, 1966; Kappagoda, Linden and Snow, 1970). If the

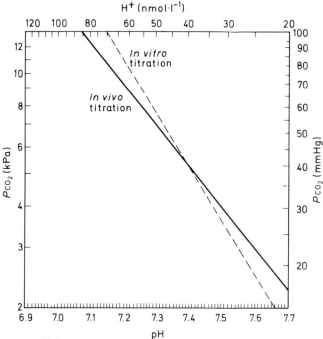

Figure 44.3
In vivo and *in vitro* CO_2 titration curves

P_{aCO_2} is either increased or decreased, and time allowed for a steady state to be reached, an *in vivo* CO_2 titration curve (straight line using a pH/log P_{CO_2} plot) is obtained (*Figure 44.3*). When such a titration is performed in animals made deliberately acid, with varying amounts of hydrochloric acid, a family of curves, approximately parallel to, and to the left of the normal curve, is found. The more acid that is added the further is the curve shifted to the left. Similarly, in man, a non-respiratory acidosis produces curves shifted to the left and a non-respiratory alkalosis to the right. Buffering capability increases with increasing non-respiratory acidosis so that left shifted curves are more vertical than the normal (*Figure 44.4*).

In vitro CO_2 titration

The early assessment of acid–base status was determined with a pH electrode. Arterial blood was tonometered with two gases of known,

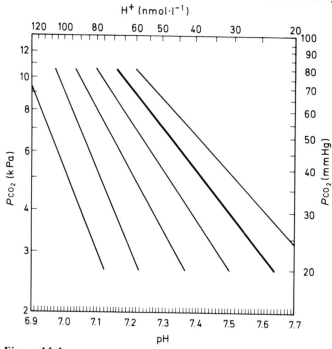

Figure 44.4
Family of *in vivo* CO$_2$ titration curves in non-respiratory acidosis
and alkalosis

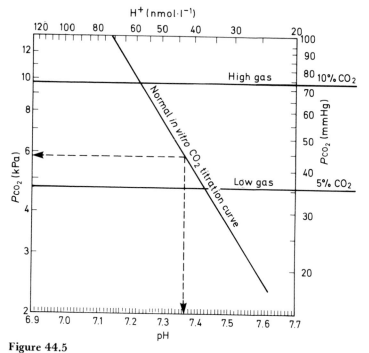

Figure 44.5
Measurement of $P\text{CO}_2$ by interpolation and construction of *in vitro*
CO$_2$ titration curve

different CO_2 concentrations. If the pH was measured after tonometry an *in vitro* blood CO_2 titration curve could be constructed (*Figure 44.5*) and the actual $P\mathrm{co}_2$ of the original blood sample determined by interpolation if its pH was measured (Astrup *et al.*, 1960).

In general, it was realized that blood from acidotic patients lay to the left of this curve and from alkalotic patients to the right. But it was appreciated that the haemoglobin concentration altered the slope of the curve and induced errors. Thus a number of indices were used to obviate these errors.

BASE EXCESS (BE) (Astrup *et al.*, 1960)

When normal blood is diluted to different haemoglobin concentrations and equilibrated with gas mixtures of different $P\mathrm{co}_2$, this yields a family of $P\mathrm{co}_2$/pH curves intersecting at pH 7.4 and $P\mathrm{co}_2$ 5.3 kPa (40 mmHg). If 10 mmol of strong acid or alkali is added, a different family of curves is produced. If the intersections of each family are joined, a base excess curve is produced (*Figure 44.6*). The value of the base excess is thus

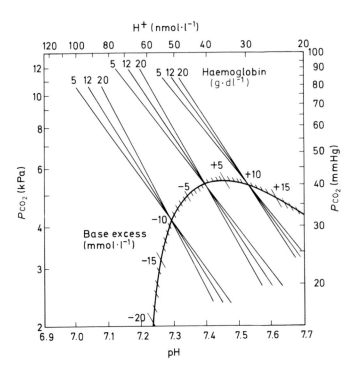

Figure 44.6
Construction of 'base excess' curve

independent of the haemoglobin concentration and is a useful index of the patient's non-respiratory acid—base status.

It was found, empirically, that correction of a metabolic acidosis could often be obtained by the infusion of $(0.3 \times BE \times$ weight in kg) mmol sodium bicarbonate. However, inaccuracy is introduced by the use of *in vitro* titration curves. The *in vivo* CO_2 titration may be considered as the titration of ECF including the blood volume which has an average haemoglobin concentration of $3-5$ g·dl^{-1} and is thus relatively unaffected by changes in the haemoglobin concentration of the blood. Various corrections have been applied to the base excess approach (Lewis and Stoddart, 1973; Severinghaus, 1976).

BUFFER BASE (Singer and Hastings, 1948)

An earlier assessment was achieved from a nomogram to calculate the sum of the concentration of the buffer anions in mmol·l^{-1}. The total included bicarbonate, plasma proteins and haemoglobin.

STANDARD BICARBONATE (Jorgensen and Astrup, 1957)

The influence of haemoglobin was eliminated by determining the $[HCO_3^-]$ in plasma, after separation from whole blood, that had been equilibrated to a $P\text{CO}_2$ of 5.33 kPa (40 mmHg) at 37°C.

All these indices may be derived from the Siggaard-Andersen (1962) nomogram. But all suffer from the inaccuracy of using *in vitro* titration curves. Linguistically the indices are far from perfect. Consequently, acid—base analysis for the remainder of this chapter is interpreted from *in vivo* titration curves.

PRIMARY ACID—BASE DISTURBANCES

Respiratory disturbances (*Table 44.3, Figure 44.7*)

RESPIRATORY ACIDOSIS

Acidosis due to CO_2 retention is due to inadequate ventilation of the lungs resulting from disturbance of neuromuscular integrity or pulmonary disease. During and after anaesthesia the commonest cause is hypo-ventilation due either to drug-induced respiratory centre depression or incomplete reversal of neuromuscular blocking drugs.

Biochemically, in acute disturbances, arterial pH falls according to the *in vivo* CO_2 titration curve. In long-standing conditions the kidney excretes an increasing proportion of the acid load producing a shift to the right of the titration curve (A → C in *Figure 44.7*), but this secondary change takes 24—48 hours.

As with all acid—base disturbances, correction should be aimed, primarily, toward treatment of the underlying cause. In chronic CO_2

TABLE 44.3. Respiratory disturbances of acid—base status

Acidosis — hypoventilation	(1)	Respiratory centre depression Opiates General anaesthesia
	(2)	Nerve conduction depression Neurological disease, e.g. poliomyelitis, peripheral neuritis
	(3)	Neuromuscular paralysis Relaxant drugs Myasthenia gravis
	(4)	Respiratory disease Obstructive lung disease Parenchymal lung disease Thoracic injury (pneumothorax)
	(5)	Inadequate IPPV
Alkalosis — hyperventilation	(1)	Cortical stimulation Pain, fear, anxiety Analeptic drugs Salicylate poisoning Head injury Hepatic failure
	(2)	Hypoxic drive Altitude Shock (cellular hypoxia)
	(3)	Cardiopulmonary disease Asthma Pulmonary oedema
	(4)	Excessive IPPV

retention, renal compensation causes an increase in plasma and CSF $[HCO_3^-]$ to return pH toward normal. This reduces the central drive to respiration, which becomes dependent upon the peripheral chemoreceptors, particularly their response to Po_2. If the $Paco_2$ is reduced rapidly in these patients the sudden increase in CSF pH will reduce cerebral blood flow and may produce unconsciousness and convulsions (Cotev and Severinghaus, 1969). Therefore, CO_2 retention in these patients should be corrected slowly over 24—48 hours.

RESPIRATORY ALKALOSIS

Alkalosis due to hyperventilation may originate from increased respiratory drive by central or peripheral afferent stimulation. The pain, anxiety and fear induced by the clumsy collection of an arterial blood sample may result in a $Paco_2$ as low as 4 kPa (30 mmHg). Mild hyperventilation is common in the pregnant patient and during labour the $Paco_2$ may fall to 3.3 kPa (25 mmHg). In hepatic failure, CO_2 depletion is common, but progressive liver failure causes lactic acid accumulation and metabolic acidosis so that the pH is normal or below. Peripheral chemoreceptor hypoxic drive occurs at high altitude and probably explains the hyperventilation of severe cardiopulmonary disease and shock, although the metabolic acidosis in the shocked patient also contributes to the respiratory drive (Freeman and Nunn, 1963). Respiratory alkalosis seen by the anaesthetist is usually due to mechanical hyperventilation.

Biochemically, during acute respiratory alkalosis, the pH increases according to the *in vivo* CO_2 titration curve. Renal compensation (B → D in *Figure 44.7*) is again slow. Sykes, McNicol and Campbell (1976) have

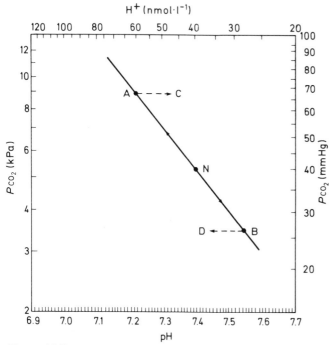

Figure 44.7
pH–P_{CO_2} changes during respiratory disturbances. Acute respiratory acidosis follows titration line N → A and alkalosis N → B. Renal compensation is slow and causes pH change A --→ C and B --→ D

drawn attention to the severe depletion of the body's CO_2 stores during hyperventilation. When hyperventilation ceases the stores are replaced during a period of hypoventilation. Because oxygen consumption is unchanged the respiratory quotient (CO_2 output/O_2 consumption) is decreased. From calculations based on the alveolar air equation the reduction in RQ causes a decrease in Pa_{O_2} and is thus another reason why patients should receive additional oxygen during weaning from mechanical ventilation.

Correction of respiratory alkalosis lies in preventing the increased central or peripheral drive if this is inappropriate. Mechanical ventilation should be controlled by monitoring of arterial or end-tidal P_{CO_2}.

Non-respiratory (metabolic) changes (*Table 44.4*)

NON-RESPIRATORY ACIDOSIS (*Figure 44.8*)

Non-respiratory acidosis may be caused by an increase in the production of non-volatile acids during anaerobic metabolism in starvation, diabetes mellitus, after cardiac arrest and following administration of large amounts of sodium nitroprusside. The administration of large volumes of stored blood, when ACD is used as the anticoagulant, produces an acute acidosis although hepatic metabolism of the lactate in the next two to three days will convert this to a non-respiratory alkalosis. A non-respiratory acidosis also accompanies excessive loss of base from diarrhoea or pancreatic and biliary fistulae. Severe renal disease or isolated distal tubular defects cause an acidosis by a net reduction in renal acid excretion. An uncommon,

TABLE 44.4. Non-respiratory disturbances of acid—base status

Acidosis	Acid load	Anaerobic metabolism
		Acid infusion
		ACD blood
		fructose
		Starvation
		Diabetes mellitus
		Sodium nitroprusside
		Lactic acidosis
	Loss of base	Diarrhoea
		Pancreatic/biliary fistula
	↓ Acid excretion	Renal acidosis
		Acetazolamide
	Dilutional	Saline excess
Alkalosis	Alkaline load	$NaHCO_3$ infusion
		ACD blood
		Oral alkali
	Acid loss	Vomiting
		Gastric fistula
	K^+ loss	Hypokalaemia
		$1°$ aldosteronism
		Diuretics

but probably overemphasized, cause of non-respiratory acidosis occurs if extracellular bicarbonate is diluted by overenthusiastic replacement with saline. Such administration only occurs during the resuscitation of the severely hypovolaemic patient in whom the restoration of circulatory volume by an isotonic fluid is an urgent requirement to restore tissue perfusion and aerobic metabolism. Lactic acidosis will be considered separately.

Biochemically, the *in vivo* CO_2 titration curve is shifted to the left in non-respiratory acidosis. Ventilation is stimulated by peripheral chemoreceptor drive so that arterial and CSF P_{CO_2} and $[HCO_3^-]$ are lowered until

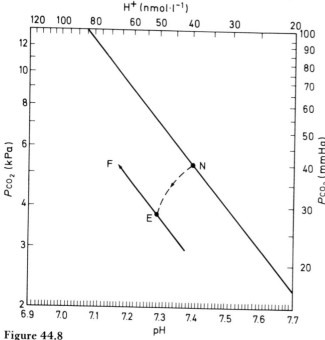

Figure 44.8

Acid–base changes during non-respiratory acidosis. Respiratory
stimulation allows pH to move N --→ E. In the absence of respiratory
compensation, pH would be F

pH returns almost to normal (*Figure 44.8*). If the pH is corrected rapidly
by the administration of bicarbonate, CSF Pco_2 will rise and pH fall
stimulating central chemoreceptors and replacing the arterial non-
respiratory acidosis with a respiratory alkalosis.

The correction of a non-respiratory acidosis is probably the commonest
therapeutic manipulation of acid–base status. Exact, single-dose, correction
could only be achieved if it were possible to determine whether the patient
was improving or deteriorating and how quickly, and also if the volume
of distribution of H^+ was known precisely. Only empirical general guidelines
can be given. Correction should be by the slow administration of sodium
bicarbonate, over ten minutes, and monitored by repeated blood gas analysis
to prevent overcorrection. A simple guide is to calculate the change in
pH which would have occurred if no respiratory compensation had taken
place. This is achieved by drawing a line parallel to the normal *in vivo* CO_2
titration curve to pass through the point at which the patient lies (E in
Figure 44.8). Point F represents the expected pH at a Pco_2 of 5.33 kPa.
For a 70 kg patient, 100 mmol $NaHCO_3$ should then be given for each 0.1
decrease in pH from 7.4. A further set of Pco_2–pH values should be
obtained in 30 minutes and the process repeated.

EXAMPLE

A 70 kg patient is admitted after a road traffic accident shocked and with
pH 7.26 and Pco_2 4 kPa (30 mmHg). The expected pH at 5.3 kPa (40 mmHg)

(called 'non-respiratory pH' by Kappagoda, Linden and Snow, 1970) would be 7.2 (see *Figure 44.4*). Thus 200 mmol sodium bicarbonate should be given initially. Blood gas assessment should be repeated 30 minutes later.

The advantage of such a method, compared with the use of 'base excess' and an exact formula is that it is based on the *in vivo* CO_2 titration curve and involves no jargon. It recognizes that the correction of non-respiratory acidosis is imprecise and that non-respiratory alkalosis must be avoided.

NON-RESPIRATORY ALKALOSIS (*Figure 44.9*)

Most of the causes of non-respiratory alkalosis are iatrogenic either by the administration of excessive alkali, sodium bicarbonate, or oral antacids, or by failing to recognize hypokalaemia due to diuretic therapy. Acid may be lost from the body either from the stomach by prolonged vomiting, or from the kidney by hypokalaemia with its paradoxical combination of acid urine and alkaline ECF. Severe non-respiratory alkalosis (pH > 7.55) has a high mortality (Wilson *et al.*, 1972).

Biochemically, the *in vivo* CO_2 titration curve is shifted to the right. There is usually some respiratory compensation, although less than in a metabolic acidosis, so that the P_{CO_2} is elevated, which reduces CSF pH and leads to an increase in CSF $[HCO_3^-]$.

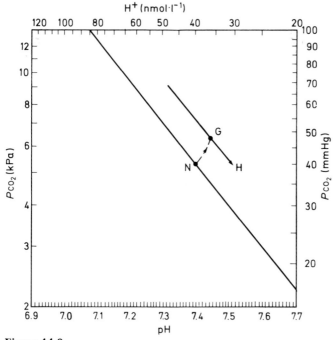

Figure 44.9
Acid—base changes during non-respiratory alkalosis. Respiratory compensation allows pH to move N --→ G. In the absence of respiratory compensation pH would be H

Correction of a non-respiratory alkalosis is achieved, predominantly, by treating the cause. In particular, potassium loss should be replaced. One-sixth molar NH_4Cl has been used as a source of acid as two molecules NH_4Cl condense to form one molecule urea and two molecules HC1. It is contraindicated in hypokalaemic patients as further K^+ loss is induced. The place of intravenous acid, as 0.3 molar HCl given by a central venous catheter, is not widely accepted. If correction is contemplated, the same criteria as those suggested for the treatment of a non-respiratory acidosis should be used. Correction should be slow and with frequent acid—base monitoring. Acid dosage should be based upon the degree of shift of the *in vivo* CO_2 titration curve.

Compensatory changes

It has been shown that primary acid—base disturbances induce secondary or compensatory changes so that the deviation of the pH from normal is limited. Secondary respiratory changes are invoked more rapidly than secondary metabolic changes. Flenley (1971) and Goldberg *et al.* (1973) have plotted the 95% confidence limits of the observed relationship between pH and $P\text{CO}_2$ in a variety of acute and chronic respiratory and metabolic acid—base disorders. This can be reconstructed on a pH/log $P\text{CO}_2$ diagram (*Figure 44.10*). Such an 'acid—base map' may be useful in providing the diagnosis from a set of acid—base results. For example,

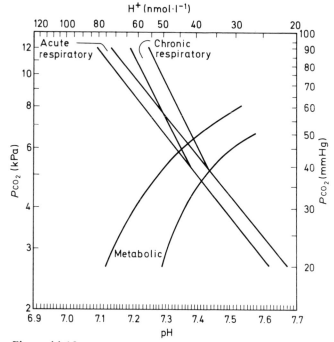

Figure 44.10
95% confidence limits of acute and chronic acid—base disturbances

Patient A, an elderly chronic bronchitis patient, before operation was found to have a pH of 7.30 and $PaCO_2$ of 8 kPa (60 mmHg). These results are compatible with a chronic respiratory acidosis.

Other authors dispute the value of such 'compensation maps' preferring to relate the pH and PCO_2 to the normal *in vivo* titration curve (*Figure 44.3*) and the patient's medical history and clinical situation.

An acid–base set (B) pH 7.2 and $PaCO_2$ 10.67 kPa (80 mmHg) could represent, using the acid–base compensation map, either a mild metabolic alkalosis and a severe acute respiratory acidosis or a mild metabolic acidosis in a patient with a severe chronic respiratory acidosis. The clinical history of such a patient is essential in reaching a correct diagnosis.

THE EFFECTS OF ACID–BASE DISTURBANCES
(see also Chapters 22 and 23)

Circulation

The effect of acid–base alteration on the cardiovascular system is difficult to elucidate. This difficulty is partly due to the attempt to separate changes of PCO_2 from changes of pH and partly from the difficulty of separating the effect of CO_2 alone from the sympathoadrenal stimulation which occurs during hypercapnia. In general, if PCO_2 is maintained constant, an increase or a decrease in pH causes depression of myocardial contractility and a fall in stroke volume and cardiac output associated with a decrease in peripheral vascular resistance. In addition, the responsiveness of the heart to catecholamines is diminished in a metabolic acidosis.

Hypercapnia produces increased stroke volume and cardiac output, by increasing sympathetic activity. The effect on the peripheral vasculature depends on the degree of sympathetic innervation. Richly innervated organs (e.g. the kidney) respond to hypercapnia by vasoconstriction, whereas poorly innervated organs (e.g. cerebral cortex) respond by vasodilatation. During hypocapnia there is generalized vasoconstriction independent of sympathetic innervation.

Respiration

Changes in acid–base status alter respiration and oxygen delivery by effects on minute ventilation and on the oxygen dissociation curve.

Hypercapnia increases ventilation by stimulating central and peripheral chemoreceptors to a maximum at 11–12 kPa (80–90 mmHg) (Sykes, McNicoll and Campbell, 1976). Above that, ventilation decreases. Carbon dioxide stimulates the respiratory centre by decreasing the pH of the ECF perfusing the central chemoreceptors on the ventrolateral surface of the medulla. This takes place slowly, over several minutes. Carbon dioxide and pH produce a more rapid effect, within seconds, on the peripheral chemoreceptors of the aortic and carotid bodies. Respiratory stimulation by

CO_2 in normal man varies widely in different individuals (0.07—1.08 $l \cdot min^{-1} \cdot kPa^{-1}$; 0.5—5 $l \cdot min^{-1} \cdot mmHg^{-1}$), but in the same individual the CO_2 response curve is similar at different times. The curve is shifted to the left by metabolic acidosis and to the right by metabolic alkalosis.

Both CO_2 and pH alter the position of the oxygen dissociation curve. An increase in CO_2 or a decrease in pH shift the curve to the right causing an increased P_{50} (P_{50} is the oxygen partial pressure of blood when haemoglobin is 50% saturated, normal value 3.5 kPa, 26.6 mmHg). Hypocapnia and alkalaemia cause a shift to the left. The P_{50} is increased by about 0.3 kPa (2 mmHg) by a reduction in pH of 0.1 units (10 $nmol \cdot l^{-1}$) (Bohr effect). When the pH is reduced by CO_2 the shift is greater, indicating a specific effect of CO_2. The right shift produced by a decrease in pH is partially antagonized by the decrease in 2,3-diphosphoglycerate (2,3-DPG) induced by a decrease in intracellular pH.

Tissue oxygen delivery is the product of cardiac output and arterial oxygen content (C.O. $\times$ Hb $\times$ SO_2% and dissolved oxygen). A metabolic acidosis decreases cardiac output which is partly compensated by the right shift of the O_2 dissociation curve, whereas a metabolic alkalosis reduces O_2 delivery by decreasing cardiac output and shifting the dissociation curve to the left. Consequently, correction of a metabolic acidosis should err towards under- and not overcorrection.

Nervous system

The effect of CO_2 on cerebral perfusion has been described. Increasing pain thresholds during hyperventilation are probably the result of this. Cerebral metabolic activity, in *in vitro* brain slices, is maximal at a pH of 7. Carbon dioxide has little direct effect on cerebral metabolism.

The tetany observed in alkalotic states results from decreased calcium ionization.

Enzymic activity

Each enzyme has its optimal pH. Cellular enzymic integrity depends upon the balance of the activity of different enzymes. If the pH varies beyond normal limits, enzymic chaos results as the activity of some enzymes is enhanced whilst that of others is reduced.

Pharmacology

Most drugs are weak acids or bases existing partly in the ionized and partly in the un-ionized state. The un-ionized form is lipid soluble and can readily diffuse across cell membranes. This is demonstrated by gastric drug absorption. Weak acids (e.g. salicylates) are mainly un-ionized at gastric pH and are more readily absorbed than weak bases (e.g. ephedrine).

Alkalinization of the gastric pH will enhance the absorption of quinidine and delay the absorption of salicylates. This pH alteration of drug absorption is made use of in the deliberate alkalinization of the urine to increase the renal excretion of weak acids, salicylates and phenobarbitone, by reducing the amount of reabsorbable un-ionized drug.

Changes in ionization also affect the protein binding of drugs and, consequently, alter the amount of active, unbound drug. Muscle relaxant activity may be altered by acid–base changes partly by an alteration in protein binding and also, for *d*-tubocurarine, by increasing its activity in acidotic conditions by structural alteration.

INTRACELLULAR pH

Attempts have been made to measure intracellular pH (pH_i) either by inserting microelectrodes with tips smaller than 1 μm diameter into the cell or by calculations from the distribution of weak acids, such as 5,5-dimethyl-1,2,4-oxazolidine (DMO) administered systemically. Rough estimates can be made after the administration of indicator drugs or by examining the rates of pH-dependent intracellular reactions. All methods, currently available, are open to methodological criticism. In addition, it is unlikely that the cells of all parts of the organism, or indeed all parts of the same cell, are at the same pH.

Nevertheless, many studies show that during health the intracellular pH is roughly related to the extracellular pH (pH_e), but lower than it. When pH_e is 7.4, pH_i is usually less than 7.

During acid–base disturbances the $pH_i:pH_e$ ratio may alter. CO_2 is freely permeable across cell membranes so that respiratory changes are reflected by similar changes in pH_e and pH_i. Within three hours of the administration of CO_2, compensating intracellular changes tend to restore pH_i towards normal. Highly ionized substances, HCl and $NaHCO_3$, do not cross the cell membrane. Changes in their extracellular concentration have a negligible effect on pH_i.

Changes in the intra-:extracellular ratio of the electrolytes sodium and potassium do alter the ratio $pH_i:pH_e$. As the concentration of H^+ is one-thousandth to one-hundred-thousandth of the concentration of K^+, the changes are not the result of a one-to-one exchange across the cell membrane. Total replacement of intracellular H^+ by extracellular K^+ would produce no measurable change in K^+ concentrations. Nevertheless, in potassium deficiency the intracellular cation deficit is partly compensated by the movement of H^+ resulting in extracellular alkalosis and intracellular acidosis.

If the chemical potential exerted by Na^+ and K^+ is expressed as the log of the concentration gradient of Na^+ or K^+ inside and outside the cell there is a relationship between changes produced in Na^+ and K^+ and changes in the pH gradient across the cell membrane.

$$(\log \frac{[Na^+]_i}{[Na^+]_e} \quad \text{or} \quad \log \frac{[K^+]_i}{[K^+]_e})$$

For instance, as the relative intracellular concentration of Na^+ or K^+ increases, there is a relative increase in pH_i. These changes were produced by a variety of methods which included electrolyte administration or depletion, or the administration of acidifying or alkalinizing agents. The change in gradient for Na^+ is about five times that for K^+ (Waddell and Bates, 1969).

CEREBROSPINAL FLUID (CSF) pH

CSF pH is controlled within narrower limits than the rest of the ECF. Compared with arterial blood the CSF pH is lower (0.1 pH units), the P_{CO_2} is higher (1–1.3 kPa; 7–9 mmHg), but the bicarbonate concentration is similar. As elevation of the P_{CO_2} increases cerebral perfusion and thus eliminates more CO_2, the blood–brain P_{CO_2} difference is decreased in hypercapnia and increased in hypocapnia.

CSF acid–base status can be modified either by changes in its P_{CO_2} or HCO_3^- (the only CSF buffer). Changes in systemic acid–base status are not mirrored in the CSF because the blood–brain barrier is relatively impermeable to H^+ and HCO_3^- although CO_2 equilibration is rapid. Consequently, respiratory disturbances cause an equivalent CSF change whilst non-respiratory disturbances cause much smaller changes in CSF. In long-standing systemic disturbances, lasting several hours or days, the CSF pH remains almost unchanged in non-respiratory disturbances whilst the change in CSF pH in respiratory acidosis or alkalosis is corrected within hours. The compensation for respiratory change is accompanied by a change in CSF HCO_3^- so that CSF pH returns towards normal values. Although occasionally incomplete, such compensation for respiratory disturbances and the minimal response to non-respiratory changes result in the relative constancy of CSF pH. The parts played by active and/or passive mechanisms in the adjustment of CSF HCO_3^- are, so far, uncertain. Similarly, the role of the brain cells in generating HCO_3^- is unclear (Leusen, 1972).

LACTIC ACIDOSIS

Lactic acidosis is best defined as the combination of a pH of less than 7.25 and a blood lactate concentration of more than 5 mmol·l^{-1} (Alberti and Nattrass, 1977). Care must be taken to exclude other conditions, e.g. renal failure and ketoacidosis, where the elevation of lactic acid is not alone responsible for the acidosis.

Biochemistry

Lactic acid is formed from pyruvic acid which is the final product in the glycolytic chain (*Figure 44.11*). Glycolysis can continue in anaerobic

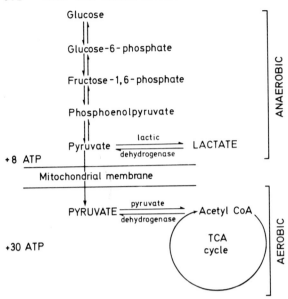

Figure 44.11
Pyruvate—lactate metabolism

conditions, but further metabolism requires its entry into the oxidative tricarboxylic acid cycle within the mitochondria. Accumulation of H^+ and pyruvate would inhibit glycolysis within seconds, but transformation to lactate allows energy production to continue for several minutes. Thus lactate accumulation occurs during anaerobic metabolism or by reduced pyruvate disposal, either by decreased gluconeogenesis in the liver or kidney or by the failure of pyruvate to enter the tricarboxylic acid (TCA) cycle. For the latter, as well as entry into the mitochondria, activation of pyruvate dehydrogenase is essential for its conversion to acetyl CoA. Hepatic utilization of lactate usually accounts for 1500 mmol per day and has the ability to rise to 3400 mmol per day.

Aetiology

Cohen and Woods (1976) have simplified the classification of lactic acidosis by defining two types: type A due to tissue hypoxia and anaerobic metabolism; type B due to other causes. This classification replaces the earlier concept of 'excess lactate' which has been shown to be a poor index of tissue hypoxia.

TYPE A LACTIC ACIDOSIS

The association of metabolic acidosis with circulatory collapse and hypoxia is well recognized. Impaired tissue perfusion may be the result of any form of shock and tissue oxygenation is further compromised by severe anaemia and hypoxaemia. Blood lactate concentration, although seldom measured, is closely correlated with mortality. There is a mortality of 73% in patients with blood lactate from 4.4 to 8.9 mmol·l^{-1}, but only 18% mortality with lactates of 1.3—4.4 mmol·l^{-1}.

Treatment entails removal of the cause and alkali therapy.

TYPE B LACTIC ACIDOSIS

There are many causes of type B lactic acidosis (*Table 44.5*) although biguanide therapy and agents used for parenteral nutrition have received recent attention.

TABLE 44.5. Aetiology of type B lactic acidosis

β_1	β_2	β_3
Common disorders	*Drugs and toxins*	*Inherited*
Diabetes mellitus	Biguanides: phenformin	Glycogen storage disease
Renal failure	metformin buformin	Fructose-1,6-diphosphate deficiency
Hepatic disease	Parenteral nutrition:	Leigh's syndrome
Infection	fructose sorbitol	Methylmalonic acidaemia
Leukaemia	xylitol ethanol	
	Salicylates	
	Methanol	

Biguanides

These drugs produce hypoglycaemia by

(1) reducing the alimentary absorption of glucose and amino acids;
(2) increasing glycolysis;
(3) decreasing hepatic gluconeogenesis.

Thus the lactic acidosis is inherent in the hypoglycaemic actions of (2) and (3). Usually blood lactate is less than 2 mmol·l^{-1}, but impaired renal excretion, hepatic dysfunction or cardiovascular disease may easily induce lactic acidosis.

Parenteral nutrition

Fructose, sorbitol and xylitol have been used as energy substances instead of glucose as they can be metabolized without insulin. This is of particular importance in the sick patient who may be insulin resistant. In addition, these agents are less irritant to veins than glucose. However, all result in the increased production of lactate (*Figure 44.12*). Thirty-five per cent of a fructose infusion is converted rapidly to lactate and pyruvate by the liver.

Ethyl alcohol infusion inhibits hepatic gluconeogenesis. In the presence of hepatic disease or when administered with fructose, sorbitol or a biguanide, lactic acidosis may result.

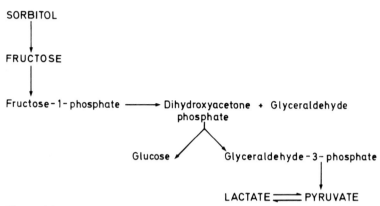

Figure 44.12
Metabolism of fructose and sorbitol

The treatment of type B lactic acidosis is difficult. If possible the cause should be removed. Large amounts of alkali are necessary due to the continuing lactate production. Attempts have been made to remove the lactate by dialysis or by stimulating pyruvate dehydrogenase to encourage conversion of lactate to pyruvate by the removal of the latter via the tricarboxylic acid cycle. Glucose and insulin seldom help as glycolysis is stimulated and gluconeogenesis inhibited. Experimental use of dichloro-acetate, a specific stimulator of pyruvate dehydrogenase, shows promise, but an intravenous preparation is not yet available for human use.

References

Alberti, K. G. M. and Nattrass, M. (1977). Lactic acidosis. *Lancet* ii, 25—29

Astrup, P., Jorgensen, K., Siggaard-Andersen, O. and Engel, K. (1960). The acid—base metabolism. A new approach. *Lancet* i, 1035—1039

Bates, R. G. (1964). *Determination of pH. Theory and Practice.* New York: Wiley

Cohen, R. D. and Woods, H. F. (1976). *Clinical and Biochemical Aspects of Lactic Acidosis.* Oxford: Blackwell

Cotev, S. and Severinghaus, J. W. (1969). Role of cerebrospinal fluid pH in management of respiratory problems. *Anesth. Analg. curr. Res.* 48, 42—47

Flenley, D. C. (1971). Another non-logarithmic acid—base diagram? *Lancet* i, 961—965

Freeman, J. and Nunn, J. F. (1963). Ventilation—perfusion relationships after haemorrhage. *Clin. Sci.* 24, 135—147

Goldberg, M., Green, S. B., Moss, M. L., Marbach, C. B. and Garfinkel, D. (1973). Computer-based instruction and diagnosis of acid—base disorders. *J. Am. med. Ass.* 223, 269—275

Hasselbalch, K. A. (1917). Die berechnung der wasserstoffzahl des blutes aus der freiend und gebunenen. Kohlensaure desselben und die sauer-stoffbindung des blutes als funktion des wasserstoffzahl. *Biochem. Z.* 78, 112—144

Henderson, L. J. (1908). The theory of neutrality regulation in the animal organism. *Am. J. Physiol.* 21, 427–450

Jorgensen, K. and Astrup, P. (1957). Standard bicarbonate, its clinical significance, and a new method for its determination. *Scand. J. clin. Lab. Invest.* 9, 122–132

Kappagoda, C. T., Linden, R. J. and Snow, H. M. (1970). An approach to the problems of acid–base balance. *Clin. Sci.* 39, 169–182

Leusen, I. (1972). Regulation of cerebrospinal fluid composition with reference to breathing. *Physiol. Rev.* 52, 1–56

Lewis, D. G. and Stoddart, J. C. (1973). Alternative measurements of the metabolic component of the acid–base status in acute clinical situations. *Clin. Sci.* 44, 297–300

Nunn, J. F. (1977). *Applied Respiratory Physiology,* 2nd edn. London and Boston: Butterworths

Pitts, R. F. (1974). *Physiology of the Kidney and Body Fluids,* 3rd edn. Chicago: Year Book Medical

Prys-Roberts, C., Kelman, G. R. and Nunn, J. F. (1966). Determination of the *in vivo* carbon dioxide titration curve of anaesthetised man. *Br. J. Anaesth.* 38, 500–509

Severinghaus, J. W. (1976). Acid–base balance nomogram — A Boston–Copenhagen detente. *Anesthesiology* 45, 539–541

Siggaard-Andersen, O. (1962). The pH–log PCO_2 blood acid–base nomogram revised. *Scand. J. clin. Lab. Invest.* 14, 598–604

Singer, R. B. and Hastings, A. B. (1948). An improved method for the estimation of disturbances of the acid–base balance of human blood. *Medicine, Baltimore* 27, 223–239

Sorensen, S. P. L. (1909). Enzymstudien: Uber die messung und die bedentung der wasser stuffiunen kaizentration bei ensymatischen prozessen. *Biochem. Z.* 21, 131–304

Sykes, M. K., McNicol, M. W. and Campbell, E. J. M. (1976). *Respiratory Failure,* 2nd edn. Oxford, London, Edinburgh, Melbourne: Blackwell

Waddell, W. J. and Bates, R. G. (1969). Intracellular pH. *Physiol. Rev.* 49, 285–329

Wilson, R. F., Gibson, D., Percinel, A. K., Ali, M. A., Baker, G., Le Blanc, L. P. and Lucas, C. (1972). Severe alkalosis in critically ill surgical patients. *Archs Surg., Chicago* 105, 197–203

45 Neurological and muscular disorders
J. A. Thornton

The incidence of medical disease in the population of surgical patients in the United Kingdom is of the order of 25–40% (Kyei-Mensah and Thornton, 1974). Cardiovascular and respiratory disease form by far the largest proportion of the total.

However, disease of the central nervous system and muscle, though representing a relatively small number of patients at risk, nevertheless, in many instances, present to the anaesthetist a considerable challenge to his basic knowledge and skills.

An understanding of the problems of the commoner neurological and muscular disorders in relation to anaesthetic management is clearly an important factor in the reduction of morbidity and mortality associated with these conditions.

AUTONOMIC FAILURE

Autonomic failure may arise from a localized lesion in the brain stem or spinal cord, or with diffuse lesions as in polyneuropathy (Johnson and Spalding, 1976). The widespread interruption of autonomic function may give rise to disturbances in the regulation of the blood pressure and the body temperature. The afferent pathways in the autonomic reflex may be affected in tabes dorsalis, diabetes mellitus and alcohol addiction. The brain stem may be involved in familial dysautonomia (Riley–Day syndrome), cerebrovascular disease, posterior fossa tumours, acute polyneuropathy, and by drugs. Involvement of efferent pathways in the spinal cord, the sympathetic chain and postganglionic nerves may also give rise to autonomic failure. Typical disturbances are trauma, transverse myelitis, syringomyelia, intramedullary tumours, and degeneration of the intermediolateral column (as part of a multiple system disease). Acute polyneuropathy, chronic polyneuropathy caused by diabetes mellitus, chronic alcoholism, tumours, renal failure, porphyria and drugs account for other causes of autonomic disturbance.

DIAGNOSIS OF AUTONOMIC DYSFUNCTION

Clinical examination may reveal disturbance of pupillary reflexes to illumination and shade, absent sinus arrhythmia, postural hypotension with absence of reflex tachycardia, and a dry skin. More specific tests can be used to test the response of the pupil to methacholine, hydroxy-amphetamine and adrenaline (Turner, 1975). The presence of an abnormal response to the Valsalva manoeuvre may be further confirmatory evidence. Many other tests have been employed and discussed in detail (Editorial, 1976).

Riley–Day syndrome

Riley *et al.* (1949) described a rare condition occurring in Jewish children which is probably transmitted as a simple autosomal recessive gene. This condition presents not only with widespread evidence of autonomic nervous system involvement including blood pressure, thermal liability, and sweating abnormalities, but also with evidence of other neurological involvement. The diagnosis is made on history, the presence of a smooth tongue with absent taste buds and filiform papillae, and postural hypotension. Preoperative residual chest infections, intraoperative cardiovascular instability, and postoperative vomiting and aspiration are the most frequent anaesthetic problems. Premedication with chlorpromazine and atropine and general anaesthesia with nitrous oxide, oxygen and controlled ventilation employing curare is advised (Meridy and Creighton, 1971). Inkster (1971) has used moderately heavy sedation with propranolol and atropine preoperatively, and nitrous oxide–oxygen–halothane and suxamethonium for anaesthesia.

Shy–Drager syndrome

In 1960 Shy and Drager described a condition which was characterized by orthostatic hypotension, Parkinsonism, urinary and bowel dysfunction, impaired libido and decreased sweating. The anaesthetic management of such a case has been discussed by Cohen (1971).

Diabetic autonomic neuropathy

Abnormality of cardiovascular innervation in diabetics has been recognized for some time (Ewing *et al.*, 1973; Wheeler and Watkins, 1973). The mortality associated with this condition is high (Ewing, Campbell and Clarke, 1976). Abnormal respiratory control in some diabetics has also been noted (Courteney-Evans, Benson and Hughes, 1971; Eisele *et al.*, 1971; Page and Watkins, 1978). Cardiorespiratory arrest appears to be a specific feature of diabetic autonomic neuropathy and may be particularly prone to occur in relation to general anaesthesia (Page and Watkins, 1978).

SPINAL CORD INJURIES

Following complete section of the spinal cord a clinical picture which can best be described as 'spinal shock' immediately develops. This clinical picture persists for one to two weeks and then passes into a phase of reflex hyperactivity. Immediately following spinal cord injury, loss of visceral and somatic sensation, and flaccid paralysis is found below the level of the lesion. Tendon reflexes, abdominal reflexes and plantar response are absent and there is retention of urine and faeces. A zone of hyperaesthesia is found above the level of the lesion. The appearance of the Babinski sign heralds development of the phase of reflex activity. If the lesion lies in the spinal cord, then flexor reflexes predominate, but if the lesion is above the pons, extensor reflexes predominate. Occasionally elicitation of the flexor reflexes is associated with evacuation of the bowel and bladder. The mass reflex can be initiated by cutaneous, proprioceptive, and visceral stimuli and results in autonomic and motor hyper-reflexia.

A transverse section of the cervical cord leaves the whole of the sympathetic outflow functionally separated from the brain stem and hypothalamus. Such loss of sympathetic integration leads to reflex autonomic activity below the site of the lesion. With a high thoracic lesion ventilation is maintained only by virtue of diaphragmatic activity and during the phase immediately following injury ventilation may have to be supported by artificial means. Long-term ventilatory support by stimulation of the diaphragm has been employed (Glenn *et al.*, 1976). Respiratory and renal infection account for the high morbidity associated with paraplegia, and in the long term, renal and adrenal amyloidosis may result. Electrolyte and metabolic disturbances may occur as a result of the frequent use of enemas. Anaemia is frequently associated with paraplegia. Thermal regulation is disturbed, the patients being essentially poikilothermic below the level of the lesion (Downey *et al.*, 1976). Wastage of muscle and skin lesions require enthusiastic management and physiotherapy. Some of these patients are hypovolaemic (Desmond and Laws, 1974) and attention should be paid to accurate control of blood loss and its replacement.

Of particular relevance to the anaesthetist is the autonomic hyper-reflexia. This condition does not develop if the lesion is below the level of the seventh thoracic segment. Commonly the condition is provoked by bladder distension and is associated with rises in blood pressure and a high incidence of cardiac irregularities. Reflex bradycardia in response to the rise in blood pressure is also frequently found. As the area of the body below the lesion is already devoid of sensation it is not always necessary to induce general anaesthesia and all that is required is control of the hypertension.

General anaesthesia in these patients is fraught with difficulties (Quimby, Williams and Greifenstein, 1973). If anaesthesia is too deep, a precipitous fall in blood pressure may occur. On the other hand too light anaesthesia is associated with hypertensive crises. Blood pressure invariably falls with induction of anaesthesia despite cautious administration of agents

(Desmond, 1970). However, when surgery commences the blood pressure tends to rise. A rise in blood pressure has been met by deepening anaesthesia and the use of halothane (Drinker and Helrich, 1963; Alderson and Thomas, 1975), spinal and epidural anaesthesia (Gilberti, Goldfein and Rovenstine, 1954; Rocco and Vandam, 1959), and sacral nerve block (Green, Grennell and Awad, 1974). Preoperative oral hexamethonium has been used to permit routine bladder and bowel care (Kurnick, 1956). However, general anaesthesia in patients so treated may lead to a catastrophic fall in blood pressure.

Pentolinium has been employed for the effective control of autonomic hyper-reflexia (Texter, Reece and Hranowsky, 1976; Basta, Niejadlik and Pallares, 1977), and the shorter acting trimetaphan (Arfonad) by Thorn-Alquist (1975) and Wedley (1976). Change in posture of the paraplegic patient under general anaesthesia may lead to cardiac arrest (Gode, 1970). Suxamethonium should be used with great caution in the patients (Stone, Beach and Hamelberg, 1970) as elevated levels of serum potassium are found after such severe injuries. Tobey (1970) and Tobey *et al.* (1972) suggest that suxamethonium should perhaps not be used after the first 24 hours following injury. The period of excessive sensitivity to suxamethonium has not been determined. It has been suggested that general anaesthesia with a small dose of thiopentone, nitrous oxide and oxygen, with *d*-tubocurarine, following premedication with promethazine, is suitable for patients undergoing bladder operations (Hassan, 1974). Reflex cardiac arrest sometimes occurs during tracheobronchial suction in these patients and atropinization with attention to oxygenation are advised (Frankel, Mathias and Spalding, 1975). IPPV in these patients may lead to a severe fall in cardiac output (Baker and Cowie, 1977).

GUILLAIN–BARRÉ SYNDROME

In this condition an acute polyneuritis gives rise to motor weakness or paralysis, abolition of tendon reflexes and sensory disturbances. There is usually an associated autonomic involvement with excessive or inadequate activity of the sympathetic and parasympathetic systems (Lichtenfeld, 1971). This may manifest itself as postural hypotension, bouts of uncontrolled hypertension, profuse sweating, changes in the ECG and arrhythmias. A personal experience of this condition is described by Henschel (1977).

The problem of anaesthesia in these patients has been discussed by Desmeules, Fournier and Sirois (1972) and Perel, Reches and Davidson (1977). It is suggested that barbiturates and phenothiazines are avoided since severe circulatory collapse can follow their administration. Changes of posture and reduction in blood volume are likely to cause hypotension. Intermittent positive pressure ventilation should be undertaken with great care as reflex venoconstriction is impaired (Elstein *et al.*, 1971).

MULTIPLE SCLEROSIS

Although multiple sclerosis is a relatively common neurological disorder there is scant reference in the literature to the effects of anaesthesia and surgery in these patients. It is well recognized that any form of stress may lead to a deterioration in the condition of these patients. Postoperative chest infection is particularly likely to occur in these patients. In certain cases autonomic dysfunction may be present and constitute a problem (see page 867). In view of the widespread muscle wasting it is probably advisable to avoid the use of suxamethonium. It would appear that there is no contraindication to the use of other anaesthetic agents (Baskett and Armstrong, 1970; Siemkowicz, 1976; Frost, 1977).

MOTOR NEURON DISEASE

This name is given to a condition of unknown aetiology, in which there is a progressive degeneration of the anterior horn cells, the motor muscles of the medulla, and the upper motor neurons of the spinal cord, brain stem and to some extent the central hemispheres. It is twice as common in males than females. Rarely occurring under the age of 20 years its greatest incidence is between 50 and 60 years. Three main groups are recognized: progressive bulbar palsy, progressive muscular atrophy and amyotrophic lateral sclerosis. Spasticity due to pyramidal tract involvement may be prominent, and all muscles may eventually develop atrophy, weakness and fasciculations secondary to neuronal degeneration. The sensory and autonomic systems are not affected (Jokelainen and Palo, 1976).

Some patients with amyotrophic lateral sclerosis show an increased sensitivity to non-depolarizing muscle relaxants (Mulder, Lambert and Eaton, 1959; Wise, 1963; Rowland, 1967; Rosenbaum, Neigh and Strobel, 1971). The use of depolarizing agents in this condition is inadvisable as hyperkalaemia and cardiac arrest may follow their administration.

EPILEPSY

The patient with a history of epilepsy poses particular problems for the anaesthetist. Before giving a general anaesthetic to such a patient the anaesthetist must ascertain what medication the patient is receiving and whether the condition is controlled. The frequency of attacks will give an indication as to the degree of control and to the timing of anaesthesia and surgery. The drugs themselves may influence the response to anaesthetic agents. Phenytoin, phenobarbitone and primidone would appear to be the best drugs available for the treatment of grand mal including temporal lobe epilepsy. Ethosuximide is particularly suitable for the management of petit mal. Recently sodium valproate (sodium salt of dipropylacetic acid) has been employed in the management of epilepsy.

Sodium valproate is a simple two-chain fatty acid, and it is suggested that it increases the cerebral concentration of the inhibitory transmitter γ-aminobutyric acid and that this may account for its therapeutic effect. Sodium valproate is completely absorbed orally and has a plasma half-life of 10—15 hours. It has, however, been demonstrated that the half-life is shorter when phenytoin is administered concurrently. It can also interact with phenobarbitone leading to a rise in plasma phenobarbitone levels. Although the drug has not yet been fully evaluated, in view of its relatively few side-effects, it should be tried if existing drug therapy is ineffective.

The patient with an epileptiform diathesis is vulnerable to certain agents employed for the induction and maintenance of general anaesthesia. Methohexitone is well recognized for its tendency to provoke convulsions in susceptible individuals (Galley, 1956; Rose, Bourne and Goldman, 1969; Thornton, 1970), and for this reason its use is contraindicated in patients with a history of epilepsy. The increased incidence of grand mal with this drug is attributed to the methylation at position 3 of this oxybarbiturate. It had been thought that propanidid did not cause convulsions but Baron (1974) has reported three patients who exhibited typical epileptiform seizures when using this agent. Convulsions have also been reported following the administration of Althesin (Uppington, 1973). These reports limit the choice of intravenous induction agent in such patients to thiopentone. Ketamine is known to cause CNS excitation and phencylidine (a closely related compound) has been known to cause convulsions (Winters *et al.*, 1967). However, Fisher (1974) and Coppel (1975) have successfully used ketamine in the treatment of convulsions, whereas Lees and MacNamara (1977) have reported convulsions in a patient with a history of epilepsy when ketamine was administered. In view of the fact that enflurane has been shown to provoke an epileptiform pattern on EEG its use should be avoided in patients with a history of epilepsy.

Prolonged therapy with phenobarbitone leads to liver microsomal enzyme induction and sudden withdrawal of such therapy in patients receiving phenytoin, digoxin, griseofulvin and certain anticoagulants may create problems. Increased biodegradation of methoxyflurane, halothane and fluroxene has also been reported in subjects pretreated with phenobarbitone (see Chapter 7). The administration of chlordiazepoxide or diazepam has also been found to increase the blood levels of phenytoin, and thereby upset the carefully balanced control. Increased sensitivity to d-tubocurarine has been reported in patients receiving phenytoin therapy (Harrah, Way and Katzung, 1970).

Management of status epilepticus

The mortality rate, which was 30—50% at the beginning of the century, has been dramatically reduced to around 3—21% (Oxbury and Whitty, 1971) by the use of anticonvulsant drugs and modern techniques of cardiorespiratory support. When treating a patient in status epilepticus, immediate steps must be taken to prevent him from causing harm to himself and to ensure an adequate airway and pulmonary ventilation. Diazepam would appear to be the drug of choice and 10 mg should be injected intravenously and the fits controlled by an intravenous infusion of 1 mg·min^{-1} of diazepam in a solution of 100 mg in 1 litre of isotonic sodium chloride. Recently clonazepam (Rivotril) has been introduced and the results of its use appear promising. Adults should be given a slow injection of 1 mg dissolved in 1 ml water: 1 mg should be given over a period of 30 seconds and repeated if necessary, control being maintained by an infusion of 3 mg in 50 ml sodium chloride (B.P.) or in 5 or 10% dextrose (B.P.).

The intramuscular administration of paraldehyde (10 ml) has also been employed, though the incidence of sterile abscess associated with this route of administration is high. Alternatively, phenytoin (200 mg in 5 ml solvent) may be infused at a rate of 50 mg per minute. Initially 150–250 mg should be given but a further 100–150 mg may be given after 30 minutes. The dosage is best controlled with continuous EEG monitoring. Subcutaneous or perivascular deposition must be carefully avoided because of the highly alkaline nature of the preparation. Phenytoin should not be added to intravenous crystalloids as precipitation is likely to occur. Chlormethiazole (Heminevrin) can be administered intravenously in a 0.8% solution at a rate of 60–100 drops per minute. A faster rate of infusion may be accompanied by hypotension; 100–500 ml may be given for an adult and 250 ml for a child. Occasionally, convulsions cannot be controlled with these agents and it may be necessary to use a thiopentone drip or even administer curare. In this latter instance respiratory control with IPPV will be required. Whatever agent is employed, it is essential to monitor the cardiovascular and respiratory state carefully and continuously, and to provide supportive measures when needed.

PARKINSON'S DISEASE (Bevan, Monks and Calne, 1973)

The characteristic clinical picture is that of a wide-eyed, unblinking patient with staring expression. The facial muscles are smoothed out and immobile, giving rise to the drooling of saliva. Muscular rigidity is frequently present and is associated with 'cog-wheel' rigidity. The patients often walk with a slow, short, shuffling gait and an involuntary tremor is usually present.

The idiopathic form tends to occur in the middle-aged and elderly but drugs such as the phenothiazines, reserpine tranquillizers and butyrophenones can produce a similar clinical picture. The idiopathic condition is thought to be due to dopamine deficiency in the basal ganglia. In the past atropine-like drugs and antihistamines have been employed to reduce the symptoms. Recently levodopa (which crosses the blood–brain interface and is converted to dopamine in the brain) has been shown to be beneficial. Levodopa has a short half-life in the body and is usually administered in a daily dose of 2–8 g in divided doses.

Adverse reactions encountered in relation to general anaesthesia are arrhythmias, and lability of the blood pressure. To reduce these complications it is advised that levodopa therapy is discontinued the night prior to operation and restarted as soon as possible postoperatively. In view of the high levels of circulating catecholamines associated with this therapy, halothane is probably best avoided and arrhythmias treated with β-adrenergic blocking agents or intravenous lignocaine.

HUNTINGTON'S CHOREA (Davies, 1966; Gualandi and Bonfanti, 1968; Farina and Rauscher, 1977)

This hereditary disorder of the central nervous system gives rise to progressive dysarthria ataxia, choreiform movements and dementia.

Although undue sensitivity to thiopentone non-depolarizing and depolarizing agents has been suggested by Davies (1966) and Gualandi and Bonfanti (1968), it would appear that the cautious administration of thiopentone and pancuronium is safe (Farina and Rauscher, 1977).

NEUROFIBROMATOSIS (Von Recklinghausen's Disease)

This condition is a rare inherited disorder characterized by multiple tumours and spots of increased skin pigmentation. As many organs are often involved in the disease process problems may be encountered which may complicate anaesthesia. Occasionally, the patients are mentally retarded. Kyphoscoliosis, honeycomb lung cysts, laryngeal stenosis and hydrocephalus may impair respiratory function. The lesions may undergo sarcomatous change and may produce bone cysts. Pulsating exophthalmos, glaucoma, spinal nerve compression, spina bifida, hypospadias and elephantiasis have been described with this condition. Renal artery stenosis has been found in a number of cases and phaeochromocytoma occurs in about 13% of patients with neurofibromatosis. Neurofibromatosis has also been found in between 10 and 25% of patients with phaeochromocytoma (Krishna, 1975). An abnormal response to neuromuscular blocking agents has also been demonstrated (Manser, 1970; Magbagbeola, 1970; Fisher, 1975; Yamashita and Matsuki, 1975). There appears to be increased sensitivity to both the non-depolarizing and depolarizing agents.

THE MYOPATHIES*

The myopathies which are genetically determined, are thought to represent inborn errors of muscle metabolism. Their onset usually occurs in childhood or early adult life (Gardner-Medwin, 1977).

* Myasthenia gravis is considered in Chapter 43.

Wasting is usually symmetrical with slow progression downhill. Some muscle fibres may be replaced by fat, giving the muscle an unduly bulky appearance (pseudohypertrophy). Kyphoscoliosis may be found. Inter-current infection, particularly of the respiratory tract, is often present. Heart muscle is also affected and clinical signs of cardiac movement such as tachycardia are sometimes found. Atrophy of the smooth muscle of the gastrointestinal tract occurs with dilation of the stomach, regurgitation and accumulation of pharyngeal secretions increasing the hazard of inhalation. Several syndromes are recognized:

(1) pseudohypertrophic muscular dystrophy (Duchenne, Erb);
(2) facioscapulohumeral dystrophy (Landouzy–Dejerine);
(3) arm and shoulder (Erb);
(4) distal myopathy (Gower).

Mild preanaesthetic sedation is advised, avoiding the use of atropine. There appears to be no contraindication to the administration of small carefully controlled doses of thiopentone (McClelland, 1960; Kaufman, 1960; Cobham and Davis, 1964). Myocardial depressants are best avoided. The patient's response to small doses of non-depolarizing neuromuscular blocking agents should be assessed. Although suxamethonium has been given to these cases (Wislicki, 1962), its use is best avoided as cardiac arrest may be induced (Genever, 1971).

THE MYOTONIC SYNDROME (Desnoyers, 1969; Coccagna *et al.*, 1975; Hook, Anderson and Noto, 1975; Suppan, 1975; Meyers and Barash, 1976)

Myotonia dystrophica (dystrophia myotonica) – Steinart's disease

This hereditary disease usually has an onset when the patient is in his early thirties. Muscular weakness may make itself apparent by difficulty in swallowing, nasal voice and weakness of the hands. Slowness is added to the weakness and stiffness of muscles develops. The latter is particularly noticeable as difficulty in releasing the grip after handshake. Other asso-ciative features are wasting of the sternomastoids and muscles of the face and hands. Sustained contraction of muscles may occur with percussion. Baldness, cataracts, testicular atrophy, dementia, diabetes mellitus, pituitary dysfunction, cardiac myopathy and conduction defects also may be found. A continuous infusion of Althesin has been employed for general anaesthesia in these cases (Muller and Suppan, 1977).

Myotonia congenita – Thomsen's disease

This condition manifests itself at birth or in early childhood. Muscle involvement is widespread with obvious muscular hypertrophy. Involve-ment of other systems is unusual.

Paramyotonia

This is a rare condition, the characteristic feature being the development of myotonia on exposure to cold.

Anaesthetic problems of the myotonic syndrome

As the myotonic syndrome tends to be a multisystem disease, complications may arise in relation to the administration of a general anaesthetic. The cardiomyopathy and conduction defects may precipitate a cardiac crisis in the presence of known myocardial depressants (thiopentone, halothane, etc.).

A generalized myotonia following the administration of suxamethonium has been reported (Paterson, 1962). Muscular damage may also predispose to high potassium levels particularly when suxamethonium is given. For these reasons suxamethonium should be avoided. It has been suggested that these patients may have an increased sensitivity to thiopentone (Dundee, 1952; Bourke and Zuck, 1957) though thiopentone has been administered with apparent impunity (Kaufman, 1960). Although it has been postulated that thiopentone may have a peripheral action on the diseased muscle (Dundee, 1952), contraindications to its use would appear to be relative rather than absolute and depend upon respiratory and cardiovascular reserve (Gillam, Heat and Kaufman, 1964; Dalal *et al.,* 1972). There would appear to be no contraindications to the use of non-depolarizing neuromuscular blocking agents though increased sensitivity may be present. Small doses should be used initially. Many of these patients receive steroid therapy and supplementation for anaesthesia and surgery may be necessary. Postoperative ventilatory support may be required (Ravin, Newmark and Saviello, 1975).

DYSTONIA MUSCULORUM DEFORMANS (Davis and Davis, 1975)

This is a rare inherited disease of the central nervous system characterized by involuntary movements and torsion spasms which may give rise to opisthotonos and hyperextension of the neck. Neither depolarizing nor non-depolarizing muscle relaxants are contraindicated in this condition. However, relaxation for intubation can be achieved by the use of inhalational agents alone.

FAMILIAL PERIODIC PARALYSIS

Transmission of this condition, which occurs predominantly in males of all races, it thought to be by an autosomal dominant trait. This rare disease is associated with hyper- and hypokalaemia and occasionally with normal levels of serum potassium, and intermittent attacks of muscle weakness or paralysis. The skeletal muscles are usually affected and the bulbar muscles spared. Cardiac arrhythmias may occur with the paralysis and abnormalities of adrenal and thyroid function may be present. Attacks may be precipitated by high carbohydrate meals, emotional excitement, severe muscular exertion, infectious disease, cold, menstruation, accidental or surgical trauma. Close attention should be paid towards minimizing stress and anxiety, maintaining a normal serum potassium and avoiding a carbohydrate load (Siler and Discavage, 1975). Thiopentone and muscle relaxants should be used with caution (Bashford, 1977; Horton, 1977). It has been suggested that the inhalation of salbutamol is of value in alleviating paralytic attacks associated with hyperkalaemia (Wang and Clausen, 1976). Facilities for intubation and respiratory assistance must be available in the postoperative period as episodes of paralysis may occur for several hours after surgery.

MALIGNANT HYPERPYREXIA (HYPERTHERMIA) – MH

Attention was first drawn to this condition by Denborough and Lovell in 1960. Ten out of 38 relatives of a patient who nearly died of hyperpyrexia during general anaesthesia with nitrous oxide, oxygen and halothane were subsequently found to have died when receiving anaesthesia. All of these patients had received either diethyl ether or ethyl chloride and these administrations were associated with sudden hyperpyrexia and convulsions. It was suggested that the patients had inherited a dominant gene that carried the susceptibility to this condition. Spinal anaesthesia subsequently administered to a member of the family who was known to be susceptible to general anaesthesia had no adverse effect (Denborough *et al.*, 1962).

Before 1960 anaesthetists had recognized that certain pyrexial patients, particularly young toxic and dehydrated children, had a tendency to develop convulsions during general anaesthesia. These convulsions, which carried a high mortality, were often associated with the administration of diethyl ether, often in humid and hot environments. However, the condition described by Denborough and Lovell would appear to be unrelated, and associated with a sudden increase of calcium ions in the myoplasm of an affected individual when exposed to the causative agent (Kalow *et al.*, 1970).

Malignant hyperthermia still carries a high mortality despite an increasing understanding of the problem involved. Two predisposing myopathies have been recognized. One, dominantly inherited, is impossible to distinguish clinically and is the most common. The other is a rare myopathy which is found in young boys who are small in stature for their age, have undescended testicles, lumbar lordosis, thoracic kyphosis, pectus carinatum, webbing of the neck and winging of the scapulae.

Diagnosis

Whittaker, Spencer and Searle (1977) have drawn attention to the apparently common association of cholinesterase variants in families of patients who have suffered malignant hyperthermia. A family history of problems associated with general anaesthesia should alert the anaesthetist to the possibility of susceptibility to malignant hyperthermia. Such susceptibility can only be confirmed by the exposure of a muscle biopsy to the agents likely to be used in the general anaesthetic technique. Muscle of patients susceptible to malignant hyperthermia contracts on exposure to the causative agent. Estimation of plasma creatine phosphokinase (CPK) is a much less reliable index of suspicion, normal levels of CPK (60 μg·l^{-1}) having been found in patients who have recovered from malignant hyperpyrexia (Ellis *et al.*, 1976).

Volatile inhalational agents, depolarizing muscle relaxants, lignocaine and possibly ketamine (Lees and MacNamara, 1977) are contraindicated in subjects susceptible to malignant hyperpyrexia. Susceptibility to suxamethonium may be sometimes associated with rigidity, and in some instances relaxation has not occurred. Agents which would appear safe to administer are thiopentone, Althesin, fentanyl, droperidol, diazepam, procaine hydrochloride, pancuronium and methylprednisolone. Doubt currently exists about the use of atropine, phenothiazines and nitrous oxide (Cain and Ellis, 1977). Work in susceptible animals also suggests that α-adrenergic agonists should be avoided (Hall, Lucke and Lister, 1977).

Treatment

It would appear that the most reliable way at the moment to detect the possible development of malignant hyperpyrexia is to monitor the patient's temperature. An abrupt rise in temperature should prompt the anaesthetist to terminate general anaesthesia immediately. Cooling should be instituted and the cardiovascular and respiratory systems supported.

Although procaine, procainamide, hydrocortisone and dexamethasone have been administered to some patients who have recovered from this condition, doubt exists as to the real value of such drugs. Large doses of procaine will inhibit halothane contracture of muscle *in vitro* but such large doses *in vivo* may produce cardiovascular collapse.

Dantrolene sodium, a skeletal muscle relaxant, administered orally, has been used successfully to prevent malignant hyperpyrexia in susceptible swine (Harrison, 1977). Austin and Denborough (1977) have demonstrated that dantrolene sodium was the most effective drug available in reversing and inhibiting drug-induced muscle contracture *in vivo*. It is thought to act by lowering the raised myoplasmic concentrations of calcium. Because of difficulties in producing a water-soluble preparation a readily injectable form has not been available fully for use in humans.

References

Alderson, J. D. and Thomas, D. G. (1975). The use of halothane anaesthesia to control autonomic hyperreflexia during trans-urethral surgery in spinal cord injury patients. *Paraplegia* 131, 183−188

Austin, K. L. and Denborough, M. A. (1977). Drug treatment of malignant hyperpyrexia. *Anaesth. Intens. Care* 5, 207−213

Baker, A. B. and Cowie, R. W. (1977). Effects of varying inspiratory flow waveform and time in intermittent positive pressure ventilation. III Blockade of the autonomic nervous system. *Br. J. Anaesth.* 49, 1235−1237

Baron, D. W. (1974). Propanidid in epilepsy. *Anaesthesia* 291, 445−447

Bashford, A. V. (1977). Anaesthesia in familial hypokalaemic periodic paralysis. *Anaesth. Intens. Care* 5, 74−75

Baskett, P. J. F. and Armstrong, R. (1970). Anaesthetic problems in multiple sclerosis. *Anaesthesia* 25, 397−401

Basta, J. W., Niejadlik, J. and Pallares, V. (1977). Automatic hyperreflexia: intraoperative control with pentolinium tartrate. *Br. J. Anaesth.* 49, 1087−1091

Bevan, D. R., Monks, P. S. and Calne, D. B. (1973). Cardiovascular reactions to anaesthesia during treatment with levodopa. *Anaesthesia* 28, 29−31

Bourke, T. and Zuck, D. (1957). Thiopentone in dystrophia myotonica. *Br. J. Anaesth.* 29, 35−38

Cain, P. A. and Ellis, F. R. (1977). Anaesthesia for patients susceptible to malignant hyperpyrexia. A study of pancuronium and methylprednisolone. *Br. J. Anaesth.* 49, 941−944

Cobham, I. G. and Davis, H. S. (1964). Anesthesia for muscular dystrophy patients. *Anesth. Analg. curr. Res.* 43, 22−29

Coccagna, G., Mantovani, M., Parchi, C., Mironi, F. and Lugaresi, E. (1975). Alveolar hypoventilation and hypersomnia in myotonic dystrophy. *J. Neurol. Neurosurg. Psychiat.* 38, 977−984

Cohen, C. A. (1971). Anesthesia management of a patient with Shy−Drager syndrome. *Anesthesiology* 35, 95−97

Coppel, D. L. (1975). Ketamine hydrochloride and convulsions. *Surv. Anesth.* 191, 554

Courtenay-Evans, R. J., Benson, M. K. and Hughes, D. T. D. (1971). Abnormal chemoreceptor response to hypoxia in patients with tabes dorsalis. *Br. med. J.* 1, 530−531

Dalal, F. Y., Bennett, E. J., Raj, P. P. and Lee, D. G. (1972). Dystrophia myotonica: a multisystem disease. *Can. Anaesth. Soc. J.* 19, 436−444

Davies, D. D. (1966). Abnormal response to anaesthesia in a case of Huntington's chorea. *Br. J. Anaesth.* 38, 490−491

Davis, N. L. and Davis, R. (1975). Anesthetic management of a patient with dystonia musculorum. *Anesthesiology* 42, 630−631

Denborough, M. A. and Lovell, R. R. H. (1960). Anaesthetic deaths in a family. *Lancet* ii, 45

Denborough, M. A., Forster, J. F. A., Lovell, R. R. H., Maplestone, P. A. and Villers, J. D. (1962). Anaesthetic deaths in a family. *Br. J. Anaesth.* 34, 395−396

Desmeules, H., Fournier, L. and Sirois, G. H. (1972). Le syndrome de Guillain−Barré: le role de l'anaesthetiste dans le traitment des complications cardiovasculaires et respiratoires. *Can. Anaesth. Soc. J.* 19, 290−298

Desmond, J. (1970). Paraplegia: Problems confronting the anaesthesiologist. *Can. Anaesth. Soc. J.* 17, 435−451

Desmond, J. W. and Laws, A. K. (1974). Blood volume and capacitance vessel compliance in the quadriplegic patient. *Can. Anaesth. Soc. J.* 21, 421−426

Desnoyers, Y. (1969). A propos de la dystrophica myotonique. *Can. Anaesth. Soc. J.* 16, 372−384

Downey, J. A., Huckaba, C. E., Kelley, P. S., Tam, H. S., Darling, R. C. and Chen, H. Y. (1976). Sweating responses to central and peripheral heating in spinal man. *J. appl. Physiol.* 40, 701−706

Drinker, A. S. and Helrich, M. (1963). Halothane anesthesia in the paraplegic patient. *Anesthesiology* 24, 399−400

Dundee, J. W. (1952). Thiopentone in dystrophia myotonia. *Anesth. Analg. curr. Res.* 31, 257−262

Editorial. (1976). The diagnosis of autonomic dysfunction. *Lancet* i, 1115−1116

Eisele, J. H., Cross, C. E., Rausch, D. C., Kurpershoek, C. J. and Zelis, R. F. (1971). Abnormal respiratory control in acquired dysautonomia. *New Engl. J. Med.* 285, 366−368

Ellis, F. R., Clarke, I. M. C., Modgill, E. M., Currie, S. and Harrison, D. G. F. (1976). Serum creatine phosphokinase and malignant hyperpyrexia. *Br. med. J.* 1, 584

Elstein, M., Legg, N. J., Murphy, M., Park, D. M. and Sutcliffe, M. M. L. (1971). Guillain−Barré syndrome in pregnancy: Respiratory paralysis by a fatal tracheo-innominate fistula. *Anaesthesia* 26, 216−224

Ewing, D. J., Campbell, I. W. and Clarke, B. F. (1976). Mortality in diabetic autonomic neuropathy. *Lancet* i, 601−603

Ewing, D. J., Campbell, I. W., Burt, A. A. and Clarke, B. F. (1973). Vascular reflexes in diabetic autonomic neuropathy. *Lancet* ii, 1354−1356

Farina, J. and Rauscher, L. A. (1977). Anaesthesia and Huntington's chorea. *Br. J. Anaesth.* 49, 1167−1168

Fisher, M. McD. (1974). Use of ketamine hydrochloride in the treatment of convulsions. *Anaesth. Intens. Care* 21, 266−268

Fisher, M. McD. (1975). Anaesthetic difficulties in neurofibromatosis. *Anaesthesia* 30, 648–650

Frankel, H. L., Mathias, C. J. and Spalding, J. M. K. (1975). Mechanisms of reflex cardiac arrest in tetraplegic patients. *Lancet* ii, 1183–1185

Frost, P. M. (1977). Anaesthesia and multiple sclerosis. *Anaesthesia* 32, 392

Galley, A. H. (1956). Unforeseen complications during dental anaesthesia. Fits and faints. *Proc. R. Soc. Med.* 59, 734–738

Gardner-Medwin, D. (1977). Children with genetic muscular disorders. *Br. J. hosp. Med.* 17, 314–340

Genever, E. E. (1971). Suxamethonium-induced cardiac arrest in unsuspected pseudohypertrophic muscular dystrophy. *Br. J. Anaesth.* 43, 984–985

Gilberti, B. J., Goldfein, J. and Rovenstine, E. A. (1954). Hypertension during anesthesia in patients with spinal cord injuries. *Anesthesiology* 15, 273–279

Gillam, P. M. S., Heat, P. J. D. and Kaufman, L. (1964). Respiration in dystrophia myotonica. *Thorax* 19, 112–120

Glenn, W. W. L., Jolcomb, W. G., Shaw, R. K., Hogan, J. F. and Holschuh, K. R. (1976). Long-term ventilatory support by diaphragm pacing in quadriplegia. *Ann. Surg.* 183, 566–577

Gode, G. R. (1970). Paraplegia and cardiac arrest: case reports. *Can. Anaesth. Soc. J.* 17, 452–455

Green, J. F., Grennell, H. J. and Awad, S. A. (1974). Selective sacral nerve blocks in the management of 'uninhibited neurogenic bladder'. *Can. Anaesth. Soc. J.* 21, 417–420

Gualandi, W. and Bonfanti, G. (1968). A case of prolonged apnoea in Huntington's chorea. *Acta anaesth., Padova* 19 (Suppl. 6), 235

Hall, G. M., Lucke, J. N. and Lister, D. (1977). Porcine malignant hyperthermia V. Fatal hyperthermia in the pie train pig associated with the infusion of α-adrenergic agonists. *Br. J. Anaesth.* 49, 855–863

Harrah, M. D., Way, W. Z. and Katzung, B. G. (1970). The interaction of *d*-tubocurarine with anti-arrhythmic drugs. *Anesthesiology* 33, 406–410

Harrison, G. G. (1977). The prophylaxis of malignant hyperthermia by oral dantrolene sodium in swine. *Br. J. Anaesth.* 49, 315–317

Hassan, H. G. (1974). Anaesthesia in paraplegic patients. *Anaesthesia* 29, 629–630

Henschel, E. O. (1977). The Guillain–Barré syndrome. A personal experience. *Anesthesiology* 47, 228–231

Hook, R., Anderson, E. F. and Noto, P. (1975). Anesthetic management of a parturient with myotonia atrophica. *Anesthesiology* 43, 689–692

Horton, B. (1977). Anesthetic experiences in a family with hypokalemic familial periodic paralysis. *Anesthesiology* 47, 308–310

Inkster, J. S. (1971). Anaesthesia for a patient suffering from familial dysautonomia (Riley–Day syndrome). *Br. J. Anaesth.* 43, 509–512

Johnson, R. H. and Spalding, J. M. K. (1976). Widespread autonomic failure. *Br. J. hosp. Med.* 15, 266–274

Jokelainen, M. and Palo, J. (1976). Amyotrophic lateral sclerosis and the autonomic nervous system. *Lancet* i, 1246

Kalow, N., Britt, B. A., Terreau, M. E. and Haist, C. (1970). Metabolic error of muscle metabolism after recovery from malignant hyperthermia. *Lancet* ii, 895–898

Kaufman, L. (1960). Anaesthesia in dystrophia myotonica. *Proc. R. Soc. Med.* 53, 183–188

Krishna, G. (1975). Neurofibromatosis, renal hypertension and cardiac dysrhythmias. *Anesth. Analg. curr. Res.* 54, 542–545

Kurnick, N. B. (1956). Hyperreflexia and its control in patients with spinal cord lesions. *Ann. intern. Med.* 44, 678–686

Kyei-Mensah, K. and Thornton, J. A. (1974). The incidence of medical disease in surgical patients. *Br. J. Anaesth.* 46, 470–574

Lees, D. E. and MacNamara, T. (1977). Ketamine-induced hyperthermia. Postictal or malignant. *Anesthesiology* 47, 390–391

Lichtenfeld, P. (1971). Autonomic dysfunction in the Guillain–Barré syndrome. *Am J. Med.* 50, 772–780

McClelland, R. M. A. (1960). The myasthenic state and the myotonic syndrome. *Br. J. Anaesth.* 32, 81–88

Magbagbeola, J. A. O. (1970). Abnormal responses to muscle relaxants in patients with von Recklinghausen's disease (multiple neurofibromatosis). *Br. J. Anaesth.* 42, 710

Manser, J. (1970). Abnormal responses in von Recklinghausen's disease. *Br. J. Anaesth.* 42, 183–184

Meridy, H. E. and Creighton, R. E. (1971). General anaesthesia in eight patients with familial dysautonomia. *Can. Anaesth. Soc. J.* 18, 563–570

Meyers, M. B. and Barash, P. G. (1976). Cardiac decompensation during enflurane anesthesia in a patient with myotonia atrophica. *Anesth. Analg. curr. Res.* 55, 433–434

Mulder, D. W., Lambert, E. H. and Eaton, L. M. (1959). Myasthenic syndrome in patients with amyotrophic lateral sclerosis. *Neurology* 9, 627–629

Muller, J. and Suppan, P. (1977). Case report: Anaesthesia in myotonic dystrophy. *Anaesth. Intens. Care* 5, 70–73

Oxbury, J. M. and Whitty, C. W. M. (1971). Causes and consequences of status epilepticus in adults. A study of 86 cases. *Brain* 94, 733–742

Page, M. McB. and Watkins, P. J. (1978). Cardiorespiratory arrest with diabetic autonomic neuropathy. *Lancet* i, 14–16

Paterson, I. S. (1962). Generalised myotonia following suxamethonium. *Br. J. Anaesth.* 34, 340–342

Perel, A., Reches, A. and Davidson, J. T. (1977). Anaesthesia in the Guillain–Barré syndrome: A case report and recommendations. *Anaesthesia* 32, 257–260

Quimby, C. W., Williams, R. N. and Greifenstein, F. E. (1973). Anesthetic problems of the acute quadriplegic patient. *Anesth. Analg. curr. Res.* 52, 333–340

Ravin, M., Newmark, Z. and Saviello, G. (1975). Myotonia dystrophica – An anesthetic hazard. Two case reports. *Anesth. Analg curr. Res.* 54, 216–218

Riley, C. M., Day, R. L., Greeley, D. McL. and Langford, W. S. (1949). Central autonomic dysfunction with defective lacrimation; report of 5 cases. *Pediatrics* 3, 468–478

Rocco, A. and Vandam, L. (1959). Problems for anesthesia for paraplegics. *Anesthesiology* 20, 348–354

Rose, J. G. M., Bourne, J. G. and Goldman, V. (1969). Methohexitone and epilepsy. *Br. dent. J.* 126, 203

Rosenbaum, K. J., Neigh, J. L. and Strobel, G. E. (1971). Sensitivity to non-depolarising muscle relaxants in amyotrophic lateral sclerosis: Report of two cases. *Anesthesiology* 35, 638–641

Rowland, L. P. (1967). Myasthenia gravis. In *Advances in Anesthesiology: Muscle Relaxants,* p. 85. L. C. Mark and E. M. Papper. (ed.). New York: Harper and Row

Shy, G. M. and Drager, G. A. (1960). A neurological syndrome associated with orthostatic hypotension. *Archs Neurol.* 2, 511–527

Siemkowicz, E. (1976). Multiple sclerosis and surgery. *Anaesthesia* 31, 1211–1216

Siler, J. N. and Discavage, W. J. (1975). Anesthetic management of hypokalaemic periodic paralysis. *Anesthesiology* 43, 489–490

Stone, W. A., Beach, T. P. and Hamelberg, W. (1970). Succinylcholine – danger in the spinal-cord-injured patient. *Anesthesiology* 32, 168–169

Suppan, P. (1975). Althesin and dystrophia myotonica. *Anaesthesia* 30, 95–96

Texter, J. H., Reece, R. W. and Hranowsky, N. (1976). Pentolinium in the management of automatic hyperreflexia. *J. Urol.* 116, 350–351

Thorn-Alquist, A-M. (1975). Prevention of hypertensive crises in patients with high spinal lesions during cystoscopy and lithotripsy. *Acta anaesth. scand. Suppl.* 57, 79–82

Thornton, J. A. (1970). Methohexitone and its application in dental anaesthesia. *Br. J. Anaesth.* 42, 255–261

Tobey, R. E. (1970). Paraplegia, succinylcholine and cardiac arrest. *Anesthesiology* 32, 359–364

Tobey, R. E., Jacobsen, P. M., Kahle, C. T., Clubb, R. J. and Dean, M. A. (1972). The serum potassium response to muscle relaxants in neural injury. *Anesthesiology* 37, 332–337

Turner, P. (1975). The human pupil as a model for clinical pharmacological investigations. *Jl R. Coll. Physns, Lond.* 9, 165–172

Uppington, J. (1973). Epileptiform convulsion with Althesin. *Anaesthesia* 28, 546–550

Wang, P. and Clausen, T. (1976). Treatment of attacks in hyperkalaemic familial periodic paralysis. *Lancet* i, 221–223

Wedley, J. R. (1976). Control of the 'mass reflex' in tetraplegia. *Anaesthesia* 31, 301–304

Wheeler, T. and Watkins, P. J. (1973). Cardiac denervation in diabetes. *Br. med. J.* 4, 584–586

Whittaker, M., Spencer, R. and Searle, J. (1977). Plasma cholinesterase and malignant hyperthermia. *Br. J. Anaesth.* 49, 393

Winters, W. D., Mori, K., Spooner, C. E. and Bauer, R. O. (1967). The neuro-physiology of anesthesia. *Anesthesiology* 28, 65–80

Wise, R. P. (1963). Muscle disorders and the relaxants. *Br. J. Anaesth.* 35, 558–564

Wislicki, L. (1962). Anaesthesia and post-operative complications in progressive muscular dystrophy. *Anaesthesia* 17, 482–487

Yamashita, M. and Matsuki, A. (1975). Muscle relaxant requirements in patients with von Recklinghausen's disease. *Br. J. Anaesth.* 47, 1032

46 Metabolic and other disorders
J. A. Thornton and R.W.E. Watts

INHERITED METABOLIC DISEASES

The inherited metabolic diseases or inborn errors of metabolism are a group of about 150 diseases in which there is an identifiable inherited biochemical lesion affecting a single protein molecule which is usually an enzyme. The inborn errors of metabolism present problems in all fields of medicine, and *The Metabolic Basis of Inherited Disease* (4th edition 1978) edited by J. B. Stanbury, J. B. Wyngaarden and D. S. Fredericksen is an authoritative and comprehensive treatise and a good source of references. *The Treatment of Inherited Metabolic Disease* edited by D. N. Raine (1975) is another useful source reference. See also Brown, Walson and Taussig (1975).

The selection of topics from such a wide field for inclusion in a work on anaesthesia must lay emphasis on diseases which may influence anaesthetic practice either from the point of view of the selection of anaesthetic, analgesic and premedication drugs, the management of the unconscious patient, or his care in the recovery suite and intensive therapy unit. The inborn errors of metabolism are individually rare, so that the personal experience of the authors and their close colleagues will inevitably influence this selection to some extent.

An inborn error of metabolism will usually be an added background complication in a patient who requires surgery for an independent disease; for example, the patient with Duchenne muscular dystrophy, extensive muscle weakness and poor respiratory reserve and an acute abdomen. Surgery is less often directly needed in relation to the diagnosis or treatment of the primary disease or its complications, but the anaesthetist may, for example, encounter the problem of an infant with suspected type 1 glycogen storage disease causing intractable hypoglycaemia and profound lactic acidosis who needs the repair of an inguinal hernia or an open liver biopsy in order to establish the diagnosis. The latter type of situation is less difficult because the operation is usually an elective one and identifiable biochemical abnormalities should be well documented and difficulties due to them foreseen. The anaesthetist may also have a special role to play in the management of major clinical aspects of the disease itself, for example the care of a patient with respiratory paralysis due to acute intermittent porphyria.

The porphyrias (Sumner, 1975)

The term porphyrias is a collective one which includes all the disorders of porphyrin metabolism. The porphyrias are broadly classified as erythropoietic, hepatic and protoporphyria (erythropoietic protoporphyria or erythrohepatic protoporphyria). The terms erythropoietic and hepatic indicate the organs in which the main accumulation of porphyrins and porphyrin precursors occur.

Erythropoietic porphyria is a well known but rare disorder which causes severe photosensitivity with ulceration and mutilation of the face and hands unless they are adequately protected, splenomegaly, haemolytic anaemia, erythrodontia and the excretion of red urine due to the presence of large amounts of porphyrins. It is inherited in an autosomal recessive manner. Protoporphyria is a more common but clinically less severe disease than congenital erythropoietic porphyria. It is inherited in an autosomal dominant manner and associated with an increased incidence of cholelithiasis. Erythopoietic porphyria and protoporphyria do *not* cause acute abdominal crises or neuropsychiatric disturbances and are only likely to cause minor anaesthetic difficulties if the nose and lips are extensively scarred or ulcerated.

The hepatic porphyrias comprise:

(1) three separate genetically determined diseases (acute intermittent porphyria, hereditary coproporphyria, variegate porphyria);
(2) cutaneous hepatic porphyria (porphyria cutanea tarda symptomatica);
(3) toxic porphyria.

Acute intermittent porphyria (Swedish porphyria) is inherited in an autosomal dominant manner. The term intermittent refers to the periodicity of the acute manifestations. The fundamental biochemical lesion is always present, and the patient excretes excessive amounts of δ-aminolaevulinic acid and porphobilinogen in the urine. These are increased during the acute episodes and form porphyrins after the urine has been secreted. Abdominal pain of variable severity is a prominent feature and acute abdominal crises may bring the patient to the anaesthetist in error, or surgery may be needed for a genuine coincidental disease. The neurological disturbances involve the peripheral, central and autonomic nervous systems. There may be a peripheral neuritic picture, sometimes of ascending (Landry) type, with flaccid motor paresis and sensory loss, cranial nerve palsies, respiratory paralysis and a history of psychiatric disability. Sinus tachycardia and hypertension occur. These patients do *not* have photosensitivity. The attacks can be precipitated by drugs which increase the activity of δ-aminolaevulinic acid synthetase, this being the enzyme which regulates the rate of porphyrin biosynthesis. Increased δ-aminolaevulinic acid synthetase activity exacerbates the accumulation of δ-aminolaevulinic acid and porphobilinogen which is caused by the metabolic lesion in acute intermittent porphyria (uroporphyrinogen I synthase deficiency) and therefore precipitates an acute episode. The mechanism which links these biochemical changes to the clinical manifestations is unknown. *Althesin, methohexitone, thiopentone and all other barbiturate drugs are totally contraindicated in these patients.* Ketamine, propanidid, phenoperidine and droperidol are said not to increase δ-aminolaevulinic acid synthetase activity (Parik and Moore, 1975) and ketamine has been used as an induction agent in these cases (Rizk, Jacobson and Silvay, 1977). Sulphonamides, griseofulvin, chloramphenicol and oestrogens and a wide range of sedatives, hypnotics and tranquillizers also precipitate attacks. The following widely used drugs which the anaesthetist may encounter appear to be *safe* from this point of view: aspirin, cephalexin, chloral hydrate, chlorpromazine, dexamethasone, diazepam, dicoumarol anticoagulants, morphine, paracetamol, pethidine, prednisolone, propranolol, tetracyclines and sodium valproate.

Variegate porphyria (South African porphyria) is also inherited in an autosomal dominant fashion. Cutaneous photosensitivity and systemic manifestations, the latter resembling those of acute intermittent porphyria, coexist. The acute attacks have the same precipitants as in the latter disease and the same restrictions with respect to anaesthetic agents and other drugs apply. Hereditary coproporphyria resembles variegate porphyria clinically except that a larger percentage of the affected individuals remain asymptomatic. It is a discrete genetic and biochemical entity, and is inherited in an autosomal dominant manner. The same restrictions with respect to the use of barbiturates and other drugs apply in this type of hepatic porphyria as in the others.

Hepatic cutaneous porphyria is generally assumed to be an acquired disorder associated with underlying liver disease. There may, however, be genetic predisposing factors. Abdominal and neurological manifestations are absent.

The term porphyria cutanea tarda has been used synonymously with both variegate porphyria and hepatic cutaneous porphyria. If this is done, the distinction should be drawn by the qualifications porphyria cutanea tarda hereditaria and porphyria cutanea tarda symptomatica respectively.

A few toxic substances (e.g. hexachlorobenzene) cause a wholly acquired type of porphyria.

Homocystinuria

This condition is transmitted in an autosomal recessive manner. It is due to cystathionine β-synthase deficiency and is characterized biochemically by increased plasma levels of homocystine and methionine and an increased excretion of homocystine in the urine. The patients may present with osteoporosis, mental handicap, the features of Marfan's syndrome, of which ectopia lentis is the most consistent, and repeated venous and/or arterial thrombotic episodes. The latter are associated with a high surgical mortality. The anaesthetist should pay particular attention to the avoidance of thrombotic episodes and hypoglycaemia by administering dextran and correcting the hypoglycaemia. The blood sugar should be estimated at 30-minute intervals during the operation. See also Crooke, Towers and Taylor (1971).

Maple syrup urine disease (Delaney and Gal, 1976)

This condition arises because of a defect in the oxidative decarboxylation of α-oxoisocaproic acid, α-oxo-β-methylvaleric acid and α-oxoisovaleric acid. These compounds and the corresponding amino acids leucine, isoleucine and valine respectively accumulate in the blood and urine. The α-oxo acids have a characteristic smell which gives the disease its name. Severe neurological and respiratory disturbances may occur. There is also a tendency towards hypoglycaemia. Blood sugar and acid—base balance should be controlled by repeated monitoring and correction with glucose and bicarbonate infusions. Maple syrup urine disease is representative of a class of inborn errors of metabolism, the organic acidopathies in which a specific inherited metabolic block causes the accumulation of a relatively highly ionized organic acid, and severe metabolic acidosis.

Gilbert's disease (Black and Sherlock, 1970; Nishimura, Jackson and Cohen, 1973)

This abnormality of bile pigment metabolism due to inadequate bilirubin conjugation is associated with jaundice. As the condition is sometimes treated with phenobarbitone in order to induce liver microsomal enzymes and enhance metabolism, problems may arise because of increased biodegradation of anaesthetic agents. Gilbert's disease is also associated with the abnormal metabolism of certain drugs including the opiates, which for this reason should not be used.

The glycogen storage diseases

The glycogen storage diseases are a series of inborn errors of metabolism in which the metabolic lesion impairs glycogen metabolism. The liver is particularly involved in types I, III, IV and VI and an open liver biopsy may be necessary in order to establish the precise diagnosis.

Type I glycogen storage disease (von Gierke's disease; glucose-6-phosphatase deficiency) causes gross hepatomegaly, stunting of growth, severe hypoglycaemia and lactic acidosis, hyperlipidaemia and hyperuricaemia. Surgical operations in these children are associated with circulatory collapse unless special care is taken to correct the main biochemical abnormalities. Continuous intragastric or intravenous glucose corrects all of the biochemical abnormalities but the children become more sensitive to the hypoglycaemia if it occurs because the possibility of using lactate as an alternative metabolic fuel to glucose has been withdrawn. The degree of hepatomegaly and abdominal distension may be sufficient to embarrass respiration, and cause herniae.

Type III glycogen storage disease (Forbe's disease, glycogen debrancher enzyme deficiency) is also associated with hepatomegaly, hypoglycaemia, hyperlipidaemia and hyperlactic acidaemia, the biochemical abnormalities are usually less severe than in the type I disease.

Type IV glycogen storage disease (Andersen's disease, glycogen brancher enzyme deficiency) causes progressive hepatic cirrhosis and death from hepatic failure.

Type VI glycogen storage disease (Hers disease, liver phosphorylase deficiency) includes several different entities. Clinically, they all resemble a mild form of type I glycogen storage disease.

Patients with type II glycogen storage (Pompé's disease, lysosomal-α-glucosidase deficiency) present with intractable congestive cardiac failure in the first few months of life or with hypotonic muscle weakness in very early childhood. These forms of disease are invariably fatal. A rare adult type presents with muscle weakness mimicking the muscular dystrophies. The anaesthetic problems will be those usually associated with cardiorespiratory failure and/or severe generalized muscle weakness.

The mucopolysaccharidoses

This group of inborn errors of metabolism is due to congenital deficiencies of one of the series of lysosomal enzymes which degrade mucopolysaccharides (glycosaminoglycans). There are six well known mucopolysaccharidoses and other rarer forms are gradually being identified. The clinical manifestations are due to neurological, visceral and skeletal involvement. Mucopolysaccharidosis I (Hurler's disease; α-iduronidase deficiency) and mucopolysaccharidosis II (Hunter's disease; iduronate sulphate sulphatase deficiency) have all three types of multisystem involvement with similar phenotypic manifestations which include mental handicap. Hurler's disease which is inherited in an autosomal recessive manner, produces the most severe disability and the patients rarely survive beyond the first decade. Hunter's disease patients more often survive to adolescence or beyond and this disorder is inherited in a sex-linked recessive fashion. Both Hurler and Hunter disease patients have respiratory tract involvement, chronic nasal obstruction and repeated respiratory infections. The provision of an adequate airway can be a major problem in their anaesthetic management. They have gross hepatosplenomegaly with abdominal distension, multiple herniae, which may rupture or obstruct, and a grossly reduced range of respiratory excursion. They may also require ophthalmic surgery for the relief of ocular complications. Cardiac involvement can make them particularly sensitive to salt and water overloading. Cases of mucopolysaccharidoses IV (Morquio's disease; hexosamine-6-sulphatase deficiency) and VI (Maroteaux–Lamy syndrome; arylsulphatase B deficiency) have mainly skeletal abnormalities with severe stunting of their stature.

The sphingolipidoses

The sphingolipidoses are another group of lysosomal diseases which are due to a series of discrete metabolic lesions involving the degradation of the oligosialogangliosides. Some of these diseases were recognized and identified by eponymous names (e.g. Gaucher, Niemann–Pick, Krabbé, Tay–Sachs, Fabry) many years before they were delineated and classified biochemically.

Patients with the usual chronic non-neuronopathic (adult) type of Gaucher's disease (glucocerebroside β-cerebrosidase deficiency) have gross splenomegaly with hypersplenism and may require splenectomy. They have a haemorrhagic tendency due to thrombocytopoenia. A minority of patients with Niemann–Pick disease (sphingomyelinase deficiency) present to the anaesthetist in a similar manner. The latter patients may also have reduced respiratory reserve because of pulmonary infiltration. Most cases of Niemann–Pick disease are of the acute neuronopathic (infantile) type with progressive neurological deterioration as well as visceral involvement and death in the early years of life. Gaucher's disease and Niemann–Pick disease are both inherited in an autosomal recessive manner.

Primary hyperoxaluria

This is an inborn error of metabolism in which there is excessive oxalate biosynthesis which causes recurrent calcium oxalate urolithiasis and extensive nephrocalcinosis. Although the surgical management of these patients involves the utmost conservatism, they usually have multiple operations for the relief of obstructive uropathy. It is essential that a high rate of urine flow is maintained during the operative and postoperative period and that they do not become hypotensive. Unless these precautions are observed calcium oxalate may precipitate in the collecting tubules of the kidney from which it cannot be mobilized, and the patients become anuric, with virtually no prospect of recovery or effective long-term treatment.

Phenylketonuria

This inborn error of metabolism is due to a deficiency of the enzyme phenylalanine hydroxylase which catalyses the conversion of phenylalanine to tyrosine. It is detected by routine biochemical screening of all infants on the sixth day of life by means of the Guthrie test, which is a micro-biological inhibition assay for plasma phenylalanine. This test also detects infants with lesser degrees of hyperphenylalaninaemia than occur in classic phenylketonuria. Some of these cases remain hyperphenylalaninaemic throughout life (persistent or essential hyperphenylalaninaemia); in others, the hyperphenylalaninaemia disappears as the child grows older (transient mild hyperphenylalaninaemia). The combined incidence of all cases of hyperphenylalaninaemia at birth is between 1 in 6000 and 1 in 12 000 in the Caucasian races. It is customary in the UK to treat all cases with plasma phenylalanine levels above 14 mg·dl^{-1} (0.85 mmol·l^{-1}). A low phenylalanine diet is given for the first 8–12 years of life and it is customary to aim to keep the phenylalanine level at about 4—6 mg·dl^{-1}; this is a little above the upper limit of normal (2 mg·dl^{-1}; 0.12 mmol·l^{-1}) because prolonged phenylalanine restriction can also cause brain damage as well as skin complications.

Surgical treatment of these patients will clearly involve interrupting their regular diet but no special problems should arise in cases where the usual type of postoperative fluid regimen involving the use of dextrose and inorganic salt solutions can be followed. Cases that require prolonged parenteral nutrition will present a more difficult problem because, if amino-acid mixtures are to be used, it will be necessary to reduce markedly the amount of the phenylalanine present in order to avoid hyperphenyl-alaninaemia. If the use of prolonged parenteral feeding with amino-acid solutions cannot be avoided, then specialized biochemical and dietetic help will be needed. It is probable that little harm will be done by allowing the plasma phenylalanine to rise as high as 10 mg·dl^{-1} (0.6 mmol·l^{-1}) for a short period if necessary. The general principle should be to use non-amino acid containing parenteral nutrients and to aim to return to the patient's preoperative low phenylalanine diet as soon as possible.

Cystic fibrosis (mucoviscidosis)

This inborn error of metabolism has an incidence of about 1 in 2000 in Caucasian populations. The nature of the fundamental biochemical defect is unknown. These patients have cystic degeneration and fibrosis of the pancreas, and pulmonary fibrosis affecting particularly the lower lobes of the lungs. The meconium is abnormally viscid and approximately 15% of cases develop a form of intestinal obstruction which is termed meconium ileus. These infants may present to the anaesthetist. Older children and young adults with pulmonary involvement will present the same respiratory problems to the anaesthetist as other patients with extensive pulmonary fibrosis, recurrent chest infections or bronchiectasis.

α^1-Antitrypsin deficiency

Deficiency of α^1-antitrypsin in the serum is associated with some cases of chronic obstructive pulmonary disease and emphysema which begin in early life and progress rapidly.

Absent or deficient cholinesterase

Shortly after the introduction of suxamethonium into clinical practice in 1951, there were reports of prolonged apnoea in association with its use. In most instances these cases of apnoea occurred in patients who were found subsequently to have a low plasma cholinesterase activity. Such diminished activity may occur in malnutrition, burns (Viby-Mogenson *et al.*, 1975), liver disease and exposure to organophosphorus compounds such as ecothiopate iodide eye-drops. However, altered activity may also occur in patients who have an atypical enzyme due to the inheritance of an abnormal gene. Though such patients may have normal quantities of cholinesterase present in the plasma there is an associated qualitative change in the enzyme resulting in abnormal activity. These cholinesterase genotypes may be distinguished by employing inhibitors of cholinesterase activity such as *n*-butyl alcohol, chloride, urea, succinyldicholine, cinchocaine, fluoride and R02–0683. The percentage inhibition (or inhibitor number) of these substances in some instances overlaps and precise phenotyping is occasionally difficult (Zsigmond, 1973; King and Griffin, 1974). The patient with a normal (usual) gene at the E_1 locus is represented by E_1^u. The pair of allelomorphic genes in the normal homozygote is therefore denoted $E_1^u E_1^u$: such a patient has a normal level of cholinesterase (2.6–7.8 units·ml^{-1}*) and an inhibition of its activity by cinchocaine of between 70 and 85%. The atypical homozygote ($E_1^a E_1^a$) has a cinchocaine number of 16–25% (16–25% inhibition) and a low plasma pseudocholinesterase. The fluoride resistant (E_1^f) and silent genes (E_1^s) are examples of other variants encountered.

Another abnormal gene (C_5^+) has been demonstrated at the E_2 locus. Due to continuing improvements in analytical techniques a number of genotypes such as the heterozygote atypical ($E_1^u E_1^a$) have subsequently been typed as fluoride resistant ($E_1^u E_1^f$) and, as a consequence, a closer correlation between the phenotype and the subsequent response has been possible. The genotypes $E_1^a E_1^a$ and $E_1^s E_1^s$ (devoid of all plasma cholinesterase) are markedly sensitive and $E_1^f E_1^f$ moderately sensitive to suxamethonium. The frequency in the population of the E_1^a allele ($E_1^a E_1^a$) is about 15–30 $\times$ 10^{-3} in Caucasians. The E_1^f allele is 3–8 $\times$ 10^{-3} and the E_1^s rarer still (1 $\times$ 10^{-5}). The heterozygote genotypes $E_1^u E_1^a$, $E_1^u E_1^s$ and $E_1^u E_1^f$ are not sensitive to suxamethonium. $E_1^a E_1^s$ is, however, markedly sensitive whilst $E_1^a E_1^f$ and $E_1^f E_1^s$ are moderately sensitive.

MANAGEMENT OF PATIENT SUSPECTED OF HAVING AN ABNORMAL OR LOW PLASMA PSEUDOCHOLINESTERASE

The failure of a patient to breathe following the administration of suxamethonium may not necessarily be on account of a low or abnormal plasma cholinesterase. Other causes of apnoea must be excluded. Whilst the process of eliminating the other causes proceeds, the patient must be artificially ventilated and maintained in an unconscious state by administering 60–75% nitrous oxide in the inspired mixture. A peripheral nerve stimulator may demonstrate a change from depolarizing block towards a non-depolarizing block (the so-called dual block). The judicious administration of 1 mg edrophonium intravenously whilst this process develops will often indicate the degree to which the block has progressed toward one of non-depolarization. However, the temptation to administer neostigmine at this stage is best resisted.

*1 unit = amount of enzyme that will hydrolyse 1 μmol of butyonyl thiocholine substrate per minute at 25°C.

The patient should continue to be ventilated until the slow hydrolysis of suxamethonium has been completed over a period of up to 12—24 hours. The infusion of fresh blood or plasma has been advocated (Vickers, 1963) as a means of providing cholinesterase. More recently suxamethonium apnoea has been terminated with commercial cholinesterase (Stovner and Stadskleiv, 1976). In all cases a sample of heparinized blood should be sent for screening. If a genetic abnormality is detected the patient's family should be investigated as the possibility of the members being at risk is great (Bauld *et al.*, 1974). All subjects found to be at risk should be adequately warned and, if possible, identification discs issued.

SICKLE HAEMOGLOBINOPATHIES

More than 100 genetically transmitted abnormal haemoglobins have been described in man, and the haemoglobin S haemoglobinopathies are particularly important in anaesthetic practice. This abnormal haemoglobin arises because of the substitution of valine for glutamic acid at the position 6 peptide on the β chain of the haemoglobin molecule. When haemoglobin S occurs in association with the normal adult haemoglobin (A) the haemoglobin genotype AS results and this heterozygote state is known as the sickle cell trait. Sickle cell anaemia (genotype SS), sickle cell haemoglobin C disease (SC), haemoglobin SD and haemoglobin SF are rarer haemoglobinopathies. When haemoglobin S is deoxygenated, the valine groups form polar bonds with adjacent haemoglobin molecules, producing long chains of haemoglobin (tactoids). Several of these polymers may twist upon each other giving rise to distortion of the red cell membrane and the characteristic shape. Because of their abnormal shape the red cells are unable to pass through small arterioles, occluding capillaries and causing thrombosis and resulting infarction. Their increased fragility leads to haemolysis and anaemia. This sickling tendency depends upon the proportion of HbS and the nature of the haemoglobin present. The order of ease with which haemoglobins protect from sickling may be ranked F, A, D and C. The tendency to sickle also depends on the proportion of haemoglobin S in the cell, the oxygen tension and the pH. The higher the pH the lower the oxygen tension at which sickling is provoked. However, small changes of pH (0.05—0.1 units) have not been found to affect sickling significantly (Cawein *et al.*, 1969).

Haemoglobin S is found in subjects of Indian, East and West African, and West Indian origin and thus it is found in American Negroes. However, it is not confined solely to coloured races, having been detected in Eastern Mediterranean subjects.

The high levels of fetal haemoglobin (HbF) in homozygous sickle cell (SS) disease are generally associated with less rapid haemolysis, less evidence of small-vessel obstruction both direct (alterations in conjunctival vasculature) and indirect (progressive splenic atrophy), more normal growth and development, and a generally milder clinical course. It has been postulated that genes exist for heterocellular hereditary persistence of

HbF, in carriers (HbAS), and marked elevation in their offspring with homozygote (HbSS) sickle cell anaemia.

Homozygote state (sickle cell anaemia) – HbSS

In sickle cell anaemia the red cell contains 95% or more haemoglobin S, the remainder being haemoglobin F (fetal haemoglobin). Patients with this condition often give a history of bone and joint pains from early childhood and present with moderate or severe anaemia. Jaundice is usually present and bossing of the skull and overgrowth of the maxilla (due to increased red cell production in the bone marrow) are associated features. Lymphadenopathy is often found but the spleen may not be felt because of recurrent splenic infarcts. Infarcts may also affect other tissues – bone (giving rise to osteomyelitis), lungs (haemoptysis), abdominal viscera (acute abdomen). Cerebral thrombosis may result in neurological deficits. Chronic punched-out ulcers may be found in the skin, commonly at the ankles.

Heterozygote state (sickle cell trait) – HbAS

The heterozygote state is characterized by the presence of between 20 and 50% sickle haemoglobin (HbS), the rest being adult haemoglobin (HbA). Although red cells are more resistant to sickling than those of sickle cell anaemia, the pathogenicity of this condition depends upon the degree of hypoxaemia in the capillary bed.

Splenic infarction has been reported in subjects with sickle cell trait when flying high in unpressurized aircraft (Smith and Conley, 1955) and in climbers at high altitude (O'Brien *et al.*, 1972). The sickle cell trait is prevalent among black populations and most carriers suffer little disability from it. However, evidence suggests that anaesthesia in these subjects is not always benign (Dalal *et al.*, 1974).

Sickle cell haemoglobin C disease – HbSC

The molecular defect in haemoglobin C is the replacement of glutamic acid by lysine at position 6 peptide on the β-chain of haemoglobin. This is primarily an infarctive disease and vitreous haemorrhage is a particular feature.

Sickle cell β-thalassaemia – HbSβT

These patients have approximately 75% haemoglobin S, with abnormal amounts of fetal haemoglobin (F) and A_2 haemoglobin (a slow-moving component of electrophoresis). Because of high proportion of haemoglobin S, patients with this condition are particularly vulnerable to hypoxaemia.

Management of patients for anaesthesia

In countries where hospital and laboratory facilities permit, all patients thought to be at risk should be screened. The Sickledex test is a useful rapid and reasonably reliable method of screening. False negatives have not been reported but the occasional false positive is found. The test relies upon the haemolysis and reduction of the red cells with the visual assessment of the insoluble precipitate of haemoglobin S (Loh, 1971). A subject found to be positive by this test should be further evaluated by haemoglobin electrophoresis to determine the haemoglobin genotype. The absence of the result of a screening test in a subject potentially at risk is regarded as a contraindication to general anaesthesia by many anaesthetists in the UK.

As there must be a certain amount of deoxygenated haemoglobin S in the red cells before sickling can occur, the amount of deoxygenated haemoglobin can be reduced by increasing oxygen tension, by increasing the affinity of oxygen for haemoglobin S, or by decreasing the intracellular concentration of haemoglobin S. The oxygen can be increased by oxygen therapy, maintenance of cardiac output, and adequate blood volume, attention to optimal respiratory function, and the achievement of a mixed venous oxygen content as high as possible. An increase in oxygen affinity for haemoglobin can be produced by shifting the oxygen dissociation curve to the left by alkalinization, alteration of the red cell pH by the use of a carbonic anhydrase inhibitor or by reducing the level of 2,3-diphosphoglycerate (2,3-DPG) in the red cell. Howells *et al.* (1972) recommend routine preoperative preparation with either oral sodium bicarbonate ($0.5-1.0$ g·kg^{-1} per day) or 3.3 mmol·kg^{-1}·h^{-1} intravenously for 90 minutes.

Searle (1973), on the other hand, recommends that alkalinization should be reserved for established metabolic acidosis. Urea in invert sugar has been employed to break down the hydrophobic bonds between HbS molecules thus reversing sickling and terminating crises. The sugar solution protects the erythrocyte from haemolysis. In order to be effective the blood urea has to be maintained between $25-34$ mmol·l^{-1} (normal range, $3-7$ mmol·l^{-1}) and, as many patients with HbS haemoglobinopathy have concurrent renal disease and associated dehydration this treatment is not without risk. As the results of such therapy have not been conclusive its use has been abandoned.

Despite the recognized hazards of blood transfusion in patients with anaemia and a high HbS, transfusion of fresh blood to patients with a haemoglobin of 5 g·dl^{-1} is regarded as essential and some authorities (Gilbertson, 1965; Green *et al.*, 1975) recommend exchange transfusion. Sodium cyanate has also been suggested as a useful form of treatment (Gilette *et al.*, 1974). The cyanate binds to haemoglobin and acts by increasing the oxygen affinity and hence, at any given oxygen tension, the haemoglobin is more saturated with oxygen and less likely to sickle. Early clinical trials of long-term oral administration are encouraging in that the incidence of crises appears to be reduced and toxic effects have not been excessive (Peterson *et al.*, 1974). The administration of low molecular weight dextran reduces blood viscosity and therefore promotes blood flow. Maduska *et al.* (1975) confirm the view that elective surgery in patients with sickle cell disease does not lead to a prohibitive morbidity and mortality.

The choice of anaesthetic is not of great importance provided that attention is paid to optimum oxygenation and maintenance of blood volume, cardiac output, blood pressure and tissue perfusion. It is suggested that epidural anaesthesia should be employed rather than general anaesthesia when circumstances permit (Crawford, 1971). Preoperative preparation should attempt to achieve an optimal medical condition. Anaemia should be corrected by blood transfusion employing exchange when considered necessary. Metabolic acidosis should be avoided and sodium bicarbonate may be administered to maintain normal acid–base status. It is stated that unnecessary hypothermia should be avoided (Gilbertson, 1967) but it should be noted that successful cardiac surgery employing profound hypothermia has been carried out (Somanathan, 1976). Although the risks from using tourniquets would appear to have been overstated, every effort should be made to exsanguinate the limb as much as possible. Postoperatively, attention should be paid to the adequacy of ventilation, oxygenation, perfusion (cardiac output, blood pressure) and the reduction of shivering.

'COLLAGEN DISEASES' (Beeson and McDermott, 1975)

Cutaneous and systemic lupus erythematosus, dermatomyositis, and polyarteritis nodosa are 'inflammatory' connective tissue disorders. Their aetiologies are incompletely understood although immunological abnormalities are clearly important. They present a large variety of symptoms and signs including myasthenia (Wolf, 1972; Davis, 1974).

Lupus erythematosus

Lupus erythematosus is associated with malaise and fever. Symptoms may arise from the involvement of any organ. Blistering and ulceration of the skin and mucous membranes may occur and complicate the management of anaesthesia. Purpura is occasionally present. Arthralgia, pneumonitis and pleurisy are common. Myocarditis may give rise to heart failure. Splenomegaly and lymphadenopathy may be found. Renal involvement occurs in the majority of patients. Leucopenia, thrombocytopenia and hyperglobulinaemia may also occur. Altered plasma protein pattern and liver involvement may influence the response to neuromuscular blocking agents. Steroid therapy and possible diminished response to stress may require special management.

Dermatomyositis

Dermatomyositis is usually associated with malaise, fever, loss of weight, erythema, painful swollen muscles and weakness. Effusions may occur into serous cavities. Myocarditis and anaemia may be found. Steroids are frequently employed in the management of this condition. Caution should be used if neuromuscular blocking agents are employed as an altered response may be encountered (Fielsen and Stovner, 1978).

Scleroderma

This is a multisystem disease which presents anaesthetic problems because of visceral as well as cutaneous disease. Typically the skin condition gives rise to lack of ready access to veins and difficulty in opening the mouth. Oesophageal involvement may cause incompetence of the gastro-oesophageal sphincter. Cardiopulmonary changes may be present and the bowel, kidney, eyes and joints are sometimes also affected by the disease process. The skin blood flow is frequently impaired, producing Raynaud's phenomenon. The patients may be receiving steroid therapy. Great care should be taken with laryngoscopy and endotracheal intubation because of the risk of lacerating the tissues around the mouth (Davidson-Lamb and Finlayson, 1977). Prolonged regional analgesia has been reported following nerve block (Eisele and Reitan, 1971; Lewis, 1974).

Rheumatoid arthritis (Gardener and Holmes, 1961; Jenkins and McGraw, 1969)

Adult rheumatoid arthritis usually involves the distal joints most severely, and it may evolve rapidly. The main anaesthetic difficulties are due to ankylosis of the costovertebral, temporomandibular and laryngeal joints (Funk and Raymon, 1975). The vital capacity is reduced, and it is difficult to intubate and to maintain an adequate airway in these patients. A pre-operative tracheostomy is occasionally necessary. Patients with chronic rheumatoid arthritis are frequently debilitated and anaemic, and the lungs and heart may be directly involved in the primary disease process. Local and intravenous anaesthetic methods are recommended in preference to inhalation anaesthesia. Pneumonia is a particularly common postoperative complication, and adrenocortical suppression by steroid therapy will be an indication to give additional intravenous steroids before and during the operation.

Juvenile chronic polyarthritis (Still's disease)

This is similar to the adult condition in most respects but the disease process tends to affect the larger joints. Splenomegaly is frequently encountered. Impairment of growth of the mandible may also be found, together with endocarditis and pleural effusion. Most patients respond well to corticosteroid therapy and complete remissions are seen in 75—80% of patients.

Ankylosing spondylitis (Wright and Moll, 1973)

This is a chronic progressive disease which causes bony ankylosis of the intervertebral and costovertebral joints with ossification of the spinal ligaments and the margins of the intervertebral discs. The sacroiliac, hip and shoulder joints are also involved. Iridocyclitis, aortitis with aortic insufficiency and cardiac conduction defects with first degree atrioventricular block are the most important extra-articular manifestations. Diminished chest expansion and impaired pulmonary function are particularly important complications from the anaesthetic viewpoint (Stewart, Ridyard and Pearson, 1976). Impaired movement of the neck may make endotracheal intubation difficult (Munson and Cullen, 1965). Ketamine has been advocated for anaesthesia in these cases (D'Arcy *et al.*, 1976).

OCULOMUCOCUTANEOUS SYNDROMES

Epidermolysis bullosa

This is a chronic non-inflammatory, inherited (usually autosomal dominant) disease involving skin and mucous membrane. The lesions are common on the lower extremities especially the feet, but the hands may also be involved. The lesions consist of bullae ranging from a few mm to several cm in size with or without a surrounding erythematous area. The bullae contain sterile fluid and rupture to form shallow ulcers. Touching the skin may be painful to the patient and the application of a blood pressure cuff, adhesive tape, electrodes and airways carries the risk of trauma. There should therefore be minimal contact with the skin. Facemasks should be avoided, and skin which is exposed to pressure during anaesthesia should be protected by the application of muslin soaked in 0.5% hydrocortisone. The anaesthetist must be aware that many of these patients receive therapy with steroids and he should ensure that extra steroid cover is prescribed. Although the mucous membrane is least commonly involved, disease of the oropharynx can produce bullae, infiltrated areas, ulceration and bleeding or patches of leucoplakia which may extend to the epiglottis and larynx. Microstomia, impaired mobility of the tongue and scar formation may make conditions very difficult for intubation, and good relaxation will be required. Endotracheal intubation should be avoided as far as possible. Unfortunately, suxamethonium is an unsuitable agent because of the associated muscle wasting and malnutrition.

Barbiturates should not be used because of the possible association of this condition with certain types of porphyria. Ketamine anaesthesia has been advocated (Lee and Nagel, 1975; Pratulas and Biezunski, 1975; LoVerme and Oropollo, 1977). The patients should be lain on their side in the head-down position when there is danger of bleeding in the oral cavity, and, if bleeding occurs, swabs soaked in adrenaline solution may be applied in an attempt to control troublesome haemorrhage. Regional anaesthesia is generally unsuitable because of infection and contractures but epidural anaesthesia may be considered in suitable circumstances.

Behçets syndrome (Turner, 1972)

This syndrome, which is often difficult to diagnose, is associated with buccal ulceration, aphthous changes in hypopharynx, eye, skin, genitourinary systems, with arthritic, central nervous and cardiovascular lesions. Thrombophlebitis may be found. Severe scarring of the oropharynx is rare but when it occurs intubation may be difficult.

Erythema multiforme (Cucchiara and Dawson, 1971)

This is an acute or subacute inflammatory eruption of the skin associated with fever, malaise and arthralgia. The skin lesions may take the form of erythematous macules or papules, weals, vesicles and sometimes bullae. The mucous membrane of the oropharynx may also be involved. The syndrome is sometimes associated with drug sensitivity and for this reason it is important to know what drugs, if any, the patient has been taking.

Stevens–Johnson syndrome

The severe type of erythema multiforme is known as Stevens–Johnson syndrome and carries a high morbidity with involvement myocarditis and pericarditis. Patients occasionally die from this disease.

Pemphigus

When occurring in elderly patients, this condition may lead to scarring with adhesions between the lips, soft palate and pharyngeal wall.

Management

When there is involvement of the upper airway, intubation should be avoided as far as possible. The use of ketamine should be considered. Many of these patients receive steroid therapy and dosage will need to be adjusted. Attention should be paid to water and electrolyte balance.

MISCELLANEOUS CONDITIONS

Obesity

The problems of anaesthesia and surgery in the obese subject are well recognized (Edelist, 1968; McIntyre, 1968; Vaughan, 1974; Fisher, Waterhouse and Adams, 1975; Fox, 1975, McKenzie *et al.*, 1975). Whereas in the past operation was avoided as far as possible, or regional techniques employed in preference to general anaesthesia, the development of intestinal bypass operations in attempts to reduce body weight (Tseuda, Pugh and Boyan, 1976) has increasingly involved the anaesthetist in the management of these patients. Many obese patients have additional pathology, affecting to a varying degree the cardiovascular and respiratory systems, thus making anaesthesia and surgery particularly hazardous. Metabolic and endocrine disorders such as diabetes mellitus and Cushing's disease may be present. Some of the patients may be receiving fenfluramine in an attempt to reduce weight. The increased incidence of potentially dangerous arrhythmias in patients receiving this drug has been reported (Bennett and Eltringham, 1977). It is suggested that such therapy should be discontinued for seven days prior to general anaesthesia and the use of halothane avoided.

CARDIOVASCULAR EFFECTS

Myocardial dysfunction arising from fatty infiltration is compounded in some instances by coronary artery disease and the associated ischaemia. Systemic and pulmonary arterial hypertension, and left ventricular hypertrophy are frequently found (Backman *et al.*, 1973).

Accurate determination of the blood pressure in these subjects is influenced by the circumference of the arm and the size of the selected cuff (Vaughan, 1973), and in order to overcome this error the Doppler technique has been employed with success in the obese (McKenzie *et al.*, 1975). Atherosclerosis may affect the central nervous and renal systems. The blood volume is low in relation to total body weight. Veins are notoriously difficult to find and venepuncture may be unreliable.

RESPIRATORY EFFECTS

Hypoxaemia is a common feature (Andersen, Rasmussen and Eriksen, 1977) and arises mainly from the increased oxygen cost of breathing and mismatch between ventilation and perfusion with the lung. Alveolar hypoventilation may occasionally be present giving rise to retention of carbon dioxide within the body, and more rarely, associated with excessive somnolence (Pickwickian syndrome), right heart failure and polycythaemia (Burwell, Robin and Whaley, 1956). The precise nature of this somnolence is not clear and some authorities have postulated that the sleepiness may be due to either a reduced sensitivity of the respiratory centre to chemical drive and to a direct effect of carbon dioxide, or to an associated hypopituitary disorder. The ventilation/perfusion abnormality found in obesity arises from the reduction of expiratory reserve volume and chest compliance (Waltemath and Bergman, 1974), and an increase in the closing volume (Farebrother and McHardy, 1974), resulting from the splinting of the chest wall and diaphragm by adipose tissues and is aggravated by general anaesthesia and artificial ventilation (Hedenstierna and Santesson, 1977).

Fortunately, the application of positive end-expiratory pressure (PEEP) reduces the degree of venous admixture in these subjects under general anaesthesia (Santesson, 1976). The maldistribution of ventilation may, however, be made worse by the sputum retention and pulmonary infection often occurring in these patients. Nevertheless, reduction in the ability of the patient to shift air through the larger air passages is not found in the obese unless infection, bronchospasm and/or sputum retention are present. The forced expiratory volume and midexpiratory flow rate are therefore usually normal.

MANAGEMENT

These patients have short, fat necks and relatively large tongues, and difficulties may arise with maintenance of the airway and endotracheal intubation in the unconscious patient. Other associated disorders often found are gall-stones, hiatus hernia and varicose veins. The large volume of intra-abdominal contents and the increased intra-abdominal pressure make surgery in the abdomen extremely difficult even though muscular relaxation may be adequate. The obese find the horizontal posture uncomfortable and if, therefore, a regional local anaesthetic technique is employed with the patient conscious, he should be permitted to lie upright or semiupright. Because of the large amount of adipose tissue, effective regional blockade may be difficult and general anaesthesia preferred. Choice of general anaesthetic technique does not appear to be critical provided immediate postoperative return to full consciousness is ensured if spontaneous ventilation is to be permitted. For this reason, residual effects of inhalational agents, potent narcotic analgesics and neuromuscular blocking agents cannot be tolerated.

Because surgery poses very great technical difficulties for the surgeon in obese subjects undergoing abdominal operations there may be a tendency for the anaesthetist to give relatively large doses of neuromuscular blocking agents in an attempt to provide the best possible conditions. Fox (1975) suggests the combination of an epidural anaesthesia with a neurolept technique and the maintenance of postoperative pain relief by the epidural route. Bromage and Fox (1976) claim that this combination of epidural blockade and light endotracheal anaesthesia is neither difficult nor unpredictable during the operative period, and postoperative management of an active co-operative patient is simpler compared to the complexities of dealing with a gross obese patient who is partially paralysed and intubated. However, obese subjects may be receiving anticoagulants as prophylaxis against postoperative phlebothrombosis and such therapy will constitute a contraindication to epidural anaesthesia. The deterioration of pulmonary function often found in the immediate postoperative period after laparotomy in the obese is due to spasm of the abdominal wall, painful abdominal distension, immobilization, posture, and increased oxygen cost of breathing (Eriksen, Andersen and Rasmussen, 1977). Post-operative mechanical ventilation has been advocated. However, Fox (1975) and Eriksen and his colleagues (1977) favour early extubation, intensive cardiopulmonary care, adoption of the semirecumbent position, humidification of inspired oxygen and chest physiotherapy. Because of the increased incidence of postoperative phlebothrombosis, early ambulation is advised.

Prader—Willi syndrome (Prader, Labhart and Willi, 1956; Milliken and Weintraub, 1975; Palmer and Atler, 1976)

This condition, which may be as common as Down's syndrome, is associated with severe neonatal hypotonia, hyperphagia in early childhood, obesity, diabetes, hypogonadism, dental caries and mental deficiency. The obesity leads to cardiorespiratory failure. The anaesthetic problem arises from the extreme obesity, hypotonia and disturbed carbohydrate metabolism. Attention should be directed towards airway protection and avoidance of postoperative pulmonary complications arising from a weak cough. Because of the decreased muscle mass and greatly increased fatty tissue, care should be exercised with all anaesthetic agents. The blood glucose should be carefully monitored and glucose administered if hypo-glycaemia develops.

Addiction

In many instances addiction is complicated by the intake of a variety of substances. Recent efforts to curb the excessive prescription of drugs has reduced the abuse of barbiturates. Drug addicts exhibit a high degree of tolerance to morphine, phenothiazines and the barbiturates (Kilpatrick, 1955; Adriani and Morton, 1968; Giuffrida *et al.*, 1970; Jenkins, 1972; Experts Opine, 1973). The abstinence syndrome is well recognized and it would seem advisable to maintain drugs preoperatively and for the patient to be allowed to continue his drugs in the postoperative period. It should be remembered that many of these patients, because of their social and economic status, are malnourished and their general health may be poor. The need for an increased amount of agents, due to tolerance and cross-tolerance, may lead to overdosage and technical difficulties during anaesthesia. Cross-tolerance is common with the barbiturates, the alcohol-type drugs and the aliphatic inhalational agents. Hypotension has been reported during anaesthesia in narcotic addicts and may be treated in some instances with intravenous morphine. The amphetamines increase the requirement for anaesthetic agents and may be associated with cardiac arrhythmias. The presence of LSD within the tissues at the time of anaesthesia may be a matter of concern because the drug manifests a certain degree of anticholinesterase activity, which potentiates narcotic activity and inhibits destruction of suxamethonium. Veins may be inaccessible and sepsis may be encountered with liver and kidney damage (Butterfield, 1972; Pollard, 1973; Geelhoed and Joseph, 1974). If a patient is receiving narcotics it may be necessary to increase the usual narcotic dose in the premedication. The withdrawal syndrome for the barbiturates can be serious and terminate fatally if not properly managed. This is in contradistinction to the morphine type where withdrawal is uncomfortable but not fatal. Pentazocine has also been demonstrated to lead to addiction (Kripke and Hechtmann, 1972) but its use in the presence of opiate addiction can cause withdrawal symptoms.

Perhaps the commonest form of addiction is found in chronic alcoholism (Lee, Cho and Dobkin, 1964; Keilty, 1969; Tammisto and Takki, 1973; Takki and Tammisto, 1974). Excessive intake leads to impaired nutrition. Vitamin deficiency may include pellagra (niacin deficiency), scurvy (vitamin C deficiency), and beriberi (vitamin B_1 deficiency). Cirrhosis of the liver, a late complication in alcoholics, possibly results from a direct hepatotoxic effect as well as specific nutritional deficiencies of proteins and vitamins. The cirrhosis leads to an irreversible impairment of liver function which prevents adequate glycogen storage and promotes a tendency to hypoglycaemia. Hypoxaemia may also be found in cirrhosis of the liver (Funahashi, Kutty and Prater, 1976). The cardiomyopathy sometimes found in these patients (Bridgen, 1977) may lead to cardiovascular instability. Acute withdrawal may lead to delirium tremens and this factor must be considered in relation to general anaesthesia and surgery.

It has long been recognized that these patients may be resistant to general anaesthesia (Tammisto and Tigerstedt, 1977a). Han (1969) has demonstrated a rise in the MAC of the chronic alcoholic. The response of the patient to neuromuscular blocking agents is sometimes modified. An increased sensitivity to suxamethonium is possibly due to the lowered level of pseudocholinesterase found in liver disease.

Typically the cirrhotic patient is resistant to curare. This is possibly due to the altered protein pattern often found in liver disease. Denial of intake of alcohol in the perioperative period may give rise to disturbances associated with acute withdrawal such as delerium tremens. This effect can be minimized by permitting a moderate intake of alcohol. Sedation can be achieved by the cautious administration of phenothiazines or benzodiazepines (Foster, 1977). Perphenazine and chlorpromazine are particularly valuable drugs. Delirium tremens should be treated by attention to fluid balance, administration of vitamins (particularly thiamine). Control can best be achieved by intravenous sedation with 0.8% chlormethiazole (Heminevrin). Barbiturates should be avoided (Kalant, Khanna and Marshmann, 1970). A nitrous oxide—oxygen—relaxant technique with analgesic supplementation is suitable for these subjects (Tammisto and Tigerstedt, 1977b).

Hereditary angioneurotic oedema (HAE)

This disorder is inherited as an autosomal dominant and is thought to be due to abnormally low levels of the plasma inhibitor for the activated first component of complement. The exact pathology is not understood but attacks are probably precipitated by local exhaustion of inhibitor by consumption by any of the plasma enzymes with which the inhibitor can react. There is no known allergic basis to HAE and antihistamines; adrenaline and steroids are ineffective. However, ε-aminocaproic acid (EACA) and fresh frozen plasma (FFP) have been reported to be of some value (Hamilton, Bosley and Bowen, 1977). Acute laryngeal oedema is the cause of the high mortality associated with this condition (Abada and Owens, 1977) and for this reason care should be taken to avoid laryngeal intubation when possible. Tracheostomy is occasionally necessary to overcome the respiratory obstruction arising from laryngeal oedema.

References

Abada, R. P. and Owens, W. D. (1977). Hereditary angioneurotic oedema. An anaesthetic dilemma. *Anesthesiology* 46, 428–430

Adriani, J. and Morton, R. C. (1968). Drug dependence: important considerations from the anaesthesiologists viewpoint. *Anesth. Analg. curr. Res.* 47, 472–482

Andersen, J., Rasmussen, J. P. and Eriksen, J. (1977). Pulmonary function in obese patients scheduled for jejuno-ileostomy. *Acta anaesth. scand.* 21, 346–351

Backman, L., Freyschuss, V., Hollberg, D. and Melcher, A. (1973). Cardiovascular function in extreme obesity. *Acta med. scand.* 193, 437–446

Bauld, H. W., Gibson, P. J., Jebson, P. J. and Brown, S. S. (1974). Aetiology of prolonged apnoea after suxamethonium. *Br. J. Anaesth.* 46, 273–281

Beeson, P. B. and McDermott, W. (1975). *Textbook Medicine.* 14th edn. Saunders: Philadelphia

Bennett, J. A. and Eltringham, R. J. (1977). Possible dangers of anaesthesia in patients receiving fenfluramine. *Anaesthesia* 32, 8–13

Black, M. and Sherlock, S. (1970). Treatment of Gilbert's syndrome with phenobarbitone. *Lancet* i, 1359–1361

Bridgen, W. (1977). Alcoholic cardiomyopathy. *Br. J. hosp. Med.* 18, 122–125

Bromage, P. R. and Fox, G. S. (1976). Obesity its relation to anaesthesia. *Anaesthesia* 31, 557–559

Brown, B. R., Walson, P. D. and Taussig, L. M. (1975). Congenital metabolic disease of pediatric patients: anesthetic implications. *Anesthesiology* 43, 197–209

Burwell, C. S., Robin, E. D. and Whaley, R. D. (1956). Extreme obesity associated with alveolar hypoventilation — a Pickwickian syndrome. *Am. J. Med.* 21, 811–818

Butterfield, W. C. (1972). Surgical complications of narcotic addiction. *Surgery Gynec. Obstet.* 134, 237–240

Cawein, M. J., O'Neill, R. A., Danzer, L. A., Lappat, E. J. and Roach, T. (1969). A study of the sickling phenomenon and oxygen dissociation curve in patients with haemoglobin S, SD, SF and SC. *Blood* 34, 682–690

Crawford, J. S. (1971). Anaesthesia for obstetric emergencies. *Br. J. Anaesth.* 43, 864–873

Crooke, J. W., Towers, J. F. and Taylor, W. H. (1971). Management of patients with homocystinuria requiring surgery under general anaesthesia: a case report. *Br. J. Anaesth.* 43, 96–99

Cucchiara, R. C. and Dawson, B. (1971). Anaesthesia in Stevens–Johnson syndrome: report of a case. *Anesthesiology* 35, 537–539

Dalal, F. Y., Schmidt, G. B., Bennett, E. J. and Ramamurthy, S. (1974). Sickle-cell trait: a report of a postoperative neurological complication. *Br. J. Anaesth.* 46, 387–388

D'Arcy, E. J., Fell, R. H., Ansell, B. M. and Arden, G. P. (1976). Ketamine and juvenile chronic polyarthritis (Still's Disease). *Anaesthesia* 31, 624–632

Davidson-Lamb, R. W. and Finlayson, M. C. K. (1977). Scleroderma — complications encountered during dental anaesthesia. *Anaesthesia* 32, 893–895

Davis, J. N. (1974). Myasthenia. *Br. J. hosp. Med.* 11, 933–940

Delaney, A. and Gal, T. J. (1976). Hazards of anesthesia and operation in maple-syrup urine disease. *Anesthesiology* **44**, 83–86

Edelist, G. (1968). Extreme obesity. *Anesthesiology* **29**, 846–847

Eisele, J. H. and Reitan, J. A. (1971). Scleroderma, Raynaud's phenomenon and local anaesthetics. *Anesthesiology* **34**, 386–387

Eriksen, J., Andersen, J. and Rasmussen, J. P. (1977). Postoperative pulmonary function in obese patients after upper abdominal surgery. *Acta anaesth. scand.* **21**, 336–341

Experts Opine (1973). What are your most important considerations in the management of the drug addict who requires general anesthesia for a surgical procedure. *Surv. Anesth.* **17**, 376–379

Farebrother, M. J. B. and McHardy, G. J. R. (1974). Respiratory complication of obesity. *Br. med. J.* **3**, 469

Fielsen, O. and Stovner, J. (1978). Dermatomyositis: Suxamethonium action and atypical plasma cholinesterase. *Can. Anaesth. Soc. J.* **25**, 63–64

Fisher, R. A., Waterhouse, T. D. and Adams, A. P. (1975). Obesity: its relation to anaesthesia. *Anaesthesia* **30**, 633–647

Foster, A. R. (1977). Sedatives for alcoholics. *Br. med. J.* **1**, 1355

Fox, G. S. (1975). Anaesthesia for intestinal short circuiting in the morbidly obese with reference to the pathophysiology of gross obesity. *Can. Anaesth. Soc. J.* **22**, 307–315

Funahashi, A., Kutty, A. V. P. and Prater, S. L. (1976). Hypoxaemia and cirrhosis of the liver. *Thorax* **31**, 303–308

Funk, D. and Raymon, F. (1975). Rheumatoid arthritis of the cricoarytenoid joints: An airway hazard. *Anesth. Analg. curr. Res.* **54**, 742–745

Gardner, D. L. and Holmes, F. (1961). Anaesthetic and postoperative hazards in rheumatoid arthritis. *Br. J. Anaesth.* **33**, 258–264

Geelhoed, G. W. and Joseph, W. L. (1974). Surgical sequelae of drug abuse. *Surgery Gynec. Obstet.* **139**, 749–755

Gilbertson, A. A. (1965). Anaesthesia in West African patients with sickle cell anaemia, haemoglobin SC disease and sickle cell trait. *Br. J. Anaesth.* **37**, 614–622

Gilbertson, A. A. (1967). The management of anaesthesia in sickle cell states. *Proc. R. Soc. Med.* **60**, 631–636

Gilette, P. N., Peterson, C. M., Lu, Y. S. and Cerami, A. (1974). Sodium cyanate as a potential treatment for sickle-cell disease. *New Engl. J. Med.* **290**, 654–660

Giuffrida, J. G., Bizzari, D. V., Saure, A. C. and Sharoff, R. L. (1970). Anesthetic management of drug abuses. *Anesth. Analg. curr. Res.* **49**, 272–278

Green, N. M., Hall, R. J. C., Huntsman, R. G., Lawson, A., Pearson, T. C. and Wheeler, P. C. G. (1975). Sickle cell oxsis treated by exchange transfusion. *J. Am. med. Ass.* **231**, 948–950

Hamilton, A. G., Bosley, A. R. J. and Bowen, D. J. (1977). Laryngeal oedema due to hereditary angioedema. *Anaesthesia* **32**, 265–267

Han, Y. H. (1969). Why do chronic alcoholics require more anaesthesia? *Anesthesiology* **30**, 341–342

Hedenstierna, G. and Santesson, J. (1977). 'Studies on intrapulmonary gas distribution in the extremely obese. Influence of anaesthesia and artificial ventilation with and without positive end-expiratory pressure. *Acta anaesth. scand.* **21**, 257–265

Howells, T. H., Huntsman, R. G., Boys, J. E. and Mahmood, A. (1972). Anaesthesia and sickle cell haemoglobin. *Br. J. Anaesth.* **44**, 975–987

Jenkins, L. C. (1972). Anaesthetic problems due to drug abuse and dependence. *Can. Anaesth. Soc. J.* **19**, 461–477

Jenkins, L. C. and McGraw, R. W. (1969). Anaesthetic management of the patient with rheumatoid arthritis. *Can. Anaesth. Soc. J.* **16**, 407–415

Kalant, H., Khanna, J. M. and Marshmann, J. (1970). Effect of chronic intake of ethanol on pentobarbital metabolism. *J. Pharmac. exp. Ther.* **175**, 318–324

Keilty, S. R. (1969). Anesthesia for the alcoholic patient. *Anesth. Analg. curr. Res.* **48**, 659–664

Kilpatrick, A. (1955). General anaesthesia for a morphine addict. *Br. J. Anaesth.* **27**, 178–180

King, J. and Griffin, D. (1974). Relationship between suxamethonium apnoea serum cholinesterase activity and dibucaine numbers. *Br. J. Anaesth.* **46**, 908–911

Kripke, B. J. and Hechtmann, H. B. (1972). Nitrous oxide for pentazocine addiction and for intractable pain: report of case. *Anesth. Analg. curr. Res.* **51**, 520–527

Lee, C. and Nagel, E. L. (1975). Anesthetic management of a patient with recessive epidermolysis bullosa dystrophica. *Anesthesiology* **43**, 122–124

Lee, K. Y. P., Cho, M. H. and Dobkin, A. B. (1964). Effects of alcoholism, morphinism and barbiturate resistance on induction and maintenance of general anaesthesia. *Can. Anaesth. Soc. J.* **11**, 354–381

Lewis, G. B. H. (1974). Prolonged regional analgesia in scleroderma. *Can. Anaesth. Soc. J.* **21**, 495–497

Loh, Wei-Ping (1971). Evaluation of a rapid test tube morbidity test for the detection of sickle cell. *Am. J. clin. Path.* **55**, 55–57

LoVerme, S. R. and Oropollo, A. T. (1977). Ketamine anesthesia in dermolytic bullous dermatosis (Epidermolysis bullosa). *Anesth. Analg. curr. Res.* **56**, 398–401

McIntyre, J. W. R. (1968). Problems for the anaesthetist in the care of the obese patient. *Can. Anaesth. Soc. J.* **15**, 317–324

McKenzie, R., Figallo, E. M., Tantisira, B., Wadhwa, R. K. and Sinchioco, C. S. (1975). Anaesthesia for jejunoileal shunt: Review of 88 cases. *Anesth. Analg. curr. Res.* **54**, 65–70

Maduska, A. L., Guinee, W. S., Heaton, J. A., North, W. C. and Barreras, L. M. (1975). Sickling dynamics of red blood cells and other physcotopic studies during anaesthesia. *Anesth. Analg. curr. Res.* **54**, 361–365

Milliken, R. A. and Weintraub, D. M. (1975). Cardiac abnormalities during anesthesia in a child with Prader–Willi syndrome. *Anesthesiology* **43**, 590–592

Munson, E. S. and Cullen, S. C. (1965). Endotracheal intubation in a patient with ankylosing spondylitis of the cervical spine. *Anesthesiology* **26**, 365

Nishimura, T. G., Jackson, S. H. and Cohen, S. N. (1973). Prolongation of morphine anaesthesia in a patient with Gilbert's disease. Report of a case. *Can. Anaesth. Soc. J.* **20**, 709–711

O'Brien, R. T., Pearson, H. A., Godley, J. A. and Spencer, R. P. (1972). Splenic infarct and sickle (cell) trait. *New Engl. J. Med.* **287**, 720

Palmer, S. K. and Atler, J. L. (III) (1976). Anesthetic management of the Prader–Willi syndrome. *Anesthesiology* **44**, 161–163

Parik, R. K. and Moore, M. R. (1975). Anaesthetics in porphyria: intravenous induction agents. *Br. J. Anaesth.* **47**, 907

Peterson, C. M., Lu, Y. S., Herbert, J. T., Cerami, A. and Gillette, P. N. (1974). Studies with intravenous sodium cyanate in patients with sickle cell anaemia. *J. Pharmac. exp. Ther.* **189**, 577–584

Pollard, R. (1973). Surgical implications of some types of drug dependence. *Br. med. J.* **1**, 784–787

Prader, A., Labhart, A. and Willi, H. (1956). Ein syndrom von adipositas Kleinwuchs kryptorchismus und oligophrenia nach myatonie artigam zustand im neugenborenalter. *Schweiz. med. Wschr.* **86**, 1260–1261

Pratulas, V. and Biezunski, A. (1975). Epidermolysis bullosa manifested and treated during anesthesia. *Anesthesiology* **43**, 581–583

Raine, D. N. (ed.) (1975). *The Treatment of Inherited Metabolic Disease.* Lancaster: Medical and Technical Publishing Co. Ltd.

Rizk, S. F., Jacobson, J. H. and Silvay, G. (1977). Ketamine as an induction agent for acute intermittent porphyria. *Anesthesiology* **46**, 305–306

Santesson, J. (1976). 'Oxygen transport and venous admixture in the extremely obese. Influence of anaesthesia and artificial ventilation with and without positive end-expiratory pressure. *Acta anaesth. scand.* **20**, 387–394

Searle, J. F. (1973). Anaesthesia in sickle cell states. *Anaesthesia* **28**, 466

Smith, E. W. and Conley, C. L. (1955). Sicklemia and infarction of the spleen during aerial flight. Electrophoresis of the haemoglobin in 15 cases. *Bull. Johns Hopkins Hosp.* **96**, 35–41

Somanathan, S. (1976). Anaesthesia and hypothermia in sickle cell disease. *Anaesthesia* **31**, 113–114

Stanbury, J. B., Wyngaarden, J. B. and Fredericksen, D. S. (ed.) (1978). *The Metabolic Basis of Inherited Disease.* 4th edn. New York: McGraw-Hill

Stewart, R. M., Ridyard, J. B. and Pearson, J. D. (1976). Regional lung infection in ankylosing spondylitis. *Thorax* **31**, 433–437

Stovner, J. and Stadskleiv, K. (1976). Suxamethonium apnoea terminated with commercial serum cholinesterase. *Acta anaesth. scand.* **20**, 211–215

Sumner, E. (1975). Porphyria in relation to surgery and anaesthesia. *Ann. R. Coll. Surg.* **56**, 81–88

Takki, S. and Tammisto, T. (1974). The effect of operative stress on plasma catacholamine levels in chronic alcoholics. *Acta anaesth. scand.* **18**, 127–132

Tammisto, T. and Takki, S. (1973). Nitrous oxide–oxygen–relaxant anaesthesia in alcoholics: a retrospective study. *Acta anaesth. scand. Suppl.* **53**, 68–75

Tammisto, T. and Tigerstedt, I. (1977a). The need for halothane supplementation of nitrous oxide–oxygen–relaxant anaesthesia in chronic alcoholics. *Acta anesth. scand.* **21**, 17–23

Tammisto, T. and Tigerstedt, I. (1977b). The need for fentanyl supplementation of nitrous oxide–oxygen–relaxant anaesthesia in chronic alcoholics. *Acta anaesth. scand.* **21**, 216–221

Tseuda, K., Pugh, S. T. and Boyan, C. P. (1976). Pattern of oxygenation during intestinal bypass for morbid obesity. *Anesthesiology* **45**, 668–670

Turner, M. E. (1972). Anaesthetic difficulties associated with Behçets syndrome. *Br. J. Anaesth.* **44**, 100–102

Vaughan, R. W. (1973). Blood pressure in obesity. *J. Am. med. Ass.* **226**, 1011

Vaughan, R. W. (1974). Anaesthetic considerations in jejunoileal small bowel bypass for morbid obesity. *Anesth. Analg. curr. Res.* **53**, 421–429

Viby-Mogenson, J., Hanel, H. K., Hansen, E., Sørensen, B. M. and Graae, J. (1975). Serum cholinesterase activity in burned patients 1. Biochemical findings. *Acta anaesth. scand.* **19**, 159–168

Vickers, M. D. A. (1963). The mismanagement of suxamethonium apnoea. *Br. J. Anaesth.* **35**, 260–268

Waltemath, C. L. and Bergman, N. A. (1974). Respiratory compliance in obese patients. *Anesthesiology* **41**, 84–85

Wolf, S. M. (1972). Myasthenia and systemic lupus erythematosus. *Br. med. J.* **1**, 380

Wright, V. and Moll, J. M. H. (1973). Ankylosing spondylitis. *Br. J. hosp. Med.* **9**, 331–341

Zsigmond, E. K. (1973). Fluoride Numbers. *Br. J. Anaesth.* **45**, 1053

Appendix:
Drug name equivalents, UK and USA

Note: The list of approved names includes some chemical names and some commonly used unofficial names

UK approved name *UK trade name(s)*	US approved name *US trade name(s)*
Acebutolol	Acebutolol
Sectral	*Sectral*
Acetazolamide	Acetazolamide
Diamox	*Diamox*
Acetohexamide	Acetohexamide
Dimelor	*Dymelor*
ACTH (*see* Corticotrophin)	
ADH (antidiuretic hormone; *see* Vasopressin)	
Adrenaline	Epinephrine
Simplene	*Adrenalin, Bronkaid Mist, Primatene Mist*
Alcohol (ethanol)	Alcohol
Alcuronium chloride	Alcuronium chloride
Alloferin	*Alloferin*
Aldosterone	Aldosterone
Aldocorten	*Electrocortin*
Alkavervir	Alkavervir
Veriloid	*Veriloid*
Allopurinol	Allopurinol
Zyloric	*Zyloprim*
Alphadolone } Alphaxalone } **Althesin*	Alfadolone Alfaxolone
Alprenolol	Alprenolol hydrochloride
Aptin	*Aptine*
Althesin (alphadolone + alphaxalone)	
Aluminium hydroxide gel	Aluminum hydroxide gel
Aludrox	*Amphojel*
Ambenonium chloride	Ambenonium chloride
Mytelase, Mysuran	*Mytelase Chloride, Mysuran*
Amethocaine hydrochloride	Tetracaine hydrochloride
Anethaine, Norgotin	*Pontocaine Hydrochloride*
Amikacin	Amikacin sulfate
Amikin	

* indicates a formulation which is a mixture.

UK approved name *UK trade name(s)*	US approved name *US trade name(s)*
Aminobenzoic acid	Aminobenzoic acid *Pabanol*

Aminoglycosides (*see* Amikacin,
  Gentamicin, Kanamycin,
  Streptomycin and Tobramycin)	

Aminophylline *Cardophylin, Phyldrox, Phyllocontin*	Aminophylline *Rectalad-Aminophylline, Somophyllin, Aminodur*
Amiodarone	Amiodarone
Amitriptyline *Domical, Lentizol, *Limbritol, Saroten, Tryptizol*	Amitriptylene hydrochloride *Elavil, Endep*
Amoxycillin *Amoxil*	Amoxicillin *Amoxil, Larotid, Polymox, Robamox, Trimox*
Amphetamine sulphate	Amphetamine sulfate *Benzedrine, *Amphedrine*
Amphotericin *Fungilin, Fungizone*	Amphotericin B *Fungizone*

Ampicillin
*Amfipen, Penbritin, Pentrexyl,
  Vidopen*
	Ampicillin
	*Alpen, Amcill, Omnipen, Pen A Oral,
	  Penbritin, Polycillin, Ponecil,
	  Principen, Totacillin, Acillin,
	  Pensyn, QIDamp*

Amyl nitrite	Amyl nitrite
Amylobarbitone *Amytal*	Amobarbital sodium *Amytal sodium*
Antidiuretic hormone (*see* Vasopressin)	
Antimycin A	Antimycin A
Apomorphine hydrochloride	Apomorphine hydrochloride
Aprotinin *Trasylol*	Aprotinin *Trasylol*
Arginine glutamate *Modumate*	Arginine glutamate *Modumate*

Ascorbic acid
Redoxon
	Ascorbic acid
	*Ascorbicap, Cebione, Cecon, Cetane-
	  Caps TD, Cenolate, Cetane,
	  Cevalin, Cevex, Ce-Vi-Sol, C-level,
	  C-Long, Meri-C, Natrascorb*

Aspirin
*Breoprin, Caprin, Claradin, Levius,
  Nu-seals, Aspirin, Solprin*
	Aspirin
	*ASA, Aceromyl, Aspergum,
	  Aspirdrops, Asteric, Crystar,
	  Ecotrin, Empirin, Entericin,
	  Extren, Measurin, Pirseal,
	  Spira-Dine*

Atenolol *Tenormin*	Atenolol
Atropine sulphate	Atropine sulfate *Allergan, Atropisol*
Azathioprine *Imuran*	Azathioprine *Imuran*
Barbitone sodium	Barbital sodium

* indicates a formulation which is a mixture.

UK approved name *UK trade name(s)*	US approved name *US trade name(s)*

Beclomethasone
  Beconase, Becotide, Propaderm
	Beclomethasone dipropionate
	  Vanceril

Bentonite	Bentonite

Benzhexol
  Artane
	Trihexyphenidyl hydrochloride
	  *Antitrem, Artane, Pipanol, Tremin
	    Hydrochloride*

Benzquinamide	Benzquinamide *Quantril*

Benztropine
  Cogentin
	Benztropine
	  Cogentin

Benzylpenicillin
  Crystapen G, Tabillin
	Penicillin G potassium
	  *Cilloral, Liquapen, Penaler, Penisem,
	    Pentids, Pfizerpen, QIDpen G,
	    Sugracillin, *TuCillin*

Betamethasone
  *Betnelan, Betnesol, Betnovate,
    Bextasol*
	Betamethasone
	  *Celestone, Benisone, Flurobate,
	    Diprosone, Valisone*

Bethanidine *Bethanidid, Esbatal*	Bethanidine sulfate

Biperiden
  Akineton
	Biperiden
	  Akineton

Biphasic insulin *Insulin Novo Rapitard*	

Bretylium tosylate
  Bretylate, Darenthin
	Bretylium tosylate
	  Bretylol

Buclizine
  Equivert, Migraleve
	Buclizine hydrochloride
	  Bucladin-S

Buformin	Buformin

Bupivacaine
  Marcain
	Bupivacaine hydrochloride
	  Marcaine Hydrochloride

Buprenorphine *Temgesic*	Buprenorphine hydrochloride
Buthalitone sodium	Buthalital sodium

Calciferol
  Sterogyl-15
	Ergocalciferol
	  Drisdol, Deltalin

Calcitonin
  Calcitare
	Calcitonin
	  Calcimar

Calcium chloride	Calcium chloride
Calcium gluconate	Calcium gluconate *Calglucon*
Capsaicin	Capsaicin
Carbachol	Carbachol *Carcholin*

Carbenicillin
  Pyopen
	Carbenicillin
	  Geopen, Pyopen

Carbimazole *Neo-Mercazole*	Carbimazole
Carbon dioxide	Carbon dioxide
Carbon tetrachloride	Carbon tetrachloride *Benzinoform*

Casein hydrolysate (*see* Protein hydrolysate)

* indicates a formulation which is a mixture.

UK approved name *UK trade name(s)*	US approved name *US trade name(s)*
Cefoxitin	Cefoxitin *Mefoxin*
Cefuroxime *Zinacef*	Cefuroxime
Cephalexin *Ceporex, Keflex*	Cephalexin *Keflex, Keforal*
Cephaloridine *Ceporin*	Cephaloridine *Kefloridin, Loridine*
Cephalosporins (*see* Cephaloridine, Cephalothin, Cephazolin, Cephra- dine, Cefoxitin, Cephamandole, Cefuroxime, Cephalexin)	
Cephalothin *Keflin*	Cephalothin *Keflin*
Cephamandole	Cefamandole nafate *Mandol*
Cephazolin *Kefzol*	Cefazolin sodium *Ancef*
Cephradine *Velosef*	Cephradine *Velosef, Anspor*
Charcoal, activated *Medicoal*	Charcoal, activated *Darco G-60*
Chloral hydrate *Noctec*	Chloral hydrate *Felsules, Lycoral, Noctec, Rectules, Lorinal, Somni Sed, Somnos*
Chloramphenicol *Chloromycetin, Kemicetine*	Chloramphenicol *Chloroptic, Chloromycetin, Cylphenicol*
Chlordiazepoxide *Librium, Tropium*	Chlordiazepoxide hydrochloride *Librium, SK-Lygen*
Chlormethiazole *Heminevrin*	Clomethiazole
m-Chlorocresol	Chlorocresol
Chloroform	Chloroform
Chlorpromazine *Largactil*	Chlorpromazine *Thorazine, Cromedazine, Chlor-PZ*
Chlorpropamide *Diabinese, Melitase*	Chlorpropamide *Diabinese*
Cimetidine *Tagamet*	Cimetidine *Tagamet*
Cinchocaine *Nupercaine*	Dibucaine *Nupercainal*
Cinnarizine *Stugeron*	Cinnarizine *Mitronal*
Clindamycin *Dalacin C*	Clindamycin *Cleocin Phosphate*
Clonazepam *Rivotril*	Clonazepam *Clonopin*
Clonidine *Catapres, Dixarit*	Clonidine *Catapres*
Cloxacillin *Orbenin*	Cloxacillin *Cloxapen, Tegopen*

* indicates a formulation which is a mixture.

UK approved name *UK trade name(s)*	US approved name *US trade name(s)*
Cocaine	Cocaine
Codeine phosphate	Codeine phosphate
Colchicine	Colchicine
Colistin	Colistin sulfate
Colomycin	*Coly-Mycin*
Copper sulphate	Cupric sulfate
Corticotrophin	Corticotropin
Acthar, Cortico-Gel, Cortrophin Zn	*Actest Gel, Acthar, Depo-Acth* *Cortrophin*
Cortisone	Cortisone acetate
Cortelan, Cortistab, Cortisyl	*Cortogen Acetate, Cortone Acetate*
Co-trimoxazole	Co-trimoxazole
Bactrim, Septrin	*Septra*
Cromoglycic acid (disodium salt)	Cromolyn
Intal, Lomusol, Nalcrom, Opticrom, *Rynacrom*	*Intal, Aarane*
Cyclizine	Cyclizine hydrochloride
Marzine, Valoid	*Marezine Hydrochloride*
Cyclobarbitone	Cyclobarbital
Phanodorm, Rapidal	*Phanodorn*
Cyclopropane	Cyclopropane
Cysteamine	Mercaptamine
Dantrolene	Dantrolene sodium
Dantrium	*Dantrium*
DDT (*see* Dicophane)	
Debrisoquine	Debrysoquin sulfate
Declinax	*Declinax*
Decamethonium iodide	Decamethonium bromide
	Syncurine
Dexamethasone	Dexamethasone
Decadron, Dexacortisyl, Maxidex, *Oradexon*	*Aeroseb-D, Deronil, Gammacorten,* *Decaderm, Decadron, Decaspray,* *Dexameth, Dexone, Maxidex*
Dextran	Dextran
Dextaven, Gentran, Lomodex, *Macrodex, Rheomacrodex*	*Gentran, Rheomacrodex, Rheotran,* *Hyskon, Macrodex, Gentran*
Dextromoramide	Dextromoramide tartrate
Palfium	*Dimorlin Tartrate*
Dextropropoxyphene	Propoxyphene hydrochloride
*Depronal SA, Doloxene, *Distalgesic*	*Darvon, Dolene, Doloxene, Proxagesic*
Dextrose	Dextrose
	Cartrose
Diamorphine hydrochloride (heroin)	Diacetylmorphine hydrochloride
Diatrizoic acid (sodium salt)	Diatrizoate sodium
Hypaque	
Diazepam	Diazepam
Atensine, Valium	*Valium*
Diazoxide	Diazoxide
Eudemine	*Hyperstat, Proglycem*
Dichloroisoprenaline	Dichloroisoprotorenol
Dicophane	Chlorophenothane
Dicoumarol	Dicumarol

* indicates a formulation which is a mixture.

UK approved name *UK trade name(s)*	US approved name *US trade name(s)*
Dicyclomine *Merbentyl*	Dicyclomine hydrochloride *Bentyl*
Diethyl ether	Ether
Digitalis	Digitalis *Digitora, Digifortis, Digiglusin*
Digoxin *Diganox Nativelle, Lanoxin*	Digoxin *SK-Digoxin*
Dihydrocodeine tartrate *DF 118*	Drocode *Rapocodin*
Dihydroxybenzene (*see* Hydroquinone)	
Di-isopropylphosphorofluoridate (*see* Dyflos)	
Dimenhydrinate *Dramamine, Gravol*	Dimenhydrinate *Dimenest, Dramamine, Eldoram*
Dinoprost	Dinoprost *Prostin F_2 Alpha*
Dinoprostone *Prostin E_2*	Dinoprostone *Prostin E_2*
Diphenhydramine *Benadryl*	Diphenhydramine hydrochloride *Benadryl, Bendylate, Eldadryl*
Diphenylhydantoin sodium (*see* Phenytoin sodium)	
Dipipanone *Pipadone*	Dipipanone hydrochloride *Pipadone*
Diquat (a herbicide) *Aquacide, Reglone*	Diquat *Reglone*
Disodium cromoglycate (*see* Cromoglycic acid)	
Disopyramide *Norpace, Rhythmodan*	Disopyramide phosphate *Norpace*
Distalgesic (dextropropoxyphene + paracetamol)	
Distigmine bromide *Ubretid*	Hexamarium bromide
Dobutamine *Dobutrex*	Dobutamine
L-Dopa (*see* Levodopa)	
Dopamine *Intropin*	Dopamine *Intropin*
Doxapram *Dopram*	Doxapram *Dopram*
Doxycycline *Vibramycin*	Doxycycline *Doxy- II, Vibramycin*
Droperidol *Droleptan, *Thalamonal*	Droperidol *Inapsine, *Innovar*
Dyflos	Isoflurophate *Floropryl*
Ecothiopate iodide *Phosphiline Iodide*	Echothiophate iodide
Edrophonium chloride *Tensilon*	Edrophonium chloride *Tensilon*
Enflurane *Ethrane*	Enflurane *Ethrane*

* indicates a formulation which is a mixture.

UK approved name *UK trade name(s)*	US approved name *US trade name(s)*
Ephedrine	Ephedrine *l-Sedrin, Mandarin*
Ergometrine	Ergonovine maleate *Ergotrate Maleate*
Erythromycin *Erythrocin, Erythromid, Erythroped,* *Ilosone, Ilotycin, Rectin*	Erythromycin estolate *Ilosone*
Ethanol (*see* Alcohol)	
Ethosuximide *Emeside, Zarontin*	Ethosuximide *Zarontin*
Ether (diethyl ether)	
Ethyl carbamate (*see* Urethane)	
Ethylene	Ethylene
Ethylene oxide	Ethylene oxide
Etidocaine	Etidocaine *Duranest*
Etomidate sulphate *Hypnomidate*	Etomidate
Eugenol	Eugenol
Fazadinium bromide *Fazadon*	Fazadinium bromide
Felypressin	Felypressin
Fenfluramine *Ponderax*	Fenfluramine hydrochloride *Ponderex, Pondimin*
Fentanyl *Sublimaze, *Thalamonal*	Fentanyl *Sublimaze, *Innovar*
Flucloxacillin *Floxapen*	Floxacillin *Floxapen*
Fludrocortisone *Florinef*	Fludrocortisone acetate *F-Cortef Acetate, Florinef*
Fluphenazine *Modecate, Moditen*	Fluphenazine hydrochloride *Permitil, Prolixin*
Flurazepam *Dalmane*	Flurazepam *Dalmane*
Flurothyl	Flurothyl *Indoklon*
Fluroxene	Fluroxene *Fluoromar*
Folic acid	Folic acid *Folvite*
Fructose (laevulose)	Fructose *Levugen*
Frusemide *Dryptal, Frusid, Lasix*	Furosemide *Lasix*
FSH (*see* Human follicle-stimulating hormone)	
Fuller's earth	Fuller's earth
Fusidic acid (sodium salt) *Fucidin*	Fusidic acid
Gallamine *Flaxedil*	Gallamine triethiodide *Flaxedil*

* indicates a formulation which is a mixture.

UK approved name *UK trade name(s)*	US approved name *US trade name(s)*
Gelatin	Gelatin
Gentamicin	Gentamicin
Cidomycin, Garamycin, Genticin	*Garamycin*
Germine diacetate	Germine
GH (*see* Growth hormone)	
Globin zinc insulin	Insulin (injection) globin zinc
Globulin insulin (*see* Globin zinc insulin)	
Glucagon	Glucagon
Glucose, liquid	Glucose, liquid
Glutethimide	Glutethimide
Doriden	*Doriden*
Glyceryl trinitrate	Nitroglycerin
Nitrocontin, Sustac	*KlaviCordal, Myocon, Nitrospan,*
	Nitrotest, Trates
Glycine	Aminoacetic acid
Griseofulvin	Griseofulvin
Fulcin, Grisovin	*Fulvicin-U/F, Grisactin, Grifulvin V*
Growth hormone	
Crescormon	
Guanethidine	Guanethidine sulfate
Ismelin	*Ismelin*
Haloperidol	Haloperidol
Haldol, Serenace	*Haldol*
Halothane	Halothane
Fluothane	*Fluothane*
Helium	Helium
Heparin	Heparin sodium
Pularin, Minihep	*Hepathrom, Heprinar, Lipo-Hepin,*
	Liquaemin Sodium, Panheprin
Heroin (*see* Diamorphine hydrochloride)	
Hetastarch	Hetastarch
	Hespan, Volex
Hexafluorenium	Hexafluorenium
	Mylaxen
Hexafluorodiethyl ether (*see* Flurothyl)	
Hexamethonium bromide	Hexamethonium bromide
Vegolysen	*Bistrium Bromide*
Hexobarbitone	Hexobarbital
Evipan	*Evipal, Sombucaps, Sombulex,*
	Somnalert
Human follicle-stimulating hormone	Menotropins
Perganol	*Perganol, Humegon, Pregova*
Human lutenising hormone	Gonadorelin hydrochloride
	Factrel
Hydrallazine	Hydralazine hydrochloride
Apresoline	*Apresoline Hydrochloride*
Hydrocortisone	Hydrocortisone
Colifoam, Corlan, Cortenema,	**Barseb HC, Cetacort, Cort-Dome,*
Efcortelan, Efcortesol,	*Cortef, Cortenema, Dermacort,*
Hydrocortisab, Hydrocortone	*Eldecort, Hydrocortone, Hytone,*
	Komed-HC
Hydroquinone	Hydroquinone
	Astra, Eldopaque, Eldoquin

* indicates a formulation which is a mixture.

UK approved name *UK trade name(s)*	US approved name *US trade name(s)*
Hydroxyamphetamine	Hydroxyamphetamine hydrobromide
Hydroxydione sodium succinate	Hydroxydione sodium succinate *Viadril*
Hydroxyethylstarch (HES; *see* Hetastarch)	
5-Hydroxytryptamine (5-HT; *see* Serotonin)	
Hyoscine methobromide	Methscopolamine bromide
Pamine	*Ampyrox, Pamine Bromide*
Imipramine	Imipramine hydrochloride
Berkomine, Norpramine, Tofranil	*Imavate, Janimine, SK-Pramine,* *Tofranil*
Insulin, biphasic (*see* Biphasic insulin)	
Insulin zinc suspension	Insulin zinc (suspension)
Insulin Lente, Lentard, Monotard MC	*Lente Insulin, Lente Iletin*
Insulin zinc suspension (amorphous)	Insulin zinc (suspension) prompt
Insulin Semilente, Semitard MC	*Semilente Insulin, Semilente Iletin*
Insulin zinc suspension (crystalline)	Insulin zinc (suspension) extended
Insulin Ultralente, Ultratard	*Ultralente Insulin, Ultralente Iletin*
Iodised oil	Iodized oil
Lipiodol, Ultrafluid	*Lipiodol*
Iothalamic acid	Iothalamic acid
Conray	*Conray, Vascoray*
Isoflurane	Isoflurane
	Forane
Isophane insulin	Insulin (suspension) isophane
Leo Retard	*NPH Iletin*
Isoprenaline	Isoproterenol hydrochloride
Aleudrin, Saventrine, Suscardia	*Isuprel Hydrochloride, Norisodrine* *Hydrochloride, Vapo-N-Iso*
Isosorbide dinitrate	Isosorbide dinitrate
Cedocard, Isordil, Sorbitrate, Vascardin	*Isordil, Sorbitrate, Sorquad*
Kanamycin	Kanamycin sulphate
Kannasyn, Kantrex	*Kantrex*
Ketamine	Ketamine
Ketalar	*Ketaject, Ketalar, Kataset*
Labetalol	Labetalol hydrochloride
Trandate	
Lactic acid	Lactic acid
Lactulose	Lactulose
Duphalac	*Duphalac, Cephulac*
Leucine	Leucine
Levallorphan	Levallorphan tartrate
Lorfan	*Lorfan*
Levodopa	Levodopa
Berkdopa, Brocadopa, Larodopa	*Bendopa, Dopar, Larodopa*
Levorphanol	Levorphanol tartrate
Dromoran	*Levo-Dromoran*
LH (*see* Human lutenising hormone)	
Lignocaine	Lidocaine hydrochloride
Lidothesin, Xylocaine, Xylocard, *Xylotox*	*Xylocaine Hydrochloride, Dolicaine*
Lincomycin	Lincomycin
Lincocin, Mycivin	*Lincocin*

* indicates a formulation which is a mixture.

UK approved name *UK trade name(s)*	US approved name *US trade name(s)*
Liothyronine sodium *Tertroxin*	Liothyronine sodium *Cytomel*
Lithium carbonate *Camcolit, Phasal, Priadel*	Lithium carbonate *Lithane, Eskalith, Lithotabs, Lithonate*
Magnesium chloride	Magnesium chloride
Magnesium sulphate	Magnesium sulfate
Magnesium trisilicate *Magsorbent*	Magnesium trisilicate *Trimax, Trisil*
Malathion (an insecticide) *Derbac, Prioderm*	Malathion *Cythion, Malamar, Malaspray, Prioderm*
Mandrax (methaqualone + diphenhydramine)	
Mannitol	Mannitol
Mecamylamine *Inversine*	Mecamylamine hydrochloride *Inversine*
Meclozine	Meclizine hydrochloride *Bonine, Antivert*
Meglumine	Meglumine
Meperidine (*see* Pethidine)	
Mephentermine	Mephentermine sulfate *Wyamine Sulfate*
Mepivacaine *Carbocaine*	Mepivacaine hydrochloride *Carbocaine Hydrochloride*
Metformin *Glucophage*	Metformin
Methacholine chloride	Methacholine chloride *Mecholyl*
Methadone *Physeptone*	Methadone hydrochloride *Adanon Hydrochloride, Althose Hydrochloride, Dolophine Hydrochloride*
Methanol (*see* Methyl alcohol)	
Methaqualone **Mandrax*	Methaqualone *Quaalude, Tuazole, Sopor, Somnaface*
Methimazole	Methimazole *Tapazole*
Methionine	Methionine *Meonine*
Methitural	Methitural sodium *Neraval Sodium*
Methohexitone *Brevital, Brietal*	Methohexital sodium *Brevital Sodium*
Methotrimeprazine *Veractil*	Methotrimeprazine *Levoprome*
Methoxamine hydrochloride *Vasoxine, Vasylox*	Methoxamine hydrochloride *Vasoxyl*
Methoxyflurane *Penthrane*	Methoxyflurane *Penthrane*
Methyldopa *Aldomet, Dopamet*	Methyldopa *Aldomet*
Methylene blue	Methylene blue

* indicates a formulation which is a mixture.

UK approved name *UK trade name(s)*	US approved name *US trade name(s)*
Methyl hydroxybenzoate	Methylparaben
Methylphenidate	Methylphenidate hydrochloride
Ritalin	*Ritalin Hydrochloride*
Methylprednisolone	Methylprednisolone sodium phosphate
Medrone, Solu-Medrone	
α-Methyltyrosine (α-MPT; αMT)	α-Methyl-*p*-tyrosine
Metoclopramide	Metoclopramide hydrochloride
Maxolon, Primperan	*Reglan*
Metoprolol	Metoprolol
Betaloc, Lopresor	
Metronidazole	Metronidazole
Flagyl	*Flagyl*
Metyrapone	Metyrapone
Metopirone	*Metopirone, Metroprione*
Mexiletine	Mexiletine
Mexitil	
Morphine	Morphine hydrochloride
Duromorph	
Nalorphine	Nalorphine hydrochloride
Lethidrone	*Nalline*
Naloxone	Naloxone
Narcan	*Narcan*
Neomycin	Neomycin sulfate
Mycifradin, Neomin, Nivemycin	*Mycifradin*
Neostigmine	Neostigmine bromide
Prostigmin	*Prostigmin*
Neutral insulin injection	Insulin, neutral
Actrapid MC	
Nicotine	Nicotine
Nitrazepam	Nitrazepam
Mogadon, Nitrados, Remnos,	*Mogadon*
Somnased, Somnite	
Nitroglycerin (*see* Glyceryl trinitrate)	
Nitrous oxide	Nitrous oxide
Noradrenaline	Levarterenol bitartrate
Levophed	*Levophed Bitartrate*
Nystatin	Nystatin
Nystan, Nystavescent	*Candex, Mycostatin, Nilstat, O-V Statin*
Oestrogens, conjugated	Estrogens conjugated
Premarin	*Premarin*
Oleic acid	Oleic acid
Orciprenaline	
Alupent	
Orgotein (superoxide dismutase)	Orgotein
	Ontosein
Orphenadrine	Orphenadrine
Norflex	
Ouabain (synonym Strophanthin-G)	Ouabain
Oxazepam	Oxazepam
Serenid D	*Serax*

* indicates a formulation which is a mixture.

UK approved name *UK trade name(s)*	US approved name *US trade name(s)*
Oxprenolol *Trasicor*	Oxprenolol *Trasicor*
Oxycodone *Proladone*	
Oxytocin *Pitocin, Syntocinon*	Oxytocin *Pitocin, Syntocinon, Uteracon*
Pancuronium *Pavulon*	Pancuronium *Pavulon*
Papaveretum *Omnopon, *Nepenthe*	
Papaverine	Papaverine hydrochloride *Vasal, Cerespan, Pavabid, Pavatest*
Paracetamol *Calpol, Panadol, Salzone, *Distalgesic*	Acetaminophen *Anapap, Apadon, Janupap, Nebs, SK-Apap, Tempra, Tylenol, Valadol*
Paraldehyde	Paraldehyde *Paral*
Paraquat (a herbicide) *Dextronex, Essram, Gramoxone*	Paraquat
Parathion (an insecticide)	Parathion *Alkron, Alleron, Amphamite, Etilon, Folidol, Fosferno, Niram, Paraphos, Rhodiatox, Thiophos*
Parathyroid *Para Thor-mone*	Parathyroid *Paroidin*
Pargyline *Eutonyl*	Pargyline *Eutonyl*
Pempidine	Pempidine
Penicillin G (*see* Benzylpenicillin)	
Pentamethonium bromide	Pentamethonium bromide
Pentazocine *Fortral*	Pentazocine *Talwin*
Pentobarbitone sodium *Nembutal*	Pentobarbital *Nembutal*
Pentolinium tartrate *Ansolysen*	Pentolinium tartrate *Ansolysen Tartrate*
Perphenazine *Fentazin*	Perphenazine *Trilafon*
Pethidine	Meperidine hydrochloride *Demeral, Mepadin*
Phenacetin	Phenacetin
Phenazocine *Narphen*	Phenazocine hydrobromide *Pyridium, Azomine*
Phencyclidine hydrochloride	Phencyclidine hydrochloride *Sernylan*
Phenformin *Dibotin, Dipar*	Phenformin hydrochloride *Meltrol-50, DBI*
Phenindione *Dindevan*	Phenindione *Hedulin, Indon*

* indicates a formulation which is a mixture.

UK approved name *UK trade name(s)*	US approved name *US trade name(s)*
Phenobarbitone *Gardenal, Luminal*	Phenobarbital *Eskabarb, Stental, Luminal, Barbivis,* *Liquital, Solfoton, Solu-Barb,* *Talpheno*
Phenol	Phenol
Phenoperidine *Operidine*	Phenoperidine
Phenoxybenzamine *Dibenyline*	Phenoxybenzamine hydrochloride *Dibenzyline*
Phentolamine *Rogitine*	Phentolamine hydrochloride *Regitine Hydrochloride*
Phenylbutazone *Butazolidin*	Phenylbutazone *Azolid, Busone, Butazolidin, Zorane*
Phenylephrine *Fenox, Neophryn*	Phenylephrine hydrochloride *Alcon-Efrin, Biomydrin, Degest,* *Synasal, Mistra D,* *Neo-Synephrine Hydrochloride,* *Prefrin Liquifilm*
Phenytoin *Epanutin*	Phenytoin *Dilantin*
Phytomenadione *Aquamephyton, Konakion*	Phytonadione *Aquamephyton, Konakion, Mephyton,* *Mono-Kay*
Pindolol *Visken*	Pindolol *Visken*
Piritramide *Dipidolar*	Piritramide
Polymyxin *Aerosporin*	Polymyxin B sulfate *Aerosporin*
Polyvinylpyrrolidone (*see* Povidone)	
Potassium chloride *Leo-K, Kay-Cee-L, Kalium Durules,* *Slow-K*	Potassium chloride *K-Lor, K-Lyte, Kaochlor, Kaon-Cl,* *Kay Ciel, Pficlor, Slow K*
Potassium phosphate	Potassium phosphate, monobasic
Povidone	Povidone *Plasdone, Vinisil*
Practolol *Eraldin*	Practolol
Pralidoxime *Protopam*	Pralidoxime *Protopam Chloride*
Prazosin *Hypovase*	Prazosin hydrochloride *Minipress*
Prednisolone *Codelcortone, Codelsol, Delta-Cortef,* *Deltacortril, Deltastab,* *Sintisone, Ultracortenol*	Prednisolone *Delta-Cortef, Hydettra, Meti-Derm,* *Paracortrol, Predne-Dome,* *Prednis, Sterane, Sterolone,* *Ulacort*
Prednisone *Decortisyl, Deltacortone*	Prednisone *Delta-Dome, Deltasone, Lisacort,* *Meticorten, Orasone, Paracort,* *Servisone*

* indicates a formulation which is a mixture.

UK approved name *UK trade name(s)*	US approved name *US trade name(s)*
Prilocaine *Citanest*	Prilocaine *Citanest Hydrochloride*
Primidone *Mysoline*	Primidone *Mysoline*
Probenecid *Benemid*	Probenecid *Benemid*
Procainamide *Pronestyl*	Procainamide hydrochloride *Pronestyl*
Procaine	Procaine hydrochloride *Neocaine, Novocain*
Prochlorperazine *Stemetil, Vertigon*	Prochlorperazine *Compazine*
Procyclidine *Kemadrin*	Procyclidine hydrochloride *Kemadrin*
Progesterone *Cyclogest, Gestone, Progestasert*	Progesterone *Colprosterone, Gesterol, Lingusorbs, Lucorteum, Lutromone, Membrettes, Nalutron, Progesterol, Proluton, Syngesterone, Syngestrets*
Prolactin	Prolactin
Promazine *Sparine*	Promazine hydrochloride *Sparine*
Promethazine *Phenergan*	Promethazine hydrochloride *Phenergan, Fellozine, Ganphen, Remsed*
Pronethalol	Pronetalol
Propanidid *Epontol*	Propanidid *Epontol*
Propantheline *Pro-Banthine*	Propantheline bromide *Pro-Banthine*
Propoxyphene (*see* Dextropropoxyphene)	
Propranolol *Inderal*	Propranolol *Inderal*
Propylene glycol	Propylene glycol
Prostaglandin E_1	Alprostadil
Prostaglandin E_2 (*see* Dinoprostone)	
Prostaglandin $F_{2\alpha}$ (*see* Dinoprost)	
Protamine zinc insulin	Insulin (suspension) protamine zinc
Protein hydrolysate *Aminosol*	Protein hydrolysate *Amigen, Aminosol, Hyprotigen, Perenamine, Travamin*
Pyridine	Pyridine
Pyridostigmine bromide *Mestinon*	Pyridostigmine bromide *Mestinon*
Quinalbarbitone sodium *Seconal Sodium*	Secobarbital sodium *Seconal Sodium, Barbosec*
Quinidine *Kinidin, Quinicardine*	Quinidine sulfate *Quinidex, Quinicardine, Cin-Quin*
Reserpine *Serpasil*	Reserpine *Rau-Sed, Roxinoid, Reserpoid, Sandril, Serpasil, Sertina, Serpiloid, Vio-Serpine*

* indicates a formulation which is a mixture.

UK approved name *UK trade name(s)*	US approved name *US trade name(s)*

Rifampicin
  Rifadin, Rimactane
	Rifampin
	  Rifadin, Rimactane

Salbutamol
  Ventolin
	Albuterol or Salbutamol
	  Proventil

Saxitoxin	Saxitonin
Serotonin	Serotonin
Sevoflurane	Sevoflurane
Silver nitrate	Silver nitrate

Silver sulphadiazine
  Flamazine
	Silver sulfadiazine
	  Silvadene

Sodium acetrizoate
  Diaginol
	Acetrizoate sodium
	  Cystokon, Pyelokon-R, Thixokon,
	    Urokon

Sodium bicarbonate	Sodium bicarbonate *Neut*
Sodium iodide	Sodium iodide
Sodium lactate	Sodium lactate
Sodium metrizoate	Metrizoate sodium

Sodium nitroprusside
  Nipride
	Sodium nitroprusside
	  Nipride

Sodium oxybate	Sodium oxybate
Sodium thiamylal	Thiamylal sodium *Surital*
Sodium valproate *Epilim*	Valproate sodium
Sorbitol	Sorbitol
Sotalol *Beta-Cardone, Sotacor*	Sotalol
Soya oil *Intralipid*	Soybean oil
Soya bean oil (*see* Soya oil)	

Spironolactone
  Aldactone
	Spironolactone hydrochloride
	  Spiro-32

Streptokinase
  Kabikinase, Streptase
	Streptokinase
	  Streptase

Streptomycin	Streptomycin sulfate *Strycin*
Strophanthin-G (*see* Ouabain)	

Sulphasalazine
  Salazopyrin
	Sulfasalazine
	  Azulfidine, Rorasul, S.A.S.-500,
	    Sulcolon

Superoxide dismutase (*see* Orgotein)	

Suxamethonium chloride
  Anectine
	Succinylcholine chloride
	  Sucostrin Chloride, Quelicin, Sux-Cert,
	    Anectine

T₃ (tri-iodothyronine; *see* Liothyronine sodium)	
Tri-iodothyronine (*see* Liothyronine sodium)	
T₄ (*see* Thyroxine)	
Tacrine *THA*	Tacrine

* indicates a formulation which is a mixture.

UK approved name *UK trade name(s)*	US approved name *US trade name(s)*
Talampicillin *Talpen*	Talampicillin hydrochloride
Tetracaine (*see* Amethocaine)	
Testosterone *Sustanon, Testoral*	Testosterone *Testrone, Andrusol, Synandrol F, Oreton, Mertestate, Malogen, Testosteroid, Virosterone*
Tetracosactrin *Cortrosyn, Synacthen*	Cosyntropin *Cortrosyn*
Tetracycline *Achromycin, Sustamycin, Tetrabid, Tetrachel, Tetracyn, Totomycin*	Tetracycline *Panmycin, Tetracyn, Robitet, T-125*
Tetraethylammonium	Tetraethylammonium chloride
Tetraethyl pyrophosphate	Tetraethyl pyrophosphate
Tetrahydroaminacrine (*see* Tacrine)	
Tetrodotoxin	Tetrodotoxin
Theophylline *Monotheamin, Nuelin, Theograd*	Theophylline *Elixophyllin, Theophyl-225*
Thialbarbitone	Thialbarbital
Thiamine *Benerva*	Thiamine hydrochloride *Bewon, Vinothiam, Betaxin, Betalin*
Thiamylal (*see* Sodium thiamyl)	
Thiethylperazine *Torecan*	Thiethylperazine maleate *Torecan Maleate*
Thiopentone sodium *Intraval Sodium, Pentothal*	Thiopental sodium *Pentothal Sodium*
Thiopropazate *Dartalan*	Thiopropazate hydrochloride
Thymoxamine *Opilon*	Moxisylyte
Thyrotrophin *Thytropar*	Thyrotropin *Thytropar*
Thyroxine sodium *Eltroxin*	Levothyroxine sodium *Roxstan, Synthroid*
L-Thyroxine (*see* Thyroxine sodium)	
Timolol *Betin, Blocadren, Timoptol*	Timolol maleate *Timoptic*
Tobramycin *Nebcin*	Tobramycin *Nebcin*
α-Tocopheral acetate (*see* Vitamin E)	
Tolazoline *Priscol*	Tolazoline hydrochloride *Priscoline Hydrochloride*
Tolbutamide *Pramidex, Rastinon*	Tolbutamide *Orinase*
Toxiferine	c-Toxiferine I
Trichloroethanol	2,2,2-Trichloroethanol
Trichloroethylene *Trilene*	Trichloroethylene *Trilene*
Triclofos *Tricloryl*	Triclofos sodium *Triclos*

* indicates a formulation which is a mixture.

UK approved name *UK trade name(s)*	US approved name *US trade name(s)*
Trifluoperazine *Stelazine*	Trifluoperazine hydrochloride *Stelazine*
Trifluopromazine hydrochloride	Trifluopromazine hydrochloride *Vesprin*
Trimeprazine *Vallergan*	Trimeprazine tartrate *Temaril*
Trimetaphan camsylate *Arfonad*	Trimethaphan camsylate *Arfonad*
Trimethoprim *Rimexolone*	Trimethoprim *Syraprim*
TSH (Thyroid-stimulating hormone, *see* Thyrotrophin)	
Tubocurarine chloride *Tubarine*	Tubocurarine chloride *Tubadil, Tubarine*
d-Tubocurarine (*see* Tubocurarine chloride)	
Urethane	Urethan
Vancomycin *Vancocin*	Vancomycin hydrochloride *Vancocin Hydrochloride*
Vasopressin (ADH) *Pitressin*	Vasopressin tannate *Pitressin Tannate*
Verapamil *Cordilox*	Verapamil *Isoptin*
Veratridine/Veratrum (*see* Alkavervir)	
Vinblastine *Velbe*	Vinblastine sulfate *Velban*
Vincristine *Oncovin*	Vincristine sulfate *Oncovin*
Vitamin A *Ro-A-Vit*	Vitamin A *Acon, Alphalin, Homogenets Aoral,* *Super A, Vi-Dom-A, Anatola,* *Aquasol A, A-Sol, A-Vitan,* *Testavol-S, Vi-Alpha, Vio-A*
Vitamin C (*see* Ascorbic acid)	
Vitamin D (*see* Calciferol)	
Vitamin E *Ephynal*	Vitamin E *Dalfatol, Epsilan-M, Tocopherex,* *Aquasol E, E-Ferol, Esorb,* *Eprolin, E-Toplex, Lan-E,* *Natopherol, Vascuals*
Vitamin H' (*see* Aminobenzoic)	
Vitamin K (*see* Phytomenadione)	
Vitamin N *Vamin N*	
Warfarin *Marevan*	Warfarin sodium *Coumadin, Panwarfin*

* indicates a formulation which is a mixture.

Index